Principles of
NEUROLOGIC
Infectious Diseases

Principles of
NEUROLOGIC
Infectious Diseases

EDITOR

Karen L. Roos, MD
John and Nancy Nelson Professor of Neurology
Department of Neurology
Indiana University School of Medicine
Indianapolis, Indiana

McGraw-Hill
Medical Publishing Division

New York   Chicago   San Francisco   Lisbon   London   Madrid   Mexico City   Milan
New Delhi   San Juan   Seoul   Singapore   Sydney   Toronto

Principles of Neurologic Infectious Diseases

1 2 3 4 5 6 7 8 9 0 KGP KGP 0 9 8 7 6 5 4 3 4

ISBN 0-07-140816-9

This book was set in Garamond by Matrix Publishing Services, Inc.
The editors were Marc Strauss, Michelle Watt, and Peter J. Boyle; the production supervisor was Richard Ruzycka; Kathrin Unger prepared the index.
Quebecor World Kingsport was printer and binder.

This book is printed on acid-free paper.

Library of Congress Cataloging-in-Publication Data

Principles of neurological infectious diseases / edited by Karen L. Roos.
    p. ; cm.
  Includes bibliographical references and index.
  ISBN 0-07-140816-9
  1. Nervous system—Infections. I. Roos, Karen L.
  [DNLM: 1. Nervous System Diseases—microbiology. 2. Communicable Diseases. WL
140 P9577 2005]
RC359.5.P77 2005
616.8′3—dc22   2004040230

To Bob, Annie, and Jan with love

CONTENTS

Color plates appear between pages 432 and 433.

CONTRIBUTORS

Latisha Ali, MD
Department of Neurology
Indiana University School of Medicine
Indianapolis, Indiana
Chapter 3

J. Andrew Alspaugh, MD
Assistant Professor
Departments of Medicine and Molecular
    Genetics/Microbiology
Division of Infectious Diseases and International
    Health
Duke University Medical Center
Durham, North Carolina
Chapter 12

Abelardo Araújo, MD, PhD
Professor
The Reference Centers for Neuroinfections and HTLV
Evandro Chagas Clinical Research Institute-FIOCRUZ
The Federal University of Rio de Janeiro, Brazil
Rio de Janeiro, Brazil
Chapter 10

James F. Bale, Jr., MD
Professor of Pediatrics and Neurology
Vice Chair of Pediatrics
Division of Pediatric Neurology
The University of Utah School of Medicine and
    Primary Children's Medical Center
Salt Lake City, Utah
Chapter 4

Russell E. Bartt, MD
Assistant Professor of Neurologic Sciences
Rush Medical College
Senior Attending Physician
Cook County Hospital and Rush University Medical
    Center
Chicago, Illinois
Chapter 22

David Chansolme, MD
Infectious Diseases Fellow
Division of Infectious Diseases, Department of
    Medicine
University of Alabama at Birmingham
Birmingham, Alabama
Chapter 14

Julio Collazos, MD
Chief, Section of Infectious Diseases
Hospital de Galdácano
Vizcaya, Spain
Chapter 7

Gregory A. Dasch, PhD
Viral and Rickettsial Zoonoses Branch
Division of Viral and Rickettsial Diseases
National Center for Infectious Diseases
Centers for Disease Control and Prevention
Atlanta, Georgia
Chapter 19

Oscar H. Del Brutto, MD
Department of Neurological Sciences
Hospital-Clinica Kennedy
Guayaquil, Ecuador
Chapter 16

Alberto J. Espay, MD
Department of Medicine
Division of Neurology
The Toronto Western Hospital
University of Toronto
Toronto, Ontario, Canada
Chapter 24

Juan Carlos Garcia-Monco, MD
Chief, Service of Neurology
Servicio de Neurologia
Hospital de Galdacano
Vizcaya, Spain
Chapter 13

Bhuwan P. Garg, MB, BS
Professor of Neurology
Department of Neurology, Section of Pediatric
    Neurology
Indianapolis, Indiana
Chapter 29

John J. Halperin, MD
Professor of Neurology
New York University School of Medicine
Chair of Neurology
North Shore University Hospital
Manhasset, New York
Chapter 15

Thiravat Hemachudha, MD
Professor of Neurology
Neurology Division, Department of Medicine
Chulalongkorn University Hospital
Bangkok, Thailand
Chapter 11

David N. Herrmann, MBBCh
Assistant Professor of Neurology and Pathology and
    Laboratory Medicine
Neuromuscular Disease Center
University of Rochester School of Medicine and
    Dentistry
Rochester, New York
Chapter 8

Edward W. Hook, III, MD
Professor of Medicine, Microbiology, and
    Epidemiology
University of Alabama at Birmingham
Medical Director, STD Control Program
Jefferson County Department of Health
Birmingham, Alabama
Chapter 14

Erik Johnson
Department of Biochemistry and Molecular Biology
Institute for Biophysical Dynamics
University of Chicago
Chicago, Illinois
Chapter 18

Anthony E. Lang, MD, FRCPC
Professor of Neurology
The Toronto Western Hospital
University of Toronto
Toronto, Ontario, Canada
Chapter 24

Justin C. McArthur, MBBS, MPH
Professor of Neurology and Epidemiology
Department of Neurology
Johns Hopkins Hospital
Baltimore, Maryland
Chapter 9

James A. Mastrianni, MD, PhD
Assistant Professor of Neurology
The University of Chicago
Co-Director, Center for Comprehensive Care and
    Memory Disorders
Committees of Neurobiology and Microbiology
Chicago, Illinois
Chapter 18

Robert M. Pascuzzi, MD
Professor and Chair, Department of Neurology
Indiana University School of Medicine
Indianapolis, Indiana
Chapter 21

Hema U. Patel, MD
Clinical Associate Professor of Neurology
Department of Neurology, Section of Pediatric
    Neurology
Indiana University School of Medicine
Indianapolis, Indiana
Chapter 29

John R. Perfect, MD
Professor, Departments of Medicine and Molecular
    Genetics/Microbiology
Division of Infectious Diseases and International
    Health
Duke University Medical Center
Durham, North Carolina
Chapter 12

Hans-Walter Pfister, MD
Professor of Neurology
Department of Neurology
Klinikum Grosshadern
Ludwig-Maximilians-University of Munich
Munich, Germany
Chapter 2

Sherry F. Queener, PhD
Associate Dean
Indiana University Graduate School
Professor of Pharmacology
Indiana University School of Medicine
Indianapolis, Indiana
Chapter 27

Karen L. Roos, MD
John and Nancy Nelson Professor of Neurology
Department of Neurology
Indiana University School of Medicine
Indianapolis, Indiana
Chapters 1, 2, 3, 5, 6, and 20

Charles E. Rupprecht, VMD, PhD
Chief of the Rabies Section
Viral and Rickettsial Zoonoses Branch
Centers for Disease Control and Prevention
Atlanta, Georgia
Chapter 11

Thomas D. Sabin, MD
Department of Neurology
New England Medical Center
Boston, Massachusetts
Chapter 23

Giovanni Schifitto, MD
Assistant Professor of Neurology
Movement and Inherited Neurological Disorders Unit
Department of Neurology
University of Rochester School of Medicine and
    Dentistry
Rochester, New York
Chapter 8

Erich Schmutzhard, MD, DTM&H
Professor of Neurology
Department of Neurology
University Hospital Innsbruck
Innsbruck, Austria
Chapter 17

Daniel J. Sexton, MD
Professor, Division of Infectious Diseases
Duke University Medical Center
Durham, North Carolina
Chapter 19

Avanee Shah, MD
Department of Radiology
Indiana University School of Medicine
Indianapolis, Indiana
Chapters 3 and 20

Marcus Tulius T. Silva, MD, MSc
The Reference Centers for Neuroinfections and HTLV
Evandro Chagas Clinical Research Institute-FIOCRUZ
The Fluminense Federal University
Brazil
Chapter 10

Riley Snook, MD
Department of Neurology
Indiana University School of Medicine
Indianapolis, Indiana
Chapter 28

Nina J. Solenski, MD
University of Viginia Health System
The Stroke Center, Department of Neurology
Charlottesville, Virginia
Chapter 26

Thomas R. Swift, MD
Professor Emeritus of Neurology
Department of Neurology
Medical College of Georgia
Augusta, Georgia
Chapter 23

Anita Venkataramana, MD
Department of Neurology
Johns Hopkins Hospital
Baltimore, Maryland
Chapter 9

Robert D. Yee, MD, FACS
Chair and Merrill Grayson Professor of
    Ophthalmology
Indiana University School of Medicine
Indianapolis, Indiana
Chapter 25

PREFACE

The inspiration for *Principles of Neurologic Infectious Diseases* developed over years of listening to the future contributors to this textbook lecture on their areas of expertise in infectious diseases of the central nervous system. I thought it would be terribly helpful to clinicians if these experts wrote about how they manage their patients. What are the pearls in the clinical presentation that suggest a specific infection? What tests are most likely to yield the diagnosis? What is the best treatment? When is therapy adjunctive to antimicrobial therapy indicated?

Scientific knowledge in the field has grown rapidly in the last few years, not only in our understanding of disease pathophysiology and ability to identify causative organisms, but also in our knowledge of the adverse effects of central nervous system inflammation and in an increased awareness of ever-emerging infectious agents. Treatment options range from antimicrobial agents to adjunctive therapy targeted at attenuating the inflammatory response and minimizing neurologic complications.

Each of the authors is a worldwide authority on a specific infection, and the best in the field. Clinicians can use this textbook to research the clinical features, diagnosis, and treatment of a given disease, to review a topic, or to learn about the most recent developments in our understanding of the pathogenesis of the infection. The textbook begins with a chapter dedicated to analysis of the cerebrospinal fluid and ends with a chapter on the prevention of infection through immunization. In-between are chapters on every important central nervous system infection—plus a number of unique chapters, including infectious etiologies of movement disorders and ophthalmic manifestations of neurologic infections. It is my hope that clinicians will find the book both informative and helpful.

I must acknowledge and thank all of the authors who contributed not only their manuscripts, but also their time and expertise to this textbook. I am very grateful to the artists Avanee Shah, MD, and Andrew Swift for their beautiful illustrations. I also want to express my heartfelt gratitude to Linda Hagan who has been my editorial assistant for more than 15 years and who worked so hard on this textbook.

Karen L. Roos, MD

Principles of
NEUROLOGIC
Infectious Diseases

CHAPTER 1
Cerebrospinal Fluid

Karen L. Roos

The majority of cerebrospinal fluid (CSF) is formed in the choroid plexus of the lateral, third, and fourth ventricles, with the remainder being formed in the capillary bed of the brain and the subarachnoid pial surface.[1] CSF flows out of the lateral ventricles through the foramina of Munro to the third ventricle and then through the cerebral aqueduct to the fourth ventricle. It exits the fourth ventricle through the lateral foramina of Luschka and the foramen of Magendie into the subarachnoid space. CSF is formed at a rate of 500 ml/day.[2] Most of the CSF is absorbed into the venous system by the arachnoid villi and granulations. Analysis of the CSF is an irreplaceable test in the diagnosis of infectious and inflammatory diseases of the central nervous system (CNS).

► LUMBAR PUNCTURE

The Technique of Lumbar Puncture

Before performing a lumbar puncture, the patient should be examined for papilledema and/or a focal neurologic deficit. A cranial computed tomographic (CT) scan or magnetic resonance imaging (MRI) is indicated prior to lumbar puncture in every patient with papilledema, an altered level of consciousness, a focal neurologic deficit, a new-onset seizure, or an immunocompromised state. A cranial MRI is indicated in every patient with a cerebellar deficit prior to lumbar puncture. The platelet count should be 50,000 or greater, and the international normalized ratio (INR) should be less than 1.5.

The patient is placed in the lateral recumbent position with the knees and the neck flexed (Fig. 1-1) or the seated position with the neck flexed. The patient's back should be as close to the edge of the table as possible. The top of the iliac crest is palpated, and the thumb of the same hand is placed in the interspace that forms a vertical line with the top of the iliac crest. This usually crosses the L3–4 interspace (see Fig. 1-1). Lumbar puncture can be performed at the L3–4, L4–5, or L5–S1 interspace. The L2–3 interspace and higher levels should be avoided because the conus medullaris terminates at the L1–2 interspace in 95 percent of individuals and the L2–3 interspace in the remainder.[2]

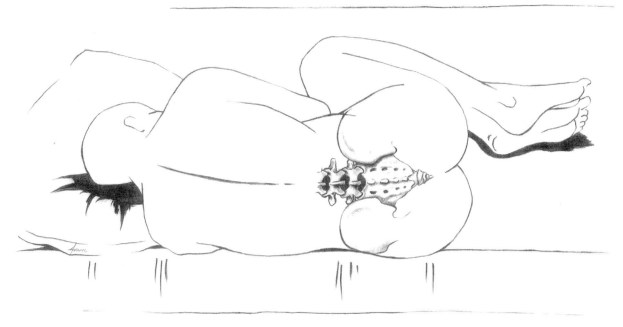

Figure 1-1. Proper positioning of the patient for lumbar puncture. The L3–4, L4–5, and L5–S1 interspaces are shown. *(Drawn by Avanee Shah M.D.)*

Heinrich Quincke developed the technique of lumbar puncture and described measurement of the opening pressure with a manometer and analysis of the CSF.[3] The standard needle used for lumbar puncture is the Quincke needle with a beveled tip. The bevel of the needle should be parallel to the longitudinal fibers of the dura. If the patient is in the lateral recumbent position, the flat portion of the bevel of the needle is pointed upward to the patient's side. When the flat portion of the bevel of the needle is positioned correctly, the notch in the hub for the stylet should point up toward the physician. If the patient is seated, the flat portion of the bevel of the needle is pointed to the patient's side, and the notch in the hub of the stylet is in the direction of the patient's side. Whether the patient is in the lateral recumbent or the seated position, the flat portion of the bevel of the needle and the notch in the hub of the stylet should point in the direction of the patient's side.[4]

Advancement of the needle may be prevented by bone. This is usually the spinous process or lamina (Fig. 1-2). The needle should be withdrawn and readvanced in a slightly different direction. A pop is often felt as the needle pierces the supraspinous ligament (Fig. 1-3*A*), and a second pop is felt as the needle enters the subarachnoid space (see Fig. 1-3*B*). If fluid does not appear when the stylet is removed, replace the stylet and rotate the needle 90 degrees. Then if fluid does not appear after the stylet is removed, insert the needle a few millimeters further slowly until fluid appears at the needle hub. If this fails, the needle should be withdrawn almost to the skin because redirection of the needle is not possible when the tip of the needle is deep in the tissue.[2]

When fluid appears at the needle hub, a three-way stopcock with manometer is attached. The fluid is allowed to rise slowly in the manometer. The upper limit of normal CSF opening pressure with a patient in the

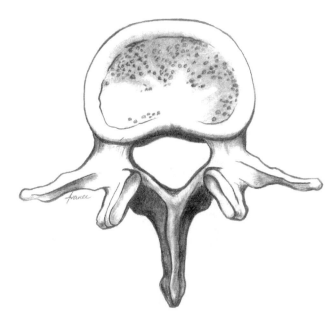

Figure 1-2. Vertebral body. When bone prevents advancement of the needle, it is most often due to failure to open the interspace adequately by proper positioning of the patient, or the needle is touching the spinous process or lamina. *(Drawn by Avanee Shah, M.D.)*

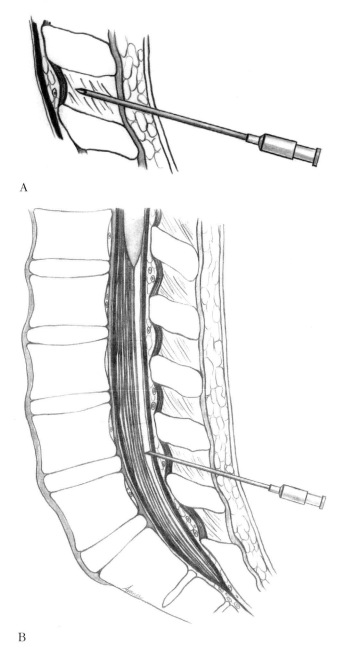

A

B

Figure 1-3. *A.* Sagittal view of lumbar puncture needle bevel position as it is advanced through the interspinous ligament prior to entering the subarachnoid space. The layers that the needle goes through are depicted from the skin are as follows: skin, subcutaneous fat, supraspinous ligament, and interspinous ligament. The needle tip has not yet gone through the ligamentum flavum. *(Drawn by Avanee Shah, M.D.) B.* Sagittal view of lumbar puncture needle tip in the subarachnoid space. The layers that the needle goes through are skin, subcutaneous fat, supraspinous ligament, interspinous ligament, ligamentum flavum, epidural fat, dura, arachnoid, and the tip in the subarachnoid space. *(Drawn by Avanee Shah, M.D.)*

lateral recumbent position is 110 mmH$_2$O in infants, 150 mmH$_2$O in children, 180 mmH$_2$O in adults, and 250 mmH$_2$O in obese adults.[5] A very slow rise of the CSF in the manometer is indicative of either a partial obstruction of the needle tip by meningeal membrane or nerve root or a low CSF pressure.[2] To determine if there is an obstruction to the outflow of CSF, firm abdominal pressure can be applied with the physician's or assistant's hands. If CSF is free to flow, firm abdominal pressure should give a rapid rise in the fluid in the manometer, and a rapid fall should occur when the pressure is released.[2]

When the flow of CSF is slow, a few techniques can be tried to increase the rate of flow of the fluid. The patient can be asked to bear down to increase intraabdominal pressure, an assistant can apply pressure to the abdomen with the palm of the hand, or CSF can be gently aspirated with a syringe. The latter technique, however, increases the risk of nerve root herniation through the opening of the needle.

When obtaining CSF for analysis, it is important to remember that adults have approximately 150 ml of CSF, but infants and children have lower amounts ranging from 30 to 60 ml in the neonate to 100 ml in the adolescent.[6] The volume of CSF in a child aged 4 to 13 years ranges from 65 to 140 ml, with an average volume of 90 ml.[1] Approximately 10 to 15 ml of CSF should be withdrawn from adults for analysis, and the withdrawal of 3 to 5 ml is recommended in neonates and children.[6]

After CSF is collected, the stylet is reinserted and the needle is withdrawn. The rationale for reinserting the stylet before removing the needle is to prevent a strand of arachnoid that may have entered the needle with the outflowing CSF from being threaded back through the dural defect when the needle is removed. If a strand of arachnoid is in the dural defect, this allows for prolonged leakage of CSF along the arachnoid. When the stylet is reinserted to the tip of the needle, any strand of arachnoid that has entered the needle will be pushed out or cut off.[7]

Contraindications to Lumbar Puncture

A lumbar puncture is contraindicated when there are clinical signs of impending uncal, central, transtentorial, or cerebellar herniation and when the needle must pass through an area of infection that could result in infection in the subarachnoid space. Spinal epidural or subdural hematoma may complicate lumbar puncture performed in patients with thrombocytopenia (platelet counts of less than 50,000) or a prolonged prothrombin time or INR. Raised intracranial pressure is an expected complication of a number of CNS infections and is not a contraindication to lumbar puncture. Patients who have an alteration in the level of consciousness, a focal neurologic deficit on examination, unilateral or bilateral sluggishly reactive or nonreactive pupils, decerebrate or decorticate rigidity, irregular respiratory patterns, oculomotor abnormalities, the Cushing reflex (bradycardia, hypertension, and irregular respirations), and/or papilledema should have a neuroimaging procedure prior to lumbar puncture. Once the neuroimaging procedure has excluded a focal intracranial mass lesion, lumbar puncture usually can be performed safely. When the presence of raised intracranial pressure is suspected based on clinical examination, a bolus dose of mannitol 1 g/kg of body weight can be given intravenously and lumbar puncture performed 20 minutes later. Alternatively, the patient can be intubated and hyperventilated in addition to being treated with intravenous mannitol prior to lumbar puncture.

▶ COMPOSITION OF NORMAL CSF

Cell Count

The number of white blood cells (WBCs) in the CSF varies somewhat with age; however, the presence of more than five WBCs/mm³ in CSF is abnormal in individuals 8 weeks of age and older.

Newborns
The upper limit of normal for CSF total WBC count is 22/mm³ in full-term neonates, 15/mm³ in infants 4 to 8 weeks of age, and 5/mm³ in those older than 8 weeks of age. In newborns, in normal uninfected CSF, about 60 percent of the cells are polymorphonuclear leukocytes and 40 percent are mononucleated cells.

Children and Adults
In children and adults, in uninfected CSF, the normal WBC count ranges from 0 to 5 mononuclear cells (lymphocytes and monocytes) per cubic millimeter. In normal uninfected CSF, there should be no polymorphonuclear leukocytes; however, with use of the cytocentrifuge, an occasional polymorphonuclear leukocyte may be seen. If the total WBC count is less than 5/mm³, the presence of a single polymorphonuclear leukocyte may be considered normal.[1,6,8]

Traumatic Tap
A *traumatic tap* refers to the introduction of blood into the subarachnoid space by the spinal tap. Blood is introduced into the CSF during lumbar puncture when the spinal needle penetrates the radicular arterial vessels and veins. When this occurs, interpretation of the results must determine if the CSF pleocytosis is real or if the WBCs were introduced into the subarachnoid space by the spinal tap. To determine the true number of WBCs in the CSF, 1 WBC/mm³ for every 700 red blood cells (RBCs) per cubic millimeter is subtracted from the total WBC count. Thus, if there are 700 RBCs and 10 WBCs, 9 WBCs were present in the CSF prior to introduction of RBCs and WBCs by the spinal tap.[9]

A traumatic tap is fairly easy to distinguish from a subarachnoid hemorrhage. When the spinal needle has penetrated a radicular artery or vein, a clot or thread of blood appears in the CSF in the collection tube. If only a small amount of blood appears, the fluid can be allowed to drip for a few seconds before a sample is collected for analysis. Tubes 1 and 4 can be sent for cell count to demonstrate that the number of RBCs has decreased in the CSF between tube 1 and tube 4, supporting the assumption that the RBCs are present because the tap was traumatic. When a subarachnoid hemorrhage has occurred, the CSF remains pink-tinged through all four tubes as it is collected. A sample of the bloody CSF should be centrifuged. In a traumatic tap, the supernatant is colorless, whereas in a subarachnoid hemorrhage, the supernatant is yellow (xanthochromic). It takes from 2 to 12 hours for xanthochromia to appear from a subarachnoid hemorrhage, and the xanthochromia persists for weeks. Xanthochromia also can be seen in the CSF of patients who have had a number of lumbar punctures during any of which the spinal needle penetrated a radicular artery or vein, introducing red blood cells into the CSF, and when the CSF protein concentration is greater than 150 mg/dl.

Glucose

The concentration of glucose in the CSF depends on the serum glucose concentration, the facilitated membrane carrier system that transfers glucose between blood and CSF, and the rate of glucose metabolism by the various cellular elements in the CSF.[9] The normal CSF glucose concentration is between 45 and 80 mg/dl when the serum glucose concentration is 70 to 120 mg/dl, or approximately 65 percent of the serum glucose level. CSF glucose concentrations below 45 mg/dl are abnormal. The differential diagnosis of a decreased CSF glucose concentration (hypoglycorrhachia) includes bacterial meningitis, herpes simplex virus encephalitis, fungal meningitis, tuberculous meningitis, carcinomatous meningitis, sarcoidosis, and hypoglycemia. A serum glucose concentration always should be obtained at the time of lumbar puncture to determine the CSF–serum glucose ratio. The normal CSF–serum glucose ratio is 0.6. The CSF glucose concentration is low when the CSF–serum glucose ratio is less than 0.6, and a CSF–serum glucose ratio of 0.31 or less is highly predictive of bacterial meningitis. Hyperglycemia increases the CSF glucose concentration, and its presence may mask a decreased CSF glucose concentration.[9]

In preterm and full-term infants, the normal CSF–serum glucose ratio is 0.81 due to the immaturity of the glucose exchange mechanisms, the greater permeability of the blood-brain barrier, and the greater rate of cerebral blood flow in infancy compared with adulthood.[8,9]

Protein

The upper range of normal for the lumbar CSF protein concentration is 50 mg/dl in adults, 45 mg/dl in children, and 150 mg/dl in neonates. The higher number for the normal neonatal CSF protein concentration is due to the immaturity of the neonatal CSF blood-brain barrier. By 1 year of age, the normal value for the lumbar CSF protein concentration is 45 mg/dl. The upper range of normal for the cisternal CSF protein concentration is 30 mg/dl in children and adults and 170 mg/dL in neonates.[10] An increased CSF protein concentration is a nonspecific abnormality that is seen in any process that increases the permeability of the blood-brain barrier. When the lumbar puncture has been traumatic, the CSF protein concentration will be increased by 1 mg/dl for every 1000 RBCs/mm^3.[6]

▶ CENTRAL NERVOUS SYSTEM INFECTIONS

Meningitis

Bacterial Meningitis

The classic CSF abnormalities in bacterial meningitis are the following: (1) an increased opening pressure, (2) a polymorphonuclear leukocytosis (>100 cells/mm^3 in 90 percent), (3) a decreased glucose concentration (<40 mg/dl and/or a CSF–serum glucose ratio of less than 0.31), and (4) an increased protein concentration (>45 mg/dl in 90 percent). The CSF should be examined by Gram's stain and culture.

Oral antimicrobial therapy prior to lumbar puncture will not alter the CSF WBC count or glucose concentration significantly but will decrease the likelihood of identifying the organism on Gram's stain or isolating the organism in culture. Gram's stain is positive in identifying the meningeal pathogen in 60 to 90 percent of patients with community-acquired bacterial meningitis. The likelihood of identifying the organism on Gram's stain depends not only on the CSF concentration of bacteria but also on the specific bacterial pathogen causing the meningitis.[11] The latex particle agglutination (LA) test detects bacterial antigens of *Hemophilus influenzae* type b (Hib), *Streptococcus pneumoniae*, *Neisseria meningitidis*, group B *Streptococcus*, and *Escherichia coli* K1 strains in CSF. The specificity of the LA test is greater than the sensitivity for common bacterial pathogens. The limulus amebocyte lysate assay is a rapid diagnostic test for the detection of gram-negative

endotoxin in CSF and thus for making a diagnosis of gram-negative bacterial meningitis. The test has a specificity of 85 to 100 percent and a sensitivity approaching 100 percent.[12] A positive limulus amebocyte lysate assay will be seen in virtually all patients with gram-negative bacterial meningitis, but false-positive results may occur.

A broad-range bacterial polymerase chain reaction (PCR) assay is available for the early detection of bacterial meningitis. The broad-range PCR assay has a sensitivity of 100 percent, a specificity of 98.2 percent, a positive predictive value of 98.2 percent, and a negative predictive value of 100 percent. Therefore, the broad-range PCR assay may be used to exclude the diagnosis of bacterial meningitis.[13] PCR assays also are available to detect DNA of all the common meningeal pathogens, but the sensitivity and specificity of these tests have not yet been defined.

The CSF Gram's stain should be negative, and culture of the CSF obtained 24 hours after initiation of antimicrobial therapy should be sterile if the infecting organism is sensitive to the antibiotic. Present recommendations are that a repeat lumbar puncture be performed in all patients with pneumococcal meningitis 24 to 36 hours after the initiation of antimicrobial therapy to document eradication of the pathogen, given the increasing incidence of penicillin- and cephalosporin-resistant strains of pneumococci.[14] In most patients, the CSF glucose concentration returns to normal within 3 days after antimicrobial therapy is initiated; however, the glucose concentration may remain low for 10 days or longer despite clinical improvement. There may be an increase in the CSF WBC count within 18 to 36 hours of initiation of antimicrobial therapy, and this should not be interpreted as an indication that the organism is not sensitive to the antibiotic.[1,15]

Blood cultures should be obtained in all patients with suspected bacterial meningitis. A serum glucose concentration should be obtained at the time of lumbar puncture to determine the CSF–serum glucose ratio.

Viral Meningitis

The classic CSF abnormalities in viral meningitis are (1) a normal opening pressure, (2) a lymphocytic pleocytosis, (3) a normal glucose concentration, and (4) a normal or slightly elevated protein concentration. The enteroviruses [coxsackieviruses, echoviruses, and the viruses identified by number (enteroviruses 68 to 71)] are the most common viruses to cause meningitis. Herpes simplex virus type 2 (HSV-2), the human immunodeficiency virus (HIV-1), and the arthropod-borne viruses are also fairly common etiologic agents of meningitis. Initially, there may be a predominance of polymorphonuclear leukocytes in enteroviral meningitis with a transition to a lymphocytic pleocytosis within 24 hours. Enteroviruses either can be isolated in CSF culture or can be detected in CSF by the reverse-transcriptase polymerase chain reaction (RT-PCR) technique. HSV-2 DNA can be detected in CSF by PCR. CSF culture is positive for HSV-2 in most cases of meningitis associated with primary genital herpes but is rarely positive in cases of meningitis associated with recurrent episodes of genital herpes. HIV-1 RNA levels can be measured in CSF, and the virus can be cultured in CSF.

In meningitis due to an arthropod-borne virus, there may be a polymorphonuclear leukocytosis early in infection with a shift to a lymphocytic or mononuclear pleocytosis later in the illness. Rarely, polymorphonuclear leukocytes may predominate in the first 48 hours of illness with West Nile virus and may persist for up to a week before there is a shift to a lymphocytic pleocytosis. La Crosse virus has not been cultured in CSF. The St. Louis encephalitis virus is rarely isolated from CSF.[16] There is a CSF PCR test available for West Nile virus, but the sensitivity and specificity have not been defined. The best diagnostic test for West Nile virus meningitis is the detection of West Nile virus IgM in CSF, but this may not be positive until 7 days after the onset of symptoms. Identification of an arthropod-borne virus as the causative agent of meningitis often depends on serology. According to the Centers for Disease Control and Prevention (CDC), a confirmed case of arboviral meningitis is defined as a febrile illness with mild neurologic symptoms during a period when arboviral transmission is likely to occur plus at least one of the following criteria: (1) a fourfold or greater increase in serum antibody titer between acute and convalescent sera, (2) viral isolation from tissue, blood, or CSF, or (3) specific immunoglobulin M (IgM) antibody to an arbovirus in the CSF. A presumptive case is defined as a compatible illness plus either a stable increased antibody titer to an arbovirus ($\geq$320 by hemagglutination inhibition, $\geq$128 by complement fixation, $\geq$256 by immunofluorescent assay, or $\geq$160 by plaque-reduction neutralization test) or specific IgM antibody in serum by enzyme immunoassay.[17]

The lymphocytic choriomeningitis virus can cause an aseptic meningitis with the CSF abnormalities of a lymphocytic pleocytosis and hypoglycorrhachia.[18] The lymphocytic choriomeningitis virus is one of the few etiologic agents of an aseptic meningitis with hypoglycorrhachia. This virus can be grown in culture of CSF. To make a diagnosis of lymphocytic choriomeningitis virus infection, IgM antibodies must be detected in blood and CSF. Acute and convalescent sera can be sent to detect a fourfold increase in IgG. The mumps virus also may cause a lymphocytic pleocytosis with a decreased CSF glucose concentration.

Meningitis may complicate acute Epstein-Barr virus (EBV) infection. Acute infection is confirmed by the detection of antiviral capsid antigen (VCA) titers of 1:320 or higher, positive IgM antibody titers to the viral capsid antigen (EBV VCA IgM antibodies), and the absence of antibodies to virus-associated nuclear antigen [antibodies to EBV nuclear antigen (anti-EBNA IgG)]. In subsequent serum specimens (collected 36 days after the onset of illness), there should be a fourfold decrease in the IgG antibody titer to the viral capsid antigen and a 16-fold increase in anti-EBNA IgG.[19,20] EBV DNA also can be detected in CSF by PCR.

In patients with CSF abnormalities classic for bacterial meningitis but in whom the CSF Gram's stain and culture are negative and in patients with a CSF polymorphonuclear leukocytosis and a normal glucose concentration in whom the clinical suspicion is viral meningitis, additional diagnostic tests are necessary to distinguish between bacterial and viral meningitis. CSF lactate concentrations are, in general, nonspecific and can be elevated in patients with bacterial meningitis, cerebral hypoxia, and cerebral ischemia or by the metabolism of CSF leukocytes. An elevated serum concentration of procalcitonin is fairly sensitive and specific for bacterial meningitis.[21,23] Enteroviruses can be isolated from throat or stool cultures. During enteroviral infections, viral shedding in stool may persist for several weeks. For this reason, the presence of an enterovirus in stool is not diagnostic but rather presumptive evidence that the enterovirus is the causative virus of the meningitis.

Fungal Meningitis

The CSF abnormalities in fungal meningitis are the following: (1) a normal or slightly elevated opening pressure, (2) a lymphocytic pleocytosis (20 to 500 cells/mm^3), (3) a decreased glucose concentration, and (4) an elevated protein concentration. Fluid should be sent for India ink stain and culture. The LA test for the cryptococcal antigen is highly sensitive and specific; the antigen can be detected in CSF in 85 to 90 percent of cases of cryptococcal meningitis and in 95 percent of cases of cryptococcal meningitis in HIV-infected individuals.[24] *Cryptococcus neoformans* also can be identified on India ink stain and grown in culture. The India ink stain is reported to be positive in 50 percent of all cases and in 75 to 88 percent of HIV-positive individuals.[25,26]

In areas endemic for *Histoplasma capsulatum*, specifically the midwestern United States in the Mississippi and Ohio River valleys and regions of Central and South America, CSF should be examined for the histoplasma polysaccharide antigen. The presence of the histoplasma polysaccharide antigen in CSF is a reliable indicator of CNS infection; however, there have been reports of cross-reactivity with *C. immitis, C. neoformans,* and *Candida* in histoplasma polysaccharide antigen tests of CSF. When fungal meningitis is suspected, large volumes of CSF (15 to 20 ml) should be cultured on at least three occasions to increase the yield for isolation of the fungus. Consideration also should be given to obtaining CSF by cisternal or high cervical puncture. In cases of fungal meningitis, one CSF culture out of several may be positive, emphasizing the need for repeated sampling of CSF to isolate the fungus.

In areas endemic for *Coccidioides immitis*, specifically California, Arizona, New Mexico, and Texas, the complement fixation antibody test for *C. immitis* is performed on CSF. The complement fixation antibody test on CSF is reported to have a specificity of 100 percent and a sensitivity of 75 percent in *C. immitis* meningitis.[25] Meningitis due to *C. immitis* may be associated with either an eosinophilic or a neutrophilic pleocytosis. Cultures are positive in only 25 percent of cases.

Meningitis due to *Blastomyces dermatitidis* may present with a CSF polymorphonuclear leukocytic pleocytosis. *B. dermatitidis* is endemic in the Piedmont area of the United States, as well as the Mississippi, Ohio, and St. Lawrence River valleys. It is rare to identify *B. dermatitidis* from CSF obtained by lumbar puncture. Culture of cisternal or ventricular CSF has a better yield.

Patients suspected of having fungal meningitis should have chest x-rays or a CT scan to evaluate for a pulmonary source of infection.

Tuberculous Meningitis

The classic CSF abnormalities in tuberculous meningitis are (1) an elevated opening pressure, (2) a lymphocytic pleocytosis of 10 to 500 cells/mm^3, (3) a decreased glucose concentration, and (4) an elevated protein concentration in the range of 100 to 500 mg/dl. The CSF glucose concentration may be only minimally decreased in the range of 35 to 40 mg/dl. The combination of a chronic CSF lymphocytic pleocytosis (for more than 4 weeks) or a persistent CSF neutrophilic pleocytosis with a minimally decreased glucose concentration is suspicious for tuberculous meningitis. The gold standard for the diagnosis of tuberculous meningitis has been the detection of acid-fast bacilli (AFB) in smears of CSF or a positive culture result. Cultures of CSF require 3 to 6 weeks for growth to be detectable and are positive in approximately 50 to 75 percent of cases of tuberculous meningitis. As is true for fungal meningitis, the yield on smear and culture increases the more samples of CSF that are studied; therefore, two or three serial samples of CSF should be obtained from the lumbar space for smear and culture, followed by examination of a CSF sample obtained from a cisternal or lateral cervical puncture, if necessary. Today, many hospital laboratories have rapid molecular diagnostic techniques for the identification of *M. tuberculosis* in CSF. The PCR technique for detection of tubercle bacilli DNA in CSF is only one of these rapid diagnostic techniques. The PCR technique for the detection of *M. tuberculosis* DNA has a reported sensitivity of 50 percent and a 10 percent false-positive rate.[28–30] The CSF abnormalities in non-HIV-infected individuals and in HIV-infected individuals with tuberculous meningitis are the same.

A nonspecific abnormality that has been reported in tuberculous meningitis is an increase in adenosine deaminase levels. The CSF chloride concentration may be decreased in tuberculous meningitis. This is, however, a nonspecific abnormality because the CSF chloride concentration typically decreases as the CSF protein concentration increases.

Syphilitic Meningitis

The classic abnormalities on examination of the CSF in syphilitic meningitis are as follows: (1) an increased opening pressure, (2) a mononuclear pleocytosis, (3) an elevated protein concentration, and (4) a positive Venereal Disease Research Laboratory (VDRL) test. A nonreactive CSF VDRL test does not rule out neurosyphilis. The VDRL test is reported to be nonreactive in 30 to 57 percent of samples of CSF from patients with neurosyphilis.[31,32] A reactive CSF VDRL test virtually confirms the diagnosis of neurosyphilis except when the CSF is tinged with blood.[33] A false-positive CSF VDRL test may be obtained when the CSF is contaminated with visible amounts of blood.[34] A nonreactive CSF fluorescent treponemal antibody absorption (FTA-ABS) test or a nonreactive microhemagglutination–*Treponema pallidum* (MHA-TP) test excludes the diagnosis; however, a reactive CSF FTA-ABS test or a reactive CSF MHA-TP test does not establish the diagnosis.[35] The CSF FTA-ABS test, the CSF MHA-TP test, or both may be falsely reactive as the result of the passive transfer of *T. pallidum*–specific IgG across the meninges from the serum into the CSF.

Lyme Disease

The most common form of neurologic Lyme disease or neuroborreliosis is headache with neck stiffness, low-grade fever, and a unilateral or bilateral (in 25 percent of cases) facial nerve palsy. There is disagreement about whether all patients with a facial nerve palsy due to Lyme disease need CSF analysis. Some experts recommend that CSF analysis be performed only in patients who have severe headache or nuchal rigidity in addition to a seventh cranial nerve palsy and that patients with only a seventh cranial nerve palsy be treated with doxycycline without CSF analysis. The classic CSF abnormalities in neuroborreliosis are (1) a lymphocytic pleocytosis, (2) an increased protein concentration, (3) a normal glucose concentration, (4) an elevated IgG index and IgG synthesis rate, and (5) oligoclonal bands. Definitive diagnosis requires demonstration of intrathecal anti–*Borrelia burgdorferi* antibody production, but the inability to detect intrathecal antibody production does not rule out infection. As with all CNS infections, CSF antibody concentrations must be compared with

▶ **TABLE 1-1.** ROUTINE CSF DIAGNOSTIC STUDIES FOR FEVER AND HEADACHE

Cell count with differential
Glucose and protein concentration
Stain and culture
   Gram's stain and bacterial culture
   India ink and fungal culture
   Viral culture
   Acid fast smear and *M. tuberculosis* culture
Antigens
   Cryptococcal polysaccharide antigen
   Histoplasma polysaccharide antigen
Polymerase chain reaction
   Broad-range bacterial PCR
   Specific meningeal pathogen PCR
   Reverse-transcriptase PCR for enteroviruses
   PCR for herpes simplex virus 2
   PCR for HIV RNA
   PCR for West Nile virus
   PCR for Epstein-Barr virus
Antibodies
   Herpes simplex virus
   Arthropod-borne viruses
   B. burgdorferi
   C. immitis complement-fixation antibody
   Lymphocytic choriomeningitis virus
Other
   Limulus amebocyte assay
   VDRL and FTA-ABS

serum antibody concentrations to determine if the observed antibody is actually being produced in the CSF. The ratio of the CSF antibody titer to the serum antibody titer must be greater the 1. PCR assay for *B. burgdorferi* in CSF is specific but insensitive. Table 1-1 provides a list of the routine studies to perform on CSF for evaluation of fever and headache when meningitis is suspected.

Viral Encephalitis

Any of a number of viruses can cause encephalitis. Table 1-2 is a list of the viral causes of encephalitis and the best diagnostic tests to identify the viruses. CSF analysis in viral encephalitis typically demonstrates a lymphocytic pleocytosis, a normal glucose concentration, and a mildly elevated protein concentration. On examination of the CSF in HSV-1 encephalitis, there is an increased opening pressure, a lymphocytic pleocytosis of 5 to 500 cells/mm^3, a mild to moderate increase in the protein concentration, and normal or mildly decreased glucose concentration. CSF viral cultures for HSV-1 are almost always negative. PCR assay has become the gold standard for making the diagnosis of HSV encephalitis. HSV DNA was detected in CSF by PCR in 53 of 54 pa-

tients (98 percent) with biopsy-proven HSV encephalitis.[36] The PCR assay may be negative if treatment has been initiated with acyclovir, if there are inhibitors of the PCR assay in the CSF such as porphyrin compounds from the degradation of heme in erythrocytes, or if CSF is examined by PCR assay too early after the onset of symptoms. The PCR test may be negative in the first 3 days following the onset of symptoms.[37,38] If a PCR test for HSV DNA in CSF that has been obtained within the first 72 hours of symptoms is negative, and if HSV encephalitis remains a good possibility, the CSF should be reexamined by PCR for HSV DNA. Cultures of CSF for HSV-1 are almost always negative in adults with HSV encephalitis, but CSF culture is positive in approximately 50 percent of patients with neonatal HSV encephalitis. CSF PCR assay may remain persistently positive for HSV DNA despite adequate therapy. Routine retesting of CSF is not recommended at the end of 21 days of acyclovir therapy.

HSV DNA in CSF precedes the appearance of HSV antibodies by several days. CSF and serum samples should be obtained to determine if there is intrathecal synthesis of antibodies against HSV. Antibodies against HSV do not appear in the CSF until approximately 8 to 12 days after the onset of disease and may increase markedly during the first 2 to 4 weeks of infection. A serum-CSF antibody ratio of 20:1 or less is considered diagnostic of HSV infection.

Definitive diagnosis of arboviral encephalitis requires one or more of the following: (1) a fourfold increase in antibody titer between acute and convalescent sera, (2) viral isolation from tissue, blood, or CSF, and (3) virus-specific IgM antibody in CSF. A presumptive case is defined as a compatible illness plus either a stable elevated antibody titer to an arboviral virus (≥320 by hemagglutination inhibition, ≥128 by complement fixation, ≥256 by immunofluorescent assay, or ≥160 by plaque-reduction neutralization test) or specific IgM antibody in serum by enzyme immunoassay.

In arboviral encephalitis, the CSF typically shows a lymphocytic pleocytosis, a normal glucose concentration, and a normal or mildly elevated protein concentration. Some features unique to the virus are that patients with La Crosse virus encephalitis may have hyponatremia or hypoosmolarity due to the syndrome of inappropriate secretion of antidiuretic hormone (SIADH). Serologic testing is the best way to make a diagnosis of La Crosse virus encephalitis by demonstrating serum IgM antibody titers of 1:10 or greater or a fourfold increase in IgG antibody titers between acute and convalescent sera. Hyponatremia and serum hypoosmolarity due to SIADH also may be seen in St. Louis encephalitis. The CSF may demonstrate an increased number of polymorphonuclear leukocytes early in infection with a subsequent shift to a lymphocytic pleocytosis. West Nile virus encephalitis also may have an

▶ **TABLE 1-2.** VIRAL CAUSES OF ENCEPHALITIS AND THE BEST DIAGNOSTIC TEST TO IDENTIFY THE VIRUS

Virus	Diagnostic Test
Herpes simplex virus type 1	CSF PCR for HSV-1 DNA CSF HSV antibodies
Herpes simplex virus type 2 (neonates)	CSF viral culture CSF PCR for HSV-1 and HSV-2 DNA CSF HSV antibodies
Mosquito-borne viruses:	CSF IgM antibody titers CSF PCR for West Nile virus Fourfold increase in IgG between acute and convalescent sera

La Crosse virus
    Snowshoe hare virus
    St. Louis encephalitis virus
    West Nile virus
    Japanese encephalitis virus
    Eastern equine encephalitis virus
    Western equine encephalitis virus
    Venezuelan encephalitis virus
    Dengue virus	

Tick-borne virus
    Tick-borne encephalitis virus
    Powassan virus
    Colorado tick fever virus
	Serum antibodies to the virus

Varicella-zoster virus	CSF IgM antibodies CSF PCR for VZV DNA CSF viral culture
Adenovirus	CSF viral culture Fourfold increase in IgG between acute and convalescent sera
Epstein-Barr virus	CSF PCR for EBV DNA CSF IgM and IgG antibodies to viral capsid antigen
Cytomegalovirus	CSF PCR for CMV DNA
Enterovirus	CSF RT-PCR for enteroviruses CSF viral culture
Measles virus	CSF antibody titers

initial predominance of polymorphonuclear leukocytes with a subsequent shift to a lymphocytic pleocytosis. The CSF glucose concentration is typically normal, and the protein concentration is usually mildly to moderately elevated. The best way to make a diagnosis of West Nile virus CNS infection is by detection of anti–West Nile virus IgM antibodies in CSF by capture enzyme-linked immunosorbent assay (ELISA), but this test may not be positive until 7 days after the onset of symptoms. A positive serologic result by ELISA can be confirmed by plaque-reduction neutralization assays. IgM antibodies may persist in both serum and CSF for several months. There is a PCR test available for West Nile virus encephalitis. It is reported to have a low sensitivity, and a negative result does not rule out infection.

St. Louis encephalitis virus, eastern equine encephalitis virus, and western equine encephalitis are rarely isolated from CSF. In eastern equine encephalitis there is typically a much more elevated leukocyte count in CSF than in the other arthropod-borne encephalitides, with 20 to 2000 cells/mm^3, 60 to 90 percent of which are neutrophils. The Powassan virus belongs to the tick-borne encephalitis complex of flaviviruses. The Colorado tick fever virus is a member of the reovirus family. Diagnosis of the tick-borne virus encephalitides is based on serology. The CSF abnormalities are typical of the arboviral encephalitides with a normal glucose concentration, a mild to moderately elevated protein concentration, and an initial polymorphonuclear pleocytosis shifting to a lymphocytic pleocytosis later in the disease course. Neutralizing antibody to the Powassan virus is usually detectable at the time of onset of illness, but brain biopsy may be necessary to make the diagnosis. Antibodies to Colorado tick fever virus are usually not detectable until 1 to 2 weeks after the onset of illness.[16]

The typical abnormalities on examination of the CSF in varicella-zoster virus (VZV) encephalitis are a mild mononuclear pleocytosis, an elevated protein concentration, and a decreased glucose concentration. The detection of VZV DNA in CSF by PCR assay can confirm the diagnosis. VZV antibody is often present in CSF, but viral culture is rarely positive. The detection of IgM against VZV in CSF suggests active infection. Positive CSF cultures occur with a higher frequency in encephalitis that occurs as a complication of reactivation of VZV than in encephalitis as a complication of primary VZV infection.

The diagnosis of adenovirus encephalitis is made by isolating the virus in cultures of CSF or by demonstrating a fourfold increase in antibody titer between acute and convalescent sera. The diagnosis of encephalitis due to EBV is made by the detection of EBV DNA in the CSF, provided that the lumbar puncture was not traumatic. EBV DNA is found in peripheral blood mononuclear cells and can contaminate the CSF if the lumbar puncture is traumatic. IgM and IgG antibodies to viral capsid antigen can be detected in CSF.

The CSF formula in cytomegalovirus (CMV) encephalitis is typical of viral infections, but in CMV myeloradiculitis, the CSF formula is atypical. There is a pleocytosis of polymorphonuclear leukocytes and a decreased CSF glucose concentration. CSF PCR assay is both sensitive and specific, but CMV viremia or retinitis may cause a false-positive result. Quantitative PCR is available in many laboratories and is used increasingly to evaluate both the severity of disease and the response to treatment.[39,40]

Human herpesvirus type 6 may cause an encephalitis with focal features resembling HSV-1 encephalitis or an encephalitis with multifocal areas of demyelination in immunosuppressed individuals. The diagnosis of human herpesvirus type 6 encephalitis requires isolation of the virus in CSF culture and a concomitant fourfold or greater increase in IgG titer between acute and convalescent sera. The detection of human herpesvirus type 6 DNA in CSF by PCR assay does not distinguish between latent infection and active viral replication associated with reactivation.

Progressive multifocal leukoencephalopathy is a demyelinating disease occurring in patients with severe cellular immunosuppression due to reactivation of a virus acquired in childhood, the JC virus. The CSF is typically noninflammatory, but there may be a mild elevation of the protein concentration. CSF PCR assay for JC virus DNA is highly specific but not very sensitive;

therefore, a positive result establishes the diagnosis, but a negative result does not exclude the diagnosis.

The diagnosis of subacute sclerosing panencephalitis is made on the basis of evidence of increased measles antibody titer in the CSF or serum (or both). Subacute measles encephalitis occurs in immunosuppressed individuals with a latent period of 1 to 10 months between the measles-like illness and the encephalitis.[41,42] Examination of the CSF reveals a mild mononuclear pleocytosis and a mild elevation in the protein concentration, but in about one-third of patients the CSF is entirely normal. Diagnosis is made by brain biopsy.

Rocky Mountain Spotted Fever

Rocky mountain spotted fever is caused by the bacteria *Rickettsia rickettsii,* which is transmitted by a tick bite. CSF abnormalities include a mild (rarely more than 100 cells/mm^3) lymphocytic pleocytosis and an elevated protein concentration. The diagnosis is made by skin biopsy of the rash with a demonstration of rickettsiae in the endothelial cells of blood vessels by immunofluorescence, by the demonstration of *R. rickettsii* IgM in serum (IgM > 1:132), or by a twofold increase in *R. rickettsii* IgG titers over a 2-week period.

Postinfectious Encephalomyelitis

Postinfectious encephalomyelitis is an acute monophasic disorder of the CNS that occurs within days to weeks of a viral illness or a vaccination and is characterized neuropathologically by perivenular inflammation and demyelination. Examination of the CSF demonstrates a mononuclear cell pleocytosis, an elevated protein concentration, and a normal glucose concentration. In about one-third of patients, the CSF analysis is normal. Myelin basic protein and oligoclonal bands may be found in the CSF.[43]

▶ 14-3-3 IMMUNOASSAY

The 14-3-3 immunoassay on CSF has been demonstrated to be useful for the diagnosis of Creutzfeldt-Jakob disease (CJD) in select patients with progressive dementia (of less than 2 years duration) and myoclonus, visual abnormalities, ataxia, and pyramidal or extrapyramidal signs.[44] False-positive results have been reported in patients with HSV encephalitis, recent cerebral infarction, degenerative dementias (including Alzheimer's disease), carcinomatous meningitis, paraneoplastic neurologic disorders, and anoxic encephalopathy. Present recommendations are that this test not be used for screening purposes and only be used in patients who meet the diagnostic criteria for CJD (classic clinical presentation and course and electroencephalographic abnormalities).[45]

REFERENCES

1. Bonadio WA: The cerebrospinal fluid: Physiologic aspects and alterations associated with bacterial meningitis. *Pediatr Infect Dis J* 11:423, 1992.

2. Fishman RA: Examination of the cerebrospinal fluid: Techniques and complications. In Fishman RA (ed): *Cerebrospinal Fluid in Diseases of the Nervous System*, 2d ed. Philadelphia: Saunders, 1992, pp 157–182.

3. Quincke H: *Uber hydrocephalus, Verhandlungen des Congressus fur innere Medizin*, Vol 10, Wiesbaden, Germany: Bergman, 1981, p 321.

4. Evans RW: Complications of lumbar puncture. *Neurol Clin North Am* 16:83, 1998.

5. Corbett JJ, Mehta MP: Cerebrospinal fluid pressure in normal obese subjects and patients with pseudotumor cerebri. *Neurology* 33:1386, 1983.

6. Dougherty JM, Roth RM: Cerebral spinal fluid. *Emerg Med Clin North Am* 4:281, 1986.

7. Strupp M, Brandt T, Muller A: Incidence of post-lumbar puncture syndrome reduced by reinserting the stylet: A randomized, prospective study of 600 patients. *J Neurol* 245:589, 1998.

8. Conley JM, Ronald AR: Cerebrospinal fluid as a diagnostic body fluid. *Am J Med* 75:102, 1983.

9. Fishman RA: Composition of the cerebrospinal fluid. In Fishman RA (ed): *Cerebrospinal Fluid in Diseases of the Nervous System*. Philadelphia: Saunders, 1992, pp 183–252.

10. Greenlee JE: Approach to diagnosis of meningitis: Cerebrospinal fluid evaluation. *Infect Dis Clin North Am* 4:583, 1990.

11. Gray LD, Fedorko DP: Laboratory diagnosis of bacterial meningitis. *Clin Microbiol Rev* 5:130, 1992.

12. Dwelle TL, Dunkle LM, Blair L: Correlation of cerebrospinal fluid endotoxin-like activity with clinical and laboratory variables in gram-negative bacterial meningitis in children. *J Clin Microbiol* 25:856, 1987.

13. Saravolatz LD, Manzor O, VanderVelde N, et al: Broad-range bacterial polymerase chain reaction for early detection of bacterial meningitis. *Clin Infect Dis* 36:40, 2003.

14. Kleiman MB, Weinberg GA, Reynolds JK, et al: Meningitis with beta-lactam-resistant *Streptococcus pneumoniae*: The need for early repeat lumbar puncture. *Pediatr Infect Dis J* 12:782, 1993.

15. Lebel M, McCracken G: Delayed cerebrospinal fluid sterilization and adverse outcome of bacterial meningitis in infants and children. *Pediatrics* 83:161, 1989.

16. Calisher CH: Medically important arboviruses of the United States and Canada. *Clin Microbiol Rev* 7:89, 1994.

17. Arboviral disease—United States, 1994. *MMWR* 44:641, 1995.

18. Roebroek RMJA, Postma BH, Dijkstra UJ: Aseptic meningitis caused by the lymphocytic choriomeningitis virus. *Clin Neurol Neurosurg* 96:178, 1994.

19. Connelly KP, DeWitt LD: Neurologic complications of infectious mononucleosis. *Pediatr Neurol* 10:181, 1994.

20. Caldas C, Bernicker E, Nogare AD, et al: Case report: Transverse myelitis associated with Epstein-Barr virus infection. *Am J Med Sci* 307:45, 1994.

21. Gendrel D, Raymond J, Assicot M, et al: Measurement of procalcitonin levels in children with bacterial or viral meningitis. *Clin Infect Dis* 24:1240, 1997.

22. Viallon A, Zeni F, Lambert C, et al: High sensitivity and specificity of serum procalcitonin levels in adults with bacterial meningitis. *Clin Infect Dis* 28:1313, 1999.

23. Schwarz S, Bertram M, Schwab S, et al: Serum procalcitonin levels in bacterial and abacterial meningitis. *Crit Care Med* 28:1828, 2000.

24. Greenlee JE: Approach to diagnosis of meningitis: Cerebrospinal fluid evaluation. *Infect Dis Clin North Am* 4:583, 1990.

25. Treseler CB, Sugar AM: Fungal meningitis. *Infect Dis Clin North Am* 4:789, 1990.

26. Chuck SL, Sande MA: Infection with *Cryptococcus neoformans* in the acquired immunodeficiency syndrome. *New Engl J Med* 321:794, 1989

27. Leonard JM, Des Prez RM: Tuberculous meningitis. *Infect Dis Clin North Am* 4:769, 1990.

28. Lin JJ, Harn HJ, Hsu YD, et al: Rapid diagnosis of tuberculous meningitis by polymerase chain reaction assay of cerebrospinal fluid. *J Neurol* 242:147, 1995

29. Macher A, Goosby E. PCR and the misdiagnosis of active tuberculosis. *New Engl J Med* 332:128, 1995.

30. Noordloek GT, van Embden JDA, Kolk AH: Questionable reliability of the polymerase chain reaction in the detection of *Mycobacterium tuberculosis*. *New Engl J Med* 329:2036, 1993.

31. World Health Organization: *Diagnosis of Neurosyphilis by Cerebrospinal Fluid Examination in Treponemal Infections*. WHO Technical Report Series 674. Geneva: WHO, 1982, pp 34–70.

32. Dans PE, Cafferty L, Otter SE, et al: Inappropriate use of the cerebrospinal fluid Venereal Disease Research Laboratory (VDRL) test to exclude neurosyphilis. *Ann Intern Med* 104:86, 1986

33. Merritt HH, Moore M: Acute syphilitic meningitis. *Medicine* 14:119, 1935.

34. Davis LE, Sperry S: The CSF-FTA test and the significance of blood contamination. *Ann Neurol* 6:68, 1979.

35. Marra CM, Critchlow CW, Hook EW: Cerebrospinal fluid treponemal antibodies in untreated early syphilis. *Arch Neurol* 52:68, 1995.

36. Lakeman FD, Whitley RJ: Diagnosis of herpes simplex encephalitis: Application of polymerase chain reaction to cerebrospinal fluid from brain-biopsied patients and correlation with disease. National Institute of Allergy and Infectious Diseases Collaborative Antiviral Study Group. *J Infect Dis* 171:857, 1995.

37. Aurelius E, Johansson B, Skoldenberg B, et al: Rapid diagnosis of herpes simplex encephalitis by nested polymerase chain reaction assay of cerebrospinal fluid. *Lancet* 337:189, 1991.

38. De Tiege X, Heron B, Lebon P, et al: Limits of early diagnosis of herpes simplex encephalitis in children: A retrospective study of 38 cases. *Clin Infect Dis* 36:1335, 2003.

39. Wildemann B, Haas J, Lynen N, et al: Diagnosis of cytomegalovirus encephalitis in patients with AIDS by

quantitation of cytomegalovirus genomes in cells of cerebrospinal fluid. *Neurology* 50:693, 1998.

40. McCutchan JA: Cytomegalovirus infections of the nervous system in patients with AIDS. *Clin Infect Dis* 20:747, 1995.

41. Budka H, Urbanits S, Liberski PP, et al: Subacute measles virus encephalitis: A new and fatal opportunistic infection in a patient with AIDS. *Neurology* 46(2):586, 1996.

42. Mustafa MM, Weitman SD, Winick NJ, et al: Subacute measles encephalitis in the young immunocompromised host: Report of two cases diagnosed by polymerase chain reaction and treated with ribavirin and review of the literature. *Clin Infect Dis* 16:654, 1993.

43. Johnson RT, Griffin DE, Gendelman HE: Postinfectious encephalomyelitis. *Semin Neurol* 5:180, 1985.

44. Zerr I, Pocchiari M, Collins S, et al. Analysis of EEG and CSF 14-3-3 proteins as aids to the diagnosis of Creutzfeldt-Jakob disease. *Neurology* 55:811, 2000.

45. Burkhard PR, Sanchez JC, Landis T, Hochstrasser DF: CSF detection of the 14-3-3 protein in unselected patients with dementia. *Neurology* 56:1528, 2001.

CHAPTER 2

Bacterial Meningitis

Hans-Walter Pfister and Karen L. Roos

Despite the improvements in antimicrobial therapy and critical care during the last decades, mortality rate and neurologic sequelae due to bacterial meningitis remain high. An unfavorable clinical course of bacterial meningitis is often due to intracranial complications, such as generalized cerebral edema, hydrocephalus, cerebrovascular arteritis and infarction, or venous sinus thrombosis. These complications can lead to increased intracranial pressure, stroke, and seizures. There is an increasing prevalence of *Streptococcus pneumoniae* and *Neisseria meningitidis* strains resistant to penicillin and cephalosporin antibiotics. With the increasing incidence of antibiotic-resistant bacteria, there is a critical need to develop new antibiotics for pneumococcal and meningococcal meningitis. The development of central nervous system (CNS) complications and brain damage during bacterial meningitis occurs via a number of mechanisms that are increasingly understood. Traditional adjunctive therapy (hyperosmolar agents, hyperventilation, ventricular drainage) and newer adjunctive agents improve the outcome of bacterial meningitis.

▶ EPIDEMIOLOGY

The incidence of bacterial meningitis is estimated at 5 to 10 cases per 100,000 persons per year. Bacterial meningitis is much more common in developing countries and in specific geographic areas, such as the "meningitis belt" of Africa, where there is an estimated incidence of 70 cases per 100,000 persons per year. There are approximately 25,000 cases of bacterial meningitis annually in the United States. An estimated 2200 to 3000 cases of invasive meningococcal infection occur every year in the United States.[1] Since 1960, the annual incidence of meningococcal disease in the United States has been 0.9 to 1.5 cases per 100,000 population. The incidence is highest among infants younger than 1 year of age, in whom 7.1 cases per 100,000 population were reported in 2001, as compared with rates of 1.8, 0.7, and 0.7 per 100,000 in persons 2 to 4 years, 5 to 17 years, and 18 to 34 years of age, respectively.[1,2] Five meningococcal serotypes—A, B, C, Y, and W-135—account for the majority of cases worldwide. In 2001, meningococcal disease due to serogroups B, C, Y, and W-135 accounted for approximately 35, 24, 34, and 2 percent, respectively, of all cases of invasive meningococcal disease in the United States. Serogroup A is the most common cause of meningococcal infection in sub-Saharan Africa but is rare in the United States.

Recent major epidemiologic trends in bacterial meningitis include a dramatic decline in the incidence of *Hemophilus influenzae* type b meningitis since the introduction of the protein-conjugated *H. influenzae* vaccines, which became available in 1988.[3] With widespread use of *H. influenzae* type b conjugate vaccines beginning in 1990, the incidence of *H. influenzae* type b invasive disease among children younger than 5 years of age declined from an estimated 100 cases per 100,000 population in the prevaccine era to an incidence of 0.3 cases per 100,000 population in 1996.[4] By 1996, the incidence of *H. influenzae* type b invasive disease, such as meningitis and sepsis, among children younger than 5 years of age had declined by more than 99 percent. Recent epidemiologic surveillance data from 1998–2000 indicate that the incidence of *H. influenzae* type b invasive disease among infants and children remains low in the United States.[4]

The causative organism of bacterial meningitis can be predicted by the age of the patient, predisposing factors, and underlying diseases. The most common etiologic agents of bacterial meningitis in adults are *N. meningitidis* and *S. pneumoniae*, followed in frequency by *Listeria* (<5 percent of cases), staphylococci (according to different clinical studies, 1 to 9 percent of cases), gram-negative enteric bacilli including *Escherichia coli*, *Klebsiella*, *Enterobacter*, and *Pseudomonas aeruginosa* (<10 percent of the cases), and rarely, *H. influenzae* (1 to 3 percent). *S. pneumoniae* and *N. meningitidis* are the major causes of meningitis in children 1 month of age or older. Among neonates, *S. agalactiae* (group B streptococcus), *E. coli*, and *Listeria monocytogenes* are the leading etiologic agents of bacterial meningitis.

The most common agents causing bacterial meningitis in the immunocompromised patient are *S. pneumoniae*, *L. monocytogenes*, and gram-negative Enterobacteriaceae, including *P. aeruginosa*. In a review of 776 previously reported and 44 new cases of CNS listeriosis outside pregnancy and the neonatal period, hematologic malignancy and kidney transplantation were the leading predisposing factors for *Listeria* meningitis/meningoencephalitis, but no underlying diseases were identified in 36 percent of cases.[5] Nosocomial bacterial meningitis is caused most often by staphylococci (*Staphylococcus aureus* and *S. epidermidis*, including methicillin-resistant staphylococci) and gram-negative Enterobacteriaceae, including *P. aeruginosa*. Gram-negative Enterobacteriaceae are the etiologic agents in 60 to 70 percent of all cases of meningitis following a neurosurgical procedure and are a common cause of meningitis in the elderly and adults debilitated by chronic illness. Anaerobic microorganisms are responsible for less than 1 percent of cases. Mixed infection with more than one bacterial microorganism is found in 1 percent of meningitis cases, in particular in patients with immunosuppression, skull fracture, a previous neurosurgical procedure, or parameningeal infectious foci (i.e., sinusitis, otitis).

More than half of adults with bacterial meningitis have underlying risk factors, including parameningeal infections [i.e., otitis, sinusitis (Fig. 2-1), mastoiditis (Fig. 2-2), brain abscess, and subdural empyema], a recent neurosurgical procedure, a history of a previous head trauma with or without a dural fistula, a remote infectious focus (e.g., pneumonia, infective endocarditis, psoas abscess), an immunodeficient state (e.g., diabetes mellitus, chronic alcoholism, previous splenectomy, therapy with immunosuppressive agents, and acquired immunodeficiency syndrome), or malignancy (Table 2-1).

Bacterial meningitis following lumbar puncture or peridural anesthesia is seen very rarely. Recurrent bacterial meningitis occurs in patients with congenital defects (i.e., meningomyelocele, dermal sinus), previous head trauma (i.e., skull fracture, dural leak), parameningeal foci (i.e., chronic mastoiditis), and immunodeficient states (i.e., due to splenectomy).

A major epidemiologic concern is an increasing prevalence of *S. pneumoniae* strains resistant to antipneumococcal antibiotics in both developing and developed countries. The occurrence of infections with

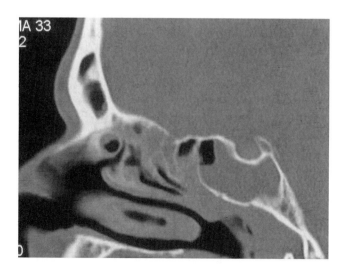

Figure 2-1. Acute purulent sphenoid sinusitis as primary infectious focus of purulent meningitis (cranial cone window technique).

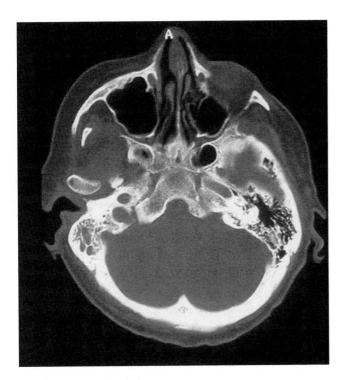

Figure 2-2. Acute purulent mastoiditis (right side) as primary infectious focus of pneumococcal meningitis in a 74-year-old patient (cranial CT bone window technique).

penicillin-resistant *S. pneumoniae* was first noted to increase in Spain, Hungary, and South Africa. Recently, antibiotic-resistant strains of *S. pneumoniae* have become prevalent in Asia and have emerged as a major problem in the United States. In the United States, the proportion of penicillin-resistant *S. pneumoniae* strains increased from 21 percent of tested isolates in 1995 to 24 percent in 1998 with substantial geographic differences in the rate of resistance.[7,8] Likewise, recent data from France show a high rate of resistance to antibiot-

▶ **TABLE 2-1.** UNDERLYING AND ASSOCIATED CONDITIONS IN 87 ADULTS WITH PNEUMOCOCCAL MENINGITIS

Underlying/Associated Conditions	*n* (%)
Ear or sinus infection	50 (57.5)
Chronic debilitating conditions	27 (31.0)
Chronic alcoholism	14 (16.1)
Malignancies	6 (6.9)
Diabetes mellitus	5 (5.7)
Chronic immunosuppressive therapy	3 (3.4)
Terminal renal failure	2 (2.3)
Chronic hepatitis (liver cirrhosis)	2 (2.3)
Pneumonia	19 (21.3)
CSF fistula	18 (20.7)
Asplenia	11 (12.6)
Endocarditis	2 (2.3)

SOURCE: Modified after Kastenbauer and Pfister.[6]

ics.[9] In 1996, 55.8 percent of the *S. pneumoniae* strains isolated from cerebrospinal fluid (CSF) were penicillin-resistant.[9] The resistance of *S. pneumoniae* is mediated by alterations in the penicillin-binding proteins involved in the synthesis of bacterial cell walls.[10] Worldwide, resistance of *S. pneumoniae* to antibiotics is largely confined to a limited number of pneumococcal serotypes, in particular to serotypes 6A, 6B, 9V, 14, 19A, 19F, and 23F.[7] Antibiotic-resistant strains of *N. meningitidis* are also emerging in some regions of the world. For example, since the 1980s, an increasing number of meningococcal isolates with reduced susceptibility to penicillin have been reported in England, Spain, South Africa, and France.[11] With increasing prevalence of penicillin-resistant bacteria, the need for alternative antibiotic therapy for pneumococcal and meningococcal meningitis is critical.

▶ PATHOPHYSIOLOGY AND PATHOGENESIS

During recent years, experimental studies using animal models and cell culture systems have substantially increased our knowledge of the complex pathophysiologic mechanisms of brain injury during bacterial meningitis.[12] A better understanding of the pathogenesis and pathophysiology will help to identify potential adjunctive agents to improve the prognosis of bacterial meningitis.[13] Once bacteria enter the subarachnoid space, they survive because immunoglobulin concentrations in the CSF are very low, and complement components appear to be virtually absent. The CSF is an area of host regional immunodeficiency. Replication and autolysis of bacteria in the CSF leads to the release of bacterial components into the CSF. Lipopolysaccharides, teichoic acids, and peptidoglycans are powerful stimuli for the release of proinflammatory host factors. In addition to cell wall components, microbial toxins (i.e., pneumolysin, pathogen-derived hydrogen peroxide) also may be involved in induction of the inflammatory host response.

Bacteria, i.e., pneumococci, may induce the activation of the transcription factor NF-κB either directly (i.e., by the release of hydrogen peroxide) or indirectly by receptor activation [e.g., interaction of cell wall components with Toll-like receptors (TLRs) or the interleukin-1-receptor and consecutive activation of the MyD 88-pathway). NF-κB activation was observed in the brain during acute pneumococcal meningitis.[14] NF-κB is a key regulator of the inducible expression of many cytokines, chemokines, adhesion molecules, acute-phase proteins, and antimicrobial peptides. During recent years, experimental and clinical studies identified a wide variety of mediators involved in the complex pathogenic network of bacterial meningitis including the proinflammatory cytokines, interleukin (IL)-1β, IL-

6, tumor necrosis factor (TNF)-α, chemokines (i.e., IL-8, Gro-α), arachidonic acid metabolites, platelet-activating factor, reactive oxygen species, and reactive nitrogen intermediates.[15]

The expression of chemotactic factors and adhesion molecules during bacterial meningitis results in a massive influx of leukocytes into the CSF. Leukocytes in the subarachnoid space are thought to be more harmful than beneficial. Due to the lack of opsonins, leukocytes are ineffective in the eradication of the microbial pathogens in the CSF. However, activated leukocytes release a complex assortment of potentially cytotoxic agents, including reactive oxygen species (i.e., superoxide) and reactive nitrogen intermediates (i.e., nitric oxide). The simultaneous production of both nitric oxide and superoxide favors the production of a potentially even more toxic species, the strong oxidant peroxynitrite. Oxidants such as peroxynitrite may contribute to the development of CNS complications and brain damage during bacterial meningitis via a variety of independent mechanisms. One of these pathways involves an attack on polyunsaturated fatty acids, thus initiating lipid peroxidation that ultimately can lead to loss of cellular membrane function and integrity. An alternative pathway involves oxidant-induced DNA strand breakage and subsequent poly-ADP-ribose-polymerase (PARP) activation, thus initiating an energy-consuming intracellular cycle that ultimately can result in cellular energy depletion and death. Both mechanisms contribute to endothelial cell injury during bacterial meningitis. Endothelial dysfunction leads to loss of cerebrovascular autoregulation, loss of carbon dioxide reactivity of cerebral vessels, and increased permeability of the blood-brain barrier. Vasogenic brain edema is the major cause of increased intracranial pressure (ICP) during bacterial meningitis. Elevated ICP is potentially harmful to patients with bacterial meningitis either by causing cerebral herniation or by decreasing cerebral perfusion (due to a reduction in cerebral perfusion pressure and/or a loss of cerebrovascular autoregulation), which ultimately can lead to cortical necrosis. In addition, neuronal apoptotic cell death in the hippocampus occurs in the course of bacterial meningitis.[16,17]

► CLINICAL FEATURES

The classic clinical presentation of bacterial meningitis includes stiff neck, headache, fever, photophobia, malaise, vomiting, irritability, and lethargy. There is a progressive deterioration in the level of consciousness from lethargy to stupor and then obtundation and coma. Meningismus is present in most patients with altered consciousness even if they are comatose. Neck stiffness may be mild or absent in children, the elderly, immunocompromised patients, and at a very early stage of the disease. Clinical symptoms and signs of bacterial meningitis usually evolve rapidly within several hours; however, meningitis also may have a more subacute presentation, evolving over 24 to 48 hours.

A petechial-purpuric rash on presentation is highly suggestive of *N. meningitidis* infection or, more rarely, *S. aureus* or pneumococcal infection. In the series of Andersen and colleagues,[18] a petechial-like rash was present in 75 percent of 255 patients with acute meningococcal meningitis. Patients older than 30 years of age had less frequent petechiae (62 percent) than younger patients (81 percent). About 10 percent of meningococcal infections have an overwhelming course, resulting in the Waterhouse-Friderichsen syndrome (i.e., fulminating meningococcal septicemia). This is characterized by fever, large petechial hemorrhages in the skin and mucous membranes, cardiovascular insufficiency, and disseminated intravascular coagulation (Fig. 2-3). The presence of peripheral cutaneous emboli (Osler's spots), especially on the fingers and toes, in a patient with bacterial meningitis should prompt an evaluation for infective endocarditis.

Focal neurologic signs (e.g., hemi- or tetraparesis, ataxia, aphasia, visual field defects) are found in approximately 10 to 15 percent of patients. Seizures occur in 20 to 40 percent of patients. Cranial nerve palsies, usually of the third, sixth, seventh, or eighth cranial nerve, are detectable in approximately 10 percent of patients. Hearing impairment due to purulent labyrinthitis is a well-known sequela of acute bacterial meningitis in children and adults in up to 30 percent of patients.[6,19,20]

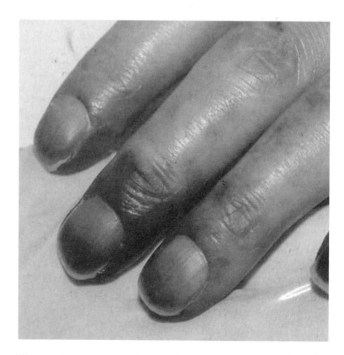

Figure 2-3. Disseminated intravascular coagulation leading to necrosis of the fingers in a 73-year-old patient with severe meningitis and sepsis.

▶ **TABLE 2-2.** MORTALITY RATES OF BACTERIAL MENINGITIS IN ADULTS

Bacterial Pathogen	Mortality Rate (%)
Pneumococcal meningitis	20–35*
Meningococcal meningitis	3–10
Listeria meningitis	20–30
Staphylococcus aureus meningitis	20–40
Gram-negative meningitis	20–30

*In a recent study, dexamethasone significantly reduced mortality rates of pneumococcal meningitis in adults to 14 percent (34 percent in the placebo-group).[24]

▶ COMPLICATIONS

The highest mortality rates, exceeding 15 to 20 percent, are found in pneumococcal and *Listeria* meningitis. Between 3 and 10 percent of patients with meningococcal meningitis die[21,22] (Table 2-2). Neurologic sequelae occur in 20 to 40 percent of patients, including sensorineural hearing loss, neuropsychological abnormalities, hemiparesis, epileptic seizures, hemianopia, ataxia, and cranial nerve palsies.[21,23]

Cerebral and systemic complications during the acute phase of the disease are responsible both for the mortality and for the long-term sequelae of bacterial meningitis[25–27] (Tables 2-3 and 2-4). About half of adult

▶ **TABLE 2-3.** CEREBRAL COMPLICATIONS IN ADULTS WITH BACTERIAL MENINGITIS

Complication	Frequency (%)
Brain edema with the risk of herniation	10–15
Cerebrovascular involvement	15–20
Cerebral arterial complications: arteritis, vasospasm, focal cortical hyperperfusion, disturbed cerebral autoregulation	
Septic sinus thrombosis (in particular of the superior sagittal sinus) and cortical venous thrombosis	
Hydrocephalus (communicating or obstructive type)	10–15
Vestibulocochlear involvement (hearing impairment, vestibulopathy)	10–30
Cranial nerve palsies (second, third, sixth, seventh, eighth cranial nerves)	~10
Cerebritis	<10
Sterile subdural effusion*	~2
Rarely as a consequence of meningitis: Brain abscess†, subdural empyema	

*Especially in infants younger than 2 years of age.
†Especially in newborn infants infected with *Citrobacter diversus* or *Proteus* species.

▶ **TABLE 2-4.** SPECTRUM OF COMPLICATIONS IN PNEUMOCOCCAL MENINGITIS (87 ADULTS)

Complication	n (%)
Diffuse brain edema	25 (28.7)
Hydrocephalus	14 (16.1)
Arterial cerebrovascular complication	19 (21.8)
Venous cerebrovascular complication	9 (10.3)
Spontaneous intracranial hemorrhage	8 (9.2)
Subarachnoid bleeding (due to vasculitis)	2 (2.3)
Subarachnoid and intracerebral bleeding (due to vasculitis)	2 (2.3)
Intracerebral bleeding (due to sinus thrombosis)	1 (0.9)
Intracerebral bleeding (unknown etiology)	3 (3.4)
Cerebritis	4 (4.6)
Seizures	24 (27.6)
Cranial nerve palsies	4 (4.6)
Spinal cord dysfunction (myelitis)	2 (2.3)
Hearing loss	17 (19.5)*
Septic shock	27 (31)
Disseminated intravascular coagulation	20 (23.0)
Renal failure requiring hemofiltration	10 (11.5)
Adult respiratory distress syndrome	6 (6.9)

*Of all patients (25.8 percent of survivors).
SOURCE: *Modified after Kastenbauer and Pfister.*[6] *Meningitis-associated intracranial complications developed in 65 (74.7 percent) and systemic complications in 33 of 87 (37.9 percent) patients.*

patients with bacterial meningitis develop complications of varying severity during the acute stage of the disease. The first week of bacterial meningitis is the critical time period, and patients with this disease should be treated in an intensive care unit during the initial phase of the disease.

The major cerebral complications are brain edema (Fig. 2-4), hydrocephalus, both obstructive and communicating types (Fig. 2-5), and cerebrovascular complications (Fig. 2-6). Cerebrovascular complications, both of arteries (arteritis, vasospasm) and veins (septic sinus venous thrombosis), may lead to infarction with severe irreversible cerebral damage and an increase in ICP due to cytotoxic edema. In one series, 19 percent of 52 adult patients with bacterial meningitis had stroke.[28] Hemorrhagic stroke as a complication of bacterial meningitis was reported in 2.1 percent of 296 adults.[29] In addition to edema, increased intracranial blood volume due to disturbed cerebrovascular autoregulation or to septic venous sinus thrombosis may lead to a life-threatening elevation of ICP with the risk of herniation. There is a risk of cortical necrosis when cerebral perfusion pressure (defined as the difference between systemic mean arterial blood pressure and ICP) decreases as a result of increased ICP and systemic

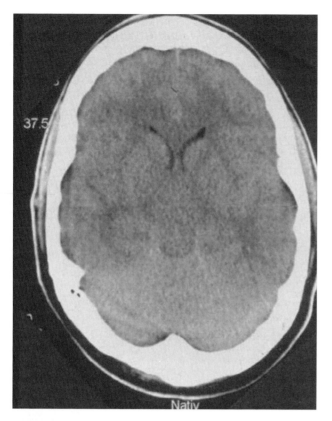

Figure 2-4. Marked brain edema in a young patient with meningococcal meningitis.

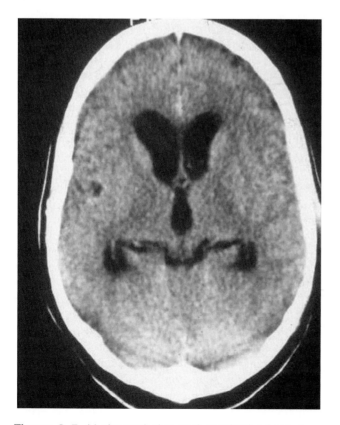

Figure 2-5. Hydrocephalus and cerebral edema in a 43-year-old patient with acute bacterial meningitis.

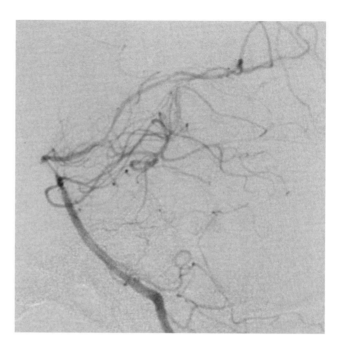

Figure 2-6. Cerebral vasculitis (vasospasm) of the posterior cerebral artery in a patient with pneumococcal meningitis (digital subtraction angiography); segmental narrowing marked by arrows.

hypotension. Interstitial edema may occur due to transependymal movement of CSF from the ventricular system into the surrounding brain parenchyma as a consequence of obstructive hydrocephalus.

The most common extracranial complications during the acute phase of bacterial meningitis include septic shock, disseminated intravascular coagulation (DIC), acute respiratory distress syndrome (ARDS), arthritis (septic or reactive), electrolyte disturbances [hyponatremia, syndrome of inappropriate antidiuretic hormone secretion (SIADH), or rarely, central diabetes insipidus and cerebral salt wasting syndrome], rhabdomyolysis, pancreatitis, septic unilateral or bilateral endophthalmitis or panophthalmitis, and blindness due to vasculitis and spinal complications (e.g., myelitis, infarction).[21,30]

▶ DIAGNOSIS

The opening pressure is elevated and the CSF appears cloudy in patients with bacterial meningitis. There is typically a polymorphonuclear leukocytic pleocytosis with more than 1000 cells/μl, a severe blood-CSF barrier disruption (elevated total protein content > 120 mg/dl), and a low CSF glucose concentration (<30 mg/dl and a ratio of CSF to blood glucose of <0.3 in most patients). In patients with extremely low CSF glucose concentrations (<5 mg/dl), usually a high number of bacterial microorganisms can be found on microscopy of the CSF. A CSF lactate concentration of greater than 3.5 mmol/liter is typical of bacterial meningitis and is helpful in the diagnosis of bacterial meningitis in postneurosurgical patients, in whom increased white blood cell counts and protein concentrations are nonspecific. A CSF white blood cell count of less than 1000 cells/μl may be found early in the disease, in partially treated bacterial meningitis, in overwhelming bacterial meningeal infection (apurulent bacterial meningitis), and in immunosuppressed and leukopenic patients. Diagnosis of acute bacterial meningitis is established by identification of the bacterial pathogen by microscopy of a Gram-stained smear (Fig. 2-7) or methylene blue–stained smear and by a positive bacterial CSF culture.

Bacterial microorganisms are detectable in the CSF in 70 to 90 percent of patients by at least one of the above-mentioned methods. Blood cultures are positive in 50 percent of patients with bacterial meningitis. They should be obtained prior to the start of antibiotic therapy. Antigen detection in the CSF using latex particle agglutination (e.g., antigen detection of *N. meningitidis, S. pneumoniae, H. influenzae,* and *S. agalactiae*) can provide diagnostic confirmation or give additional information if there are suspected bacterial pathogens on a microscopically stained smear. The use of antigen detection tests to detect classic meningeal pathogens is indicated (1) to confirm unclear microscopic CSF results, (2) if the CSF shows marked pleocytosis but a negative microscopic bacterial result, and (3) if there is a history of antibiotic pretreatment.

If there is a clinical suspicion of meningococcal disease but negative microscopic and culture results, then the polymerase chain reaction (PCR) assay to detect meningococcal DNA in the CSF should be done. A broad-range PCR can detect small numbers of viable and nonviable organisms in CSF. When the broad-range PCR is positive, a PCR that uses specific bacterial primers to detect the nucleic acid of *S. pneumoniae, N. meningitidis, E. coli, L. monocytogenes, H. influenzae,* and *S. agalactiae* should be done.

The peripheral white blood cell count, C-reactive protein, and sedimentation rate are usually elevated in patients with bacterial meningitis, with the possible exception of immunosuppressed patients. Recent data suggest that measurement of plasma procalcitonin may be of value in the differential diagnosis of meningitis due to either bacteria or viruses.[31,32] Procalcitonin is a polypeptide that increases in patients with severe bacterial infections. Neuroimaging demonstrates a variety of abnormalities in patients with bacterial meningitis (Table 2-5). Cerebrovascular complications may be detected by magnetic resonance imaging (T$_2$-weighted, perfusion and diffusion MRI).[33] Magnetic resonance (MR) angiography and transcranial Doppler sonography (TCD) are useful in diagnosing and monitoring involvement of the great arteries at the base of the brain.[34] In addition, MRI or venous computed tomographic (CT) angiography may reveal septic sinus thrombosis.

To detect vestibulocochlear functional abnormalities in the acute phase of bacterial meningitis, the following methods are recommended: audiometry, brain stem auditory evoked potentials, otoacoustic emissions, and electronystagmography including caloric testing. Recently, high-resolution MRI was used to demonstrate inner ear involvement in adults with bacterial meningitis.[20] The structures involved most frequently were the cochlear nerve, the first cochlear turn, the vestibulum, and the semicircular canals.

▶ **TABLE 2-5.** POSSIBLE FINDINGS ON CT OR MRI IN PATIENTS WITH BACTERIAL MENINGITIS

Cerebral edema

Hydrocephalus (obstructive or communicating type)

Ventriculitis (ventricular empyema)

Brain infarction (bland and hemorrhagically transformed) due to cerebral vasculitis or septic embolism or infarction in case of venous sinus thrombosis

Intracerebral hemorrhage (due to disseminated intravascular coagulation or hemorrhage due to venous sinus thrombosis)

Cerebritis

Signs of venous sinus thrombosis (e.g., empty delta sign)

Parameningeal infectious foci (bone window technique), e.g., sinusitis, mastoiditis

Intracranial free air due to a dural leak

Meningeal and ventricular ependymal enhancement

Basilar purulent exudate

Brain abscess or subdural empyema (leading secondarily to bacterial meningitis)

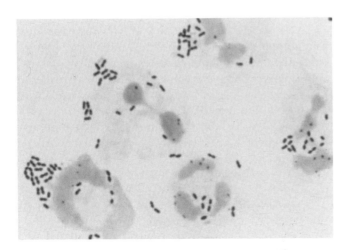

Figure 2-7. Detection of gram-positive diplococci on Gram staining of the cerebrospinal fluid from a patient with acute bacterial meningitis (later identified by culture as *S. pneumoniae*).

► DIFFERENTIAL DIAGNOSIS

Differential diagnosis of bacterial meningitis includes viral meningitis, viral encephalitis (e.g., herpes simplex virus encephalitis), tuberculous meningitis, fungal meningitis, *Naegleria* meningoencephalitis, carcinomatous meningitis, rickettsial infection, parameningeal purulent infectious foci (brain abscess, epidural abscess, subdural empyema), acute basilar artery thrombosis, subarachnoid hemorrhage, venous sinus thrombosis, and tumor in the posterior fossa.[27]

► TREATMENT

General Management of a Patient with Bacterial Meningitis

In patients with clinical signs and symptoms suggestive of acute bacterial meningitis, antibiotic therapy is started immediately after drawing a single blood culture.[35] In patients who have an altered level of consciousness, a focal neurologic deficit (e.g., hemiparesis), or a seizure, a CT scan should be performed prior to lumbar puncture to detect conditions associated with an increase in ICP (e.g., hydrocephalus, brain edema, brain abscess). In the absence of these, lumbar puncture can be performed without CT. To avoid a therapeutic delay while waiting on the CT scan, antibiotics should be administered immediately after drawing blood for culture. Thereafter, a CT scan should be performed as soon as possible, and then, if there is no contraindication, a lumbar puncture should be done. Contraindications to lumbar puncture are clinical signs of cerebral herniation (i.e., unconsciousness, a unilaterally dilated and unreactive pupil, decerebrate posturing) or a focal mass lesion (i.e., large, space-occupying brain abscess) on CT. However, a clinically significant increase of ICP cannot be ruled out by CT.[36,37] The presence of a parameningeal infectious focus such as sinusitis or mastoiditis also should be investigated by CT, including the bone window technique (see Table 2-5). In addition, clinical examination by an otolaryngologist should be performed. If a parameningeal focus (i.e., otitis, mastoiditis, sinusitis) is identified as a possible origin of bacterial meningitis, drainage is required as soon as possible. Depending on the history and clinical findings, other infectious foci should be searched for (i.e., by x-ray examination of the thorax, abdominal ultrasound or CT, echocardiography). Surgical correction of a CSF dural leak (i.e., in a patient with previous head trauma) is usually performed after the meningeal bacterial infection is treated, typically after 10 to 14 days, rather than during the acute stage of meningitis.

Initial Empirical Antibiotic Therapy

Since antibiotic therapy has to be started without microbiologic confirmation, empirical therapy is initiated with consideration of the patient's age, predisposing factors, underlying diseases, and the most probable meningeal pathogen (Table 2-6).

The most common bacterial microorganisms in *neonates* with bacterial meningitis are enteric gram-negative bacilli, *S. agalactiae*, and *L. monocytogenes* (see Table 2-6). A third-generation cephalosporin (e.g., cefotaxime) plus ampicillin is recommended as empirical therapy in this age group. Alternatively, some authors recommend ampicillin combined with an aminoglycoside. In *infants, children,* and *adults* with community-acquired bacterial meningitis, the recommended initial empirical antibiotic therapy is a combination of a third-generation cephalosporin (most commonly ceftriaxone or cefotaxime) or a fourth-generation cephalosporin (cefepime) plus vancomycin. In patients with risk factors for *L. monocytogenes* meningitis (immunosuppression, alcoholism, corticosteroids, pregnancy), ampicillin is added to cover *L. monocytogenes*.

Importantly, the sensitivity of the causative pathogen to the antibiotic regimen must be confirmed by in vitro testing, and antibiotic coverage should be adjusted based on the sensitivity results. Penicillin G should not be given as monotherapy until it is confirmed that the CSF isolates of *S. pneumoniae* or *N. meningitidis* are sensitive to penicillin G. For penicillin-resistant meningococci or relatively penicillin-resistant pneumococci, a third-generation cephalosporin is recommended. Highly-resistant pneumococci typically also have reduced sensitivity or resistance to third-generation cephalosporins, and in areas where these highly-resistant organisms are commonly isolated, the addition of vancomycin (or rifampin) is necessary until the organism and its antibiotic susceptibilities are known (see Table 2-7).

Empirical antibiotic therapy of bacterial meningitis as a complication of a recent head trauma or a neurosurgical procedure should include a cephalosporin (e.g., ceftazidime) combined with an antistaphylococcal antibiotic (e.g., vancomycin). Ventriculitis associated with an external intraventricular drainage device or a ventriculoperitoneal shunt should be treated with antibiotics that cover *S. epidermidis*, *S. aureus*, and enteric gram-negative bacilli. In this clinical setting, a combination of vancomycin plus ceftazidime (or meropenem) is recommended.

The administration of intraventricular gentamicin (Refobacin-L; adults: 5 to 10 mg/d; children: 1 to 2 mg/d) is reserved for special cases of gram-negative meningitis if (1) a gentamicin-sensitive microorganism has been identified, (2) external intraventricular drainage has to be done because of ventricular en-

▶ **TABLE 2-6.** INITIAL EMPIRICAL ANTIBIOTIC THERAPY OF BACTERIAL MENINGITIS

Age Group, Clinical Setting	Typical Pathogen	Recommended Initial Antibiotics
Newborns	Gram-negative Enterobacteriaceae (*Escherichia coli, Klebsiella, Enterobacter, Proteus*) Group B streptococci (*S. agalactiae*) *Listeria monocytogenes*	Cefotaxime plus ampicillin
Infants and children	*N. meningitidis, S. pneumoniae, Hemophilus influenzae**	Ceftriaxone or cefotaxime plus vancomycin‡
Adults: healthy, immunocompetent, community-acquired	*S. pneumoniae, N. meningitidis, L. monocytogenes*	Third- or fourth-generation cephalosporin† plus ampicillin plus vancomycin‡
Nosocomial (e.g., postneurosurgery or posttraumatic brain injury)	Gram-negative Enterobacteriaceae, *P. aeruginosa*, staphylococci	Meropenem plus vancomycin§
Ventriculitis, shunt infection	*S. epidermis, S. aureus*, gram-negative Enterobacteriaceae, *P. aeruginosa*	Meropenem plus vancomycin§
Immunocompromised or older patients (impaired cellular immunity)	*L. monocytogenes*, gram-negative Enterobacteriaceae, *P. aeruginosa*, pneumococci	Third or fourth generation cephalosporin plus ampicillin plus vancomycin‡

*Incidence has declined since the introduction of *H. influenzae* type b vaccine.
†For example, ceftriaxone or cefotaxime or cefepime.
‡In some areas increasing resistance rates of pneumococci against penicillin and the cephalosporins have been reported during recent years, in particular, in Hungary, Spain, Australia, South Africa, and some areas of the United States. The initial treatment in these areas consists of ceftriaxone plus vancomycin or ceftriaxone plus rifampin.
§There are no uniform recommendations in the literature. Antibiotics as an alternative to vancomycin (according to susceptibility tests): fosfomycin, rifampin, and linezolid.

▶ **TABLE 2-7.** ANTIBIOTIC THERAPY OF BACTERIAL MENINGITIS (KNOWN BACTERIAL PATHOGEN)

Bacterial Pathogen	Antibiotic*
N. meningitidis	**Penicillin G or ampicillin** Ceftriaxone or cefotaxime for penicillin-resistant strains
S. pneumoniae Penicillin-susceptible Penicillin-tolerant (MIC 0.1–1 μg/ml) Penicillin-resistant (MIC > 1 μg/ml)	Penicillin G or ceftriaxone (or cefotaxime or cefepime) Ceftriaxone (or cefotaxime or cefepime) or meropenem **Ceftriaxone (or cefotaxime or cefepime) plus vancomycin** or Cefotaxime (or ceftriaxone or cefepime) plus rifampin or meropenem
H. influenzae	**Ceftriaxone or cefotaxime** Ampicillin plus chloramphenicol
S. agalactiae (group B streptococci)	Penicillin G or ampicillin plus an aminoglycoside or Cefotaxime
Gram-negative Enterobacteriaceae (i.e., *Klebsiella, E. coli, Proteus*)	**Ceftriaxone or cefotaxime or cefepime** or meropenem
Pseudomonas aeruginosa	**Meropenem** or cefepime
Staphylococci Methicillin-susceptible	**Nafcillin or oxacillin** or cefazolin or fosfomycin or vancomycin or linezolid†
Methicillin-resistant	**Vancomycin**
Listeria monocytogenes	**Ampicillin plus gentamicin** or trimethoprim-sulfamethoxazole or meropenem

*Recommended therapy is in bold. The choice of antibiotic depends on the results of the susceptibility tests.
†Linezolid (Zyvoxid) has activity comparable to that of vancomycin; it has excellent CSF penetration. Reports on the use of linezolid in staphylococcal infections of the CNS are rare.[39]

largement, (3) CSF analysis shows clear signs of ventriculitis, (4) the clinical findings document a severe clinical picture (e.g., comatose patient), and (5) there is no clinical and microbiologic improvement despite intravenous antibiotic therapy.

Intraventricular vancomycin (10 mg/d in children and 20 mg/d in adults) is used for catheter-associated ventriculitis caused by staphylococci.[38] Intraventricular vancomycin is beneficial in patients with highly resistant pneumococcal meningitis and staphylococcal meningitis not responding to parenteral vancomycin. A combination of a third- or fourth-generation cephalosporin plus vancomycin plus ampicillin is recommended for immunocompromised adults to cover *L. monocytogenes*, *S. pneumoniae*, and gram-negative Enterobacteriaceae.

Specific Antibiotic Therapy

Once the bacterial microorganism causing meningitis is known, antibiotic coverage should be modified to provide highly active but narrow coverage against the microorganism causing meningitis (Tables 2-7 and 2-8). High systemic (intravenous) doses of antibiotics are needed in order to provide adequate CSF concentrations because the blood-brain barrier limits access of antibiotic to the site of infection; other factors, such as the acidic environment in the inflamed CSF and the slow rate of bacterial growth, also may reduce antibiotic efficacy. Experimental and clinical studies have suggested that the best therapeutic response is achieved with CSF antibiotic concentrations that exceed by 10- to 20-fold the in vitro minimal bactericidal concentration for a particular organism.

Duration of Antibiotic Treatment

The recommended duration of antibiotic treatment depends on the response to antibiotic therapy and the specific bacterial pathogen. Bacterial meningitis due to *S. pneumoniae*, *H. influenzae*, and group B streptococci is usually treated with intravenous antibiotics for 10 to 14 days. Shorter courses of 4 to 7 days may be adequate for uncomplicated meningococcal meningitis. For treatment of meningitis due to *L. monocytogenes* and Enterobacteriaceae, a 3- to 4-week course of therapy is required.

Monitoring Treatment

The CSF usually becomes sterile within 24 to 48 hours after beginning therapy if the organism is susceptible

▶ **TABLE 2-8.** ANTIBIOTICS COMMONLY USED IN THE TREATMENT OF BACTERIAL MENINGITIS IN CHILDREN AND ADULTS

Antibiotic Agent	Total Daily Dosage (Dosing Interval)*
Ampicillin	Child: 300–400 mg/kg/d (every 4 h) Adult: 12–15 g/d (every 4–6 h)
Ceftriaxone	Child: 80–100 mg/kg/d (every 12 h) Adult: 4 g/d (every 12 h)
Cefotaxime	Child: 300 mg/kg/d (every 6 h) Adult: 12 g/d (every 4 h)
Ceftazidime	Adult: 6 g/d (every 8 h)
Cefepime	Adult: 4 g/d (every 12 h)
Fosfomycin	15 g/d (every 8 h)
Meropenem	6 g/d (every 8 h)
Penicillin G	250,000 U/kg/d or 20–24 million units/d (every 4–6 h)
Nafcillin	Child: 200–300 mg/kg/d (every 4 hours) Adult: 9–12 g/d
Rifampin	600–1200 mg/d (every 12 h)
Gentamicin,[†,‡] tobramycin[‡]	6 mg/kg/d (every 8 h)
Trimethoprim (TMP) plus sulfamethoxazole (SMZ)	15–20 mg/kg/d of TMP component (every 8 h)
Metronidazole	1500–2000 mg (every 8 h)
Vancomycin[‡]	Child: 60 mg/kg/d (every 6 h) Adult: 2–3 g/d (every 6–12 h)

*Reduction of dose of the antibiotics (with the exception of ceftriaxone) in case of renal failure is necessary.
†Dose in case of intraventricular administration: children 1–2 mg/day, adults 5–10 mg/day.
‡Determination of the serum concentrations are required; recommended peak levels 1 h after intravenous administration: gentamicin and tobramicin 5 to 10 μg/ml; vancomycin, 25 μg/ml.

to the antimicrobial therapy. However, in bacterial meningitis due to Enterobacteriaceae (including *P. aeruginosa*), CSF cultures may remain positive for 2 to 3 days after the start of therapy. In general, if the patient's clinical condition does not improve despite antibiotic therapy within 24 to 48 hours, the following should be considered:

- Development of cerebral edema, arteritis or infarction, or venous sinus thrombosis
- Persistent infectious focus (e.g., an incompletely surgically treated parameningeal focus such as mastoiditis, sinusitis, or otitis media)
- Inadequate antibiotic regimen or too low a dosage

Complications of bacterial meningitis should be investigated (e.g., repeat CT scan or MRI, ENT examination), and additional sources of infection should be sought (e.g., endocarditis). If the causative organism has not been isolated, broadening or changing the antibiotic coverage should be considered in the patient who fails to respond to initial therapy. Repeat lumbar puncture is usually recommended if a resistant pneumococcus has been isolated from the initial CSF culture and if the patient's clinical condition does not improve during antibiotic therapy.[40]

Patient Isolation

Patients with clinically suspected meningococcal meningitis (e.g., petechial rash, gram-negative diplococci on Gram-stained smear of the CSF) have to be isolated for the first 24 hours after initiation of antibiotic therapy. Close contacts should be identified and informed about the increased risk and clinical signs of meningococcal disease (e.g., fever, chills, headache, stiff neck). Chemoprophylaxis is recommended (Table 2-9). Patients with bacterial meningitis due to bacterial microorganisms other than meningococci do not require isolation.

Adjunctive Therapy

Corticosteroids

Corticosteroids have been shown to be beneficial in animal models of bacterial meningitis and in clinical trials of children and adults with bacterial meningitis. Corticosteroids decrease ICP, reduce brain edema and meningeal inflammation, improve abnormalities in CSF hydrodynamics, and prevent changes in cerebral blood flow. In prospective, placebo-controlled clinical studies in infants and children with bacterial meningitis (*H. influenzae* type b was the causative organism in the majority), dexamethasone reduced the incidence of sensorineural hearing loss[41] and neurologic sequelae.[42,43] A 4-day regimen of dexamethasone was demonstrated to be equally effective in children with bacterial meningitis as a 2-day dexamethasone regimen.[44] In a retrospective data analysis of children with pneumococcal meningitis, neurologic sequelae were detected less frequently in children treated with dexamethasone than in those treated with antibiotics alone.[45] In a prospective, randomized study it was shown for the first time that dexamethasone may reduce mortality of pneumococcal meningitis.[46] However, criticisms of this study were that an extraordinarily high percentage of patients presented in a comatose state, the majority of patients (370 of 429) received inadequate therapy for 3 to 5 days prior to hospitalization, the antibiotics were administered intramuscularly, and no differences in mortality were noted in patients with meningococcal or Hib meningitis.

In a multicenter, double-blind, randomized trial in France and Switzerland, the clinical benefit of early adjunctive dexamethasone therapy (10 mg qid for 3 days) was investigated in adults with bacterial meningitis.[47] Unfortunately, the study had to be stopped prematurely because of a new national recommendation to use a third-generation cephalosporin and vancomycin as a result of the increasing incidence of penicillin-resistant *S.*

▶ **TABLE 2-9.** CHEMOPROPHYLAXIS OF MENINGOCOCCAL MENINGITIS*

Antibiotic, Age Group	Dosage
Rifampin (Rifa)	
Adults	600 mg every 12 h for 2 days PO
Infants ≥ 1 month	10 mg/kg every 12 h for 2 days PO
Infants < 1 month	5 mg/kg every 12 h for 2 days PO
Ciprofloxacin (Ciprobay)	
Adults	500 mg as single dose PO
Ceftriaxone (Rocephin)	
Adults and children ≥ 15 years	250 mg as single dose IM (or IV)
Children < 15 years	125 mg as single dose IM (or IV)

*Rifampin and ciprofloxacin should not be prescribed during pregnancy. Furthermore, the use of ciprofloxacin is not recommended for children and adolescents (<18 years).

pneumoniae in France. The difference in the rate of cure without any neurologic sequelae was not statistically significant between the dexamethasone group (74.2 percent, $n = 31$) and the placebo group (51.7 percent, $n = 29$).

A meta-analysis of 11 randomized clinical trials since 1988 using dexamethasone as adjunctive therapy in bacterial meningitis was performed.[48] In pneumococcal meningitis, only studies in which dexamethasone was given early suggested protection, which was significant for severe hearing loss and approached significance for any neurologic or hearing deficit. In *H. influenzae* meningitis in children, dexamethasone reduced severe hearing loss overall.

In contrast, a prospective, randomized, double-blind study in 598 children with bacterial meningitis did not show superiority of dexamethasone compared with placebo.[49] Dexamethasone was given for 2 days, and it was started 5 to 10 minutes before antibiotic therapy. There was no significant difference between the dexamethasone and the placebo groups. Dexamethasone did not reduce mortality rates and the incidence of neurologic deficits, but the evaluation of hearing loss was suboptimal and still suggested a steroid benefit. However, in this study, a considerable number of patients were malnourished and had human immunodeficiency virus (HIV) infection or inappropriate or delayed antibiotic therapy; thus there are limitations on interpretation of the results of this study.

A very recent systematic review of 18 studies examining the efficacy and safety of adjunctive corticosteroid therapy in 1853 patients revealed that in children, corticosteroids reduced severe hearing loss in *H. influenzae* meningitis as well as in meningitis caused by other bacteria.[50] The American Academy of Pediatrics recommends consideration of dexamethasone therapy (0.15 mg/kg of body weight intravenously every 6 hours for 2 to 4 days) in infants and children 2 months of age and older with proven or suspected bacterial meningitis.[51] The first dose of dexamethasone should be administered several minutes before the first dose of antibiotic in order to achieve maximal inhibition of the inflammatory cascade, which is initiated by antibiotic-induced bacteriolysis and the release of cell wall components. When using short-term therapy with dexamethasone, the risk of delayed CSF sterilization and the number of serious side effects are likely to be low. Corticosteroids are not recommended for newborns with bacterial meningitis.

Recently a prospective, randomized, multicenter, double-blind trial of adjuvant therapy with dexamethasone as compared with placebo in 301 adults with acute bacterial meningitis was performed.[24] Dexamethasone (10 mg) or placebo was administered 15 to 20 minutes before or with the first dose of antibiotic and was given every 6 hours for 4 days. The primary outcome measure was the score on the Glasgow Outcome Scale at 8 weeks (a score of 5 indicating a favorable outcome, a score of 1 to 4 indicating an unfavorable outcome). Treatment with dexamethasone was associated with a significant reduction in the risk of an unfavorable outcome and also was associated with a significant reduction in mortality. The mortality rate was 7 percent for dexamethasone-treated patients versus 15 percent in the placebo group and 14 percent versus 34 percent for pneumococcal meningitis. Among the patients with pneumococcal meningitis, there were unfavorable outcomes in 26 percent of the dexamethasone group, as compared with 52 percent of the placebo group. Gastrointestinal bleeding occurred in two patients in the dexamethasone group and in five patients in the placebo group. Based on these data, the use of dexamethasone is recommended in adult patients with suspected bacterial meningitis (e.g., clinical suspicion plus cloudy CSF, detection of bacteria in the CSF by microscopy of a Gram-stained smear, or a CSF cell count of more than 1000 cells/μl). The subgroup analyses revealed that dexamethasone was protective only for patients with pneumococcal meningitis but not for others (i.e., meningococcal meningitis).[24] Thus, in patients with bacterial meningitis not caused by *S. pneumoniae*, dexamethasone therapy may be discontinued.[52]

The patient's level of consciousness may be an important guide to a decision to administer corticosteroids because the beneficial effect of dexamethasone was limited to the group of more severely ill patients (Glasgow Coma Scale score < 12). The question of whether to administer adjunctive dexamethasone to less severely ill patients or to patients who are strongly suspected to have meningococcal meningitis is important because animal studies of experimental meningitis have shown that adjuvant dexamethasone causes aggravation of hippocampal neuronal apoptosis and learning deficits.[53,54] This concern should be studied scientifically by neuropsychological testing of survivors of meningitis.

When using dexamethasone, the concomitant use of an intravenous H_2 receptor antagonist to prevent gastrointestinal bleeding and low-dose heparin to prevent deep venous thrombosis of the legs is recommended.

In animal models of penicillin- and cephalosporin-resistant pneumococcal meningitis, the penetration of both ceftriaxone and vancomycin into the CSF was reduced with dexamethasone therapy, resulting in a delay in CSF sterilization.[55] In a prospective study of 11 adults with community-acquired pneumococcal meningitis who were treated with a combination of dexamethasone and vancomycin at a dose of 15 mg/kg every 8 hours or 7.5 mg/kg every 6 hours, there were 4 therapeutic failures.[56] The dose of vancomycin was well below the recommended dose of 60 mg/kg per day. In a prospective, randomized clinical trial of the bactericidal activity of vancomycin against cephalosporin-resistant pneumococci in children with acute bacterial meningitis, vancomycin at a dose of 60 mg/kg per day penetrated reliably into the CSF when the children were treated concomitantly with dexamethasone (0.6 mg/kg per day divided into four doses for 4 days).[57] Thus, in areas with high rates of resistant pneumococcal strains, initial empirical therapy should include two antibiotics, ceftriaxone and vancomycin, and the dose of vancomycin should be 60 mg/kg per day.

Other Symptomatic Treatment Options

Generalized brain edema causing increased ICP is managed by *elevation of the head* of the bed to 30 degrees and intravenous *administration of hyperosmolar agents* (e.g., 20% mannitol). Mannitol can be given either as a bolus intravenous injection of 1 g/kg over 10 to 15 minutes or in small frequent doses of 0.25 g/kg every 2 to 3 hours. A bolus injection can be repeated at 3- to 4-hour intervals in order to maintain the serum osmolality between 315 and 320 mosmol/liter. Other therapeutic measures to reduce increased ICP include *hyperventilation* to maintain a P_{CO_2} concentration between 32 and 35 mmHg in ventilated patients, administration of tris-hydroxy-methyl-aminomethane (THAM) buffer, and high-dose barbiturate (e.g., pentobarbital or thiopental) therapy. The effect of moderate hypothermia (33 to 36°C) to lower ICP has not been investigated systematically in patients with bacterial meningitis. Stuporous or comatose patients benefit from an ICP monitoring device to guide therapy.[58] ICP exceeding 20 mmHg is abnormal and should be treated; however, outcome may be improved if pressures greater than 15 mmHg are treated. If meningitis-associated hydrocephalus is diagnosed, CT scan follow-up investigations or ventricular drainage should be performed depending on the patient's level of consciousness and the degree of ventricular dilatation on CT scan.

Anticoagulation of septic venous sinus thrombosis in bacterial meningitis is controversial.[59] There are no prospective, controlled clinical studies. However, a retrospective study showed a beneficial effect of heparin in patients with septic cavernous sinus thrombosis.[59] Anticoagulation with dose-adjusted intravenous heparin should be considered in patients with meningitis-associated septic venous sinus thrombosis proven by MR or cerebral angiography. In patients with meningitis-associated thrombosis of the transverse sinus, an increased risk of bleeding was reported.[59]

There are no proven treatments for arterial cerebrovascular complications (arteritis, vasospasm). MR angiographic studies and transcranial Doppler sonographic recordings in patients with bacterial meningitis and focal neurologic deficits may reveal vasospasm of the large arteries at the base of the brain resembling vasospasm following subarachnoid hemorrhage. In these patients, *hypervolemic therapy* or *nimodipine therapy* (i.e., 1 to 2 mg/h intravenously in adults) should be considered; however, these therapeutic approaches have not been investigated systematically in clinical tri-

als. *Anticonvulsants* are used when the course is complicated by seizures, e.g., rapid intravenous fosphenytoin administration (i.e., 20 mg/kg, no faster than 150 mg per minute in adults). Sterile subdural effusion usually resolves spontaneously and does not require surgical therapy. CT-guided stereotactic aspiration is recommended initially for cases of subdural empyema, but open surgical procedures may be necessary. Currently, no data exist that justify the experimental procedure of *CSF filtration* in patients with bacterial meningitis.

The efficacy of *activated protein C* has been studied in patients with severe meningococcal septicemia.[60,61] In addition to its antithrombotic and profibrinolytic properties, activated protein C has anti-inflammatory actions, e.g., by downregulating lipopolysaccharide-induced tumor necrosis factor α (TNF-α) and interleukin 1β production in monocytes. As discussed earlier, these proinflammatory cytokines have a significant role in the pathogenesis of the neurologic complications of bacterial meningitis. Thus activated protein C may have a role not only in the management of thrombosis in meningococcal septicemia but also in downregulating the inflammatory response. A large randomized, double-blind, placebo-controlled, multicenter trial showed a significant reduction in mortality in patients with severe sepsis treated with activated protein C.[62] However, treatment with activated protein C was associated with a higher incidence of serious bleeding.[62] Whether there is a role for activated protein C in the treatment of bacterial meningitis is questionable because the CSF penetration of activated protein C is poor, and severe intracranial bleeding complications such as subarachnoid hemorrhage have been reported.[63]

Several therapeutic agents that may limit meningeal inflammation have shown beneficial effects in animal models of bacterial meningitis. Aside from dexamethasone, these anti-inflammatory agents include nonsteroidal anti-inflammatory drugs (e.g., indomethacin), pentoxifylline, antagonists of leukocyte–endothelial cell adhesion molecules, monoclonal antibodies against cytokines, platelet-activating factor receptor antagonists, free radical scavengers, nitric oxide synthase inhibitors, inhibitors of matrix metalloproteinases, and caspases.[12,15] Aside from dexamethasone, these agents have not yet been investigated in humans with bacterial meningitis, but some (e.g., antioxidants such as *N*-acetyl-L-cysteine) show very promising beneficial effects in experimental models.

▶ PREVENTION

Chemoprophylaxis

Eradication of bacterial pathogens from the nasopharynx by chemoprophylaxis prevents secondary cases of *H. influenzae* meningitis and meningococcal meningitis.

Meningococcal Meningitis

Prophylaxis for meningococcal meningitis is recommended for every person sleeping in the same household and engaging in saliva-exchanging contacts and all persons who may have had contact with oropharyngeal secretions of the index patient. Rifampin is the drug most often recommended for chemoprophylaxis of meningococcal meningitis (see Table 2-9); alternative drugs are ceftriaxone and ciprofloxacin. A single dose of ciprofloxacin (e.g., 500 mg in a single oral dose) is as effective as rifampin. Rifampin and ciprofloxacin should not be prescribed during pregnancy. Furthermore, the use of ciprofloxacin is not recommended for children and adolescents (<18 years of age). Pregnant and lactating women and children under 2 years of age may be given intravenous or intramuscular ceftriaxone (e.g., a single injection of 250 mg for adults and 125 mg for children). If the index patient was treated with penicillin G, chemoprophylaxis with rifampin is recommended before discharge from the hospital. Since meningococci may not be eradicated from the upper respiratory tract by penicillin G despite successful systemic antibiotic therapy, the index patient could remain a potential carrier.

H. Influenzae Meningitis

Chemoprophylaxis with rifampin is recommended for the index case and all household contacts of the patient with *H. influenzae* meningitis when there is at least one child (other than the index case) under 48 months of age.

Vaccination

The *H. influenzae* type b conjugate vaccine series (bacterial polysaccharide conjugated to protein) should begin at age 2 to 6 months. There is no effective vaccine against meningococci of serogroup B. The tetravalent (Men A/C/Y/W-135) meningococcal polysaccharide vaccine is recommended for patients older than 2 years with terminal complement component deficiency or dysfunction, asplenic patients, and travelers to areas with hyperendemic or epidemic meningococcal disease (e.g., Nigeria, Cameroon). The Advisory Committee on Immunization Practices also recommends that college freshmen be vaccinated against meningococcal meningitis with the meningococcal polysaccharide vaccine. In response to the recent Hajj-associated outbreak of W-135 meningococcal disease, quadrivalent meningococcal vaccine became a visa requirement.[64] A meningococcal serogroup C conjugate vaccine was licensed in the United Kingdom in 1999 for routine childhood immunization and has already decreased dramatically the incidence of serogroup C disease.[65] This meningococcal conjugate vaccine was subsequently licensed in other countries such as Canada, the Netherlands, and Australia. The meningococcal polysaccharide vaccine is not effective in young children. In contrast, the meningococcal conjugate vaccine induces high concentrations of bactericidal antibodies and is highly effective in preventing meningococcal disease in infants, young children, and adults. Meningococcal conjugate vaccines against one or more serogroups probably will be available in the United States within the next few years.[2]

Candidates for *S. pneumoniae* immunoprophylaxis with the 7-valent pneumococcal conjugate (Prevnar) or the 23-valent pneumococcal polysaccharide (Pneumovax and Pnu-Imune) vaccine are individuals with asplenic states (e.g., splenectomy, sickle cell anemia), chronic debilitating diseases (e.g., diabetes, congestive heart failure), or HIV infection. In addition, the Centers for Disease Control and Prevention recommend that all persons with cochlear implants receive age-appropriate vaccination against pneumococcal disease because cochlear implant recipients have an increased risk of pneumococcal meningitis.[66]

REFERENCES

1. Rosenstein NE, Perkins BA, Stephens DS, et al: Meningococcal disease. *New Engl J Med* 344:1378, 2001.
2. Offit PA, Peter G: The meningococcal vaccine: Public policy and individual choices. *New Engl J Med* 349:2353, 2003.
3. Schuchat A, Robinson K, Wenger JD, et al: Bacterial meningitis in the United States in 1995. Active Surveillance Team. *New Engl J Med* 337:970, 1997.
4. Centers for Disease Control and Prevention: Progress toward elimination of *Hemophilus influenzae* type b invasive disease among infants and children—United States, 1998–2000. *MMWR* 51:234, 2002.
5. Mylonakis E, Hohmann EL, Calderwood SB: Central nervous system infection with *Listeria monocytogenes*: 33 years' experience at a general hospital and review of 776 episodes from the literature. *Medicine* 77:313, 1998.
6. Kastenbauer S, Pfister HW: Pneumococcal meningitis in adults: Spectrum of complications and prognostic factors in a series of 87 cases. *Brain* 126:1015, 2003.
7. Whitney CG, Farley MM, Hadler J, et al: Increasing prevalence of multidrug resistant *Streptococcus pneumoniae* in the United States. *New Engl J Med* 343:1917, 2000.
8. McCormick AW, Whitney CG, Farley MM, et al: Geographic diversity and temporal trends of antimicrobial resistance in *Streptococcus pneumoniae* in the United States. *Nature Med* 9:424, 2003.
9. Doit C, Bourrillon A, Bingen E: Childhood bacterial meningitis: Bacterial epidemiology and antibiotic resistance. *Presse Med* 27:1177, 1998.
10. Tomasz A: Antibiotic resistance in *Streptococcus pneumoniae*. *Clin Infect Dis* 24:S85, 1997.

11. Antignac A, Ducos-Galand M, Guiyoule A, et al.: *Neisseria meningitidis* strains isolated from invasive infections in France (1999–2002): Phenotypes and antibiotic susceptibility patterns. *Clin Infect Dis* 37:912, 2003.

12. Koedel U, Scheld WM, Pfister HW: Pathogenesis and pathophysiology of pneumococcal meningitis. *Lancet Infect Dis* 2:721, 2002.

13. Roos KL: Bacterial meningitis. In Roos KL (ed): *Central Nervous Infectious Diseases and Therapy.* New York: Marcel Dekker, 1997, p 99.

14. Koedel U, Bayerlein I, Paul R, et al: Pharmacological interference with NFκB activation attenuates central nervous system complications in experimental pneumococcal meningitis. *J Infect Dis* 182:1437, 2000.

15. Koedel U, Pfister HW: Oxidative stress in bacterial meningitis. *Brain Pathol* 9:57, 1999.

16. Zysk G, Brück W, Gerber J, et al: Anti-inflammatory treatment influences neuronal apoptotic cell death in the dentate gyrus in experimental pneumococcal meningitis. *J Neuropathol Exp Neurol* 55:722, 1996.

17. Braun JS, Novak R, Herzog KH, et al: Neuroprotection by a caspase inhibitor in acute bacterial meningitis. *Nature Med* 5:298, 1999.

18. Andersen J, Backer V, Voldsgrard P, et al: Acute meningococcal meningitis: Analysis of features of the disease according to the age of 255 patients. *J Infect* 34:227, 1997.

19. Dodge PR, Davis H, Feigin RD, et al: Prospective evaluation of hearing impairment as a sequela of acute bacterial meningitis. *New Engl J Med* 311:869, 1984.

20. Dichgans M, Jäger L, Mayer T, et al: Bacterial meningitis in adults: Demonstration of inner ear involvement using high-resolution MRI. *Neurology* 52:1003, 1999.

21. Durand ML, Calderwood SB, Weber DJ, et al: Acute bacterial meningitis: A review of 493 episodes. *New Engl J Med* 328:21, 1993.

22. Hussein AS, Shafran SD: Acute bacterial meningitis in adults: A 12-year review. *Medicine* 79:360, 2000.

23. Pomeroy SL, Holmes SJ, Dodge PR, et al: Seizures and other neurologic sequelae of bacterial meningitis in children. *New Engl J Med* 323:1651, 1990.

24. De Gans J, van de Beek D, for the European Dexamethasone in Adulthood Bacterial Meningitis Study Investigators: Dexamethasone in adults with bacterial meningitis. *New Engl J Med* 347:1549, 2002.

25. Pfister HW, Feiden W, Einhäupl KM: The spectrum of complications during bacterial meningitis in adults: Results of a prospective clinical study. *Arch Neurol* 50:575, 1993.

26. Roos KL: Acute bacterial meningitis. *Semin Neurol* 20:293, 2000.

27. Pfister HW, Roos KL: Bacterial meningitis. In Noseworthy JH (ed): *Neurological Therapeutics: Principles and Practice,* Vol 1. London: Dunitz, 2003, p 863.

28. Weststrate W, Hijdra A, De Gans J: Brain infarcts in adults with bacterial meningitis. *Lancet* 347:399, 1996.

29. Gironell A, Domingo P, Mancebo J, et al: Hemorrhagic stroke as a complication of bacterial meningitis in adults: Report of three cases and review. *Clin Infect Dis* 21:1488, 1995.

30. Kastenbauer S, Winkler F, Fesl G, et al: Acute severe spinal cord dysfunction in bacterial meningitis in adults: MRI findings suggest extensive myelitis. *Arch Neurol* 58:806, 2001.

31. Gendrel D, Raymond J, Assicot M, et al: Measurement of procalcitonin levels in children with bacterial and viral meningitis. *Clin Infect Dis* 24:1240, 1997.

32. Viallon A, Zeni F, Lambert C, et al: High sensitivity and specificity of serum procalcitonin levels in adults with bacterial meningitis. *Clin Infect Dis* 28:1313, 1999.

33. Jan W, Zimmerman RA, Bilaniuk LT, et al: Diffusion-weighted imaging in acute bacterial meningitis in infancy. *Neuroradiology* 45:634, 2003

34. Haring HP, Rötzer HK, Reindl H, et al: Time course of cerebral blood flow velocity in central nervous system infections. *Arch Neurol* 50:98, 1993.

35. Pfister HW, Bleck TP: Bacterial infections. In Brandt T, Caplan LR, Dichgans J, Diener HC, Kennard C (eds): *Neurological Disorders: Course and Treatment,* 2d ed. Amsterdam: Academic Press, 2003, p 529.

36. Heyderman RS, Lambert HP, O'Sullivan I, et al: Early management of suspected bacterial meningitis and meningococcal septicaemia in adults. *J Infect* 46:75, 2003.

37. Oliver WJ, Shope TC, Kuhns LR: Fatal lumbar puncture: Fact versus fiction—an approach to a clinical dilemma. *Pediatrics* 112:174, 2003.

38. Pfausler B, Spiss H, Beer R, et al: Treatment of staphylococcal ventriculitis associated with external cerebrospinal fluid drains: A prospective, randomized trial of intravenous compared with intraventricular vancomycin therapy. *J Neurosurg* 98:1040, 2003.

39. Viale P, Pagani L, Cristini F, et al: Linezolid for the treatment of central nervous system infections in neurosurgical patients. *Scand J Infect Dis* 34:456, 2002.

40. Saez-Llorens X, McCracken GH Jr: Bacterial meningitis in children. *Lancet* 361:2139, 2003.

41. Lebel MH, Freji BJ, Syrogiannopoulos GA, et al: Dexamethasone therapy for bacterial meningitis: Results of two double-blind, placebo-controlled trials. *New Engl J Med* 319:964, 1988.

42. Odio CM, Faingezicht I, Paris M, et al: The beneficial effects of early dexamethasone administration in infants and children with bacterial meningitis. *New Engl J Med* 324:1525, 1991.

43. Schaad UB, Lips U, Gnehm HE, et al: Dexamethasone therapy for bacterial meningitis in children. *Lancet* 342:457, 1993.

44. Syrogiannopoulos GA, Lourida AN, Theodoridou MC, et al: Dexamethasone therapy for bacterial meningitis in children: 2- versus 4-day regimen. *J Infect Dis* 169:853, 1994.

45. Kennedy WA, Hoyt MJ, McCracken GH Jr: The role of corticosteroid therapy in children with pneumococcal meningitis. *Am J Dis Child* 145:1374, 1991.

46. Girgis NI, Farid Z, Mikhail IA, et al: Dexamethasone treatment for bacterial meningitis in children and adults. *Pediatr Infect Dis J* 8:848, 1989.

47. Thomas R, Le Tulzo Y, Bouget J, et al: Trial of dexamethasone treatment for severe bacterial meningitis in adults. Adult Meningitis Study Group. *Intensive Care Med* 25:475, 1999.

48. McIntyre PB, Berkey CS, King S, et al: Dexamethasone as adjunctive therapy in bacterial meningitis. *JAMA* 278:925, 1997.

49. Molyneux EM, Walsh AL, Forsyth H, et al: Dexamethasone treatment in childhood bacterial meningitis in Malawi: A randomised, controlled trial. *Lancet* 360:211, 2002.

50. Van de Beek D, de Gans J, McIntyre P, et al: Corticosteroids in acute bacterial meningitis. *Cochrane Database Syst Rev* CD004305, 2003.

51. Kaplan SL, Fishman MA: Supportive therapy for bacterial meningitis. *Pediatr Infect Dis J* 6:670, 1987.

52. Tunkel AR, Scheld WM: Corticosteroids for everyone with meningitis? *New Engl J Med* 347:1613, 2002.

53. Nau R, Brück W: Neuronal injury in bacterial meningitis: Mechanisms and implications for therapy. *Trends Neurosci* 25:38, 2002.

54. Meli DN, Christen S, Leib SL, et al: Current concepts in the pathogenesis of meningitis caused by *Streptococcus pneumoniae*. *Curr Opin Infect Dis* 15:253, 2002.

55. Paris MM, Hickey SM, Uscher MI, et al: Effect of dexamethasone on therapy of experimental penicillin- and cephalosporin-resistant pneumococcal meningitis. *Antimicrob Agents Chemother* 38:1320, 1994.

56. Viladrich PF, Gudiol F, Linares J, et al: Evaluation of vancomycin for therapy of pneumococcal meningitis. *Antimicrob Agents Chemother* 35:2467, 1991.

57. Klugman KP, Friedland IR, Bradley JS: Bactericidal activity against cephalosporin-resistant *Streptococcus pneumoniae* in cerebrospinal fluid of children with acute bacterial meningitis. *Antimicrob Agents Chemother* 39:1988, 1995.

58. Winkler F, Kastenbauer S, Yousry TA, et al: Discrepancy between cranial CT scan and clinically relevant raised intracranial pressure (ICP) in adults with pneumococcal meningitis: Should ICP monitoring be performed early? *J Neurol* 249:1292, 2002.

59. Southwick FS: Septic thrombophlebitis of major dural venous sinuses. *Curr Clin Top Infect Dis* 15:179, 1995.

60. White B, Livingstone W, Murphy C, et al: An open-label study of the role of adjuvant hemostatic support with protein C replacement therapy in purpura fulminans–associated meningococcemia. *Blood* 96:3719, 2000.

61. Weisel G, Joyce D, Gudmundsdottir A, et al: Human recombinant activated protein C in meningococcal sepsis. *Chest* 121:292, 2002.

62. Bernard GR, Vincent JL, Laterre PF, et al: Efficacy and safety of recombinant human activated protein C for severe sepsis. *New Engl J Med* 344:699, 2001.

63. King D, Higgins D: Subarachnoid haemorrhage following activated protein C for bacterial meningitis. *Anaesthesia* 58:911, 2003.

64. Wilder-Smith A, Memish Z: Meningococcal disease and travel. *Int J Antimicrob Agents* 21:102, 2003.

65. Balmer P, Borrow R, Miller E: Impact of meningococcal conjugate vaccine in the UK. *J Med Microbiol* 51:717, 2002.

66. Centers for Disease Control and Prevention: Notice to readers: Pneumococcal vaccination for cochlear implant recipients. *MMWR* 51:931, 2002.

CHAPTER 3

Bacterial Brain Abscess, Epidural Abscess, and Subdural Empyema

Latisha Ali, Avanee Shah, and Karen L. Roos

► BACTERIAL BRAIN ABSCESS

Overview

A brain abscess is a focal suppurative process in the brain parenchyma. In 1893, Sir William Macewen was the first surgeon to describe cranial surgical anatomy in detail, and he published his experiences in treating patients with brain abscess.[1,2] He stated, "The uncomplicated cerebral abscess early recognized, accurately localized and promptly operated on is one of the most satisfactory of the intracranial lesions."[1–3] Significant advances were made in the diagnosis of cerebral abscess with the advent of radiologic studies such as computed tomographic (CT) scanning and magnetic resonance imaging (MRI). This is reflected by the fact that mortality and morbidity rates for this disease have decreased significantly in the last 30 years.

Epidemiology

Bacterial brain abscesses occur in approximately 1500 to 2500 patients each year in the United States; multi-ple abscesses occur in 10 to 50 percent of these patients. The mortality rate reported in the literature prior to antibiotics was between 60 to 80 percent.[4–6] Prior to CT scanning, the mortality rate among patients with brain abscess was 30 to 50 percent despite treatment with antibiotics.[7–9] Population studies over five decades determined an incidence rate of 1.3 per 100,000 person-years. There is a male-to-female ratio of 2:1 to 3:1. Most cases of brain abscess are seen during the third and fourth decades of life, but they may occur at any age.[10,11]

The epidemiology of the disease is also changing in the postantibiotic era. There has been a decrease in the incidence of brain abscess due to traditional causes, such as acute or chronic sinusitis, chronic otitis media, penetrating cranial trauma, and dental infections, and a rise in the incidence seen in immunocompromised patients with organ and bone marrow transplants, human immunodeficiency virus (HIV) infection and AIDS, and patients receiving cancer chemotherapy.[10] In immuno-compromised patients, most brain abscesses are due to *Nocardia* spp., *Toxoplasma gondii, Entamoeba his-*

tolytica, Acanthamoeba spp., *Balamuthia mandrillaris,* and fungi (*Blastomyces dermatitidis, Candida* spp., *Aspergillus* spp., the dermatiaceous molds, and the zygomycetes). With the exception of *Nocardia* spp. brain abscesses, which are covered in this chapter, brain abscess in immunocompromised patients due to amebas, fungi, and parasites are covered in Chaps. 7, 12, and 17.

Etiology

Most brain abscesses in immunocompetent patients are bacterial in origin. The most common etiologic organisms are microaerophilic streptococci and anaerobic bacteria (anaerobic streptococci and *Bacteroides* spp.).[10,12] Other common organisms include *Staphylococcus aureus* (after trauma or craniotomy), *Clostridium* spp., Enterobacteriaceae, *Pseudomonas aeruginosa,* and *Hemophilus* spp. In brain abscess associated with cyanotic congenital heart disease, the predominant organisms are viridans, microaerophilic, or anaerobic streptococci. Approximately 20 to 40 percent of brain abscess cases are referred to as *cryptic* because no obvious source can be identified.[2,13]

Pathophysiology

The brain is very resistant to bacteria because of the calvarium, the dura, and the relatively impermeable blood-brain barrier formed by the capillary-endothelial tight junctions.[2] A brain abscess may develop in any of the three following ways: (1) by direct spread from a contiguous cranial site of infection, (2) following cranial trauma, either surgical or accidental, and (3) as a result of hematogenous spread from a remote site of infection. Those which develop by direct spread from a contiguous cranial site of infection can arise from paranasal sinusitis, mastoiditis, otitis media, or dental infections. When the underlying source of infection is an otitis media or mastoiditis, the brain abscess typically develops in the inferior temporal lobe or cerebellum, and the most common pathogens are streptococci, *Bacteroides* spp., *Pseudomonas* spp., *Hemophilus* spp., and Enterobacteriaceae. Infection that arises in the frontal or ethmoid sinus and dental infections usually are associated with brain abscess in the frontal lobes and typically are caused by streptococci, staphylococci, *Bacteroides* spp., *Hemophilus* spp., and *Fusobacterium* spp. Foreign bodies such as bullet fragments, trauma (open skull fracture or penetrating trauma), and neurosurgical procedures also can serve as a nidus for infection. In this setting, brain abscesses typically are due to *S. aureus*, coagulase-negative staphylococci, streptococci, enterobacteria, and *Clostridium* spp.[14] Hematogenous seeding that leads to a brain abscess arises in a primary infection elsewhere in the body, most typically a pulmonary or cardiac disease (cyanotic congenital heart disease, infective endocarditis) but also urinary tract infections, wound and skin infections, intraabdominal infections, and osteomyelitis. Infection with *Nocardia asteroides*, which is found in soil and decaying vegetables, is acquired primarily by inhalation of airborne spores, with hematogenous dissemination from the lungs to the central nervous system (CNS). The risk of CNS infection is increased in organ transplant recipients and in patients receiving cytotoxic chemotherapy and chronic corticosteroid therapy.

For bacterial invasion of brain parenchyma to occur, there must be preexisting or concomitant areas of ischemia, necrosis, or hypoxia in brain tissue. The intact brain parenchyma is relatively resistant to infection. Once bacteria have established infection, brain abscess formation evolves through four stages regardless of the infecting organism. These stages are early cerebritis, late cerebritis, early capsule formation, and late capsule formation. The early cerebritis stage (days 1–3) is characterized by perivascular infiltration of inflammatory cells composed of polymorphonuclear leukocytes, plasma cells, and mononuclear cells that surround a central core of coagulative necrosis. During this stage, the margin of the inflammatory infiltrate is ill-defined.[14] In the second stage, the late cerebritis stage (days 4–9), the necrotic center has reached its maximal size and is surrounded at its border by an inflammatory infiltrate of macrophages and fibroblasts. The appearance of fibroblasts and the marked increase in new vessel formation around the developing abscess set the stage for capsule formation. A thin capsule of fibroblasts and reticular fibers develops gradually, and the surrounding area of cerebral edema becomes more distinct than in the previous stage. In the third stage, the stage of early capsule formation (days 10–13), the necrotic center begins to decrease in size, and the inflammatory infiltrate changes in character, containing an increasing number of fibroblasts and macrophages. Mature collagen evolves from reticulin precursors, forming a capsule that is better developed on the cortical than on the ventricular side of the lesion. The final stage, the stage of late capsule formation (day 14 and on), is characterized by a well-formed necrotic center with a peripheral zone of inflammatory cells and a dense collagenous capsule. The surrounding area of cerebral edema has regressed, but marked gliosis with large numbers of reactive astrocytes has developed outside the capsule.[15–17]

Clinical Presentation

The clinical presentation of a brain abscess is influenced by a number of factors, most important of which are the size and location of the abscess.[2] The triad of fever, headache, and focal neurologic deficit is the classic presentation of a brain abscess. Headache is present in two-thirds of patients with brain abscess. Fever and leukocytosis are more common during the suppurative phase of cerebral abscess formation but may resolve once the abscess becomes encapsulated. Approximately 50 percent of patients have fever. Seizures occur in approximately 25 to 50 percent. As the cerebral edema and mass effect of the abscess increase, signs of raised intracranial pressure (ICP) develop, including an altered level of consciousness and papilledema.

Diagnosis

The diagnosis of a brain abscess usually is made by neuroimaging, either cranial CT scanning with contrast administration or MRI. On CT scan after contrast administration, a brain abscess in the early cerebritis stage has the appearance of a low-density lesion with faint contrast enhancement at the lesion's edge. Delayed scans obtained 30 minutes after the infusion of intravenous contrast material show diffusion of contrast into the low-density center. An abscess in the late cerebritis stage has the appearance on CT scan after contrast administration of a low-density lesion that is larger than in the early cerebritis stage with prominent ring enhancement following contrast administration. Delayed scans continue to reveal diffusion of contrast material into the low-density center. An abscess in the early capsule-formation stage has the appearance on cranial CT after contrast administration of an area of low density, and the diameter of ring contrast enhancement has decreased in size compared with the abscess in the late cerebritis stage. There is no significant inward diffusion of contrast material on delayed scans in an abscess in the early capsule-formation stage. On cranial CT scan, an abscess in the late capsule-formation stage has the appearance of a low-density lesion surrounded by a sharply demarcated dense ring of contrast enhancement.[16] On MRI, an abscess that is in the cerebritis stage appears as a hyperintense lesion on T_2-weighted scans; as the abscess develops a capsule, the capsule is iso- or hyperintense on T_1-weighted scans and hypointense on T_2-weighted images. On T_2-weighted scans, the hyperintense abscess cavity is surrounded by a hypointense capsule and surrounding edema that is hyperintense as well (Fig. 3-1*A*). On T_1-weighted MRI after the administration of intravenous gadolinium, the abscess appears as a central area of hypointensity surrounded by a ring of contrast enhancement (see Fig. 3-1*B*). The radiographic appearance of a brain abscess is similar to that of primary brain tumors, brain metastases, lymphoma, ischemic infarction, and resolving hematomas.[14]

MR spectroscopy (MRS) may be helpful in confirming the diagnosis of cerebral abscess by demonstrating the presence of amino acids such as acetate in the MRS spectra of the abscess, a quality not seen in

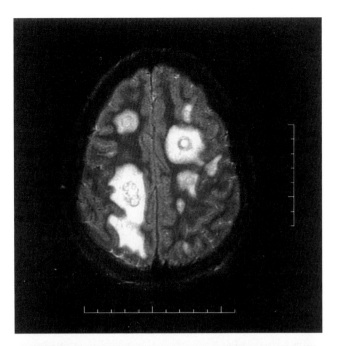

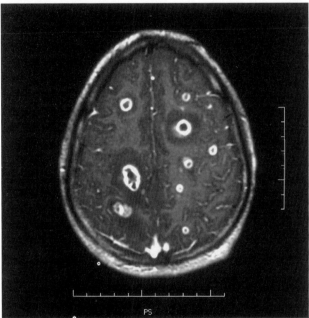

Figure 3–1. *A.* Brain abscess. T_2-weighted MRI. The hyperintense abscess cavity is surrounded by a hypointense capsule and surrounding edema that is hyperintense as well. *B.* T_1-weighted MRI after gadolinium administration. The abscess appears as a central area of hypointensity surrounded by a ring of contrast enhancement.

necrotic or cystic tumors.[18,19] Additionally, diffusion-weighted MRI (DWI) may be helpful in differentiating between brain abscess and tumor. The data suggest that the combination of high signal and reduced apparent diffusion coefficients (ADC) within a lesion on DWI is characteristic of but not pathognomonic for cerebral abscess.[20–25] On DWI, brain tumors or metastases usually give a low signal (and high apparent-diffusion coefficients).[14]

A lumbar puncture generally is contraindicated in the setting of cerebral abscess because it can lead to herniation. It is not a useful method of confirming the presence of an abscess or in identifying the pathogen because the cerebrospinal fluid (CSF) abnormalities typically are nonspecific, and culture is often negative. A careful physical examination should be performed to determine the source of the brain abscess. Echocardiography and chest CT scan can be obtained to determine a pulmonary or cardiac source of infection. A panoramic view of the mouth is helpful in determining a dental source of infection. Aerobic and anaerobic blood cultures can be obtained but are fairly insensitive for the detection of the organism causing the brain abscess. To establish a definitive diagnosis and identify the causative organism(s), CT- or MRI-guided stereotactic aspiration is recommended.

Treatment

Successful treatment of a cerebral abscess requires a combination of medical and surgical therapy.

In the early stage of cerebritis, before an abscess has become encapsulated and localized, there may be a response to antimicrobial therapy without surgical drainage. In addition, an initial trial of antimicrobial therapy is recommended in patients who are poor surgical candidates or have multiple abscesses or abscesses in deep or eloquent locations in the brain.[26] In general, once an abscess has formed, CT-guided stereotactic aspiration through a burr hole, drainage, or excision combined with a prolonged course of antibiotics is the management of choice.

Preoperative antibiotics should not be administered if surgery can be performed without delay. An abscess beyond the cerebritis stage should be managed by aspiration or excision. The advantages of aspiration are (1) it decreases the size of the intracranial mass and in this way decreases increased ICP, and (2) by removal of the purulent material in the core of the abscess, antibiotics are less likely to be inactivated by bacterial or leukocytic enzymes in the pus. Aspiration may provide only temporary benefit. External drainage of an abscess through an intracavitary catheter can be done by irrigating the abscess cavity with 10 ml sterile saline solution, and when the aspirate is clear, the drain is removed. This typically takes 5 days.[14] Excision is the definitive procedure when antibiotics and aspiration cannot control infection and when there are lesions greater than 3 cm in size on neuroimaging. Excision is contraindicated in the early stages of the abscess, before a capsule has formed, and where an abscess is deep in the brain or in vital structures. A major complication of excision is the likelihood of a permanent neurologic deficit.

Empirical antimicrobial therapy typically is started before the result of Gram's stain and culture is known. Empirical therapy should include a combination of a third- or fourth-generation cephalosporin (e.g., cefotaxime, ceftriaxone, or cefepime) with vancomycin and metronidazole. The predisposing conditions associated with a brain abscess help to predict the etiologic organism and can be used in decisions regarding initial empirical therapy. A brain abscess that arises from sinusitis is usually due to streptococci and anaerobic organisms. *Hemophilus* spp. also may be the causative organisms. Empirical therapy of a sinusitis-associated brain abscess should include a combination of penicillin G or a third- or fourth-generation cephalosporin and metronidazole. Penicillin has excellent activity against streptococci; metronidazole has excellent bactericidal activity against anaerobes. Microaerophilic streptococci are resistant to metronidazole. A third- or fourth-generation cephalosporin is added to provide coverage for *Hemophilus* spp. The most common organisms isolated in a brain abscess from an otitic source are *Streptococcus* spp., enterobacteriaeceae, *Bacteroides* spp., and *P. aeruginosa*. Empirical therapy of an otogenic abscess should include a combination of penicillin G, metronidazole, and ceftazidime. A brain abscess as a result of penetrating head trauma is most often due to *S. aureus*, *Clostridium* spp., or enterobacteriaeceae. Empirical therapy should include a combination of a third- or fourth-generation cephalosporin plus vancomycin. When a brain abscess complicates a neurosurgical procedure, staphylococci, enterobacteriaeceae, and *Pseudomonas* spp. are the usual etiologic organisms. Empirical therapy should include a combination of ceftazidime or meropenem plus vancomycin. Once the organism has been identified, antimicrobial therapy can be modified according to Table 3-1. A 6- to 8-week course of intravenous antimicrobial therapy is recommended. During antimicrobial therapy, CT scan or MRI is recommended biweekly or at any time when there are clinical signs of neurologic deterioration. If an abscess enlarges after a 2-week course of antimicrobial therapy or fails to diminish in size after 3 to 4 weeks of antimicrobial therapy, further surgical drainage is recommended.[14]

A brain abscess due to *Nocardia* spp. requires surgical excision and at least 6 to 12 months of therapy with trimethoprim-sulfamethoxazole (15 to 20 mg/kg per day of the trimethoprim component and 75 to 100 mg/kg per day of the sulfamethoxazole component). Complete excision of a brain abscess due to *Nocardia* usually is required for cure.

The use of corticosteroids is recommended in patients with significant edema, mass effect, and signs of increased ICP. Steroids can alter the clinical and radio-

▶ **TABLE 3-1.** RECOMMENDED ANTIMICROBIAL AGENT BASED ON PATHOGEN

Pathogen	Antimicrobial Agent Total Daily Adult Dose (Dosing Interval)
Streptococcus spp.	Penicillin G 20–24 million units/d (every 4 h) *or* Ceftriaxone 4 g/d (every 12 h) *or* Cefotaxime 12 g/d (every 4 h) *or* Cefepime 4 g/d (every 12 h)
Staphylococci	
Methicillin-susceptible	Nafcillin or oxacillin 12 g/d (every 4–6 h)
Methicillin-resistant	Vancomycin 2–3 g/d (every 6 h)
Gram-negative enterobacteriaeceae (*E. coli, Proteus* spp., *Klebsiella* spp.)	Ceftriaxone or cefotaxime or cefepime
Bacteroides fragilis	Metronidazole 2000 mg/d (every 6 h)
Hemophilus influenzae	Ceftriaxone or cefotaxime
Pseudomonas aeruginosa	Ceftazidime 6 g/d (every 8 h) *or* Meropenem 6 g/d (every 8 h) *or* Cefepime
Nocardia asteroides	Trimethoprim-sulfamethoxazole

graphic findings and lead to decreased antibiotic penetration into the abscess; therefore, once the edema and mass effect have improved, corticosteroids should be tapered to avoid retardation of abscess wall formation.[27] The recommended corticosteroid dose is intravenous or oral dexamethasone given in a dose of 10 mg q6h and tapered over 3 to 7 days.[2]

Seizures are a frequent complication of brain abscess and may occur in as many as 50 percent of patients during the initial period of hospitalization and 70 percent in the subsequent months.[2] Patients should be treated empirically with anticonvulsant therapy at the time of diagnosis and for the following 2 years. If the patient is seizure-free 2 years after therapy, the antiepileptic drug may be discontinued.

▶ CRANIAL EPIDURAL ABSCESS

A cranial epidural abscess or cranial epidural empyema develops in the space between the dura and the inner table of the skull (Fig. 3-2). A cranial epidural abscess

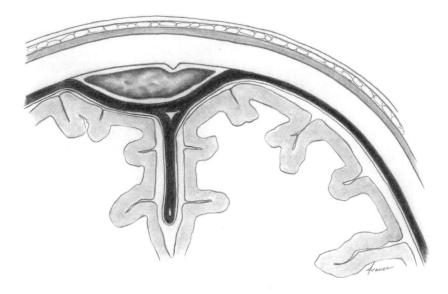

Figure 3–2. Cranial epidural abscess. (*Drawn by Avanee Shah, M.D.*)

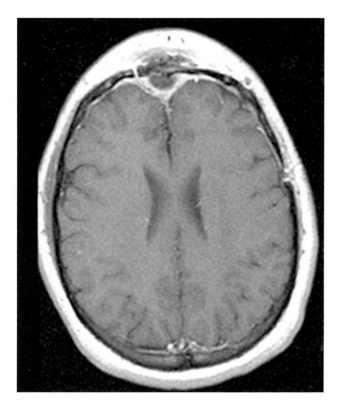

Figure 3–3. Axial T₁-weighted MRI after gadolinium administration demonstrating a cranial epidural abscess due to contiguous osteomyelitis. *(Courtesy of Vincent Mathews, M.D.)*

develops when infection in the frontal sinuses, middle ear, mastoid, or orbit reach the epidural space through the retrograde spread of infection in the emissary veins that drain these areas, by direct spread of infection through bone, or through direct infection of the epidural space during craniotomy.

The clinical presentation of a cranial epidural abscess is an unrelenting hemicranial headache with fever. Cranial MRI is the procedure of choice to demonstrate an epidural abscess. An epidural abscess appears as a crescentic purulent fluid collection that is of higher signal intensity on T₁-weighted images than the CSF. Following the administration of gadolinium, enhancement of the dura is seen (Fig. 3-3).

The definitive step in the management of cranial epidural abscess is immediate neurosurgical drainage. At surgery, Gram's stain and culture of the purulent material are performed. Empirical antimicrobial therapy should include a combination of a third- or fourth-generation cephalosporin, metronidazole, and vancomycin. Antibiotic coverage can be modified when the results of bacterial culture and sensitivities are known. Intravenous antibiotic therapy is continued for 4 to 6 weeks after surgical drainage of the epidural abscess, followed by 2 to 3 months of oral antibiotic therapy.

▶ SUBDURAL EMPYEMA

A subdural empyema is a collection of pus in the space between the dura and the arachnoid (Fig. 3-4). Paranasal sinusitis is the most common predisposing condition associated with a subdural empyema, and less commonly, infection in the inner ear and mastoid can be complicated by a subdural empyema. A subdural empyema also may complicate a neurosurgical procedure. In infants, a subdural empyema usually represents an infected subdural effusion associated with bacterial meningitis.

Most subdural empyemas develop over the convexity of the cerebral hemispheres. Once infection is established in the subdural space, evolution of an empyema tends to be remarkably rapid. The empyema,

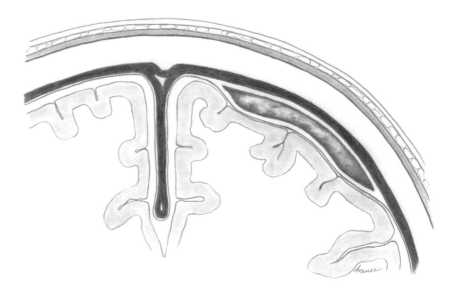

Figure 3–4. Cranial subdural empyema. *(Drawn by Avanee Shah, M.D.)*

aided by gravity, extends mainly in a posterior direction but also extends medially over the tentorium toward the falx. Aerobic, microaerophilic, and anaerobic streptococci are the predominant organisms isolated in empyemas complicating sinusitis, otitis, and mastoiditis. Staphylococci are found in subdural empyemas that complicate neurosurgical procedures.

The initial signs and symptoms of a subdural empyema are those of infection, increased ICP from an expanding mass lesion, and focal brain ischemia or infarction. Most patients complain of headache. This is followed by a change in the level of consciousness progressing from confusion to stupor and coma. Focal neurologic deficits are present in 80 to 90 percent of patients. Most patients have fever. Seizures may begin as focal motor seizures but then secondarily generalize. Patients with subdural empyemas are quite ill and may have a rapid progression of neurologic deficits and altered level of consciousness. T_1-weighted MRI after gadolinium administration and the FLAIR sequence are the best studies to demonstrate a subdural empyema (Figs. 3-5 and 3-6). A lumbar puncture is contraindicated in a patient with a subdural empyema due to the risk of herniation from mass effect and increased ICP.

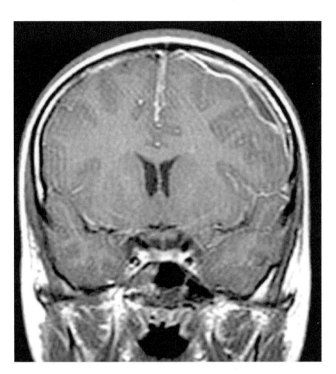

Figure 3–6. Coronal T_1-weighted MRI after gadolinium administration demonstrating cranial subdural empyema. *(Courtesy of Vincent Mathews, M.D.)*

Neurosurgical evacuation of the empyema through burr-hole drainage or craniotomy is the definitive step in the management of this infection and should be done emergently. The etiologic organism of the subdural empyema is identified by Gram's stain and culture of pus obtained either via burr-hole drainage or craniotomy. Empirical therapy should include a combination of penicillin G or a third- or fourth-generation cephalosporin, metronidazole, and vancomycin. Antibiotic therapy can be modified when the results of the Gram's stain and bacterial cultures and sensitivities are known. Intravenous antibiotics should be continued for 3 or 4 weeks after surgical drainage, and then oral antibiotic therapy can be substituted to complete a 6-week course of therapy.

REFERENCES

1. Macewen W: *Pyogenic Infective Diseases of the Brain and Spinal Cord.* Glasgow: James Maclehose and Sons, 1983, pp 105–111.
2. Mathisen GE, Johnson JP: Brain ascess. *Clin Infect Dis* 25:763, 1997.
3. Stephanov S: Surgical treatment of brain abscess. *Neurosurgery* 22:724, 1988.
4. Morgan H, Wood MW, Murphey F: Experience with 88 consecutive cases of brain abscess. *J Neurosurg* 38:698, 1973.
5. Mamelak AN, Mampalam TJ, Obana WG, et al: Im-

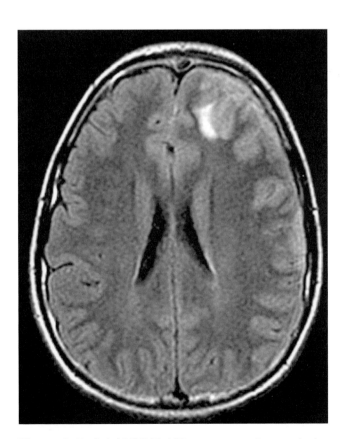

Figure 3–5. Axial MRI FLAIR sequence demonstrating cranial subdural empyema with subjacent cerebritis and edema. *(Courtesy of Vincent Mathews, M.D.)*

proved management of multiple brain abscesses: A combined surgical and medical approach. *Neurosurgery* 36:76, 1995.

6. Alderson D, Strong AJ, Ingham HR, et al: Fifteen-year review of the mortality of brain abscess. *Neurosurgery* 8:1, 1981.

7. Mampalam TJ, Rosenblum ML: Trends in the management of bacterial brain abscesses: A review of 102 cases over 17 years. *Neurosurgery* 23:451, 1988.

8. Carey ME, Chan SN, French LA: Experience with brain abscesses. *J Neurosurg* 36:1, 1972.

9. Jooma OV, Pennybacker JB, Tutton GD: Brain abscess: Aspiration, drainage or excision. *J Neurol Neurosurg Psychiatry* 14:308, 1951.

10. Calfee D, Wispelwey B: Brain abscess. *Semin Neurol* 20:353, 2000.

11. Nicolosi A, Hauser WA, Musicco M, et al: Incidence and prognosis of brain abscess in a defined population: Olmsted County, Minnesota, 1935–1981. *Neuroepidemiology* 10:122, 1991.

12. Gortvai P, De Louvois J, Hurley R: The bacteriology and chemotherapy of acute pyogenic brain abscess. *Br J Neurosurg* 1:189, 1987.

13. Svanteson B, Nordström CH, Rausing A: Non-traumatic brain abscess. *Acta Neurochir* 94:57, 1988.

14. Kastenbauer S: Infectious intracranial mass lesions, in Noseworthy JH (ed): *Neurological Therapeutics: Principles and Practice*. London: Martin Dunitz, 203, pp 874–888.

15. Garvey G: Current concepts of bacterial infection of the central nervous system: Bacterial meningitis and bacterial brain abscess. *J Neurosurg* 59:735, 1983.

16. Britt RH, Enzmann DR, Yeager AS: Neuropathological and computerized tomographic findings in experimental brain abscess. *J Neurosurg* 55:590, 1981.

17. Enzmann DR, Britt RR, Obana WG, et al: Experimental *Staphylococcus aureus* brain abscess. *AJNR* 7:395, 1986.

18. Martínez-Pérez I, Moreno A, Alonso J, et al: Diagnosis of brain abscess by magnetic resonance spectroscopy. *J Neurosurg* 86:708, 1997.

19. Kim SH, Chang KH, Song IC, et al: Brain abscess and brain tumor: Discrimination in vivo H-1 MR spectroscopy. *Radiology* 204:239, 1997.

20. Noguchi K, Watanabe N, Nagayoshi T, et al: Role of diffusion-weighted echo planar MRI in distinguishing between brain abscess and tumour: A preliminary report. *Neuroradiology* 41:171, 1999.

21. Guo AC, Provenzale JM, Cruz JR, et al: Cerebral abscess: Investigation using apparent diffusion coefficient maps. *Neuroradiology* 43:370, 2001.

22. Chang SC, Lai PH, Chen WL, et al: Diffusion-weighted MRI features of brain abscess and cystic or necrotic brain tumors: A comparison with conventional MRI. *J Clin Imag* 26:227, 2002.

23. Tung GA, Evangelista P, Rogg JM, et al: Diffusion-weighted MR imaging of rim-enhancing brain masses: Is markedly decreased water diffusion specific for brain abscess? *AJR* 177:709, 2001.

24. Tung G, Rogg J: Diffusion weighted imaging of cerebritis. *AJNR* 24:1110, 2003.

25. Hartmann M, Jansen O, Heiland S, et al: Restricted diffusion within ring enhancement is not pathognomonic for brain abscess. *AJNR* 22:1738, 2001.

26. Rosenblum ML, Hoff JT, Norman D, et al: Nonoperative treatment of brain abscesses in selected high-risk patients. *J Neurosurg* 52:217, 1980.

27. Schroeder KA, McKeever PE, Schaberg DR, et al: Effect of dexamethasone on experimental brain abscess. *J Neurosurg* 66:264, 1987.

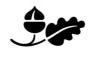

CHAPTER 4

Congenital and Perinatal Viral Infections

James F. Bale, Jr.

► HISTORICAL OVERVIEW

The physicians of the 1850s knew of congenital syphilis, but the concept that other infectious pathogens, especially viruses, could damage the developing fetus or the newborn did not emerge until the twentieth century. The observations of E. E. Southard, contained in the 1910 edition of *Osler's Modern Medicine,* illustrate the meager scope of knowledge regarding congenital and perinatal infections at the turn of the last century.[1] "There is a form of encephalitis in the newborn which is at times a cause of stillbirth or of death soon after birth, and is due to various factors (sometimes to pyogenic infection, sometimes to syphilis, and sometimes to unknown intoxications), perhaps more often maternal than non-maternal."

Reports in the early 1900s relied entirely on detailed histopathologic examinations of fetal or neonatal tissues. Among the earliest was the description of cytomegalic inclusion disease, a disorder producing intracellular and intracytoplasmic inclusions in the spleen, liver, and other tissues.[2] Although the designation "owl eye" inclusions fit the pathologic findings well, an early pathologist, perhaps intrigued by novel observations regarding congenital toxoplasmosis, erroneously attributed the abnormalities to infection with a protozoa (*Entamoeba mortinatalium*). Physicians apparently ignored potential cases of intrauterine infection because the placenta was considered to be an effective barrier to infectious agents, including viruses.

The pace of discovery regarding congenital and perinatal viral infections remained sluggish until 1941, when Norman McAlister Gregg, an ophthalmologist from Sydney, Australia, described the association of congenital cataracts and maternal rubella virus infection.[3] Gregg's observations stimulated clinical studies that ultimately led to the prevention of congenital rubella through compulsory immunization. His landmark report also would motivate clinician-scientists throughout the world to determine if other maternal viral infections were teratogenic for human infants.

In the 1940s, investigators identified perinatal herpes simplex virus infection as a cause of disseminated disease and death in infancy. Further discoveries, however, would await the development of cell culture methods, which provided a means by which viruses could be propagated and classified. In 1949, Enders, Weller, and Robbins observed that the poliovirus could be grown in tissue cultures of human cells and discovered that infection produced characteristic changes in cell monolayers, termed the *cytopathic effect.* This discovery led not simply to the Nobel prize for Enders, Weller, and Robbins in 1954[4] but directly to laboratory methods by which several viruses, including the varicella-zoster virus and cytomegalovirus (CMV), could be identified as important neonatal pathogens. In the mid-1950s, Weller isolated CMV in cell culture and correctly linked this agent to cytomegalic inclusion disease.[5]

During the latter half of the twentieth century, physician-scientists focused on categorizing congenital and perinatal infections, identifying the cause(s) of infection more rapidly, and devising more effective means of therapy and prevention. Investigators at Emory University and the Centers for Disease Control and Prevention (CDC) in the early 1970s introduced the concept of TORCH, an acronym referring to *To*xoplasma gondii, *r*ubella, *c*ytomegalovirus, and *h*erpes simplex virus. This popular acronym underscored the clinical observation that these agents produce similar clinical manifestations in congenitally infected newborns.[6]

Since the 1970s, the Collaborative Antiviral Study Group (CASG), supported by the National Institutes of Allergy and Infectious Diseases, has evaluated potential antiviral therapies for infants with congenital or perinatal infections. Current strategies for managing neonatal herpes simplex virus[7] and varicella-zoster virus infections with acyclovir and cytomegalovirus infections with ganciclovir directly reflect the concerted efforts of the CASG.[8,9] In the 1990s, investigators discovered that the polymerase chain reaction (PCR) can be an exceedingly sensitive and specific method for detecting many viruses, especially herpes simplex viruses and nonpolio enteroviruses.[10]

The twenty-first century brings optimism and challenge. Certain vaccines have fulfilled their promise; Gregg's congenital rubella syndrome has virtually disappeared in nations with compulsory immunization programs.[11] Using advanced cell culture and molecular methods, clinicians can rapidly identify the agents causing congenital and perinatal infections. Current antiviral agents are better tolerated and more effective. However, certain congenital disorders, including congenital CMV infection, the most frequent intrauterine infection, cannot be prevented. Others, such as perinatal enteroviral infections and congenital lymphocytic choriomeningitis virus infection, await effective antiviral therapy.

► EPIDEMIOLOGY

Arboviruses

Several RNA viruses transmitted to humans by ticks, mosquitoes, or biting flies have been grouped historically as the arboviruses, a designation that reflects their arthropod-borne origin.[12] In rare instances, a few of the arboviruses, including Venezuelan equine encephalitis (VEE) virus (an alphavirus), Western equine encephalitis (WEE) virus (an alphavirus), Japanese encephalitis (JE) virus (a flavivirus), and West Nile virus (WNV) (a flavivirus), produce intrauterine or perinatal infections.[13–15] The reported cases of fetal and neonatal infections generally have occurred during epidemics, such as the massive 2002 U.S. epidemic of WNV.[16]

As their names imply, these viruses tend to display distinct geographic predilections. JE virus infects persons living throughout Asia from Japan to India.[12] VEE virus periodically affects equines and humans living in Latin America, whereas cases of WEE virus cluster in the plains and agricultural valleys of the western United States and Canada.[12] Although originally detected in North Africa, WNV has now been reported in several regions, including eastern Europe and the United States.[12,16] Persons of all ages can be infected with these viruses; fortunately, subclinical infections greatly outnumber disease cases. The overall incidence of intrauterine or perinatal infections with these agents is very low.

Cytomegalovirus

Cytomegalovirus (CMV), a betaherpesvirus, remains the most common cause of congenital or perinatal virus infection among infants in developed nations. In the United States, for example, 0.4 to 2.5 percent of newborn infants shed CMV at birth.[17] The majority of humans become infected with the virus during childhood or adulthood, usually without recognizable symptoms.[18] The incidence of acquired CMV infection among children and adults, including women of childbearing age, averages 1 to 2 percent annually. By adulthood, 40 to 100 percent of the population has been infected with CMV.[17]

Congenitally infected newborn infants acquire CMV transplacentally during maternal viremia. Nursing infants can become infected postnatally via their mother's breast milk, and young children can become infected through direct contact with CMV-excreting playmates. Group child care plays a major role in the transmission of CMV among young children, their parents, and their care providers.[19,20] Adults acquire CMV via blood transfusion, sexual contact, organ transplantation, or contact with young children.[21–23] Adults with multiple sexual partners have increased rates of CMV acquisition.[18] Young children in child care environments and adults with multiple partners can be infected with new CMV strains, indicating that reinfection is possible.[24]

Acutely infected children or adults have CMV viremia that lasts up to 3 months, and within 1 month of acute infection, infectious virus appears in the urine, saliva, semen (if male), and cervical fluids (if female). The virus can be found in these fluids for 1 year or more, even among immunocompetent hosts. Congenitally infected infants can shed CMV in urine for several years.[25] Seropositive breast-feeding women begin to secrete infectious virus in breast milk within 1 month of lactation as a consequence of reactivated CMV infections.[26]

As with most of the agents discussed in this chapter, host immunity plays a major role in determining the risk of congenital or perinatal infection.[27] Nonimmune seronegative women have the greatest risk of transmitting CMV to their unborn infants. Approximately 40 percent of women who acquire primary CMV infection during pregnancy transmit CMV to the fetuses, and approximately 10 percent of the infected infants have CMV disease.[28] Although seropositivity to CMV provides an important protective effect for most pregnant women, CMV-seropositive women can be reinfected with new CMV strains, and these new CMV strains can cause disease in their offspring.[29]

Nonpolio Enteroviruses

The nonpolio enteroviruses (EVs), a group of more than 60 small RNA viruses [coxsackieviruses, echoviruses, and viruses identified by number (e.g., EV71)], colonize the upper respiratory and gastrointestinal tracts of humans and spread by direct contact with infected material.[30,31] Infected persons shed EVs for extended periods in oral secretions and feces. The EVs characteristically exhibit seasonal outbreaks in the northern hemisphere, June through early November, but occur year round in tropical climates, suggesting that environmental factors facilitate viral transmission.

During peak EV season, neonates frequently acquire infections vertically from their mothers in the perinatal period or horizontally from contact with infected persons. Less commonly, EVs can be transmitted *in utero*. In a study of approximately 600 infants cultured during an EV season in Rochester, New York, Jenista and colleagues found no examples of congenital infection (isolation of an EV within 1 day of delivery) but observed a 12.6 percent incidence of EV acquisition during the first month of life.[32] The overall rate of neonatal coxsackievirus infections was found to be 50 per 100,000 on Long Island, New York, approximately fourfold greater than the frequency of perinatally acquired herpes simplex virus infection.[33]

Herpes Simplex Viruses Type 1 and Type 2

Herpes simplex virus types 1 (HSV-1) and 2 (HSV-2) infect approximately 1000 infants in the U.S. annually.[34] HSV-2 causes approximately two-thirds of neonatal HSV infections, with the remainder due to HSV-1. Millions of persons harbor HSV latently, and many thousands acquire primary HSV-1 or HSV-2 infections annually.[35] Although HSV-1 usually causes oral lesions and HSV-2 typically produces genital lesions, either virus can be found at either site. HSV-1 and HSV-2 display approximately 50 percent nucleotide homology.

In most regions of the world, children acquire HSV-1 between 6 months and 4 years of age.[35] The actual rates of infection depend on socioeconomic status (SES), with rates being inversely related to SES. Primary HSV-1 infections are usually inapparent, but young children can have gingivostomatitis, a disorder associated with fever and mucosal ulceration. Recurrent oral herpes infection with HSV-1, herpes labialis, occurs endemically, although as many as 90 percent of reactivated infections are subclinical. Neonates acquire HSV-1 during delivery by contact with infected cervical secretions or postnatally by contact with persons with active oral HSV-1 infections.

The incidence of HSV-2 infection is highest among women of childbearing age, when approximately 2 percent acquire the virus each year. Primary HSV-2 infections, like those of HSV-1, usually occur without recognizable symptoms. Epidemiologic studies from several regions of the world indicate that approximately 30 percent of 30-year-old women have serologic evidence of prior HSV-2 infection.[36,37] The seroprevalence of HSV-2 infection among women in the United States has risen steadily during the past three decades.[36] HSV-2 seropositivity among U.S. women is associated with African-American race, lower income, greater number of lifetime sexual partners, earlier age of sexual intercourse, and drug use.[38]

When primary HSV-2 infection occurs during pregnancy, spontaneous abortion, stillbirth, or premature labor can occur.[39] By contrast, the risk of intrauterine transmission of HSV-2 to the fetus appears to be very low. Women can shed HSV-2 in the cervix asymptomatically after primary or recurrent (reactivated) infections, exposing infants to HSV-2 during passage through infected birth canals. Neonatal disease is more likely when mothers have active genital HSV infection near the time of delivery.

Varicella-Zoster Virus

The varicella-zoster virus (VZV) causes chickenpox (varicella) and shingles (herpes zoster). The incidence of chickenpox, the clinical manifestation of symptomatic primary VZV infection, peaks between 5 and 9 years of age among nonimmunized children in temperate climates.[40] Common during the winter and spring, chickenpox results from respiratory transmission of virus-contaminated droplets. VZV-infected persons are contagious for approximately 4 days before and 5 days after onset of the rash.

Chickenpox develops in approximately 0.05 percent of pregnant women.[41] Women who acquire VZV before the twentieth week of gestation have a 2 percent risk of delivering an infant with the fetal varicella syndrome.[42–44] This risk is greatest during first-trimester infections, whereas the fetal varicella syndrome is highly unlikely in women who have chickenpox during the last half of pregnancy. Maternal shingles, the clinical manifestation of VZV reactivation, poses little or no risk to the developing fetus. By contrast, neonatal varicella, a life-threatening disorder, develops commonly in the infants of women who have chickenpox during the 5 days before and the 2 days after delivery.[45]

Lymphocytic Choriomeningitis Virus

Lymphocytic choriomeningitis (LCM) virus, first identified as a cause of human infection in the 1930s, naturally infects the feral house mouse, *Mus musculus,* and also can infect golden hamsters.[46] Infected rodents shed LCM virus chronically in urine, feces, and respiratory secretions. Humans become infected when they inhale infected aerosols, touch infected animals, or ingest material contaminated by infected excreta. Occasional outbreaks of human illness have been associated with occupational contact with infected laboratory mice or the purchase of pet hamsters.[47,48] Recognized human infections in temperate climates often present during the winter months, but infections can occur throughout the year.

Seroprevalence studies suggest that the incidence of LCM virus infection is low in the general population. Approximately 5 percent of the adults attending a sexually transmitted disease clinic in Baltimore had serologic evidence of prior LCM virus infection.[49] Trapping of mice from urban sites in Baltimore disclosed considerable variation in LCM virus infection rates among mouse colonies, a factor that influences the risk of human LCM virus infection. A seroepidemiologic study from Birmingham, Alabama, indicated that persons over 30 years were more likely to have serologic evidence of prior LCM virus infection (5.4 percent seroprevalence among persons older than 30 years of age versus 0.3 percent among persons younger than 30 years of age).[50] Seroprevalence rates of 2.4 and 4 percent were observed among adults in Argentina and Nova Scotia, respectively.[51,52] Intrauterine LCM virus infection is presumed to be a rare condition, but the exact incidence of the disorder is undetermined.[53]

Rubella Virus

The epidemiology of congenital rubella syndrome (CRS), the consequence of maternal rubella (German measles) infection, has changed considerably since Gregg's 1941 report.[3] In the prevaccine era, epidemics of rubella appeared every 6 to 9 years, causing numerous cases of CRS, but after licensure of the rubella vaccine in 1969 and aggressive immunization programs targeting adolescents and adults in the 1980s, the incidence of the CRS in many regions of the world declined dramatically.[11,54] In the United States, only 1 to 3 cases of CRS were reported to the CDC annually during the middle to late 1980s, an overall incidence of less than 0.1 case of CRS per 100,000 live births.[55]

In the early 1990s, the CDC received reports of 56 CRS cases in the United States, a rate of 0.6 to 0.8 case per 100,000 live births, a substantial increase over the preceding several years.[55] This resurgence of CRS reflected rubella outbreaks among unimmunized persons in California, New York, and Pennsylvania, as well as sporadic indigenous cases in several other locations. The incidence of rubella and CRS subsequently reached record lows in the late 1990s, indicating that CRS is nearing elimination in the United States.[11] Approximately 10 percent of young adults in the United States remain susceptible to rubella virus, however, and rubella continues to pose a threat to infants born in countries without compulsory immunization programs.

▶ PATHOGENESIS

With the exception of LCM and rubella viruses, which produce neonatal disease only after intrauterine infection, each of the viruses described in this chapter can produce disease in neonates after either intrauterine or perinatal acquisition. Each of the agents also can infect humans without producing symptoms, a feature common to many viruses. Rubella, CMV, and LCM virus typically cause severe disease as a consequence of intrauterine infection. CMV can be acquired postnatally, especially via the breast milk of nursing mothers. Although postnatal infections can cause hepatosplenomegaly, pneumonia, thrombocytopenia, anemia, and occasionally death in small premature infants,[60] perinatally acquired CMV infections do not typically damage the brain, inner ear, or retina. By contrast, most symptomatic HSV-2, VZV, and EV infections occur as a result of perinatal transmission during delivery or shortly thereafter. Intrauterine infections with these agents are rare but nonetheless important events.

The complications of intrauterine and perinatal viral infection are influenced by the complex interaction of the mother, the placenta, the fetus, and the viral pathogen. The immune status of the mother is a major factor in determining the likelihood of maternal infection and the consequences of infection. Women who possess antibodies to a specific pathogen (seropositive) have been infected with the agent previously and have substantially reduced risks of transmitting infection to their infants. Infants with CRS, for example, are born rarely to women with anticipated or proven immunity to rubella virus. The same principle holds true for VZV.

The relationship between previous maternal infection and the risk of congenital or perinatal disease is slightly less clear for CMV. Although maternal seropositivity protects most infants from intrauterine infection and permanent organ damage,[27] occasional infants with CMV disease are born to mothers with preexisting immunity to CMV.[29] This appears to be due to maternal reinfection with new CMV strains, implying that maternal seropositivity may not confer absolute protection.

Women who are seronegative for HSV-2 have the greatest likelihood of transmitting HSV-2 to the fetus when primary infection occurs during pregnancy. However, seropositive women can experience genital reactivations of HSV-2 and transmit HSV-2 to their infants during delivery. HSV-1 or HSV-2 also can be acquired postnatally by the infant through contact with infected persons other than the mother, including hospital personnel.

During intrauterine infections, viruses such as CMV or rubella reach the placenta during maternal viremia. There, the viruses replicate, enter the fetal circulation, and disseminate hematogenously to the target organs of the developing fetus. For certain viruses, such as rubella and VZV, the fetal consequences of infection relate directly to the timing of maternal infection.[41,56] Maternal rubella infection during the initial 8 weeks of pregnancy, for example, produces cataracts and congenital heart lesions, whereas sensorineural hearing loss correlates with infection during the first 16 weeks. Stillbirth or spontaneous abortion also can occur during this time interval. By contrast, rubella infections after the sixteenth week of gestation usually leave no sequelae.

For other viruses, such as CMV, the relationship between the timing of infection and the likelihood of fetal damage is less clearcut.[18] Although CMV infection during critical stages of *in utero* development can produce severe central nervous system (CNS) malformations, such as lissencephaly or schizencephaly,[57,58] damage to other organs, including the eye, inner ear, liver, and spleen, seems to occur irrespective of the timing of maternal infection. Less than 10 percent of primary maternal CMV infections produce fetal damage. This observation implies that additional factors, such as variations in host immune responses, host polymorphisms in viral receptors, or variations in virus strains, contribute to the potential for fetal tissue damage and postnatal sequelae.

Perinatal virus infections usually result from vertical transmission of viral pathogens from mothers to newborn infants during or shortly before delivery. Contact with virus-infected maternal secretions may occur during vaginal delivery, and this mechanism accounts for most cases of neonatal HSV and EV infections. The viruses replicate at the site of inoculation, usually the skin, conjunctivae, or oropharynx, and if replication continues unabated by the infant's immune responses, viremia ensues. Viremia then disseminates the pathogen to target organs, such as the liver, spleen, bone marrow, retina, and brain. Tissue damage generally reflects lytic infection of target cells, but host immune responses, especially induction of cytokines, have dual roles in limiting virus infection and inducing damage to host tissues.

Ascending infection, i.e., direct transmission of viruses to the fetus from the cervix or vagina, can contribute to perinatal infection, especially for HSV-2. Perinatal transmission of viral pathogens is influenced by such factors as the maternal virus load, maternal-fetal immunity, and the route of delivery. Although cesarean section prior to rupture of the amniotic membranes reduces the infant's chances for contact with HSV in women with active genital herpes, infections can still occur, indicating that ascending infection or viremia participates in the pathogenesis of perinatal infection.[59] Infections with HSV, VZV, CMV, or nonpolio EV after the immediate neonatal period can result from postnatal contact with the virus-infected secretions of hospital personnel, siblings, and other family members.

▶ CLINICAL MANIFESTATIONS

Arboviruses

The arboviruses have been associated with intrauterine infection, resulting in stillbirth or severe CNS damage, and neonatal infection, causing meningoencephalitis of varying severity. Intrauterine infection with VEE virus causes stillbirth and hydranencephaly that resembles VZV embryopathy.[61] Intrauterine JE virus infection also can lead to fetal death. Vertical transmission of WEE virus occasionally produces neonatal meningoencephalitis with fever, irritability, lethargy, and bulging fontanels.[15] A single case of intrauterine WNV infection was associated with bilateral chorioretinitis and cystic encephalomalacia.[14]

Cytomegalovirus

Most CMV-infected neonates (90 percent or more) with intrauterine CMV infections have no apparent signs of CMV infection at birth.[17,28] The silently infected infants have a 10 to 15 percent lifetime risk of sensorineural hearing loss, but these infants do not have permanent damage to other tissues or organs. Approximately 10 percent of the infected newborns have systemic abnormalities (Table 4-1) that consist of jaundice, hepatomegaly, splenomegaly, petechial or purpuric rash, intrauterine growth retardation, or respiratory distress.[17,62] Neurologic features of intrauterine CMV infection include microcephaly, chorioretinitis, seizures, sensorineural hearing loss, and hypo- or hypertonia. Approximately 5 percent of infants with congenital CMV disease die in the perinatal period.

Perinatal CMV infections can occur via transfusion of CMV-seropositive blood or ingestion of CMV-infected breast milk. These infections pose little or no risk to healthy full-term infants. However, disseminated infections with hepatitis, gastroenteritis, pneumonia, thrombocytopenia, and anemia can develop in premature in-

▶ **TABLE 4-1.** NEONATAL CLINICAL FEATURES IN INFANTS WITH INTRAUTERINE CYTOMEGALOVIRUS OR RUBELLA VIRUS INFECTIONS

Feature	Approximate Prevalence	
	CMV*	Rubella†
Petechiae	50%	35%
Microcephaly	50%	25%
Hydrocephalus	5%	—
Intrauterine growth retardation	50%	60%
Hepatomegaly	45%	35%
Splenomegaly	45%	35%
Jaundice at birth	40%	15%
Sensorineural hearing loss	40%	60%
Abnormal tone	25%	ND
Chorioretinitis	10%	10%
Seizures	10%	ND
Death	5%	ND
Pneumonitis	5%	ND
Congenital heart disease	—	70%

*Modified from data of the National Congenital Cytomegalovirus Disease Registry.[112]
†Modified from data of Schlutter et al.[54]
ND = no data.

fants. Occasionally, disseminated perinatal CMV infections can be fatal in small premature infants.[60]

Nonpolio Enteroviruses

Neonates infected perinatally with the nonpolio EVs usually become symptomatic during the first 2 weeks of life.[63] The early features of EV disease consist of fever, poor feeding, jaundice, irritability, and lethargy and mimic those of bacterial and HSV infections. Neonatal illnesses with nonpolio EVs are often mild, but infected infants can have severe, invasive disease with encephalitis, hepatitis, myocarditis, and disseminated intravascular coagulopathy (DIC).[63] Disseminated neonatal EV disease, especially that due to echovirus 11, occasionally can be fatal.[64]

Infrequently, infants exhibit signs at birth compatible with the intrauterine transmission of nonpolio EVs. The clinical manifestations of congenital EV infections include papulovesicular, bullous, or exanthematous skin lesions, as well as hepatitis, hepatic calcifications, myocarditis, and meningoencephalitis.[65,66] The latter manifestations are comparable with those seen in perinatally acquired infections. In one reported case, the skin lesions mimicked those of the congenital varicella syndrome.[65]

A single case report indicates that enterovirus 71 (EV71), a particularly neurovirulent EV strain, can cause congenital infection.[67] Ultrasonography at 25 weeks identified hepatosplenomegaly, hepatic calcifications, ascites, and mild ventricular enlargement in an infant whose mother had a confirmed EV71 infection at 17 weeks' gestation. Postmortem examination of the stillborn infant at 26 weeks revealed marked hepatosplenomegaly, fibrotic peritonitis, and meconium staining. EV71 antigens were detected by immunohistochemistry in the infant's liver and midbrain.

Herpes Simplex Viruses Type 1 and Type 2

Neonatal HSV infections historically have been divided into three clinical syndromes: (1) mucocutaneous (skin-eye-mouth) infection, (2) disseminated disease, and (3) encephalitis.[7,34] Infants with mucocutaneous or disseminated infections usually become symptomatic at approximately 10 days of age, whereas infants with encephalitis usually become symptomatic on average at 17 days of age.[7] However, any form of perinatal HSV disease can be seen as early as the first day of life.[7,68]

Infants with mucocutaneous infections have conjunctivitis, keratitis, or a vesicular rash. The early symptoms of disseminated HSV infection or neonatal HSV encephalitis consist of poor feeding, irritability, lethargy, or high-pitched cry. These nonspecific features also can be seen in infants with benign EV infections or invasive bacterial disease. Systemic signs suggesting HSV infection include fever, jaundice, tachypnea, petechiae, and vesicular rash, although the absence of rash or fever does not eliminate HSV from consideration.[69] Neurologic manifestations, such as seizures (partial or generalized), hypotonia, hypertonia, and coma, can be early or late manifestations of neonatal HSV encephalitis. HSV-infected infants also can have hepatitis, pneumonitis, adrenalitis, or DIC.[70]

Approximately 5 percent of HSV-infected neonates acquire HSV *in utero*.[59,71,72] These infants, usually infected with HSV-2, have skin lesions at birth, ocular abnormalities (e.g., chorioretinitis, cataracts, and/or microphthalmia), and microcephaly or hydranencephaly. Infants with congenital HSV disease closely resemble neonates with other intrauterine infections, especially the fetal varicella syndrome.[73] Such infants almost always have parenchymal brain abnormalities, typically cystic encephalomalacia, and dense intracranial calcifications involving the thalamus and basal ganglia.

Lymphocytic Choriomeningitis Virus

The clinical features of congenital LCM virus infection mimic those of intrauterine CMV disease and congenital toxoplasmosis.[53,74] Among 26 reported cases reviewed by Wright and colleagues in 1997, 88 percent had chorioretinopathy, 43 percent had macrocephaly at birth, and 13 percent were microcephalic.[53] Virtually all infants were born at term and had normal birth weights. Occasional infants have vesicular or bullous skin lesions, but other signs of disseminated infection, such as hepatosplenomegaly or jaundice, are absent. Given that there have been no prospective studies of congenital LCM virus infection, the spectrum of disease associated with this virus has not been determined. A recent review by Barton indicated that 10 to 15 percent of infants with intrauterine LCM virus infections also have hearing loss, illustrating further the similarities with congenital CMV infection.[74] Approximately one-half the mothers who give birth to infants with congenital LCM virus infection have influenza-like illnesses during pregnancy, and one-fourth recall contact with mice.[53]

Rubella Virus

In 1941, Gregg linked maternal rubella virus infection to cataracts, hearing loss, and heart disease in young infants.[3] Later reports, especially those describing infants born during the rubella pandemic of the early 1960s, described additional features associated with maternal rubella virus infections.[56,75,76] Neonates with CRS have a spectrum of abnormalities that includes cataracts, retinopathy, microphthalmia, microcephaly, and sensorineural hearing loss, as well as meningoencephalitis, osteopathy, pneumonitis, hepatitis, hepatosplenomegaly, thrombocytopenia, and jaundice (see Table 4-1). The propensity of the rubella virus to infect the developing heart causes myocarditis, patent ductus arteriosus, valvular stenosis, and septal defects at the atrial or ventricular level.[56]

Varicella-Zoster Virus

Chickenpox in healthy young children typically causes a mild illness with fever, malaise, and rash that evolves from maculopapular to vesicular lesions. By contrast, neonates can experience severe, disseminated varicella with pneumonitis, hepatitis, and DIC.[40,41] The risk of varicella infection is highest in infants whose mothers have the onset of chickenpox from 5 days before until 2 days after delivery. Neonatal fatalities can occur as a result of perinatal vertical transmission, particularly among premature infants. Term infants exposed to VZV after birth usually have a relatively benign illness.

Infants with varicella embryopathy, a rare disorder with approximately 100 reported cases, have skin lesions, chorioretinitis, microphthalmia, cataracts, paralysis, microcephaly, hydrocephalus, congenital Horner's syndrome, and limb hypoplasia.[41,43,73] The cicatrix, a feature of congenital varicella infection affecting approximately 75 percent of reported infants, consists of skin scarring and new skin formation that conforms to a dermatomal distribution. Neurologic and ophthalmologic abnormalities are present in approximately 50 percent of infants with varicella embryopathy.

▶ DIAGNOSIS

Arboviruses

Arbovirus infections generally are diagnosed by detecting agent-specific serologic responses in infants and their mothers. Identifying arbovirus-specific IgM in neonatal serum confirms infection and strongly implicates the agent as the cause of the fetal or neonatal disease. Reverse transcription (RT)–PCR can detect these viruses, but the sensitivity of RT-PCR in diagnosing congenital or perinatal arbovirus infection is unknown.

Cerebrospinal fluid (CSF) analysis in infants with intrauterine or perinatal arbovirus infections usually reveals a lymphocytic or mixed pleocytosis, elevated protein concentration, and a normal glucose concentration. Cranial computed tomography (CT) or magnetic resonance imaging (MRI) of infants with meningoencephalitis will be normal or reveal meningeal enhancement. Infants with intrauterine arbovirus infections can have imaging abnormalities consisting of cystic encephalomalacia, hydrocephalus, or hydranencephaly.[14,61]

Cytomegalovirus

The diagnosis of intrauterine CMV infection is made by detecting the virus in urine or saliva samples collected during the first 3 weeks of life.[17] Although PCR allows rapid detection of CMV DNA,[77] the shell vial cell culture assay remains the gold standard for diagnosis of intrauterine infection. Detecting CMV-specific IgM in neonatal blood samples supports intrauterine infection. Intrauterine infection also can be established by detecting infectious virus in amniotic fluid or CMV-specific IgM in fetal blood,[78] but detection of CMV prenatally does not distinguish symptomatic from asymptomatic fetal infections. Detecting CMV in urine or saliva samples obtained after 4 weeks of age supports infection, but intrauterine infection cannot be distinguished from infection acquired postnatally via breast feeding, blood transfusion, or horizontal transmission.

Infants with symptomatic intrauterine CMV infections commonly have thrombocytopenia, direct hyperbilirubinemia, and elevated serum transaminases.[62] Hemolytic anemia also can be observed. The CSF can be normal or show a mixed or lymphocytic pleocytosis with an increased protein concentration.[62,79] Cranial CT shows periventricular calcifications (Fig. 4-1) in approximately 50 percent of symptomatic CMV infections. When infection occurs during periods of neuronal cell migration, infants can have lissencephaly, schizencephaly, polymicrogyria, and cortical dysplasia[80] (Fig. 4-2). The latter abnormalities can be confirmed by performing MRI, but MRI can miss small calcifications (Fig. 4-3).

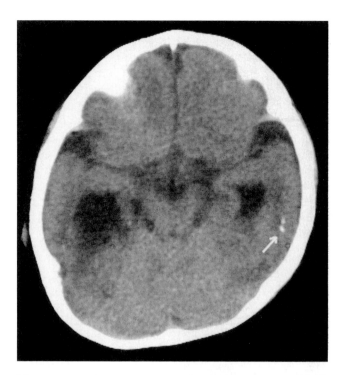

Figure 4-1. Unenhanced head CT scan in an infant with confirmed congenital CMV disease shows punctate calcifications (*arrow*) adjacent a dilated temporal horn of the lateral ventricle.

Nonpolio Enteroviruses

The diagnosis of perinatal EV infections can be confirmed by isolating infectious virus from CSF, tissues, or throat or rectal swabs. The diagnosis of perinatal EV in-

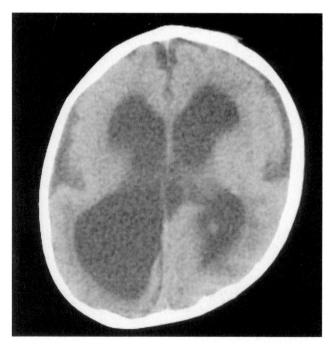

Figure 4-2. Unenhanced head CT scan from the same child shows a lissencephalic-like appearance of the cortical surface.

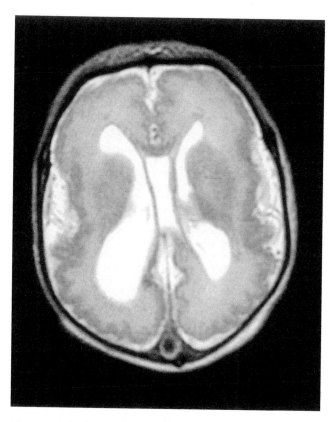

Figure 4-3. T_2-weighted axial MRI from the same child demonstrates more clearly the extensive cortical dysplasia, as well as revealing passive ventriculomegaly and a cavum vergae.

fection can be established rapidly by detecting EV RNA in CSF or stool samples by using RT-PCR.[81]

Infants with neonatal nonpolio EV infections often have thrombocytopenia, elevated serum transaminases, and laboratory evidence of DIC, particularly when infections are severe. The CSF can be normal or show a lymphocytic pleocytosis, elevated protein concentration, and a normal glucose concentration. Imaging studies, whether CT or MRI, are usually normal, but severe infections producing DIC, shock, and cerebral hypoperfusion can be associated with cerebral edema, multifocal ischemia, and cystic encephalomalacia.[82] Cardiomyopathy may be evident by electrocardiogram (ECG) and echocardiography. Calcifications of the liver can be observed as a consequence of intrauterine EV infections.[66]

Herpes Simplex Viruses Type 1 and Type 2

Neonatal HSV infections can be confirmed by isolating HSV-1 or HSV-2 from any of several sites, including the conjunctiva, throat, rectum, circulating leukocytes, CSF, and skin. HSV can be detected in CSF samples by cell culture in approximately 50 percent of infants with HSV encephalitis.[68] HSV-1 and HSV-2 grow rapidly, usually enabling a specific diagnosis within 72 to 96 hours. The diagnosis of HSV infection can be established rapidly

and specifically by studying CSF or vesicle fluid using PCR,[10] but not all infants with neonatal HSV encephalitis have positive CSF PCR results. Thus negative PCR results must be interpreted cautiously.

HSV-infected infants can have thrombocytopenia, hemolytic anemia, elevated serum transaminases, metabolic acidosis, or CSF abnormalities consisting of a mixed pleocytosis, xanthochromia, modest hypoglycorrachia, and an elevated protein concentration.[68] Chest radiographs may reveal pneumonitis.[70] Because neonatal HSV encephalitis results from hematogenous dissemination of HSV to the brain rather than virus reactivation, neurodiagnostic studies (e.g., electroencephalogram, CT, or MRI) usually reveal diffuse or multifocal abnormalities (Fig. 4-4). Infants who acquire HSV after the neonatal period may have localization of disease to the temporal lobes (Fig. 4-5). Cystic encephalomalacia is a common sequela, given the lytic nature of HSV infection (Fig. 4-6).

Lymphocytic Choriomeningitis Virus

Currently, the diagnosis of intrauterine LCM virus infection is established by serologic studies of the mother and infant.[53,74] Antibodies against LCM virus can be detected in the infant's serum or CSF. Because of the low

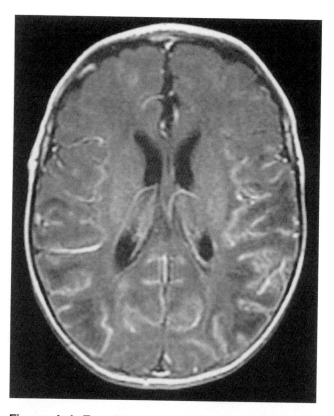

Figure 4-4. T_1-weighted axial MRI with gadolinium shows extensive cortical enhancement and abnormal cortical signal, especially in the temporal-parietal regions, in an infant with perinatal HSV encephalitis.

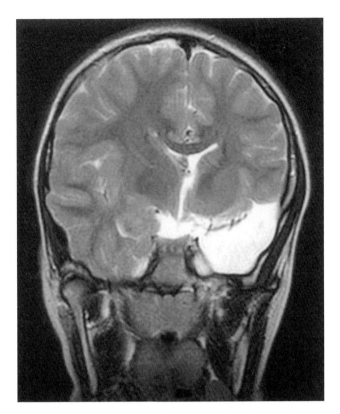

Figure 4-5. T$_2$-weighted coronal MRI shows cystic degeneration of the left temporal lobe and volume loss of the left hemisphere in a young child who recovered from HSV encephalitis.

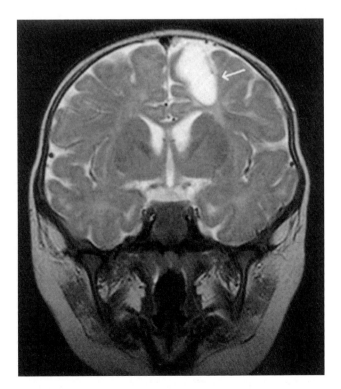

Figure 4-6. T$_2$-weighted coronal MRI shows cystic encephalomalacia (*arrow*) in an infant who survived perinatal HSV encephalitis.

seroprevalence of LCM virus infection in the general population, detection of LCM virus–specific antibodies, particularly LCM virus–specific IgM, strongly supports the diagnosis of congenital infection. The virus can be detected by RT-PCR, but this method does not, as yet, have diagnostic utility in human infections. The CSF can be normal but frequently shows a mixed pleocytosis and an elevated protein concentration. Imaging studies in infants with congenital LCM virus infections show hydrocephalus, intracranial calcifications, and cortical dysplasia.[53]

Varicella-Zoster Virus

Infection can be confirmed by detecting VZV-specific IgM in serum, VZV antigens or infectious virus in skin lesions, or VZV DNA in amniotic fluid, CSF, or skin lesions using PCR.[40,41,83] Persistence of VZV-specific IgG in the infant's serum postnatally supports congenital varicella infection.

Infants with congenital varicella syndrome often have CT or MRI evidence of cystic encephalomalacia and intracranial calcifications.[73,84] Porencephaly and hydranencephaly also can be detected. Examination of the CSF may reveal a lymphocytic pleocytosis and an elevated protein concentration.

Rubella Virus

The diagnosis of CRS can be confirmed by detecting infectious virus in body fluids (e.g., nasal secretions, urine, or CSF) or rubella-virus specific IgM in the infant's serum.[85,86] Postnatal persistence of rubella-specific IgG supports the diagnosis of CRS. Infants with CRS can have thrombocytopenia and elevated serum transaminases. Imaging studies (CT or MRI) reveal periventricular calcifications, subependymal cysts, or periventricular leukomalacia.

▶ DIFFERENTIAL DIAGNOSIS

As the acronym TORCH implies, congenital toxoplasmosis deserves consideration when neonates have clinical, laboratory, or radiographic features suggesting intrauterine viral infection.[6,87] When compared with intrauterine CMV infection, infants with congenital toxoplasmosis usually have hydrocephalus and high rates (~75 percent) of chorioretinitis, whereas CMV-infected infants often have microcephaly and low rates (~10 percent) of chorioretinitis. The intracranial calcifications in infants with congenital toxoplasmosis tend to be diffuse rather than periventricular (Fig. 4-7). Congenital toxoplasmosis closely resembles intrauterine LCM virus infection, and microbiologic studies may be the only effective means to differentiate these disorders.

Intrauterine transmission of *Plasmodium* species produces congenital malaria, a neonatal disorder with

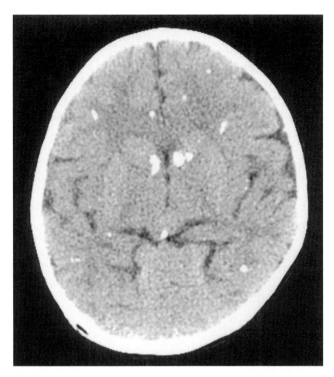

Figure 4-7. Unenhanced head CT shows diffuse parenchymal calcifications in an infant with congenital toxoplasmosis.

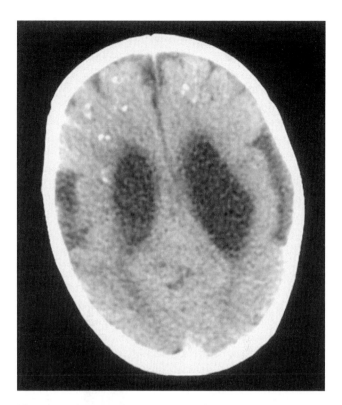

Figure 4-8. Unenhanced head CT scan in an infant with pseudo-TORCH syndrome shows punctate calcifications of the frontal lobes bilaterally and an anomalous cortex.

fever, jaundice, hepatosplenomegaly, thrombocytopenia, and hemolytic anemia.[88] Thus congenital malaria can resemble disseminated HSV, CMV, and EV infections. The diagnosis of neonatal malaria can be suspected on the basis of sociodemographic data (mothers born or living for extended periods in endemic regions), and the disorder can be confirmed by detecting parasites in Wright's- or Giemsa-stained blood smears.

Infants with congenital Chagas' disease, a disorder endemic in Latin America and caused by intrauterine infection with *Trypanosoma cruzi*, have hepatosplenomegaly, petechiae, jaundice, hemolytic anemia, and seizures. Such infants closely resemble those with congenital CMV infection, as well as congenital toxoplasmosis. The diagnosis of congenital Chagas' disease can be established by detecting parasitemia or serologic responses using enzyme-linked immunosorbent assay (ELISA) or indirect hemagglutination.[89]

Certain noninfectious disorders produce clinical features that overlap those of intrauterine viral infections. Aicardi syndrome and Walker-Warburg syndrome, for example, produce brain malformations that initially may suggest intrauterine CMV infection. The rash of incontinentia pigmenti can be mistaken for the "blueberry muffin" rash of CRS, and neonatal Graves' disease produces jaundice and hepatosplenomegaly, features common to many intrauterine viral infections.

The most intriguing of the noninfectious conditions are Aicardi-Goutieres and pseudo-TORCH syndromes,

disorders that appear to be autosomal recessive.[90–92] Infants with either disorder have microcephaly and intracranial calcifications. The calcifications involve the basal ganglia in Aicardi-Goutieres syndrome but tend to be more diffuse in pseudo-TORCH syndrome, thus closely mimicking intrauterine CMV and LCM virus infections, as well as congenital toxoplasmosis[91] (Fig. 4-8).

Infants with Aicardi-Goutieres syndrome often have CSF lymphocytosis and progressive abnormalities of white matter evident by MRI.[90] Approximately one-half the infants with pseudo-TORCH syndrome have jaundice, hyperbilirubinemia, thrombocytopenia, and hepatomegaly, further emphasizing the similarities between this disorder and intrauterine virus infection. Recent data suggest that Aicardi-Goutieres and pseudo-TORCH syndromes may represent allelic disorders.[92]

▶ TREATMENT

Arboviruses

Intrauterine or perinatal arboviral infections do not respond to the currently available antiviral agents.

Cytomegalovirus

The National Institutes of Allergy and Infectious Diseases and the Collaborative Antiviral Study Group

(CASG) conducted a prospective, controlled clinical trial of postnatal ganciclovir therapy in symptomatic newborns with evidence of CNS disease or chorioretinitis.[8,9] Ganciclovir was given at doses of 8 or 12 mg/kg intravenously for 6 weeks. Therapy with ganciclovir transiently reduces viral shedding and has a modest beneficial effect on hearing outcomes. Infants who receive prolonged ganciclovir therapy can have thrombocytopenia (attributable, in part, to CMV infection) and neutropenia. The effect of postnatal ganciclovir therapy on long-term neurologic outcomes of CMV-infected infants is unknown, although one study reported more favorable outcomes in treated infants.[93]

Nonpolio Enteroviruses

Pleconaril, a novel antiviral agent, has activity against several RNA viruses, including members of the EV group.[94,95] Therapeutic trials in human EV infections are ongoing (additional details can be obtained from the CASG, University of Alabama, Birmingham, 205-934-5316). Given the currently available data, pleconaril should be considered for severe, invasive EV infections in neonates.

Infants with perinatal EV infections require meticulous attention to fluid and electrolyte status and should be monitored closely for arrhythmias or congestive heart failure. Seizures require therapy with standard doses of lorazepam, phenobarbital, or phenytoin. Transfusion of platelets, fresh-frozen plasma, and other blood products may be required for DIC. Because the clinical features of severe nonpolio EV infections mimic those of bacterial and perinatal HSV infections, neonates require empirical therapy with broad-spectrum antibiotics and acyclovir until culture and PCR results are known.

Herpes Simplex Viruses Type 1 and Type 2

Infants with suspected HSV infection should receive acyclovir at 60 mg/kg per day intravenously in evenly divided doses every 8 hours.[96] Given that improved outcome of neonatal HSV infections corresponds, in part, to early initiation of acyclovir therapy, parenteral treatment should be started as soon as the diagnosis of neonatal HSV infection is considered. For maximum sensitivity, cultures should be obtained prior to acyclovir treatment, but HSV CSF PCR remains positive for 24 to 48 hours or longer after initiation of acyclovir therapy. Therapy should be continued for a minimum of 14 days in infants with uncomplicated mucocutaneous infections and for a minimum of 21 days in infants with disseminated infections or HSV encephalitis.[96]

Infants who recover from neonatal HSV infections often have mucocutaneous reactivations. Infants who initially have skin-eye-mucous membrane infections only and later experience three or more cutaneous re-

activations have an increased risk of long-term neurodevelopmental sequelae. Neurologic sequelae presumably occur because viremia develops during reactivations, and the virus invades and damages the developing CNS. The CASG is currently investigating the role of suppressive antiviral therapy after treatment of neonatal HSV infections in a placebo-controlled trial using oral acyclovir for 6 months. Information regarding this and other current drug trials for infants with intrauterine or perinatal viral infections can be obtained from the CASG (University of Alabama, Birmingham, 205-934-5316).

Lymphocytic Choriomeningitis Virus

There is currently no specific antiviral therapy for infants with congenital LCM virus infections. However, such infants require supportive care and shunting of progressive hydrocephalus.

Rubella Virus

Because CRS cannot be treated effectively with postnatal antiviral therapy, prevention through vaccination is critical. All children should have rubella virus immunization during early childhood (12 to 15 months of age) and again at school entry (4 to 6 years of age).[85] Serologic screening of women should be performed prior to pregnancy and in pregnant women exposed to rubella. The presence of maternal antibody prior to conception or at the time of exposure to rubella indicates that the fetus is not at risk.

Varicella-Zoster Virus

Therapy with acyclovir should be considered for neonates with chickenpox using 60 mg/kg per day intravenously divided every 8 hours.[97] Therapy should be continued for 7 to 14 days, and renal function and hematologic parameters should be monitored. Hospitalized infants with varicella should be maintained in standard, airborne, and contact isolation. Exposed, asymptomatic infants should be discharged, when possible, or cohorted and maintained in airborne and contact isolation for 21 days if they did not receive varicella-zoster immune globulin (VZIG) or for 28 days if they received VZIG because VZIG may delay the presentation of VZV in the neonate.[45] Infants with the congenital varicella syndrome do not require acyclovir therapy or isolation.[73]

► COMPLICATIONS

Cytomegalovirus

Infants who survive symptomatic congenital CMV infections have a substantial risk (~90 percent) of having disabling sequelae affecting vision, hearing, cognition, and motor abilities.[98] The spectrum ranges from children with severe cognitive and motor delays to children who have subtle cognitive or behavioral problems. Approximately 20 percent of the infants who survive congenital CMV infections have epilepsy. Infants with intracranial calcifications are more likely to have permanent neurologic sequelae.[99,100] Because infants with congenital CMV infections can experience progressive sensorineural hearing loss, audiograms should be obtained biannually for the first 2 to 3 years of life and annually thereafter into late childhood.

Nonpolio Enteroviruses

Severe infections, especially with echovirus 11, can cause death from DIC, cardiomyopathy, hemorrhage, and hepatic failure.[64] Most infants who survive perinatal EV infections have no permanent neurodevelopmental, visual, or hearing abnormalities.[101]

Herpes Simplex Viruses Type 1 and Type 2

The prognosis of neonatal HSV infection depends on the severity of the organ involvement and the response to acyclovir therapy. Infants who are detected early and treated aggressively with acyclovir generally fare better. Adverse neurologic sequelae occur rarely in infants with disease restricted to the skin, eyes, and mucous membranes; approximately 5 percent of such infants have neurodevelopmental sequelae.[102] By contrast, infants with encephalitis or disseminated disease have high rates of mortality and morbidity even with appropriate antiviral therapy.[102] Approximately 10 percent of infants with invasive HSV infections die despite acyclovir therapy, and as many as 50 percent have permanent neurologic deficits. Sequelae include epilepsy, developmental delay, vision loss, cerebral palsy, and recurrent cutaneous reactivation of HSV. With few exceptions, infants with congenital HSV infection have poor prognoses.[71,73]

Lymphocytic Choriomeningitis Virus

Approximately 35 percent of infants reported to date have died from complications of congenital LCM virus infection.[53] Most surviving infants have neurodevelopmental sequelae, consisting of cerebral palsy, epilepsy, vision loss, and mental retardation. Due to aqueductal obstruction from the intense inflammatory reaction in CSF pathways, congenitally infected infants can have progressive hydrocephalus and require shunt placement.

Rubella Virus

Neurologic sequelae of CRS include microcephaly, hearing loss, language delay, autism, and developmental or mental retardation.[103–105] Progressive sensorineural hearing loss can develop in survivors of CRS, indicating the need for serial audiometry. Cardiac lesions may require surgical correction. Survivors of CRS have increased risks of diabetes mellitus, thyroid disorders, and if women, early menopause, complications that usually appear in the third or fourth decades of life.[105] Postrubella panencephalitis, a progressive neurodegenerative disorder associated with seizures, ataxia, and dementia, is a rare potential complication of CRS.[106]

Varicella-Zoster Virus

Approximately 30 percent of infants with congenital VZV infection die within the first few months of life.[107] Infants who survive varicella embryopathy have visual, motor, cognitive, or orthopedic sequelae.[84,107]

► PREVENTION

Arboviruses

Infection with the JE virus can be prevented by vaccination, and the CDC recommends immunization of travelers to endemic regions.[108] On theoretical grounds, minimizing maternal contact with mosquitoes can reduce the risk of intrauterine or perinatal WEE virus, VE virus, and WNV infections. Pregnant women should avoid wetland areas and limit outdoor activities when mosquitoes are active. Protective clothing, headnets, and repellants containing N,N-diethyl-m-toluamide (DEET) can lessen the risk of mosquito contact.

Cytomegalovirus

Congenital CMV infection currently cannot be prevented by vaccination, but trials of whole-virus and subunit vaccines are ongoing.[109] Seronegative women have the greatest risk of acquiring CMV and delivering CMV-infected infants. Hygienic measures may diminish the risk of maternal infection,[110] although the ability of these strategies to prevent fetal infection has not been studied rigorously.

While pregnant, women should avoid contact with the secretions or excretions of young children, including their own, who may be infected silently with CMV. Women who are pregnant or anticipating pregnancy within 6 months should wash their hands well after contact with the urine or saliva of children and should refrain from kissing or sharing food or eating utensils with young children. Women who work in child care centers or have toddler-aged children attending group child care centers have increased risks of becoming infected with CMV.[21–23] CMV infection is also more likely in women with multiple sexual partners.

Hospitalized CMV-infected infants require excretion-secretion precautions to prevent inadvertent trans-

▶ **TABLE 4-2.** STRATEGIES FOR THE PREVENTION AND TREATMENT OF INTRAUTERINE AND PERINATAL INFECTIONS

Infectious Disorder	Preventive Measures	Treatment
Arboviruses	Avoid contact with mosquitoes during pregnancy	None
Cytomegalovirus	Avoid contact with young children during pregnancy; practicing monogamy	Ganciclovir*
Enteroviruses	Good handwashing	None/Pleconaril†
Herpes simplex virus	None established	Acyclovir‡
Lymphocytic choriomeningitis virus	Avoiding contact with mice and hamsters during pregnancy	None
Rubella	Immunization in childhood	None
Varicella-zoster virus	Avoiding contact with persons with chickenpox	None
	Immunization§	Acyclovir¶

*Experimental; see text.
†Considered experimental for invasive neonatal enteroviral disease; see text for details.
‡Acyclovir therapy will diminish viral shedding but will not affect neurologic outcome in congenitally infected infants. However, acyclovir is mandatory therapy for infants with neonatal HSV infections.
§Presumptive benefit of childhood immunization.
¶Acyclovir therapy is required for infants with perinatal chickenpox.

mission to seronegative pregnant women. However, many infants and young children excrete CMV asymptomatically, indicating that medical personnel should practice standard precautions during contact with all young children. The risk of CMV infection among health care workers does not exceed that of the general population.[111]

Nonpolio Enteroviruses

Neonatal EV infections cannot be prevented by vaccination. Horizontally transmitted neonatal EV infections can be prevented, in theory, by discouraging postnatal contact between young infants and persons with viral syndromes, especially during the summer months. Often infection cannot be prevented because infection occurs vertically during the week prior to delivery or horizontally after contact with asymptomatic children or adults. Hospital personnel must practice meticulous hygiene to prevent outbreaks among hospitalized newborns and others.

Herpes Simplex Viruses Type 1 and Type 2

In neonatal HSV infections, 20 to 30 percent of mothers report genital HSV during pregnancy.[102] However, most women (>80 percent) who have infants with HSV infection lack evidence of cervical HSV during labor and delivery. Neonates also can acquire HSV infection after cesarean section in women with genital herpes and intact amniotic membranes. These epidemiologic characteristics indicate that neonatal HSV infections will remain difficult to prevent by obstetrical management.

HSV infections currently cannot be prevented by vaccination.

Lymphocytic Choriomeningitis Virus

No vaccine exists to prevent infection with LCM virus, but pregnant women can reduce their risk of LCM virus infection by avoiding mice and pet hamsters during their pregnancies.

Rubella Virus

The Committee on Infectious Diseases of the American Academy of Pediatrics (AAP) recommends that serologic studies be repeated in 2 to 3 weeks in women who are exposed to rubella and initially seronegative. Serologic studies should be obtained again 6 weeks after exposure if the second sample also was negative.[85] Seroconversion indicates infection and potential risk to the fetus, whereas persistently seronegative samples indicate that maternal infection did not occur. Termination of pregnancy is a consideration for women who have confirmed primary infections early in gestation. When termination is not an option, immune globulin can be considered, although the efficacy of this approach is unproven.

The management of an infant with suspected CRS should include (1) an ophthalmologic examination for cataracts or pigmentary retinopathy, (2) audiometry to detect sensorineural hearing loss, and (3) a cardiac evaluation. Infants with suspected rubella require standard and droplet isolation (i.e., private room; masks, gowns, and gloves for persons having patient contact). Infants with confirmed infections should be considered contagious for at least 12 months, unless nasopharyngeal and urine cultures are negative on serial samples obtained after 3 months of age.[85] Nonimmune pregnant women must not have contact with infants with CRS.

Varicella-Zoster Virus

The Committee on Infectious Diseases of the AAP recommends that VZIG (125 units) be given as soon as possible to neonates, term or preterm, whose mothers experience chickenpox during the 5 days before or 2 days after delivery.[45] Varicella can develop despite VZIG, although the illness is usually mild. Term infants exposed outside this interval do not require VZIG, and VZIG is not indicated if the mother has zoster.

VZIG should be administered after postnatal VZV exposure to hospitalized preterm infants born before 28 weeks' gestation and/or weighing 1000 g or less at birth regardless of the maternal history or VZV serologic status.[45] VZIG should be administered to exposed hospitalized premature infants of 28 weeks' or more gestation whose mothers have negative varicella histories or serologies. Screening for VZV antibodies using the whole-cell enzyme immunofluorescence antibody assay can determine the risk status of exposed infants.

Varicella vaccine, licensed for use in the United States since 1995, may prevent congenital or perinatal varicella. Varicella vaccination is recommended for all children between 12 and 15 months of age who have not had varicella. Cell-mediated and humoral immunity develop in more than 95 percent of immunized young children; approximately 5 percent of vaccinees have mild VZV after vaccination. In contrast to the potentially damaging effects of primary VZV infection in pregnant women, reactivated VZV infections (i.e., zoster) appear to pose no risk to the developing fetus.[41]

REFERENCES

1. Southard EE: Acute encephalitis and brain abscess. In Osler W (ed): *Modern Medicine*. Philadelphia: Lea and Feibiger, 1910, p 638.
2. Ribbert H: Veber protozoenartige Zellen in der Niere eines syphilitischen Negeborenen und in der Parotis von Kindern. *Zentralbl Allg Pathol* 15:945, 1904.
3. Gregg NM: Congenital cataract following German measles in the mother. *Trans Ophthalmol Soc Aust* 3:35, 1941.
4. Gard S: *http://www.nobel.se/medicine/laureates/1954/press.html.*
5. Weller TH, Macauley JC, Craig JM, et al: Isolation of intranuclear inclusion producing agents from infants with illnesses resembling cytomegalic inclusion disease. *Proc Soc Exp Biol Med* 94:4, 1957.
6. Nahmias AJ: The TORCH complex. *Hosp Pract* May:65, 1974.
7. Kimberlin DW, Lin CY, Jacobs RF, et al: Natural history of neonatal herpes simplex virus infections in the acyclovir era. *Pediatrics* 108:223, 2001.
8. Whitley RJ, Cloud G, Gruber W, et al: Ganciclovir treatment of symptomatic congenital cytomegalovirus infection: Results of a phase II study. *J Infect Dis* 175:1080, 1996.
9. Kimberlin DW, Lin CY, Sanchez P, et al: Ganciclovir (GCV) treatment of symptomatic congenital cytomegalovirus (CMV) infection: results of a phase III randomized trial. Presented at the 40th Interscience Conference on Antimicrobial Agents and Chemotherapy, Toronto, Canada, September 2000 (abstract no 1942).
10. Kimberlin DW, Lakeman, Arvin AM, et al: Application of the polymerase chain reaction to the diagnosis and management of neonatal herpes simplex virus disease. *J Infect Dis* 174:1162, 1996.
11. Reef SE, Plotkin S, Cordero JF, et al: Preparing for elimination of congenital rubella syndrome (CRS): Summary of a workshop on CRS elimination in the United States. *Clin Infect Dis* 31:85, 2000.
12. Bale JF Jr: Virus encephalitis. In Joynt RJ, Griggs RE (eds): *Baker's Clinical Neurology*. 2004, Philadelphia: Lippincott-Raven.
13. Charuvedi UC, Mathur A, Chandra SK, et al: Transplacental infection with Japanese encephalitis virus. *J Infect Dis* 141:712, 1980.
14. Nguyen Q, Morrow C, Novick L, et al: Intrauterine West Nile Virus Infection—New York, 2002. *MMWR* 51:1135, 2002.
15. Shinefield HR, Townsend TE: Transplacental transmission of western equine encephalomyelitis. *J Pediatr* 43:21, 1953.
16. CDC. Provisional surveillance summary of the West Nile virus epidemic—United States, November 2002. *MMWR* 51:1129, 2002.
17. Demmler GJ:. Summary of a workshop on surveillance of congenital cytomegalovirus disease. *Rev Infect Dis* 13:315, 1991.
18. Britt WJ, Alford CA: Cytomegalovirus. In Fields BN, Knipe DM, Howley JM (eds): *Fields Virology*, 3d ed. Philadelphia: Lippincott-Raven, 1996, pp 2493–2523.
19. Pass RF, August AM, Dworsky M, et al: Cytomegalovirus infection in a day care center. *New Engl J Med* 307:477, 1982.
20. Murph JR, Bale JF, Murray JC, et al: Cytomegalovirus transmission in a Midwest day care center: Possible relationship to child care practices. *J Pediatr* 109:35, 1986.
21. Pass RF, Hutto C, Ricks R, et al: Increased rate of cytomegalovirus infection among parents of children attending day care centers. *New Engl J Med* 314:366, 1986.
22. Adler SP: Cytomegalovirus and child day care: Evidence for an increased infection rate among day care workers. *New Engl J Med* 321:1290, 1989.
23. Murph JR, Baron JC, Brown CK, et al: The occupational risk of cytomegalovirus among day care providers. *JAMA* 265:603, 1991.
24. Bale JF Jr, Petheram SJ, Souza IE, et al: Cy-

tomegalovirus reinfection in children. *J Pediatr* 128:347, 1996.

25. Noyola DE, Demmler GJ, Williamson WD, et al: Cytomegalovirus urinary excretion and long term outcome in children with congenital cytomegalovirus infection. *Pediatr Infect Dis J* 19:505, 2000.

26. Hamprecht K, Mashmann J, Vochem M, et al: Epidemiology of cytomegalovirus from mother to preterm infant by breastfeeding. *Lancet* 357:513, 2001.

27. Fowler KB, Stagno S, Pass RF, et al: The outcome of congenital cytomegalovirus infection in relation to maternal antibody status. *New Engl J Med* 326:664, 1992.

28. Stagno S, Pass RF, Cloud G, et al: Primary cytomegalovirus infection in pregnancy: Incidence, transmission to fetus, and clinical outcome. *JAMA* 256:1904, 1986.

29. Boppana SB, Rivera LB, Fowler KB, et al: Intrauterine transmission of cytomegalovirus to infants of mothers with preconceptional immunity. *New Engl J Med* 344:1366, 2001.

30. Modlin JF: Update on enterovirus infection in infants and children. *Adv Pediatr Infect Dis* 12:155, 1996.

31. Sawyer MH: Enterovirus infections: Diagnosis and treatment. *Curr Opin Pediatr* 13:65, 2001.

32. Jensita JA, Powell KR, Menegus MA: Epidemiology of neonatal enterovirus infection. *J Pediatr* 104:685, 1984.

33. Kaplan MH, Klein SW, McPhee J, et al: Group B coxsackievirus infections in infants younger than three months: A serious childhood illness. *Rev Infect Dis* 5:1019, 1983.

34. Jacobs RF: Neonatal herpes simplex virus infections. *Semin Perinatol* 24:64, 1998.

35. Corey L, Spear PG: Infections with herpes simplex viruses. *New Engl J Med* 314:686, 749, 1986.

36. Buchacz K, McFarland W, Hernandez M, et al: Prevalence and correlates of herpes simplex virus type 2 infection in a population-based survey of young women in low-income neighborhoods of northern California. The Young Women's Survey Team. *Sex Transm Dis* 27:393, 2000.

37. Patrick DM, Dawar M, Cook DA, et al: Antenatal seroprevalence of herpes simplex virus type 2 (HSV-2) in Canadian women: HSV-2 prevalence increases throughout the reproductive years. *Sex Transm Dis* 28:424, 2001.

38. Sucato G, Celum C, Dithmer D, et al: Demographic rather than behavioral risk factors predict herpes simplex virus type 2 infection in sexually active adolescents. *Pediatr Infect Dis J* 20:422, 2001.

39. Brown ZA, Selke S, Zeh J, et al: The acquisition of herpes simplex virus during pregnancy. *New Engl J Med* 337:509, 1997.

40. Arvin A: Varicella-zoster virus. *Clin Microbiol Rev* 9:361, 1996.

41. Brunell P: Varicella in pregnancy, the fetus, and the newborn: Problems in management. *J Infect Dis* 166:42, 1992.

42. Paryani SG, Arvin AM: Intrauterine infection with varicella-zoster virus after maternal varicella. *New Engl J Med* 14:1542, 1986.

43. Pastuszak A, Levy M, Schick B, et al: Outcome after maternal varicella infection in the first 20 weeks of pregnancy. *New Engl J Med* 330:901, 1994.

44. Jones KL, Johnson KA, Chambers CA: Offspring of women infected with varicella during pregnancy: A prospective study. *Teratology* 49:29, 1994.

45. American Academy of Pediatrics: Varicella zoster virus. In Pickering LK (ed): *2000 Red Book: Report of the Committee on Infectious Diseases,* 25th ed . Elk Grove Village, IL: American Academy of Pediatrics, 2000, pp. 630–631.

46. Lehmann-Grube F: Portrait of viruses: Arenaviruses. *Intervirology* 22:121, 1984.

47. Deibel R, Woodall JP, Becher WJ, et al: Lymphocytic choriomeningitis virus in man: Serologic evidence of association with pet hamsters. *JAMA* 232:501, 1975.

48. Dykewicz CA, Dato VM, Fisher-Hoch SP, et al: Lymphocytic choriomeningitis outbreak associated with nude mice in a research institute. *JAMA* 267:1349, 1992.

49. Childs JE, Glass GE, Ksiazek TG, et al: Human-rodent contact and infection with lymphocytic choriomeningitis and Seoul viruses in an inner-city population. *Am J Trop Med Hyg* 44:117, 1991.

50. Park JY, Peters CJ, Rollin PE, et al: Age distribution of lymphocytic choriomeningitis virus serum antibody in Birmingham, Alabama: Evidence of a decreased risk of infection. *Am J Trop Med Hyg* 57:37, 1997.

51. Ambrosio AM, Feuillade MR, Gamboa GS, et al: Prevalence of lymphocytic choriomeningitis virus infection in a human population in Argentina. *Am J Trop Med Hyg* 50:381, 1994.

52. Marie TJ, Saron MF: Seroprevalence of lymphocytic choriomeningitis virus in Nova Scotia. *Am J Trop Med Hyg* 58:47, 1998.

53. Wright R, Johnson D, Neumann M, et al: Congenital lymphocytic choriomeningitis virus syndrome: A disease that mimics congenital toxoplasmosis or cytomegalovirus infection. *Pediatrics* 100:9, 1997.

54. Schluter WW, Reer SE, Redd SC, et al: Changing epidemiology of congenital rubella syndrome in the United States. *J Infect Dis* 178:636, 1998.

55. Cochi Sl, Edmonds LE, Dyer K, et al: Congenital rubella syndrome in the United States, 1970–1985. *Am J Epidemiol* 129:349, 1989.

56. Ueda K, Nishida Y, Oshmia K, et al: Congenital rubella syndrome: Correlation of gestational age at time of maternal rubella with type of defect. *J Pediatr* 94:763, 1979.

57. Iannetti P, Nigro G, Spalice A, et al: Cytomegalovirus infection and schizencephaly: Case reports. *Ann Neurol* 43:123, 1998.

58. Hayward JC, Titelbaum DS, Clancy RC, et al: Lissencephaly-pachygyria associated with congenital cytomegalovirus infection. *J Child Neurol* 6:109, 1991.

59. Baldwin S, Whitley RJ: Intrauterine herpes simplex virus infections. *Teratology* 39:1, 1989.

60. Maschmann J, Hamprecht K, Dietz K, et al: Cytomegalovirus infection of extremely low-birth weight infants via breast milk. *Clin Infect Dis* 33:1998, 2001.

61. Wenger F: Venezuelan equine encephalitis. *Teratology* 16:358, 1977.
62. Boppana SB, Pass RF, Britt WJ, et al: Symptomatic congenital cytomegalovirus infection: neonatal morbidity and mortality. *Pediatr Infect Dis J* 11:93, 1992.
63. Lake AM, Lauer BA, Clark JC, et al: Enterovirus infections in neonates. *J Pediatr* 89:787, 1976.
64. Modlin JF: Fatal echovirus 11 disease in premature infants. *Pediatrics* 66:775, 1980.
65. Sauerbrei A, Gluck G, Jung K, et al: Congenital skin lesions caused by intrauterine infection with coxsackievirus B3. *Infection* 28:326, 2000.
66. Konen O, Rathaus V, Bauer S, et al: Progressive liver calcifications in neonatal coxsackievirus infection. *Pediatr Radiol* 30:343, 2000.
67. Chow KC, Lee CC, Lin TY, et al: Congenital enterovirus 71 infection: A case study with virology and immunohistochemistry. *Clin Infect Dis* 31:509, 2000.
68. Koskiniemi M, Happonen JM, Jarvenpaa AL, et al: Neonatal herpes simplex virus infection: A report of 43 patients. *Pediatr Infect Dis J* 8:30, 1989.
69. Arvin Am, Yeager AS, Bruhn FW, et al: Neonatal herpes simplex virus infection in the absence of mucocutaneous lesions. *J Pediatr* 100:715, 1982.
70. Anderson RD: Herpes simplex virus infection of the neonatal respiratory system. *Am J Dis Child* 141:274, 1987.
71. Hutto C, Arvin A, Jacobs R, et al: Intrauterine herpes simplex virus infections. *J Pediatr* 110:97, 1987.
72. Hoppen T, Eis-Hubinger AM, Schild RL, et al: Intrauterine herpes simplex virus infection. *Klin Padiatr* 213:63, 2001.
73. Grose C: Congenital infections caused by varicella-zoster virus and herpes simplex virus. *Semin Pediatr Neurol* 1:43, 1994.
74. Barton LL, Mets MB: Congenital lymphocytic choriomeningitis virus infection: Decade of rediscovery. *Clin Infect Dis* 33:370, 2001.
75. Dudgeon J: Congenital rubella. *J Pediatr* 87:1078, 1975.
76. Givens KT, Lee DA, Jones T, et al: Congenital rubella syndrome: Ophthalmic manifestations and associated systemic disorders. *Br J Ophthalmol* 77:358, 1993.
77. Demmler G, Buffone G, Schimbor C, et al: Detection of cytomegalovirus in urine from newborns by using polymerase chain reaction DNA amplification. *J Infect Dis* 58:1177, 1988.
78. Lazzarotto T, Varani S, Gabrielli L, et al: New Advances in the diagnosis of congenital cytomegalovirus infection. *Intervirology* 42:390, 1999.
79. Bale JF, Bell WE, Bray PF: The spectrum of neuroradiographic abnormalities in symptomatic congenital cytomegalovirus infection. *Pediatr Neurol* 1:42, 1985.
80. Barkovich A, Lindan C: Congenital cytomegalovirus infection of the brain: Imaging analysis and embryologic considerations. *Am J Neuroradiol* 15:703, 1994.
81. Schlesinger Y, Sawyer MH, Storch GA: Enteroviral meningitis in infancy: Potential role for polymerase chain reaction in patient management. *Pediatrics* 94:157, 1994.
82. Haddad J, Messer J, Gut JP, et al: Neonatal echovirus encephalitis with white matter necrosis. *Neuropediatrics* 21:215, 1990.
83. Isada NB, Paar DP, Johnson MP, et al: In utero diagnosis of congenital varicella-zoster virus infection by chorionic villus sampling and polymerase chain reaction. *Am J Obstet Gynecol* 165:1727, 1991.
84. Alkalay AL, Pomerance JJ, Rimoin DL: Fetal varicella syndrome. *J Pediatr* 111:320, 1987.
85. American Academy of Pediatrics: Rubella. In Pickering LK (ed): *2000 Red Book: Report of the Committee on Infectious Diseases,* 25th ed. Elk Grove Village, IL: American Academy of Pediatrics, 2000, p 497.
86. Souza I, Bale JF Jr: The diagnosis of congenital infections: Contemporary strategies. *J Child Neurol* 10:271, 1995.
87. Swisher C, Boyer K, McLeod R: Congenital toxoplasmosis. *Semin Pediatr Neurol* 1:4, 1994.
88. Hulbert T: Congenital malaria in the United States: Report of a case and review. *Clin Infect Dis* 14:922, 1992.
89. Bittencourt AL: Congenital Chagas' disease. *Am J Dis Child* 130:97, 1975.
90. Aicardi J, Goutieres F: A progressive familial encephalopathy in infancy with calcifications of the basal ganglia and chronic cerebrospinal fluid lymphocytosis. *Ann Neurol* 15:49, 1984.
91. Vivarelli R, Grosso S, Cioni M, et al: Pseudo-TORCH syndrome or Baraitser-Reardon syndrome: Diagnostic criteria. *Brain Dev* 23:18, 2001.
92. Crow YJ, Black DN, Ali M, et al: Cree encephalitis is allelic with Aicardi-Goutieres syndrome: Implications for the pathogenesis of interferon alpha metabolism. *J Med Genet* 40:183, 2003.
93. Nigro G, Scholz H, Bartmann U: Ganciclovir therapy for symptomatic congenital cytomegalovirus infection in infants: A two-regimen experience. *J Pediatr* 124:318, 1994.
94. Pevear DC, Tull TM, Seipel ME, et al: Activity of pleconaril against enteroviruses. *Antimicrob Agents Chemother* 43:2109, 1999.
95. Schiff GM, Sherwood J: Clinical activity of pleconaril in an experimentally induced coxsackievirus A21 respiratory infection. *J Infect Dis* 181:20, 2000.
96. Whitley RJ: Herpes simplex virus infection. *Semin Pediatr Infect Dis* 13:6, 2002.
97. Whitley RJ: Approaches to the treatment of varicella-zoster virus infections. *Contrib Microbiol* 3:158, 1999.
98. Pass RF, Stagno S, Meyers GJ, et al: Outcome of symptomatic congenital cytomegalovirus infection: Results of long-term, longitudinal follow-up. *Pediatrics* 66:758, 1980.
99. Boppana SB, Fowler KB, Vaid Y, et al: Neuroradiographic findings in the newborn period and long-term outcome in children with symptomatic congenital cytomegalovirus infection. *Pediatrics* 99:409, 1997.
100. Noyola DE, Demmler GJ, Nelson CT, et al: Early predictors of neurodevelopmental outcome in symptomatic congenital cytomegalovirus infection. *J Pediatr* 138:325, 2001.

101. Bergman I, Painter M, Wald E, et al: Outcome in children with enteroviral meningitis during the first year of life. *J Pediatr* 110:705, 1987.

102. Whitley R, Arvin A, Prober C, et al: Predictors of morbidity and mortality in neonates with herpes simplex virus infections. *New Engl J Med* 324:450, 1991.

103. Desmond MM, Fisher ES, Vorderman AL, et al: The longitudinal course of congenital rubella syndrome in nonretarded children. *J Pediatr* 93:584, 1979.

104. Desmond MM, Wilson CW, Vorderman AL: The health and educational status of adolescents with the congenital rubella syndrome. *Dev Med Child Neurol* 27:721, 1985.

105. Forrest JM, Turnbull FM, Sholler GF, et al: Gregg's congenital rubella patients 60 years later. *Med J Aust* 177:664, 2002.

106. Townsend JJ, Baringer JR, Wolinsky JS, et al: Progressive rubella panencephalitis: Late onset after congenital rubella. *New Engl J Med* 292:990, 1975.

107. Sauerbrie A, Wutzler P: The congenital varicella syndrome. *J Periatol* 20:548, 2000.

108. ACIP: Inactivated Japanese encephalitis virus vaccine: Recommendations of the Advisory Committee on Immunization Practices. *MMWR Recomm Rep* 42(RR-1):1, 1993.

109. Plotkin SA: Vaccination against cytomegalovirus. *Arch Virol Suppl* 17:121, 2001.

110. Adler SP, Finney JW, Manganello AM, et al: Prevention of child-to-mother transmission of cytomegalovirus by changing behaviors: A randomized controlled trial. *Pediatr Infect Dis J* 15:240, 1996.

111. Bale J, Murph J: The risk of cytomegalovirus infection in hospital personnel and child care providers: A review. *Pediatr Rev Commun* 4:233, 1991.

112. Istas AS, Demmler GJ, Dobbins JG, Stewart JA: Surveillance for congenital cytomegalovirus disease: A report from the National Congenital Cytomegalovirus Disease Registry. *Clin Infect Dis* 20:665, 1995.

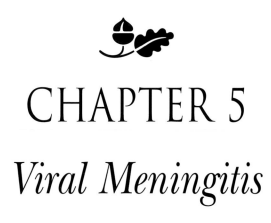

CHAPTER 5
Viral Meningitis

Karen L. Roos

Viral meningitis is a syndrome of fever, headache, photophobia, and stiff neck. The headache is usually frontal or retroorbital and often is associated with pain on moving the eyes. Nausea and vomiting, anorexia, rash, diarrhea, cough, and myalgias may precede or accompany the symptoms of viral meningitis. The neurologic examination is normal except for meningismus. Focal neurologic deficits and seizure activity do not occur in viral meningitis, with the exception of febrile seizures that may complicate viral meningitis in children. The viruses that cause meningitis are the nonpolio enteroviruses [coxsackieviruses A and B, echoviruses (E11, E13, and E30), and the viruses identified by numbers (enteroviruses 68 to 71)], arthropod-borne viruses (arboviruses), herpes simplex virus type 2 (HSV-2), Epstein-Barr virus, human immunodeficiency virus (HIV), and the lymphocytic choriomeningitis virus. Less commonly, varicella-zoster virus, mumps virus, and adenovirus cause meningitis.

▶ EPIDEMIOLOGY

Enteroviruses are the most common cause of viral meningitis. The enteroviruses include the coxsack-ieviruses, echoviruses, polioviruses, and human enteroviruses 68 to 71. Infection with these viruses is acquired primarily by fecal-oral contamination and less commonly by respiratory droplets. The association of a maculopapular erythematous rash beginning on the face and trunk with symptoms of meningitis suggests that the causative organism is either a coxsackievirus or an echovirus. Although enteroviral infections are more common in the summer months, infection occurs year-round.

Arboviral infections are acquired by a mosquito or tick bite. St. Louis encephalitis virus, La Crosse virus, western equine encephalitis virus, Colorado tick fever virus, West Nile virus, and tick-borne encephalitis virus cause a viral meningitis syndrome.[1]

Herpes simplex virus type 2 (HSV-2) may cause a viral meningitis at the time of or shortly after primary genital infection, or it may cause recurrent episodes of meningitis with or without genital herpetic lesions. Meningitis may complicate acute Epstein-Barr virus (EBV) infection. Human immunodeficiency virus type 1 (HIV-1) seeds the meninges and cerebrospinal fluid (CSF) early during the course of infection and may cause an aseptic meningitis syndrome at the time of seroconversion and episodes of acute and chronic meningitis during the course of HIV infection.[2] Cranial nerve palsies are more common in HIV meningitis than in other viral infections. Meningitis due to the lymphocytic choriomeningitis virus occurs in the late fall or winter in individuals who are exposed to house mice or laboratory rodents. The mumps virus was previously a fairly common cause of viral meningitis, but with widespread use of the attenuated Jeryl-Lynn mumps vaccine, mumps meningitis is now rare. Varicella-zoster virus (VSV) meningitis may occur in association with chicken pox or shingles.

▶ PATHOPHYSIOLOGY AND PATHOGENESIS

Enteroviral infections are acquired primarily by fecal-oral contamination. The viral inoculum is swallowed, and the enterovirus binds to specific receptors on enterocytes. The virus then transverses the intestinal lining cells and reaches Peyer's patches in the lamina propria mucosae, where viral replication occurs. This is followed by a viremia, during which the central nervous system (CNS) is seeded.[3] Unlike other viruses that are cleared by cellular immune mechanisms, enteroviruses are cleared from the host by antibody-mediated mechanisms. The usual course of viral meningitis due to an enterovirus is benign in an immunocompetent host, but a protracted course of enteroviral meningitis or encephalitis can occur in persons with hypogammaglobulinemia or agammaglobulinemia.[4]

Arboviral infections are introduced into the host by subcutaneous inoculation by a mosquito or tick, and local replication occurs in tissue and lymph nodes, followed by a viremia and seeding of the CNS. The La Crosse virus is a bunyavirus that is transmitted to the host by the bite of an *Aedes triseriatus* or an *Aedes albopictus* mosquito. These mosquitoes breed in tree holes in the woods and in standing water in discarded automobile tires.[1] The La Crosse virus was first isolated in 1964 from brain tissue from a young girl who died of meningoencephalitis in La Crosse, Wisconsin. West Nile virus is a member of the Japanese encephalitis antigenic complex of the genus *Flavivirus*, and infection is transmitted to humans by the bite of a *Culex* species (*Culex pipiens, C. restuans,* and *C. tarsalis*) mosquito. West Nile virus infection also has been transmitted through blood transfusions and organ transplantation. St. Louis encephalitis is also a flavivirus, and it is transmitted to the host by subcutaneous inoculation of virus by the bite of a *C. tarsalis* or a *C. pipiens* mosquito. Aseptic meningitis accounts for 35 to 60 percent of symptomatic cases of St. Louis encephalitis virus infection in children.[5] The western equine encephalitis, a member of Togaviridae, is transmitted to the host by the bite of a *C. tarsalis* mosquito. Colorado tick fever

virus, an orbivirus, is a less common cause of aseptic meningitis. It is transmitted by the bite of a *Dermacentor andersoni* tick.

HSV-2 may cause a meningitis at the time of or shortly after primary genital infection, and it may cause recurrent episodes of meningitis. HSV establishes latent infection in sensory neurons of sacral dorsal root ganglia and periodically reactivates to cause genital lesions, radiculitis, and meningitis. HSV is the major causative agent of benign recurrent lymphocytic meningitis, historically known as *Mollaret's meningitis*.[6]

Humans acquire the lymphocytic choriomeningitis virus from mice or hamsters through ingestion of food contaminated by animal urine or exposure of open wounds. EBV infections are acquired by contact with oral secretions or by allogeneic bone marrow transplantation. B cells are thought to be the site of persistent EBV within the body. Meningitis may complicate acute EBV infection.[7]

VZV causes the disease chickenpox (varicella). Vesicles develop primarily over the face and trunk. The virus is transported along sensory nerves to the sensory ganglia, where the virus establishes latent infection within neurons. A decline in cell-mediated immunity allows the virus to reactivate, causing shingles (zoster). In addition to shingles and meningitis, VZV also can cause encephalitis and an acute cerebellar ataxia.

▶ CLINICAL FEATURES

The clinical features of viral meningitis are fever (38 to 40°C), headache, photophobia, nuchal rigidity, and chills. There also may be constitutional signs and symptoms of viral infection, including nausea and vomiting, anorexia, rash, diarrhea, cough and upper respiratory symptoms, and myalgias.[8] There may be a mild degree of lethargy or drowsiness, but the presence of more profound alterations in consciousness, such as stupor, coma, or confusion, should prompt consideration of alternative diagnoses. Focal neurologic deficits and seizure activity do not occur in viral meningitis, with the exception of febrile seizures that may complicate viral meningitis in children.

Some unique clinical features are virus-specific. The association of a maculopapular erythematous rash with symptoms of meningitis suggests that the causative organism is an enterovirus. Coxsackievirus and enterovirus 71 can cause vesicular lesions on the hands and feet and in the oropharynx (hand-foot-mouth).[9] Genital vesicular lesions may occur in patients who have symptoms of meningitis due to a primary HSV-2 genital infection. In recurrent meningitis due to HSV-2, genital lesions may not be seen at the time of meningitis. Patients also may complain of lumbosacral dysesthesias and urinary retention. Aseptic meningitis due to VZV may be associated with lesions typical of shingles or may occur without the rash of zoster but with dermatomal distribution pain (zoster sine herpetic).[10]

Infectious mononucleosis is a 4-day to 3-week acute illness consisting of fever, pharyngitis, lymphadenopathy, splenic enlargement (in 50 percent of patients), and fatigue.[11] Symptoms of meningitis may develop at any time in the course of the illness.

Clinical features of infection with lymphocytic choriomeningitis are typical of an influenza-like illness, and symptoms of fever, myalgias, and cough may be accompanied by symptoms of orchitis, parotitis, myopericarditis, arthritis, headache, fever, and stiff neck.[12]

▶ DIAGNOSIS

Examination of the CSF is the most important laboratory test in the diagnosis of viral meningitis. There is typically a lymphocytic pleocytosis, a normal or mildly decreased glucose concentration, and a normal or mildly increased protein concentration. Rarely, polymorphonuclear leukocytes may predominate in the first 48 hours of the illness, especially in patients with infections due to echovirus 9, West Nile virus, eastern equine encephalitis virus, or mumps. Despite these exceptions, the presence of a CSF polymorphonuclear leukocytosis requires empirical therapy for bacterial meningoencephalitis until this can be ruled out. The CSF glucose concentration is typically normal in viral meningitis, although it may be decreased in cases of meningitis due to enteroviruses, HSV-2, VZV, and lymphocytic choriomeningitis virus. As a rule, the presence of a lymphocytic pleocytosis with a decreased glucose concentration should raise consideration of fungal, listerial, tuberculous, or noninfectious disorders, especially carcinomatous meningitis.

Enteroviruses can be grown in culture of CSF, and enteroviral RNA can be detected with the reverse-transcriptase polymerase chain reaction (RT-PCR) assay. Enteroviruses can be isolated from throat and stool cultures. Isolation of an enterovirus from a throat or stool culture in the setting of fever, headache, stiff neck, and CSF lymphocytic pleocytosis is presumptive evidence of enteroviral meningitis; it is not diagnostic. Enteroviruses can be isolated from throat and stool cultures for several weeks after a systemic enteroviral infection has resolved.

According to the Centers for Disease Control and Prevention (CDC), a confirmed case of arboviral meningitis is defined as a febrile illness with mild neurologic symptoms during a period when arboviral transmission is likely to occur plus at least one of the following criteria: (1) a fourfold or greater increase in serum antibody titer between acute and convalescent sera, (2) viral isolation from tissue, blood, or CSF, or (3) specific

immunoglobulin M (IgM) antibody to an arbovirus in the CSF. A presumptive case is defined as a compatible illness plus either a stable increased antibody titer to an arbovirus ($\geq$320 by hemagglutination inhibition, $\geq$128 by complement fixation, $\geq$256 by immunofluorescent assay, or $\geq$160 by plaque reduction neutralization test) or specific IgM antibody in serum by enzyme immunoassay.[13] An arthropod-borne viral infection may be asymptomatic, and many healthy individuals have serum antibodies to arboviruses. A positive serologic test result alone is insufficient to attribute a neurologic illness to an arbovirus. In order to do so, viral nucleic acid must be detected in CSF or viral IgM antibodies by enzyme-linked immunosorbent assay (ELISA), or there must be a fourfold increase in IgG between acute and convalescent sera obtained 4 weeks later, or the virus must be isolated from the brain or spinal cord.

West Nile virus IgM and IgG antibody titers that are positive by ELISA should be confirmed by the more specific plaque-reduction neutralization assay in cell culture. Serum IgM antibodies may persist for 6 to 12 months or longer after an individual has been infected with West Nile virus.[14] The diagnostic test of choice at the present time for West Nile virus CNS infection is CSF IgM antibody. IgM in CSF appears within 7 days of onset of symptoms in 80 percent of patients.[15] The detection of IgM antibodies in CSF may require at least a second lumbar puncture 7 or 8 days after the onset of symptoms.

In patients with acute EBV infection, the heterophil antibody may be positive and/or atypical lymphocytes may be present. In acute infection there is a serologic response to EBV. Acute infection is confirmed by the detection of antiviral capsid antigen (VCA) IgG titers of 1:320 or higher, positive IgM antibody titers to the viral capsid antigen (EBV VCA IgM antibody), and the absence of antibodies to virus-associated nuclear antigen [antibodies to EBV nuclear antigen (anti-EBNA IgG)]. In subsequent serum specimens (collected 36 days after the onset of illness), there should be a fourfold decrease in the IgG antibody titer to the VCA and a 16-fold increase in anti-EBNA IgG.[11,16] IgG antibody titers to the VCA may persist at low titers for life. A combination of IgG VCA antibodies and EBNA antibodies is consistent with past infection or long-term latent infection. EBV DNA can be detected in CSF by PCR assay. EBV DNA is found in peripheral blood mononuclear cells; as such, EBV nucleic acid can be introduced into the CSF if the CSF is contaminated by blood during the lumbar puncture.

A diagnosis of meningitis due to HSV can be made by detecting HSV DNA in CSF. Table 5-1 provides a list of CSF studies for viral meningitis. Table 5-2 provides diagnostic studies that can be done in addition to CSF analysis for viral meningitis.

▶ **TABLE 5-1.** CEREBROSPINAL FLUID ROUTINE STUDIES FOR VIRAL MENINGITIS

Cell count with differential
Glucose and protein concentration
Gram's stain and bacterial culture
India ink and fungal culture
Viral culture
Acid-fast smear and *M. tuberculosis* culture
Cryptococcal polysaccharide antigen
Histoplasma polysaccharide antigen
Complement fixation antibody titers for *C. immitis*
Virus-specific IgM antibodies (HSV, West Nile virus, VZV)
B. burgdorferi antibodies
B. henselae antibodies
VDRL, FTA-ABS
RT-PCR for enteroviruses
PCR for West Nile virus RNA
PCR for HSV-2 DNA
PCR for EBV DNA
PCR for HIV-1 RNA

▶ DIFFERENTIAL DIAGNOSIS

The differential diagnosis of the aseptic meningitis syndrome characterized by headache, fever, stiff neck, fatigue, and anorexia in association with a CSF lymphocytic pleocytosis can be divided into infectious and noninfectious etiologies. The most common infectious etiologies of fever, headache, and a CSF lymphocytic pleocytosis are fungal meningitis, *Mycobacterium tuberculosis* meningitis, and Lyme disease. Fungal meningitis can occur in both immunocompetent and immunosuppressed individuals. Fungal meningitis is usually secondary to infection elsewhere in the body; commonly, there is a primary pulmonary focus of infection. The most common fungal pathogen causing meningitis is *Cryptococcus neoformans.* Cryptococcal

▶ **TABLE 5-2.** DIAGNOSTIC STUDIES IN ADDITION TO CSF FOR VIRAL MENINGITIS

Throat and stool cultures for enteroviruses
Paired acute and convalescent sera for IgG antibodies to
 • Enteroviruses
 • Arthropod-borne viruses
Virus-specific IgM antibodies
Heterophil antibody (EBV)
Antiviral capsid antigen (VCA) titer (EBV acute infection)
EBV VCA IgM antibodies
Anti-Epstein-Barr virus nuclear antigen (EBNA) IgG antibodies
HIV serology
VDRL, FTA-ABS
Genital lesions

meningitis is the most common life-threatening opportunistic fungal infection in patients with the acquired immune deficiency syndrome (AIDS). The use of corticosteroids is also a risk factor for cryptococcal meningitis; specifically, prednisone doses of greater than 10 mg/day increase the risk for cryptococcal meningitis. Patients who are immunosuppressed for stem cell or solid-organ transplantation are also at increased risk for cryptococcal meningitis. *Histoplasma capsulatum* is endemic to the Ohio and Mississippi River valleys of the central United States and to parts of Central and South America. *Coccidioides immitis* is endemic to the desert areas of the southwestern United States, specifically California, Arizona, New Mexico, and Texas, as well as northern Mexico and Argentina. In most instances, this fungus causes a subclinical or limited pulmonary infection. An increased risk for disseminated coccidioidomycosis is associated with pregnancy, certain racial groups (African-American, Hispanic, and Filipino), immunosuppressive therapy, HIV infection, organ transplantation, and hemodialysis.

In addition to *C. neoformans, H. capsulatum* and *C. immitis, Candida albicans, Sporothrix schenckii,* and rare fungi can cause meningitis in immunosuppressed patients from solid-organ or bone marrow transplantation or cancer and cancer chemotherapy. The typical clinical presentation of fungal meningitis is headache and low-grade fever that have developed over 1 to 2 weeks or longer. Cryptococcal meningitis may present with cognitive difficulty, and lower extremity spasticity and difficulty with gait may develop during the course of the illness. The characteristic CSF abnormalities are a mononuclear or lymphocytic pleocytosis, an increased protein concentration, and a decreased glucose concentration. *C. immitis* is unique among the common fungal pathogens in that it may cause a CSF eosinophilia. Microscopy and culture of CSF are often negative in fungal meningitis. To increase the yield of a positive fungal culture, large volumes of CSF (approximately 10 to 15 ml) should be cultured on at least three occasions. CSF obtained by cisternal tap has a higher yield for positive fungal culture than CSF obtained by lumbar puncture. The cryptococcal polysaccharide antigen test is a highly sensitive and specific test for cryptococcal meningitis. A reactive CSF cryptococcal polysaccharide antigen test establishes the diagnosis. Detection of the histoplasma polysaccharide antigen in CSF can be used to make a diagnosis of histoplasma meningitis. This test may be falsely positive in coccidioidal and candidal meningitis. Complement fixation antibody titers should be obtained on CSF to make a diagnosis of coccidioidal meningitis. The complement fixation antibody test on CSF is reported to have a specificity of 100 percent and a sensitivity of 75 percent in the setting of active disease. Measurement of antibodies against a 33-kDa antigen from spherules of *C. im-*

mitis in CSF is also a sensitive indicator of coccidioidal meningitis. Detection of antibodies to *S. schenckii* in CSF is helpful in making the diagnosis of meningitis due to this fungus.

The combination of a CSF lymphocytic pleocytosis and a mildly decreased glucose concentration that on serial lumbar punctures continues to decrease is suggestive of meningitis due to *M. tuberculosis*. The diagnosis is made by acid-fast smear and culture of CSF. *M. tuberculosis* also may be the etiology of a persistent neutrophilic meningitis. There may be a shift in the cell type in the CSF following the initiation of antituberculous therapy from an initial lymphocytic pleocytosis to a predominance of polymorphonuclear leukocytes. Although CSF culture for *M. tuberculosis* remains the gold standard for diagnosis, it is insensitive. The last tube of CSF collected at lumbar puncture is the best sample to use to detect acid-fast bacilli. There may be a pellicle in the CSF or a cobweb-like clot on the surface of the fluid. Acid-fast bacilli can be demonstrated best in a smear of the clot or sediment. If no clot forms, the addition of 2 ml of 95% alcohol results in a heavy protein precipitate that, on centrifuging, draws bacilli to the bottom of the tube. The centrifuged deposit of CSF can then be examined on a glass slide for the bacilli. The amount of time spent searching for the organisms by direct examination of CSF under the microscope is critical to making the diagnosis.[17,18]

Repeat examination of the CSF most likely will demonstrate a progressive increase in the protein concentration, a progressive decrease in the glucose concentration, and a shift to a mononuclear pleocytosis. The CSF chloride concentration may be decreased in tuberculous meningitis to less than 110 meq/liter. However, this is a nonspecific abnormality because the CSF chloride concentration typically decreases as the CSF protein concentration increases and does not have diagnostic value. Mycobacterial DNA can be detected in CSF by PCR assay. PCR for *M. tuberculosis* has not yet reached its potential due to problems with false-positive results and inconsistent standards and variability between laboratories.

The most common form of CNS Lyme disease is headache with mild neck stiffness, low-grade fever, photophobia, and CSF lymphocytic pleocytosis. Most patients have other neurologic abnormalities in addition to the meningeal symptoms, most often a unilateral or bilateral facial nerve palsy. CSF should be analyzed for anti–*Borrelia burgdorferi* antibodies, oligoclonal bands, and IgG index.

Bartonella henselae, the causative organism of cat-scratch disease, may cause an aseptic meningitis syndrome with fever, stiff neck, and CSF lymphocytic pleocytosis. The diagnosis is made by detection of *B. henselae* IgG or IgM in the CSF or *B. henselae* nucleic acid by PCR assay.

Acute syphilitic meningitis should be included in the differential diagnosis. The most common symptoms are headache, nausea and vomiting, and neck stiffness. There also may be cranial nerve palsies. The meningeal symptoms typically develop within 1 year of the initial infection, most often within 3 to 7 months of the appearance of the chancre. Examination of the CSF reveals a mononuclear pleocytosis, an elevated protein concentration, and a positive Venereal Disease Research Laboratory (VDRL) test. A positive CSF VDRL test establishes the diagnosis of neurosyphilis. The specificity of the CSF VDRL test for neurosyphilis is 100 percent, and the sensitivity is 50 percent. A nonreactive test does not exclude the diagnosis, however. A nonreactive CSF fluorescent treponemal antibody absorption test (FTA-ABS) or microhemagglutination *Treponema pallidum* (MHA-TP) test excludes the diagnosis of neurosyphilis. However, a reactive CSF FTA-ABS test or a reactive MHA-TP test does not establish the diagnosis.[19]

The noninfectious etiologies of a CSF lymphocytic pleocytosis are listed in Table 5-3 and include lymphoma, carcinomatous meningitis, sarcoidosis, Behçet's disease, Wegener's granulomatosis, and medications. Non-Hodgkin's lymphoma is the leading cause of cancer-related deaths for people between 20 and 40 years of age.[20] Patients present with B symptoms (i.e., fever, night sweats, or loss of more than 10 percent of body weight). Approximately 10 percent of patients with non-Hodgkin's lymphoma will develop leptomeningeal infiltration of tumor cells.[21] Examination of the CSF demonstrates a lymphocytic pleocytosis. CSF should be sent for cytology, flow cytometry, and cytokine analysis. Interleukin 10 (IL-10), a B-cell growth and differentiation factor, is normally undetectable in CSF. IL-10 is produced by systemic lymphoma cells. Elevated levels of IL-6, an inflammatory cytokine produced by B- and T-lymphocytes, has been found in infectious and noninfectious, nonmalignant inflammatory disorders. An elevated IL-10 level with an IL-10:IL-6 ratio greater than 1 is a strong predictor of the presence of lymphoma cells in the CSF. Alternatively, an IL-10:IL-6 ratio of less than

▶ **TABLE 5-3.** NONINFECTIOUS ETIOLOGIES OF A CSF LYMPHOCYTIC PLEOCYTOSIS

Lymphoma
Carcinomatous meningitis
Sarcoidosis
Behçet's disease
Wegener's granulomatosis
Medications
    Nonsteroidal anti-inflammatory agents
    Sulfa-containing antibiotics
    Intravenous immunoglobulin
    Muromonab-CD3 (OKT3)
    Isoniazid

1 is characteristic of an infectious or noninfectious nonmalignant inflammatory disorder.[22] CSF can be sent for immunophenotyping by flow cytometry. CD-10 may be found in lymphoblastic leukemia, undifferentiated lymphomas, and follicular low-grade lymphomas. The presence of CD-1 signifies lymphoblastic lymphoma or, when seen in conjunction with a mature T-cell phenotype, represents an "aberrant" retention of an immature T-cell marker (T-cell leukemia or lymphoma). Coexpression of CD-5 and CD-20 is usually associated with well-differentiated lymphocytic lymphomas.[23]

Headache, nausea, and vomiting may be early signs of leptomeningeal carcinomatosis. By definition, the dissemination of malignant cells through the leptomeninges is referred to as *carcinomatous meningitis* when leptomeningeal metastases develop from solid tumors and *lymphomatous* or *leukemic meningitis* when the meninges are seeded during the course of these diseases. Adenocarcinoma and malignant melanoma are the most common solid tumors to metastasize to the leptomeninges. Headache may be associated with or followed by cranial nerve abnormalities and signs of spinal nerve root involvement. Examination of the CSF shows an increased opening pressure and a moderately to markedly increased protein concentration. A striking increase in protein concentration is often the best clue to this diagnosis. The glucose concentration is either normal or decreased. A nonspecific pleocytosis consisting of lymphocytes, monocytes, and polymorphonuclear leukocytes is seen. The gold standard for the diagnosis of leptomeningeal carcinomatosis is the cytologic identification of malignant cells in the CSF.[24]

Sarcoidosis is a multisystem granulomatous disorder of unknown etiology characterized by noncaseating epithelioid cell granulomas in more than one organ. Any organ in the body can be affected, but the most commonly affected organ is the lung. Intrathoracic lymphadenopathy, typically in the form of bilateral, symmetric hilar and mediastinal lymphadenopathy, is present in up to 90 percent of patients with sarcoidosis at some time during the course of the illness.[25] Fifty percent develop permanent pulmonary abnormalities. Patients typically are between 20 and 40 years of age. As many as 17 percent of patients with sarcoidosis have clinical or pathologic evidence of CNS involvement. Meningeal involvement in sarcoidosis is a common pathologic finding. Cranial neuropathy is the most frequent manifestation of sarcoidosis of the nervous system, and a facial nerve palsy is the single most common abnormality.[26] Aseptic meningitis characterized by headache, meningismus, and CSF lymphocytic pleocytosis may be a recurrent problem in patients with neurosarcoidosis.[26]

The CSF abnormalities in sarcoidosis are nonspecific and are as follows: (1) lymphocytic pleocytosis, (2) increased protein concentration, (3) decreased glucose concentration, (4) elevated IgG index and synthesis rate indicative of intrathecal immunoglobulin production,[27,28] (5) oligoclonal banding,[28,29] and (6) elevated CSF angiotensin-converting enzyme (ACE). ACE is produced in the epithelioid and giant cells of sarcoid granulomas. The sensitivity of the CSF ACE level for neurosarcoidosis is 24 percent, and the specificity is 95 percent.[30] To make a diagnosis of neurosarcoidosis, the following is recommended: (1) chest radiography for bilateral, symmetric hilar and mediastinal lymphadenopathy, (2) serum and CSF ACE determination, and (3) lymph node, skin, or transbronchial lung biopsy. Biopsy evidence of a noncaseating epithelioid cell granulomatous inflammatory process is mandatory to make a definitive diagnosis of sarcoidosis.[31]

Behçet's disease is a chronic relapsing inflammatory vasculitic syndrome. HLA B51 is the main allele associated with Behçet's disease. This disease is endemic to the Middle East and the Mediterranean basin. The international diagnostic definition of Behçet's disease requires the presence of recurrent oral ulcerations and at least two of the following: (1) recurrent genital ulcerations, (2) skin lesions, either erythema nodosum, pseudofolliculitis, papulopustular lesions, or acneiform nodules, (3) eye lesions, either anterior uveitis, posterior uveitis, cells in the vitreous, or retinal vasculitis, and (4) a positive pathergy test.[32] The pathergy test consists of pricking a sterile needle into the patient's forearm to detect an erythematous nodule that is more than 2 mm in diameter at 24 to 48 hours.[33] CNS involvement in Behçet's disease may be in the form of inflammatory parenchymal lesions, an aseptic meningitis, or due to increased intracranial pressure from venous sinus thrombosis.[34] When Behçet's disease is complicated by the aseptic meningitis syndrome, examination of the CSF shows a lymphocytic or polymorphonuclear pleocytosis, an increased protein concentration, and an increased IgG level. Oligoclonal bands and antibodies against myelin basic protein are not found in patients with Behçet's disease.[34]

Wegener's granulomatosis also may present as an aseptic meningitis syndrome. Wegener's granulomatosis is characterized by necrotizing, granulomatous vasculitis of the upper or lower respiratory tracts (or both) with or without focal necrotizing glomerulitis and variable degrees of small-vessel vasculitis.[35,36] Presenting symptoms are typically cough, chest pain, hemoptysis, epistasis, purulent nasal discharge, or sinus pain. Neurologic abnormalities occur either by proximity to a granulomatous lesion or by ischemia or hemorrhage from the inflammatory vascular disease. Cranial neuropathies are typically due to erosion of the bony structures at the base of the brain from contiguous extension of granulomas.[35] The second, sixth, seventh, and eighth cranial nerves are affected most frequently. Hearing loss, proptosis, ophthalmoplegias, and facial paresis are prominent features.[35] Antibodies reactive with the cytoplasma of human neutrophils can be detected in patients with active Wegener's granulomatosis. The autoantibodies produce a characteristic cytoplasmic staining and are referred to as *cytoplasmic antineutrophil cytoplasmic autoantibodies* (c-ANCAs). In classic Wegener's granulomatosis, as defined by granulomatous inflammatory disease of the respiratory tract and active glomerular nephritis, more than 90 percent of patients have a positive c-ANCA level. In the absence of active renal disease, however, the sensitivity of the c-ANCA test may be as low as 65 to 70 percent.[37] CSF may be normal or demonstrate a mild pleocytosis with an elevated protein concentration.[38] c-ANCAs also can be detected in CSF.[39] The diagnosis is suggested by the combination of pulmonary symptoms, positive c-ANCAs, cranial neuropathies, and CSF pleocytosis. Table 5-4 provides a list of the diagnostic studies for noninfectious etiologies of a CSF lymphocytic pleocytosis.

Patients with medication-induced aseptic meningitis present with headache, fever, meningismus, and occasionally, altered mental status. They also may have a rash, arthralgias, myalgias, or liver test abnormalities. There is a CSF pleocytosis with negative results on CSF Gram's stain; CSF cultures for bacteria, fungi, and virus; and PCR and a negative CSF cryptococcal antigen. The CSF glucose concentration is normal, and the protein concentration may be mildly increased. Eosinophils are seen occasionally. Several medications have been associated with this syndrome, including nonsteroidal anti-inflammatory agents; sulfa-containing antibiotics, specifically trimethoprim-sulfamethoxazole; intravenous immunoglobulin, OKT3 monoclonal antibodies, and isoniazid.[40–43] The meningitis typically is self-limited, and there may be resolution of symptoms despite continuation of therapy.[40–43] Systemic lupus erythematosus is the most common underlying condition associated with medication-induced aseptic meningitis. To distinguish lupus aseptic meningitis from medication-induced aseptic meningitis in association with systemic lupus erythematosus, the CSF cellular response in lupus meningitis is usually lymphocytic, and the signs and symptoms of meningitis are accompanied by other clinical and laboratory abnormalities indicative of a lupus flareup.[43]

When the lumbar puncture has been traumatic, the question arises as to whether the CSF pleocytosis is real or the white blood cells (WBCs) were introduced into the CSF by the lumbar puncture itself. One way to resolve this issue is to obtain a red blood cell (RBC) count on tubes 1 and 4. The number of red blood cells in the CSF will decrease between tubes 1 and 4 if a traumatic puncture occurred. Alternatively, a two-step calculation using the peripheral blood and CSF cell count can be performed: (1) a ratio of WBCs per cubic millimeter to RBCs per cubic millimeter is determined for CSF and for peripheral blood, and then (2) a ratio of CSF WBCs

▶ **TABLE 5-4.** DIAGNOSTIC STUDIES FOR NONINFECTIOUS ETIOLOGIES OF A CSF LYMPHOCYTIC PLEOCYTOSIS

Lymphoma and carcinomatous meningitis
CSF
  Cell count with differential
  Glucose and protein concentration
  Cytology
  Flow cytometry
  Cytokine analysis
Imaging
  Gadolinium-enhanced cranial and spinal MRI
  Abdominal and pelvic CT scan for lymph nodes for biopsy
  Mammogram
  Chest CT scan
Sarcoidosis
CSF
  Cell count with differential
  Glucose and protein concentration
  IgG index
  Oligoclonal bands
  Angiotensin-converting enzyme
Imaging
  Chest CT scan
Serum
  Angiotensin-converting enzyme
Biopsy
  Lymph node, skin, or transbronchial
Behçet's disease
Serum
  HLA B51
Physical examination
  Oral and genital ulcerations
  Eye lesions
  Skin lesions
  Pathergy test
CSF
  Cell count with differential
  Glucose and protein concentration
  IgG
Wegener's granulomatosis
Serum
  Cytoplasmic antineutrophil cytoplasmic autoantibodies (c-ANCA)
  Creatinine
CSF
  Cell count with differential
  Glucose and protein concentration
  c-ANCA

to RBCs to peripheral blood WBCs to RBCs is determined. The calculation is based on the assumption that if the ratio of WBCs to RBCs in the CSF is the same as the ratio of WBCs to RBCs in the blood, then the WBCs were most likely introduced by the lumbar puncture.

If, however, the ratio of WBCs to RBCs in the CSF is higher than the ratio of WBCs to RBCs in the blood, then the excess of WBCs is due to the presence of WBCs in the CSF prior to lumbar puncture.[44,45] A simpler way to determine if the WBCs in CSF were introduced by a traumatic puncture is to subtract 1 WBC per cubic millimeter for every 700 RBCs per cubic millimeter from the total WBC count. Thus, if a bloody fluid reveals 700 RBCs and 10 WBCs, 1 WBC could be accounted for by the blood present, and 9 WBCs are either due to infectious or inflammatory CNS disorders.[46]

▶ TREATMENT

Patients with viral meningitis often have relief of their headache with the removal of CSF. The headache may then return 28 to 48 hours later. Nonsteroidal anti-inflammatory agents and amitriptyline are the best medications to treat the headache. Patients with enteroviral meningitis often have headache lasting for weeks to months. Pleconaril is an antipicornavirus agent that blocks the viral encoding process by binding to the virus protein capsid, thus blocking the release of viral DNA. In a double-blind, placebo-controlled trial, 130 patients with enteroviral meningitis between the ages of 14 and 65 years were given either 200 mg pleconaril three times daily or placebo. Those receiving pleconaril had a shorter duration of headache and returned to work or school earlier than those receiving placebo.[47] Pleconaril has good oral bioavailability and excellent CNS penetration. There are ongoing clinical trials in patients with enteroviral meningitis.

Therapy for HSV-2 meningitis has not been defined by clinical trials. The current practice is to use either acyclovir or valacyclovir as recommended for primary and recurrent genital HSV-2 infections depending on whether the meningitis is associated with a primary HSV-2 infection or with recurrent HSV-2 infection. Oral acyclovir has been shown to shorten the duration of viral shedding and local and constitutional symptoms. When meningitis complicates a primary genital HSV-2 infection, acyclovir 200 mg orally five times daily or valacyclovir 1000 mg orally twice daily or famciclovir 500 mg three times daily is given for a 10-day course of therapy. For meningitis associated with recurrent genital herpes, acyclovir 200 mg orally five times daily or valacyclovir 1000 mg orally twice daily or famciclovir 500 mg three times daily is recommended for 5 days of therapy. Patients with HIV meningitis should receive potent antiretroviral therapy. The treatment of meningitis associated with zoster has not been defined by clinical trials. Antiviral therapy has been demonstrated clearly by clinical trials to be efficacious in the treatment of acute herpes zoster. In clinical trials using acyclovir 800 mg five times daily for 7 to 10 days in immunocompetent patients with acute herpes zoster, the drug significantly shortened the duration of the rash (measured in the time to last new lesion formation and full scab formation) and alleviated pain during the acute illness.[48,49] Similarly, famciclovir 500 mg three times daily for 7 days reduces viral shedding, accelerates the rate of lesion resolution, and decreases acute pain.[50] Valacyclovir 1000 mg three times daily for 7 to 10 days has been demonstrated to be superior to acyclovir in speeding resolution of zoster-associated pain.[51] Although acyclovir inhibits EBV replication and reduces viral shedding, it has not been recommended for patients with infectious mononucleosis because the symptoms primarily are due to the immune response to the virus.[7,52]

▶ CONCLUSION

Certainty about the diagnosis of viral meningitis often takes 2 to 3 days as the patient's symptoms improve. Repeat lumbar puncture is recommended in patients whose fever and headache fail to resolve after a few days, in patients with an initial polymorphonuclear leukocytosis or decreased glucose concentration, or if there is doubt about the initial diagnosis. As molecular diagnostic studies on CSF continue to improve and are readily available, the etiologic agent of viral meningitis will be identified more commonly.

REFERENCES

1. Calisher CH: Medically important arboviruses of the United States and Canada. *Clin Microbiol Rev* 7:89, 1994.
2. Di Stefano M, Gray F, Leitner T, Chiodi F: Analysis of ENV V3 sequences from HIV-1-infected brain indicates restrained virus expression throughout the disease. *J Med Virol* 49:41, 1996.
3. Rothbart HA: Enteroviral infections of the central nervous system. *Clin Infect Dis* 20:971, 1995.
4. Connolly KJ, Hammer SM: The acute aseptic meningitis syndrome. *Clin Infect Dis* 20:971, 1995.
5. Johnston RE, Peters CJ: Alphaviruses. In Fields BN, Knipe DM, Howley PM (eds): *Fields' Virology*, Vol 1, 3d ed. Philadelphia: Lippincott Raven, 1996, pp 843–898.
6. Mollaret P: La méningite endothélio-leucocytaire multi-récurrente bénigne: Syndrome nouveau ou maladie nouvelle? *Rev Neurol (Paris)* 76:57, 1994.
7. Cohen JI: Epstein-Barr virus infection. *New Engl J Med* 343:481, 2000.
8. Rotbart HA: Viral meningitis. *Semin Neurol* 20:277, 2000.
9. Alexander JP Jr, Baden L, Pallansch MA, Anderson LJ: Enterovirus 71 infections and neurologic disease—United States, 1977–1991. *J Infect Dis* 169:905, 1994.

10. Echevarria JM, Casas I, Tenorio A, et al: Detection of varicella-zoster virus–specific DNA sequences in cerebrospinal fluid from patients with acute aseptic meningitis and no cutaneous lesions. *J Med Virol* 43:331, 1994.

11. Connelly KP, DeWitt LD: Neurologic complications of infectious mononucleosis. *Pediatr Neurol* 10:181, 1994.

12. Jahrling PB, Peters CJ: Lymphocytic choriomeningitis virus: A neglected pathogen of man (editorial). *Arch Pathol Lab Med* 116:486, 1992.

13. Arboviral disease— United States, 1994. *MMWR* 44:641, 1995.

14. Peterson LR, Marfin AA: West Nile virus: A primer for the clinician. *Ann Intern Med* 137:173, 2002.

15. Tardei G, Ruta S, Chitu V, et al: Evaluation of immunoglobulin M (IgM) and IgG enzyme immunoassays in serologic diagnosis of West Nile virus infection. *J Clin Microbiol* 38:2232, 2000.

16. Caldas C, Bernicker E, Nogare AD, Luby JP: Case report: Transverse myelitis associated with Epstein-Barr virus infection. *Am J Med Sci* 307:45, 1994.

17. Molavi A, LeFrock JL: Tuberculous meningitis. *Med Clin North Am* 69:315, 1985.

18. Berenguer J, Moreno S, Laguna S, et al: Tuberculous meningitis in patients infected with the human immunodeficiency virus. *New Engl J Med* 326:668, 1992.

19. Marra CM, Critchlow CW, Hook EW III, et al: Cerebrospinal fluid treponemal antibodies in untreated early syphilis. *Arch Neurol* 52:68, 1995.

20. Theodossiou C, Schwarzenberger P: Non-Hodgkin's lymphomas. *Clin Obstet Gynecol* 45(3):820, 2002.

21. Recht LD: Neurologic complications of systemic lymphoma. *Neurol Clin* 9:1001, 1999.

22. Faller DV, Mentzer SJ, Perrine SP: Induction of the Epstein-Barr virus tymidine kinase gene with concomitant nucleoside antivirals as a therapeutic strategy for Epstein-Barr virus–associated malignancies. *Curr Opin Oncol* 13(5):360, 2001.

23. Moriarty AT, Wiersema L, Snyder W, et al: Immunophenotyping of cytologic specimens by flow cytometry. *Diagn Cytopathol* 9:252, 1993.

24. Glantz MJ, Cole BF, Glantz LK, et al: Cerebrospinal fluid cytology in patients with cancer: Minimizing false-negative results. *Cancer* 82:733, 1998.

25. Case records of the Massachusetts General Hospital (case 35-1998). *New Engl J Med* 339:1534, 1998.

26. Stern BJ, Krumholz A, Johns C, et al: Sarcoidosis and its neurologic manifestations. *Arch Neurol* 42:909, 1985.

27. Borucki SJ, Nguyen BD, Ladoulis CT, McKendall RR: Cerebrospinal fluid immunoglobulin abnormalities in neurosarcoidosis. *Arch Neurol* 46:270, 1989.

28. Scott TF, Seay AR, Goust JM: Pattern and concentration of IgG in cerebrospinal fluid in neurosarcoidosis. *Neurology* 39:1637, 1989.

29. Kinnman J, Link H: Intrathecal production of oligoclonal IgM and IgG in CNS sarcoidosis. *Acta Neurol Scand* 69:97, 1984.

30. Dale JC, O'Brien JF: Determination of angiotensin-converting enzyme levels in cerebrospinal fluid is not a useful test for the diagnosis of neurosarcoidosis. *Mayo Clin Proc* 74:535, 1999.

31. Crystal RG: Sarcoidosis. In Braunwald B, Fauci AS, Kasper DL, et al (eds): *Harrison's Principles of Internal Medicine*, 15th ed. New York: McGraw-Hill, 2001, pp 1969–1974.

32. International Study Group for Behçet's Disease: Criteria for diagnosis of Behçet's disease. *Lancet* 335:1078, 1990.

33. Sakane T, Takeno M, Suzuki N, Inaba G: Behçet's disease. *New Engl J Med* 341:1284, 1999.

34. Yazici H, Yurdakul S, Hamuryudan V: Behçet disease. *Curr Opin Rheumatol* 13:18, 2001.

35. Moore PM: Neurological manifestations of vasculitis: Update on immunopathogenic mechanisms and clinical features. *Ann Neurol* 37(S1):S131, 1995.

36. Nishino H, Rubino FA, DeRemee RA, et al: Neurological involvement in Wegener's granulomatosis: An analysis of 324 consecutive patients at the Mayo Clinic. *Ann Neurol* 33:4, 1993.

37. Sneller MC, Fauci AS: Pathogenesis of vasculitis syndrome. *Med Clin North Am* 81:221, 1997.

38. Jinnah HA, Dixon A, Brat DJ, Hellmann DB: Chronic meningitis with cranial neuropathies in Wegener's granulomatosis. *Arthritis Rheum* 40:573, 1997.

39. Spranger M, Schwab S, Meinck HM, et al: Meningeal involvement in Wegener's granulomatosis confirmed and monitored by positive circulating antineutrophil cytoplasm in cerebrospinal fluid. *Neurology* 48:263, 1997.

40. Martin MA, Massanari RM, Nghiem DD, et al: Nosocomial aseptic meningitis associated with administration of OKT3. *JAMA* 259:2002, 1988.

41. Haas EJ: Trimethoprim-sulfamethoxazole: Another cause of recurrent meningitis (letter). *JAMA* 252:346, 1984.

42. Garagusi VF, Neefe LI, Mann O: Acute meningoencephalitis: Association with isoniazid administration. *JAMA* 235:1141, 1976.

43. Moris G, Garcia-Monco JC: The challenge of drug-induced aseptic meningitis. *Arch Intern Med* 159:1185, 1999.

44. Bonadio WA: The cerebrospinal fluid: Physiologic aspects and alterations associated with bacterial meningitis. *Pediatr Infect Dis J* 11:423, 1992.

45. Mayefsky JH, Roghmann KJ: Determination of leukocytosis in traumatic tap specimens. *Am J Med* 82:1175, 1987.

46. Fishman RA: Composition of the cerebrospinal fluid. In Fishman RA (ed): *Cerebrospinal Fluid in Diseases of the Nervous System*. Philadelphia: Saunders, 1992, pp 183–252.

47. Shafran SD, Halota W, Gilbert D, et al: Pleconaril is effective for enteroviral meningitis in adolescents and adults: A randomized, placebo-controlled multicenter trial (abstract). In *Abstracts of the 39th Interscience Conference on Antimicrobial Agents and Chemotherapy, 1999*. San Francisco: American Society for Microbiology, 1999, p 436.

48. Huff JC, Bean B, Balfour HH Jr, et al: Therapy of herpes zoster with acyclovir. *Am J Med* 85:84, 1988.

49. Wood MJ, Ogan PH, McKendrick MW, et al: Efficacy of oral acyclovir treatment of acute herpes zoster. *Am J Med* 85:79, 1988.

50. Tyring S, Nahlik J, Cunningham A, et al: Efficacy and safety of famciclovir in the treatment of patients with herpes zoster: Results of the first placebo-controlled study (abstract). In *Programs and Abstracts of the 33d Interscience Conference on Antimicrobial Agents and Chemotherapy, October 17–20, 1993.* Washington: American Society for Microbiology, 1993, p 400.

51. Wood MJ, Shukla S, Fiddian AP, Crooks RJ: Treatment of acute herpes zoster: Effect of early (<48 h) versus late (48–72 h) therapy with acyclovir and valaciclovir on prolonged pain. *J Infect Dis* 178(suppl 1):S81, 1998.

52. van der Horst C, Joncas J, Ahronheim G, et al: Lack of effect of peroral acyclovir for the treatment of acute infectious mononucleosis. *J Infect Dis* 164:788, 1991.

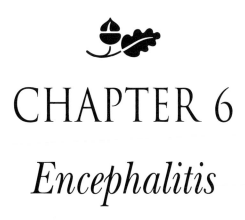

CHAPTER 6
Encephalitis

Karen L. Roos

Encephalitis is a syndrome of fever, headache, and an altered level of consciousness. In addition, there may be focal neurologic deficits and/or new-onset seizure activity. The signs and symptoms of encephalitis are due to inflammation of brain parenchyma. Encephalitis may be due to acute viral infection, a postinfectious immune-mediated process, or a paraneoplastic syndrome.

Herpes simplex virus type 1 (HSV-1) is the most common viral cause of acute sporadic encephalitis in the Western world. The arthropod-borne viruses La Crosse virus, St. Louis encephalitis virus, West Nile virus, Japanese encephalitis virus, eastern equine encephalitis virus, western equine encephalitis virus, Venezuelan equine encephalitis virus, dengue, tickborne encephalitis virus, Powassan virus, and Colorado tick fever virus all cause encephalitis during the time of the year when mosquitoes and ticks are biting. Rocky Mountain spotted fever and the ehrlichioses are tick-borne bacterial infections that also may cause encephalitis.

A number of viruses, in addition to HSV-1, acquired in childhood may reactivate to cause encephalitis. Epstein-Barr virus causes infectious mononucleosis. Encephalitis was the first described neurologic complication of infectious mononucleosis.[1] Encephalitis may be the result of direct central nervous system (CNS) invasion by the virus or a parainfectious immune disorder. In immunocompromised patients, the acquisition of or the reactivation of latent Epstein-Barr virus infection can cause a syndrome of altered mental status with or without focal neurologic deficits.[2] Varicella-zoster virus causes chickenpox and then establishes latent infection in the CNS. The most common sign of varicella-zoster virus reactivation is shingles. Chickenpox, shingles, or disseminated zoster eruption may be complicated by encephalitis. Varicella-zoster virus encephalitis is reported increasingly in immunocompromised patients. Human herpesvirus type 6 (HHV-6) is an infection acquired in childhood that, similar to varicella-zoster virus, establishes latent infection in the CNS and can reactivate in the setting of immunosuppression. Approximately 30 to 45 percent of bone marrow transplant recipients develop HHV-6 viremia within the first several weeks following transplantation.[3] HHV-6 also has been shown to reactivate following hematopoietic stem cell transplantation.[4] HHV-6 reactivation may be asymptomatic or present as a pneumonitis, graft-versus-host disease, or an encephalitis.[3] HHV-6 may cause an encephalitis with focal features resembling HSV-1 encephalitis or an encephalitis with multifocal areas of demyelination.[5,6] The JC virus, which is acquired in childhood, can reactivate and cause a multifocal demyelinating disease, progressive multifocal leukoencephalopathy. Although cytomegalovirus (CMV) may cause encephalitis in both immunocompetent and immunocompromised individuals, it is more often a causative agent of encephalitis in immunosuppressed individuals, including organ transplant recipients and HIV-infected individuals, than it is in immunocompetent individuals. The prevention of CMV disease in solid organ transplant recipients is critical to the prevention of CMV encephalitis; CMV-seronegative organ transplant recipients who receive an organ from a CMV-seropositive donor are at the greatest risk for CMV disease.

Postinfectious encephalomyelitis is an acute monophasic disorder of the CNS that occurs within days to weeks of a viral illness or a vaccination and is characterized neuropathologically by perivenular inflammation and demyelination. Postinfectious encephalomyelitis is distinguished from acute viral encephalitis by its pathology. Postinfectious encephalomyelitis is predominantly a disease of white matter, but gray matter also may be affected, particularly basal ganglia, thalami, and brainstem.[7] Acute viral encephalitis is predominantly a disease of gray matter. Although postinfectious encephalomyelitis has a clear temporal relationship to infection or immunization, it is not the result of primary neural tissue invasion by an organism. Infectious agents are identified or recovered rarely from neural tissue.[8] Postinfectious encephalomyelitis is instead an autoimmune disease triggered by an infectious agent or an immunization.

Limbic encephalitis is one of the classic paraneoplastic syndromes. The term *paraneoplastic syndromes,* by definition, refers to symptoms or signs resulting from disorders of organs remote from the site of a malignant neoplasm or its metastases. The tumor typically is found months or even a few years after the appearance of the neurologic disorder.[9] Limbic encephalitis has been associated with small cell lung cancer, breast cancer, testicular germ cell tumors, and non-small cell lung cancer.

Nonvasculitic autoimmune meningoencephalitis refers to a syndrome of a progressive fluctuating encephalopathy associated with a cerebrospinal fluid (CSF) pleocytosis that responds to high-dose intravenous corticosteroid therapy.

▶ ACUTE VIRAL ENCEPHALITIS

Pathophysiology

HSV-1 is the most common viral cause of acute sporadic encephalitis. Humans acquire herpes simplex virus infection from other humans. The virus is transmitted from infected to susceptible persons during close personal contact. The virus must come in contact with mucosal surfaces or abraded skin for infection to be initiated.[10] Primary infection with HSV-1 usually occurs in the oropharyngeal mucosa and typically is asymptomatic. Symptomatic disease is characterized by fever, pain, and inability to swallow because of lesions on the buccal and gingival mucosa. The duration of illness is 2 to 3 weeks.[10] After primary infection, HSV-1 is transported to the CNS by retrograde axoplasmic flow of virus in the axons of a division of the trigeminal nerve. The trigeminal ganglion becomes colonized, and the virus establishes latent infection in the ganglion. Reactivation of latent ganglionic infection with replication of virus leads to encephalitis, with infection in the temporal cortex and limbic system structures. HSV-1 encephalitis also may be the result of primary infection from intranasal inoculation of virus, with direct invasion of the olfactory bulbs and spread via the olfactory pathways to the orbitofrontal and temporal lobes.[11,12] Whether infection is the result of reactivation or primary infection, inflammatory and necrotizing lesions are seen in the inferior and medial temporal lobes, the orbital frontal cortex, and the limbic structures.[11,12]

The arthropod-borne viruses (arboviruses) are inoculated into the host subcutaneously by a mosquito or tick bite and then undergo local replication at the skin site. A viremia follows, and if there is a large enough inoculum of virus, invasion and infection of the CNS occur. Most arboviruses are small and thus are cleared less efficiently than other microorganisms by the reticuloendothelial system.[13] Initial CNS infection by arboviruses appears to occur via cerebral capillary endothelial cells with subsequent infection of neurons. Virus also may spread from the choroid plexus to the intraventricular CSF and then infect ventricular ependymal cells with subsequent spread to subependymal periventricular brain tissue. Virus spreads from cell to cell typically along dendritic or axonal processes. Arboviral encephalitis is primarily a disease of cortical gray matter and brainstem and thalamic nucleii. There also may be a mild inflammatory meningeal exudate composed of lymphocytes, polymorphonuclear leukocytes, plasma cells, and macrophages.[13] Japanese encephalitis virus, West Nile virus, and eastern equine encephalitis in particular have a predilection for the basal ganglia. Neuroimaging evidence of involvement of the basal ganglia and thalami can be helpful in differentiating arboviral encephalitis from herpes simplex virus encephalitis.

The first arbovirus isolated in the United States was vesicular stomatitis Indiana virus in 1925; since then, more than 400 other arboviruses have been isolated. La Crosse virus is a member of the California serogroup of the bunyavirus family, was first isolated in 1965, and is one of the most important causes of arthropod-borne viral encephalitis in the pediatric age group.[14] St. Louis encephalitis virus, West Nile virus, Japanese encephalitis virus, and Murray Valley encephalitis virus are all members of the flavivirus family. In addition to encephalitis virus, West Nile virus may cause weakness due to involvement of the anterior horn cells of the spinal cord, a "poliomyelitis-like syndrome." Poliomyelitis-like acute flaccid paralysis also has been described in other flavivirus infections, including Japanese encephalitis, Murray Valley encephalitis, St. Louis encephalitis, and tick-borne encephalitis.[15] In addition to a mosquito bite, West Nile virus can be transmitted through blood transfusion and organ transplantation.

As stated earlier, a number of herpesviruses can reactivate, especially in the setting of cell-mediated immunosuppression, and cause encephalitis. These are HHV-6, Epstein-Barr virus, JC virus, and varicella-zoster virus. In addition, immunosuppressed patients are at particular risk for encephalitis due to CMV.

The classic histopathologic signs of encephalitis are perivascular mononuclear cell inflammation, neuronophagia, and microglial nodules.

Clinical Features

The classic clinical presentation of HSV-1 encephalitis is a subacute progression of fever, hemicranial or generalized headache, behavioral abnormalities, focal seizure activity, and focal neurologic deficits, most often dysphasia or hemiparesis.

The clinical presentation of arthropod-borne viral encephalitis is nonspecific, but the specific virus can be predicted based on the geographic location where the infection was acquired and some unique clinical features. The largest number of cases of La Crosse virus encephalitis occur in wooded areas of the midwestern United States (i.e., Wisconsin, Minnesota, Illinois, Indiana, Iowa, and Ohio). Transmission typically involves *Aedes triseriatus* mosquitoes. These mosquitoes breed in tree holes in the woods and in discarded automobile tires and other stagnant water containers.[16] Clinically recognizable disease occurs primarily in children aged 4 to 11 years. Clinical manifestations of symptomatic infection range from a mild febrile illness to aseptic meningitis, a mild encephalitic illness, and severe encephalitis. A distinct prodromal phase characterized by fever, chills, headache, nausea and vomiting, and abdominal pain lasting 1 to 4 days commonly precedes the onset of symptoms of encephalitis.[17] Diarrhea is rare. These symptoms are followed by increasing

lethargy and behavior changes or brief single seizures (or both). Symptoms last for 3 to 4 days, and then the child's condition improves over the next 3 to 4 days. The less common form of La Crosse virus encephalitis is a fulminant presentation of fever, headache, disorientation, and seizures progressing to coma. Status epilepticus and focal neurologic deficits may be part of the presentation.[14] Focal neurologic deficits occur in 16 to 25 percent of children (suggesting the possibility of herpes simplex virus encephalitis) and focal and generalized seizures in 42 to 62 percent.[18] In the summertime, children also may have enteroviral meningitis, and mild cases of La Crosse virus encephalitis may resemble enteroviral meningitis. Children with La Crosse virus encephalitis, however, do not have a rash and typically do not have meningeal signs. Seizures occur in 50 percent of patients with La Crosse virus encephalitis, and the occurrence of seizures helps to distinguish La Crosse virus encephalitis from enteroviral meningitis.[14] In adults, infection is either asymptomatic or causes a benign febrile illness or aseptic meningitis. Snowshoe hare virus, considered a variant of La Crosse virus, and one of five other viruses in the California serogroup that are pathogenic to humans, causes rare but severe neurologic infections in Canada, the Rocky Mountains, and Montana.[18]

Meningitis or encephalitis develops in approximately in 1 in 150 individuals infected with the West Nile virus.[19] Older individuals, individuals with chronic illness, and individuals who are immunosuppressed are at greatest risk for encephalitis. West Nile virus fever begins with a febrile, influenza-like illness with headache, sore throat, malaise, myalgias, fatigue, and conjunctivitis. There may be a maculopapular or roseolar rash. This is associated with or followed by nausea, abdominal pain and diarrhea, and symptoms of encephalitis. Tremor is a prominent feature of West Nile virus encephalitis. Patients with West Nile virus encephalitis also may have other parkinsonian features.[20] There also may be a mild carditis, hepatitis, or pancreatitis. Patients with West Nile virus infection may develop an acute asymmetric flaccid weakness, a poliomyelitis-like syndrome.

St. Louis encephalitis virus is found in central and southeastern United States (particularly Florida), western and central Canada, and Mexico. St. Louis encephalitis virus may cause a mild febrile illness with headache, an aseptic meningitis, or an encephalitis. Most symptomatic infections in adults older than 50 years of age present as encephalitis. In younger patients, most symptomatic infections present as an aseptic meningitis syndrome. The onset of encephalitis symptoms may be preceded by an influenza-like prodrome of malaise, myalgias, and fever. This is followed by symptoms of headache, nausea and vomiting, confusion, disorientation, irritability, stupor, tremors, and occasionally, convulsions. St. Louis encephalitis has a mortality of 10 to 20 percent, and approximately 10 percent of survivors experience sequelae of memory loss, chronic fatigue, sleeplessness, headache, and occasionally, seizures or motor deficits.[21,22] A unique clinical feature of St. Louis virus encephalitis is the syndrome of inappropriate antidiuretic hormone secretion with hyponatremia and serum hypoosmolarity that can complicate this infection. Patients also may have urinary incontinence or retention.[21,22]

Japanese encephalitis virus is the most common cause of arthropod-borne human encephalitis worldwide. Epidemic disease occurs in China, northern parts of Southeast Asia, northeast India, Nepal, and Sri Lanka. The principal vector for Japanese encephalitis virus is the *Culex tritaeniorhynchus* mosquito, which breeds in the rice fields of Asia. The virus reaches the brain through hematogenous dissemination and infects the thalamus, brainstem, basal ganglia, substantia nigra, spinal cord, cerebral cortex, and cerebellum. The clinical presentation reflects the involvement of these areas. In epidemic areas, the disease primarily affects children (almost all adults have antibodies), but nonimmune adults who enter an epidemic area are susceptible to severe encephalitis. Infection with Japanese encephalitis virus may be asymptomatic, or it may appear as an influenza-like illness with headache or low-grade fever that resolves over 4 to 5 days or evolves into a more serious illness. Encephalitis due to Japanese encephalitis virus is characterized by fever, vomiting, convulsions, and coma. During the acute illness, patients may have restricted eye movements, opsoclonus, upbeating nystagmus, cogwheel rigidity (due to lesions in the substantia nigra), or flaccid paralysis (due to lesions in the spinal cord).[23–24]

Eastern equine encephalitis virus causes the most severe arboviral encephalitis, and in the United States, most cases occur along the East Coast from Massachusetts to Florida.[22] The first human case of eastern equine encephalitis occurred in Massachusetts in the summer of 1938.[25] Disease in horses or pheasants precedes human disease by 2 to 3 weeks. The clinical manifestations of eastern equine encephalitis do not differ significantly from those of other arthropod-borne viral encephalitides except in the severity of symptoms. Symptoms of encephalitis may be preceded by an influenza-like prodrome with fever, headache, vomiting, malaise, and lethargy, but more typically patients with eastern equine encephalitis have an abrupt onset of high fever and convulsions and a rapid progression from stupor to coma. Eastern equine encephalitis may present with focal signs or focal seizure activity and thus mimic herpes simplex virus encephalitis.

Western equine encephalitis is a much milder encephalitis than eastern equine encephalitis. However, neurologic sequelae are common in children who develop the disease when they are younger than 6 months of age.[26] Western equine encephalitis virus infects horses and humans in western North America, with most cases occurring between April and September and peak activity in July and August. Asymptomatic infections with western equine encephalitis virus are more common than symptomatic cases, and attack rates are highest in young children. Western equine encephalitis, like the other arboviral encephalitides, begins with an influenza-like prodrome of fever, malaise, myalgias, pharyngitis, and vomiting. As the disease progresses, lethargy, irritability, convulsions, and coma develop.[22] Postencephalitis parkinsonism is reported occasionally in adults who survive western equine encephalitis.[22,27] Venezuelan equine encephalitis virus causes encephalitis in Central and South America, and cases have been reported in Texas. Symptoms of encephalitis typically are preceded by fever, headache, myalgias, vomiting, and sometimes diarrhea.

Dengue fever is one of the world's major emerging infectious diseases.[28] Dengue virus causes dengue fever in Hawaii, Asia, Africa, the Caribbean, and Central and South America and is transmitted by the bite of a *Aedes aegypti* or *Aedes albopictus* mosquito. There is a short incubation period, with travelers to endemic areas becoming symptomatic shortly after they return home. The global incidence of dengue infection is estimated to be 50 to 100 million per year.[28,29] Dengue fever begins as an acute febrile illness with rigors, headache, retroorbital pain, myalgias, arthralgias, rash, and fatigue. Most dengue infections result in relatively mild illness, but some patients will have a course complicated by cerebral edema, hemorrhagic diathesis, hypoperfusion, hyponatremia, and liver and renal failure.[30] Infection with one of any of the four serotypes of dengue virus can predispose an individual to dengue hemorrhagic fever and/or dengue shock syndrome on reinfection with another serotype.[28]

Nipah virus caused an outbreak of encephalitis in Malaysia primarily among pig farmers and their families in September of 1998. Many of the pigs were ill with respiratory disease. Five months later, a similar disease in pigs and humans appeared in an area south of the original site after the transport of large numbers of pigs. Shortly thereafter, in March of 1999, a virus was recovered from CSF of three fatal human cases that proved to be a newly recognized virus with characteristics of the family Paramyxoviridae. These viruses are spread by respiratory routes and are not arthropod-borne. The illness began with fever, headache, dizziness, vomiting, and decreased consciousness. The encephalitis had focal clinical signs of segmental myoclonus, cerebellar ataxia, and prominent signs of brain stem and cervical cord involvement.[31]

Colorado tick fever generally is benign, and most patients have only headache, myalgias, and a maculopapular rash. Children may have more severe disease, with symptoms beginning with high fever, chills, myalgias and arthralgias, severe headache, ocular pain, conjunctival injection, nausea, and occasionally, vomiting. A transitory petechial or maculopapular rash is seen in about 50 percent of patients. Hemorrhagic manifestations ranging from rash to disseminated intravascular coagulopathy, gastrointestinal tract bleeding, and intracerebral hemorrhages may occur.[15]

Powassan virus encephalitis may begin with symptoms of sore throat and lethargy, followed by headache, fever, and convulsions. Patients may have focal neurologic deficits.[16]

Tick-borne encephalitis viruses enter the body through either a tick bite or the ingestion of infected unpasteurized goat milk or cheese.[32] The several strains of tick-borne encephalitis virus include the Central European encephalitis strain, the Eastern European encephalitis strain, and the louping-ill strain. The Central European encephalitis subtype causes disease in central and eastern Europe. The far eastern (Siberian) strains (formally called *Russian spring-summer encephalitis virus*) cause severe encephalitis in Russia and eastern Europe, often with bulbar and cervical cord involvement. The Central European encephalitis virus causes a biphasic illness. During the first phase, fever develops and persists for 2 to 7 days. This is followed by an afebrile and relatively asymptomatic period, and then in the second phase, fever recurs with symptoms and signs of meningitis or meningoencephalitis. Illness caused by the Eastern European strain is similar to that caused by the Central European encephalitis virus except that it has a monophasic course without an intervening asymptomatic period.[32] The louping-ill strain causes disease primarily in sheep with a characteristic cerebellar ataxia. Human infections are rare.

Encephalitis can complicate chickenpox or occur as a parainfectious immune-mediated demyelinating disorder after varicella infection, follow the cutaneous eruption of zoster, or occur in association with or following the eruption of a diffuse varicella-like rash (in immunocompromised patients). The encephalitis also may occur without a varicella rash or a recent history of shingles. The characteristic clinical presentation of varicella-zoster virus encephalitis is headache, malaise, confusion, and focal neurologic symptoms and signs. A large-vessel arterial disease, a granulomatous arteritis, or a small-vessel arteritis may cause acute focal neurologic deficits, and this may be combined with demyelinating lesions. When the carotid–middle cerebral artery territory is involved in the vasculopathy, hemiparesis is a frequent finding.

Encephalitis can complicate acute Epstein-Barr virus infection (infectious mononucleosis), occur as a parainfectious immune-mediated demyelinating disorder, or present as an encephalomyeloradiculitis with signs of both brain and spinal cord involvement. Patients have headache, seizures, and multifocal neurologic deficits.

HHV-6 may cause an encephalitis with focal features resembling HSV-1 encephalitis or an encephalitis with multifocal deficits typical of demyelination, i.e., spastic gait, dysmetria, and ataxia.[5,6]

CMV encephalitis presents as a diffuse encephalopathy with confusion, disorientation, apathy, psychomotor slowing, and cranial nerve palsies. There may be an associated retinitis.

Progressive multifocal leukoencephalopathy, due to reactivation of the JC virus acquired in childhood, presents with hemianopia when lytic destruction of oligodendrocytes and demyelination occurs in an occipital lobe and behavioral changes from frontal lobe involvement.

Diagnosis

The diagnosis of HSV-1 encephalitis is made by a combination of findings on magnetic resonance imaging (MRI), examination of the CSF, and electroencephalography (EEG). The characteristic MRI abnormality of HSV-1 encephalitis is a high-signal-intensity lesion on T_2-weighted and fluid-attenuated inversion recovery (FLAIR) images in the medial and inferior temporal lobe extending up into the insula (Fig. 6-1). A normal T_2-

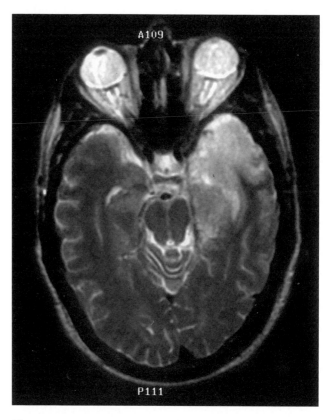

Figure 6–1. T_2-weighted MRI demonstrating classic lesion of HSV-1 encephalitis.

weighted and FLAIR MRI is evidence against the diagnosis of HSV-1 encephalitis. Examination of the CSF shows an increased opening pressure, a lymphocytic pleocytosis of 5 to 500 cells/mm³, a mild to moderate increase in the protein concentration, and a normal or mildly decreased glucose concentration. CSF viral cultures for HSV-1 are almost always negative. Herpes simplex virus nucleic acid can be detected by polymerase chain reaction (PCR). If the CSF PCR is negative and HSV-1 encephalitis is strongly suspected, the test should be repeated on CSF. CSF HSV-1 PCR has been reported to be negative in the first few days of infection. Porphyrin compounds from the degradation of heme and erythrocytes may inhibit the PCR, and a false-positive HSV-1 PCR may be obtained from bloody or xanthochromic CSF specimens. Since HSV-1 encephalitis is a hemorrhagic encephalitis, this alone may account for a false-negative PCR. CSF and serum samples should be obtained to determine if there is intrathecal synthesis of antibodies against herpes simplex virus. Antibodies against herpes simplex virus do not appear in the CSF until approximately 8 to 12 days after the onset of disease, and they can increase markedly during the first 2 to 4 weeks of infection. A serum:CSF antibody ratio of less than 20:1 is considered diagnostic of herpes simplex virus infection (Table 6-1).

HSV-1 encephalitis has a distinctive EEG pattern of periodic stereotyped sharp- and slow-wave complexes that occur at regular intervals of 2 to 3 seconds and are expressed maximally over the involved temporal lobes.

The laboratory diagnosis of arboviral encephalitis has been established by the Centers for Disease Control and Prevention (CDC) and is listed in Table 6-2. A confirmed case of arboviral encephalitis is defined as a febrile illness with encephalitis during a period when arboviral transmission is likely to occur plus at least one of the following criteria: (1) fourfold or greater increase in viral antibody titer between acute and convalescent sera, (2) viral isolation from tissue, blood, or CSF, or (3) specific IgM antibody in the CSF. A presumptive case is defined as a compatible illness plus either a stable elevated antibody titer to an arbovirus (≥320 by hemagglutination inhibition, ≥128 by complement fixation, ≥256 by immunofluorescent assay, or ≥160 by plaque-reduction neutralization test) or specific IgM antibody in serum by enzyme immunoassay.[33]

The identification of West Nile virus antibodies in serum is not sufficient to attribute the neurologic illness to West Nile virus infection. West Nile virus antibodies may be detected in the sera of asymptomatic individuals. In order to attribute the neurologic illness to West Nile virus infection, one of the following criteria must be met: (1) West Nile virus IgM antibody in CSF detected by enzyme-linked immunosorbent assay (ELISA), (2) West Nile virus nucleic acid in CSF, (3) a fourfold increase in neutralizing immunoglobulin G antibody

▶ **TABLE 6-1.** DIAGNOSTIC STUDIES FOR VIRAL ENCEPHALITIS

Herpes simplex virus
  CSF lymphocytic pleocytosis, normal glucose concentration
  CSF PCR HSV DNA
  CSF and serum antibodies (serum: CSF antibody ratio of less than 20:1)
Arboviruses
  CSF pleocytosis*
  CSF PCR for West Nile virus RNA
  CSF IgM antibody capture ELISA
  Paired acute and convalescent sera
Varicella-zoster virus
  CSF PCR VZV DNA
  CSF VZV IgG antibodies (serum:CSF ratio)
  CSF VZV IgM antibodies
Epstein-Barr virus
  CSF PCR EBV DNA
  Serology
    Heterophil antibody
    Antiviral capsid antigen (VCA)
    EBV VCA IgM antibodies
    Anti-EBNA IgG antibodies
Human herpesvirus type 6
  Isolation of virus in CSF culture + paired acute and convalescent sera
Cytomegalovirus
  PCR CMV DNA
Rocky Mountain spotted fever
  IgG and IgM by indirect immunofluorescence
  CSF lymphocytic or polymorphonuclear pleocytosis
  PCR for rickettsial DNA
Ehrlichioses
  Pancytopenia
  Elevated hepatic aminotransferases
  Wright's or Giemsa staining of blood smears
  Antibody titers
  Serum PCR for coccobacilli nucleic acid
Paraneoplastic syndromes
  Oligoclonal bands
  Myelin basic protein
  Antineuronal antibodies

*Polymorphonuclear leukocytes predominate early in infection followed in 12 to 24 hours by a predominance of lymphocytes.

titer between acute and convalescent sera obtained 4 weeks later, or (4) isolation of the virus from the brain or spinal cord. West Nile virus IgM and IgG antibody titers that are positive by ELISA should be confirmed by the more specific plaque-reduction neutralization assay and cell culture. If West Nile virus is strongly suspected as the causative agent of the CNS infection, serial samples of CSF should be collected over a number of days because it may take a number of days to detect West Nile virus antibodies in CSF.

Examination of the CSF in arboviral encephalitis demonstrates a lymphocytic pleocytosis, a normal glu-

► **TABLE 6-2.** LABORATORY DIAGNOSIS OF ARBOVIRAL ENCEPHALITIS

Definitive diagnosis of arboviral encephalitis:
   One or more of the following:
      Fourfold increase in antibody titer between acute and convalescent sera
      Viral isolation from tissue, blood, or CSF
      Viral-specific IgM antibody in CSF
Presumptive diagnosis of arboviral encephalitis:
   Stable increased antibody titer to arbovirus
      ≥320 by hemagglutination inhibition
      ≥128 by complement fixation
      ≥256 by immunofluorescent assay
      ≥160 by plaque reduction neutralization test
             or
Positive serum IgM capture enzyme immunoassay

cose concentration, and a moderately increased protein concentration. Polymorphonuclear leukocytes may predominate early in infection with a shift to a lymphocytic pleocytosis early in the disease course. The recommended neuroimaging for encephalitis is MRI with T_2-weighted and FLAIR images. In arboviral encephalitis, on T_2-weighted and FLAIR MRI, there are often small areas of hyperintensity that are focal areas of encephalitis. Hyperintense lesions in the substantia nigra, basal ganglia, and thalamus on T_2-weighted images are seen in all the flavivirus infections (West Nile virus, St. Louis encephalitis virus, and Japanese encephalitis virus). Eastern equine encephalitis virus also may cause areas of increased T_2 signal abnormalities in the thalamus and basal ganglia.

The diagnosis of varicella-zoster virus encephalitis is suggested by neuroimaging abnormalities and is confirmed by the detection of varicella-zoster virus DNA in the CSF, varicella-zoster virus IgM antibodies in the CSF, or a CSF culture that is positive for the virus. Neuroimaging may show large and small ischemic and hemorrhagic infarctions of the cortical and subcortical gray matter and white matter, as well as spherical subcortical white matter lesions with the typical appearance of demyelination.

The diagnosis of encephalitis due to Epstein-Barr virus is made by the detection of Epstein-Barr virus DNA in the CSF, provided that the lumbar puncture was not traumatic. Epstein-Barr virus DNA is found in peripheral blood mononuclear cells and can contaminate the CSF if the lumbar puncture is traumatic. When encephalitis due to Epstein-Barr virus occurs during acute mononucleosis, atypical lymphocytes or a positive heterophil antibody may be detected. Acute infection is confirmed by the detection of antiviral capsid antigen (VCA) titers of 1:320 or higher, positive IgM antibody titers to the viral capsid antigen (Epstein-Barr virus VCA IgM antibodies), and the absence of antibodies to virus-

associated nuclear antigen [antibodies to Epstein-Barr virus nuclear antigen (anti-EBNA IgG)]. In subsequent serum specimens (collected 36 days after the onset of illness), there should be a fourfold decrease in the IgG antibody titer to the VCA and a 16-fold increase in anti-EBNA IgG.[1]

The diagnosis of HHV-6 encephalitis requires both isolation of the virus in CSF culture and a concomitant fourfold or greater increase in IgG titer between acute and convalescent sera. The detection of HHV-6 DNA in CSF by PCR does not distinguish between latent infection and active viral replication associated with reactivation. HHV-6 DNA has been detected in normal brain tissue, as well as in cellular components of CSF collected from patients with noninflammatory neurologic diseases.[34,35]

The diagnosis of encephalitis due to CMV can be made by the detection of CMV DNA in CSF by PCR. The diagnosis of progressive multifocal leukoencephalopathy can be made by the detection of JC virus DNA in CSF by PCR. A positive result establishes the diagnosis, but a negative result does not exclude the diagnosis.

Treatment

The antimicrobial therapy of viral encephalitis is listed in Table 6-3. HSV-1 encephalitis is treated with intravenous acyclovir 10 mg/kg every 8 hours for 3 weeks. A positive CSF PCR for HSV-1 DNA is not required to treat for HSV-1 encephalitis. If the clinical course and abnormalities on MRI are typical for HSV-1 encephalitis, the patient should be treated. When the CSF PCR is negative, the CSF can be reexamined for HSV-1 DNA and for HSV-1 antibodies. Herpes simplex virus antibodies typically cannot be detected until 8 days after the onset of symptoms but then can be detected for at least 30 days and sometimes as long as 3 months.

The therapy of arboviral encephalitis is primarily supportive care with management of the neurologic complications of seizures and increased intracranial pressure. Ribavirin has been investigated for the therapy of La Crosse virus encephalitis. Intravenous ribavirin is begun at a dose of 25 mg/kg over the first 24 hours (in divided doses every 8 hours) and then is decreased to 15 mg/kg per day (divided every 8 hours) for 2 to 10 days.[36]

A mouse model of West Nile virus infection was studied to determine the efficacy of prophylactic and therapeutic treatment with human intravenous immunoglobulin (IgIV) prepared from pooled blood from healthy Israeli donors.[37] Full protection was achieved when the infected mice were treated with pooled plasma or IgIV within 4 hours of inoculation. This protection decreased to 64 percent when a single injection of IgIV was administered 1 day after West Nile virus in-

▶ **TABLE 6-3.** ANTIMICROBIAL THERAPY OF ENCEPHALITIS

Organism	Antimicrobial Agent
Herpes simplex virus	
Acyclovir-sensitive	Acyclovir 10 mg/kg every 8 hours for 3 weeks
Acyclovir-resistant	Foscarnet 60 mg/kg every 8 hours for 3 weeks
Varicella-zoster virus	Acyclovir 10 mg/kg every 8 hours for a minimum of 14 days
Epstein-Barr virus	Acyclovir 10 mg/kg every 8 hours
Cytomegalovirus	Induction therapy (for 2–3 weeks):
	Ganciclovir 5 mg/kg every 12 hours
	Foscarnet 60 mg/kg every 8 hours
	Maintenance therapy:
	Ganciclovir 5 mg/kg/d
	Foscarnet 60–120 mg/kg/d
HHV-6, variant A	Foscarnet 60 mg/kg every 8 hours
HHV-6, variant B	Foscarnet or ganciclovir 5 mg/kg every 12 hrs
Rocky Mountain spotted fever	Doxycycline 100 mg every 12 hours
Ehrlichiosis	Doxycycline 100 mg every 12 hours

oculation. The mice were fully protected from infection when given daily injections of IgIV on days 1 through 5 after virus inoculation. A multicenter trial is presently underway in the United States to evaluate the efficacy of an IgIV preparation from Israeli donors collected in the years 1999–2000 (Omr-IgG-am, Omrix Biopharmaceuticals SA, Rehovot, Israel).

Varicella-zoster virus encephalitis is treated with intravenous acyclovir 10 mg/kg every 8 hours for a minimum of 14 days. The newer antiviral agents with activity against varicella-zoster virus, namely, valacyclovir and famciclovir, have been shown to be efficacious in the treatment of zoster but have not been studied in clinical trials of varicella-zoster virus meningoencephalitis. Foscarnet and ganciclovir have been shown to be efficacious in individual case reports of varicella-zoster virus meningoencephalitis and myelitis in immunosuppressed patients associated with human immunodeficiency virus infection.[38,39]

HHV-6 variant A is susceptible to foscarnet in vitro but less susceptible to ganciclovir. HHV-6 variant B is inhibited by ganciclovir and foscarnet. The dose of foscarnet is 60 mg/kg intravenously every 8 hours; the dose of ganciclovir is 5 mg/kg intravenously twice daily. HHV-6, like CMV, lacks the thymidine kinase for acyclovir; as such, acyclovir has no effect on HHV-6 CNS infection as either prophylaxis or treatment.[40]

Epstein-Barr virus encephalitis is treated with acyclovir.

Present recommendations are that CMV encephalitis be treated with a combination of ganciclovir and foscarnet. No data on the efficacy of this combination therapy are available, but therapy with ganciclovir or foscarnet alone has not improved survival. The dose of ganciclovir is 5 mg/kg intravenously every 12 hours for a minimum of 2 to 3 weeks, followed by maintenance

therapy of 5 mg/kg per day for an indefinite period. The dose of foscarnet is 60 mg/kg intravenously every 8 hours for a minimum of 2 to 3 weeks, followed by maintenance therapy (60 to 120 mg/kg per day).

In approximately 70 percent of cases of viral encephalitis, an etiologic organism cannot be identified despite the availability of PCR.[41] Empirical therapy with acyclovir often is initiated based on the possibility that an acyclovir-sensitive virus may be the causative organism of the encephalitis. Acyclovir-resistant herpes simplex virus isolates have been identified as the cause of encephalitis in organ transplant recipients and in HIV-infected individuals but not yet in immunocompetent patients. Patients with acyclovir-resistant HSV-1 encephalitis have been treated successfully with foscarnet or ganciclovir. For this reason, foscarnet can be used in the treatment of patients with a viral encephalitis of undetermined etiology who continue to deteriorate neurologically or fail to improve on acyclovir therapy. Foscarnet inhibits viral DNA polymerases by binding to the pyrophosphate-binding site. The recommended dose for CNS infections is 60 mg/kg every 8 hours administered over 1 hour. Induction therapy for 14 to 21 days is followed by maintenance therapy (60 to 120 mg/kg per day). The limitation in therapy usually occurs with elevations in serum creatinine. This is reversible when foscarnet is discontinued.

▶ TICK-BORNE BACTERIAL INFECTIONS

Rocky Mountain spotted fever is caused by the bacteria *Rickettsia rickettsii,* which is transmitted by the bite of a *Dermacentor* sp. tick. Within 6 to 10 days of the tick bite, illness begins abruptly with fever, malaise, headache, myalgias, and vomiting. The skin rash appears, on average, 2 to 4 days after the onset of illness. The rash begins with macules on the wrists and ankles that subsequently spread to involve the trunk, face, palms, and soles. The rash progresses from a maculopapular rash to a petechial and then a purpuric rash. In the majority of patients, the diffuse rash is not present during the initial 3 days of illness, but 90 percent of patients develop a rash eventually. Neurologic manifestations of Rocky Mountain spotted fever include severe bifrontal headache, delirium, confusion, seizures, coma, and hyperreflexia. The combination of delirium and confusion with hyperreflexia and the presence of the characteristic rash should suggest the diagnosis. Abdominal pain, hepatosplenomegaly, diarrhea, conjunctivitis, lymphadenopathy, renal insufficiency, respiratory insufficiency, and myocarditis may develop during the course of the illness.[42]

Two human ehrlichioses may cause encephalitis. The ehrlichiae are small gram-negative pleomorphic coccobacilli. *Ehrlichia chaffeenis* causes human monocytic ehrlichiosis (HME) and infects mononuclear phagocytes in blood and tissue. An organism closely resembling *E. phagocytophila* and *E. equi* infects granulocytes and causes human granulocytic ehrlichioses (HGE). HGE is endemic to the northeastern United States.[43] The infectious agents of human ehrlichioses and Lyme disease are both transmitted by *Ixodes* sp. tick bites, and coinfection with *Borrelia burgdorferi* and ehrlichiae can occur. Symptoms of ehrlichioses begins 7 days after a tick bite with fever, chills, headache, myalgias, malaise, and in 50 percent or less, a maculopapular or petechial rash. The most characteristic clinical features are high fever and intense headache that may be associated with confusion, hyperreflexia, and ataxia.[42–44]

Diagnosis

Indirect immunofluorescent assay is the recommended serologic test for Rocky Mountain spotted fever. IgG titers greater than 1:64 and IgM titers greater than 1:32 are diagnostic, as is seroconversion with a twofold increase in titers over a 2-week period. It is important to obtain serial serologic studies because antibodies may not be present early in the disease course. Examination of the CSF in Rocky Mountain spotted fever demonstrates a lymphocytic or polymorphonuclear pleocytosis, an increased protein concentration, and a normal glucose concentration. In a small percentage of patients, the glucose concentration may be decreased.

The diagnosis of human ehrlichioses is made by demonstrating morulae (ehrlichial inclusion bodies) in leukocytes after Wright's or Giemsa staining of blood smears. The diagnosis also can be made by demonstrating a fourfold or greater rise or fall in antibody titer

by indirect immunofluorescence assay or by PCR amplification of HGE or HME nucleic acid from blood. The ehrlichioses are also associated with leukopenia with a leftward shift, lymphopenia, thrombocytopenia, and elevated hepatic aminotransferases.

Treatment

Rocky Mountain spotted fever and human monocytic and granulocytic ehrlichiosis are treated with doxycycline 100 mg intravenously every 12 hours. Rocky Mountain spotted fever is treated for at least 7 days and until the patient has been afebrile for at least 2 days. Human monocytic and granulocytic ehrlichioses are treated for a minimum of 5 to 7 days and for at least 3 days after defervescence.[43]

▶ POSTINFECTIOUS ENCEPHALOMYELITIS

Pathophysiology

Postinfectious encephalomyelitis is an acute monophasic disorder of the CNS that occurs within days to weeks of a viral illness or a vaccination. The viral illness typically is either an upper respiratory tract infection, varicella, or a nonspecific febrile illness. Postinfectious encephalomyelitis is not the result of primary neural tissue invasion by an organism; it is instead an autoimmune disease triggered by an infectious agent or an immunization.[8] The animal model of experimental allergic encephalomyelitis closely resembles the pathology of postinfectious encephalomyelitis. Experimental allergic encephalomyelitis is a demyelinating disorder of the CNS induced in animals by immunization with myelin extract proteins or peptides found in myelin. Experimental allergic encephalomyelitis can be transferred passively to normal animals by immune lymphocytes. These activated T cells assume a novel functional phenotype after transfer into a recipient animal that allows them to migrate to the CNS and pass through the blood-brain barrier. This migration briefly precedes the onset of clinical experimental allergic encephalomyelitis. There is a minimal interval of 3 days between the intravenous administration of pathogenic T cells and the onset of clinical experimental allergic encephalomyelitis.[46] Cells in the peripheral lymphoid tissues of individuals with postinfectious encephalomyelitis become immunologically committed to specific encephalitogenic antigens in the CNS.[47] Encephalitogenic CD4 and CD8 T-lymphocytes can be found in the blood, thymus, and secondary lymphoid tissues of apparently normal individuals that through the action of suppressive cytokines usually do not attack the CNS. T cells only become pathogenic if activated. One possibility is that an antigenic epitope from a microbe with a peptide that is structurally similar to myelin basic protein can trigger the activation of these self-reactive T cells by a mechanism known as *molecular mimicry*. Once activated, these cells expand in number and mature into effector T cells, producing mediators and cytokines that can react to normal self antigens, most importantly myelin.[46]

The lesions characteristic of postinfectious encephalomyelitis are around small veins in the cerebral white matter, brainstem, and spinal cord and are composed of mononuclear cells and lymphocytes. Luxol-fast blue stains that stain myelin reveal well-demarcated areas of loss of myelin. Staining for axons in the same area where there is loss of myelin reveals that the axon cylinders are relatively preserved. The neurons in the area show minor changes.[48]

Clinical Features

Postinfectious encephalomyelitis presents with the abrupt onset of neurologic symptoms 2 to 31 days after a viral illness or vaccination. Due to widespread areas of demyelination, there are often multifocal neurologic deficits, including bilateral optic neuritis, visual field deficits, ataxia, hemiparesis, paraparesis, aphasia, movement disorders, and sensory deficits. These signs may be associated with an altered level of consciousness ranging from lethargy to coma.[49] Maximum deficits are reached, on average, in 4 to 5 days, and then the patient begins to recover.[49,50] The extent of recovery depends on the preservation of axon cylinders and neurons.

Diagnosis

The diagnosis of postinfectious encephalomyelitis is based on clinical history, the presentation of a monophasic illness, evidence of multifocal neurologic deficits on neurologic examination, neuroimaging abnormalities of demyelination, and CSF analysis. T_2-weighted and FLAIR MRI images demonstrate areas of increased signal abnormality in the subcortical white matter, brainstem, cerebellum, and periventricular white matter[50] (Fig. 6-2). The lesions enhance with gadolinium during the acute illness. The lesions are bilateral, asymmetric, vary in size and number, and enhance in a nodular, spotty ring, or heterogeneous pattern after the administration of intravenous gadolinium DTPA . There may be lesions in gray matter as well. Involvement of the deep gray matter may help in distinguishing postinfectious encephalomyelitis from multiple sclerosis.[50]

This is a monophasic illness; therefore, partial resolution of existing lesions without new lesions during the recovery phase of the disease is critical in distinguishing postinfectious encephalomyelitis from other demyelinating diseases. CSF abnormalities include a mononuclear pleocytosis, an elevated protein concentration, and a normal glucose concentration. Myelin basic protein and oligoclonal bands may be detected in CSF.

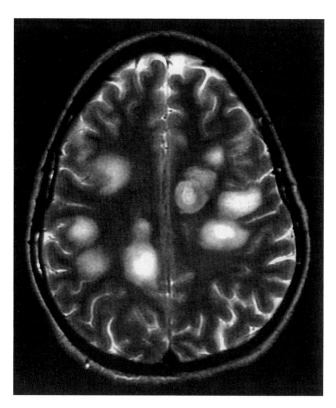

Figure 6–2. T_2-weighted MRI demonstrating multiple hyperintensities in subcortical white matter in postinfectious encephalomyelitis.

Treatment

High-dose corticosteroid therapy has been the standard of care for postinfectious encephalomyelitis for a long time, even though there are no double-blind, placebo-controlled clinical trials demonstrating the efficacy of this therapy. Typically, intravenous methylprednisolone in a daily dose of 1000 mg/d is given for 3 to 5 days. There are no firm guidelines on whether or not intravenous methylprednisolone therapy should be followed by an oral prednisone taper. A randomized, sham-controlled clinical trial of plasma exchange in patients with either multiple sclerosis (12 patients) or other inflammatory demyelinating diseases of the CNS (10 patients) was performed.[51] The 10 patients with other inflammatory demyelinating diseases than multiple sclerosis had transverse myelitis, postinfectious encephalomyelitis, neuromyelitis optica, and focal cerebral demyelinating lesions. The patients were randomly assigned to receive either true or sham plasma exchange every other day for 2 weeks. All patients had a severe clinical deficit and had failed to improve over a period of 2 weeks from the initiation of high-dose intravenous corticosteroid therapy. Eight patients who were treated with true plasma exchange experienced moderate to marked improvement at the end of 14 days. One patient who was given sham treatment had a moderate to marked improvement.[51] Based on the results of this study, the investigators recommended that plasma exchange be administered to patients with acute attacks of CNS inflammatory demyelinating diseases who failed treatment with intravenous high-dose corticosteroids.[51] There are a number of case reports of intravenous immunoglobulin therapy in acute disseminated encephalomyelitis.[52–54]

▶ PARANEOPLASTIC SYNDROMES

The possibility of paraneoplastic limbic encephalitis is considered in the patient who presents with confusion and/or seizures. Limbic encephalitis has been associated with small cell lung cancer, breast cancer, testicular germ cell tumors, and other solid tumors. The tumor may not be found for months or even years after the appearance of the neurologic disorder.[9] On MRI, there may be high signal abnormalities in the temporal lobes on T_2-weighted and FLAIR imaging having an appearance somewhat similar to HSV-1 encephalitis.

Examination of the CSF typically reveals a mild pleocytosis (30 to 40 white blood cells/mm[3]), a slightly elevated protein concentration (50 to 100 mg/dl), and an elevated IgG concentration. Approximately 60 percent of patients with paraneoplastic syndromes have antineuronal antibodies in their serum and CSF. The most common antineuronal antibodies associated with limbic encephalitis are anti-Hu, anti-Ma2, and anti-CRMP5.[55–57] Patients with suspected limbic encephalitis should have a chest CT scan, abdominal and pelvic CT scans, and a total-body fluorodeoxyglucose positron-emission tomographic (PET) scan.

Treatment is directed at identification and treatment of the tumor, as well as immunosuppressive therapy with intravenous corticosteroid therapy, plasma exchange, or IgIV.

▶ AUTOIMMUNE MENINGOENCEPHALITIS

Autoimmune meningoencephalitis refers to a syndrome of progressive fluctuating encephalopathy associated with a CSF lymphocytic or neutrophilic pleocytosis that responds to corticosteroid therapy.[58] This is primarily a diagnosis of exclusion supported by a clinical response to corticosteroid therapy. Chronic low-dose oral steroid therapy typically is required to prevent relapse. Antithyroglobulin antibodies and/or anti-thyroid peroxidase antibodies sometimes can be detected in serum. There is controversy about whether or not the detection of these antibodies is indicative of thyroid disease (Hashimoto's encephalopathy). Leptomeningeal biop-

sies of patients with nonvasculitic autoimmune meningoencephalitis show a perivascular lymphocytic infiltration that does not invade the vessel wall. A similar condition has been seen in association with other autoimmune diseases, including sarcoidosis, Sjögren's syndrome, and systemic lupus erythematosus.[59,60]

REFERENCES

1. Connelly KP, DeWitt LD: Neurologic complications of infectious mononucleosis. *Pediatr Neurol* 10:181, 1994.
2. Patchell RA: Neurological complications of organ transplantation. *Ann Neurol* 36:688, 1994.
3. Caserta MT, Mock DJ, Dewhurst S: Human herpesvirus 6. *Clin Infect Dis* 33:829, 2001.
4. Zerr DM, Gupta D, Huang ML, et al: Effect of antivirals on human herpesvirus 6 replication in hematopoietic stem cell transplant recipients. *Clin Infect Dis* 34:309, 2002.
5. McCullers JA, Lakeman FD, Whitley RJ: Human herpesvirus 6 is associated with focal encephalitis. *Clin Infect Dis* 21:571, 1995.
6. Kamei A, Ichinohe S, Onuma R, et al: Acute disseminated demyelination due to primary human herpesvirus-6 infection. *Eur J Pediatr* 156:709, 1997
7. Hartung HP, Grossman RI: ADEM: Distinct disease or part of the MS spectrum. *Neurology* 56:1257, 2001.
8. Gurvich EB, Vilesova IS: Vaccinia virus in postvaccinial encephalitis. *Acta Virol* 27(2):154, 1983.
9. Darnell RB, Posner JB: Paraneoplastic syndromes involving the nervous system. *New Engl J Med* 349:1543, 2003
10. Whitley RJ, Kimberlin DW, Roizman B: Herpes simplex viruses. *Clin Infect Dis* 26:541, 1998.
11. Barnett EM, Jacobsen G, Evans G, et al: Herpes simplex encephalitis in the temporal cortex and limbic system after trigeminal nerve inoculation. *J Infect Dis* 169:782, 1994.
12. Stroop WG, Schaefer DC: Production of encephalitis restricted to the temporal lobes by experimental reactivation of herpes simplex virus. *J Infect Dis* 153:721, 1986.
13. Johnson RT: The pathogenesis of acute viral encephalitis and postinfectious encephalomyelitis. *J Infect Dis* 155:359, 1987.
14. McJunkin JE, de los Reyes EC, Irazuzta JE, et al: La Crosse encephalitis in children. *New Engl J Med* 344:801, 2001.
15. Solomon T: Exotic and emerging viral encephalitides. *Curr Opin Neurol* 16:411, 2003.
16. Calisher CH: Medically important arboviruses of the United States and Canada. *Clin Microbiol Rev* 7:89, 1994.
17. Johnson KP, Lepow ML, Johnson RT: California encephalitis: I. Clinical and epidemiological studies. *Neurology* 18:250, 1968.
18. McJunkin JE, Khan RR, Tsai TF: California–La Crosse encephalitis. *Infect Dis Clin North Am* 12:83, 1998.
19. Petersen LR, Roehrig JT, Hughes JM: West Nile virus encephalitis. *New Engl J Med* 347:1225, 2002.
20. Sejvar JJ, Haddad MB, Tierney BC, et al: Neurologic

manifestations and outcome of West Nile virus infection. *JAMA* 290:511, 2003.

21. Whitley RJ: Viral encephalitis. *New Engl J Med* 323:242, 1990.

22. Bale JF: Viral encephalitis. *Med Clin North Am* 77:25, 1993.

23. Pradhan S, Pandey N, Shashank S, et al: Parkinsonism due to predominant involvement of substantia nigra in Japanese encephalitis. *Neurology* 53:1781, 1999.

24. Johnson RT, Burke DS, Elwell M, et al: Japanese encephalitis: Immunocytochemical studies of viral antigen and inflammatory cells in fatal cases. *Ann Neurol* 18:567, 1985.

25. Feemster RF: Equine encephalitis in Massachusetts. *New Engl J Med* 257:701, 1957.

26. Hanley DF, Ray G: Viral encephalitis: When it's likely. *Patient Care* (June 15):293, 1992.

27. Schultz DR, Barthal JS, Garrett C. Western equine encephalitis with rapid onset of parkinsonism. *Neurology* 27:1095, 1972.

28. Jelinek T, Muhlberger N, Harms G, et al: Epidemiology and clinical features of imported dengue fever in Europe: Sentinel surveillance data from Trop Net Europ. *Clin Infect Dis* 35:1047, 2002.

29. Gubler DJ: Dengue and dengue hemorrhagic fever. *Clin Microbiol Rev* 11:480, 1998.

30. Rigau-Perez JG, Gubler DJ, Zorndam AZ, et al: Dengue: A literature review and case study of travelers from the United States 1986–1994. *J Travel Med* 4:65, 1997.

31. Johnson RT: Emerging viral infections of the nervous system. *J Neurovirol* 9:140, 2003.

32. Dumpis U, Crook D, Oksi J: Tick-borne encephalitis. *Clin Infect Dis* 28:882, 1999.

33. Arboviral disease—United States, 1994. *MMWR* 44:641, 1995.

34. Caserta MT, Hall CB, Schnabel K, et al: Neuroinvasion and persistence of human herpesvirus 6 in children. *J Infect Dis* 170:1586, 1994.

35. Luppi M, Barozzi P, Maiorana A, et al: Human herpesvirus-6: A survey of presence and distribution of genomic sequences in normal brain and neuroglial tumors. *J Med Virol* 47:105, 1995.

36. McJunkin JE, Kahn R, de los Reyes EC, Parsons DL, et al: Treatment of severe LaCrosse encephalitis with intravenous ribavirin following diagnosis by brain biopsy. *Pediatrics* 99(2):261, 1997.

37. Ben-Nathan D, Lustig S, Tam G, et al: Prophylactic and therapeutic efficacy of human intravenous immunoglobulin in treating West Nile virus infection in mice. *J Infect Dis* 188:5, 2003.

38. Breton G, Fillet AM, Katlama C, et al: Acyclovir-resistant herpes zoster in human immunodeficiency virus–infected patients: Results of foscarnet therapy. *Clin Infect Dis* 27:1525, 1998.

39. Poscher ME: Successful treatment of varicella-zoster virus meningoencephalitis in patients with AIDS. *AIDS* 8:1115, 1994.

40. Cole PD, Stiles J, Boulad F, et al: Successful treatment of human herpesvirus 6 encephalitis in a bone marrow transplant recipient. *Clin Infect Dis* 27:653, 1998.

41. Studahl M, Bergstrom T, Hagberg L. Acute viral encephalitis in adults: A prospective study. *Scand J Infect Dis* 30:215, 1998.

42. Spah DH, Liles WC, Campbell GL, et al: Tick-borne diseases in the United States. *New Engl J Med* 329:936, 1993.

43. Dumler JS, Bakken JS: Ehrlichial diseases of humans: Emerging tick-borne infections. *Clin Infect Dis* 20:1102, 1995.

44. Ratnasamy N, Eberett ED, Roland WE, et al: Central nervous system manifestations of human ehrlichioses. *Clin Infect Dis* 23:314, 1996.

45. Orgad S, Cohen IR: Autoimmune encephalomyelitis: Activation of thymus lymphocytes against syngeneic brain antigens in vitro. *Science* 183:1083, 1974.

46. Wekerle H: Immune protection of the brain: efficient and delicate. *J Infect Dis* 186(2):140, 2002.

47. de Vos AF, van Meurs M, Brok HP, et al: Transfer of central nervous system autoantigens and presentation in secondary lymphoid organs. *J Immunol* 5415, 2002.

48. Scott TF: Postinfectious and vaccinal encephalitis. *Med Clin North Am* 51:701, 1967.

49. Hartung HP, Grossman RI: ADEM: Distinct disease or part of the MS spectrum. *Neurology* 56:1257, 2001.

50. Hynson JL, Kornberg AJ, Coleman LT, et al: Clinical and neuroradiologic features of acute disseminated encephalomyelitis in children. *Neurology* 56:1308, 2001.

51. Weinshenker BG: Plasma exchange for severe attacks of inflammatory demyelinating diseases of the central nervous system. *J Clin Apheresis* 16:39, 2001.

52. Marchioni E, Marinou-Aktipi K, Uggeti C, et al: Effectiveness of intravenous immunoglobulin treatment in adult patients with steroid-resistant monophasic or recurrent acute disseminated encephalomyelitis. *J Neurol* 249:100, 2002.

53. Nishikawa M, Ichiyama T, Hayashi T, et al: Intravenous immunoglobulin therapy in acute disseminated encephalomyelitis. *Pediatr Neurol* 21:583, 1999.

54. Kleiman M, Brunquell P: Acute disseminated encephalomyelitis: Response to intravenous immunoglobulin. *J Child Neurol* 10:481, 1995.

55. Alamowitch S, Graus F, Uchuya M, et al: Limbic encephalitis and small cell lung cancer: Clinical and immunological features. *Brain* 120:923, 1997.

56. Voltz R, Gultekin SH, Rosenfeld MR, et al: A serologic marker of paraneoplastic limbic and brainstem encephalitis in patients with testicular cancer. *New Engl J Med* 340:1788, 1999.

57. Kinirons P, Fulton A, Keoghan M, et al: Paraneoplastic limbic encephalitis (PLE) and chorea associated with CRMP-5 neuronal antibody. *Neurology* 61:1623, 2003.

58. Caselli RJ, Boeve BF, Scheithauer BW, et al: Nonvasculitic autoimmune inflammatory meningoencephalitis (NAIM): A reversible form of encephalopathy. *Neurology* 53(7):1579, 1999.

59. Ho SU, Berenberg RA, Kim KS, Dal Canto MC: Sarcoid encephalopathy with diffuse inflammation and focal hydrocephalus shown by sequential CT. *Neurology* 29(8):1161, 1979.

60. Caselli RJ, Scheithauer BW, Bowles CA, et al: The treatable dementia of Sjögren's syndrome. *Ann Neurol* 39(1):98, 1991.

CHAPTER 7

Opportunistic Infections of the Central Nervous System in HIV-Infected Individuals

Julio Collazos

TOXOPLASMIC ENCEPHALITIS

PROGRESSIVE MULTIFOCAL
   LEUKOENCEPHALOPATHY

CRYPTOCOCOCCAL MENINGITIS

PRIMARY CENTRAL NERVOUS SYSTEM LYMPHOMA

CYTOMEGALOVIRUS INFECTIONS

The central nervous system (CNS) is the second most frequently affected organ in patients with human immunodeficiency virus (HIV) infection, surpassed only by the lung. Symptoms of CNS disease were reported by one-third to two-thirds of patients with the acquired immunodeficiency syndrome (AIDS) before the introduction of highly active antiretroviral therapy (HAART), and pathologic evidence of CNS involvement was found in 60 to 75 percent of these patients at autopsy.[1–6]

However, the epidemiology of the opportunistic conditions associated with HIV infection has changed due to the availability of HAART in the past few years, resulting in a considerable reduction in the morbidity and longer survival periods for most of these conditions in comparison with the pre-HAART values.[7–10] However, all the classic CNS opportunistic infections still occur, usually in patients with severe depression in their CD4 lymphocyte counts. The most common opportunistic neurologic infections according to a recent series were toxoplasmic encephalitis in 31 percent of patients, HIV encephalitis in 18 percent, progressive multifocal leukoencephalopathy (PML) in 15 percent, cryptococcal meningitis in 11 percent, primary CNS lymphoma (PCNSL) in 4 percent, tuberculosis in 3 percent, and cytomegalovirus infections in 2 percent.[11] HIV encephalitis and tuberculosis are discussed elsewhere in this book, and toxoplasmic encephalitis, PML, cryptococcal meningitis, PCNSL, and cytomegalovirus infection are reviewed in this chapter.

▶ TOXOPLASMIC ENCEPHALITIS

Etiology and Epidemiology

Toxoplasma gondii is a ubiquitous obligate intracellular parasite that exists in nature in three forms: the oocyst; the tissue cyst, which contains bradyzoites; and the tachyzoite or invasive form. The definitive hosts are members of the feline family, which eliminate oocysts in their feces. *Toxoplasma* infection is prevalent worldwide. Seroprevalence in the general population varies greatly from country to country, being higher in certain European countries (70 to 90 percent) than in the United States (10 to 40 percent).[3,12,13] This protozoan usually does not cause significant disease in immunocompetent individuals, but it produces a serious illness in HIV-infected patients.

Toxoplasmic encephalitis is the most common cause of a CNS mass lesion in patients infected with HIV. Before the introduction of HAART, toxoplasmic encephalitis occurred in 3 to 50 percent of patients with AIDS who had latent infection,[1–4,13–15] but the incidence of the disease has decreased substantially in recent years owing to the combined effect of primary prophylaxis

of the population at risk and especially to the introduction of HAART.[9,16,17] Although a history of other AIDS-defining conditions is present in many patients at the time of presentation with toxoplasmic encephalitis, this infection constitutes the first opportunistic infection in 30 to 50 percent of patients.[12,14]

Pathogenesis and Pathology

Humans become infected with *T. gondii* by ingesting oocysts or by ingesting raw or undercooked meat, mainly pork and lamb, containing tissue cysts. After ingestion, the cysts release the parasites in the intestine. The parasites are then disseminated via lymphatics and the bloodstream. As the immune response develops, the parasites encyst in different tissues, mainly the brain, skeletal muscle, myocardium, and retina. The protozoan remains in a state of latency indefinitely, usually for life, unless there is a decrease in the cellular immune response of the host.[3,4,13,18] Consequently, most cases of toxoplasmic encephalitis in AIDS patients result from reactivation of a latent brain infection.[1,3,12,14] This reactivation occurs in severely immunosuppressed patients with CD4 counts below 100 cells/μl, although some patients may develop the infection with higher CD4 counts.[3,12,19,20]

The lesion begins as a single focus or, more commonly, multiple foci of encephalitis at the site of infection that progress toward the formation of abscesses of different sizes with necrosis and surrounding inflammation and edema. Uncommonly, diffuse encephalitis without any identifiable focal lesion may be found. The foci of encephalitis may involve the gray and the white matter and are mainly located in the frontal and parietal lobes, especially at the corticomedullary junction, although they can develop anywhere within the CNS.[1,3,13]

Clinical Features

Toxoplasmic encephalitis may present with focal symptoms and signs or as a subacute encephalopathy. Often focal neurologic disturbances are superimposed on a global encephalopathy. The clinical manifestations depend mainly on the number and location of the lesions and on the intensity of the surrounding edema. Fever, present in about 40 to 70 percent of patients, and headache, present in 50 to 60 percent of patients, dating from several days to a few weeks earlier constitute the most common presenting symptoms. Focal manifestations such as hemiparesis, hemianopsia, and aphasia are observed in 20 to 80 percent, cranial nerve palsies in 10 to 20 percent, and visual disturbances in 10 to 15 percent of patients at presentation. Encephalopathy, manifested as the subacute onset of confusion, loss of concentration and orientation, behavioral changes, and lethargy, may be part of the clinical presentation in 15 to 45 percent of patients, and it may be difficult to differentiate from other infections, such as HIV encephalitis, although the onset of symptoms is more recent in toxoplasmic encephalitis. Other common manifestations are seizures and ataxia, which are seen in about 15 to 30 percent of patients. Cerebellar signs and symptoms, speech disturbances, chorea, and nausea and vomiting also may be present.[2–4,12,15,19–22]

Diagnosis

IgG antibodies against *T. gondii* are detected in the serum of the vast majority of patients with toxoplasmic encephalitis, whereas IgM antibodies are uncommon.[3,12,14,19,23] Although the antibody titers are commonly high, a fourfold increase in the IgG titer is rarely detected; therefore, changes in this titer are unreliable for diagnostic purposes.[12] A major drawback of serologic studies for the diagnosis of toxoplasmic encephalitis is that seroprevalence among the general population is very high, particularly in some European countries, a fact that limits considerably the predictive value of the test. In addition, negative serologic findings are observed in a small fraction of patients with toxoplasmic encephalitis, usually fewer than 6 percent,[3,12,19] although values as high as 17 percent have been reported.[20] Consequently, the finding of *Toxoplasma*-specific antibodies in serum is not helpful for the diagnosis, but their absence is evidence against the diagnosis of toxoplasmic encephalitis, and other conditions, mainly PCNSL, should be considered.

Routine cerebrospinal fluid (CSF) studies are not useful because they lack sensitivity and specificity. CSF findings may be normal in almost 50 percent of patients or may show only mild inflammatory changes, with different combinations of mild mononuclear pleocytosis, elevated protein concentrations, or slightly decreased glucose concentrations.[3,4,12,13,20] The findings on electroencephalography (EEG) are nonspecific, usually showing focal abnormalities at the site of the lesions, as well as general changes in the background activity.[4] The value of the determination of intrathecal antibodies specific against *T. gondii* is limited, mainly due to its low sensitivity (in the range of 60 to 70 percent).[3,24,25] The usefulness of the polymerase chain reaction (PCR) for *Toxoplasma* DNA in CSF is also limited by a sensitivity of about 50 to 60 percent, although it may be improved if the test is performed within the first week of therapy before the parasite is cleared from the CSF. The specificity and positive predictive value of the DNA detection test are higher than 95 percent, and the negative predictive value is about 90 percent.[3,13,24,26] Therefore, a positive test is highly suggestive of the diagnosis, but a negative test does not exclude it. The sensitivity

of the PCR in blood is very low, and isolation of the parasite from blood is uncommon. Consequently, these procedures may be useful only in cases of disseminated disease.[24]

Imaging studies, mainly computed tomography (CT) and magnetic resonance imaging (MRI), should be performed in all patients in whom toxoplasmic encephalitis is considered because they are very helpful for diagnosis (Fig. 7-1). The typical findings on CT scan are those of one or, more commonly, multiple hypodense lesions with surrounding edema, mass effect, and ring enhancement after the infusion of contrast material, although nodular homogeneous enhancement or no enhancement also may be seen.[2–4,12,14,20] However, most of the cases in which there is no immediate enhancement after the infusion of contrast material demonstrate enhancement in late scans obtained after a double dose of contrast material.[12] MRI, which is more sensitive than CT scan, allowing for the detection of lesions overlooked by the latter, shows lesions with low signal intensity and ring enhancement with gadolinium on T_1-weighted imaging and relatively high signal intensity on T_2-weighted imaging.[1–3,12–14]

The main differential diagnosis of toxoplasmic encephalitis is PCNSL, the other major cause of CNS mass lesions in patients with AIDS. Thallium-201 single-photon-emission CT (SPECT) and positron-emission tomography (PET) have been reported to be helpful in the differentiation of toxoplasmic encephalitis and PCNSL. The absence of increased uptake in mass lesions on SPECT and decreased activity on PET are the most characteristic findings in toxoplasmic encephalitis.[3,13] In addition, the combined use of SPECT with serum *Toxoplasma* serology yields an improved diagnostic accuracy.[23]

The histopathologic demonstration of tachyzoites in the involved tissue obtained through brain biopsy is the only unequivocal method to establish the diagnosis of toxoplasmic encephalitis. Although stereotactic biopsy seems to be a relatively safe technique,[3,14,27] it carries certain risks, does not always yield the diagnosis, and may be misleading by showing other concomitant pathogens. Therefore, an empirical diagnosis based on a compatible clinical and radiologic picture and the response to therapy is used commonly in clinical practice.[3,4,24] A favorable clinical and radiologic response is expected to occur in about 80 to 90 percent of the patients by the second week of therapy. Consequently, a patient with positive *T. gondii* serology and ring-enhancing lesions on imaging studies should be treated with anti-*Toxoplasma* drugs for 1 to 2 weeks. If there is a response, it can be assumed that the lesions are due to toxoplasmic encephalitis, and brain biopsy should be considered only for patients who do not respond to this regimen.[1,3,13,14,20] However, an etiologic

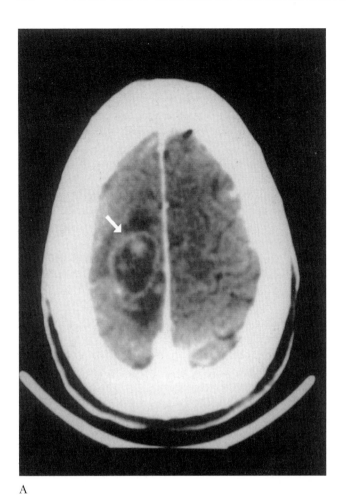

A

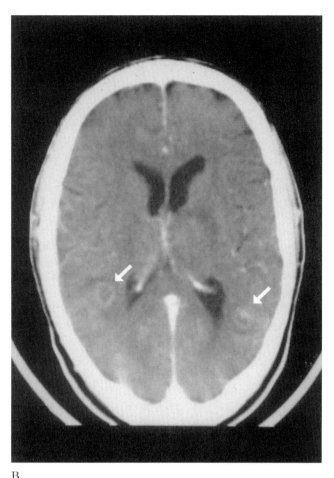

B

Figure 7-1. Toxoplasmic encephalitis. CT scan revealing multiple hypodense lesions with surrounding edema and ring enhancement after the infusion of contrast material (*arrows*).

diagnosis also may be reached without brain biopsy in patients who do not respond to empirical anti-*Toxoplasma* therapy. Figure 7-2 shows a diagnostic algorithm for HIV-infected patients who present with CNS manifestations based on the radiologic appearance of the lesions and the relative frequency of each condition.

Treatment and Outcome

The current anti-*Toxoplasma* therapy is active against the tachyzoites, but it does not eradicate the tissue cysts, which may be responsible for later episodes of reactivation.[12,13] Therefore, treatment for this condition includes an induction phase to control the active disease and a maintenance phase or secondary prophylaxis to avoid relapses. The first-choice regimen for toxoplasmic encephalitis in HIV-infected patients is the combination of pyrimethamine, an inhibitor of dihydrofolate reductase, and sulfadiazine, an inhibitor of tetrahydrofolate synthetase, which act synergistically against *T. gondii* when used in combination. Since these drugs act through the blockade of folate metabolism, folinic acid should be added to reduce the bone marrow tox-

icity of the treatment. The efficacy of this regimen has been demonstrated in many studies, with response rates greater than 80 percent, usually within the first 1 to 2 weeks.[1,3,12,14,20–22] This induction treatment should be continued for 6 weeks, although shorter treatment periods are acceptable for patients in whom there is complete resolution or marked improvement of the lesions. Common side effects of this regimen include bone marrow suppression, rash, and fever. These adverse effects occur in more than 50 percent of patients treated with pyrimethamine and sulfadiazine and lead to a change in the initial regimen in most of them.[12,20,22]

The combination of pyrimethamine and clindamycin seems to have a more favorable toxicity profile than pyrimethamine and sulfadiazine, its most common side effects in HIV-infected patients being rash and diarrhea. Although clindamycin inhibits the protein synthesis in bacteria, the mechanism of action against *T. gondii* is unknown. The response to this combination is similar to the response to pyrimethamine and sulfadiazine in the induction phase, although its long-term efficacy may be somewhat lower.[14,15,20,22] Therefore, this combination is considered the main alternative to

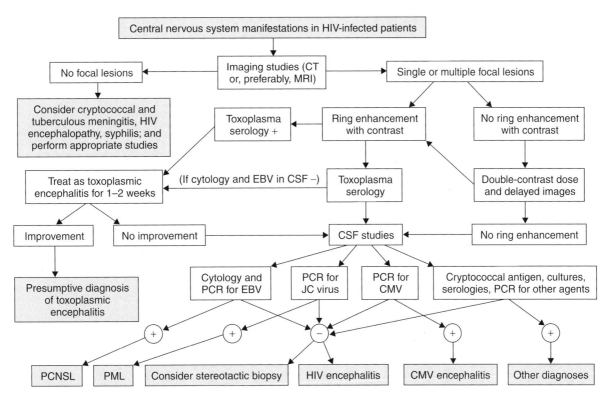

Figure 7-2. Diagnostic algorithm for the management of HIV-infected patients with CNS manifestations. (CT = computed tomography; MRI = magnetic resonance imaging; + = positive result; − = negative result; CSF = cerebrospinal fluid; PCR = polymerase chain reaction; EBV = Epstein-Barr virus; CMV = cytomegalovirus; PC-NSL = primary central nervous system lymphoma; PML = progressive multifocal leukoencephalopathy.)

the pyrimethamine-sulfadiazine regimen. Many other drugs have activity against *T. gondii* and also may be used in patients unresponsive or intolerant to the preceding regimens. These drugs include trimethoprim-sulfamethoxazole, macrolides, azalides, tetracyclines, trimetrexate, atovaquone, and dapsone, among others.[10,13,15,21,28] The therapeutic regimens commonly used for the induction treatment of toxoplasmic encephalitis are shown in Table 7-1.

The use of corticosteroids to treat the accompanying edema is controversial if the diagnosis of toxoplasmic encephalitis is presumptive. Corticosteroids also may improve the clinical and radiologic manifestations of PCNSL; therefore, this response may be falsely attributed to the effect of anti-*Toxoplasma* therapy. In the absence of a definitive diagnosis, the use of corticosteroids probably should be avoided.[2,3]

Relapses are very common if anti-*Toxoplasma* therapy is discontinued after induction therapy.[8,10,12] A maintenance phase of treatment should be initiated after the induction phase. This secondary prophylaxis is usually carried out with the same drugs that were used successfully for the induction phase, although at lower doses.

Before the HAART era, the median duration of survival for patients with toxoplasmic encephalitis was approximately 10 to 13 months[3,12]; the course in these se-

verely immunosuppressed patients was characterized by relapses of the infection, even in the presence of maintenance therapy, or development of other opportunistic infections. HAART not only has reduced the incidence of the infection but also has considerably improved its outcome. The immune recovery induced by the antiretroviral therapy has been associated with restoration of *T. gondii*–specific T-cell responses.[29,30] Therefore, antiretroviral therapy should be initiated as soon as possible in all patients with toxoplasmic encephalitis.

Prophylaxis and Prevention

For patients who have serologic evidence of *T. gondii* infection and who are severely immunocompromised with CD4 counts below 100 cells/μl, primary prophylaxis is indicated, and the drug of choice is trimethoprim-sulfamethoxazole. Primary prophylaxis should be maintained until the CD4 counts are higher than 200 cells/μl, and this increase is sustained for at least 3 months.[3,8,10]

As discussed earlier, maintenance therapy is necessary after completion of the induction phase to try to prevent relapses. Although maintenance therapy should be continued for life in the absence of antiretroviral therapy, in patients who reach a certain degree of im-

▶ **TABLE 7-1.** REGIMENS USED FOR THE TREATMENT AND PROPHYLAXIS OF *TOXOPLASMA* ENCEPHALITIS

	Primary Prophylaxis	Induction Therapy	Maintenance Therapy
First-choice regimens	TMP-SMZ (160/800 mg daily PO)	Pyrimethamine (100–120 mg loading dose, then 50–100 mg daily PO) + sulfadiazine (1–1.5 g q6h PO) + folinic acid (10–20 mg daily PO) all for 6 weeks	Pyrimethamine (25–50 mg daily PO) + sulfadiazine (0.5–1 g q6h PO) + folinic acid (10–25 mg daily PO)
Alternative regimens	TMP-SMZ (80/400 mg daily PO) Pyrimethamine (50 mg weekly PO) + dapsone (50 mg daily PO) + folinic acid (25 mg weekly PO) Pyrimethamine (75 mg weekly PO) + dapsone (200 mg weekly PO) + folinic acid (25 mg weekly PO) Atovaquone (1.5 g daily PO) Pyrimethamine (25 mg daily PO) + atovaquone (1.5 g daily PO) + folinic acid (10 mg daily PO) Pyrimethamine (25 mg twice a week PO) + sulfadoxine (500 mg twice a week PO) + folinic acid (15 mg twice weekly PO)	Pyrimethamine and folinic acid as above + clindamycin (600–900 mg q6h PO or IV) all for 6 weeks Pyrimethamine and folinic acid as above + clarithromycin (1 g q12h PO) all for 6 weeks Pyrimethamine and folinic acid as above + azithromycin (1.2–1.5 g daily PO) all for 6 weeks Pyrimethamine and folinic acid as above + dapsone (100 mg daily PO) all for 6 weeks Pyrimethamine and folinic acid as above + atovaquone (750 mg q6h PO) for 6 weeks Sulfadiazine (1–1.5 g q6h PO) + atovaquone (1.5 g q12h PO) for 6 weeks TMP-SMZ (5/25 mg/kg q12h PO or IV) for 30 days	Pyrimethamine (25–50 mg daily PO) + clindamycin (300–450 mg q6–8h PO) + folinic acid (10–25 mg daily PO) Atovaquone (750 mg q6–12h PO) Pyrimethamine (25 mg daily PO) + atovaquone (750 mg q6–12 h PO) + folinic acid (10 mg daily PO)

SOURCE: *Adapted from Collazos J: Opportunistic infections of the central nervous system in patients with acquired immunodeficiency syndrome: Diagnosis and management. CNS Drugs 17:869, 2003.*

mune reconstitution, as measured by a sustained increase in CD4 counts above 200 cells/μl for at least 6 months, discontinuation of the otherwise lifelong suppressive therapy may be accomplished safely.[3,8,10,31] The regimens used for primary and secondary prophylaxis are described in Table 7-1.

Since the mechanism of infection in humans is through ingestion and contact with oocysts from cat feces and tissue cysts from contaminated meat or other products, preventive measures in seronegative HIV-infected individuals should be based on avoidance of these risk factors. Contact with material potentially contaminated with cat feces should be avoided, and the use of gloves is advisable if this contact is unavoidable. Since oocysts require 1 to 5 days to become infective, the cat litter box should be cleaned daily, and the cats should be kept inside and not fed raw or undercooked meat. The cysts become noninfectious by heating the meat above 70°C or by freezing it below -20°C. Meat should be cooked sufficiently to eliminate any pink meat inside. Ingestion of raw eggs and unpasteurized milk should be avoided, and fruits and vegetables should be washed carefully before eating. Contact of mucous membranes with raw meat also should be avoided, and the hands should be washed thoroughly after such contact.[10,18]

▶ PROGRESSIVE MULTIFOCAL LEUKOENCEPHALOPATHY

Etiology and Epidemiology

JC virus, so named for the initials of the patient from whom it was first isolated in 1971, is the causative agent of progressive multifocal leukoencephalopathy (PML). JC virus is a ubiquitous DNA-containing polyomavirus that infects up to 80 to 90 percent of the general population, mainly during childhood or early adulthood.[1,3,13] The epidemiology of this infection is unclear. It is thought that transmission of JC virus requires close contact, and the virus is most likely transmitted through respiratory droplets. JC virus causes a silent or minimally symptomatic infection that is followed by a state of latency in lymphoid tissue, kidney, and possibly brain until immunosuppression develops and the virus reactivates, causing PML.[3,13,32]

Initially, PML was associated mainly with lymphoproliferative malignancies, but the incidence of the disease increased abruptly shortly after emergence of the HIV pandemic. Since then, HIV infection has constituted the underlying condition in the vast majority of cases of PML. PML was diagnosed in 1 to 10 percent of patients with AIDS in the pre-HAART era[2,3,13,14,33–35] and although its incidence seems to have decreased somewhat during the past few years, the decrease has

not been as marked as for other opportunistic conditions.[3,9,16,36,37] PML occurs in severely immunosuppressed patients with CD4 counts usually below 100 cells/μl, although cases in patients with higher CD4 counts also occur.[3,13,34,38–41] This entity represents the first AIDS-defining illness in 25 to 60 percent of HIV-infected patients.[2,13,14,34,42,43]

Pathogenesis and Pathology

It is unclear whether PML is the consequence of reactivation of latent JC virus infection in brain or whether the virus is transported from other infected organs to the brain.[14,32] Regardless of the pathogenetic mechanism, data suggest that the relationship between PML and HIV infection is not casual but the result of a cooperative interaction between the two pathogens. In fact, HIV infection is associated with a disruption of the blood-brain barrier and with a lack of JC virus–specific cytotoxic T-lymphocytes; in addition, the regulatory tat protein of HIV favors JC virus replication.[3,13,44–46] Therefore, patients with HIV infection have a special predisposition for the development of PML.

PML is characterized by multiple asymmetric foci of demyelinating lesions in different stages of evolution that result from a lytic infection of oligodendrocytes and astrocytes by JC virus.[2,3,47] These lesions occur mainly in the white matter of the frontal, parietal, and occipital lobes, although the cerebellum and brain stem also may be involved, and the gray matter may be affected in advanced cases. Viral inclusions can be demonstrated in the enlarged, hyperchromatic, and bizarre nuclei of oligodendrocytes and astrocytes by electron microscopy, in situ hybridization, or immunocytochemistry.[2,3,13,14]

Clinical Features

The signs and symptoms of PML at presentation are quite varied because they depend on the extent of the lesions and the areas of the brain that are involved. Altered mental status and/or focal neurologic deficits of subacute presentation and progressive course are the most common manifestations. Cognitive deficits and memory loss evolving to progressive dementia are seen in about 30 to 60 percent of patients, and 50 to 70 percent of patients may present with focal or generalized weakness. Visual disturbances, such as homonymous hemianopsia, other visual field deficits, and cortical blindness, are present in 20 to 50 percent of patients, as well as speech disturbances in 20 to 50 percent. Gait abnormalities occur in 30 to 65 percent and incoordination in 20 to 45 percent of patients. Sensory deficits, seizures, vertigo, and headache are less common manifestations.[1–3,13,33,34,40,43] If untreated, the neurologic abnormalities usually evolve over the course of weeks or months to coma and death,[1,13,33] although spontaneous fluctuations in the clinical course and prolonged survival are observed in some patients.[3,33,42]

The possibility of asymptomatic infection has been suggested by the finding of JC virus genomic sequences in the brains of some patients who did not have clinical evidence of PML.[48] The significance of these findings is unclear. This may indicate that JC virus is not invariably associated with clinical disease or that these patients were in the very earlier phases of the infection before development of the clinical manifestations. It also should be stressed that PML may develop concurrently with other CNS infections, mainly HIV encephalopathy, in the same or other areas of the brain.[33,49]

Diagnosis

A definitive diagnosis of PML can be obtained only by brain biopsy with demonstration of the typical histopathologic findings and the presence of JC virus in tissue by the appropriate techniques. However, as indicated earlier, brain biopsy has some drawbacks, and the diagnosis in clinical practice usually is made by noninvasive methods.

The typical findings on CT scan are multiple foci of low attenuation in the white matter of both cerebral hemispheres, mainly in the parieto-occipital lobes, that do not exhibit mass effect and do not enhance after the infusion of contrast media.[2,3,13,33,43] Lesions, however, may be single and may involve the gray matter and structures of the posterior fossa; occasionally, they may

exhibit minimal mass effect. MRI is more sensitive than CT scan for the detection of PML lesions,[40] and characteristically, the lesions of PML are hypointense on T_1-weighted images and hyperintense on T_2-weighted sequences without gadolinium enhancement[2,3,13,33,43] (Fig. 7-3). An abnormal MRI pattern has been described and may be related to the existence of inflammatory changes, as demonstrated by histopathologic studies,[50,51] characterized by rim enhancement with gadolinium in patients with relatively preserved immunity or in those in whom immune reconstitution is being achieved with antiretroviral therapy.[52–54]

CSF analysis may reveal normal or nonspecific findings, with a mildly elevated protein concentration and a mild mononuclear pleocytosis in some patients.[2,3,33] Measurement of the intrathecal synthesis of JC virus–specific antibodies has been found to be 76 percent sensitive and 97 percent specific for PML in one study.[55] However, the most commonly used method for the diagnosis of lesions suspicious of PML is the investigation of JC virus DNA in CSF by PCR. Although the method used and the biologic sensitivity of the different assays may influence the accuracy of this procedure, the sensitivity of the PCR for this purpose is usually greater than 70 to 80 percent as values increase with the progression of the disease. The specificity is greater than 90 percent, and the positive and negative predictive values are higher than 85 to 90 percent.[3,13,24,35]

Therefore, a patient who presents with a compatible clinical and radiologic picture and in whom JC virus

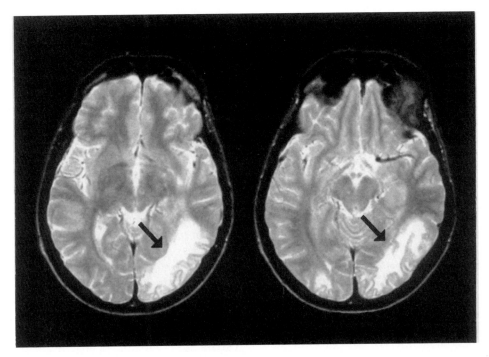

Figure 7-3. Progressive multifocal leukoencephalopathy. T_2-weighted MRI showing an ill-defined increased signal intensity in the left occipitotemporal subcortical white matter (*arrows*).

DNA is detected in CSF can be assumed to have PML. Conversely, a negative test does not exclude PML, although it suggests that other diagnoses should be considered. The significance of the detection of JC virus DNA in some asymptomatic patients is unclear. It is possible that this detection could constitute an early sign of the infection, indicating that these patients should be followed up carefully to identify the clinical manifestations of the disease as early as possible in order to take the appropriate measures in the earliest phases of the infection.[35]

The amount of JC virus DNA in CSF can be measured by quantitative PCR. This quantification seems to be of some help for evaluating the response to therapy, and it also may have prognostic implications because the amount of DNA has been related to patient survival.[3,36–39,41] Finally, JC virus DNA also may be detected in other body fluids, such as blood or urine, although the usefulness of detecting JC virus DNA in other body fluids is limited owing to its low sensitivity and specificity.[56,57]

Treatment and Outcome

The efficacy of any specific treatment for this condition has not been proven definitively. Many drugs, including cytosine arabinoside, amantadine, vidarabine, acyclovir, and interferon alpha, have been used generally in anecdotal cases or small series with varied but usually unsatisfactory results.[1,3,21,34,58] In addition, interpretation of the response to a particular drug is hampered by the fact that some patients may experience spontaneous improvement and longer-than-expected survival periods.[3,33,42] Therefore, the response to treatment should be evaluated in terms of disease activity as evaluated by the sum of clinical, radiologic, and virologic data.[59]

Another drug that has been used for the treatment of PML is cidofovir, a nucleotide analogue developed mainly for the treatment of cytomegalovirus infections that is also active against polyomaviruses in vitro.[60] Again, the small sample size of most studies, the lack of randomization and adequate controls, the different study designs and characteristics of the patients, and the interference of other interventions, such as the use of antiretroviral therapy, may have had a significant impact on the diverse results observed.[37–40,61,62]

A study that included 40 patients reported that JC virus was undetectable in CSF after 2 months of therapy in 82 percent of the patients treated with HAART plus cidofovir as compared with 42 percent of those treated only with HAART.[39] Worsening of the clinical manifestations occurred in 43 percent of the HAART plus cidofovir group and in 76 percent of the HAART group; the 1-year cumulative probability of survival was 67 versus 31 percent, respectively. Multivariate analysis

revealed that the use of cidofovir was independently predictive of longer survival periods.

In contrast, a prospective study of 24 patients, many of whom also were receiving antiretroviral therapy, failed to find a beneficial effect of cidofovir on neurologic examination scores at week 8, and the survival rate at 12 weeks was only 54 percent.[38] An observational study that included 46 patients found that patients treated with HAART plus cidofovir had a clearance rate of JC virus DNA in CSF after 6 months of 33 percent as compared with 39 percent in the patients who received only HAART. The 1-year cumulative probability of survival was 62 and 53 percent for the HAART plus cidofovir and the HAART groups, respectively, without significant differences between them.[62] Finally, a large study of 118 patients did not find survival advantages with the use of cidofovir.[40] Therefore, the efficacy of cidofovir for the treatment of PML is currently unclear.

Although the initiation of HAART has been associated with the appearance of PML lesions as another immune reconstitution phenomenon,[37,40,63,64] patients who are diagnosed with PML should receive antiretroviral therapy because such a treatment has resulted in clear survival benefits.[36,37,41,42,65] This observation is not unexpected considering the beneficial effects of antiretroviral therapy on other opportunistic infections, the relationship between JC virus and HIV,[44,46] the concomitant infection of both viruses on the same cell,[66] and the fact that higher CD4 counts are associated with better outcomes in PML patients.[34,38,40,61] Moreover, antiretroviral therapy exerts additional beneficial effects by restoring the specific T-cell responses[67] and the intrathecal synthesis of antibodies[41] against JC virus, therefore helping to reduce viral replication. In fact, antiretroviral therapy has resulted in a reduction of JC virus load in CSF below the detectable level in some patients, a decrease that also has been related to longer survival periods.[41,65] However, one-third of patients receiving antiretroviral therapy in a large multicenter study died, usually from aspiration pneumonia, a median of 12 weeks after the diagnosis of PML, stressing the severity of the illness even in the presence of antiretroviral therapy.[40] The two-thirds of patients who survived in this series remained alive for a median of 2.2 years, and one-half of them experienced an improvement in their symptoms.[40]

Therefore, despite its limitations, antiretroviral therapy constitutes the mainstay of treatment for PML. The use of other therapies in combination with HAART is debatable, and no firm recommendations can be made regarding the use of any particular drug. However, the best candidate currently seems to be cidofovir, which can be used at least in patients with severe lesions and high JC virus load in CSF or in those who fail to improve with antiretroviral therapy. The usual regimen for cidofovir is 5 mg/kg weekly for 2 weeks and then the same dose at alternate weeks. A major drawback of cidofovir is the significant rate of adverse events associated with this drug, mainly nephrotoxicity, despite the concomitant use of probenecid and, less commonly, uveitis, hematologic abnormalities, and nausea and vomiting. Therefore, cidofovir should be stopped if major toxicity develops or if the patient does not experience an improvement in the neurologic symptoms. In the case of improvement, cidofovir could be continued, if tolerated, until an appreciable immune reconstitution occurs, as measured by a sustained increase in CD4 counts. The beneficial role of quantitative PCR for the evaluation of JC virus load in CSF has not been established unquestionably, but it may be helpful to guide therapy.

Traditionally, the outcome of PML has been poor because the disease progressed inexorably to death. The median survival period is about 1 to 6 months in the absence of any intervention, although a small fraction of patients experience more benign courses with clinical and radiologic remissions and prolonged survival even in the absence of antiretroviral therapy.[2,3,13,14] Patients who are most likely to have better outcomes are those who experience a clear immunologic response as a consequence of antiretroviral therapy and those who have a low JC virus load in CSF, clearance of JC virus following therapy, younger age, absence of prior AIDS-defining conditions, absence of severe neurologic impairment, and higher CD4 counts at the time of diagnosis.[3,34,37,38,40,42,61]

▶ CRYPTOCOCOCCAL MENINGITIS

Etiology, Epidemiology, and Pathology

Cryptococcus neoformans is an encapsulated yeastlike fungus of worldwide distribution. *C. neoformans* is inhaled and produces disseminated disease, including CNS infection, in immunocompromised patients. Extraneural sites of infection are common in patients with cryptococcal meningitis. The fungus is recovered from pigeon droppings and, less frequently, from the excreta of other birds, soil, and a variety of sources. Cryptococcal meningitis represents either a reactivation of latent infection or occurs as a result of dissemination of a newly acquired infection.[13,68]

The capsule of the fungus inhibits phagocytosis and macrophage and T-cell responses, and it also may impair leukocyte migration, all of which may be responsible for the minimal inflammatory reaction that is characteristic of cryptococcal infections.[2,4,13] Consequently, the pathologic correlate of this infection is a nonexudative, chronic basilar meningitis with brain edema and microabscesses distributed mainly in the superficial layers of the cerebral cortex, which occasionally are

large enough to constitute brain masses called *cryptococcomas*.[2,13] Similar to other opportunistic infections associated with AIDS, cryptococcal meningitis is also seen in other immunocompromised patients, although the AIDS pandemic has resulted in a dramatic increase in the incidence of this condition.[70]

Cryptococcal meningitis is the most common systemic fungal infection in HIV-infected patients and the third most frequent opportunistic infection of the CNS.[11,13,14] Although the incidence of the infection varies among countries,[4,69] 2 to 11 percent of all HIV-infected patients are affected.[1,2,4,13,21,69,71] Similar to other opportunistic infections, the incidence of cryptococcal meningitis has decreased markedly since the introduction of HAART, although it is yet a relatively common infection in this population.[9,72,16]

Cryptococcal meningitis usually occurs in severely immunosuppressed patients with fewer than 100 CD4 cells/μl,[13,69,71,74–76] and it may coexist with other opportunistic illnesses.[13] Cryptococcal meningitis is the initial AIDS-defining condition in 25 to 50 percent of patients;[2,13,71,74,77–79] occasionally, it may develop as a consequence of the initiation of antiretroviral therapy as another phenomenon of immune reconstitution.[15]

Clinical Features

Despite the presence of cryptococci in other locations, cryptococcal infection in HIV-infected patients usually presents only with neurologic manifestations without evidence of systemic infection. However, patients also may present with extraneural symptoms and signs of the infection involving virtually any organ, although the main locations are the lung, skin, and genitourinary system.[71,78]

The onset and duration of neurologic symptoms are variable, usually beginning 2 to 4 weeks prior to presentation. The presenting symptoms are often subtle and nonspecific. Increasing headache and fever are the most common symptoms at presentation, reported by 75 to 90 percent of patients, accompanied by nausea and vomiting in 40 to 50 percent. Photophobia, blurred vision, and other visual disturbances are experienced by 20 to 30 percent of patients, as well as mental status changes, behavioral abnormalities, confusion, lethargy, obtundation, memory loss, and psychiatric abnormalities in 10 to 30 percent. Less common manifestations are seizures and focal neurologic signs, such as hemiparesis or cranial nerve palsies, seen in about 10 to 20 percent of patients. Despite the existence of meningitis, the minimal inflammation elicited by cryptococci, which seems to be lower in AIDS patients than in patients without HIV infection, is responsible for the frequent absence of the classic meningeal signs, such as neck stiffness, that are observed in only 20 to 50 percent of patients.[2,4,13,14,21,70,71,74,76–78] Elevated intracranial pressure is very common in cryptococcal meningitis and develops in 50 to 75 percent of patients in the absence of hydrocephalus or cerebral edema. This complication has important prognostic implications.[13,72,80]

Diagnosis

Routine CSF studies are not very useful for the diagnosis. However, after excluding the existence of a mass lesion or lesions by neuroimaging studies, lumbar puncture should be performed in all patients in whom the diagnosis of cryptococcal meningitis is considered in order to obtain CSF for microbiologic studies and to measure the CSF pressure. Due to the minimal inflammation caused by cryptococci in AIDS patients, the CSF protein concentration, glucose concentration, and leukocyte counts may be normal or near normal in about 50 percent of patients. Most patients who have an abnormal CSF have only a mild mononuclear pleocytosis, usually fewer than 20 cells/μl, and slightly increased protein and decreased glucose concentrations.[1,2,13,71,78,79] A very helpful diagnostic procedure is determination of the serum and CSF cryptococcal capsular polysaccharide antigen titer, which is positive in more than 90 percent of patients, and the titers are usually very high.[1,2,13,21,71,74,76–79,81] The sensitivity and specificity of

the cryptococcal antigen test is such that a positive result in a patient without suggestive symptoms of cryptococcal disease should be considered an early sign of the infection, which may precede the clinical manifestations by days, weeks, and even months.[76,81] This observation suggests that all patients with a positive cryptococcal capsular polysaccharide antigen test should undergo antifungal therapy irrespective of the absence or presence of symptoms, even though unnecessary therapy would be administered to some patients with false-positive antigen tests.

The India ink smear of CSF demonstrates the typical round morphology of *C. neoformans* in 75 to 90 percent of patients,[2,13,21,71,74,77–79] and the CSF culture yields the pathogen in more than 90 percent of patients.[1,2,21] The sensitivity of extraneural cultures, such as of bronchoalveolar lavage fluid and urine, is lower than that of CSF, yielding positive results in one-third to two-thirds of patients.[74,77–79,82]

Imaging studies, such as CT scan and MRI, are not very helpful in cryptococcal meningitis because they are either normal or demonstrate nonspecific abnormalities. In some cases ventricular enlargement, cerebral edema, brain atrophy, dilated perivascular Virchow-Robin spaces, or cryptococcomas may be seen (Fig. 7-4).[1,2,4,71,78]

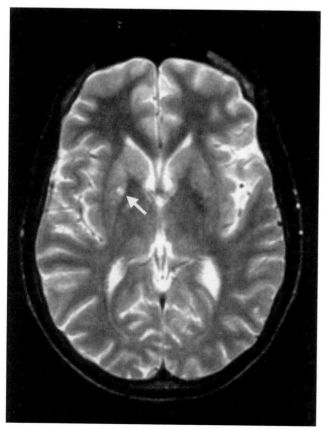

A

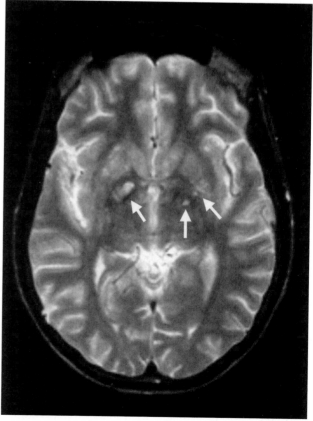

B

Figure 7-4. Cryptococcal meningitis. T_2-weighted MRI revealing bilateral small foci of increased signal in the basal ganglia (*arrows*) that may represent either cryptococcomas or dilated Virchow-Robin spaces distended with fungus and mucoid material.

Treatment

Similar to other CNS opportunistic infections in HIV-infected patients, the treatment for cryptococcal meningitis consists of an induction phase followed by maintenance therapy or secondary prophylaxis to prevent recurrence of the disease. In the era before HAART, this suppressive therapy would be continued for life. However, the improvement in immunologic status of patients treated with antiretroviral therapy allows for safe discontinuation of maintenance therapy in patients who reach a sustained immune reconstitution.

Amphotericin B constitutes the mainstay of initial therapy for cryptococcal meningitis. A large double-blind, randomized study evaluated the efficacy of amphotericin B alone or associated with flucytosine for 2 weeks followed by fluconazole or itraconazole. Sterilization of CSF cultures at 2 weeks was obtained in 60 percent of patients treated with amphotericin B plus flucytosine and in 51 percent of those receiving amphotericin B alone. At 10 weeks, there was no growth of organisms in CSF culture in 72 percent of the patients treated with fluconazole and 60 percent of those treated with itraconazole. In this study, both flucytosine and fluconazole were independent predictors of sterilization of CSF cultures in a multivariate analysis. The fatality rate was 5.5 percent during the initial 2 weeks and 4 percent during the next 8 weeks, without significant differences among the different therapeutic groups.[74] This rate was substantially lower than that observed by the same authors in an earlier study using lower doses of both amphotericin B and fluconazole[77] and lower than that reported in a retrospective study of patients treated with amphotericin B plus flucytosine, in which the mortality rate at the end of the induction period was 26 percent.[79] Interestingly, the absence of flucytosine treatment during the induction phase was the main factor associated with relapse in another study.[75]

Other formulations of amphotericin B, such as liposomal amphotericin B and amphotericin B–lipid complex, are also efficacious and have a more favorable toxicity profile than conventional amphotericin B,[82,83] although the cost of therapy with these agents is substantially higher. The use of intrathecal or intraventricular amphotericin B may be considered in refractory cases in which systemic administration of the drug has failed to eradicate the infection.

Small studies have evaluated the efficacy of high doses of fluconazole alone[73] and of fluconazole combined with flucytosine[84] with acceptable results. However, fluconazole alone seems to be inferior to fluconazole plus flucytosine,[85] as well as to amphotericin B plus flucytosine.[86] A major concern of the amphotericin B plus flucytosine regimen is the high rate of adverse effects associated with amphotericin B, mainly infusion-associated reactions and nephrotoxicity, and with flucytosine, mainly hematologic toxicity. Voriconazole, a recently introduced antifungal agent, has good activity against *C. neoformans*; therefore, it may become an additional therapeutic option, although there is no published experience of voriconazole in the treatment of cryptococcal meningitis. Another new antifungal agent, caspofungin, cannot be used for cryptococcal meningitis because of its relatively poor activity against the fungus.

In summary, the best therapeutic regimen for the induction phase of treatment currently consists of amphotericin B administered for 2 weeks, with or without flucytosine, followed by oral fluconazole for 8 to 10 weeks. The recommended doses of these drugs, as well as alternative regimens, are shown in Table 7-2.

As mentioned earlier, suppressive therapy is needed to reduce the probability of relapse after completion of a successful induction therapy because the rate of relapse in those treated only with induction therapy is high.[13,14,68,69,71] Although several drugs may be used for this purpose, fluconazole constitutes the mainstay of maintenance therapy because it is well tolerated and has proven to be better than itraconazole[75] and weekly amphotericin B[87] to prevent relapse of cryptococcal meningitis. However, positive cultures may persist or reappear in some patients despite ongoing antifungal therapy.

The efficacy of the induction and maintenance therapies may be evaluated with serial measurement of the cryptococcal capsular polysaccharide antigen in CSF because CSF titers, but not serum titers, have been related to mycologic and clinical failure.[71,88] However, the need for repeated lumbar punctures during follow-up to measure the CSF antigen titers should be questioned because relapses usually are associated with symptoms. Therefore, from a practical point of view, clinical monitoring for symptoms and signs of relapse during follow-up may be an alternative, and CSF studies could be reserved only for patients in whom there is a clinical suspicion of relapse. Samples of CSF and urine should be cultured following prostatic massage, as well as any other potentially infected tissue, at the end of the induction phase of therapy because recovery of the fungus has been related to a higher probability of relapse.[89]

As with other opportunistic infections, antiretroviral therapy should be initiated in patients diagnosed with cryptococcal meningitis. Besides the expected beneficial effects of immune reconstitution, allowing for discontinuation of the otherwise lifelong maintenance therapy,[10] antiretroviral therapy also contributes to restoration of the antimicrobial and secretory function of polymorphonuclear leukocytes against the fungus.[90]

Outcome and Complications

Several factors have been related to poor outcomes in patients with cryptococcal meningitis, including levels

▶ **TABLE 7-2.** REGIMENS USED FOR THE TREATMENT AND PROPHYLAXIS OF CRYPTOCOCCAL MENINGITIS

	Primary Prophylaxis*	Induction Therapy	Maintenance Therapy
First-choice regimens	Fluconazole (100–200 mg daily PO)	Amphotericin B (0.7–1 mg/kg daily IV) + flucytosine (25 mg/kg q6h PO) both for 2 weeks, followed by fluconazole (400 mg daily PO) for 8–10 weeks	Fluconazole (200 mg daily PO)
Alternative regimens	Itraconazole (200 mg daily PO)	Amphotericin B (0.7–1 mg/kg daily IV) + flucytosine (25 mg/kg q6h PO) both for 6–10 weeks Amphotericin B (0.7–1 mg/kg daily IV) for 6–10 weeks Lipid formulations of amphotericin B (3–6 mg/kg daily IV) for 2 weeks followed by fluconazole (400 mg daily PO) for 8–10 weeks Lipid formulations of amphotericin B (3–6 mg/kg daily IV) for 6–10 weeks Fluconazole (400–800 mg daily PO) + flucytosine (25–37 mg/kg q6h PO) both for 6 weeks Fluconazole (400–800 mg daily PO) for 10–12 weeks Itraconazole (400 mg daily PO) for 10–12 weeks	Amphotericin B (0.6–1 mg/kg once to thrice weekly IV) Itraconazole (200 mg daily PO)

*Not routinely indicated.

SOURCE: *Adapted from Collazos J: Opportunistic infections of the central nervous system in patients with acquired immunodeficiency syndrome: Diagnosis and management. CNS Drugs 7:869, 2003.*

of cryptococcal capsular polysaccharide antigen in CSF higher than 1:1024, lack of an adequate inflammatory reaction in CSF as measured by normal or low leukocyte counts, a positive CSF India ink stain, impaired mental status, hyponatremia, diastolic hypertension, positive cultures of samples other than CSF, and especially, increased intracranial pressure.[13,14,71,72,74,79,91,92] The high rates of intracranial hypertension in patients with cryptococcal meningitis are thought to be due, at least partially, to a blockade in the reabsorption of CSF in the arachnoid villi owing to high levels of cryptococcal antigen or to large amounts of cryptococci.[72,80,91,92] The degree of intracranial hypertension, which may be higher than 500 mmH$_2$O, has been related not only to death but also to visual loss, severe neurologic manifestations, poorer responses to therapy, and higher levels of cryptococcal antigen and cryptococcal proliferation in CSF.[72,74,80,91–93]

The measurement of CSF opening pressure is essential in HIV-infected patients with cryptococcal meningitis, and reduction of the elevated intracranial pressure is of the utmost importance to reduce the mortality and morbidity of the disease. This is best accomplished by daily lumbar punctures and drainage of a sufficient quantity of CSF to reduce the opening pressure by 50 percent until a normal opening pressure is reached consistently. In some patients, placement of a ventriculoperitoneal shunt or lumbar drain may be necessary to lower the intracranial pressure.[68,71,72,91] The

value of adjunctive measures such as mannitol, acetazolamide, or corticosteroids is questionable, and their usefulness, if any, is probably limited.[68,72,80] The successful use of granulocyte-macrophage colony-stimulating factor has been reported in anecdotal cases, suggesting the appealing, but unproved, hypothesis of the removal of cryptococcal antigen by stimulating the number and phagocytic function of macrophages and leukocytes in CSF.[92] Despite the successful treatment of cryptococcal meningitis and its associated complications, sequelae, such as visual disturbances, personality and mental status changes, and cranial nerve palsies, are common in these patients.

Prophylaxis and Prevention

Pharmacologic prophylaxis to prevent the first episode of cryptococcal meningitis in persons at risk, although potentially efficacious, is questionable and cannot be recommended routinely, especially in patients who are receiving antiretroviral therapy in whom an immune recovery is expected. Patients who benefit most from primary prophylaxis are those with CD4 counts lower than 50 cells/μl, until a sustained increase in CD4 counts has been reached (i.e., >100 CD4 cells/μl for more than 2 months). However, major drawbacks that limit the advisability of primary prophylaxis are concerns about the development of antimicrobial resistance to azoles by cryptococcal and candidal organisms, potential for drug interactions, costs, and absence of evidence of any survival advantage.[8,10,68,69] In contrast, secondary prophylaxis to prevent relapses after induction therapy are clearly worthwhile and should be initiated in all patients, at least until a sustained response in CD4 counts (i.e., >100 to 200 cells/μl for at least 6 months) and diminished HIV viral load are attained with antiretroviral therapy.[10,13,31,94] The recommended regimens for primary prophylaxis and maintenance therapy of cryptococcal meningitis are shown in Table 7-2.

Considering that exposure to cryptococci cannot be avoided completely, there are no effective preventive measures. HIV-infected patients probably should not keep birds as pets or have contact with their excreta, although the value of these recommendations has not been defined.[4,10]

▶ PRIMARY CENTRAL NERVOUS SYSTEM LYMPHOMA

Epidemiology

Primary central nervous system lymphoma (PCNSL), which may be defined as a lymphoma limited to the cranial-spinal axis without systemic disease, represents about one-third of all lymphomas in patients with AIDS.[95] Although this tumor also may present in immunocompetent individuals or in other non-HIV-infected immunocompromised patients, its incidence increased dramatically with the appearance of the HIV pandemic.[95] In fact, HIV infection is the condition most commonly associated with PCNSL, and this tumor is the most common brain malignancy in HIV-infected patients.[13,95]

The prevalence of PCNSL in AIDS patients before the HAART era was 0.5 to 7 percent,[1–4,13,96–99] although these values could be an underestimation. It was estimated that up to 40 percent of patients with AIDS surviving 4 years would develop non-Hodgkin's lymphoma, 25 to 50 percent of which would be PCNSL.[97] However, since the introduction of HAART, the incidence of PCNSL has dropped to 30 to 50 percent of the incidence in the pre-HAART era.[9,16,98,99]

PCNSL may be the first AIDS-defining illness in about 20 to 40 percent of patients[95,98] and characteristically occurs in patients with far-advanced HIV infection with CD4 counts at the time of diagnosis lower than 100 cells/μl and usually below 50 cells/μl.[95,98–102]

Pathogenesis

The pathogenesis of PCNSL remains speculative. However, the etiologic role of Epstein-Barr virus (EBV) in HIV-infected patients seems clear because, as opposed to immunocompetent patients, almost all PCNSLs in AIDS patients contain EBV genomic sequences.[95,97,103,104]

EBV-infected B cells undergo monoclonal expansion favored by the profound immune dysregulation associated with AIDS and the loss of EBV-specific CD8 cells, proliferation that also could be favored by the immunologic sanctuary of the CNS.[2,3,95,105] From a molecular point of view, expression of the latent membrane protein 1, one of the key effector proteins of virus-induced B-cell oncogenesis, frequently has been found in the tumor cells.[104,106] An unexpected expression of p27(Kip1) protein has been detected recently in most, although not all, AIDS-related diffuse large-cell lymphomas, either in PCNSL or in systemic lymphomas. This protein is a negative regulator of cell-cycle progression. The high proliferative rate of the lymphoma clone suggests a failure of p27(Kip1) to inhibit the cell cycle.[106]

Pathology

PCNSL is a very aggressive lymphoma of B-cell lineage,[13,97,107] although anecdotal cases of T-cell lymphoma related to human T-cell lymphotropic virus type I also have been described.[103] The most common subtypes of PCNSL are immunoblastic (30 to 70 percent) and small-cell noncleaved (25 to 60 percent) according to different series.[95–97,101,102,107,108] In 60 to 80 percent of cases the lymphomas are high grade, and in about 30 to 40 percent they are intermediate grade, mainly large-cell diffuse lymphoma (25 to 35 percent) and the mixed large- and small-cell diffuse lymphoma (3 to 7 percent). Low-grade lymphomas are virtually nonexistent.[95,97,107]

Autopsy studies have demonstrated that PCNSL is virtually always multifocal, even when solitary lesions are seen on imaging studies,[13,96,102,107] and the presence of necrosis seems to be more common than in lymphomas from patients without AIDS.[3,102] Supratentorial locations occur three times as often as infratentorial locations; in about 75 percent of patients, the lesions are located close to the cortical convexities or ventricular surfaces, usually involving the corpus callosum, basal ganglia, or thalamus. In less than 25 percent, PCNSL presents infratentorially in cerebellum, brain stem, or spinal cord.[3,13,95,102]

Clinical Features

The clinical picture depends on the type and location of the lesions. PCNSL may manifest as brain mass lesions or as an infiltrative process located mainly in the supratentorial area. Although some lesions are limited in their extension, the aggressive behavior of the tumor and its infiltrative tendency commonly result in a clinical picture that exceeds the expected focal manifestations.

Most patients are in poor condition at the time of presentation, and there is usually a history of prior opportunistic conditions.[97,109] The onset of symptoms is often 2 to 4 weeks before presentation,[3,95,100,109] and fever, night sweats, and weight loss are more common in HIV-infected than in immunocompetent patients, which may be due to the tumor itself or to uncontrolled HIV replication or associated conditions.[3,102]

More than 50 percent of patients have encephalopathic, nonfocal manifestations, such as lethargy, confusion, obtundation, and loss of attention and memory. Patients also may present with neuropsychiatric symptoms, with a change in behavior and personality, apathy, psychosis, and dementia. In 30 to 60 percent of patients, PCNSL may present with focal symptoms such as hemiparesis, dysphasia, or cranial nerve alterations. About 15 to 30 percent of patients have intracranial hypertension, and 10 to 40 percent have seizures.[1,3,4,13,14,95–97,102] Cerebellar or spinal cord manifestations are relatively uncommon. Lymphomatous meningitis, as well as ocular involvement, occurs in about 25 percent of patients.[13,97,110,111] Systemic dissemination of PCNSL is seen in about 7 to 8 percent of patients, and it occurs mainly in the final stages of the disease.[3,111] The clinical course of these patients is usually torpid, with progressive deterioration and evolution to coma and death.

Diagnosis

Routine CSF studies are nonspecific. The most common finding is an elevated protein concentration, followed by mononuclear pleocytosis and, less frequently, low glucose concentration.[13,96,102,107] Higher concentrations of soluble CD23 in CSF have been found in patients with brain lymphoma than in patients with systemic lymphoma or other CNS opportunistic infections, with a sensitivity and specificity for the diagnosis of 77 and 94 percent, respectively.[112] Although soluble CD23 concentrations could represent a noninvasive marker for the diagnosis, their usefulness in clinical practice remains to be established. The detection of malignant cells in CSF is highly specific, but these cells are found in only 10 to 25 percent of patients, usually late in the course of the disease.[13,95,97,102,107]

Lesions of PCNSL in AIDS patients are usually hypodense or isodense on CT scan, and 90 percent enhance with contrast material.[96,97,102,107] This enhancement is irregular in about 40 percent and homogeneous in the remaining 60 percent. Ring enhancement is seen in 50 percent of patients who have enhancement, a finding virtually absent in PCNSL of immunocompetent patients.[3,13,95,97,102] Solitary lesions are seen in 30 to 50 percent of patients.[95,96,101,113] The lesions have a predilection for basal ganglia, thalami, corpus callosum, and the periventricular system; the amount of edema is variable; and the mass effect is less than expected.[2,3,95–97]

Although not more specific, conventional MRI is more sensitive than CT scan because about 10 percent

of the lesions not seen on CT scan can be detected by MRI.[3,13,95,97,113] MRI is superior to CT scan particularly for small lesions, with the additional advantage of allowing a clearer definition of the leptomeninges and spinal cord. The images on MRI (Fig. 7-5) correspond to single or multiple poorly defined lesions, hypointense on T_1-weighted images and hyperintense on T_2-weighted sequences, usually with gadolinium enhancement.[3,13,97,113] Dynamic studies with MRI have revealed that the kinetics of captation of gadolinium is faster and more intense than in toxoplasmosis, therefore increasing the specificity of MRI for the diagnosis.[97]

Brain SPECT may be a useful adjunctive diagnostic tool, although it is not generally available.[97,101,114] Thallium-201 SPECT has been considered unreliable for differentiating lymphoma from nonmalignant lesions analyzing the uptake ratio.[115,116] However, a review of the published studies found a mean sensitivity and specificity of brain SPECT for the differentiation of lymphoma and toxoplasmosis of 92 and 89 percent, respectively,[3] and the thallium-201 retention index, calculated from delayed images, has been found to have a sensitivity of 96 percent and a specificity of 100 percent for the differentiation of PCNSL from nonmalignant lesions.[115]

PET, which analyzes the metabolic activity of the lesion through the use of [^{18}F]fluorodeoxyglucose as a tracer, may be useful for the differentiation of lymphoma from nonmalignant conditions.[3,13,14,97] However, it is very expensive and not widely available, and PML lesions occasionally may show increased metabolic activity, simulating, therefore, lymphomatous lesions. Another imaging technique, sequential thallium and gallium scintigraphy, has been reported to be helpful in the differentiation of tumors from some nonmalignant intracranial mass lesions.[117]

Considering the relationship between EBV and PCNSL, a major diagnostic tool is determination of EBV DNA in CSF by the PCR. The sensitivity of this technique for the diagnosis of PCNSL is higher than 80 percent, and the specificity and positive and negative predictive values are higher than 90 percent in most series.[3,24,114,118] The detection of EBV DNA may precede the diagnosis of lymphoma by months, and EBV DNA may be detected in patients without focal lesions and only microscopic lymphoma foci at autopsy.[24,119] In addition, the diagnostic value of the technique can be improved by combining its results with PET or SPECT.[24,119] Finally, quantitation of DNA levels in CSF may be useful in assessing the response to treatment and, therefore, also could have prognostic implications.[118,120]

Thus the evaluation of EBV DNA by the PCR should be considered the standard of care for the diagnosis of PCNSL. In addition, combined use of the PCR-based assays for other agents, such as *T. gondii*, JC virus, cy-

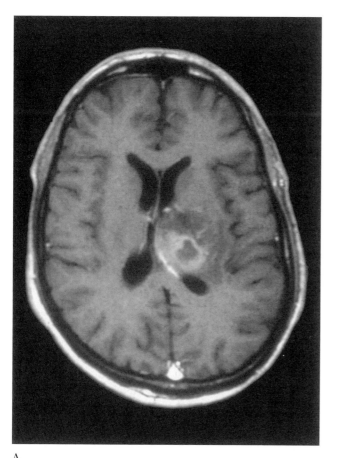
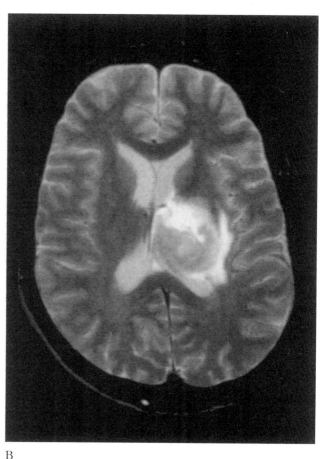

A   B

Figure 7-5. Primary CNS lymphoma. T_1- (*A*) and T_2-weighted (*B*) MRI showing a left deep gray matter mass that displays mainly low intensity and enhances partially after application of gadolinium contrast material.

tomegalovirus, and herpesviruses, may allow a rapid and reliable diagnosis of CNS lesions in HIV-infected patients with sensitivities in the range of 75 to 100 percent and specificities in the range of 90 to 100 percent.[24,121]

However, a definitive diagnosis is obtained only through biopsy. Stereotactic biopsy has proved to be efficacious and safe, yielding the diagnosis in 85 to 95 percent of patients with relatively few complications, mainly hemorrhagic.[3,12,27,97] An important point is that steroids should be avoided before biopsy because they may reduce the size of the lesions and therefore may decrease the diagnostic yield. Since the main differential diagnosis of PCNSL is toxoplasmic encephalitis, it is considered acceptable in clinical practice to initiate an empirical course of anti-*Toxoplasma* therapy for 1 to 2 weeks.[3,13,97] A stereotactic biopsy should be considered only in patients in whom a noninvasive diagnosis is not feasible. Figure 7-2 shows a diagnostic algorithm for the differentiation of PCNSL from other CNS opportunistic conditions, mainly toxoplasmic encephalitis.

Treatment

The treatment options are limited considering the usually poor clinical condition of these patients. Surgical resection is not recommended because of the multicentric and infiltrative characteristics of these lymphomas, as well as the deep locations of the lesions. In addition, surgery does not improve survival.

PCNSL is usually responsive to steroids, at doses of 16 to 24 mg/d of dexamethasone, due to the cytotoxic effect on lymphoid cells and reduction of the surrounding edema. In 30 to 70 percent of patients, steroids may reduce the size of the lesions, which may even disappear,[95,97] although improvement is always transient.

PCNSL is sensitive to radiation therapy. This is the most commonly used treatment for this condition.[2,3,13,95,97,101,108] However, 40 to 70 percent of patients are not treated with radiation therapy, and not all patients who begin radiation therapy complete a full course of therapy because of death or the appearance of other opportunistic conditions.[95,97,101] Although the optimal doses have not been established, 4000 to 5000 cGy is recommended.[3,95,97,108] The dose should be tailored to each individual patient. In patients with good performance status, more than 100 CD4 cells/μl, absence of a history of opportunistic infections, and single lesions, it may be advisable to administer higher doses, in the range of 5000 to 6000 cGy, whole brain to obtain the best possible results. In patients with poor clinical and immunologic conditions, multiple lesions, and opportunistic infections, the aim of therapy should be palliative, and the doses should be lower, in the range of 3000 to 4000 cGy.[95,97] The overall response rate in HIV-infected individuals is poorer than in immunocompetent patients. A complete response is obtained in 20 to 60 percent of patients, a partial response in 10 to 40 percent, and no response in 25 to 50 percent.[97]

The role of chemotherapy, with or without radiation therapy, in PCNSL in AIDS patients is controversial because of concerns for causing a greater degree of immunosuppression in patients already severely immunocompromised, often with associated opportunistic infections, and the usually poor performance status and poor outcome of these patients. Therefore, chemotherapy has been used only rarely.[95] Methotrexate, either by intrathecal or systemic administration, has been the drug used most commonly, although other drugs such as doxorubicin, bleomycin, vincristine, cytosine arabinoside, cyclophosphamide, procarbazine, and CCNU, among others, also have been used with modest results.[97] Some series reported better results with chemotherapy than with radiation therapy.[95,100,110] Better results with chemotherapy than with radiation therapy alone have been observed in PCNSL in immunocompetent patients,[95,102] which may be explained by the distinctive morphology and different kinetic profiles in AIDS and non-AIDS lymphomas.[122] It would be expected that a better control of HIV disease with antiretroviral therapy and the use of chemotherapy in patients with more favorable clinical and immunological profiles would result in better outcomes than in the past.

Zidovudine at high doses is active against EBV-related lymphomas, and this drug in combination with ganciclovir and interleukin-2 has been used with good results.[123,124] Hydroxyurea also has been tried for therapy based on its in vitro anti-EBV activity, resulting in survival periods in excess of 2 years.[125]

The role of antiretroviral therapy is unclear, although some benefit would be expected considering the influence that HIV-associated complications have on the outcome of these patients and the improvement in immunocompetence that might be achieved with antiretroviral therapy. In fact, as mentioned below, several reports found considerably better outcomes in patients treated with HAART than in those not receiving such therapy, which was attributed to the immune recovery experienced by the patients.[98,105,126] In addition, it also has been suggested that survival of AIDS patients with PCNSL may be improved by the radiosensitizing effects of the antiretroviral therapy.[127]

Outcome

In most series the outcome of PCNSL in AIDS patients is considerably worse than in non-AIDS patients, with median survival periods of 1 to 3 months for the former and 7 to 18 months for the latter.[95,101–103] PCNSL is a terminal condition in AIDS patients[1,4]; the mean or median survival periods are 0.5 to 3 months in the absence of treatment[3,14,95,101,108,109] and 1 to 6 months in those receiving radiation therapy.[95–97,101,102,108–110] In contrast, the mean or median survival period for patients treated with chemotherapy, with or without radiation therapy, was 7 to 18 months.[97,100,110] The combination of parenteral zidovudine, ganciclovir, and interleukin-2 has resulted in survival periods longer than 1 to 2 years in some patients.[123] However, these results should be interpreted with caution because the patients were not randomized, and a bias toward a more intensive treatment in patients with a better clinical condition may have occurred.

In addition to the influence of different therapeutic interventions on outcome, the most important factors related to survival are the clinical condition of the patient, CD4 counts, and the absence of opportunistic infections. In a review of published cases, the survival of patients with a history of opportunistic infections was 2 months as compared with 12 months for those without a history of opportunistic infections.[102] Death is the result of progression of the lymphoma or a consequence of concomitant infections.[2,3,13,95,96,107]

Since the incidence of PCNSL has decreased since the introduction of HAART, the impact of antiretroviral therapy has not been studied extensively. However, the median survival of six patients treated with HAART and radiation therapy in a small series was 3 years, with two patients still alive at the time of reporting, as compared with 4.4 months for those treated with radiation therapy and 1 month for those untreated.[126] Other anecdotal reports also had encouraging results.[98,105] Not unexpectedly, favorable outcome is related to immune recovery.[98,105,126] Although a selection bias also could have had an influence on the results, the beneficial effect of antiretroviral therapy on other AIDS-associated conditions, including systemic lymphoma, suggests that a benefit also could be expected; therefore, all patients with PCNSL should receive antiretroviral therapy.

► CYTOMEGALOVIRUS INFECTIONS

Etiology and Epidemiology

Cytomegalovirus (CMV) is a β herpes virus of worldwide distribution, as evidenced by the fact that most adults have serologic evidence of latent infection. CMV typically causes subclinical or mildly symptomatic infections in immunocompetent patients, but it also may cause life-threatening infections in immunosuppressed individuals, mainly transplant and HIV-infected patients. CMV is the most common viral pathogen in HIV-infected patients, and the reactivation of latent infection results mainly in retinitis and gastrointestinal tract involvement. CNS infection is less frequent and manifests primarily as encephalitis and polyradiculomyelitis.[13,14,128,129] Of note, some patients may develop encephalitis while they are being treated with maintenance therapy for a prior CMV retinitis,[128,130–132] an observation that underscores the difficult management of CMV CNS infections.

Clinically evident CMV encephalitis represented about 2 percent of all neurologic complications in AIDS patients in the pre-HAART era, although evidence of subclinical CNS CMV infection was found in 5 to 40 percent of autopsies.[3,13,14,129–133] However, the incidence of CMV disease, including CNS infections, has decreased substantially since the introduction of HAART[8,129,133] because antiretroviral therapy has improved considerably the immunologic condition of AIDS patients, and CMV disease characteristically occurs in very advanced stages of HIV infection, usually in patients with CD4 counts below 50 cells/μl.[128–131]

Pathology

CMV CNS infections take a variety of histopathologic forms. The most common is that of a microglial nodular encephalitis, which is characterized by multifocal, diffusely scattered micronodules composed of aggregates of glial cells and macrophages, commonly associated with the typical intranuclear Cowdry B inclusions, the so-called owl eyes, in cytomegalic cells. These nodules are observed predominantly in the gray matter and are distributed widely in the cortex, basal ganglia, and subtentorial structures. The second most common histopathologic pattern is ventriculoencephalitis, which results from infection of the ependymal cells lining the ventricles with areas of focal necrosis in the periventricular region. Other types of pathology include necrotizing focal encephalitis, isolated cytomegalic cells, meningitis, myelitis, polyradiculitis, and various combinations of these.[3,4,13,14,128–133]

In addition, simultaneous infection with other pathogens, mainly HIV encephalitis, also may occur,[1,2,12] an aspect that complicates the neuropathologic picture and interpretation of the relative contribution of each pathogen to the clinical presentation. Finally, involvement of other organs by CMV is found commonly at necropsy in HIV-infected patients with CMV CNS infections.[130,131]

Clinical Features

Many patients have a previous history of CMV disease, mainly retinitis, adrenalitis, esophagitis, or colitis, at the time of development of the neurologic manifestations.[3,13,14,131] The clinical picture of CMV encephalitis is similar to that caused by other viral infections of the CNS, especially HIV encephalitis. In addition, the common coexistence of other pathogens in the CNS such as HIV, herpes simplex, *Toxoplasma,* PML, or cryptococcal meningitis may complicate the clinical picture.[3,4,14,131,132]

The most common neuropathologic finding, diffuse micronodular encephalitis, is characterized clinically by the acute or subacute development of dementia with delirium, apathy, confusion, loss of attention, lethargy, and occasionally, focal neurologic deficits.[3,13,21,129,131] Ventriculoencephalitis usually presents as a rapidly progressive syndrome of delirium, cranial nerve deficits, nystagmus, and ataxia and fewer neuropsychological abnormalities than in diffuse micronodular encephalitis.[3,13,129–132,134] However, overlapping symptoms among these two entities are common, and the differentiation between them, and even between CMV and HIV encephalitis, may be very difficult on clinical grounds. CMV encephalitis seems to have a more rapid onset and evolution of symptoms, as well as higher degrees of delirium, confusion, apathy, and focal neurologic deficits, as well as lower CD4 counts, than HIV encephalitis.[14,128–131]

CMV infection also may present as necrotizing myelitis or radiculomyelitis, with diverse degrees of motor and sensory deficits and sphincter disturbances. A clinical picture of ascending weakness with hypotonic paresis, areflexia, hypoesthesia, and urinary retention that may progress to the upper limbs and cranial nerves also has been described.[2,129,133–135] Characteristically, there is a CSF polymorphonuclear pleocytosis, which may be a clue to the diagnosis, and CSF cultures may be positive, findings that are unusual in other CNS infections caused by CMV.[2]

Diagnosis

The diagnosis of CMV CNS infections should be considered in severely immunocompromised patients who present with neurologic signs and symptoms and who have a history of CMV infection elsewhere, even though the extraneurologic disease is controlled with therapy. In this regard, optic fundi should be examined for undetected signs of CMV retinitis in all HIV-infected patients presenting with dementia. Given the high prevalence of latent CMV infection in the general population, measurement of serum antibodies against the pathogen is not helpful for diagnostic purposes. In patients with concomitant CMV adrenalitis, electrolyte disturbances characteristic of adrenal insufficiency also may be a clue to the diagnosis.[13,14,131]

CSF examination usually shows variable and non-specific changes consisting of different degrees of pleocytosis, elevated protein concentrations, and decreased glucose concentrations. Characteristically, pleocytosis in CMV encephalitis is mononuclear, whereas in radiculomyelitis there is a pleocytosis of polymorphonuclear leukocytes.[3,13,129–132,135] CSF examination is, however, essential for the diagnosis. Although CSF cultures of CMV are usually negative, and the intrathecal production of specific antibodies against CMV appears to be of little help,[3,4,13,128–131,133,136] investigation of CMV genomic sequences by PCR is very useful. Although the different methodology used and the criteria for sample selection may account for some discrepancies in the reported results, the sensitivity, specificity, and predictive values of the detection of CMV DNA are usually in excess of 80 percent.[3,13,24,128–130,133,134] From a practical point of view, a negative PCR result excludes CMV infection and warrants investigation of other entities.

Although detection of CMV DNA in CSF is highly correlated with symptomatic CNS infection, CMV DNA also may be detected in cases of uncertain clinical significance.[24,130] Quantitation of DNA levels may be helpful because the CMV load is related to the extent of the lesions and the type of infection, with higher values observed in patients with polyradiculopathy. This measurement also may be useful for monitoring the response to therapy because the titers decrease or disappear following successful anti-CMV therapy.[3,13,24,130,133,137] Another potentially useful test is determination of the pp65 antigen in polymorphonuclear leukocytes in blood[129,137] and CSF,[129,138] which denotes ongoing CMV infection.

Imaging studies usually are nonspecific for the diagnosis of CMV infection, although the findings in ventriculoencephalitis are relatively characteristic. CT scan may show areas of low attenuation in brain parenchyma, as well as ventricular enlargement and periventricular enhancement in cases of ventriculoencephalitis. MRI, which is more sensitive than CT scan, reveals areas of increased signal intensity in cortical regions on T_2-weighted images and in the subependymal regions in patients with ventriculoencephalitis (Fig. 7-6) and also may show enhancement in the meninges, spinal cord, or lumbosacral rootlets in patients with polyradiculomyelitis.[1,3,13,129,131,135] In rare instances, CMV infection may present as a ring-enhancing mass with surrounding edema, which may be confused with other etiologies of CNS mass lesions in HIV-infected patients, such as *Toxoplasma* and lymphoma lesions.[129,139]

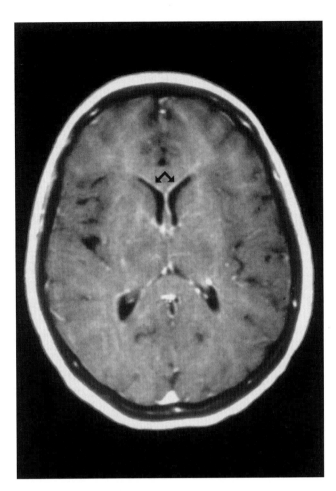

Figure 7-6. Cytomegalovirus ventriculoencephalitis. T_1-weighted MRI obtained after gadolinium contrast material administration that reveals subtle subependymal enhancement along the ventricles (*arrows*).

Brain biopsy is the only definitive method to establish the diagnosis. Due to the common absence of focal lesions in CMV CNS infections, brain biopsy is performed only in selected patients. Cytologic examination of CSF also may show the typical cytomegalic cells, especially in patients with polyradiculitis, but its sensitivity is low.[24] Therefore, the diagnosis in clinical practice is established by a compatible clinical and neuroimaging picture, especially in the setting of CMV outside the CNS, and the detection of CMV DNA and/or pp65 antigen in CSF.

Treatment and Outcome

Three drugs are currently available for the treatment of systemic CMV infections: ganciclovir, a nucleoside analogue of guanosine; foscarnet, a pyrophosphate analogue; and cidofovir, a nucleotide analogue of cytosine. All three drugs are virostatic and exert their action by competitively inhibiting the viral DNA polymerase, resulting in inhibition of DNA synthesis. However, these drugs have major limitations, mainly due to inconvenience of administration and the high incidence of adverse effects. All these drugs need to be administered by the intravenous route because there is no oral formulation, except for ganciclovir. The bioavailability of the oral formulation of ganciclovir, however, is very poor, precluding its use for induction therapy; in addition, the pill burden is substantial. A prodrug of ganciclovir, valganciclovir, has been introduced recently and has improved bioavailability of the parent compound, achieving similar plasma concentrations as intravenous ganciclovir.[140] The efficacy of valganciclovir in the treatment of CNS CMV infections has not been established. The toxicity of these agents is considerable, manifested primarily as bone marrow suppression for ganciclovir and nephrotoxicity for foscarnet and cidofovir, resulting in discontinuation of therapy in many patients.

Similar to the therapy of other opportunistic conditions, current anti-CMV agents do not eradicate the infection, and therefore, maintenance therapy is required. The regimens used for CNS CMV infections have been extrapolated from experience with other CMV infections, mainly retinitis, an extrapolation that may not be completely appropriate. Furthermore, the development of drug resistance, the possible irreversibility of the lesions, and the penetration of the drugs into the CNS are additional limitations to successful treatment of this infection.

In addition to these major drawbacks, another substantial shortcoming is that the optimal therapeutic regimens have not been established because of the lack of randomized, controlled trials and the small sample size of the published studies, a problem that presumably will not be solved in the near future due to the current low incidence of the disease. For these reasons, the recommendations for the treatment and prophylaxis of CNS CMV infections that are described in Table 7-3 should be taken with caution.

In the largest series published, a combination of ganciclovir and foscarnet was used both as induction and maintenance therapy in 31 patients with encephalitis or myelitis. Although clinical improvement or stabilization was observed in 74 percent of the patients, 32 percent developed adverse reactions of enough severity to require discontinuation of treatment during the induction phase. The median time to relapse in those who received maintenance therapy was 18 weeks, and the median survival period for all patients was only 3 months.[141] It should be noted that these poor results were obtained with a synergistic combination regimen, a fact that underscores the limitations in the treatment of this condition. Likewise, the response in cases of polyradiculitis is disappointing, with mean survival periods in those treated with ganciclovir of only 15 weeks.[135]

The role of cidofovir in the treatment of CMV CNS infections is not established. Anecdotal case reports support the usefulness of this drug,[143,142] but there are no published studies evaluating the efficacy of cidofovir in CMV CNS infections. Taking into account the severity of CMV CNS infections and the poor prognosis, aggressive therapy with a combination of ganciclovir and foscarnet, if tolerated, is recommended, especially if the patient has received any of these drugs for the treatment of extraneurologic CMV disease.[21,130,133,144] In ad-

▶ **TABLE 7-3.** REGIMENS USED FOR THE TREATMENT AND PROPHYLAXIS OF CYTOMEGALOVIRUS CNS INFECTIONS

	Primary Prophylaxis*	Induction Therapy	Maintenance Therapy
First-choice regimens	Valganciclovir (900 mg daily PO)	Ganciclovir (5 mg/kg q12h IV) + foscarnet (90 mg/kg q12h IV) both for 3–6 weeks	Ganciclovir (5–6 mg/kg 5–7 days weekly IV) Foscarnet (90–120 mg/kg daily IV)
Alternative regimens	Ganciclovir (1 g q8h PO)	Ganciclovir (5 mg/kg q12h IV for 3–6 weeks) Foscarnet (90 mg/kg q12h IV for 3–6 weeks) Cidofovir (5 mg/kg weekly IV for 2 weeks, then every 2 weeks) + probenecid (2 g PO 3 hours before the dose of cidofovir and 1 g 2 and 8 hours after the dose) Valganciclovir (900 mg q12h PO)†	Cidofovir (5 mg/kg every 2 weeks IV) + probenecid (2 g PO 3 hours before the dose of cidofovir and 1 g 2 and 8 hours after the dose) Valganciclovir (900 mg daily? q12 h? PO)†

*Not specifically indicated for CNS infections; questionable for any location (see text).
†There is no experience in CNS infections; currently not approved for this indication.
SOURCE: Adapted from Collazos J: Opportunistic infections of the central nervous system in patients with acquired immunodeficiency syndrome: Diagnosis and management. CNS Drugs 7:869, 2003.

dition to clinical and radiologic evaluations of the response to therapy, monitoring the CMV load in CSF by quantitative PCR may be helpful in evaluating the virologic response to therapy.[13]

The prognosis of CNS CMV infection in HIV-infected patients in the absence of treatment is very poor, with death usually occurring within a few weeks of presentation. The use of specific anti-CMV therapy usually results in only a slightly better prognosis, with survival periods of a few months.[130–133,135]

Clearly, an improvement in the immunologic competence of the patient is crucial for control of the disease, especially considering the poor prognosis even with specific anti-CMV therapy. Therefore, it is essential that all patients with CNS CMV infections be treated with antiretroviral therapy. Although there are no published clinical trials demonstrating the efficacy of antiretroviral therapy in CNS CMV infections, the experience with other opportunistic infections supports the usefulness of antiretroviral therapy. In addition, some anecdotal cases suggest that the outcome of patients treated with antiretroviral therapy plus anti-CMV therapy is substantially better than in those receiving only anti-CMV therapy.[141] Furthermore, antiretroviral treatment has resulted in a normalization of the previously increased CMV-specific CD4 T cells, a finding that is thought to be due to a better control of the CMV infection by successful restoration of the immune response against the virus.[145] Therefore, antiretroviral therapy probably constitutes the most efficacious measure to improve the dismal outcome of these patients.

Prophylaxis and Prevention

Maintenance therapy is necessary to decrease recurrences of the disease in all patients with CNS CMV infections who have responded to the induction therapy. This therapy should be maintained at least until a significant and sustained increase in CD4 counts (i.e., >100 to 150 cells/μl for 3 to 6 months or more) has been reached with antiretroviral treatment.[8,10,31] Maintenance therapy may be with the same drugs that were used successfully for the induction therapy but at lower doses. However, in addition to toxicity and the possible development of drug resistance, a major limitation of these regimens is the schedule of administration, requiring daily intravenous doses, except for cidofovir, which offers a much more convenient dosing regimen. Although valganciclovir may be used for maintenance therapy of CMV retinitis, there are no data about the efficacy of this agent in CNS infections.

The routine use of primary drug prophylaxis for the prevention of first episodes of CMV infection is debatable, and it should be used only in selected patients. Table 7-3 summarizes the regimens for primary and secondary prophylaxis for CNS CMV infections. Patients potentially eligible for primary prophylaxis would be those with serologic evidence of CMV infection who have fewer than 50 CD4 cells/μl. This prophylaxis should be discontinued if the CD4 counts increase to at least 100 cells/μl during 3 or more months. The cost of therapy should be considered, as should the adverse effects of these drugs, the possibility of the development of drug resistance, the absence of demonstrated survival benefits, and the immunologic improvement expected within a few months in those patients who begin antiretroviral therapy.[8,10,146] The monitoring of CMV DNA, pp65 antigen, or CMV-specific interferon gamma production in blood may be helpful for the selection of patients who could best benefit from preventive therapy by identifying individuals at the highest risk for the disease.[147,148]

As mentioned earlier, most patients already have been infected with CMV when first seen, and therefore, no specific measures to prevent the infection should be taken. In those who are seronegative, some precautions should be taken to minimize exposure to the pathogen, including the use of latex condoms in all sexual contacts, observing good hygiene when caring for children, and avoidance of CMV-seropositive blood or unfiltered blood products in the treatment of these patients.[8,10]

REFERENCES

1. McArthur JC: Neurologic manifestations of AIDS. *Medicine* 66:407, 1987.
2. Berger JR, Levy RM: The neurologic complications of human immunodeficiency virus infection. *Med Clin North Am* 77:1, 1993.
3. Skiest DJ: Focal neurological disease in patients with acquired immunodeficiency syndrome. *Clin Infect Dis* 34:103, 2002.
4. Fischer PA, Enzensberger W: Neurological complications in AIDS. *J Neurol* 234:269, 1987.
5. Masliah E, DeTeresa RM, Mallory ME, et al: Changes in pathological findings at autopsy in AIDS cases for the last 15 years. *AIDS* 14:69, 2000.
6. Gray F, Gherardi R, Scaravilli F: The neuropathology of the acquired immune deficiency syndrome (AIDS): A review. *Brain* 111:245, 1988.
7. Vago L, Bonetto S, Nebuloni M, et al: Pathological findings in the central nervous system of AIDS patients on assumed antiretroviral therapeutic regimens: Retrospective study of 1597 autopsies. *AIDS* 16:1925, 2002.
8. Kovacs JA, Masur H: Prophylaxis against opportunistic infections in patients with human immunodeficiency virus infection. *New Engl J Med* 342:1416, 2000.
9. Sacktor N, Lyles RH, Skolasky R, et al: HIV-associated neurologic disease incidence changes: Multicenter AIDS Cohort Study, 1990–1998. *Neurology* 56:257, 2001.
10. Kaplan JE, Masur H, Holmes KK: Guidelines for preventing opportunistic infections among HIV-infected persons—2002. *MMWR* 51(RR-8):1, 2002.

11. Ammassari A, Cinque P, Lorenzini P, et al: HAART exposure influences distribution and characteristics of HIV-associated neurologic disorders: Data from Italian Registry Investigation Neuro AIDS (IRINA). XIV International AIDS Conference, Barcelona, Spain, July 7–12, 2002 (abstract no ThPeB7370).

12. Renold C, Sugar A, Chave JP: *Toxoplasma* encephalitis in patients with the acquired immunodeficiency syndrome. *Medicine* 71:224, 1992.

13. Mamidi A, DeSimone JA, Pomerantz RJ: Central nervous system infections in individuals with HIV-1 infection. *J Neurovirol* 8:158, 2002.

14. Simpson DM, Tagliati M: Neurologic manifestations of HIV infection. *Ann Intern Med* 121:769, 1994.

15. Luft BJ, Remington JS: Toxoplasmic encephalitis in AIDS. *Clin Infect Dis* 15:211, 1992.

16. Sacktor N: The epidemiology of human immunodeficiency virus–associated neurological disease in the era of highly active antiretroviral therapy. *J Neurovirol* 8(suppl 2):115, 2002.

17. Abgrall S, Rabaud C, Costagliola D: Incidence and risk factors for toxoplasmic encephalitis in human immunodeficiency virus–infected patients before and during the highly active antiretroviral therapy era. *Clin Infect Dis* 33:1747, 2001.

18. Kravetz JD, Federman DG: Cat-associated zoonoses. *Arch Intern Med* 162:1945, 2002.

19. Raffi F, Aboulker JP, Michelet C, et al: A prospective study of criteria for the diagnosis of toxoplasmic encephalitis in 186 AIDS patients. *AIDS* 11:177, 1997.

20. Porter SB, Sande MA: Toxoplasmosis of the central nervous system in the acquired immunodeficiency syndrome. *New Engl J Med* 327:1643, 1992.

21. Bartlett JG, Gallant JE: *Medical Management of HIV Infection,* 2001–2002 ed. Baltimore: Johns Hopkins University Press, 2001

22. Katlama C, De Wit S, O'Doherty E, et al: Pyrimethamine-clindamycin vs pyrimethamine-sulfadiazine as acute and long-term therapy for toxoplasmic encephalitis in patients with AIDS. *Clin Infect Dis* 22:268, 1996.

23. Skiest DJ, Erdman W, Chang WE, et al: SPECT thallium-201 combined with *Toxoplasma* serology for the presumptive diagnosis of focal central nervous system mass lesions in patients with AIDS. *J Infect* 40:274, 2000.

24. Cinque P, Scarpellini P, Vago L, et al: Diagnosis of central nervous system complications in HIV-infected patients: Cerebrospinal fluid analysis by the polymerase chain reaction. *AIDS* 11:1, 1997.

25. Potasman I, Resnick L, Luft BJ, et al: Intrathecal production of antibodies against *Toxoplasma gondii* in patients with toxoplasmic encephalitis and the acquired immunodeficiency syndrome (AIDS). *Ann Intern Med* 108:49, 1988.

26. Novati R, Castagna A, Morsica G, et al: Polymerase chain reaction for *Toxoplasma gondii* DNA in the cerebrospinal fluid of AIDS patients with focal brain lesions. *AIDS* 8:1691, 1994.

27. Gildenberg PL, Gathe JC Jr, Kim JH: Stereotactic biopsy of cerebral lesions in AIDS. *Clin Infect Dis* 30:491, 2000.

28. Chirgwin K, Hafner R, Leport C, et al: Randomized phase II trial of atovaquone with pyrimethamine or sulfadiazine for treatment of toxoplasmic encephalitis in patients with acquired immunodeficiency syndrome: ACTG 237/ANRS 039 study. *Clin Infect Dis* 34:1243, 2002.

29. Alfonzo M, Blanc D, Troadec C, et al: Temporary restoration of immune response against *Toxoplasma gondii* in HIV-infected individuals after HAART, as studied in the hu-PBMC-SCID mouse model. *Clin Exp Immunol* 129:411, 2002.

30. Miró JM, Lejeune M, Claramonte X, et al: Timing of reconstitution of *Toxoplasma gondii*–specific T-cell responses in AIDS patients with acute toxoplasmic encephalitis after starting HAART: A prospective multicenter longitudinal study. 10th Conference on Retroviruses and Opportunistic Infections, Boston, MA, February 10–14, 2003 (abstract no 796).

31. Kirk O, Reiss P, Uberti-Foppa C, et al: Safe interruption of maintenance therapy against previous infection with four common HIV-associated opportunistic pathogens during potent antiretroviral therapy. *Ann Intern Med* 137:239, 2002.

32. Sabath BF, Major EO: Traffic of JC virus from sites of initial infection to the brain: the path to progressive multifocal leukoencephalopathy. *J Infect Dis* 186(suppl 2):S180, 2002.

33. Berger JR, Kaszovitz B, Post JD, et al: Progressive multifocal leukoencephalopathy associated with human immunodeficiency virus infection: A review of the literature with a report of sixteen cases. *Ann Intern Med* 107:78, 1987.

34. Fong IW, Toma E: The natural history of progressive multifocal leukoencephalopathy in patients with AIDS. *Clin Infect Dis* 20:1305, 1995.

35. McGuire D, Barhite S, Hollander H, et al: JC virus DNA in cerebrospinal fluid of human immunodeficiency virus–infected patients: Predictive value for progressive multifocal leukoencephalopathy. *Ann Neurol* 37:395, 1995.

36. Antinori A, Ammassari A, Giancola ML, et al: Epidemiology and prognosis of AIDS-associated progressive multifocal leukoencephalopathy in the HAART era. *J Neurovirol* 7:323, 2001.

37. De Luca A, Giancola ML, Ammassari A, et al: The effect of potent antiretroviral therapy and JC virus load in cerebrospinal fluid on clinical outcome of patients with AIDS-associated progressive multifocal leukoencephalopathy. *J Infect Dis* 182:1077, 2000.

38. Marra CM, Rajicic N, Barker DE, et al: A pilot study of cidofovir for progressive multifocal leukoencephalopathy in AIDS. *AIDS* 16:1791, 2002.

39. De Luca A, Giancola ML, Ammassari A, et al: Cidofovir added to HAART improves virological and clinical outcome in AIDS-associated progressive multifocal leukoencephalopathy. *AIDS* 14:F117, 2000.

40. Berenguer J, Miralles P, Arrizabalaga J, et al: Clinical course and prognostic factors of progressive multifocal leukoencephalopathy in patients treated with highly active antiretroviral therapy. *Clin Infect Dis* 36:1047, 2003.

41. Giudici B, Vaz B, Bossolasco S: Highly active antiretro-

viral therapy and progressive multifocal leukoencephalopathy: Effects on cerebrospinal fluid markers of JC virus replication and immune response. *Clin Infect Dis* 30:95, 2000.

42. Tassie JM, Gasnault J, Bentata M, et al: Survival improvement of AIDS-related progressive multifocal leukoencephalopathy in the era of protease inhibitors. *AIDS* 13:1881, 1999.

43. Whiteman MLH, Post MJD, Berger JR, et al: Progressive multifocal leukoencephalopathy in 47 HIV-seropositive patients: Neuroimaging with clinical and pathologic correlation. *Radiology* 187:233, 1993.

44. Valle LD, Croul S, Morgello S, et al: Detection of HIV-1 Tat and JCV capsid protein, VP1, in AIDS brain with progressive multifocal leukoencephalopathy. *J Neurovirol* 6:221, 2000.

45. Berger JR: Progressive multifocal leukoencephalopathy in acquired immunodeficiency syndrome: Explaining the high incidence and disproportionate frequency of the illness relative to other immunosuppressive conditions. *J Neurovirol* 9(suppl 1):38, 2003.

46. Koralnik IJ, Du Pasquier RA, Letvin NL: JC virus-specific cytotoxic T lymphocytes in individuals with progressive multifocal leukoencephalopathy. *J Virol* 75:3483, 2001.

47. Richardson-Burns SM, Kleinschmidt-DeMasters BK, DeBiasi RL, et al: Progressive multifocal leukoencephalopathy and apoptosis of infected oligodendrocytes in the central nervous system of patients with and without AIDS. *Arch Neurol* 59:1930, 2002.

48. Quinlivan EB, Norris M, Bouldin TW, et al: Subclinical central nervous system infection with JC virus in patients with AIDS. *J Infect Dis* 166:80, 1992.

49. Vazeux R, Cumont M, Girard PM, et al: Severe encephalitis resulting from coinfections with HIV and JC virus. *Neurology* 40:944, 1990.

50. Woo HH, Rezai AR, Knopp EA, et al: Contrast-enhancing progressive multifocal leukoencephalopathy: radiological and pathological correlations: Case report. *Neurosurgery* 39:1031, 1996.

51. Kotecha N, George MJ, Smith TW, et al: Enhancing progressive multifocal leukoencephalopathy: An indicator of improved immune status? *Am J Med* 105:541, 1998.

52. Miralles P, Berenguer J, Lacruz C, et al: Inflammatory reactions in progressive multifocal leukoencephalopathy after highly active antiretroviral therapy. *AIDS* 15:1900, 2001.

53. Pasquier RA, Koralnik IJ: Inflammatory reaction in progressive multifocal leukoencephalopathy: Harmful or beneficial? *J Neurovirol* 9(suppl 1):25, 2003.

54. Collazos J, Mayo J, Martinez E, et al: Contrast-enhancing progressive multifocal leukoencephalopathy as an immune reconstitution event in AIDS patients. *AIDS* 13:1426, 1999.

55. Weber T, Trebst C, Frye S, et al: Analysis of the systemic and intrathecal humoral immune response in progressive multifocal leukoencephalopathy. *J Infect Dis* 176:250, 1997.

56. Andreoletti L, Lescieux A, Lambert V, et al: Semiquantitative detection of JCV-DNA in peripheral blood leukocytes from HIV-1-infected patients with or without progressive multifocal leukoencephalopathy. *J Med Virol* 66:1, 2002.

57. Andréoletti L, Dubois V, Lescieux A, et al: Human polyomavirus JC latency and reactivation status in blood of HIV-1-positive immunocompromised patients with and without progressive multifocal leukoencephalopathy. *AIDS* 13:1469, 1999.

58. Hall CD, Dafni U, Simpson D, et al: Failure of cytarabine in progressive multifocal leukoencephalopathy associated with human immunodeficiency virus infection. *New Engl J Med* 338:1345, 1998.

59. Cinque P, Koralnik IJ, Clifford DB: The evolving face of human immunodeficiency virus–related progressive multifocal leukoencephalopathy: Defining a consensus terminology. *J Neurovirol* 9(suppl 1):88, 2003.

60. Andrei G, Snoeck R, Vandeputte M, et al: Activities of various compounds against murine and primate polyomaviruses. *Antimicrob Agents Chemother* 41:587, 1997.

61. Antinori A, Cingolani A, Lorenzini P, et al: Clinical epidemiology and survival of progressive multifocal leukoencephalopathy in the era of highly active antiretroviral therapy: Data from the Italian Registry Investigative Neuro AIDS (IRINA). *J Neurovirol* 9(suppl 1):47, 2003.

62. Gasnault J, Kousignian P, Kahraman M, et al: Cidofovir in AIDS-associated progressive multifocal leukoencephalopathy: A monocenter observational study with clinical and JC virus load monitoring. *J Neurovirol* 7:375, 2001.

63. Cinque P, Bossolasco S, Brambilla AM, et al: The effect of highly active antiretroviral therapy–induced immune reconstitution on development and outcome of progressive multifocal leukoencephalopathy: Study of 43 cases with review of the literature. *J Neurovirol* 9(suppl 1):73, 2003

64. Mayo J, Collazos J, Martínez E: Progressive multifocal leukoencephalopathy following initiation of highly active antiretroviral therapy. *AIDS* 12:1720, 1998.

65. Miralles P, Berenguer J, García de Viedma D, et al: Treatment of AIDS-associated progressive multifocal leukoencephalopathy with highly active antiretroviral therapy. *AIDS* 12:2467, 1998.

66. Brack-Werner R: Astrocytes: HIV cellular reservoirs and important participants in neuropathogenesis. *AIDS* 13:1, 1999.

67. Gasnault J, Kahraman M, de Goere MG, et al: Analysis of anti-JC virus CD4 T-cell response in healthy subjects and in HIV+ patients with or without progressive multifocal leukoencephalopathy. 9th Conference on Retrovirus and Opportunistic Infections, Seattle, WA, February 24–28, 2002 (abstract no 727-W).

68. Powderly WG: Recent advances in the management of cryptococcal meningitis in patients with AIDS. *Clin Infect Dis* 22(suppl 2):S119, 1996.

69. Pinner RW, Hajjeh RA, Powderly WG: Prospects for preventing cryptococcosis in persons infected with human immunodeficiency virus. *Clin Infect Dis* 21(suppl 1):S103, 1995.

70. Sepkowitz KA: Opportunistic infections in patients with and patients without acquired immunodeficiency syndrome. *Clin Infect Dis* 34:1098, 2002.

71. Dismukes WE: Cryptococcal meningitis in patients with AIDS. *J Infect Dis* 157:624, 1988.

72. Graybill JR, Sobel J, Saag M, et al: Diagnosis and management of intracranial pressure in patients with AIDS and cryptococcal meningitis. *Clin Infect Dis* 30:47, 2000.

73. Menichetti F, Fiorio M, Tosti A, et al: High-dose fluconazole therapy for cryptococcal meningitis in patients with AIDS. *Clin Infect Dis* 22:838, 1996.

74. van der Horst CM, Saag MS, Cloud GA, et al: Treatment of cryptococcal meningitis associated with the acquired immunodeficiency syndrome. *New Engl J Med* 337:15, 1997.

75. Saag MS, Cloud GA, Graybill JR, et al: A comparison of itraconazole versus fluconazole as maintenance therapy for AIDS-associated cryptococcal meningitis. *Clin Infect Dis* 28:291, 1999.

76. French N, Gray K, Watera C, et al: Cryptococcal infection in a cohort of HIV-1-infected Ugandan adults. *AIDS* 16:1031, 2002.

77. Saag MS, Powderly WG, Cloud GA, et al: Comparison of amphotericin B with fluconazole in the treatment of acute AIDS-associated cryptococcal meningitis. *New Engl J Med* 326:83, 1992.

78. Powderly WG: Cryptococcal meningitis in AIDS. *Clin Infect Dis* 17:837, 1993.

79. Robinson PA, Bauer M, Leal MAE, et al: Early mycological treatment failure in AIDS-associated cryptococcal meningitis. *Clin Infect Dis* 28:82, 1999.

80. Saag MS, Graybill RJ, Larsen RA, et al: Practice guidelines for the management of cryptococcal disease. *Clin Infect Dis* 30:710, 2000.

81. Feldmesser M, Harris C, Reichberg S, et al: Serum cryptococcal antigen in patients with AIDS. *Clin Infect Dis* 23:827, 1996.

82. Leenders ACAP, Reiss P, Portegies P, et al: Liposomal amphotericin B (AmBisome) compared with amphotericin B both followed by oral fluconazole in the treatment of AIDS-associated cryptococcal meningitis. *AIDS* 11:1463, 1997.

83. Sharkey PK, Graybill JR, Johnson ES, et al: Amphotericin B lipid complex compared with amphotericin B in the treatment of cryptococcal meningitis in patients with AIDS. *Clin Infect Dis* 22:315, 1996.

84. Larsen RA, Bozzette SA, Jones BE, et al: Fluconazole combined with flucytosine for treatment of cryptococcal meningitis in patients with AIDS. *Clin Infect Dis* 19:741, 1994.

85. Mayanja-Kizza H, Oishi K, Mitarai S, et al: Combination therapy with fluconazole and flucytosine for cryptococcal meningitis in Ugandan patients with AIDS. *Clin Infect Dis* 26:1362, 1998.

86. Larsen RA, Leal MA, Chan LS: Fluconazole compared with amphotericin B plus flucytosine for cryptococcal meningitis in AIDS: A randomized trial. *Ann Intern Med* 113:183, 1990.

87. Powderly WG, Saag MS, Cloud GA, et al: A controlled trial of fluconazole or amphotericin B to prevent relapse of cryptococcal meningitis in patients with the acquired immunodeficiency syndrome. *New Engl J Med* 326:793, 1992.

88. Powderly WG, Cloud GA, Dismukes WE, et al: Measurement of cryptococcal antigen in serum and cerebrospinal fluid: value in the management of AIDS-associated cryptococcal meningitis. *Clin Infect Dis* 18:789, 1994.

89. Larsen RA: A comparison of itraconazole versus fluconazole as maintenance therapy for AIDS-associated cryptococcal meningitis. *Clin Infect Dis* 28:297, 1999.

90. Monari C, Casadevall A, Baldelli F, et al: Normalization of anti-cryptococcal activity and interleukin-12 production after highly active antiretroviral therapy. *AIDS* 14:2699, 2000.

91. Denning DW, Armstrong RW, Lewis BH, et al: Elevated cerebrospinal fluid pressures in patients with cryptococcal meningitis and acquired immunodeficiency syndrome. *Am J Med* 91:267, 1991.

92. Price DA, Klein JL, Fisher M, et al: Potential role of granulocyte-macrophage colony-stimulating factor in the treatment of HIV-associated cryptococcal meningitis. *AIDS* 11:693, 1997.

93. Rex JR, Larsen RA, Dismukes WE, et al: Catastrophic visual loss due to *Cryptococcus neoformans* meningitis. *Medicine* 72:207, 1993.

94. Mussini C, Pezzotti P, Meda JM, et al: Discontinuation of maintenance therapy for cryptococcal meningitis in patients treated with HAART: A multicenter observational study. 10th Conference on Retroviruses and Opportunistic Infections, Boston, MA, February 10–14, 2003 (abstract no 799).

95. Fine HA, Mayer RJ: Primary central nervous system lymphoma. *Ann Intern Med* 119:1093, 1993.

96. Rosenblum ML, Levy RM, Bredesen DE, et al: Primary central nervous system lymphomas in patients with AIDS. *Ann Neurol* 23(suppl):S13, 1988.

97. Rubio Rodríguez MC, Rubio García R, Calvo Manuel FA: Linfoma cerebral primario asociado al SIDA: Espectro clínico, criterios diagnósticos y desarrollo terapéutico. *Rev Clin Esp* 199:161, 1999.

98. Rigolet A, Bossi P, Caumes E, et al: Caracteristiques epidemiologiques et evolution de l'incidence des lymphomes cerebraux primitifs observes chez 80 patients infectes par le VIH entre 1983 et 1999. *Pathol Biol* 49:572, 2001.

99. Inungu J, Melendez MF, Montgomery JP: AIDS-related primary brain lymphoma in Michigan, January 1990 to December 2000. *AIDS Patient Care STDs* 16:107, 2002.

100. Jacomet C, Girard PM, Lebrette MG, et al: Intravenous methotrexate for primary central nervous system non-Hodgkin's lymphoma in AIDS. *AIDS* 11:1725, 1997.

101. Raez L, Patel P, Feun L, et al: Natural history and prognostic factors for survival in patients in patients with acquired immunodeficiency syndrome (AIDS)–related primary central nervous system lymphoma (PCNSL). *Crit Rev Oncog* 9:199, 1998.

102. Remick SC, Diamond C, Migliozzi JA, et al: Primary central nervous system lymphoma in patients with and without the acquired immune deficiency syndrome: A retrospective analysis and review of the literature. *Medicine* 69:345, 1990.

103. Nuckols JD, Liu K, Burchette JL, et al: Primary central

nervous system lymphomas: A 30-year experience at a single institution. *Mod Pathol* 12:1167, 1999.

104. MacMahon EME, Glass JD, Hayward SD, et al: Epstein-Barr virus in AIDS-related primary central nervous system lymphoma. *Lancet* 338:969, 1991.

105. McGowan JP, Shah S: Long-term remission of AIDS-related primary central nervous system lymphoma associated with highly active antiretroviral therapy. *AIDS* 12:952,1998.

106. Gloghini A, Gaidano G, Larocca LM, et al: Expression of cyclin-dependent kinase inhibitor p27(Kip1) in AIDS-related diffuse large-cell lymphomas is associated with Epstein-Barr virus–encoded latent membrane protein 1. *Am J Pathol* 161:163, 2002.

107. So YT, Beckstead JH, Davis RL: Primary central nervous system lymphoma in acquired immune deficiency syndrome: A clinical and pathological study. *Ann Neurol* 20:566, 1986.

108. Baumgartner JE, Rachlin JR, Beckstead JH, et al: Primary central nervous system lymphomas: Natural history and response to radiation therapy in 55 patients with acquired immunodeficiency syndrome. *J Neurosurg* 73:206, 1990.

109. Khoo VS, Wilson PC, Sexton MJ, et al: Acquired immunodeficiency syndrome–related primary cerebral lymphoma: response to irradiation. *Australas Radiol* 44:178, 2000.

110. Chamberlain MC, Kormanik PA: AIDS-related central nervous system lymphomas. *J Neurooncol* 43:269, 1999.

111. Herrlinger U: Primary CNS lymphoma: Findings outside the brain. *J Neurooncol* 43:227, 1999.

112. Bossolasco S, Nilsson A, de Milito A, et al: Soluble CD23 in cerebrospinal fluid: a marker of AIDS-related non-Hodgkin's lymphoma in the brain. *AIDS* 15:1109, 2001.

113. Thurnher MM, Rieger A, Kleibl-Popov C, et al: Primary central nervous system lymphoma in AIDS: A wider spectrum of CT and MRI findings. *Neuroradiology* 43:29, 2001.

114. Antinori A, De Rossi G, Ammassari A, et al: Value of combined approach with thallium-201 single-photon emission computed tomography and Epstein-Barr virus DNA polymerase chain reaction in CSF for the diagnosis of AIDS-related primary CNS lymphoma. *J Clin Oncol* 17:554, 1999.

115. Lorberboym M, Wallach F, Estok L, et al: Thallium-201 retention in focal intracranial lesions for differential diagnosis of primary lymphoma and nonmalignant lesions in AIDS patients. *J Nucl Med* 39:1366, 1998.

116. Licho R, Litofsky NS, Senitko M, et al: Inaccuracy of Tl-201 brain SPECT in distinguishing cerebral infections from lymphoma in patients with AIDS. *Clin Nucl Med* 27:81, 2002.

117. Lee VW, Antonacci V, Tilak S, et al: Intracranial mass lesions: Sequential thallium and gallium scintigraphy in patients with AIDS. *Radiology* 211:507, 1999.

118. Bossolasco S, Cinque P, Ponzoni M, et al: Epstein-Barr virus DNA load in cerebrospinal fluid and plasma of patients with AIDS-related lymphoma. *J Neurovirol* 8:432, 2002.

119. al-Shahi R, Bower M, Nelson MR, et al: Cerebrospinal fluid Epstein-Barr virus detection preceding HIV-associated primary central nervous system lymphoma by 17 months. *J Neurol* 247:471, 2000.

120. Antinori A, Cingolani A, De Luca A, et al: Epstein-Barr virus in monitoring the response to therapy of acquired immunodeficiency syndrome–related primary central nervous system lymphoma. *Ann Neurol* 45:259, 1999.

121. Tachikawa N, Goto M, Hoshino Y, et al: Detection of *Toxoplasma gondii,* Epstein-Barr virus, and JC virus DNAs in the cerebrospinal fluid in acquired immunodeficiency syndrome patients with focal central nervous system complications. *Intern Med* 38:556, 1999.

122. Christov C, Adle-Biassette H, Lechapt E, et al: Primary brain lymphoma cell turnover differs in patients with and without AIDS: Relationships to *bcl-2* expression and host cell reaction. *J Neuropathol Exp Neurol* 58:1069, 1999.

123. Raez L, Cabral L, Cai JP, et al: Treatment of AIDS-related primary central nervous system lymphoma with zidovudine, ganciclovir, and interleukin 2. *AIDS Res Hum Retroviruses* 15:7139, 1999.

124. Aboulafia DM: Interleukin-2, ganciclovir and high-dose zidovudine for the treatment of AIDS-associated primary central nervous system lymphoma. *Clin Infect Dis* 34:1660, 2002.

125. Slobod KS, Taylor GH, Sandlund JT, et al: Epstein-Barr virus-targeted therapy for AIDS-related primary lymphoma of the central nervous system. *Lancet* 356:1493, 2000.

126. Hoffmann C, Tabrizian S, Wolf E, et al: Survival of AIDS patients with primary central nervous system lymphoma is dramatically improved by HAART-induced immune recovery. *AIDS* 15:2119, 2001.

127. Pajonk F, McBride WH: Survival of AIDS patients with primary central nervous system lymphoma may be improved by the radiosensitizing effects of highly active antiretroviral therapy. *AIDS* 16:1195, 2002.

128. McCutchan JA: Cytomegalovirus infections of the nervous system in patients with AIDS. *Clin Infect Dis* 20:747, 1995.

129. Maschke M, Kastrup O, Diener HC: CNS manifestations of cytomegalovirus infections: Diagnosis and treatment. *CNS Drugs* 16:303, 2002.

130. Arribas JR, Storch GA, Clifford DB, et al: Cytomegalovirus encephalitis. *Ann Intern Med* 125:577, 1996.

131. Holland NR, Power C, Mathews VP, et al: Cytomegalovirus encephalitis in acquired immunodeficiency syndrome (AIDS). *Neurology* 44:507, 1994.

132. Kalayjian RC, Cohen ML, Bonomo RA, et al: Cytomegalovirus ventriculoencephalitis in AIDS: A syndrome with distinct clinical and pathologic features. *Medicine* 72:67, 1993.

133. Cinque P, Lazzarin A: Management strategies for herpesvirus infections of the CNS: Immunocompetent and immunocompromised patients. *CNS Drugs* 14:95, 2000.

134. Anders HJ, Goebel FD: Neurological manifestations of cytomegalovirus infection in the acquired immunodeficiency syndrome. *Int J STD AIDS* 10:151, 1999.

135. Anders HJ, Goebel FD: Cytomegalovirus polyradicu-

lopathy in patients with AIDS. *Clin Infect Dis* 27:345, 1998.

136. Weber T, Beck R, Stark E, et al: Comparative analysis of intrathecal antibody synthesis and DNA amplification for the diagnosis of cytomegalovirus infection of the central nervous system in AIDS patients. *J Neurol* 241:407, 1994.

137. Cinque P, Baldanti F, Vago L, et al: Ganciclovir therapy for cytomegalovirus (CMV) infection of the central nervous system in AIDS patients: monitoring by CMV DNA detection in cerebrospinal fluid. *J Infect Dis* 171:1603, 1995.

138. Revello MG, Percivalle E, Sarasini A, et al: Diagnosis of human cytomegalovirus infection of the nervous system by pp65 detection in polymorphonuclear leukocytes of cerebrospinal fluid from AIDS patients. *J Infect Dis* 170:1275, 1994.

139. Moulignier A, Mikol J, Gonzalez-Canali G, et al: AIDS-associated cytomegalovirus infection mimicking central nervous system tumors: A diagnostic challenge. *Clin Infect Dis* 22:626, 1996.

140. Cocohoba JM, McNicholl IR: Valganciclovir: An advance in cytomegalovirus therapeutics. *Ann Pharmacother* 36:1075, 2002.

141. Anduze-Faris BM, Fillet AM, Gozlan J, et al: Induction and maintenance therapy of cytomegalovirus central nervous system infection in HIV-infected patients. *AIDS* 14:517, 2000.

142. Blick G, Garton T, Hopkins U, et al: Successful use of cidofovir in treating AIDS-related cytomegalovirus retinitis, encephalitis, and esophagitis. *J Acquir Immune Defic Syndr Hum Retrovirol* 15:84, 1997.

143. Sadler M, Morris-Jones S, Nelson M, et al: Successful treatment of cytomegalovirus encephalitis in an AIDS patient using cidofovir. *AIDS* 11:1293, 1997.

144. Whitley RJ, Jacobson MA, Friedberg DN, et al: Guidelines for the treatment of cytomegalovirus diseases in patients with AIDS in the era of potent antiretroviral therapy: Recommendations of an international panel. *Arch Intern Med* 158:957, 1998.

145. Grosse V, Schulte A, Weber K, et al: Normalization of cytomegalovirus-specific CD4 T cells in HIV-infected individuals receiving antiretroviral therapy. *AIDS* 16:1075, 2002.

146. Yazdanpanah Y, Goldie SJ, Paltiel AD, et al: Prevention of human immunodeficiency virus–related opportunistic infections in France: A cost-effectiveness analysis. *Clin Infect Dis* 36:86, 2003.

147. Tsertsvadze T, Gochitashvili N, Sharvadze L: Cytomegalovirus infection in HIV patients. XIV International AIDS Conference, Barcelona, Spain, July 7–12, 2002 (abstract ThPeB7304).

148. Weinberg A, Wohl DA, Whinney SM, et al: CMV-specific IFN gamma production correlates with protection against CMV reactivation in HIV-infected patients on HAART. 10th Conference on Retroviruses and Opportunistic Infections, Boston, MA, February 10–14, 2003 (abstract no 786).

CHAPTER 8

HIV-Associated Neuropathy and Myelopathy

David N. Herrmann and Giovanni Schifitto

Neurologic complications remain common with human immunodeficiency virus (HIV) infection, although the spectrum, frequency, and course of nervous system complications have changed in the era of highly active antiretroviral therapy (HAART).[1,2] HIV-infected individuals may develop a polyneuropathy from HIV infection, cytomegalovirus (CMV) or hepatitis C infection, impaired glucose tolerance, or antiretroviral therapy[3] (Table 8-1). HIV-associated distal sensory polyneuropathy (HIV-DSP) is the most common neurologic complication of HIV infection, affecting over 30 percent of patients during their lifetime,[4,5] with pathologic evidence of neuropathy in most patients at autopsy.[6] It is of relevance because its cardinal symptom, pain, is commonly disabling and difficult to manage, and the presence of HIV-DSP limits options for antiretroviral treatment. HIV-1-associated myelopathy causes a subacute progressive weakness, sexual dysfunction, and urinary

urgency or incontinence. Like HIV-DSP, HIV-1-associated myelopathy is more prevalent in autopsy series than symptomatic during life. Therapy for both disorders includes optimizing antiretroviral therapy.

▶ HIV-ASSOCIATED DISTAL SENSORY POLYNEUROPATHY (HIV-DSP)

Clinical and Laboratory Features and Differential Diagnosis (see Table 8-1)

HIV-DSP is a symmetric and frequently painful, predominantly sensory axonal polyneuropathy.[7,8] Symptoms are usually insidious in onset and start in a distal fashion in the feet with varying combinations of numbness, paresthesias, dysesthesias, burning pain, deep pain, lightening pains, spontaneous pain, and stimulus-

▶ **TABLE 8-1.** PERIPHERAL NEUROPATHIES ASSOCIATED WITH HIV INFECTION

	Early	Late
Polyneuropathy or polyradiculoneuropathy	ATN (dideoxynucleoside agents) Guillain-Barré syndrome (AIDP) Mononeuritis multiplex related to vasculitis (less likely in early stage) Cranial neuropathies (esp. facial)	HIV-associated DSP ATN (dideoxynucleoside agents) Guillain-Barré syndrome (AIDP) (less likely in late stage) Chronic inflammatory demyelinating polyneuropathy Autonomic neuropathy CMV-associated mononeuropathy multiplex Mononeuritis multiplex related to vasculitis Diffuse infiltrative Lymphocytosis syndrome
Polyradiculopathy or plexopathy	Usually not seen	CMV-associated lumbosacral polyradiculopathy Polyradiculopathy related to other infectious meningitides (e.g., cryptococcal infection or neoplastic meningitis) HIV-associated lumbosacral plexopathy
Anterior horn cells disorders	Usually not seen	Motor neuron disease–like illness

ATN = acute toxic neuropathy; AIDP = acute inflammatory demyelinating polyneuropathy.

evoked pain (hyperalgesia, allodynia). Patients uncommonly report paresthesias in the hands early in the course of HIV-DSP, and this symptom raises a differential diagnosis of acute toxic neuropathies (ATNs), superimposed carpal tunnel syndrome, ulnar neuropathy, cervical radiculopathy, or an alternate or coexisting cause for polyneuropathy (e.g., vitamin B_{12} deficiency or diabetes mellitus). Complaints of focal weakness are not a feature of HIV-DSP and usually suggest an associated or superimposed process, e.g., HIV-associated myopathy, mononeuritis multiplex, or inflammatory demyelinating polyneuropathy. Neurologic examination reveals a symmetric sensory loss in a distal-to-proximal gradient in the feet and legs. The frequency of abnormalities on bedside sensory testing vary with the clinical case definition of HIV-DSP. In one large study, ankle reflexes were absent or reduced in 66 percent of patients, abnormal pinprick sensation was found in 71 percent, and vibration thresholds were elevated in 65 percent, whereas loss of proprioception was less frequent (19 percent), being seen mainly in advanced cases.[8] Muscle wasting and weakness are infrequent with HIV-DSP and, when present, are confined to toe flexors and extensors and foot intrinsic muscles.[7]

Based on these clinical features, research criteria for probable HIV-DSP have been developed and include the following[9]:

Probable (must have all the following):
1. Symptoms of pain, burning, dysesthesia, and paresthesia in feet > hands

2. Neurologic examination consistent with a distal predominantly sensory polyneuropathy (decreased or absent ankle jerks, decreased vibration distally, decreased pain and temperature sensation in a stocking > glove distribution)
3. No other etiology, including exposure to zalcitabine (ddC), didanosine (ddI), and stavudine (d4T)

Possible:
1. Must meet criteria 1 and 2 above
2. Another contributing factor cannot be excluded, including a history of prior or current use of ddC, ddI, and d4T.

There are no characteristic laboratory abnormalities in HIV-DSP. Cerebrospinal fluid (CSF) studies are not performed unless there are other atypical clinical features that suggest an opportunistic infectious, autoimmune, or neoplastic process. In individuals with HIV-DSP alone, the CSF cell count is usually normal, and the protein concentration is either normal or mildly increased. The presence of pleocytosis raises the possibility of central nervous system (CNS) infection or a neoplastic process.[8]

Epidemiology

Estimates of the prevalence of symptomatic DSP (SDSP) (prior to the advent of HAART) ranged from 1.5 percent of HIV-infected individuals to about 48 percent of patients with acquired immune deficiency syndrome

(AIDS).[8,10] These disparate prevalence estimates reflect differences in the cohorts used in the study of DSP. Most studies in the pre-HAART era estimated the prevalence of HIV-DSP to be about 30 to 35 percent.[4] Since the advent of HAART, the incidence of neurologic disorders in HIV-infected individuals in general has shown a steep decline.[1] The incidence of SDSP also appears to have declined. The 1-year incidence of SDSP was 36 percent in the pre-HAART Dana cohort of HIV-infected subjects with moderate to severe immunosuppression versus 21 percent in a similarly constituted HAART era cohort.[4] By contrast, as HIV-infected patients live longer with the disease, the overall prevalence of SDSP appears to be increasing.

Large epidemiologic studies in HIV infection before the advent of HAART identified several risk factors for SDSP.[4,11] These include a history of AIDS diagnoses, worse physical function scores, advanced immunosuppression, higher HIV plasma viral load, and older age.[4,8,11] Gender does not appear to be a risk factor for SDSP.[4] The relationship between antiretroviral therapy (ART) and SDSP is complex.[12] In the pre-HAART era, the incidence of SDSP was associated with a history of ART use in the Multicenter AIDS Cohort Study (MACS), and widespread use of dideoxynucleoside reverse-transcriptase inhibitors (DDNs) has been suggested to account for the increased incidence of SDSP seen in this cohort in the years 1988–1992.[12] Dideoxynucleoside reverse-transcriptase inhibitors ddC, ddI, and d4T have been associated with a characteristic syndrome of a subacute-onset painful distal sensory neuropathy in patients with HIV infection. Symptoms typically occur within weeks or months of initiation of DDN.[3,13] Symptoms subside in most patient's after discontinuation of DDNs, although neurologic signs typically persist.[3] Acute toxic neuropathies have been seen mainly in patients with more advanced immunosuppression and with higher dosing regimens of DDNs. In an analysis of the Johns Hopkins Hospital AIDS Clinic database, Moore and colleagues found that the incidence of DSP was 8 percent with d4T, 20 percent with ddI, 21 percent with ddI + d4T, and 26 percent with ddI + d4T + hydroxyurea.[14] Hydroxyurea alone has not been associated with a sensory neuropathy but is felt to enhance the toxicity of DDN.[12] More recently, with changing patient selection and dosing of DDNs, DDN use within 6 months of study enrollment was not found to be a risk factor for SDSP in the DANA and North East AIDS dementia (NEAD) cohorts.[4,15] Indeed, although DDNs have been shown to be toxic to dorsal root ganglion (DRG) neurons in culture via mechanisms of mitochondrial toxicity, they have failed to produce SDSP in animal models, and current opinion is that DDNs probably in most instances unmask an asymptomatic neuropathy in the susceptible HIV-infected host rather than causing a de novo peripheral neurotoxicity.[12]

Recent data suggest that a state of asymptomatic DSP (ADSP), as defined by neuropathic deficits on clinical examination, may be a risk factor for progression to SDSP.[15] Use of alcohol or intravenous drugs and associated hepatitis C infection are also potential risk factors for SDSP that require further study.

Pathology

Pathologic changes have been observed at multiple levels of the peripheral nervous system in HIV-DSP.[6,16] At autopsy, peripheral nervous system pathology is observed in almost all HIV-infected patients irrespective of whether they had SDSP in life.[6] Studies demonstrate pathology that is distally accentuated and affects sensory more than motor nerves.[6,16] Dorsal root ganglia have a slight loss of neurons.[16] Axonal degeneration of the central and peripheral projections of DRG neurons is evident with a distal greater than proximal severity gradient.[6,16,17] Sural nerve biopsies show predominant loss of unmyelinated fibers, although myelinated fiber dropout is evident to some degree.[18] Sural nerve biopsies show degenerating axon profiles and axonal atrophy with few regenerative axonal clusters.[19] Demyelination, although reported, is a minor feature.[7,16] Perivascular mononuclear inflammatory collections may be seen in the epineurium or endoneurium on sural nerve biopsy; however, vasculitis is not a feature of HIV-DSP. Electron microscopy additionally discloses tubuloreticular inclusions in endothelial cells and macrophages. Skin biopsies confirm a loss of nociceptive C fibers in the epidermis in most patients, although milder cases may demonstrate a normal density of epidermal nerve fibers but the presence of morphologic changes within these fibers and in the subepidermal nerve fiber plexus.[20] These morphologic changes include focal intraaxonal swellings and an excessively segmented or tortuous appearance of surviving nerve fibers.[21]

Studies in DSP have shown infiltration of activated macrophages and T-lymphocytes (CD8 predominance) at multiple levels within the peripheral nervous system. Increased levels of proinflammatory cytokines occur in areas of axonal degeneration and in DRG neurons.[16,22] Immunohistochemical and in situ hybridization studies, in contrast, generally have failed to demonstrate productive infection of peripheral neuronal tissue by the HIV virus,[22,23] although HIV virus occasionally has been cultured from peripheral nerve tissue and HIV mRNA and protein have been observed in inflammatory cells (most likely macrophages) in peripheral nerve and DRG neurons.[22,24,25]

Pathogenesis

The exact pathogenesis of HIV-DSP has not been established. The currently held hypothesis is of dysregulated immune activation with activated macrophage infiltration of the peripheral nervous system, production of proinflammatory cytokines, and cytokine-mediated neurotoxicity.[22] These events are triggered by HIV infection or HIV proteins, e.g., GP120 envelope protein, which has been shown in experimental models to produce DRG neurotoxicity. Although this hypothesis remains to be proven in vivo, several lines of evidence favor an indirect cytokine-mediated or HIV protein–mediated neurotoxicity over a direct viral neurotoxicity. Productive HIV infection replication does not occur in DRG neurons according to most investigations.[12,22,26] In contrast, macrophage infiltration and upregulation of cytokines [in particular, tumor necrosis factor α (TNF-α)] is well established in the setting of HIV-DSP, with HIV-infected individuals without neurologic manifestations showing lower levels of proinflammatory cytokine and macrophage activation.[12,22,27] In a recent study,[15] CSF levels of the cytokine macrophage colony-stimulating factor (M-CSF) were found to be predictive of SDSP. M-CSF has been associated with active HIV replication.[28,29] In addition, M-CSF may modulate other macrophage inflammatory mediators. Recent studies also have shown in a DRG culture model that GP120 is neurotoxic to DRG neurons and that this neurotoxicity is mediated by binding of GP120 to chemokine receptors on Schwann cells with release of RANTES (regulated on activation, normal T-cell expressed and secreted), which in turn results in TNF-α-mediated neurotoxicity via caspase 3–dependent pathways.[30] Peripheral nerve injury is hypothesized to lead to a neuropathic pain cascade with peripheral sensitization of nociceptors, changes in transcription of proteins (including voltage-gated sodium channels), and central sensitization.

Diagnosis

The diagnosis of HIV-SDSP is generally a clinical one. In typical cases, electrodiagnostic studies, quantitative sensory testing, and skin or sural nerve biopsy are not mandatory. Formal assessments of peripheral nerve function and pathology are discussed below. HIV-DSP should be distinguished from a superimposed ATN related to DDNs (i.e., ddI, ddC, and d4T). ATN is generally more acute in onset and occurs within weeks to a few months of beginning therapy with a DDN.[3,12]. A combination of DDNs increases the risk for ATN.[14] A diagnosis of superimposed ATN can be supported by clinical improvement with discontinuation of the DDN. The finding on clinical examination of brisk knee reflexes, increased tone, or bladder disturbance should prompt consideration of an associated myelopathy (e.g., HIV-associated myelopathy; see next section).

In addition to a clinical evaluation, laboratory testing in suspected HIV-DSP should include screening for impaired glucose tolerance (IGT) and diabetes, vitamin B_{12} deficiency, and hypothyroidism. IGT and diabetes have become increasingly prevalent among HIV-infected patients since the introduction of protease inhibitors, and this may contribute to SDSP. Screening for vitamin B_{12} deficiency is best accomplished with a serum vitamin B_{12} determination and a methylmalonic acid determination. A careful history also should be taken for alcohol abuse or malnutrition with thiamine deficiency because these may manifest with a qualitatively similar painful sensory polyneuropathy.[8] Hepatitis C infection is being recognized increasingly in patients with HIV infection in part because of similar epidemiologic risk factors for infection, including intravenous drug abuse and unprotected sexual activity.[31] Hepatitis C infection has an expanding spectrum of peripheral neuropathies either directly associated with the infection or related to cryoglobulinemia. Hepatitis C infection may produce a distal painful predominantly sensory polyneuropathy. Thus the possibility of hepatitis C infection always should be considered in the setting of HIV infection.

Spinal fluid analysis, electrophysiologic testing, or objective measures of small sensory nerve fiber function (e.g., skin biopsy) do not need to be obtained routinely when the history and examination findings are typical. If there are atypical clinical features or uncertainty as to the presence of DSP, obtain nerve conductions studies and electromyography. These may disclose features of a distal sensory greater than motor axonal polyneuropathy. Atypical features on nerve conduction studies (e.g., the presence of a diffuse demyelinating polyneuropathy) should prompt consideration of an alternative cause for the neuropathic symptoms. However, nerve conduction studies may remain normal in approximately 50 percent of patients with HIV-DSP because of predominant small sensory nerve fiber involvement, in which instance skin biopsy with assessment of epidermal fiber (ENF) density and morphology can be helpful to support the diagnosis[20,32,33] (Fig. 8-1). Skin biopsy from the distal leg in HIV-DSP show a reduced ENF density in about 50 percent of cases and morphologic changes (e.g., axonal swellings) in most cases of SDSP.

Quantitative sensory testing (QST) has been used largely in a research setting in HIV infection. Several studies have shown presymptomatic QST abnormalities of cooling, warm, vibration, and heat pain thresholds in some HIV-infected individuals.[19] However, although QST is being incorporated increasingly in a clinical peripheral neuropathy setting, it is not used alone in HIV neuropathy to support a putative diagnosis of SDSP. There are several reasons for this. QST is nonlocalizing as to whether the sensory deficit is in the central or peripheral nervous system. In HIV-infected individuals who may have coexisting myelopathy or other neurologic complications, this dilemma is amplified. In addi-

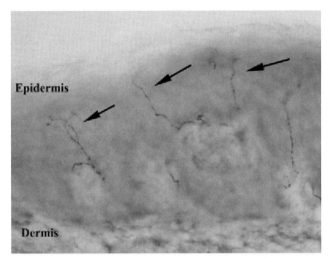

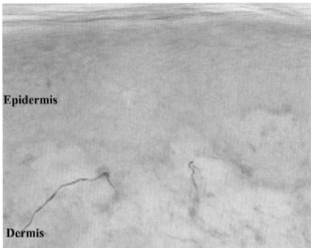

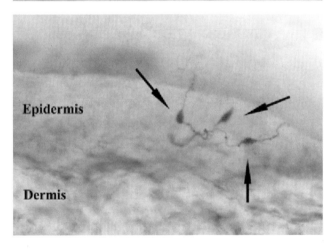

Figure 8-1. *Top:* Normal epidermal innervation (*arrows*) in a patient with HIV infection and no neuropathy. *Center:* Loss of epidermal innervation in a patient with symptomatic DSP. *Bottom:* Axon swellings (*arrows*) in a patient with DSP. *(Reprinted with permission from Herrmann DN, McDermott MD, Henderson D, Chen L, Akowuah K, Schifitto G and the North East AIDS Dementia (NEAD) Consortium: epidermal innervation, QST and development of HIV-associated distal neuropathy muscle nerve. 29:420, 2004.)*

tion, QST is a psychophysical test that, while an aid in the diagnosis of sensory disorders, should not be employed as the sole piece of "objective" testing to support a clinical suspicion of peripheral neuropathy.[34]

Treatment

Disease-Modifying Therapy

There are no therapies proven to limit progression or reverse the course of HIV-DSP. The efficacy of establishing virologic control of the HIV infection and specifically the effects of HAART on SDSP progression are uncertain and require longitudinal investigation. A pilot study has suggested that virologic control following a change in or institution of ART improves thermal thresholds.[35] Studies in the HAART era[15] suggest that the incidence of progression to HIV-DSP has decreased; however, since the lifespans of HIV-infected subjects have increased, it is expected that the prevalence of SDSP will increase. Protease inhibitors also have increased the incidence of impaired glucose tolerance and diabetes in HIV infection,[36] which may independently contribute to painful sensory neuropathy or exacerbate underlying SDSP. The focus of SDSP management thus is currently on symptomatic therapy.

Symptomatic Therapy (Table 8-2)

Review the patient's comorbidities, looking for factors (e.g., excess alcohol use) that may be compounding, and encourage lifestyle modification. If there is any question of onset of neuropathic symptoms in relation to initiation of a DDN drug, make a change in the regimen, if possible, while still maintaining an optimal virologic control.

The control of neuropathic pain is a primary objective. The approaches used are largely from studies and experience with painful diabetic neuropathies because only a limited number of compounds have been assessed in randomized, double-blind studies in HIV-DSP.

Amitriptyline, a mainstay of neuropathic pain regimens, is used widely in HIV-DSP, but to date it has not been found to be effective in double-blind, randomized, controlled trials in HIV-DSP, although the power of these studies to detect a benefit may have been limited.[37,38] Trials of mexiletine (modestly effective in some studies in diabetic neuropathy) and topical capsaicin have not been effective in HIV-DSP.[37,39] Lamotrigine (an anticonvulsant), which is a second- or third-line agent in most neuropathic pain regimens, in contrast, has been found to be effective in a double-blind, randomized study in HIV infection, although this effect was noticeable only in subjects who were exposed to ddN.[40] Studies using nerve growth factor showed improvement in neuropathic pain but no clear improvement in clinical, QST, and epidermal innervation measures of HIV-DSP.[41] Commonly used neuro-

▶ **TABLE 8-2.** SUMMARY OF THERAPEUTIC AGENTS COMMONLY USED FOR PAINFUL HIV-DSP*

Drug	Mechanism of Action	Daily Dose(mg)	Major Side Effects
Antidepressants	Na channel inhibition		Anticholinergic effects
Tricyclics/tetracyclic	5-HT/Nor inhibition		Cardiac effects
Amitriptyline (useful with concurrent insomnia)		10–150	
Nortriptyline (least cardiac effects)		10–150	
Desipramine (least anticholinergic side effects)		25–200	CNS stimulation
Anticonvulsants			
Gabapentin (generally well tolerated)	Ca channel agonist	200–3600	Sedation
Lamotrigine (to be slowly titrated)	NA channel stabilization Glutamate release inhibition	25–500	Stevens-Johnson syndrome
Opioids			
Tramadol	Mu receptor agonist	50–400	Constipation; lowers seizure threshold when used in combination with tricyclic agents
Morphine sulfate (extended release)	Opioid agonists	15–120	Respiratory depression; constipation; sedation
Fentanyl patch	Opioid agonists	25 μg/h patch (72-h application)	Respiratory depression; constipation; sedation; hypotension
Topicals			
Lidocaine patch (5%) (suitable for localized pain)	Na channel blocker	May use up to 3 patches/24 h; only use for 12 h in a 24-h period	Local irritation; CNS effect (rare)

5-HT = 5-hydroxytryptamine; Nor = noradrenaline; DA = dopamine.

pathic pain agents, such as gabapentin and tramadol, both effective in double-blind, randomized, controlled studies in diabetic neuropathy, have not been studied systematically in HIV-DSP.[42,43]

Given the limited number of controlled studies in HIV-DSP, patients with HIV-DSP can be treated in a manner similar to those with painful diabetic polyneuropathy. Tricyclic antidepressants and gabapentin generally are used as first-line agents. If either of these agents is ineffective or insufficient at a maximally tolerated dose (see Table 8-2), use a combination of these or add tramadol or lamotrigine. Do not use lamotrigine as a first-line agent because of the potential for rash, although this can be reduced significantly by a slow titration schedule. The lidocaine 5% patch may be helpful as adjunctive therapy in patients in whom the neuropathic pain is restricted to the feet or is particularly symptomatic in a focal area. Randomized, controlled studies are lacking at the present time for the lidocaine 5% patch outside of postherpetic neuralgia.[44] Long-acting narcotics, e.g., long-acting morphine preparations, and the fentanyl patch are helpful in some patients with refractory pain.

▶ HIV-1-ASSOCIATED MYELOPATHY

HIV-1-associated myelopathy is a well-described clinical entity affecting patients with advanced immune suppression. Typically, the condition follows a subacute progression of difficulty walking, fatigue, sexual dysfunction, and urinary urgency or incontinence. The neurologic examination reveals spastic tone and weakness in the lower extremities associated with hyperreflexia at the knees and bilateral Babinski signs. Ankle reflexes may be normal or decreased if there is a coexisting sensory neuropathy. The diffuse involvement of the spinal cord likely explains the fact that a sensory level is often absent. However, when present, a sensory level usually is reported in the middle to lower thoracic dermatomes, which are also the areas most affected histologically.[45,46]

Epidemiology

In the pre-HAART era, evidence of myelopathy was found at autopsy in up to 50 percent of all AIDS patients. However, a far smaller proportion of patients was ever diagnosed clinically during life.[45–47] Several opportunistic conditions may coexist and primarily be responsible for the myelopathy. For example, in a recent series from South Africa[48] of 33 patients presenting with myelopathic signs, only one patient did not have other confounding coinfections such as HTLV-I, tuberculosis, herpes simplex, herpes zoster, or syphilis. In countries where ART is available, the clinical diagnosis of myelopathy has become quite rare.

Pathology

Macroscopically, spongiform changes involve the spinal cord diffusely (Fig. 8-2) with some resemblance to that seen in subacute combined degeneration associated with vitamin B_{12} deficiency. On microscopic examination, there is vacuolation of the spinal cord white matter associated with lipid-laden macrophages, primarily affecting the thoracic cord.[45,47,49] The vacuolation involves the posterior and lateral columns, although as the process progresses the anterolateral tracts can be affected (see Fig. 8-2). In areas of severe vacuolation, axonal spheroids and activated astrocytes are present as well.[50]

Pathogenesis

The role of HIV in vacuolar myelopathy is not well understood. A few case reports[51,52] suggest clinical improvement with HAART treatment. However, the current data are suggestive of an as yet incompletely elucidated indirect mechanism of neurotoxicity that is likely linked to immune activation triggered and maintained by HIV infection.[22,53] It is possible that macrophage-released immune mediators may interfere with neuronal metabolism, e.g., transmethylation.[54] In this regard, an open-label pilot trial with L-methionine suggested some benefit in patients with HIV-1-associated myelopathy.[55]

Diagnosis

The diagnosis of HIV-1-associated myelopathy depends on the ability to exclude other confounding etiologies that can affect the spinal cord. When the myelopathic signs are equivocal, somatosensory evoked potentials can be useful in supporting the diagnosis of myelopathy.[56] Contrast-enhanced magnetic resonance imaging (MRI) of the entire spinal cord and lumbar puncture should be performed routinely to exclude infections with the herpesviruses, *Toxoplasma,* tuberculosis, CMV, syphilis, and carcinomatous meningitis.[57–65] Occasionally, non-HIV conditions such as vertebral fractures and herniated disks may be responsible for the clinical presentation. More acute presentations are suggestive of intradural or extradural mass lesions or vascular abnormalities.[66] Additional laboratory studies should include a vitamin B_{12} determination, syphilis serology, and HTLV-I tests.

Treatment

Currently, there is no treatment that modifies the course of HIV-1-associated myelopathy. Since HIV infection triggers the condition, patients should be maximized in their ART regimen to achieve undetectable virus levels. As mentioned earlier, case reports have suggested that some patients may improve when ART regimens effectively control virus replication. However, for the most part, the therapeutic effort is aimed at treating the associated spasticity and bladder dysfunction. Therefore, symptomatic treatment similar to that in other myelopathic conditions includes the use of benzodiazepines and baclofen to reduce the muscle tone and anticholinergic or cholinergic drugs in the presence of a spastic or flaccid bladder, respectively.

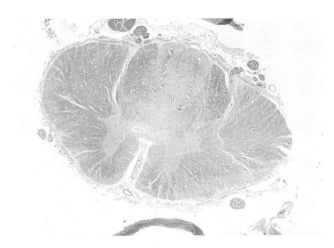

Figure 8-2. Vacuolation of the spinal cord white matter in a patient with HIV-1-associated myelopathy (luxol fast blue stain). Note the diffuse involvement of the spinal cord with near-complete myelin loss of the fasciculus gracilis. *(Reprinted with permission from Holloway R, Kieburtz K, Schifitto G. HIV-1 infection and the Nervous System in Clinical Neurology. Editors RJ Joynt, MD PhD, RC Griggs, MD. Lippincott-Raven. 1996;26B:1–45.)*

REFERENCES

1. Palella FJ, Delaney KM, Moorman AC, et al: Declining morbidity and mortality among patients with advance human immunodeficiency virus infection. *New Engl J Med* 338(13):853, 1998.
2. Sacktor N, Lyles RH, Skolasky R, et al: HIV-associated neurologic disease incidence changes: Multicenter AIDS Cohort Study, 1990–1998. *Neurology* 56:257, 2001.
3. Blum AS, Dal Pan GJ, Feinberg J, et al: Low-dose zalcitabine-related toxic neuropathy: Frequency, natural history, and risk factors. *Neurology* 46:999, 1996.

4. Schifitto G, McDermott MP, McArthur JC, et al: Incidence of and risk factors for HIV-associated distal sensory polyneuropathy. *Neurology* 58:1764, 2002.

5. So YT, Holtzman DM, Abrams DI, Olney RK: Peripheral neuropathy associated with acquired immunodeficiency syndrome: Prevalence and clinical features from a population-based survey. *Arch Neurol* 45:945, 1988.

6. Pardo CA, McArthur JC, Griffin JW: HIV neuropathy: Insights in the pathology of HIV peripheral nerve disease. *J Peripher Nerv Syst* 6(1):21, 2001.

7. Cornblath DR, McArthur JC: Predominantly sensory neuropathy in patients with AIDS and AIDS-related complex. *Neurology* 38:794, 1988.

8. Tagliati M, Grinnell J, Godbold J, Simpson DM: Peripheral nerve function in HIV infection: Clinical, electrophysiologic and laboratory findings. *Arch Neurol* 56:84, 1999.

9. Janssen RS, Cornblath DR, Epstein LG, et al: Human immunodeficiency virus (HIV) infection and the nervous system: Report from the American Academy of Neurology AIDS Task Force. *Neurology* 39(1):119, 1989.

10. Barohn RJ, Gronseth GS, LeForce BR, et al: Peripheral nervous system involvement in a large cohort of human immunodeficiency virus–infected individuals. *Arch Neurol* 50:167, 1993.

11. Childs EA, Lyles RH, Selnes OA, et al: Plasma viral load and CD4 lymphocytes predict HIV-associated dementia and sensory neuropathy. *Neurology* 52:607, 1999.

12. Cherry CL, McArthur JC, Hoy JF, Wesselingh SL: Nucleoside analogues and neuropathy in the era of HAART. *J Clin Virol* 26:195, 2003.

13. Berger AR, Arezzo JC, Schaumburg HH, et al: 2',3'-Dideoxycytidine (ddC) toxic neuropathy: A study of 52 patients. *Neurology* 43:358, 1993.

14. Moore RD, Wong W-ME, Keruly JC, McArthur JC: Incidence of neuropathy in HIV-infected patients on monotherapy versus those on combination therapy with didanosine, stavudine and hydroxyurea. *AIDS* 14:273, 2000.

15. Schifitto G, McDermott MP, McArthur JC, et al: HIV-associated painful neuropathy in the era of highly active antiretroviral therapy. *Ann Neurol* 54(suppl 7):S50, 2003.

16. Bradley WG, Shapshak P, Delgado S, et al: Morphometric analysis of the peripheral neuropathy of AIDS. *Muscle Nerve* 21(9):1188, 1998.

17. Rance NE, McArthur JC, Cornblath DR, et al: Gracile tract degeneration in patients with sensory neuropathy and AIDS. *Neurology* 38:265, 1988.

18. Luciano CA, Pardo CA, McArthur JC: Recent developments in the HIV neuropathies. *Curr Opin Neurol* 16(3):403, 2003.

19. Fuller GN, Jacobs JM, Guiloff RJ: Nature and incidence of peripheral nerve syndrome in HIV infection. *J Neurol Neurosurg Psychiatry* 56:372, 1993.

20. Polydefkis M, Yiannoutsos C, Cohen B, et al: Reduced intraepidermal nerve fiber density in HIV-associated sensory neuropathy. *Neurology* 58:115, 2002.

21. Griffin JW, McAthur JC, Polydefkis M: Assessment of cutaneous innervation by skin biopsies. *Curr Opin Neurol* 14(5):655, 2001.

22. Tyor WR, Wesselingh SL, Griffin JW, et al: Unifying hypothesis for the pathogenesis of HIV-associated dementia complex, vacuolar myelopathy, and sensory neuropathy (review). *J Acquir Immune Defic Syndr Hum Retrovirol* 9:379, 1995.

23. Brannagan TH, Nuovo GJ, Hays AP, Latov N: Human immunodeficiency virus infection of dorsal root ganglion neurons detected by polymerase chain reaction in situ hybridization. *Ann Neurol* 42(3):368, 1997.

24. de la Monte SM, Gabuzda DH, Ho DD, et al: Peripheral neuropathy in the acquired immunodeficiency syndrome. *Ann Neurol* 23(5):485, 1988.

25. Rizzuto N, Cavallaro T, Monaco S, et al: Role of HIV in the pathogenesis of distal symmetrical peripheral neuropathy. *Acta Neruopathol* 90(3):244, 1995.

26. Anonymous: Thalidomide neuropathy. *Lancet* 1(7597):713, 1969.

27. Wesselingh SL, Glass J, McArthur JC, et al: Cytokine dysregulation in HIV-associated neurological disease. *Adv Neurolimmunol* 4(3):199, 1994.

28. Kutza J, Fields K, Grimm TA, Clouse KA: Inhibition of HIV replication and macrophage colony-stimulating factor production in human macrophages by antiretroviral agents. *AIDS Res Hum Retroviruses* 18(9):619, 2002.

29. Hori K, Burd PR, Kutza J, et al: Human astrocytes inhibit HIV-1 expression in monocyte-derived macrophages by secreted factors. *AIDS* 13(7):751, 1999.

30. Keswani SC, Polley M, Pardo CA, et al: Schwann cell chemokine receptors mediate HIV-1 gp120 toxicity to sensory neurons. *Ann Neurol* 54(3):287, 2003.

31. Klein MB, Lalonde RG, Suissa S: The impact of hepatitis C virus coninfection on HIV progression before and after highly active antiretroviral therapy. *AIDS* 33(3):365, 2003.

32. McCarthy BG, Hsieh S-T, Stocks A, et al: Cutaneous innervation in sensory neuropathies: Evaluation by skin biopsy. *Neurology* 45:1848, 1995.

33. Herrmann DN, Griffin JW, Hauer P, et al: Epidermal nerve fiber density and sural nerve morphometry in peripheral neuropathies. *Neurology* 53:1634, 1999.

34. Dyck PJ, Dyck PJ, Kennedy WR, et al: Limitations of quantitative sensory testing when patients are biased toward a bad outcome (see comments). *Neurology* 50(5):1213, 1998.

35. Martin C, Solders G, Sonnerborg A, Hansson P: Antiretroviral therapy may improve sensory function in HIV-infected patients: a pilot study. *Neurology* 54(11):2120, 2000.

36. Justman JE, Benning L, Danoff A, et al: Protease inhibitor use and the incidence of diabetes mellitus in a large cohort of HIV-infected women. *J AIDS* 32(3):298, 2003.

37. Kieburtz K, Simpson D, Yiannoutsos C, et al: A randomized trial of amitriptyline and mexiletine for painful neuropathy in HIV infection. *Neurology* 51:1682, 1998.

38. Shlay JC, Chaloner K, Max M, et al: Acupuncture and amitriptyline for pain due to HIV-related peripheral neuropathy. *JAMA* 280:1590, 1998.

39. Paice JA, Ferrans CE, Lashley FR, et al: Topical capsaicin in the management of HIV-associated peripheral neuropathy. *J Pain Sympt Manag* 19(1):45, 2000.

40. Simpson DM, McArthur JC, Olney R, et al: Lamotrigine for HIV-associated painful sensory neuropathies: A placebo-controlled trial. *Neurology* 60(9):1508, 2003.

41. McArthur JC, Yiannoutsos C, Simpson DM, et al: A phase II trial of nerve growth factor for sensory neuropathy associated with HIV infection. AIDS Clinical Trials Group Team 291. *Neurology* 54(5):1080, 2000.

42. Harati Y, Gooch C, Swenson M, et al: Double-blind, randomized trial of tramadol for the treatment of the pain of diabetic neuropathy. *Neurology* 50(6):1842, 1998.

43. Backonja M, Beydoun A, Edwards KR, et al: Gabapentin for the symptomatic treatment of painful neuropathy in patients with diabetes mellitus: A randomized, controlled trial. *JAMA* 280(21):1831, 1998.

44. Rowbotham MC, Davies PS, Verkempinck C, Galer BS: Lidocaine patch: Double-blind, controlled study of a new treatment method for post-herpetic neuralgia. *Pain* 65(1):39, 1996.

45. Bergmann M, Gullotta F, Kuchelmeister K, et al: AIDS-myelopathy: A neuropathological study. *Pathol Res Pract* 189:58, 1993.

46. DalPan GJ, Glass JD, McArthur JC: Clinicopathologic correlations of HIV-1-associated vacuolar myelopathy: An autopsy-based case-control study. *Neurology* 44:2159, 1994.

47. Petito CK, Navia BA, Cho E-S, et al: Vacuolar myelopathy pathologically resembling subacute combined degeneration in patients with the acquired immunodeficiency syndrome. *New Engl J Med* 312:874, 1985.

48. Bhigjee AI, Madurai S, Bill PLA, et al: Spectrum of myelopathies in HIV seropositive South African patients. *Neurology* 57:348, 2001.

49. Artigas J, Grosse G, Niedobitek F: Vacuolar myelopathy in AIDS: A morphological analysis. *Pathol Res Pract* 186:228, 1990.

50. Rottnek M, DiRocco A, Laudier D, Morgello S: Axonal damage is a late component of vacuolar myelopathy. *Neurology* 58:479, 2002.

51. Eyer-Silva WA, Couto-Fernandez JC, Caetano MR, et al: Remission of HIV-associated myelopathy after initiation of lopinavir in a patient with extensive previous exposure to highly active antiretroviral therapy. *AIDS* 15(17):2367, 2002.

52. Staudinger R, Henry K: Remission of HIV myelopathy after highly active antiretroviral therapy (comment). *Neurology* 54(1):267, 2000.

53. Tyor WR, Glass JD, Baumrind N, et al: Cytokine expression of macrophages in HIV-1-associated vacuolar myelopathy. *Neurology* 43:1002, 1993.

54. Tan SV, Guiloff RJ: Hypothesis on the pathogenesis of vacuolar myelopathy, dementia, and peripheral neuropathy in AIDS. *J Neurol Neurosurg Psychiatry* 65(1):23, 1998.

55. DiRocco A, Tagliati M, Danisi F, et al: A pilot study of L-methionine for the treatment of AIDS-associated myelopathy. *Neurology* 51(1):266, 1998.

56. Tagliati M, Di Rocco A, Danisi F, Simpson DM: The role of somatosensory evoked potentials in the diagnosis of AIDS-associated myelopathy. *Neurology* 54:1477, 2000.

57. Vinters HV, Kwok MK, Ho HW, et al: Cytomegalovirus in the nervous system of patients with the acquired immune deficiency syndrome. *Brain* 112:245, 1989.

58. Jacobson MA, Mills J, Rush J, et al: Failure of antiretroviral therapy for acquired immunodeficiency syndrome–related cytomegalovirus myelitis. *Arch Neurol* 45:1090, 1988.

59. Tucker T, Dix RD, Katzen C, et al: Cytomegalovirus and herpes simplex virus ascending myelitis in a patient with acquired immune deficiency syndrome. *Ann Neurol* 18:74, 1985.

60. Britton CB, Mesa-Tejada J, Fenoglio CM, et al: A new complication of AIDS: Thoracic myelitis caused by herpes simplex virus. *Neurology* 35:1071, 1985.

61. Herskovitz S, Siegel SE, Schneider AT, et al: Spinal cord toxoplasmosis in AIDS. *Neurology* 39:1552, 1989.

62. Overhage JM, Greist A, Brown DR: Conus medullaris syndrome resulting from toxoplasma gondii infection in a patient with the acquired immunodeficiency syndrome. *Am J Med* 89:814, 1990.

63. Harris TM, Smith RR, Bognanno JR, Edwards MK: Toxoplasmic myelitis in AIDS: Gadolinium-enhanced MR. *J Comput Assist Tomogr* 14:809, 1990.

64. Woolesy RM, Chambers TJ, Chung HD, McGarry JD: Mycobacterial meningomyelitis associated with human immunodeficiency virus infection. *Arch Neurol* 45:691, 1988.

65. Berger JR: Spinal cord syphilis associated with human immunodeficiency virus infection: A treatable myelopathy. *Am J Med* 92:101, 1992.

66. Fenelon G, Gray F, Scaravilli F, et al: Ischaemic myelopathy secondary to disseminated intravascular coagulation in AIDS. *J Neurol* 238:51, 1991.

CHAPTER 9

HIV Dementia

Anita Venkataramana and Justin C. McArthur

The widespread use of highly active antiretroviral therapy (HAART) in developed countries since its introduction in the mid-1990s has led to a substantial reduction in morbidity and mortality in patients infected with the human immunodeficiency virus (HIV). There has been a 50 percent decline in the acquired immunodeficiency syndrome (AIDS) death rate, significantly decreased maternal-infant transmission rates, reductions in incidence rates of opportunistic infections, and a 40 to 50 percent decrease in the incidence of HIV-associated dementia (HIV-D).[1,2] Nonetheless, AIDS-associated neurologic diseases, including HIV-D and sensory neuropathies (HIV-SN), continue to be major causes of morbidity and mortality. This suggests that HAART does not provide complete protection against neurologic damage in HIV/AIDS.[3] In addition, the blood-brain barrier may prevent central nervous system (CNS) penetration of antiretroviral agents, and the brain may serve as a sanctuary for HIV, with persistent HIV replication within perivascular macrophages, the principal target in the CNS. These cells may allow reseeding of the periphery, making the CNS both a sanctuary *and* a reservoir. This chapter will review the clinical features and pathophysiology of HIV-D.

▶ EPIDEMIOLOGY OF HIV INFECTION AND AIDS

Global Epidemiology

Geographic Distribution

The HIV/AIDS epidemic has become a global tragedy. Over 95 percent of all AIDS cases occur in developing countries, with seroprevalence rates among adults ranging from less than 1 percent in India and Europe to more than 10 to 20 percent in several African countries. The epidemic is growing most rapidly in China, India, eastern Europe, and particularly in the sub-Saharan African countries, where the epidemic has had a major impact on societal health and development. Approximately 3.5 million new infections with HIV-1 were reported in 2002, with 2.4 million people dying from AIDS in 2001. Countries contributing to the high infection rates in Africa include Botswana (38.8 percent seroprevalence rates), Zimbabwe (33.7 percent), Swaziland (33.4 percent), and Lesotho (31 percent). In eastern Europe and central Asia, the number of people estimated to be living with HIV was 1.2 million in 2002. The World Health Organization (WHO) estimates that the total number of people living with HIV/AIDS worldwide is 42 million. By 1995, AIDS had surpassed cancer as the predominant cause of death in young Americans (25 to 44 years of age).[4] An overwhelming majority of HIV-positive individuals worldwide are infected as a result of unprotected sexual intercourse, and specifically about 70 percent have acquired infection through heterosexual contact. While some countries are experiencing increased prevalence rates, other countries, such as Cambodia, Uganda, Thailand, and Australia, have reported stabilizing or even falling rates of infection due to less high-risk behavior. Certain epidemiologic and clinical patterns of HIV infection vary by region, country, and race. Asia and the Pacific have a large and growing population of people living with HIV due to the growing epidemic in China of injection-drug users, plasma donors, and sex workers. In Korea, by contrast, the most common route of disease acquisition is from heterosexual contact, followed by homosexual contact.[5] There are millions of people not receiving antiretroviral therapy or even medications to treat opportunistic infections. For the majority of HIV-infected persons worldwide, these expensive treatments remain out of reach and will be available only with financial support from developed countries.

High-risk Behaviors

The acquisition of HIV has long been attributed to certain behaviors. Blood products are now an infrequent source of infection in developed countries because of careful screening measures introduced in the 1980s.

The risk of HIV infection is estimated at 1 in 493,000 blood transfusions.[6] In a recent U.S. study, 50 percent of men who had sex with men reported that they were continuing to have unprotected anal intercourse.[7] There is considerable potential for spread of new HIV infections among these men. Sharing of contaminated needles among injection-drug users (IDUs) also poses a serious threat in disease propagation not only for HIV-1 but also for HTLV-1 and hepatitis C. However, in some geographic areas, the incidence rates of HIV infection among IDUs has declined. For example, since 1995 in Australia incidence rates have dropped through needle-exchange and harm-reduction programs. There is a great need to implement more effective intervention strategies that address relationship status, serostatus of partners, and drug and alcohol use that may contribute to the risk of being infected. One such project was Children's Health and Responsible Mothering (CHARM), an HIV prevention program for adolescent mothers. The group was comprised of young women, predominantly of low socioeconomic status and of Latina background. Through educational intervention, a statistically significant improvement was seen in AIDS knowledge, intention to use condoms, and fewer sex partners.[8]

In the United States, women are the fastest growing population affected by HIV/AIDS. The proportion of women with AIDS has increased from 8 to 23 percent since the early 1980s. In the past 11 years, the cumulative number of AIDS cases reported to the Centers for Disease Control and Prevention (CDC) in adults aged 50 years or older quintupled, from 16,288 in 1990 to 90,513 by the end of December 2001.[9] There are currently more than 60,000 persons with AIDS in this age group in the United States.[10] Persons from lower socioeconomic backgrounds are less likely to be treated with HAART compared with wealthier individuals. Survival is also worse for people with AIDS who live in poverty.[11] Hepatitis C infection has emerged as an important cause of comorbidity and mortality in HIV-infected individuals as antiretroviral therapy has become more effective.[12] The prevalence of syphilis and HIV is highest in the African-American community. HIV may affect the transmission of the spirochete and accelerate the clinical course and response to treatment.[13] Tuberculosis (TB) is the most important coinfection with HIV worldwide.

Clinical Manifestations of AIDS

AIDS/HIV produces profound cellular immunodeficiency with progressive depletion of CD4+ (T-helper) cells. This leads to a propensity to develop specific *AIDS-defining* infections, neoplasms, or illnesses. The CDC has developed a staging system based on systemic

▶ **TABLE 9-1.** CDC CLASSIFICATION SYSTEM FOR HIV-1 INFECTION AND EXPANDED AIDS SURVEILLANCE CASE DEFINITION FOR ADOLESCENTS AND ADULTS

CD4+ Cell Categories	(A) Asymptomatic or PGL	(B) Symptomatic Not (A) or (C) Conditions	(C) AIDS-Indicator Conditions
(1) 500/mm^3	A1	B1	C1
(2) 200–499/mm^3	A2	B2	C2
(3) <200/mm^3 (AIDS-indicator cell count)	A3	B3	C3

Category A: Asymptomatic HIV-1 infection, persistent generalized lymphadenopathy (PGL). Acute (primary) HIV-1 infection with accompanying illness or history of acute HIV-1 infection

Category B: Symptomatic conditions occurring in an HIV-1-infected adolescent or adult, excluding those in category C, included but are not limited to bacterial endocarditis, meningitis, pneumonia, or sepsis; candidiasis, vulvovaginal persisting (>1 month duration) or poorly responsive to therapy; candidiasis, oropharyngeal (thrush); cervical dysplasia; constitutional symptoms such as fever (>38.5°C) or diarrhea lasting >1 month; hairy leukoplakia, oral; herpes zoster (shingles) involving at least two distinct episodes or more than one dermatome; idiopathic thrombocytopenia purpura; listeriosis; nocardiosis; pelvic inflammatory disease; peripheral neuropathy

Category C: Bacterial pneumonia, recurrent; candidiasis of bronchi, trachea, or lungs; candidiasis, esophageal; cervical cancer, invasive; coccidioidomycosis disseminated or extrapulmonary; cryptococcosis extrapulmonary; cryptosporidiosis, chronic intestinal (>1 month duration); cytomegalovirus disease (other than liver, spleen, or nodes); cytomegalovirus retinitis (with loss of vision); HIV-1 encephalopathy; herpes simplex: chronic ulcer(s) (>1 month duration) or bronchitis, pneumonitis, or esophagitis; histoplasmosis, disseminated or extrapulmonary; isosporiasis, chronic intestinal (>1 month duration); Kaposi's sarcoma; lymphoma, Burkitt's (or equivalent); lymphoma, immunoblastic (or equivalent term); lymphoma, primary in brain; *Mycobacterium avium* complex or *M. kansasii,* disseminated or extrapulmonary; *Mycobacterium tuberculosis,* disseminated, extrapulmonary, or pulmonary; *Mycobacterium,* other species or unidentified species, disseminated or extrapulmonary; *Pneumocystis carinii* pneumonia; progressive multifocal leukoencephalopathy; *Salmonella* sp. septicemia, recurrent; toxoplasmosis of brain; wasting syndrome due to HIV-1.

SOURCE: Neumann et al.,[18] with permission.

illnesses and CD4 count, and a wide range of illnesses are now included as AIDS-defining illnesses.

Table 9-1 lists the CDC classification system for HIV-1 infection and AIDS-indicator conditions. Worldwide, tuberculosis and hepatitis C are the most common coinfections with HIV and can lead to significant comorbidity. Tables 9-2 and 9-3 list some of the typical clinical features of HIV/AIDS and their frequencies, respectively. In some areas, unusual opportunistic infections (OIs) predominate over the "typical" OIs that traditionally have been labeled as AIDS-defining illnesses. For example, in Korea, *Candida* was the most prevalent opportunistic infection, followed by *Pneumocystis carinii* pneumonia, tuberculosis, and cytomegalovirus (CMV) infection in descending order. The most common cause of death was tuberculosis.[5]

The results of clinical trials of combinations of potent antiretrovirals and the subsequent widespread introduction of HAART have produced a new era of optimism for HIV-infected people[14] because the incidence of AIDS-associated cancers is decreasing in Western countries. In developed countries, the use of antiretro-

▶ **TABLE 9-2.** COMPLICATIONS OF HIV-AIDS: NEWER FEATURES IN HAART ERA

HIV-1-Associated	Opportunistic Infections	Neoplasms	Immune Restoration Disease	Toxicities of Treatment
HIV encephalopathy	Cerebral toxoplasmosis	Primary CNS lymphoma	Parvoviral B19 infection	Lipodystrophy
HIV meningitis	Cytomegalovirus retinitis/encephalitis	Metastatic systemic lymphoma	Inflammatory forms of PML	Hyperglycemia
Vacuolar myelopathy	Cryptococcal meningitis		Other immune events	Peripheral neuropathy
Peripheral neuropathy	Tuberculosis			Accelerated atherosclerosis
HIV-associated polymyositis	Progressive multifocal leukoencephalopathy			
HIV dementia	Other fungal/bacterial CNS infections			

▶ **TABLE 9-3.** FREQUENCY OF AIDS-DEFINING ILLNESSES IN THE UNITED STATES, 1997 (EXCLUDING LOW CD4 COUNTS)

Condition	1997
Pneumocystis carinii pneumonia	
Candida esophagitis	38
HIV wasting syndrome	14
HIV-associated encephalopathy (HIV-associated dementia)	18
Cerebral toxoplasmosis	5
Cytomegalovirus infection	4
Mycobacterium avium or *M. kansasii*, disseminated or extrapulmonary	7
Cryptococcosis, extrapulmonary	5
Herpes simplex infection with esophagitis, pneumonitis, or chronic mucocutaneous ulcers	4
Extrapulmonary tuberculosis	2
Cryptosporidiosis	1
Lymphoma, primary brain	1
Kaposi's sarcoma	7

SOURCE: *From Nolan et al.,[17] with permission.*

viral drugs during pregnancy has reduced substantially the risk of perinatal HIV transmission from mother to infant.[15] The development of resistance mutations to antiretroviral medications may lead to virologic escape with further CD4 depletion and a rise in HIV-associated neurologic diseases. With restoration of the immune response, new clinical manifestations reflecting immune activation can be observed in the initial months after beginning HAART. This has been termed *immune restoration disease* (IRD) and can include unusual inflammatory forms of progressive multifocal leukoencephalopathy (PML).[16] Reactivations of parvovirus B19 infection,[17] CMV retinitis, and Reiter's syndrome have been reported after the initiation of therapy with HAART.[18] Antiretroviral therapy also can have negative effects, with significant metabolic and toxic abnormalities, both systemic and neurologic. For example, the protease inhibitors are known to cause hyperlipidemia, lipodystrophy, insulin resistance, and diabetes. The lipodystrophy in HIV-positive patients is characterized by a marked reduction of subcutaneous fat in the face, extremities, and buttocks. The use of nucleoside analogues has been associated with lactic acidosis and hepatic steatosis through inhibition of mitochondrial DNA polymerase gamma.[19] The epidemiology of neoplasia in HIV/AIDS also has been altered. The incidence of Kaposi's sarcoma in people receiving combination therapy has fallen significantly, but cervical cancer, anal cancer, and conjunctival cancers are occurring at increased rates in some populations. Hodgkin's disease develops in long-term survivors of HIV infection as a result of prolonged immune suppression and B-cell stimulation.[20]

Neuroepidemiology

In developed countries with high rates of HAART usage, patients with AIDS are living substantially longer, and HIV/AIDS has become a manageable chronic disease. There is a declining trend in the incidence rates of HIV-D, CNS opportunistic infections, and HIV-associated distal sensory polyneuropathy, whereas that of antiretroviral drug–induced toxic neuropathy has increased.[1,21–22] The prevalence rates for both HIV-D and HIV-SN have, by contrast, increased dramatically, reflecting longer survival in the HAART era (Fig. 9-1). In a recent clinical study it was observed that older age, cognitive impairment, and cerebral atrophy were independently associated with an increased probability of HIV-D, whereas focal signs were related to a decreased risk.[23] Recent autopsy series in HAART-treated cohorts have shown that the rates of HIV encephalitis remain as high as 20 to 25 percent.[24,25]

The incidence rates of CNS opportunistic infections such as cryptococcal meningitis, toxoplasmosis, PML, and primary CNS lymphoma have decreased substantially during the 1990s[1,22] partly because of the use of primary prophylaxis (i.e., trimethoprim-sulfamethoxazole for toxoplasmosis) and partly because of immune reconstitution with HAART regimens. As an example, survival data for primary CNS lymphoma (PCNSL) has increased with HAART.[26] Since the introduction of HAART in 1996, the incidence of HIV-D has decreased by approximately 50 percent. The mean CD4 count for new cases of HIV-D is increasing, but it generally remains as a complication of moderately advanced immunosuppression.[27]

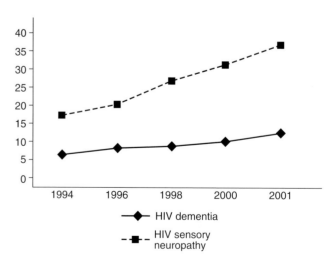

Figure 9-1. Rising prevalence of HIV-associated neurologic disorders in the Johns Hopkins University HIV clinic reflecting increasing survival.

► BIOLOGY OF HIV INFECTION RELEVANT FOR CNS DISEASE

Structure of HIV

The HIV virion has a lipid bilayer made up of envelope spikes that are comprised of gp120 and a transmembrane portion, gp41. The core of the virus is formed from four nucleic capsid proteins, p24, p17, p9, and p7. Certain genes of HIV code for structural proteins, and others code for regulatory proteins. The three groups of genes encoding structural proteins are *gag, pol,* and *env.* The *gag* region encodes for the core proteins, the nucleoid shell, and other smaller proteins. The *pol* region is important because it encodes for the enzymes, reverse transcriptase, endonuclease, and protease. Finally, *env* is responsible for coding the major envelope proteins, gp120 and gp41. The HIV replication process involves certain regulatory genes, *tat, rev, nef, vif,* and *vpr.* The protein vpr assists with binding to the nuclear pores or may disrupt the nuclear membrane by inducing blebs, rupture, and the eventual influx of cytoplasmic components. It is part of the HIV-1 preintegration complex (PIC) along with two other nucleophilic proteins, matrix and integrase. The HIV PIC enters the nucleus by traversing the central nuclear pore complex. The vpr–nuclear export signal (NES) complex is necessary for HIV replication. A mutation in the NES impairs the incorporation of vpr into newly formed virions. It was described recently as a nucleocytoplasmic shuttling protein that contains two novel nuclear proteins and exportin-1-dependent NES.[28] The *nef* gene increases viral multiplication in infected hosts and accelerates clinical progression to AIDS. It exhibits a wide range of biologic activities that include alteration of T-cell activation, enhancement of the infectivity of viral particles, and downregulation of surface expression of CD4,[29] the primary cellular receptor for HIV attachment.

With millions of replicative cycles daily and a high error rate in RNA transcription, mutants readily arise unless HIV replication is suppressed completely. This rapid replication leads to the establishment of a *cluster* of related HIV quasi-species within an individual and the selection of drug-resistant variants. The genetic variability of HIV is partly due to the strength of local selective pressures (immunologic, target-cell availability, pharmacologic), complexity of the preexisting genetic pool, and rate of viral turnover.[30,31] The relationship between the production of HIV virions and CD4 cells is very dynamic. There is a very rapid turnover of CD4 lymphocytes (approximately 2 billion daily), with an estimated total release of approximately 10 billion new virions daily.[32,33] Quiescent memory CD4+ T-lymphocytes and macrophages may serve as long-lived reservoirs for latent HIV infection.[34,35] The resting memory T-lymphocyte has been shown to be a particularly important systemic reservoir that prevents eradication because HIV remains either latent or maintains a low level of replication for years.[35] Follicular dendritic cells also may serve as another potential reservoir and have been demonstrated to sequester infectious virions for up to 9 months.[36]

While CD4+ cells are the principal target for infection with HIV, CD8+ T-lymphocytes can inhibit HIV replication by secreting a soluble factor known as *CD8 T-lymphocyte antiviral factor* (CAF). CAF action is thought to be at the step of the long terminal repeat (LTR)–driven gene expression leading to inhibition of HIV RNA transcription. It acts in conjunction with alpha-defensin 1 and stimulates the production of signal transducer and activator of transcription 1 (STAT-1), which, in turn, leads to expression of interferon regulatory factor 1 (IRF-1), thereby inhibiting HIV RNA transcription.[37]

The viral invasion of the nervous system by HIV is unique when compared with other virus-related encephalitides. HIV may enter the brain transiently in the early stage of infection, but productive infection is rarely detectable before immunosuppression has developed. The virus resides predominantly in a limited number of perivascular macrophages, microglia, and astrocytes, although most productive infection is within the perivascular macrophages. Macrophage infection, however, does not explain the significant neuronal damage seen in HIV-D. It therefore has been suggested that certain factors released from the infected cells trigger a cascade of events leading to neurodegeneration. Toxic viral proteins have been implicated, including tat, which is a nonstructural viral protein that functions as a *trans*-acting nuclear regulatory protein and is essential for viral replication. Tat may damage neighboring uninfected cells by transcellular means.[38] Even in the absence of productive neuronal infection, there is neuronal cell damage and eventual loss. This occurs by indirect mechanisms, including the release of viral proteins from infected glial cells with ensuing activation of uninfected glial cells.[39] Proinflammatory cytokines play an important role in the neuronal and astrocytic damage resulting from macrophage-microglial activation leading to apoptosis, oxidative stress, and glutamate-mediated neurotoxicity.[40] Glutamate, an excitotoxic amino acid, has been involved in degeneration of neurons and may accumulate because of reduced uptake by damaged astrocytes that downregulate excitatory amino acid transporters (EAATs).[41–43]

The progression of HIV-associated pathology in the CNS is initially dependent on parenchymal viral replication, followed by aberrant macrophage activation. Viral replication in the brain may be controlled by numerous factors, including viral binding, entry, and regulation of viral expression by the LTR portion of the genome. The LTR promotes viral expression in conjunction with viral and cellular regulatory proteins that alter its activity at certain binding sites. These sites are necessary for HIV replication. The binding affinity of cellular regulatory proteins correlates with LTR activity and may be used as a molecular marker for disease progression.[44]

Receptors and Chemokines

The principal receptor for HIV-1 is the CD4 molecule, and the chemokine receptors serve as critical "secondary" receptors.[45,46] HIV-1 strains have been divided into T-tropic (preferring to replicate in neoplastic T-cell lines) and M-tropic (in macrophages) on the basis of their use of chemokine receptors. T-tropic viruses make use of CD4 and CXCR4 (or fusin, the receptor for SDF-1), and M-tropic viruses make use of CD4 and CCR5 (the receptor for MIP-1α, MIP-1β, and RANTES). The majority of brain isolates are M-tropic and are likely to use the CCR5 receptor predominantly[45] and thus are classified as R-5 viruses. A genetic variant of the CCR5 receptor, delta32, has been found to be protective against HIV infection and to delay disease progression.[47,48] Most research has focused on HIV-1 clade B, whereas clade C is far more prevalent worldwide and is almost exclusively R-5; hence it may have important effects in the brain. A recent study revealed a novel HIV receptor on dendritic cells, the dendritic cell (DC)–specific intracellular adhesion molecule-grabbing nonintegrin (DC-SIGN), that plays a key role in the dissemination of HIV. Dendritic cells represent a major reservoir of HIV. They are located in the germinal centers of secondary lymphoid tissues, where they trap and retain antigens in the form of immune complexes.[49,50] Dendritic cells and the antigens they retain persist for many months. DC-SIGN on dendritic cells efficiently transmits low amounts of HIV to T cells, thereby enhancing infection. It exhibits its action by adhering to cell receptors mediating both DC migration and T-cell activation.[51]

Chemokines are involved in the migration of leukocytes and have been implicated in HIV-D pathogenesis. They are classified into four classes based on the positions of key cysteine residues C, CC, CXC, and CX3C. Several members of the beta chemokine subfamily of cytokines, namely, MIP-1α, MIP-1β, RANTES, and fractalkine (FKN), are part of the pathogenesis. Chemokines act through both specific and shared receptors that all belong to the superfamily of G-protein-coupled receptors. The expression of both chemokines and their receptors may be upregulated by inflammatory mediators.[52] HIV replication is under continuous regulation by a complex network of cytokines and chemokines, cell migration–inducing cytokines in cells of myeloid lineage, and can be inhibitory, stimulatory, or both.

Genetic polymorphisms in the promoter for MCP-1, as well as in CCR5 and CCR2 (the receptor for MCP-1), have been shown to influence the development of HIV-D.[53] Both neurons and microglia express FKN released in response to proinflammatory stimuli. Ligand binding to the receptor CX3CR1 induces adhesion, chemoattraction, and activation of microglia and macrophages in the brain, leading to neurodegeneration. High levels of FKN has been detected in the cerebrospinal fluid (CSF) of HIV-infected patients.[54] FKN may be involved in other neuroinflammatory processes implicated in neuronal damage.[55]

Several other cytokines may be produced by reactive astrocytes, including interferon gamma (IFN-γ), interleukin 1 (IL-1), IL-6, and transforming growth factor beta (TGF-β).[56] In addition, these reactive astrocytes release neurotoxins, including nitric oxide (NO), arachidonic acid metabolites, and reactive oxygen intermediates.[57] Activated glial cells release tumor necrosis factor alpha (TNF-α), which also plays a role in neuronal damage in HIV-D. Production of iNOS, Fas, and other inflammatory mediators may be stimulated within astrocytes or neurons by proinflammatory cytokines in HIV-D. The dopamine system also may be damaged in HIV/AIDS, and the clinical manifestations of dopaminergic dysfunction can be prominent.

The urokinase-type plasminogen activator (uPA) and its receptor (uPAR) may also play an important role in extracellular matrix degradation and cell migration in the CNS.[49,50,58] Soluble uPAR (SuPAR) concentrations were measured in both CSF and plasma[58] and were significantly higher in HIV-infected patients compared to controls. Patients with HIV-D and opportunistic infections also had elevated SuPAR levels. This supports a role for the uPA and uPAR pathway in the mechanisms leading to tissue injury and neurodegeneration in HIV-D. Moreover, SuPAR levels in CSF could represent an additional marker of both tissue damage and immune activation in HIV-related CNS complications.

Course of Systemic HIV Infection

After acute infection with HIV, the immune system is stimulated to control the virus, and a lower level of HIV viremia is established following the initial peak viremia. The level of this viral set point appears to be an important predictor of neurologic disease progression.[59] Interestingly, this is not the case for some simian immunodeficiency virus (SIV) models of encephalitis.[60] HIV-specific immune responses, both humoral and cellular (cytotoxic T cells), develop to a variable degree. Some individuals appear to be able to control HIV replication even without antiretroviral agents and have no or a very slow progression of disease. These *long-term nonprogressors* comprise about 10 to 15 percent of chronically infected individuals. The major direct effect of HIV infection on the immune system is the profound loss of CD4 lymphocytes. This leads to impaired cellular immunity and the development of reactivated latent infections or infections with organisms that are normally not pathogenic (*opportunistic*). In addition, loss of the regulatory CD4 subset appears to lead to a dysregulation of macrophages, with the overproduction of a variety of proinflammatory cytokines and chemokines. Antimicrobial peptides (*defensins*) are an area of active research as potential determinants of the control of chronic infection in these individuals and may be important for vaccine development. Specific defensins (α-1, α-2m, and α-3) may be the elusive antiviral factors derived from CD8 and T-lymphocytes that control HIV replication.[61]

▶ CLINICAL FEATURES OF HIV-ASSOCIATED DEMENTIA

HIV-1-infected individuals are susceptible to developing a progressive and frequently fatal dementia. This syndrome was added as an AIDS-indicator illness in 1987 and termed *HIV-1 encephalopathy* [or *HIV-associated dementia* (HIV-D)]. Occasionally, HIV-D develops before profound immunosuppression, but in general, it is rare among healthy HIV-1-infected persons. HIV-D constitutes about 5 percent of new AIDS-defining illnesses in developed countries, but this actually may be lower in some developing countries because individuals die of opportunistic infections before HIV-D can develop. Better epidemiologic data are essential for developing countries because of the variability in reports. For example, Howlett reported HIV-D in 54 percent of cases of HIV infection in the northern zone of Tanzania.[62]

HIV-D occurs in all groups at risk for HIV-1 infection, including children. While the *incidence* has decreased due to HAART, the cumulative *prevalence* actually has risen with improved survival in AIDS. The cumulative prevalence of HIV-D during the lifetime of an HIV-positive individual is estimated at 15 percent, and risk factors include high plasma HIV RNA levels, low CD4+ counts,[59] anemia, low body mass index, older age, more constitutional symptoms before AIDS,[63] injection-drug use,[64] and female sex.[65] More subtle

forms of cognitive impairment, termed *minor cognitive/motor disorder* (MC/MD), exist in 20 percent of symptomatic HIV-seropositive adults.[66] MC/MD has a functional impact on work and medication adherence[67] and is predictive of HIV-D and poorer survival but does not always progress inexorably to frank dementia. In adults, the clinical manifestations of HIV-D are often stereotypic, developing over a few months; occasionally, the course is more fulminant. A typical presentation includes cognitive, behavioral, and motor dysfunction and has been characterized as a *subcortical* dementia. The initial symptoms may be subtle and therefore overlooked and can be misdiagnosed as depression. In the early stages memory loss, mental slowing, reading and comprehension difficulties, and apathy are frequent complaints. Conditions that may mimic HIV-D include cryptococcal meningitis, CMV encephalitis, PML, primary CNS lymphoma, and depression. Table 9-4 illustrates some of the salient features that differentiate HIV-D from CMV encephalitis and PML. The cardinal features of HIV-D include disabling cognitive impairment accompanied by motor dysfunction and behavioral change.[68] The typical cognitive deficits of HIV dementia are characterized primarily by (1) memory loss that is selective for impaired retrieval, (2) impaired ability to manipulate acquired knowledge, (3) personality changes that are characterized by apathy, inertia, and irritability, and (4) general slowing of all thought processes. However, considerable individual variability in presentation has been reported.[69] Children also can be affected by a progressive encephalopathy with an estimated prevalence of 30 percent[70] and a typical survival of 6 to 24 months before HAART.[71,72] Clinical features in pediatric cases include microcephaly, developmental delay, and then progressive loss of developmental milestones. The prominence of motor slowing and impaired movements adds to the concern that dopaminergic dysfunction is prominent in HIV/AIDS[73] (Fig. 9-2). Gait disturbance with nonspecific complaints of stumbling and tripping is frequent. Tremor and myoclonus are uncommon but have been reported.[74] Examination findings include impaired rapid movements of eyes and limbs, diffuse hyperreflexia, frontal release signs, and sometimes parkinsonism.[75] A simple bedside test, the HIV Dementia

▶ **TABLE 9-4.** DIFFERENTIATION OF HIV DEMENTIA FROM OPPORTUNISTIC INFECTIONS

HIV Dementia	CMV Encephalitis	PML
Memory, mental slowing, gait	Delirium, seizures, brain stem signs	Focal neurologic signs
Several months	Days to weeks	Weeks to months
Diffuse atrophy, deep white matter hyperintensities	Normal or periventriculitis	Subcortical white matter lesions
Nonspecific immune activation	PCR positive for CMV DNA in 90%	PCR positive for JC virus in 60%

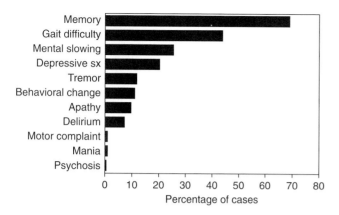

Figure 9-2. Frequency of symptoms in HIV-D among 300 subjects personally examined at the Johns Hopkins University HIV Neurology Program.

Scale, has been developed for screening for HIV-D. This nonspecific instrument has been validated in U.S. populations and can identify individuals with possible HIV-D who may need further evaluation with additional neuropsychological tests[76] (Fig. 9-3).

Score Max

MEMORY-REGISTRATION
Give four words to recall (dog, hat, green, peach)- 1 second to say each. Then ask the patient all 4 after you have said them.

( ) 4 **ATTENTION**
Anti-saccadic eye movements: 20 (twenty) trials. Record errors.
> errors= 4; 4 errors = 3; 5 errors = 2; 6 errors= 1; > 6 errors = 0

( ) 6 **PSYCHOMOTOR SPEED**
Ask patient to write the alphabet in upper case letters horizontally across and record time in seconds.
> 21 sec = 6; 21.1-24 sec = 5; 24.1- 27 sec = 4; 27.1 - 30 sec = 3; 30.1-33 sec = 2; 33.1 - 36 sec = 1; >36 sec = 0

( ) 4 **MEMORY-RECALL**
Ask for 4 words from Registration above. Give 1 point for reach correct. For words not recalled, prompt with a cue (see instructions).

( ) 2 **CONSTRUCTIONAL**
Copy 3D cube below - record time in seconds.
<25 sec = 2; 25 - 35 sec = 0

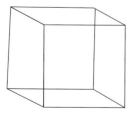

Figure 9-3. HIV dementia scale (Johns Hopkins University Neurology Program).

New-onset mania or a heightened sensitivity to neuroleptic agents also can be seen in some patients.[77] These need to be distinguished from the frequent CNS toxicities of the nonnucleoside RT inhibitor efavirenz, which can include agitation, disturbed sleep, and even catatonia.[78] Neuropsychological abnormalities include a preferential impairment of psychomotor speed and memory. As the dementia advances, more widespread deficits develop, including a global dementia, often accompanied by myelopathy and neuropathy. The course of HIV-D is variable, and some individuals remain stable for prolonged periods of time, particularly with HAART. The less severe form, HIV-associated minor cognitive-motor disorder, frequently heralds the later development of HIV-D. Different forms of neurologic involvement in chronic HIV infection have been described recently. For example, "pure" cerebellar syndromes, which could be atypical forms of HIV encephalitis,[79] and a relapsing-remitting illness not unlike multiple sclerosis have been reported, albeit rarely.[80] A form of "CNS escape" presenting as acute meningoencephalitis in patients with very high CSF HIV RNA levels but low or undetectable plasma HIV RNA levels has been observed.[81] The University of California, San Diego, group recently has reported a series of patients with a severe form of leukoencephalopathy.[82] The syndrome developed in patients failing HAART, and the neuropathologic features included intense perivascular infiltration by HIV-gp41 immunoreactive monocytes-macrophages and lymphocytes, widespread myelin loss, axonal injury, microgliosis, and astrogliosis. It is uncertain whether this is, in fact, a new pathologic entity or simply a more severe version of the HIV leukoencephalopathy that was described in one-third of demented subjects.[83] A form of leukoencephalopathy has been identified recently that appears *not* to be a form of progressive multifocal leukoencephalopathy because CSF JCV polymerase chain reaction (PCR) is persistently negative. This may in fact be a form of immune restoration disease.

▶ PATHOLOGY OF HIV-D

HIV probably gains access to the CNS from the bloodstream by the ingress of infected or activated monocytes.[84] Productive HIV-1 infection occurs principally in perivascular macrophages (Fig. 9-4) and rarely in astrocytes, in which the infection is nonproductive.[56] Infection of endothelial cells or neurons is a vanishingly rare event,[56] although endothelial infection has been reported with SIV encephalitis. The pathologic features include multinucleated giant cells, which represent the fusion of HIV-infected macrophages, and a marked activation of macrophages and astrocytes.

Immunocytochemical studies show a preponderance of productive HIV infection within the basal gan-

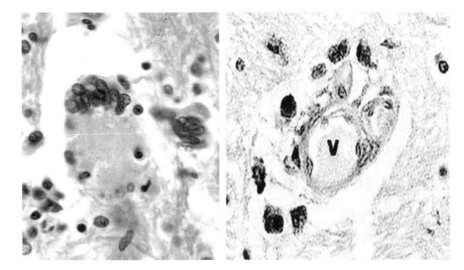

Figure 9-4. Photomicrograph of multinucleated giant cells in HIV-D (*left*) and HIV antigens in perivascular macrophages (*right*).

glia, brain stem, and deep white matter.[56,85,86] These observations suggest that initial infection occurs in the deep brain regions, probably from infection of perivascular macrophages by trafficking monocytes. Diffuse rarefaction of white matter occurs commonly. There is breakdown of the blood-brain-barrier with astrocyte apoptosis[87] and eventually dendritic simplification and neuronal loss. Morphometric studies have shown an approximate 40 percent reduction in neuronal densities within frontal and temporal areas[88,89] and reduced densities of large pyramidal neurons that correlate with dementia severity.[90] Even more prominent are the reductions in the complexity of synapses and dendritic connections.[91] These pathologic changes appear to correlate with both central atrophy on magnetic resonance imaging (MRI) and reductions in magnetic resonance spectroscopy (MRS) *N*-acetyl aspartate concentrations.[92–94] The clinical severity of HIV-D is associated most strongly with increased numbers of activated macrophages within the brain and with the quantity of activated astrocyte- and macrophage-derived products. Brain levels of HIV RNA also correlate with dementia severity but show more variability, and some individuals with severe HIV-D may have relatively low HIV RNA levels.[94] The density of apoptotic astrocytes correlates with the rapidity of progression of HIV-D.[87] With the use of in situ PCR, a greater number of astrocytes containing HIV DNA in individuals with rapidly progressing dementia can be detected. This suggests that there is both an increased rate of astrocyte apoptosis in rapidly progressive dementia and increased rates of astrocyte infection.

HIV-1 Infection and the Blood-Brain Barrier

Disruption in blood-brain barrier may contribute to the enhanced ingress of HIV-infected monocytes into the CNS. The blood-brain barrier is key in regulating cell trafficking through the CNS because of a unique anatomic feature, interendothelial tight junctions, that normally form impermeable seals between the cells. Examination of brain tissue from patients who died from HIV-D revealed a notable disruption of these tight junctions within vessels of subcortical white matter, basal ganglia, and to a lesser extent, cortical gray matter. Tight-junction disruption is associated with perivascular accumulation of activated HIV-infected monocytes, serum protein extravasation, and marked astrocytosis.[95] Imaging studies have demonstrated blood-brain barrier disruption.[96] The structural basis of these permeability changes and their relationship to enhanced infiltration of HIV-infected monocytes, a crucial event in the pathogenesis of the disease, remains unclear. It has been proposed that circulating activated monocytes bearing the markers CD14+/CD16+ are the predominant trafficking cells into the brain in HIV-D. Recent work in non-CNS tissues has shown that there may be increased monocyte-macrophage infiltration in renal tissue.[97] Increased numbers of CD14+/CD16+ macrophages in the blood will actively traffic into the brain, cross the blood-brain barrier, and induce pathologic changes within the brain. The demonstration of elevated proportions of CD14+ cells in HIV-D led to the analysis of soluble CD14+ (sCD14) levels in CSF. Higher sCD14 levels were found in patients with moderate to severe dementia. CD14+/CD16+ monocytes also may play a role in other neurologic disorders for which the measurement of sCD14 levels can be used.[98]

Monocyte/microglia and astrocytes are capable of producing matrix metalloproteases, which may lead to breakdown of the blood-brain barrier and exposure of the brain to circulating substances. Locally produced chemokines may stimulate the ingress of additional activated monocytes. Importantly, this inflammatory cascade may become "self-sustaining" so that even if HIV replication is suppressed, there may be continuing macrophage-mediated damage.

The pathophysiologic mechanisms involved in the production of HIV-D remain uncertain, although it seems most plausible that the parenchymal release of viral toxins and various proinflammatory substances impairs cellular functioning leading to various pathological changes described earlier.[99,100] A very wide range of inflammatory mediators has been implicated in the pathogenesis of HIV-D, and it is unlikely that any one "factor" is directly causative. These products include proinflammatory cytokines, eicosanoids, nitric oxide, and extracellular matrix-degrading proteases.[100,102] Platelet-activating factor, nitric oxide, and matrix metalloproteases can be neurotoxic[103] and also may have important effects on synaptic structure and function.[104–106] Monocytes may contribute to the development of HIV-D through multiple mechanisms. Activated and/or HIV-infected monocytes release a number of potent toxins, including viral gene products such as tat and gp120, as well as cellular gene products such as TNF-α, nitric oxide, and platelet-activating factor.[107] The precise role of viral proteins in pathogenesis is uncertain and is reviewed in detail elsewhere.[108] Tat may be released into the extracellular space[109] and both in vitro and in vivo may be neurotoxic for selected neuronal populations,[110] probably acting through the NMDA receptor and glutamate. Tat also stimulates the release of proinflammatory cytokines in the brain[111] and induces migration of monocytes in a blood-brain-barrier model.[73,112,113] The envelope glycoprotein gp120 is also a potent neurotoxin in vitro, and it has been proposed that its neurotoxicity is mediated indirectly through actions on glial cells.

The products of activated monocytes can activate astrocytes, leading to the release of astrocyte-derived cytokines and chemokines, as well as altered neurotransmitter uptake. These products may sensitize astrocytes and neurons to the effects of glutamate.[114] Astrocytes participate in the inactivation of neurotoxins, particularly excess excitatory amino acids such as glutamate and aspartate, and their loss may perturb the regulation of extracellular glutamate, leading to neuronal injury. Interestingly, in situ studies have shown that monocyte-macrophages are the dominant source of toxins including TNF-α and that apoptotic neurons generally are detected in close proximity to activated macrophages.[115]

Chemokines, as established previously, regulate macrophage function and can be measured in the CSF. Monocyte chemotactic protein 1 (MCP-1), RANTES, macrophage inflammatory protein 1 (MIP-1) alpha and beta, and interleukin 8 (IL-8) are significantly higher in HIV-D.[116] In addition, CSF levels of MCP-1 increase over time in patients who subsequently develop dementia, as well as in SIV AIDS macaques who develop encephalitis.[117] MCP-1 levels correlate with CSF viral load measurements. Activated macrophages and microglia release quinolinic acid, a neurotoxin and NMDA (*N*-methyl-D-aspartate) receptor agonist synthesized from L-tryptophan via the kynurenine pathway and is hypothesized to contribute to neuronal injury and cerebral volume loss. Elevated CSF quinolinic acid levels worsened brain activity, corroborated by MRI findings. Moreover, the striatum and limbic cortex were the main targets of these excitotoxic insults. CSF quinolinic acid concentrations correlated with CSF HIV RNA levels.[118] Various other CSF markers of immune activation, such as neopterin and β_2-microglobulin,[119] also correlated with the severity of HIV-D and decline with HAART treatment. β_2-Microglobulin, a nonspecific and nonexcitotoxic marker, was unrelated to regional brain volume loss. Neopterin concentrations were higher in both CSF and serum in persons with HIV than in those who were seronegative. Neopterin is also elevated in bacterial and viral meningitis and therefore is a nonspecific marker, but it may be used as a guide to monitor the clinical course of patients.[120] The levels of soluble Fas (sFas) and soluble Fas ligand (sFasL) in CSF and serum of HIV-infected patients with dementia were elevated. Fas usually is not expressed in normal individuals but is expressed in patients with HIV encephalitis by astrocytes. sFas is produced during cellular activation by macrophages. The sFasL is predominantly expressed on activated T-lymphocytes and macrophages. These are nonspecific markers of CNS apoptosis. With HAART, the levels declined.[121] CSF levels of protein tau, a marker of axonal degeneration, may be useful but cannot discriminate between HIV-D and neurologic complications of HIV.[122] Prostaglandin F2α and thromboxane B2, products of the cyclooxygenase pathway of arachidonic acid metabolism, also were elevated and contributed to neurologic dysfunction.[123]

Immune Activation in the Pathogenesis of HIV-D

The brain may serve as a sanctuary for unchecked HIV replication both because the blood-brain-barrier may prevent CNS penetration of antiretrovirals and also because perivascular macrophages, one of the principal targets within the CNS, may serve as long-lived sequestered sites for HIV.[35,98,124] Within the brain, most of the virus is unintegrated, and it is unknown whether it can give rise to infectious particles.[125,126] Most investigators believe that neurons are rarely, if ever, the site of productive HIV infection and that perivascular macrophages are the primary target. However, astrocytes may serve as important targets for restricted HIV infection[56] and, while nonproductive, nonetheless could affect astrocytic and neuronal function. The loss of homeostasis caused by astrocytosis that is induced during HIV brain infection indeed may be a critical event in HIV-D. Astrocytes are responsible for neuronal maintenance and function by buffering the extracellular milieu, providing cytoskeletal support, and protecting neurons during injury and infection. The restricted infection of astrocytes may have important pathophysiologic consequences. Astrocytes react to CNS injury or infection by increasing their size, density, and expression of GFAP.[127] The mechanisms of neuronal injury in HIV-D are *indirect;* i.e., apoptotic neurons do not appear to colocalize with infected macrophages[128]: (1) There is impaired reuptake or enhanced release of glutamate, an excitotoxic amino acid involved in degeneration of neurons, a concept strengthened by recent observations of elevated glutamate in CSF in HIV-D[129,130]; (2) viral proteins such as tat may be directly toxic to neurons and also may stimulate the production of chemokines including MCP-1, thus facilitating more monocyte ingress; (3) production of iNOS, Fas, fractalkine, and other inflammatory mediators may be stimulated within astrocytes or neurons by proinflammatory cytokines; and (4) the dopamine system also may be damaged in HIV/AIDS, and the clinical manifestations of dopaminergic dysfunction can be prominent.[73]

Utility of CSF Immune Activation Markers and Resistance Patterns in HIV-D

In the pre-HAART era, CSF immune activation markers including β_2-microglobulin, neopterin, and eicosanoids were significantly elevated in HIV-D.[123,131,132] Levels or activity of MMP-2, MMP-7, and MMP-9 were all increased in CSF from patients with HIV-D.[133] In the Northeastern AIDS Dementia (NEAD) cohort, where HAART was used in more than 70 percent, there was no correlation between neurologic status and CSF levels of TNF-α, MCP-1, or M-CSF, suggesting that immune activation markers are less frequently elevated in contemporary HAART-using cohorts compared with studies from 5 to 10 years ago. These markers are used rarely in clinical practice.

The role of measuring viral resistance patterns in either plasma or CSF remains to be established and has not yet entered clinical practice for the treatment of HIV-D. The detection of resistance mutations generally requires an HIV RNA level of greater than 400 copies/ml, so for CSF, where levels are often lower, resistance testing is frequently not technically feasible. Some studies have shown that there can be discordance between plasma and CSF resistance patterns (Ellis R, personal communication, 2002; Cinque P, personal communication, 2002).[134] Further studies are needed to determine the clinical relevance of these observations, but at this point, the determination of resistance mutations has not entered clinical practice.

Interpretation of CSF HIV RNA Assays in HIV-D

The quantification of plasma HIV RNA has become a critical tool for monitoring levels of replicating HIV.

Studies using reverse transcriptase (RT)–PCR, branched DNA techniques, or enzymatic amplification assays have demonstrated that HIV RNA quantification is a powerful predictor of decreases in CD4+ lymphocyte count, progression to AIDS, and death.[135–137] Plasma viral load strongly predicts the prognosis of HIV/AIDS,[136] and the combined measurement of plasma HIV RNA and CD4+ lymphocytes provides an even more accurate prognosis.[138] A higher plasma HIV RNA set point is predictive of HIV-D.[59]

In contrast to plasma surrogate markers, the utility and predictive value of CSF analysis is less clear. Certainly CSF abnormalities are common in HIV-D, with elevated CSF levels of HIV RNA and immune activation markers occurring in most demented individuals. CSF levels of HIV RNA correlate with the severity of neurologic deficits[139–141]; at least this was so in the pre-HAART era. CSF HIV RNA levels may be predictive of subsequent neurologic deterioration and transition into HIV-D.[142] The correlation between CSF HIV RNA levels and neurologic status in HAART-treated individuals appears to be much weaker now than in the pre-HAART era. While a significant correlation has been demonstrated in HAART-treated patients,[143] the much larger NEAD cohort, which also had high rates of HAART usage, showed no such relationship[144] (Fig. 9-5). The inference can be made that HAART can effectively suppress both HIV levels and immune activation markers among individuals with advanced HIV disease and that the introduction of HAART actually may have attenuated the severity of neurologic disease.

The measurement of CSF HIV RNA has ill-defined utility in the clinical setting. However, there are situations where the comparison of paired plasma and CSF HIV RNA levels can be useful. For example, in the situation of CNS escape where an acute encephalopathic picture develops, CSF HIV RNA levels substantially higher than plasma levels may indicate compartmentalized CNS infection (Wendell K, Clinical Infectious Diseases, 2003). For a patient with established dementia who is beginning a new HAART regimen, monitoring the decline in CSF HIV RNA levels with treatment can provide information about the CNS efficacy of that particular regimen. Finally, although less precise in HAART-treated individuals, the determination of CSF HIV RNA levels may help distinguish MC/MD or early HIV-D from psychiatric conditions.

HAART and CSF HIV RNA

Several studies have shown conclusively that either dual therapy or HAART can suppress CSF HIV RNA levels rapidly, particularly in antiretroviral-naive individuals. An early study comparing patients on monotherapy, dual therapy, and HAART showed a significant difference in the proportion of patients with suppressed CSF viral load between the different regimens. Of those pa-

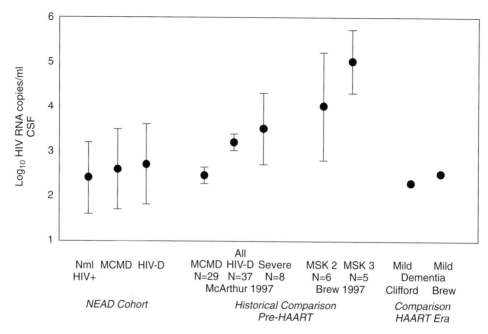

Figure 9-5. Comparison of CSF HIV RNA values in contemporary treated NEAD cohort (>70 percent HAART) with earlier untreated cohorts.

tients on one nucleoside reverse transcriptase inhibitor (NRTI), only one patient had a CSF viral load below 20 copies/ml, compared with 41 percent of patients on dual NRTIs and 69 percent of those on HAART. Declines in CSF HIV RNA with HAART appear to coincide with the successful reversal of neurologic deficits[145,146] and with subsequent improvements in neuropsychological test performance. Higher HIV RNA levels correlated with increased levels of quinolinic acid, which, in turn, correlated with worsening brain atrophy quantified by MRI in regions vulnerable to excitotoxic damage, the striatum, and the limbic cortex. Despite these overall cohort effects, on an individual basis CSF virologic failures remain common, especially in community-based settings. For example, in an uncontrolled open-label study of 21 patients initiating antiretroviral therapies, 50 percent had persistently detectable HIV RNA (limit of detection 100 copies/ml) even after 8 months of triple antiretroviral therapy.[147] Several groups have examined the dynamics of HIV replication after the initiation or interruption of HAART. Ellis et al.[146] and Price[148] both suggested that CSF and plasma HIV replication dynamics are relatively independent in advanced HIV disease, with a compartmental discrepancy in HIV-D. For example, after stopping HAART, both plasma and CSF HIV RNA levels can rebound rapidly within days, and levels actually may be higher within the CSF.[149] To date, the determinants of virologic failure in the CSF have not been fully defined, and the clinical significance of CSF virologic persistence remains uncertain. The concern is that it may indicate persistence of CNS HIV replication, and Ellis' recent ob-

servations suggest a high rate of subsequent neurologic deterioration in those with high CSF HIV RNA levels.[142,150]

▶ RADIOLOGIC MARKERS FOR HIV-D

MRI is the initial study of choice for evaluating brain pathology. This modality excludes opportunistic infections that can mimic HIV-D. MRI in HIV-D typically demonstrates both cortical and central atrophy with characteristic confluent signal abnormalities within the deep white matter (Fig. 9-6). These changes represent an increased brain water content, and not demyelination, and are reversible with HAART.[151] Perfusion studies have indicated that there is an increased degree of permeability of the blood-brain-barrier in HIV-D[152,153] corresponding to the pathologic changes described earlier. Some of the opportunistic infections and their characteristic MRI patterns are depicted in Table 9-5.

Proton MRS[154] is a noninvasive tool with high reproducibility that measures the concentrations of specific brain metabolites that reflect CNS function. In HIV-D, MRS shows increases in choline and myoinositol, reflecting inflammation and astrocytosis, with reductions in N-acetyl aspartate, indicating neuronal injury. NAA/creatine (Cr) and N-acetyl aspartate/choline (Cho) ratio reductions were seen in both centrum semiovale and thalamic areas. The difference of NAA/Cr was more pronounced in the white matter than in the gray matter.[155] More recently, neurologically asymptomatic HIV-infected patients were found to have early metabolic

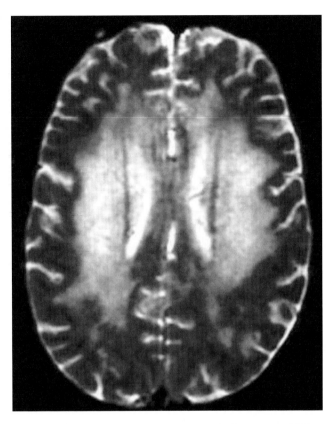

Figure 9-6. T_2-weighted cranial MRI in severe HIV-D. Note symmetrical white matter intensities.

changes by proton MRS, the NAA/Cho ratio was significantly lower in HIV patients, and no changes were found in the NAA/Cr ratio. There was also a statistically significant reduction in NAA/H$_2$O and Cr/H$_2$O ratios. These results indicate neuronal loss and gliosis in patients with HIV[156] (Fig 9-7). Brain metabolite levels correlate strongly with various clinical and biochemical indices of neurologic progression in HIV-positive individuals, such as severity of HIV-D, overall functional level, CD4 cell count, plasma viral load, and CSF viral load.[93] Cerebral metabolite levels can normalize after 9 months of treatment with HAART, although the changes appear to lag behind improvements in CD4 count and CSF HIV RNA levels.[157] Furthermore, there may be dif-

ferent patterns of MRS abnormalities. A so-called basal ganglia pattern with elevated myoinositol in the basal ganglia is potentially indicative of inflammation, and a neuronal pattern with reduced NAA levels in subcortical and cortical regions corresponding to diffuse neuronal injury can be seen.[158] Proton MRS has been shown to be sensitive to changes in brain cellular metabolism in patients with HIV-D, and this may be useful as a marker of regional brain injury.[159–164] However, most of these studies were performed before the introduction of HAART. It is likely that MRS abnormalities may be attenuated by HAART, as has been observed for CSF HIV RNA (Pomper and Sacktor, Neurology, 2002).

Critical questions relating to the use of MRS as a noninvasive surrogate marker for HIV-D include (1) What is the frequency of MRS abnormalities in HIV-D in the era of HAART? (2) What are the confounding factors (e.g., duration of HIV-D, medication adherence to HAART, depression) that may alter MRS metabolite concentrations in HIV-D patients? (3) Do abnormalities of MRS markers of inflammation and neuronal injury predict progression of clinical disease?

Magnetization transfer imaging (MTI) has been used in evaluating brain pathology. It is a new magnetic resonance (MR) technique for improving image contrast and is based on application of off-resonance radiofrequency pulses and observing their effects on MR images, as well as measuring the signal intensity with and without application of the pulses, termed *magnetization transfer ratio* (MTR). MTRs can be used to detect changes in the structural status of brain parenchyma that may or may not be visible with standard MR techniques. In addition to HIV and the accompanying opportunistic infections, MTI can evaluate lesions of multiple sclerosis, tumors, Alzheimer's disease, and mild cognitive impairment (MCI).[165] MTR values were compared in HIV patients with PML and normal-appearing white matter (NAWM) in age-matched controls, and it was found that there was a strong and significant decrease in the values in PML. In another study, MTR has been helpful in distinguishing HIV encephalitis from PML, where MTR values were noted to be dramatically lower in PML lesions. Furthermore, MTI allowed a quantification of the degree of demyelination that can be

▶ **TABLE 9-5.** RADIOLOGIC PATTERN OF HIV-RELATED CNS DISEASE

Disorder	Number	Pattern	Enhancement	Location
HIV dementia	Diffuse	Ill-defined	0	Deep white matter
Toxoplasmosis	1–many	Ring mass	++	Basal ganglia
Primary CNS lymphoma	1–several	Solid mass	+++	Periventricular
PML	1–several	No mass effect	0	Subcortical white matter
Cryptococcus	1–many	"lacunar"	0	Basal ganglia
CMV encephalitis	1–several	Confluent	++	Periventricular

SOURCE: Modified from Price RW: American Academy of Neurology Course, 1991.

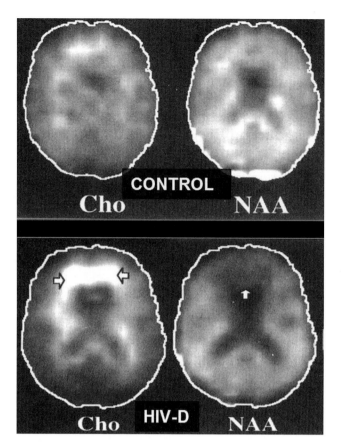

Figure 9-7. Magnetic spectroscopic imaging in HIV-D. Left panel indicates increased choline (CHO) and right panel reduced NAA in frontal lobes (*arrow*) compared with control subject. *(From Barker et al.[92] with permission.)*

helpful in other demyelinating diseases of the CNS, as stated previously.[166] Studies involving fMRI had demonstrated increased brain activation in HIV-positive patients who did not demonstrate neuropsychological impairment on clinical testing. It may be a tool for detecting early HIV-associated brain pathology.[167]

▶ THERAPY OF HIV-D

General Principles of Antiretroviral (ARV) Therapy

Recent advances in the application and monitoring of ARV therapy have produced major improvements in the care and prognosis of HIV-infected individuals. Suppression of viral replication is a priority even in early disease when CD4 lymphocyte counts are relatively preserved. The effectiveness of HAART can be monitored by laboratory assays measuring HIV RNA levels, an index of ongoing viral replication. Combining different ARV agents is a beneficial therapeutic strategy because this raises the threshold for HIV to acquire effective re-

sistance through mutations. Currently, typical ARV regimens consist of at least three agents: one to two HIV protease inhibitors (PIs) or a nonnucleoside reverse transcriptase inhibitor combined with two nucleoside analogues. The objective of therapy is to reduce measurable plasma viral burden to below the level of detection. Even with combination ARV agents, some degree of resistance is common. It is possible to evaluate for the presence of resistance in individual patients by using genotypic and phenotypic assays, which in turn help the clinician decide on which ARV agents to use.

HIV encephalopathy is associated with high levels of viral RNA in the CNS.[139] Combining various ARV agents has led to reduced plasma RNA levels. HAART effectively reduces viral replication in both plasma and CSF. A recent study in 40 HIV-positive patients in whom CSF and plasma were collected found that delayed virus decay from the CSF during HAART was associated with late-stage symptomatic HIV infection in the brain.[168] Penetration through the blood-brain barrier is different for various ARV agents. Among these agents, PIs appear to have the lowest CSF levels. Pure protease-containing regimens have resulted in failure of viral suppression in CSF.

Planned interruptions of HAART, referred to as a *structured treatment interruption,* were thought to represent a new strategy in ARV therapy. This approach may be seen as counterintuitive and potentially harmful because treatment interruptions often result in a resurgence of viral replication and a risk of immunologic decline and selection for drug resistance. The overall therapeutic benefits and risks of structured treatment interruption have not been outlined clearly, and recent studies have suggested that they may lead to virologic rebound and more rapid CD4 declines.[169] Structured treatment interruption therefore is not recommended for general clinical use.

CNS Penetration of ARV Agents

Complete suppression of viral replication in the CNS is critical in preventing the emergence of a reservoir of resistant strains of virus and subsequent brain impairment in the later stages of infection. Variable penetration of the ARV agents into sanctuary sites may contribute to the differential evolution of HIV and the emergence of drug resistance. It remains controversial whether the available ARV agents have adequate parenchymal penetration. Table 9-6 indicates the CSF-plasma ratio for available agents, which is a surrogate for their CNS penetration. In general, the higher the ratio, the higher is the CSF penetration. However, the CSF levels of a drug are not necessarily directly related to its parenchymal penetration. There are inadequate human data on the actual parenchymal penetration of ARV agents, with only a very few animal experiments quan-

▶ **TABLE 9-6.** ANTI-HIV DRUGS. CSF-PLASMA CONCENTRATION RATIOS

	Date Approved	CSF-Plasma Ratio
Nucleos/tide RT inhibitors		
Retrovir (zidovudine, AZT)	3/87	0.3–1.35
Zerit (stavudine, d4T)	6/94	0.16–0.97
Ziagen (abacavir)	12/98	0.3–0.42
Videx (didanosine, ddI)	10/91	0.16–0.19
Epivir (lamivudine, 3TC)	11/95	0.11
Hivid (zalcitabine, ddC	6/92	0.09–0.37
Viread (tenofovir)	10/01	Unknown
Nonnucleoside RT inhibitors		
Viramune (nevirapine)	6/96	0.28–0.45
Rescriptor (delavirdine)	7/97	0.02
Sustiva (efavirenz)	11/98	0.01
Protease inhibitors		
Crixivan (Indinavir)	3/96	0.02–0.06
Fortovase (saquinavir)	12/95	<0.05
Viracept (nelfinavir)	4/97	<0.05
Norvir (ritonavir)	3/96	<0.05
Kaletra (lopinavir + ritonavir)	11/00	<0.05
Agenerase (amprenavir)	3/99	<0.05
Membrane fusion inhibitors		
Fuzeon (enfuviritide)	5/03	Unknown

tifying tissue penetration.[170,171] ARV drugs differ greatly in their ability to penetrate the blood-CSF-CNS barriers. Among the different classes of ARV agents, the PIs appear to achieve the lowest CSF levels relative to plasma. The PI indinavir appears to have the highest CNS penetration of this class.[172] In contrast, the nonnucleoside reverse transcriptase inhibitors (NNRTIs), specifically nevaripine, are the drug class with the best overall ability to penetrate the CNS. Potential benefits are limited by the fact that the virus can develop high-level resistance to them quickly. On a theoretical basis, some of the nucleoside analogues may be anticipated to penetrate the brain parenchyma more effectively than others.[173] Among the NRTIs, zidovudine has the highest penetration, followed by stavudine. The CNS penetration of NRTIs occurs primarily by passive diffusion, governed by such properties as lipophilicity, molecular weight, and charge. On theoretical grounds, both the NRTIs and the PIs may achieve only low levels within the brain parenchyma either because the blood-brain barrier limits their entry or active efflux mechanisms exist. For example, the PIs may be eliminated from the brain through the actions of *p*-glycoprotein, which is expressed at the blood-brain barrier.[173,174] For the NRTIs, organic acid transport systems also may eliminate NRTIs from the brain.[170,175] Inhibitors of these efflux systems, verapamil or nifedipine, and for the organic acid transporters, uricosuric compounds probenecid, benzylpenicillin, or benzbromarone) have been proposed for the treatment of established HIV encephali-

tis. To date, neither the selective inhibition of these efflux systems nor the monitoring of ARV levels in CSF has entered clinical practice.

Another unanswered issue is whether specific HAART regimens can provide superior CNS virologic suppression compared with other regimens. Relevant to this, one study of a regimen containing only PIs failed to suppress CSF viral load effectively,[176] raising the clinical concern that PIs used alone without NRTIs or NNRTIs may not be effective for the prevention or treatment of CNS infection. In a recently reported study of 50 subjects on HAART, better viral load reductions from baseline CSF (1.14 $\log_{10}$ copies/ml) were observed in those receiving "CNS-penetrating" HAART regimens than those with theoretically less penetrant regimens (a reduction of only 0.05 $\log_{10}$ copies/ml). This suggests that CSF virologic suppression is correlated with predicted CNS ARV drug penetrance. In contrast, neurocognitive improvement with HAART appears to be independent of this variable, and it remains to be determined whether specific HAART regimens are more efficacious for treatment of established HIV-D.[177]

We now believe that the principal effect of HAART may occur outside the CNS, perhaps by reducing the proportion of circulating activated monocytes, the cells presumed to carry HIV into the brain.[157,163–166,174] From a practical point of view, in selecting ARV agents for treatment of HIV-D, first select a regimen that is most likely to reduce plasma HIV RNA levels rapidly and that can lead to durable virologic suppression. A secondary consideration is the theoretical CNS penetration of the agent. The agents zidovudine, stavudine, lamuvidine, efavirenz, nevaripine, and indinavir have most consistently had the best CNS penetration[178] and could be included in regimens where feasible. For some patients this may require supervised HAART administration, either at home with family support or with daily observed therapy. Occasionally, when this cannot be arranged, a patient will be institutionalized (nursing home placement) to receive HAART in a controlled environment.

Treatment of HIV-D

Neuropsychological batteries have been used to track improvements in neurologic and neuropsychological deficits of HIV-D and MC/MD and have been included as the primary outcome measure in all the placebo-controlled trials of ARV therapy, as well as for trials of adjunctive agents.[179–181] While specific neuropsychological instruments that measure psychomotor speed may indeed be sensitive to HIV-D, the relationship of changes in neuropsychological performance to improvements in function has not yet been demonstrated.[181,182] A substantial proportion of individuals with HIV-D or MC/MD actually show partial reversal of neuropsychological deficits with ARV therapy. For example, Cohen and colleagues[183] reported that women taking HAART for 18 months had significant improvements in psychomotor and executive functions, whereas those not taking HAART declined. Tozzi and colleagues[184] also found sustained improvements in neurocognitive performance after 6 months of HAART, as did Ferrando's group.[185] There is no longer any role for monotherapy in the treatment of HIV-D. The effect of more potent ARV regimens was examined in a multicenter trial of 1313 adult HIV-positive subjects with CD4 counts of less than 50cells/μl. Four combinations consisting of AZT, alternating monthly with ddl, or AZT plus ddC, AZT plus ddl, or AZT plus ddl plus nevirapine were tested, and a four-item quantitative neurologic performance battery score was administered. Triple therapy and the AZT-ddl combination preserved or improved neurologic performance compared with the alternating-dual-therapy zidovudine (ZDV)–ddl and ZDV-ddC regimens ($p < 0.001$), paralleling their impact on survival.[154] More recent studies also have confirmed the effects of HAART in reversing the neurocognitive deficits of HIV-D, showing improvements in motor and psychomotor speed.[185,186]

Only one placebo-controlled trial of HAART in HIV-D has been conducted, a trial of high-dose ZDV monotherapy in the late 1980s.[180] Significant improvements on neurocognitive performance were observed. In the era of HAART, there have been no placebo-controlled trials for HIV-D. However, instructive results were derived from an "add-on" study of high-dose abacavir to background HAART.[187] One hundred and five HIV-1 infected subjects with mild to moderate HIV-D were randomized to receive abacavir (600 mg twice daily) or matched placebo added to a stable HAART regimen. The primary outcome measure was the change over 12 weeks in a composite score derived from the mean of eight neuropsychological tests. The median change from baseline was comparable between the two groups (+0.76 SD units for the abacavir group and +0.63 for placebo) (Fig. 9-8). Those receiving abacavir had greater decreases in CSF HIV-1 RNA. The unanticipated results from this study were as follows: (1) the augmentation of HAART with one drug provided no additional improvement in neuropsychological performance and (2) neuropsychological improvements continued even after 8 or more weeks of HAART. These findings suggest that a reversal of neurologic deficits may be slow. Interestingly, 83 percent of the subjects enrolled in this study had normal CSF levels of CSF β_2-microglobulin at baseline, suggesting that active CNS inflammation in this group was not present.

Some individuals fail to respond to HAART, which may be due to an irreversible stage of pathology with prominent neuronal loss and "burnt out" inflammation. The measurement of CSF HIV RNA levels, combined with markers of CNS inflammation and apoptosis, may provide critical information regarding the persistence of CNS infection and damage. The identification of predictive factors of treatment response will be of great importance to better understand the course of HIV-D and its pathogenetic mechanisms. Determinants of treatment response are still unclear but obviously would be useful in selecting individuals with established dementia, perhaps for more aggressive regimens. A recent observational study of 28 patients who were followed longitudinally after HAART initiation suggests that a history

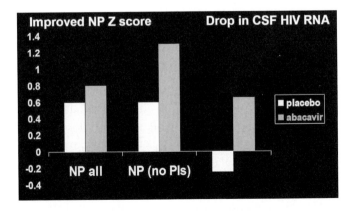

Figure 9-8. Abacavir add-on trial for HIV-D. Neuropsychological improvement was observed both for those receiving abacavir and for those in stable HAART. CSF HIV RNA levels dropped for abacavir recipients. NP, neuropsychological; PI, protease inhibitors. *(Courtesy of Dr. B. Brew.)*

of IDU, incomplete plasma virologic suppression, and the type of ARV regimen predicted a lack of neurologic response.[188] Levels of CSF β_2-microglobulin were twofold higher in those who showed neurologic response with HAART, suggesting that higher initial levels of CNS inflammation correlate with reversible neurologic deficits. Differences in neurologic response to therapy were not dependent on the initial severity of dementia, self-reported medication adherence, CD4 counts, or baseline plasma HIV RNA levels.[188] Systemic virologic response to HAART appears to predict neurologic response, suggesting that the effects of HAART are mediated both in the CNS and in the systemic compartment, presumably by reducing the activation levels and subsequent CNS ingress of circulating cells.[189]

The role of genetic differences in determining treatment response is of great interest, especially with the observations from psychiatry of genetic differences in response to antidepressants.[190] As one example of genetic susceptibility in HIV/AIDS, HLA-B57 positivity correlates with a heightened risk of abacavir sensitivity.[191] Specific polymorphisms in the *mdr-1* gene correlate with lower plasma levels of specific PIs and better virologic response, putatively through enhanced cellular penetration of the drug.[192] The relationship between ARV drug concentrations in plasma and CSF and polymorphisms in the *mdr-1* gene controlling the expression of *p*-glycoprotein at the blood-brain barrier are being explored and may have therapeutic importance.

▶ ADJUVANT THERAPIES FOR HIV-D

Given that immune activation is likely to play a pivotal role in sustaining or magnifying the CNS damage induced by HIV-1, attention has focused on *adjunctive* therapies targeted at attenuating the CNS effects of in-flammatory products. At this point, the most promising available adjunctive agent is selegiline. This MAO-B inhibitor has been shown to improve memory in two separate placebo-controlled studies.[193,194] Although its mechanism of action is speculative and may involve an antioxidant effect, a larger phase II trial is underway in the United States, with results expected within a year. Other agents under investigation as adjunctive agents for HIV-D include the platelet-activating factor antagonist lexipafant, the TNF-α antagonists pentoxifylline and CPI1189, and an experimental antioxidant, thioctic acid. The results of most trials (Table 9-7) have been disappointing, with either no or only modest effects on neuropsychological function. One agent recently evaluated for the treatment of HIV-D was memantine, and a controlled trial has suggested some benefit on neurocognitive performance (Navia B, 2003, under review). Memantine is a noncompetitive inhibitor of the NMDA receptor. Since excitotoxicity has been implicated in neurodegeneration, this medication may act as a neuroprotective agent. Memantine has virtually no undesirable side effects, and its safety and efficacy have been established by clinical experience in humans. Memantine is considered to be a promising drug for treatment of other types of dementias, and it has been approved in Germany for the treatment of dementia for over 10 years.

Lithium salts are used widely in psychiatry as mood-stabilizing agents. Lithium ions have regulatory effects on the protein kinase glycogen synthase kinase 3β (GSK3β). GSK3β may play a role in cellular regulation by regulating oncoproteins, including β-catenin. Boosting the activity of GSK3β may stimulate the body's natural defenses against viral infections and facilitate neuroprotection against tat- or gp120-mediated toxicity. With these properties, lithium (or valproic acid, which has similar effects on GSK3β) may be considered in the

▶ TABLE 9-7. PLACEBO-CONTROLLED TRIALS OF ADJUNCTIVE AGENTS FOR HIV DEMENTIA

Agent	Action	Conclusions
Nimodipine[195]	Calcium channel	Trend for improvement in neuropsychological performance (NP) at highest dose only
Peptide T[196]	Uncertain, possibly chemokine receptor blockade	No effect
OPC14117[197]	Antioxidant, neuroprotectant	Positive NP performance
Thioctic acid versus selegiline[193]	Antioxidant, neuroprotectant	Selegiline + effect on NP performance
Lexipafant[198]	PAF antagonist	Trend for improvement in verbal learning and timed gait
Memantine (Navia B, in press)	NMDA antagonist	Positive effect on NP performance (but only after completion of double-blind phase)
CPI-1189[199]	TNF-α antagonist	Minimal effect on NP performance; improvement in peg board test at highest dose
Selegiline	Antioxidant, neuroprotectant	Improvement in verbal learning; trend for improvement in recall and psychomotor speed

SOURCE: From Turchan.[200]

Figure 9-9. Model of different patterns of HIV-D in the era of HAART.

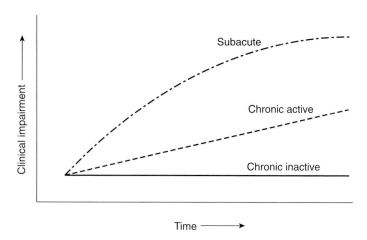

treatment of HIV-associated cognitive impairment as a novel therapeutic choice. Another strategy for adjunctive therapy is the use of neurotrophic agents. For example, fibroblast growth factor 1 (FGF1) may be a neurotrophic factor capable of protecting neurons against the deleterious effects of HIV. FGF1 levels were found to be mild to moderately elevated in patients without HIV encephalitis and neurodegeneration, whereas low levels were found in HIV encephalitis and neurodegeneration.[120,131,132,134,167] Various agents studied in clinical trials are summarized in Table 9-7.

► CHANGING FEATURES OF HIV-D IN THE ERA OF HAART

While the prevalence of HIV-D in contemporary cohorts is actually increasing, the severity of neurologic disease appears to be milder since the introduction of HAART. For example, in our own referral cohort, the percentage of newly diagnosed moderate or severe dementias (MSK 2 or 3) has fallen very dramatically: from about 6.6 percent in 1989 to 1.0 percent in 2000. Prior to the introduction of HAART, the course of HIV-D usually was progressive over 6 to 9 months, leading in a stereotypic manner to severe neurologic deficits and death.[69,201] Since the introduction of HAART in 1996, however, the course of HIV-D appears to be much more variable. Most HAART-treated individuals with HIV-D remain neurologically stable or may show some partial reversal of neurologic deficits for years after starting HAART.

We hypothesize that HIV-D in the era of HAART may now have three distinct subtypes: (1) a "subacute progressive" dementia in untreated patients with a clinical syndrome of severe, progressive dementia similar to that seen in the pre-HAART era, (2) a "chronic active" dementia in patients on HAART with poor adherence or with viral resistance who are at risk for neurologic progression, and (3) a "chronic inactive" dementia in patients on HAART with good drug ad-

herence and effective virologic suppression who have had some recovery from neuronal injury and remain neurologically stable (Fig. 9-9).

The development of surrogate markers to identify these three HIV-D subtypes would be of great importance in understanding the clinical course and pathogenetic mechanisms of HIV-D and in planning future treatments. Currently available clinical and laboratory markers of HIV-D may be less useful in the era of HAART. Neuroimaging markers, in concert with clinical and laboratory markers, may be necessary to identify patients with HIV-D who are at risk for progression.

Several independent contemporary studies have shown that the levels of CSF HIV RNA appear to be significantly lower in untreated subjects with HIV-D than those seen in pre-HAART studies.[144,199] This might suggest that under the pressure of HAART, the HIV envelope may have evolved toward a less virulent type (Wong J, personal communication, 2002). These observations suggest that both the phenotype and the biologic markers of HIV-D have undergone an evolution, and perhaps the virus has become attenuated under the influence of HAART.

REFERENCES

1. Brodt HR, Kamps BS, Gute P, et al: Changing incidence of AIDS-defining illnesses in the era of antiretroviral combination therapy. *AIDS* 11:1731, 1997.

2. Sacktor N, Lyles RH, Skolasky R, et al: HIV-associated neurologic disease incidence changes: Multicenter AIDS Cohort Study, 1990–1998. *Neurology* 56(2):257, 2001.

3. Bouwman FH, Skolasky R, Hes D, et al: Variable progression of HIV-associated dementia. *Neurology* 50:1814, 1998.

4. Centers for Disease Control and Prevention: *HIV/AIDS Surveillance Report* 7(2):1, 1995.

5. Kim JM, Cho GJ, Hong SK, et al: Epidemiology and clinical features of HIV infection/AIDS in Korea. *Yonsei Med J* 44(3):363, 2003.

6. Schreiber GB, Busch MP, Kleinman SH, Korelitz JJ: The risk of transfusion-transmitted viral infections. The Retrovirus Epidemiology Donor Study. *New Engl J Med* 334:1685, 1996.

7. Koblin BA, Chesney MA, Husnik MJ, et al: High-risk behaviors among men who have sex with men in six U.S. cities: Baseline data from the EXPLORE Study. *Am J Public Health* 93(6):926, 2003.

8. Koniak-Griffin D, Lesser J, Nyamathi A, et al: Project CHARM: An HIV prevention program for adolescent mothers. *Fam Commun Health* 26(2):94, 2003.

9. Centers for Disease Control and Prevention: *HIV/AIDS Surveillance Report* 13, 2002.

10. Mack KA, Ory MG: AIDS and older Americans at the end of the twentieth century. *J Acquir Immune Defic Syndr* 33(suppl 2):S68, 2003.

11. McFarland W, Chen S, Hsu L, et al: Low socioeconomic status is associated with a higher rate of death in the era of highly active antiretroviral therapy, San Francisco. *J Acquir Immune Defic Syndr* 33(1):96, 2003.

12. Gonzalez SA, Talal AH: Hepatitis C virus in human immunodeficiency virus–infected individuals: An emerging comorbidity with significant implications. *Semin Liver Dis* 23(2):149, 2003.

13. Funnye AS, Akhtar AJ: Syphilis and human immunodeficiency virus coinfection. *J Natl Med Assoc* 95(5):363, 2003.

14. Shapiro MF, Morton SC, McCaffrey DF, et al: Variations in the care of HIV-infected adults in the United States: Results from the HIV Cost and Services Utilization Study. *JAMA* 281(24):2305, 1999.

15. Connor EM, Sperling RS, Gelber R, et al: Pediatric AIDS Clinical Trials Group Protocol 076 Study Group. Reduction of maternal-infant transmission of human immunodeficiency virus type 1 infection with zidovudine treatment. *New Engl J Med* 331:1173, 1994.

16. Safdar A, Rubocki RJ, Horvath JA, et al: Fatal immune restoration disease in human immunodeficiency virus type 1–infected patients with progressive multifocal leukoencephalopathy: impact of antiretroviral therapy–associated immune reconstitution. *Clin Infect Dis* 35(10):1250, 2002.

17. Nolan RC, Chidlow G, French MA: Parvovirus B19 encephalitis presenting as immune restoration disease after highly active antiretroviral therapy for human immunodeficiency virus infection. *Clin Infect Dis* 36(9):1191, 2003.

18. Neumann S, Kreth F, Schubert S, et al: Reiter's syndrome as a manifestation of an immune reconstitution syndrome in an HIV-infected patient: successful treatment with doxycycline. *Clin Infect Dis* 36(12):1628, 2003.

19. Carr A: Lactic acidemia in infection with human immunodeficiency virus. *Clin Infect Dis* 36(suppl 2):S96, 2003.

20. Grulich AE, Wan X, Law MG, et al: B-cell stimulation and prolonged immune deficiency are risk factors for non-Hodgkin's lymphoma in people with AIDS. *AIDS* 14(2):133, 2000.

21. Keswani S, Pardo CA, Cherry CL, et al: HIV-associated sensory neuropathies. *AIDS* 16:1, 2002.

22. Bacellar H, Munoz A, Miller EN, et al: Temporal trends in the incidence of HIV-1 related neurologic diseases: Multicenter AIDS Cohort Study, 1985–1992. *Neurology* 44:1892, 1994.

23. Tozzi V, Uccella I, Larussa D, et al: Characteristics and factors associated with HIV-1-related neurocognitive disorders during HAART era (abstract H.64). *J Neurovirol* 9(suppl 3):82, 2003.

24. Masliah E, DeTeresa RM, Mallory ME, Hansen LA: Changes in pathological findings at autopsy in AIDS cases for the last 15 years. *AIDS* 14(1):69, 2000.

25. Grant I, Gelman BB, Morgello S, Singer EJ: National NeuroAIDS Tissue Consortium (abstract I.67). *J Neurovirol* 9(suppl 3):113, 2003.

26. Hoffmann C, Tabrizian S, Wolf E, et al: Survival of AIDS patients with primary central nervous system lymphoma is dramatically improved by HAART-induced immune recovery. *AIDS* 15(16):2119, 2001.

27. Sacktor N: The epidemiology of human immunodeficiency virus–associated neurological disease in the era of highly active antiretroviral therapy. *J Neurovirol* 8(S2):115, 2002.

28. Sherman MP, de Noronha CM, Eckstein LA, et al: Nuclear export of Vpr is required for efficient replication of human immunodeficiency virus type 1 in tissue macrophages. *J Virol* 77(13):7582, 2003.

29. Stoddart CA, Geleziunas R, Ferrell S, et al: Human immunodeficiency virus type 1 Nef-mediated downregulation of CD4 correlates with Nef enhancement of viral pathogenesis. *J Virol* 77(3):2124, 2003.

30. Bassiri A, Holden J, Wong M: A case of fulminant human immunodeficiency virus dementia. *Clin Infect Dis* 21:1313, 1995.

31. Wong JK, Gunthard HF, Havlir DV, et al: Reduction of HIV-1 in blood and lymph nodes following potent antiretroviral therapy and the virologic correlates of treatment failure. *Proc Natl Acad Sci USA* 94:12574, 1997.

32. Coffin JM: HIV population dynamics in vivo: Implications for genetic variation, pathogenesis, and therapy. *Science* 267:483, 1995.

33. Saag M: Use of HIV viral load in clinical practice: Back to the future (editorial). *Ann Intern Med* 26:983, 1997.

34. Saag MS, Holodniy M, Kuritzkes DR, et al: HIV viral load markers in clinical practice. *Nature Med* 2:625, 1996.

35. Finzi D, Hermankova M, Pierson T, et al: Identification of a reservoir for HIV-1 in patients on highly active antiretroviral therapy. *Science* 278:1295, 1997.

36. Burton G, Keele B, Estes J, et al: Follicular dendritic cell contributions to HIV pathogenesis. *Semin Immunol* 14(4):275, 2002.

37. Chang TL, Francois F, Mosoian A, Klotman ME: CAF-mediated human immunodeficiency virus (HIV) type 1 transcriptional inhibition is distinct from alpha-defensin-1 HIV inhibition. *J Virol* 77(12):6777, 2003.

38. Peruzzi F, Gordon J, Darbinian N, Amini S: Tat-induced deregulation of neuronal differentiation and survival by nerve growth factor pathway. *J Neurovirol* 8(S2):91, 2002.

39. Nath A: Human immunodeficiency virus (HIV) proteins in neuropathogenesis of HIV dementia. *J Infect Dis* 86(S2):S193, 2002.

40. Gras G, Chretien F, Vallat-Decouvelaere AV, et al: Regulated expression of sodium-dependent glutamate transporters and synthetase: A neuroprotective role for activated microglia and macrophages in HIV infection? *Brain Pathol* 13(2):211, 2003.

41. Vallat-Decouvelaere AV, Chretien F, Gras G, et al: Expression of excitatory amino acid transporter-1 in brain macrophages and microglia of HIV-infected patients: A neuroprotective role for activated microglia? *J Neuropathol Exp Neurol* 62(5):475, 2003.

42. Choi SY, Kim S-Y, Chao W, et al: Differential expression of EAAT1 and EAAT2 glutamate transporters by human fetal astrocytes and their response to HIV-1 infection or gp120 (abstract I.25). *J Neurovirol* 9(suppl 3):98, 2003.

43. Kim S-Y, Choi S-Y, Chao W, Volsky DJ: Cloning and characterization of the human excitatory amino acids transporter 1 (EAAT1) promoter region that regulates expression of a key glutamate transporter in human astrocytes (abstract I.86). *J Neurovirol* 9(suppl 3):118, 2003.

44. Hogan TH, Stauff DL, Krebs FC, et al: Structural and functional evolution of human immunodeficiency virus type 1 long terminal repeat CCAAT/enhancer binding protein sites and their use as molecular markers for central nervous system disease progression. *J Neurovirol* 9(1):55, 2003.

45. He J, Chen Y, Farzan M, et al: CCR3 and CCR5 are coreceptors for HIV-1 infection of microglia. *Nature* 385:645, 1997.

46. Premack BA, Schall TJ: Chemokine receptors: Gateways to inflammation and infection. *Nature Med* 2:1174, 1996.

47. Martin MP, Dean M, Smith MW, et al: Genetic acceleration of AIDS progression by a promoter variant of CCR5. *Science* 282(5395):1907, 1998.

48. van Rij RP, Roda Husman AM, Brouwer M, et al: Role of CCR2 genotype in the clinical course of syncytium-inducing (SI) or non-SI human immunodeficiency virus type 1 infection and in the time to conversion to SI virus variants. *J Infect Dis* 178(6):1806, 1998.

49. Mandel TE, Phipps RP, Abbot A, Tew JG: The follicular dendritic cell: Long-term antigen retention during immunity. *Immunol Rev* 53:29, 1980.

50. Szakal AK, Kosco MH, Tew JG: Microanatomy of lymphoid tissue during humoral immune responses: Structure-function relationships. *Annu Rev Immunol* 7:91, 1989.

51. Estes JD, Keele BF, Tenner-Racz K, et al: Follicular dendritic cell-mediated upregulation of CXCR4 expression on CD4 T cells and HIV pathogenesis. *J Immunol* 169(5):2313, 2002.

52. Bajetto A, Bonavia R, Barbero S, et al: Chemokines and their receptors in the central nervous system. *Front Neuroendocrinol* 22(3):147, 2001.

53. Gonzalez E, Rovin BH, Sen L, et al: HIV-1 infection and AIDS dementia are influenced by a mutant MCP-1 allele linked to increased monocyte infiltration of tissues and MCP-1 levels. *Proc Natl Acad Sci USA* 99(21):13795, 2002.

54. Erichsen D, Lopez AL, Peng H, et al: Neuronal injury regulates fractalkine: Relevance for HIV-1-associated dementia. *J Neuroimmunol* 138(1–2):144, 2003.

55. Cotter R, Williams C, Ryan L, et al: Fractalkine (CX3CL1) and brain inflammation: Implications for HIV-1-associated dementia. *J Neurovirol* 8(6):585, 2002.

56. Takahashi K, Wesselingh SL, Griffin DE, et al: Localization of HIV-1 in human brain using polymerase chain reaction/in situ hybridization and immunocytochemistry. *Ann Neurol* 39:705, 1996.

57. Kaul M, Garden GA, Lipton SA: Pathways to neuronal injury and apoptosis in HIV-associated dementia. *Nature* 410(6831):988, 2001.

58. Sidenius N, Nebulonin M, Santovito M, et al: The urokinase plasminogen activator receptor is highly expressed in brain tissue and cerebrospinal fluid of patients with AIDS dementia complex and other HIV-related neurological manifestations (abstract H.59). *J Neurovirol* 9(suppl 3):11, 2003.

59. Childs EA, Lyles RH, Selnes OA, et al: Plasma viral load and CD4 lymphocytes predict HIV-associated dementia and sensory neuropathy. *Neurology* 52:607, 1999.

60. Zink MC, Suryanarayana K, Mankowski JL, et al: High viral load in the cerebrospinal fluid and brain correlates with severity of simian immunodeficiency virus encephalitis. *J Virol* 73(12):10480, 1999.

61. Zhang L, Yu W, He T, et al: Contribution of human alpha-defensin 1, 2, and 3 to the anti-HIV-1 activity of CD8 antiviral factor. *Science* 298(5595):995, 2002.

62. Howlett WP, Nkya WM, Mmuni KA, Missalek WR: Neurological disorders in AIDS and HIV disease in the northern zone of Tanzania. *AIDS* 3:289, 1989.

63. McArthur JC, Hoover DR, Bacellar H, et al: Dementia in AIDS patients: Incidence and risk factors. *Neurology* 43:2245, 1993.

64. Janssen RS, Nwanyanwu OC, Selik RM, Stehr-Green JK: Epidemiology of human immunodeficiency virus encephalopathy in the United States. *Neurology* 42:1472, 1992.

65. Chiesi A, Seeber AC, Dally LG, et al: AIDS dementia complex in the Italian National AIDS Registry: Temporal trends (1987–1993) and differential incidence according to mode of transmission of HIV-1 infection. *J Neurol Sci* 144:107, 1996.

66. Janssen RS, Saykin AJ, Cannon L, et al: Neurological and neuropsychological manifestations of HIV-1 infection: Association with AIDS-related complex but not asymptomatic HIV-1 infection. *Ann Neurol* 26:592, 1989.

67. Ammassari AA, Starace F, Aloisi MS, et al: Medication adherence among HIV+ adults: Effects of cognitive dysfunction and regimen complexity. *Neurology* 61(5):723, 2003.

68. Janssen RS, Cornblath DR, Epstein LG, et al: Nomenclature and research case definitions for neurological manifestations of human immunodeficiency virus type-1 (HIV-1) infection: Report of a working group of the American Academy of Neurology AIDS Task Force. *Neurology* 41:778, 1991.

69. Navia BA, Jordan BD, Price RW: The AIDS dementia complex: I. Clinical features. *Ann Neurol* 19:517, 1986.

70. Belman AL, Ultmann MH, Horoupian D, et al: Neurological complications in infants and children with acquired immune deficiency syndrome. *Ann Neurol* 18:560, 1985.

71. Epstein LG, Sharer LR, Joshi VV, et al: Progressive encephalopathy in children with acquired immune deficiency syndrome. *Ann Neurol* 17:488, 1985.

72. Mintz M, Epstein LG, Koenigsberger MR: Neurological manifestations of acquired immunodeficiency syndrome in children. *Int Pediatr* 4:161, 1989.

73. Nath A, Anderson C, Jones M, et al: Neurotoxicity and dysfunction of dopaminergic systems associated with AIDS dementia. *J Psychopharmacol* 14(3):222, 2000.

74. Maher J, Choudhri S, Halliday W, et al: AIDS dementia complex with generalized myoclonus. *Mov Disord* 12:593, 1997.

75. Mirsattari SM, Power C, Nath A: Parkinsonism with HIV infection. *Mov Disord* 13(4):684, 1998.

76. Davis HF, Skolasky RL Jr, Selnes OA, et al: Assessing HIV-associated dementia: Modified HIV dementia scale versus the Grooved Pegboard. *AIDS Read* 12(1):29, 38, 2002.

77. Hriso E, Kuhn T, Masdeu JC, Grundman M: Extrapyramidal symptoms due to dopamine-blocking agents in patients with AIDS encephalopathy. *Am J Psychiatry* 148:1558, 1991.

78. Sabato S, Wesselingh S, Fuller A, et al: Efavirenz-induced catatonia. *AIDS* 16(13):1841, 2002.

79. Tagliati M, Simpson D, Morgello S, et al: Cerebellar degeneration associated with human immunodeficiency virus infection. *Neurology* 50:244, 1998.

80. Berger JR, Sheremata WA, Resnick L, et al: Multiple sclerosis–like illness occurring with human immunodeficiency virus infection. *Neurology* 39:324, 1989.

81. Wendel KA, McArthur JC: Acute meningoencephalitis in chronic human immunodeficiency virus (HIV) infection: Putative central nervous system escape of HIV replication. *Clin Infect Dis* 37(8):1107, 2003.

82. Langford TD, Letendre SL, Marcotte TD, et al: Severe, demyelinating leukoencephalopathy in AIDS patients on antiretroviral therapy. *AIDS* 16(7):1019, 2002.

83. Glass JD, Wesselingh SL, Selnes OA, McArthur JC: Clinical-neuropathologic correlation in HIV-associated dementia. *Neurology* 43:2230, 1993.

84. Gartner S: HIV infection and dementia (see comments). *Science* 287(5453):602, 2000.

85. Kure K, Llena JF, Lyman WD, et al: Human immunodeficiency virus-1 infection of the nervous system: An autopsy study of 268 adult, pediatric, and fetal brains. *Hum Pathol* 22:700, 1991.

86. Brew BJ, Rosenblum M, Cronin K, Price RW: AIDS dementia complex and HIV-1 brain infection: Clinical-virological correlations. *Ann Neurol* 38:563, 1995.

87. Thompson KA, McArthur JC, Wesselingh SL: Correlation between disease progression and astrocyte apoptosis in HIV-associated dementia. *Ann Neurol* 49:745, 2001.

88. Ketzler S, Weis S, Haug H, Budka H: Loss of neurons in the frontal cortex in AIDS brains. *Acta Neuropathol (Berl)* 80:92, 1990.

89. Masliah E, Ge N, Achim CL, et al: Selective neuronal vulnerability in HIV encephalitis. *J Neuropathol Exp Neurol* 51:585, 1992.

90. Asare E, Dunn G, Glass J, et al: Neuronal pattern correlates with the severity of human immunodeficiency virus–associated dementia complex: Usefulness of spatial pattern analysis in clinicopathological studies. *Am J Pathol* 148:31, 1996.

91. Masliah E, Heaton RK, Marcotte TD, et al: Dendritic injury is a pathological substrate for human immunodeficiency virus-related cognitive disorders. *Ann Neurol* 42:963, 1997.

92. Barker PB, Lee RR, McArthur JC: AIDS dementia complex: Evaluation with proton MR spectroscopic imaging. *Radiology* 195:58, 1995.

93. Chang L, Ernst T, Leonido-Yee M, et al: Cerebral metabolic abnormalities correlate with clinical severity of HIV-1 cognitive motor complex. *Neurology* 52:100, 1999.

94. McClernon DR, Lanier R, Gartner S, et al: HIV in the brain: RNA levels and patterns of zidovudine resistance. *Neurology* 57(8):1396, 2001.

95. Dallasta LM, Pisarov LA, Esplen JE, et al: Blood-brain barrier tight junction disruption in human immunodeficiency virus-1 encephalitis. *Am J Pathol* 155(6):1915, 1999.

96. Berger JR, Nath A, Greenberg RN, et al: Cerebrovascular changes in the basal ganglia with HIV dementia (in process citation). *Neurology* 54(4):921, 2000.

97. Fischer-Smith T, Croul S, Haxhistasa O, et al: Perivascular macrophages represent the predominant reservoir of CNS HIV infection in HIV associated dementia complex: Comparison of CNS and visceral organ tissues reveals systemic abnormalities in monocyte/macrophage trafficking and organ invasion (abstract H.22). *J Neurovirol* 9(suppl 3):5, 2003.

98. Fischer-Smith T, Croul S, Sverstiuk AE, et al: CNS invasion by CD14+/CD16+ peripheral blood-derived monocytes in HIV dementia: Perivascular accumulation and reservoir of HIV infection. *J Neurovirol* 7(6):528, 2001.

99. Glass JD, Fedor H, Wesselingh SL, McArthur JC: Immunocytochemical quantitation of HIV in the brain: Correlations with HIV-associated dementia. *Ann Neurol* 38:755, 1995.

100. Wesselingh SL, Takahashi K, Glass JD, et al: Cellular localization of tumor necrosis factor mRNA in neurological tissue from HIV-infected patients by combined reverse transcriptase polymerase chain reaction in situ hybridization and immunohistochemistry. *J Neuroimmunol* 74:1, 1997.

100. Griffin DE: Cytokines in the brain during viral infection: clues to HIV-associated dementia. *J Clin Invest* 100(12):2948, 1997.

102. Adamson DC, McArthur JC, Dawson TM, Dawson VL: Rate and severity of HIV-associated dementia: Correlations with gp41 and iNOS. *Mol Med* 5:98, 1999.

103. Epstein LG, Gendelman HE: Human immunodeficiency virus type 1 infection of the nervous system: Pathogenetic mechanisms. *Ann Neurol* 33:429, 1993.

104. Yong VW, Krekoski CA, Forsyth PA, et al: Matrix metalloproteinases and diseases of the CNS. *Trends Neurosci* 21(2):75, 1998.

105. Vos CM, Sjulson L, Nath A, et al: Cytotoxicity by matrix metalloprotease-1 in organotypic spinal cord and dissociated neuronal cultures. *Exp Neurol* 163(2):324, 2000.

106. Patton BL, Chiu AY, Sanes JR: Synaptic laminin prevents glial entry into the synaptic cleft. *Nature* 393(6686):698, 1998.

107. Lipton SA, Gendelman HE: Dementia associated with the acquired immunodeficiency syndrome. *New Engl J Med* 332:934, 1995.

108. Nath A, Geiger J: Neurobiological aspects of human immunodeficiency virus infection: Neurotoxic mechanisms (review). *Prog Neurobiol* 54:19, 1998.

109. Ensoli B, Buonaguro L, Barillari G, et al: Release, uptake, and effects of extracellular human immunodeficiency virus type 1 Tat protein on cell growth and viral transactivation. *J Virol* 67(1):277, 1993.

110. Hayman M, Arbuthnott G, Harkiss G, et al: Neurotoxicity of peptide analogues of the transactivating protein tat from Maedi-Visna virus and human immunodeficiency virus. *Neuroscience* 53(1):1, 1993.

111. Chen P, Mayne M, Power C, Nath A: The Tat protein of HIV-1 induces tumor necrosis factor-alpha production: Implications for HIV-1-associated neurological diseases. *J Biol Chem* 272(36):22385, 1997.

112. Nath A, Conant K, Chen P, et al: Transient exposure to HIV-1 Tat protein results in cytokine production in macrophages and astrocytes: A hit and run phenomenon. *J Biol Chem* 274(24):17098, 1999.

113. Magnuson DSK, Knudsen BE, Geiger JD, et al: Human immunodeficiency virus type 1 tat activates non-*N*-methyl-D-aspartate excitatory amino acid receptors and causes neurotoxicity. *Ann Neurol* 37:373, 1995.

114. Conant K, Garzinodemo A, Nath A, et al: Induction of monocyte chemoattractant protein-1 in HIV-1 tat-stimulated astrocytes and elevation in AIDS dementia. *Proc Natl Acad Sci USA* 95:3117, 1998.

115. Gelbard HA, James H, Sharer L, et al: Identification of apoptotic neurons in postmortem brain tissue with HIV-1 encephalitis and progressive encephalopathy. *Neuropathol Appl Neurobiol* 21:208, 1995.

116. Kelder W, McArthur JC, Nance-Sproson T, et al: Beta-chemokines MCP-1 and RANTES are selectively increased in cerebrospinal fluid of patients with human immunodeficiency virus–associated dementia. *Ann Neurol* 44:831, 1998.

117. Zink MC, Coleman GD, Mankowski JL, et al: Increased macrophage chemoattractant protein-1 in cerebrospinal fluid precedes and predicts simian immunodeficiency virus encephalitis. *J Infect Dis* 184(8):1015, 2001.

118. Heyes MP, Brew BJ, Martin A, et al: Quinolinic acid in cerebrospinal fluid and serum in HIV-1 infection: Relationship to clinical and neurologic status. *Ann Neurol* 29:202, 1991.

119. Brew BJ, Bhalla RB, Fleisher M, et al: Cerebrospinal fluid beta-2 microglobulin in patients infected with human immunodeficiency virus. *Neurology* 39:830, 1989.

120. Hagberg L, Dotevall L, Norkrans G, et al: Cerebrospinal fluid neopterin concentrations in central nervous system infection. *J Infect Dis* 168(5):1285, 1993.

121. Sabri F, De Milito A, Pirskanen R, et al: Elevated levels of soluble Fas and Fas ligand in cerebrospinal fluid of patients with AIDS dementia complex. *J Neuroimmunol* 114:197, 2001.

122. Andersson L, Blennow K, Fuchs D, et al: Increased cerebrospinal fluid protein tau concentration in neuro-AIDS. *J Neurol Sci* 171(2):92, 1999.

123. Griffin DE, Wesselingh SL, McArthur JC: Elevated central nervous system prostaglandins in HIV-associated dementia. *Ann Neurol* 35:592, 1994.

124. Williams KC, Corey S, Westmoreland SV, et al: Perivascular macrophages are the primary cell type productively infected by simian immunodeficiency virus in the brains of macaques: implications for the neuropathogenesis of AIDS. *J Exp Med* 193(8):905, 2001.

125. Shaw GM, Harper ME, Hahn BH, et al: HTLV-III infection in brains of children and adults with AIDS encephalopathy. *Science* 227:177, 1985.

126. Pang S, Koyanagi Y, Miles S, et al: High levels of unintegrated HIV-1 DNA in brain tissue of AIDS dementia patients. *Nature* 343:85, 1990.

127. Brack-Werner R: Astrocytes: HIV cellular reservoirs and important participants in neuropathogenesis. *AIDS* 13(1):1, 1999.

128. Shi B, De Girolami U, He J, et al: Apoptosis induced by HIV-1 infection of the central nervous system. *J Clin Invest* 98:1979, 1996.

129. Ferrarese C, Aliprandi A, Tremolizzo L, et al: Increased glutamate in CSF and plasma of patients with HIV dementia. *Neurology* 57(4):671, 2001.

130. Ferrarese C, Riva R, Dolara A, et al: Elevated glutamate in the cerebrospinal fluid of patients with HIV dementia. *JAMA* 277(8):630, 1997.

131. Brew BJ, Bhalla RB, Paul M, et al: Cerebrospinal fluid neopterin in human immunodeficiency virus type-I infection. *Ann Neurol* 28:556, 1990.

132. Griffin DE, McArthur JC, Cornblath DR: Neopterin and interferon-gamma in serum and cerebrospinal fluid of patients with HIV-associated neurologic disease. *Neurology* 41:69, 1991.

133. Conant K, McArthur JC, Griffin DE, et al: Cerebrospinal fluid levels of MMP-2, -7, and -9 are elevated in association with human immunodeficiency virus dementia (in process citation). *Ann Neurol* 46(3):391, 1999.

134. Wendell KA, McClernon DR, Lanier ER, McArthur JC: Discordant HIV-1 drug resistance mutations in paired CSF and plasma. Infectious Disease Society of America Meeting, 2001.

135. Schooley RT: Correlation between viral load measurements and outcome in clinical trials of antiviral drugs. *AIDS* 9(suppl 2):S15, 1995.

136. Mellors JW, Munoz A, Giorgi JV, et al: Plasma viral load and CD4+ lymphocytes as prognostic markers of HIV-1 infection. *Ann Intern Med* 126:946, 1997.

137. Hogervorst E, Jurriaans S, Dewolf F, et al: Predictors for non- and slow progression in human immunodeficiency virus (HIV) type 1 infection: Low viral RNA copy numbers in serum and maintenance of high HIV-1 p24-specific but not V3-specific antibody levels. *J Infect Dis* 171:811, 1995.

138. Mellors JW, Rinaldo CR, Gupta P, et al: Prognosis in HIV-1 infection predicted by the quantity of virus in plasma. *Science* 272:1167, 1996.

139. McArthur JC, McClernon DR, Cronin MF, et al: Relationship between human immunodeficiency virus–associated dementia and viral load in cerebrospinal fluid and brain. *Ann Neurol* 42:689, 1997.

140. Ellis RJ, Hsia K, Spector SA, et al: Cerebrospinal fluid human immunodeficiency virus type 1 RNA levels are elevated in neurocognitively impaired individuals with acquired immunodeficiency syndrome. *Ann Neurol* 42:679, 1997.

141. Brew BJ, Pemberton L, Cunningham P, Law MG: Levels of human immunodeficiency virus type 1 RNA in cerebrospinal fluid correlate with AIDS dementia stage. *J Infect Dis* 175:963, 1997.

142. Ellis RJ, Moore DJ, Childers ME, et al: Progression to neuropsychological impairment in human immunodeficiency virus infection predicted by elevated cerebrospinal fluid levels of human immunodeficiency virus RNA. *Arch Neurol* 59(6):923, 2002.

143. De Luca A, Ciancio BC, Larussa D, et al: Correlates of independent HIV-1 replication in the CNS and of its control by antiretrovirals. *Neurology* 59(3):342, 2002.

144. McArthur JC, McDermott MP, McClernon D, et al: Attenuated CNS infection and immune activation in advanced HIV/AIDS. *Arch Neurol,* in press.

145. Marra CM, Coombs RW, Collier AC: Changes in CSF and plasma HIV-1 RNA and in neuropsychological test performance after starting HAART (abstract 408). Sixth Conference on Retroviruses and Opportunistic Infections, January 31–February 4, 1999.

146. Ellis RJ, Gamst AC, Capparelli E, et al: Cerebrospinal fluid HIV RNA originates from both local CNS and systemic sources (in process citation). *Neurology* 54(4):927, 2000.

147. McArthur JC, McClernon DR, Nance-Sproson L, et al: Factors associated with durable suppression of HIV in the cerebrospinal fluid (abstract P03.005). *Neurology* 52:A191, 1999.

148. Price RW, Paxinos EE, Grant RM, et al: Cerebrospinal fluid response to structured treatment interruption after virological failure. *AIDS* 15(10):1251, 2001.

149. Price RW, Paxinos EE, Grant RM, et al: Cerebrospinal fluid response to structured treatment interruption after virological failure. *AIDS* 15(10):1251, 2001.

150. Tyler KL, McArthur JC: Through a glass, darkly: Cerebrospinal fluid viral load measurements and the pathogenesis of human immunodeficiency virus infection of the central nervous system. *Arch Neurol* 59(6):909, 2002.

151. Filippi CG, Sze G, Farber SJ, et al: Regression of HIV encephalopathy and basal ganglia signal intensity abnormality at MR imaging in patients with AIDS after the initiation of protease inhibitor therapy. *Radiology* 206:491, 1998.

152. Berger JR, Avison MJ: Diffusion tensor imaging in HIV infection: What is it telling us? *AJNR* 22(2):237, 2001.

153. Chang L, Rooney W, Carasig D, et al: Abnormal blood-brain barrier permeability in human immunode-

ficiency virus patients (abstract 282). American Neurological Association Meeting, New York, October 13–16, 2002.

154. Price RW, Yiannoutsos CT, Clifford DB, et al: Neurological outcomes in late HIV infection: Adverse impact of neurological impairment on survival and protective effect of antiviral therapy. AIDS Clinical Trial Group and Neurological AIDS Research Consortium Study Team. *AIDS* 13(13):1677, 1999.

155. Suwanwelaa N, Phanuphak P, Phanthumchinda K, et al: Magnetic resonance spectroscopy of the brain in neurologically asymptomatic HIV-infected patients. *Magn Reson Imaging* 18(7):859, 2000.

156. Tarasow E, Wiercinska-Drapalo A, Kubas B, et al: Cerebral MR spectroscopy in neurologically asymptomatic HIV-infected patients. *Acta Radiol* 44(2):206, 2003.

157. Chang L, Witt M, Eric M, et al: Cerebral metabolite changes during the first nine months after HAART (abstract S63.001). *Neurology* 56:A474, 2001.

158. Yiannoutsos C: Patterns of regional brain metabolism and diagnostic utility of proton MRS in AIDS dementia complex. Unpublished work, 2002.

159. Menon DK, Ainsworth JG, Cox IJ, et al: Proton MR spectroscopy of the brain in AIDS dementia complex. *J Comput Assist Tomogr* 16:538, 1992.

160. Menon DK, Baudouin CJ, Tomlinson D, Hoyle C: Proton MR spectroscopy and imaging of the brain in AIDS: Evidence of neuronal loss in regions that appear normal with imaging. *J Comput Assist Tomogr* 14:882, 1990.

161. Chong WK, Sweeney B, Wilkinson ID, et al: Proton spectroscopy of the brain in HIV infection: Correlation with clinical, immunologic, and MR imaging findings. *Radiology* 188:119, 1993.

162. Chong WK, Paley M, Wilkinson ID, et al: Localized cerebral proton MR spectroscopy in HIV infection and AIDS. *AJNR* 15:21, 1994.

163. Confort-Gouny S, Vion-Dury J, Nicoli F, et al: Metabolic characterization of neurological diseases by proton localized NMR spectroscopy of the human brain. *CR Acad Sci* 315(7):287, 1992.

164. Jarvik JG, Lenkinski RE, Grossman RI, et al: Proton MR spectroscopy of HIV-infected patients: Characterization of abnormalities with imaging and clinical correlation. *Radiology* 186:739, 1993.

165. Van Der Flier WM, Van Den Heuvel DM, Weverling-Rijnsburger AW, et al: Magnetization transfer imaging in normal aging, mild cognitive impairment, and Alzheimer's disease. *Ann Neurol* 52(1):62, 2002.

166. Armand JP, Dousset V, Franconi JM, et al: Progressive multifocal leukoencephalopathy: Study of the demyelination by magnetization transfer. *J Radiol* 78(2):131, 1997.

167. Ernst T, Chang L, Jovicich J, et al: Abnormal brain activation on functional MRI in cognitively asymptomatic HIV patients. *Neurology* 59(9):1343, 2002.

168. Eggers C, Hertogs K, Sturenburg HJ, et al: Delayed central nervous system virus suppression during highly active antiretroviral therapy is associated with HIV en-

cephalopathy, but not with viral drug resistance or poor central nervous system drug penetration. *AIDS* 17(13):1897, 2003.

169. Lawrence J, Mayers DL, Hullsiek KH, et al: Structured treatment interruption in patients with multidrug-resistant human immunodeficiency virus. *New Engl J Med* 349(9):837, 2003.

170. Thomas SA, Segal MB: The passage of azido-deoxythymidine into and within the central nervous system: Does it follow the parent compound, thymidine? *J Pharmacol Exp Ther* 281(3):1211, 1997.

171. Yang Z, Brundage RC, Barbhaiya RH, Sawchuk RJ: Microdialysis studies of the distribution of stavudine into the central nervous system in the freely-moving rat. *Pharm Res* 14(7):865, 1997.

172. Solas C, Lafeuillade A, Halfon P, et al: Discrepancies between protease inhibitor concentrations and viral load in reservoirs and sanctuary sites in human immunodeficiency virus-infected patients. *Antimicrob Agents Chemother* 47(1):238, 2003.

173. Groothuis DR, Levy RM: The entry into antiviral and antiretroviral drugs into the central nervous system. *J Neurovirol* 3:387, 1997.

174. Pardridge WM: Targeting neurotherapeutic agents through the blood-brain barrier. *Arch Neurol* 59(1):35, 2002.

175. Schaner ME, Gerstin KM, Wang J, Giacomini KM: Mechanisms of transport of nucleosides and nucleoside analogues in choroid plexus. *Adv Drug Deliv Rev* 39(1–3):51, 1999.

176. Gisolf EH, Enting RH, Jurriaans S, et al: Cerebrospinal fluid HIV-1 RNA during treatment with ritonavir/saquinavir or ritonavir/saquinavir/stavudine. *AIDS* 14(11):1583, 2000.

177. Sacktor N, Tarwater PM, Skolasky RL, et al: CSF antiretroviral drug penetrance and the treatment of HIV-associated psychomotor slowing. *Neurology* 57(3):542, 2001.

178. Wynn HE, Brundage RC, Fletcher CV: Clinical implications of CNS penetration of antiretroviral drugs. *CNS Drugs* 16(9):595, 2002.

179. Sacktor NC, McArthur JC: Prospects for therapy of HIV-associated neurologic disease. *J Neurovirol* 3:89, 1997.

180. Sidtis JJ, Gatsonis C, Price RW, et al: Zidovudine treatment of the AIDS dementia complex: results of a placebo-controlled trial. *Ann Neurol* 33:343, 1993.

181. Schifitto G, Kieburtz K, McDermott MP, et al: Clinical trials in HIV-associated cognitive impairment: Cognitive and functional outcomes. *Neurology* 56(3):415, 2001.

182. Price RW, Sidtis JJ: Evaluation of the AIDS dementia complex in clinical trials. *J Acquir Immune Defic Synd* 3(suppl 2):S51, 1990.

183. Cohen RA, Boland R, Paul R, et al: Neurocognitive performance enhanced by highly active antiretroviral therapy in HIV-infected women. *AIDS* 15(3):341, 2001.

184. Tozzi V, Balestra P, Galgani S, et al: Positive and sustained effects of highly active antiretroviral therapy on HIV-1-associated neurocognitive impairment. *AIDS* 13(14):1889, 1999.

185. Ferrando S, van Gorp W, McElhiney M, et al: Highly active antiretroviral treatment in HIV infection: Benefits for neuropsychological function. *AIDS* 12(8):F65, 1998.

186. Sacktor NC, Skolasky RL, Lyles RH, et al: Improvement in HIV-associated motor slowing after antiretroviral therapy including protease inhibitors. *J Neurovirol* 6(1):84, 2000.

187. Brew BJ, Halman M, Catalan J, et al: Abacavir in AIDS dementia complex: Efficacy and lessons for future trials. Unpublished work, 2000.

188. Dougherty RH, Skolasky RL, McArthur JC: Progression of HIV-associated dementia treated with HAART. *AIDS Read* 12:69, 2002.

189. Sacktor N, Skolasky RL, Tarwater PM, et al: Response to systemic HIV viral load suppression correlates with psychomotor speed performance. *Neurology* 61(4):567, 2003.

190. Hahn MK, Blakely RD: Monoamine transporter gene structure and polymorphisms in relation to psychiatric and other complex disorders. *Pharmacogenom J* 2(4):217, 2002.

191. Mallal S, Nolan D, Witt C, et al: Association between presence of HLA-B*5701, HLA-DR7, and HLA-DQ3 and hypersensitivity to HIV-1 reverse-transcriptase inhibitor abacavir. *Lancet* 359(9308):727, 2002.

192. Fellay J, Marzolini C, Meaden ER, et al: Response to antiretroviral treatment in HIV-1-infected individuals with allelic variants of the multidrug resistance transporter 1: A pharmacogenetics study. *Lancet* 359(9300):30, 2002.

193. The Dana Consortium on the Therapy of HIV Dementia and Related Cognitive Disorders: A randomized, double-blind, placebo-controlled trial of deprenyl and thioctic acid in human immunodeficiency virus–associated cognitive impairment. *Neurology* 50:645, 1998.

194. Sacktor N, Schifitto G, McDermott MP, et al: Transdermal selegiline in HIV-associated cognitive impairment: Pilot, placebo-controlled study. *Neurology* 54(1):233, 2000.

195. Navia BA, Dafni U, Simpson D, et al: A phase I/II trial of nimodipine for HIV-related neurologic complications. *Neurology* 51:221, 1998.

196. Heseltine PNR, Goodkin K, Atkinson JH, et al: Randomized, double-blind, placebo-controlled trial of peptide T for HIV-associated cognitive impairment. *Arch Neurol* 55:41, 1998.

197. The Dana Consortium on Therapy of HIV Dementia and Related Cognitive Disorders: Safety and efficacy of the antioxidant OPC-14117 in HIV-associated cognitive impairment. *Neurology* 49:142, 1997.

198. Schifitto G, Sacktor N, Marder K, et al: Randomized trial of the platelet-activating factor antagonist lexipafant in HIV-associated cognitive impairment. *Neurology* 53:391, 1999.

199. Clifford DB, McArthur JC, Schifitto G, et al: A randomized clinical trial of CPI-1189 for HIV-associated cognitive-motor impairment. *Neurology* 59(10):1568, 2002.

200. Turchan J: Neuroprotective therapy for HIV dementia. *Curr HIV Res* 1:373, 2003.

201. McArthur JC: Neurologic manifestations of AIDS. *Medicine* 66:407, 1987.

CHAPTER 10

Neurologic Manifestations of HTLV-I Infection

Abelardo Araújo and Marcus Tulius T. Silva

▶ OVERVIEW

The year 2004 celebrates the twenty-fifth anniversary of the discovery of the first human retrovirus: the human T-cell lymphotropic virus type I (HTLV-I), the etiologic agent of adult T-cell leukemia (ATL) and HTLV-I-associated myelopathy/tropical spastic paraparesis (HAM/TSP). Although the importance of this discovery was overshadowed by the advent of acquired immunodeficiency syndrome (AIDS) in the next year, its discovery has had several remarkable implications. First, it provided clear proof of a relationship between viruses and cancer. Second, the discovery of antibodies against HTLV-I in patients with TSP, a puzzling neurologic disease of unknown etiology, uncovered a new field of research for virologists and neurologists. Finally, the laboratory tools employed in the discovery of HTLV-I clearly facilitated the detection and isolation of HIV.

HTLVs are ancient infectious agents of humans, and some related retroviruses were found in Old World primates. Transmission of the simian T-cell leukemia virus type I (STLV-I) from nonhuman primates to humans in Africa[1] is the most probable origin of HTLV-I. However, the means by which the virus was disseminated are controversial. Phylogenetically, HTLV-I can be classified into three major groups: cosmopolitan, Central African, and Melanesian. There is a strong correlation between the viral genotype and the geographic area of virus carriers between the Central African and Melanesian groups. The cosmopolitan group can be further subdivided into four subgroups: transcontinental (type A), Japanese (type B), West African (type C), and North African (type D). Subgroup B prevails mostly in Japan, subgroup C is found in West Africa and the Caribbean, and subgroup D is found in North Africa. Subgroup A is distributed worldwide. There are two main hypotheses of how HTLV was disseminated from Africa to the New World. One is that dissemination to the New World and Japan occurred during the slave trade, during the period of great travels by ocean. The second theory is based on ancient movements of HTLV carriers and the observation of HTLV prevalence among Amerindians.

It is possible that some Amerindian populations were infected on arrival in South America. Mongoloid populations carrying HTLV-I subgroup A, which prevailed in East Asia, brought the virus both to Japan and, about 10,000 to 20,000 years ago, to the New World via the land bridge of Bering. The same could apply to HTLV-II, which is endemic in different populations of Amerindians and can be found in Mongolia. Therefore, it is possible that the spread of HTLVs to the rest of the world occurred in the pre-Colombian period, before discovery of the Americas and the slave trade. In South America these two hypotheses are not mutually exclusive because HTLVs do not necessarily have a single origin. In fact, although the majority of HTLV-I in South America spread from Amerindians, it would not be surprising that some of them found their way to Latin America from Africa via the Atlantic Ocean.[2] Figure 10-1 shows the worldwide distribution of HTLVs and the probable routes of dissemination.

Since 1956, a spastic paraparetic syndrome initially known as *Jamaican neuropathy* has been reported in Jamaica. Similar cases of chronic progressive paraparesis of unknown etiology were described by neurologists from tropical regions in diverse designations. In 1969, Mani and colleagues, recognizing the clinical and histopathologic similarities among these patients, coined the term *tropical spastic paraparesis* (TSP). The etiology of this medical myelopathy remained obscure until 1985, when Gessain and colleagues discovered that most TSP patients from Martinique had antibodies against HTLV-I in their sera. A couple of months later, Osame and colleagues, in Japan, observed the presence of atypical lymphocytes in the cerebrospinal fluid (CSF) of some individuals with chronic spastic paraparesis. They also described the association of antibodies against HTLV-I with this myelopathy and suggested the term *HTLV-I-associated myelopathy* (HAM) because Japan is not a tropical country. Soon it became clear that both diseases were in fact the same, and in 1989, a consensus conference sponsored by the World Health Organization (WHO) suggested the hybrid designation HAM/TSP.

At the present time, the role of HTLV-II in human disease remains poorly defined. This retrovirus is more prevalent among intravenous drug users (IDUs) and some native Amerindian groups. There also has been sparse evidence of its role in some neurologic abnormalities and rare lymphoproliferative disorders. It has been difficult to establish a definitive role of HTLV-II in a specific disease because most published cases come from either IDUs or HIV–infected individuals. However, there have been some reports of ataxia, spasticity, peripheral neuropathy, and cognitive dysfunction in HTLV-II-infected patients.[3,4] Because of this uncertainty, only the HTLV-I-associated neurologic diseases will be discussed here.

▶ EPIDEMIOLOGY

Like HIV, the HTLVs can be transmitted by sexual contact with an infected individual, through sharing of contaminated needles and syringes by IDUs, following transfusion of contaminated blood (mainly from cellular products), and from mother to child through perinatal exposure or breast feeding (intrauterine transmission is very rare).

The real prevalence of HTLV-I is still unknown, but it is estimated that 10 to 20 million individuals carry the virus worldwide. The seroprevalence increases with age and is twice as high in females. This gender difference usually emerges after 30 years of age and probably reflects a more efficient transmission of the virus from males to females in the sexually active years (see below).[5]

Foci of HTLV-I infection are found in geographic clusters (see Fig. 10-1). The infection is endemic in southern Japan, the Caribbean, sub-Saharan Africa, the Middle East, South America, the Pacific Melanesian Islands, and Papua New Guinea. Population-based studies have shown that HTLV-I seroprevalence ranges from 3 to 6 percent in Trinidad, Jamaica, and other Caribbean islands to 30 percent in rural Miyazaki, southern Japan.[6,7] In Brazil, the largest South American country, prevalence rates are highly variable according to the region studied (from 0.08 percent in the southern region to 1.8 percent in Salvador in the northeastern region).[8] In the United States and Europe, HTLV-I infection has been identified primarily among IDUs (9 versus 41 percent for HIV prevalence), female sex workers, recipients of multiple blood transfusions, and immigrants from endemic areas.[9,10]

Blood transfusion is perhaps the most efficient means of virus transmission. The probability of seroconversion after a transfusion of contaminated blood is 40 to 60 percent, and the median time to seroconversion is estimated to be around 51 days.[11] A study of 39,898 random blood donors in eight U.S. cities identified 10 HTLV-I-seropositive donors (0.025 percent).[12] Since 1988, routine screening of donors has been done in the United States, and the risk of transfusion-associated HTLV-I infection is less than 1:50,000.[13] *Breast feeding* for more than 6 months has been associated with a probability of mother-to-child transmission of 10.5 to 39.6 percent. The main maternal risk factors for virus transmission are a high proviral load, a high percentage of mononuclear cells infected by HTLV-I in the breast milk, and high antibodies levels.[14,15] The immunodominance of epitopes Env1/5 and RE3, two viral envelope glycoprotein antibodies, may confer some protection against breast-feeding transmission.[16] Interventional studies in Japan have found that infection still occurs in 3 to 12.8 percent of children who were not breast-fed, suggesting an alternative means of transmission.[17,18] *Sexual transmission* has the potential to in-

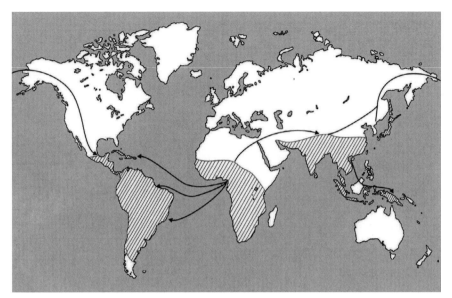

Figure 10-1. World distribution of HTLV-I and probable routes of its dissemination. Marked areas are endemic foci of HTLV-I, with population prevalence ranging from 0.45 percent (as in Rio de Janeiro, Brazil) to 30 percent (as in Miyazaki, Japan). The lines represent the probable routes of HTLV dissemination to the New World.

troduce infection into previously unexposed groups. HTLV-I is transmitted four times more effectively from males to females than the inverse, at a rate of 4.9 per 100 person-years among females married to an infected male compared with 1.2 among males married to infected females.[19] More recently, HTLV-I transmission by *infected organ donors* has been reported. In all organ recipients, a rapid development of a subacute myelopathy was observed, possibly due to a large virus inoculum or a high proviral load favored by the lack of a CD8+ cytotoxic T-lymphocyte (CTL) response as a result of the immunosuppressed status (see below).[20,21] These reports raise the question of whether potential organ donors should be screened routinely for HTLV-I. By using blood transfusion as an analogy, the probability of infection in recipients of a contaminated organ should be between 13 and 60 percent. Although there are some concerns about the time that confirmatory serologic tests for HTLV-I usually take, there should be an ethical discussion before transplantation is endorsed, mainly in endemic areas.

▶ PATHOPHYSIOLOGY AND PATHOGENESIS

The human T-cell lymphotropic viruses are enveloped RNA, type C viruses, belonging to the Retroviridae family and the Oncorvirus subfamily (Fig. 10-2*A*). They are single-stranded RNA retroviruses with reverse transcriptase activity that leads to DNA transcription of the virus and random integration into the host genome. Once integrated, such proviruses can persist latently, escaping immune surveillance. The genetic structure of HTLV-I is similar to that of other retroviruses, and it shares about 60 percent genetic homology with HTLV-

II. Its genome contains *gag, pol,* and *env* genes flanked by two long terminals repeats (LTRs) (see Fig. 10-2*B*). HTLV-I has a unique region in the LTR 3′ region referred to as the *p*X region. It encodes two crucial proteins, both for the activation of host genes and virus replication: tax and rex (Table 10-1). The CD8+ CTL response to tax, the main viral antigen, plays a decisive role in the pathogenesis of HTLV-I infection (see below).

The life cycle of HTLV-I is similar to that of other retroviruses. Infection requires the interaction between the viral envelope and a cellular receptor, following which the nuclear content is released into the cytoplasm and transported to the nucleus (Fig. 10-3). Unlike HIV, HTLV-I does not use the CD4+ molecule as a receptor. Indirect evidence suggests that its receptor may be encoded on chromosome 17.[22] As with other retroviruses, the hallmark of HTLV is reverse transcription of viral RNA to produce proviral DNA that is then integrated into the host genome. HTLV is also able to replicate without the use of reverse transcription by infectious spread; after integration, transactivation of cellular genes results in cell proliferation, and at each cell division, a new copy of the integrated HTLV provirus is made (mitotic transmission). The relative sequence stability of HTLV-I suggests that the high proviral load is maintained mainly by mitotic transmission because this route is associated with a much lower rate of mutation.[23]

The main target of HTLV-I is the T cell. About 10 to 15 percent of T cells in the peripheral blood of patients with HAM/TSP are infected with HTLV-I. The phenotype of these cells is predominantly CD4+CD45R0+. In contrast, HTLV-II preferentially infects peripheral blood CD8+ T cells.[24] Glial, dendritic, and endothelial cells also may be infected with HTLV-I. The hallmark of T cells infected with HTLV-I is the expression of ac-

Figure 10-2. Viral (*A*) and genomic (*B*) structures of HTLV-I. Between the two long terminal repeat (LTR) sequences lies the provirus genome. It contains regulatory elements that control virus expression and virion production. The encoding genes of the virus are *gag*, *pol*, *env*, and a series of accessory genes that regulate virus expression. Tax, an important viral protein, is coded in the *p*X region.

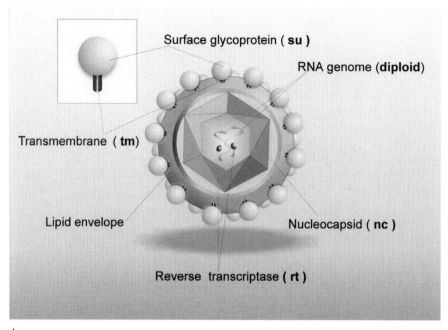

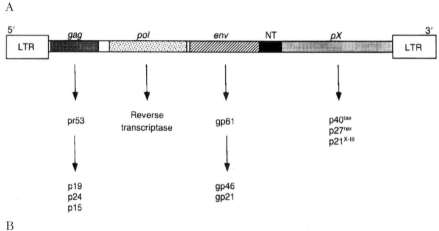

TABLE 10-1. CELLULAR TRANSCRIPTION FACTORS AND GENES ACTIVATED BY HTLV-I TAX PROTEIN

Cellular transcription factors
Cyclic AMP responsive element binding (CREB)
Nuclear transcriptional factor kappa B (NF-κB)
Transactivated cellular genes
Interleukin 2 (IL-2)
Interleukin 2 receptor α chain (IL-2 Rα)
β-Globulin
Vimentin
Major histocompatibility complex class I (MHC-I)
Granulocytic-macrophage colony-stimulating factor (GM-CSF)
Nerve growth factor (NGF)
TGF-β1
Parathyroid hormone–related protein (PTHrP)
Cellular oncogenes (c-*fos*, c-*sis*, c-*myc*)

tivation markers, such as the p55 chain of the interleukin 2 (IL-2) receptor and the major histocompatibility complex (MHC) class II antigens.[25] The result of cell activation by HTLV-I is proliferation of peripheral blood mononuclear cells (PBMCs) in vitro. T cells transformed by HTLV-I have been reported to induce and secrete a variety of cytokines.

The real mechanisms of HTLV-I-induced diseases such as HAM/TSP remain unknown. There are three major hypotheses regarding the pathogenesis of the myelopathy (Fig. 10-4). In the first hypothesis (*direct toxicity theory*), HTLV-I-infected glial cells present viral antigens on their cell surfaces. CD8+ CTLs specific against HTLV-I antigens (mainly tax) cross the blood-brain barrier (BBB), attack the infected cells, and release cytokines, which destroy the glial cells. In the second hypothesis (*autoimmunity theory*), there would be a glial cell "self" antigen similar to a viral antigen. As a

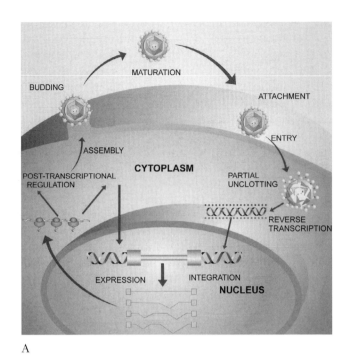

A

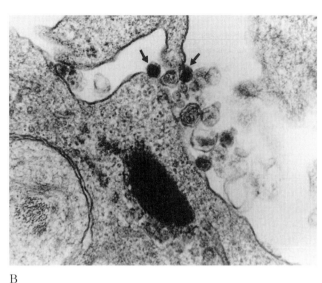

B

Figure 10-3. *A.* The life cycle of HTLV-I. Infection requires the interaction between the viral envelope and a cellular receptor, which is followed by the release of the nuclear contents into the cytoplasm and their transport to the nucleus. Once the proviral DNA is integrated into the cellular genome, the cellular infection is everlasting. *B.* Electron microscopy shows the exact moment of virus budding from a cultured lymphocyte. *(Courtesy, Dr. M. J. Andrada-Serpa.)*

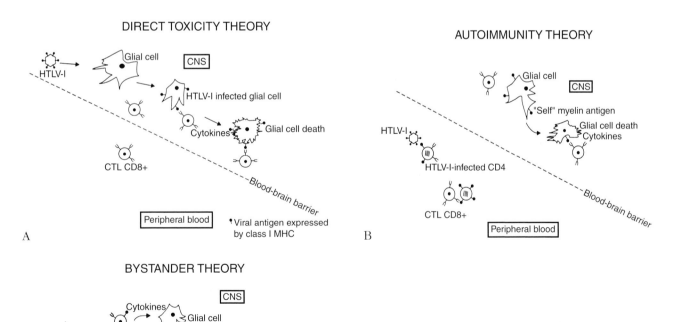

C

Figure 10-4. Major hypotheses regarding the pathogenesis of the myelopathy. (CNS = central nervous system; CTL CD8+ = cytotoxic T-lymphocyte; MHC = major histocompatibility complex.) See text for details.

result, activated CD4+ T-helper cells cross the BBB, confuse the glial cell with an infected cell, and react against it in an autoimmune reaction that results in glial cell death. Recently, a role for molecular mimicry also has been suggested as a hypothesis that links infection with autoimmune diseases.[26] Molecular mimicry is characterized by an immune response to an environmental agent that cross-reacts with a host antigen, resulting in disease. There are antibodies against the HTLV-I tax protein that cross-react with the neuronal self antigen heterogeneous nuclear ribonucleic protein A1 (hnRNP-A1), an intracellular neuronal protein. Such antibodies have been detected in serum, CSF, and the central nervous system (CNS). Antibodies can cross the BBB at sites of inflammation, and perivascular inflammation is one of the features of HAM/TSP. Therefore, molecular mimicry between the viral tax protein and the neuronal hnRNP-A1 could be responsible for the chronic neurologic deficit in HAM/TSP. The last hypothesis (*bystander damage theory*) assumes that HTLV-I-infected CD4+ and anti-HTLV-I-specific CD8+ CTLs migrate across the BBB and interact inside the CNS. This interaction results in release of cytokines and subsequent glial damage. There has been no in vivo evidence so far to support the direct toxicity theory. Yet the remaining theories could still play a role in the CNS damage. It is still possible that CD8+ CTLs recognize viral products presented by HTLV-I-infected vascular endothelial cells or other infected T cells.[25] This would result in activation of CD8+ CTLs and subsequent cytokine secretion.

Although HTLV-I persists notwithstanding a strong immune response, only 2 to 3 percent of infected individuals will develop HAM/TSP. Most genotypic studies of HTLV-I fail to demonstrate any association between HTLV-I variants and the risk of developing HAM/TSP.[27] The factors unequivocally associated with an increased risk of HAM/TSP are a high anti-HTLV-I antibody titer, a high proviral load, and female gender.[28] The proviral load in PBMCs of HAM/TSP patients is very high when compared with that of asymptomatic carriers. In a recent study, the proviral load in PBMCs of 202 HAM/TSP individuals was about 16-fold higher than in 200 asymptomatic carriers. Furthermore, in 43 asymptomatic carriers genetically related to HAM/TSP patients, the proviral load also was higher than that of nonrelated asymptomatic carriers, suggesting a possible genetic factor.[29] Perhaps host factors that determine the "strength" or "efficiency" of the CD8+ CTL response to HTLV-I might in turn determine an individual's proviral load and the risk of HAM/TSP.[23] "Strong CTL responders" to tax maintain a low equilibrium concentration of the tax protein, whereas the equilibrium concentration exceeds the threshold needed to elicit proinflammatory cytokines in "weak CTL responders."[23] The role of CD8+ CTLs in the pathogenesis of HAM/TSP is corroborated by

other studies. Specific CD8+ CTLs to tax are detected in higher frequency both in PBMCs and CSF of HAM/TSP patients when compared with asymptomatic carriers.[30] Moreover, histopathologic analysis revealed a high number of activated CD8+ CTLs in spinal cord lesions of HAM/TSP patients.[31,32]

Regarding immunogenetics, Japanese studies have shown a reduction in both the proviral load and the risk of HAM/TSP in individuals with the class I gene HLA-A*02.[33] Previous studies showed a predisposition to myelopathy in carriers of HLA-DRB1*0101,[34,35] but this only happens in the absence of the "protective gene," HLA-A*02.[33] Maybe HLA-A*02-restricted CD8+ CTLs are particularly efficient in eliminating HTLV-I-infected lymphocytes, which determines a lower proviral load. Probably genetic polymorphism outside the MHC also influences the susceptibility to HAM/TSP.[23] A recent study from Japan demonstrated that the promoter TNF-863A allele predisposed to HAM/TSP, whereas SDF-1+801A, 3'UTR, and IL-15 191C alleles conferred protection. Knowledge of HTLV-I-infected individuals' ages, sex, provirus load, HTLV-I subgroup, and genotypes at the loci HLA-A, HLA-C, SDF-1, and TNF-α allowed for the correct identification of 88 percent of cases of HAM/TSP in this Japanese cohort.[36]

▶ CLINICAL FEATURES

The diagnosis of HAM/TSP is based on clinical and laboratory data. The patient should present unequivocal signs and symptoms of a myelopathy along with clear evidence of HTLV-I infection. The WHO's diagnostic criteria for HAM/TSP are summarized in Table 10-2. These criteria should not be followed strictly but only as general guidelines.

HAM/TSP is a disease with a slow onset and a chronic and steady progression. However, occasionally it can show a rapid progression. Spontaneous improvement is very rare.[37] The risk for development of HAM/TSP among HTLV-I carriers ranges from 0.25 percent among Japanese patients to 2.4 percent among HTLV-I-infected blood donors from the United States.[38,39] Young age at onset of the disease has been associated with a rapid clinical deterioration. Patients with lower anti-HTLV-I antibody titers in the CSF had, on average, an older age of onset, milder clinical symptoms, and a lower neopterin level (an inflammatory marker) in the CSF than those in the high-titer subgroup, regardless of the mode of HTLV-I transmission. The progression of the neurologic disability occurs mainly during the first or second year of the disease and then becomes relatively stable. This could reflect an initial inflammatory phase, with a theoretical therapeutic window lying in this first or second year of the disease (see below).

▶ **TABLE 10-2.** WHO GUIDELINES FOR THE DIAGNOSIS OF HAM/TSP

Clinical Data	Guidelines
Age and sex	Mostly sporadic and adult; female predominates
Onset	Usually insidious
Main neurologic manifestations	Chronic spastic paraparesis, which usually progresses slowly, sometimes remains static after an initial progression
	Weakness of the lower limbs, more marked proximally
	Bladder disturbances usually an early feature; constipation usually occurs later; impotence and decreased libido is common
	Sensory symptoms are more prominent than objective physical signs
	Low lumbar pain with radiation to the legs is common
	Vibration sense is frequently impaired
	Hyperreflexia of lower limbs, often with clonus and Babinski's sign
	Hyperreflexia of upper limbs frequently with positive Hoffmann's and Tromner signs
	Exaggerated jaw jerk in some patients
Less frequent neurologic findings	Cerebellar signs, optic atrophy, deafness, nystagmus, other cranial nerve deficits, hand tremor, absent or depressed ankle jerks
Other neurologic manifestations that may be associated	Muscular atrophy, fasciculations, polymyositis, peripheral neuropathy, polyradiculopathy, cranial neuropathy, meningitis, encephalopathy
Systemic nonneurologic manifestations that may be associated	Pulmonary alveolitis, uveitis, Sjögren's syndrome, arthropathy, vasculitis, ichthyosis, cryoglobulinemia, monoclonal gammopathy, adult T-cell leukemia/lymphoma
Laboratory findings	
Blood	Presence of HTLV-I antibodies* or antigens
	Lobulated lymphocytes may be present
	Viral isolation when possible
CSF	Presence of HTLV-I antibodies or antigens*
	Lobulated lymphocytes may be present
	Mild to moderate increase of protein may be present
	Viral isolation when possible

*Present in blood *and* CSF.

About 60 percent of HAM/TSP patients have weakness of the lower limbs as the first symptom.[40] This steadily progresses to an abnormal spastic gait. There is no definitive way to predict when or who will need a wheelchair in the future. In the course of the disease, bladder dysfunction is very common, with frequency, urgency, incontinence, or retention, as well as impotence in males. Other frequently reported symptoms are back pain, paresthesias in the lower limbs, xerosis, xerophthalmia, and xerostomia (sicca syndrome).

On neurologic examination, these patients have a spastic gait along with spastic weakness of the lower extremities, hyperreflexia, and extensor plantar responses. Although the strength in the arms is usually preserved, deep tendon reflexes tend to be brisk in the upper extremities, and a Hoffmann's sign and a brisk jaw jerk can be elicited occasionally. Sometimes, a Romberg sign and abnormal deep or superficial sensory signs also can be observed.

HAM/TSP can be associated with other HTLV-I-related manifestations such as pulmonary alveolitis, uveitis, arthritis, dermatitis, Sjögren's syndrome, Behçet's disease, thyroid disease, crusted scabies, and cystitis and prostatitis. Although the coincidence of ATL and HAM/TSP in the same patient is considered rare, it has been reported increasingly.[41]

In addition to typical HAM/TSP, other neurologic manifestations have been described in association with HTLV-I, evidence that the neurologic spectrum of HTLV-I may be broader than previously thought. The association of *polymyositis* with HTLV-I was first described in 1988 in Jamaica. Since then, other reports have appeared in the literature.[42] Although isolated HTLV-I-associated polymyositis has been described, most published cases are associated with HAM/TSP. Therefore, inflammatory myopathy is an important diagnosis to consider if a patient with HAM/TSP develops a new pattern of muscular weakness (proximal weakness), myalgias, and increased creatine kinase (CK) levels. The muscle biopsy may show a mononuclear inflammatory infiltrate, a variation in fiber size, and evidence of regeneration. Immunohistochemistry and in situ polymerase chain reaction (PCR) analysis demonstrated that HTLV-I infects mainly CD4+ lymphocytes and not the muscle cells.[43] Although there has been some controversy regarding the importance of the involvement of peripheral nerves in HTLV-I-infected individuals, *peripheral neuropathies* (PNs) have been described in association with this virus.[44] The clinical picture is characterized by paresthesias, burning sensations, and abnormal superficial sensation distally in a stocking and glove distribution, generally associated with absent ankle jerks. In most cases, the peripheral nerve involvement is associated with HAM/TSP, although isolated PN associated with HTLV-I infection also is observed.[45] The sural nerve biopsy shows a mixed axonal or demyelinating multifocal neuropathy with perineural and perivascular infiltrates. Moderate axonal loss, wallerian degeneration, and demyelinating lesions of isolated fibers also have been described. Teased-fiber analysis demonstrated the globule-like changes (Dyck's G change) accompanied by the formation of adjacent demyelinated segments. Because they have seldom been found in other demyelinating neuropathies, the demyelinating process with globule formation in HAM/TSP could be somewhat specific.[46] *Autonomic disturbances* in HAM/TSP patients are characterized by impairment of cardiovascular and sweat control and clearly indicate dysfunction of the sympathetic nervous system. The dysautonomia may be more frequent than previously suggested,[47] and in some cases it may be severe enough to warrant specific treatment. An *amyotrophic lateral sclerosis–like* picture has been described infrequently as a manifestation of HTLV-I infection.[48] In one autopsied case, the brain and spinal cord were atrophic, with prominent infiltration of inflammatory cells.[49] The prevalence of magnetic resonance imaging (MRI) abnormalities in the brain white matter (*encephalomyelitis*) is significantly higher in HAM/TSP (66 percent) when compared with normal controls (23 percent) and seronegative spastic paraparesis patients (11 percent).[50] These brain MRI abnormalities (Fig. 10-5) may reflect a chronic perivascular inflammation with progressive gliosis (chronic disseminated encephalomyelitis) and could be the cause of the mild cognitive disturbance reported in some HTLV-I-infected individuals. Psychomotor slowing and deficits in verbal and visual memory, attention, and visuomotor abilities can be observed in formal neuropsychological testing.[51] Although *ataxia* has been described more frequently in HTLV-II-infected patients,[52] some cases of cerebellar involvement have been described in HTLV-I-infected patients either associated with the typical picture of HAM/TSP or as a more distinct clinical syndrome.[53] *Meningeal signs* in HTLV-I-infected patients always should raise the suspicion of infiltration of the nervous system by leukemic cells.[54] *Chronic hypertrophic cranial pachymeningitis* associated with HTLV-I has been described in two patients presenting with recurrent multiple cranial neuropathies. Their brain MRIs showed diffuse thickening and gadolinium enhancement of the dura mater.[55]

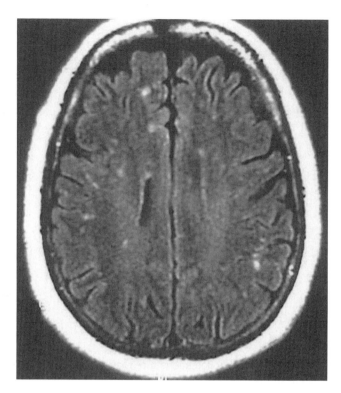

Figure 10-5. Cranial MRI (FLAIR image) of a HAM/TSP patient showing multiple hyperintense foci in the cerebral white matter.

▶ DIAGNOSIS

The diagnosis of HTLV-I infection and its associated diseases usually requires some additional studies besides the clinical picture. Enzyme-linked immunosorbent assays (ELISA) using disrupted whole-virus lysate or particle agglutination assays are the most commonly used screening tests for HTLV-I infection. The WHO guidelines recommend that newly identified seropositive individuals have additional blood collected for repeat testing to eliminate possible technical errors. Confirmatory criteria require Western blot (WB) assay reactivity to *gag* (p19 or p24) and *env* (gp21 or gp46) gene products. Because HTLV-II shares 60 percent genomic homology with HTLV-I, it is sometimes difficult to distinguish between the two unless virus-specific reagents are used. The PCR also can be used on PBMCs from infected individuals to distinguish HTLV-I from HTLV-II and to detect DNA in tissue or other biologic specimens.

The first specific antibodies to appear after HTLV-I infection are directed against the gag protein, and these predominate in the first 2 months after infection. Later, antienvelope antibodies appear, and finally, about 50 percent of infected individuals produce a detectable concentration of antibodies against the tax protein. Patients suspected of having HAM/TSP but with persistently negative ELISAs or indeterminate WBs should undergo a PCR analysis for different genomic regions of HTLV-I. Long-term cocultivation of white blood cells from patients, although a time-consuming and more expensive method, is an alternative way to detect infection. An in vitro characteristic of infected lymphocytes, spontaneous proliferation, also can be used as a laboratory tool for studying some individuals.

A number of systemic laboratory abnormalities can be found in patients with HAM/TSP, such as the presence of "flowers cells" in peripheral blood smears (Fig. 10-6), hypergammaglobulinemia, increased proportion of CD4+ cells, false-positive VDRL and Lyme serology, and the presence of autoantibodies such as the rheumatoid factor. The most common CSF findings are a moderate pleocytosis and modestly elevated protein concentration. In addition, oligoclonal IgG bands, increased levels of some cytokines such as neopterin, tumor necrosis factor α (TNF-α), IL-6, and IL-γ and increased intrathecal antibody synthesis specific for both HTLV-I core and envelope antigens also have been described. Cerebral white matter lesions (see Fig. 10-5) and spinal cord abnormalities have been observed in HAM/TSP patients. Early in the course of the myelopathy, there is evidence of spinal cord edema, reflecting an active inflammatory process (Fig. 10-7).

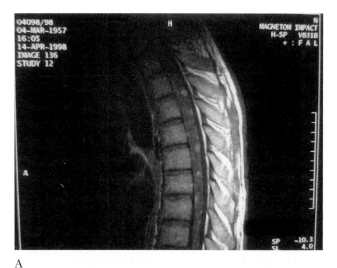

Figure 10-7. *A.* Thoracic spinal MRI (T$_1$-weighted section) of a HAM/TSP patient in the early course of the disease. Notice spinal cord edema along with multiple enhanced foci after contrast material injection. *B.* Spinal cord atrophy seen 5 months afterwards.

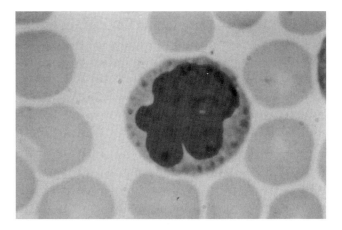

Figure 10-6. The typical "flower cell" seen in the peripheral blood of a HAM/TSP patient is a morphologically abnormal infected lymphocyte.

▶ DIFFERENTIAL DIAGNOSIS

The main neurologic conditions in the differential diagnosis are the spinal form of multiple sclerosis (MS), the vacuolar myelopathy of AIDS, familial spastic paraparesis, primary lateral sclerosis, spinal cord compression, vitamin B$_{12}$ deficiency (subacute combined degeneration of the spinal cord), Lyme disease, syphilis, and HTLV-I-negative TSP.[56]

The *isolated spinal form of MS* is rare and more often associated with optic nerve involvement and brain stem or cerebral lesions, as shown by MRI. Moreover, apart from the progressive form of MS, the typical temporal profile of this demyelinating disease is periods of relapses and remissions, which is not seen in typical HAM/TSP. *Vacuolar myelopathy* is a late manifestation of AIDS. This may represent a real diagnostic challenge in patients with HIV–HTLV-I coinfection. *Familial spastic paraparesis*, also known as *Strümpell-Lorrain syndrome*, is less frequent than HAM/TSP, has a strong familial trait, tends to affect younger patients, and sometimes is associated with mental retardation, optic atrophy, ataxia, dystonia, dysarthria, and peripheral neuropathy. *Primary lateral sclerosis* is a rare motor neuron disease presenting with spastic tetraparesis, pseudo-bulbar signs, and normal bladder function. Spinal MRI easily excludes *spinal cord compression from a mass lesion. B_{12} deficiency, Lyme disease,* and *syphilis* are diagnosed easily by specific blood tests.

There are also so-called *HTLV-I-seronegative TSPs.* Approximately 40 to 65 percent of suspected HAM/TSP patients in some endemic regions are HTLV-I-seronegative. Although both conditions are similar clinically, the etiology of HTLV-I-seronegative TSP is still unknown. Molecular and PCR studies show divergent results, and a putative role of a defective HTLV-I virus as the etiologic agent of this condition has been postulated.[57] The lack of viral sequences detected by PCR analysis may be explained by replication incompetence and the absence of HTLV-I antigens for an immune response. There is the possibility that HTLV-I-seronegative TSP patients carry a defective virus as a consequence of a vigorous immune response early in the infection that eradicated the infected cells, leaving only cells with defective viral sequences. HTLV-I-seronegative TSPs remain a scientific challenge, and another exogenous virus could be responsible for these cases.

► TREATMENT

Unfortunately, no effective treatment for HAM/TSP has been found. Most cases have not been the subject of a proper placebo-controlled, double-blind study. A meta-analysis of therapeutic trials in 200 HAM/TSP patients showed that the best results were obtained with the administration of steroids, plasmapheresis, and interferon-alpha (IFN-α). Less impressive results were achieved with azathioprine, pentoxifylline, and high-dose vitamin C.[58] Although these results were a compilation of different treatments in open trials, they suggest that immunomodulatory therapies may have some beneficial effects in HAM/TSP, particularly early in the disease. This can be explained by the pathophysiology of the disease. It is reasonable to suggest that anti-inflammatory or immunomodulatory drugs should be tried in selected patients. These drugs may be especially useful in cases of 1 or 2 years' duration or in individuals with

clear signs of active inflammation in their CSF or on MRI. A reasonable proposal for treating HAM/TSP patients fulfilling these requirements would be oral prednisone, 1 mg/kg for 2 months, followed by a slow tapering until a minimum effective dose is reached. This can be preceded by intravenous methylprednisolone (1 g/day for 5 consecutive days). In cases of steroid failure or contraindication, intramuscular interferon-alpha (3 million units/day), oral azathioprine (2.5 mg/kg per day), oral methotrexate (7.5 to 15 mg weekly), or high-dose intravenous gammaglobulin (400 mg/kg per day for 5 consecutive days) could be tried.

Patients with HAM/TSP typically have a high HTLV-I proviral load in the peripheral blood along with mononuclear cells and abundant activated HTLV-I-specific CTLs. Nucleoside reverse transcriptase inhibitors, including lamivudine (3TC) and zidovudine (ZDV), have been evaluated for the treatment of HAM/TSP. 3TC and ZDV, which are able to control HTLV-I replication in vitro, have been studied in a few small, uncontrolled series.[59,60] Although 3TC and ZDV could reduce the proviral load, their real efficacy in HAM/TSP patients awaits confirmation.

As adjunctive treatments, oral vitamin C (1 to 2 g/day) and pentoxifylline (400 to 1200 mg/day) could be offered to these patients in accordance with some series that reported good results.[61,62] Spasticity can be treated with oral baclofen (10 to 80 mg/day), oral tizanidine (4 to 16 mg/day), oral diazepam (5 to 40 mg/day), or botulinum toxin injection in selected muscles. Oral oxybutynin (5 to 15 mg/day) may be useful for neurogenic bladder. Since many HAM/TSP patients may have a Sjögren-like syndrome, skin emollients, artificial tears, and artificial saliva can be used to treat the sicca symptoms.

► COMPLICATIONS

In general, life expectancy is not diminished in HAM/TSP. Major complications are related to bladder disturbances (urinary tract infection, hydronephrosis), chronic constipation, decubitus ulcers, and venous thrombosis in wheelchair-bound patients. As in most chronic diseases, major depression is a concern and should be treated. Although rare in clinical practice, the combination of ATL and HAM/TSP is described in a few patients.[41] Disseminated strongyloidiasis has been described, mainly in ATL, although it may be seen in HAM/TSP patients and in asymptomatic carriers.[63] It is postulated that HTLV-I infection in certain individuals may selectively impair immune responses that are critical in controlling strongyloidiasis. Nowadays, it is unclear if concomitant HIV-1 infection alters the natural history of HAM/TSP or if HTLV-I influences the development of HIV-1-associated neurologic diseases. Because HTLV-I induces lymphocyte proliferation, CD4 counts may not be a good surrogate marker for AIDS in these patients.

▶ PREVENTION

Compulsory screening of donors in many countries has eliminated transmission of HTLV-I through blood transfusion. Although difficult, the same should apply to organ donors. Vertical transmission can be halted through avoidance of breast feeding by infected mothers. Since breast feeding is very important for public health, especially in underdeveloped countries, breast feeding for a period of less than 6 months would be acceptable in these settings. Sexual transmission may be prevented by the use of condoms. Infection in IDUs remains unabated in many areas of the world. The policy of avoidance of needle sharing should be strengthened.

REFERENCES

1. Yamashita M, Miura T, Ibuki K, et al: Phylogenetic relationships of HTLV-I/STLV-I in the world. *Leukemia* 11(S3):50, 1997.
2. Yamashita M, Ido E, Miura T, et al: Molecular epidemiology of HTLV-I in the world. *J Acquir Immune Defic Syndr Hum Retrovirol* 13(suppl 1):S124, 1996.
3. Araujo AQ, Sheehy N, Takahashi H, et al: Concomitant infections with human immunodeficiency virus type 1 and human T-lymphotropic virus types 1 and 2. In Brodgen A, Guthmiller JM (eds): *Polymicrobial Diseases.* Washington: ASM Press, 2002.
4. Dooneief G, Marlink R, Bell K, et al: Neurologic consequences of HTLV-II infection in injection-drug users. *Neurology* 46(6):1556, 1996.
5. Manns A, Hisada M, La Grenade L: Human T-lymphotropic virus type I infection. *Lancet* 353:1951, 1999.
6. Murphy EL, Figueroa JP, Gibbs WN, et al: Human T-lymphotropic virus type I (HTLV-I) seroprevalence in Jamaica: I. Demographic determinants. *Am J Epidemiol* 133(11):1114, 1991.
7. Mueller N, Okayama A, Stuver S: Findings from the Miyazaki cohort study. *J Acquir Immune Defic Syndr* 13:S2, 1996.
8. Galvao-Castro B, Loures LA, Rodrigues LG: Distribution of HTLV-I among blood donors: A nationwide Brazilian study. *Transfusion* 37:242, 1997.
9. Robert-Guroff M, Weiss JH, Giron JA: Prevalence of antibodies to HTLV-I, -II, and -III in intravenous drug abusers an AIDS endemic region. *JAMA* 255:3133, 1986.
10. Khabbaz RF, Darrow WW, Hartley TM, et al: Seroprevalence and risk factors for HTLV-I/II infection among female prostitutes in the United States. *JAMA* 263(1):60, 1990.
11. Manns A, Wilks RJ, Murphy EL, et al: A prospective study of transmission by transfusion of HTLV-I and risk factors associated with seroconversion. *Int J Cancer* 51(6):886, 1992.
12. Williams AE, Fang CT, Slamon D: Seroprevalence and epidemiological correlates of HTLV-I infection in U.S. blood donors. *Science* 240:643,1988.
13. Dood RY: Current viral risks of blood and blood products. *Ann Med* 2:469, 2000.
14. Yoshinaga M, Yashiki S, Oki T, et al: A maternal risk factor for mother-to-child HTLV-I transmission: Viral antigen-producing capacities in culture of peripheral blood and breast milk cells. *Jpn J Cancer Res* 86(7):649, 1995.
15. Ureta-Vidal A, Angelin-Duclos C, Tortevoye P, et al: Mother-to-child transmission of human T-cell-leukemia/lymphoma virus type I: Implication of high antiviral antibody titer and high proviral load in carrier mothers. *Int J Cancer* 82(6):832, 1999.
16. Hino S, Katamine S, Miyamoto T, et al: Association between maternal antibodies to the external envelope glycoprotein and vertical transmission of human T-lymphotropic virus type I: Maternal anti-env antibodies correlate with protection in non-breast-fed children. *J Clin Invest* 95(6):2920, 1995.
17. Oki T, Yoshinaga M, Otsuka H, et al: A sero-epidemiological study on mother-to-child transmission of HTLV-I in southern Kyushu, Japan. *Asia Oceania J Obstet Gynaecol* 18(4):371, 1992.
18. Hino S, Katamine S, Miyata H, et al: Primary prevention of HTLV-I in Japan. *J Acquir Immune Defic Syndr Hum Retrovirol* 13(suppl 1):S199, 1996.
19. Stuver S, Tachibana K, Okayama A: Heterosexual transmission of HTLV-I among married couples in southwestern Japan: An initial report from the Miyasaki cohort study. *J Infect Dis* 167:57, 1993.
20. Toro C, Rodés B, Poveda E, et al: Rapid development of subacute myelopathy in three organ transplant recipients after transmission of HTLV-I from a single donor. *Transplantation* 75(1):102, 2003.
21. Remesar MC, del Pozo AE, Pittis MG: Transmission of HTLV-I by kidney transplant. *Transfusion* 40:1421, 2000.
22. Sommerfelt MA, Williams BP, Clapham PR, et al: Human T-cell leukemia viruses use a receptor determined by human chromosome 17. *Science* 242(4885):1557, 1988.
23. Bangham CR: The immune response to HTLV-I. *Curr Opin Immunol* 12(4):397, 2000.
24. Ijichi S, Ramundo MB, Takahashi H, et al: In vivo cellular tropism of human T-cell leukemia virus type II (HTLV-II). *J Exp Med* 176(1):293, 1992.
25. Hollsberg P, Hafler DA: Pathogenesis of diseases induced by HTLV-I infection. *New Engl J Med* 328(16): 1173, 1992.
26. Levin MC, Lee SM, Kalume F, et al: Autoimmunity due molecular mimicry as a cause of neurological disease. *Nature Med* 8(5):509, 2002.
27. Bangham CR, Kermode AG, Hall SE: The cytotoxic T-lymphocyte response to HTLV-I: The main determinant of disease? *Semin Virol* 7:41, 1996.

28. Bangham CR: HTLV-I infections. *J Clin Pathol* 53:581, 2000.

29. Nagai M, Usuku K, Matsumoto W, et al: Analysis of HTLV-I proviral load in 202 HAM/TSP patients and 243 asymptomatic HTLV-I carriers: High proviral load strongly predisposes to HAM/TSP. *J Neurovirol* 4(6):586, 1998.

30. Jacobson S, Shida H, McFarlin DE, et al: Circulating CD8+ cytotoxic T-lymphocytes specific for HTLV-I *pX* in patients with HTLV-I-associated neurological disease. *Nature* 348(6298):245, 1990.

31. Umehara F, Izumo S, Nakagawa M, et al: Immunocyto-chemical analysis of the cellular infiltrate in the spinal cord lesions in HTLV-I-associated myelopathy. *J Neuropathol Exp Neurol* 52(4):424, 1993.

32. Levin MC, Jacobson S: Cellular and humoral immune responses associated with HTLV-I-associated myelopathy/tropical spastic paraparesis. *Ann NY Acad Sci* 835:142, 1997.

33. Jeffery KJ, Usuku K, Hall SE, et al: HLA alleles determine human T-lymphotropic virus-I (HTLV-I) proviral load and the risk of HTLV-I-associated myelopathy. *Proc Natl Acad Sci USA* 96(7):3848, 1999.

34. Usuku K, Nishizawa M, Matsuki K, et al: Association of a particular amino acid sequence of the HLA-DR beta 1 chain with HTLV-I-associated myelopathy. *Eur J Immunol* 20(7):1603, 1990.

35. Usuku K, Sonoda S, Osame M, et al: HLA haplotype-linked high immune responsiveness against HTLV-I in HTLV-I-associated myelopathy: Comparison with adult T-cell leukemia/lymphoma. *Ann Neurol* 23(suppl):S143, 1988.

36. Vine A, Witkover A, Lloyd A, et al: Polygenic control of human T-lymphotropic virus type I (HTLV-I) provirus load and the risk of HTLV-I-associated myelopathy/tropical spastic paraparesis. *J Infect Dis* 186:932, 2002.

37. Araujo AQ, Leite AC, Dultra SV, et al: Progression of neurological disability in HTLV-I-associated myelopathy/tropical spastic paraparesis (HAM/TSP). *J Neurol Sci* 129(2):147, 1995.

38. Kaplan JE, Osame M, Kubota H, et al: The risk of development of HTLV-I-associated myelopathy/tropical spastic paraparesis among persons infected with HTLV-I. *J Acquir Immune Defic Syndr* 3(11):1096, 1990.

39. Murphy EL, Fridey J, Smith JW, et al: HTLV-associated myelopathy in a cohort of HTLV-I- and HTLV-II-infected blood donors. The REDS investigators. *Neurology* 48(2):315, 1997.

40. Araujo AQ, Andrade-Filho AS, Castro-Costa CM, et al: HTLV-I-associated myelopathy/tropical spastic paraparesis in Brazil: A nationwide survey. HAM/TSP Brazilian Study Group. *J Acquir Immune Defic Syndr Hum Retrovirol* 19(5):536, 1998.

41. Tamiya S, Matsuoka M, Takemoto S, et al: Adult T-cell leukemia following HTLV-I-associated myelopathy/tropical spastic paraparesis: Case reports and implication to the natural course of ATL. *Leukemia* 9(10):1768, 1995.

42. Gabbai AA, Wiley CA, Oliveira ASB: Skeletal muscle involvement in tropical spastic paraparesis/HTLV-I-associated myelopathy. *Muscle Nerve* 17:923, 1994.

43. Higuchi I, Hashimoto K, Kashio N, et al: Detection of HTLV-I provirus by in situ polymerase chain reaction in mononuclear inflammatory cells in skeletal muscle of viral carriers with polymyositis. *Muscle Nerve* 18(8):854, 1995.

44. Kiwaki T, Umehara F, Arimura Y, et al: The clinical and pathological features of peripheral neuropathy accompanied with HTLV-I-associated myelopathy. *J Neurol Sci* 206:17, 2003.

45. Leite ACC, Silva MTT, Almay AH, et al: Peripheral neuropathy in HTLV-I infected individuals without tropical spastic paraparesis/HTLV-I-associated myelopathy. *J Neurol,* in press.

46. Bhigjee AI, Bill PL, Wiley CA, et al: Peripheral nerve lesions in HTLV-I associated myelopathy (HAM/TSP). *Muscle Nerve* 16(1):2126, 1993.

47. Alamy AH, Menezes FB, Leite AC, et al: Dysautonomia in human T-cell lymphotrophic virus type I–associated myelopathy/tropical spastic paraparesis. *Ann Neurol* 50(5):681, 2001.

48. Hanakawa T, Nakamura M, Suenaga T, et al: Response to corticosteroid therapy in a patient with HTLV-I-associated motor neuron disease. *Neurology* 50(4):1188, 1998.

49. Kuroda Y, Sugihara H: Autopsy report of HTLV-I-associated myelopathy presenting with ALS-like manifestations. *J Neurol Sci* 106(2):199, 1991.

50. Kira J, Fujihara K, Itoyama Y, et al: Leukoencephalopathy in HTLV-I-associated myelopathy/tropical spastic paraparesis: MRI analysis and a two-year follow-up study after corticosteroid therapy. *J Neurol Sci* 106(1):41, 1991.

51. Silva MTT, Mattos P, Alfano A, Araújo AQ-C: Neuropsychological assessment in HTLV-I infection: A comparative study among TSP/HAM, asymptomatic carriers and healthy controls. *J Neurol Neurosurg Psychiatry* 74:1085, 2003.

52. Peters AA, Oger JJ, Coulthart MB, et al: An apparent case of human T-cell lymphotropic virus type II (HTLV-II)– associated neurological disease: A clinical, molecular, and phylogenetic characterisation. *J Clin Virol* 14(1):37, 1999.

53. Sato Y, Honda Y, Ohshima Y, et al: Acute myelopathy and cerebellar signs associated with uveitis with positive serum and cerebrospinal fluid antibodies to HTLV-I. *Kurume Med J* 41(4):193, 1994.

54. Imaizume R, Fujiwara H, Matsumoto T: Syndrome of inappropriate antidiuretic hormone secretion associated with meningeal infiltration of tumor cells and elevated IL-1 beta and IL-6 in CSF of a patient with adult T-cell leukemia. *Rinsho Ketsueki* 4:140, 2000.

55. Kawano Y, Kira J: Chronic hypertrophic cranial pachymeningitis associated with HTLV-I infection. *J Neurol Neurosurg Psychiatry* 59(4):435, 1995.

56. Castro-Costa CM, Carton H, Santos TJT: HTLV-I-negative tropical spastic paraparesis: A scientific challenge. *Arq Neuropsiquiatr* 59(2A):289, 2001.

57. Ramirez E, Fernandes J, Cartier L, et al: Defective HTLV-I provirus in seronegative tropical spastic paraparesis/HTLV-I–associated myelopathy (TSP/HAM) patients. *Virus Res* 91:231, 2003.

58. Nakagawa M, Nakahara K, Maruyama Y, et al: Therapeutic trials in 200 patients with HTLV-I-associated myelopathy/ tropical spastic paraparesis. *J Neurovirol* 2(5):345, 1996.

59. Taylor GP: Pathogenesis and treatment of HTLV-I-associated myelopathy. *Sex Transm Infect* (5):316, 1998.

60. Machuca A, Rodes B, Soriano V: The effect of antiretroviral therapy on HTLV infection. *Virus Res* 78(1–2):93, 2001.

61. Kataoka A, Imai H, Inayoshi S, et al: Intermittent high-dose vitamin C therapy in patients with HTLV-I-associated myelopathy. *J Neurol Neurosurg Psychiatry* 56(11):1213, 1993.

62. Nakamura T, Shirabe S, Ichinose K, et al: Pentoxifylline treatment in HTLV-I-associated myelopathy. *Intern Med* 34(5):460, 1995.

63. Newton RC, Limpuangthip P, Greenberg S, et al: *Strongyloides stercoralis* hyperinfection in a carrier of HTLV-I virus with evidence of selective immunosuppression. *Am J Med* 92(2):202, 1992.

CHAPTER 11
Rabies

Thiravat Hemachudha and Charles E. Rupprecht

Rabies is an acute progressive encephalitis with the highest case to fatality ratio of any infectious disease. The causative agents are neurotropic RNA viruses in the family Rhabdoviridae, genus *Lyssavirus*, of seven putative genotypes. Rabies has been recognized since antiquity and is the most significant viral zoonosis today. At present, rabies kills more people than yellow fever, dengue fever, and Japanese encephalitis.[1] Despite millions of human exposures and thousands of human deaths, primarily in developing countries in Asia, Africa, and Latin America, the World Health Organization (WHO) ranks rabies low on its list of important infectious diseases. In contrast, rabies virus infections in humans in the United States and other developed countries are uncommon, accounting for no more than a few cases each year. Mammalian reservoirs include species in the Carnivora and Chiroptera, but rabid dogs still pose the greatest hazard worldwide.

Clinical symptomatology, once believed to be unique, may be more variable, particularly in bat-related cases. This causes diagnostic confusion. Differences in cellular tropism either at the inoculation site or in the nervous system, as well as differences in routes of spread, viral variants, and participation of host factors, may account for this diversity. Unreliable epidemiologic data and the complexity of clinical manifestations are compounded by limitations in diagnostic laboratories. With rapid movement of people and animals, cases can appear in regions where rabies has been eliminated or never recorded. Strict adherence to WHO guidelines for rabies prophylaxis has proven effective, and deviations should not be allowed. Physicians should diagnose and differentiate rabies from other neurologic conditions and understand how to provide proper postexposure prophylaxis (PEP).

► HISTORY

Rabies is one of the oldest recognized infectious diseases. Few other maladies possess the mythical linkage with animals, exposures, and ensuing dramatic illness. Although the annual disease burden is less than direct human contagions such as smallpox, influenza, and acquired immunodeficienct syndrome (AIDS), the striking clinical manifestations and inevitably fatal progression of rabies have secured its place to the present as the most important viral zoonosis.[2] Ancient civilizations were aware of the disease.[3–5] Passages described in the pre-Mosaic Eshnunna Code of Mesopotamia from the twenty-third century B.C. harken to the dangers of bites from the "mad dog," as well as the ensuing legal penalties to the dog's owner. Familiarity with rabies is apparent from Greek, Roman, Hebrew, and Chinese literary, religious, and medical writings. Careful observers surmised that a poison or a "virus" was present in saliva. Inquisitive scholars rightly noted clinical aspects of infection, including that the patient seemed tortured by thirst and the concomitant repulsion toward water. Early suggestions for treatment included excision of tissue and cauterization of the wound, as well as dunking victims into water, and all manner of ingested potions and apothecary concoctions. Throughout the ages, various talismans were believed to be curatives, as was the need for divine intervention. Although superstitions and supposed cures would persist to the present day in several cultures (including the suggestion for salves of hot chili peppers or animal venoms applied directly to the wounds), many examples from the classical periods to the Renaissance contained otherwise remarkable moments of clarity and pragmatism. For example, the Italian physician Fracastoro, in a treatise of 1546 entitled,

The Incurable Wound, vividly described a human case: " . . . its incubation is so stealthy, slow and gradual that the infection is very rarely manifest before the 20th day, in most cases after the 30th, and in many cases not until four or six months have elapsed . . . cases recorded in which it became manifest a year after the bite . . . the patient can neither stand nor lie down; like a madman he flings himself hither and thither, tears his flesh with his hands, and feels intolerable thirst . . . the most distressing symptom, for he so shrinks from water and all liquids that he would rather die than drink or be brought near to water; it is then that they bite at other persons, foam at the mouth, their eyes look twister, and finally they are exhausted and painfully breathe their last."[6]

Despite its widespread occurrence and recognition in the Old World for apparently thousands of years, the history of rabies in the New World is complicated by a paucity of written records prior to European colonization. Likely, it was present well before Columbus' arrival in the fifteenth century. For example, as cited by Koprowski in an allusion to vampire bats, the bishop Petrus Martyr-Anglerius wrote: " . . . in places bats not much smaller than turtle doves used to fly at them in the early evening with brutal fury and with their venomous bites brought those injured to madness, . . . bats . . . come in from the marshes on the river and attack our men with deadly bite." Several hundred years would elapse before the major role of bats in rabies was better appreciated.[7] Elsewhere in North America, a rabid wolf was reported by the Reverend Lucio Marmolejo in Mexico during 1709, and some 200 years after initial Spanish invasion, canine rabies was described in 1753 from the Virginia Colony and later among foxes.[3,8] Human migration had left its mark, and the risk posed by translocation of animals as viral portals continues to this day.

For centuries, the bite of a rabid animal was thought to be the likely source of rabies infection, but it was Zinke (1804) who demonstrated experimental disease transmission using dog saliva.[9] In 1879, Galtier experimented with rabies in rabbits as a model and transmission from rabbit to rabbit.[5] Clinical descriptions, paired with animal inoculation, formed the basis for rabies diagnosis until the advent of light microscopy and observation of microscopic lesions. Negri (1903) described the cytoplasmic inclusions that bear his name (Negri bodies) in neurons of rabid animals.[10] While the value of Negri bodies was appreciated and debated throughout the twentieth century, their nature and composition awaited development of electron microscopy in the 1960s (when virions actually were visualized). Laboratory-based diagnostics did not improve significantly until development of the immunofluroscent technique.[11]

Pasteur's collected work on rabies is probably the best known historical achievement in the field.[12] Building on the knowledge that preceded them, Pasteur and his colleagues in their cramped Parisian quarters adapted the virus to animals and succeeded in altering its properties. This remarkable French team applied basic scientific concepts and approaches toward the first protective protocol against rabies. Desiccated spinal cords from infected rabbits formed the raw material for the vaccine. Progressive inoculations of material, from oldest to freshest, amounted to increased doses of infectious viral inocula. Despite severe reservations over preparedness for human experimentation, on July 6, 1885, a young boy, Joseph Meister, who was bitten at multiple sites by a rabid dog 3 days earlier, received the first of multiple inoculations of vaccine and, to everyone's relief, became the first registered survivor.

After considerable medical debate, Pasteur's method became the accepted approach throughout the world in the early twentieth century as other vaccine evolutions began.[13] Gradual improvements to the technique included the addition of chemical fixation and adaptation to duck embryos and suckling mice to improve vaccine safety.[14–17] Continual modifications were needed because improperly inactivated virus could cause rabies, and brain tissue induced neuroparalytic accidents.[18] Also, vaccine alone was not totally effective in cases of severe bites, such as those inflicted on the face and head by rabid wolves. Postexposure prophylaxis (PEP) against rabies through the simultaneous administration of antirabies serum and vaccine was suggested as early as the late 1800s.[19] The combined approach found few adherents until the 1940s, when international interest was revived. After a WHO-sponsored trial in 1954, analysis of the combined use of serum and vaccine was found to be more effective than vaccine alone.[20,21] Today, the combination approach is the recommended standard for human rabies prophylaxis.

Additional adaptation of the virus to primary and, later, continuous cell lines removed the need for animal vaccine production.[22,23] In the 1960s and 1970s, a rabies virus grown in human diploid cells was used as a source of purification and concentration for production of a safe and efficacious vaccine[24] and eliminated many of the problems connected with neuronal tissue and poor potency from other cultures. The human diploid cell vaccine (HDCV) is used widely throughout the world, although for economic reasons several developing countries still use nervous tissue vaccines. After demonstration of the primary utility of HDCV, other cell-culture vaccines were developed, including those produced in Vero cells and avian embryos.[25] Newer generations of vaccines throughout the twenty-first century have an impressive legacy to exceed and will carry the considerable burden of maximum purity, potency, efficacy, and safety while still being affordable in those regions afflicted with enzootic dog rabies.

▶ EPIDEMIOLOGY

A better understanding of the epidemiology of this complex zoonosis requires an appreciation of the agent, its hosts, and the environmental facets that will shape its distribution over time.[26] At one point only a single agent was believed to cause rabies. However, in the 1960s and 1970s, various serotypes were suggested between rabies virus and what were then termed *rabies-related viruses* before use of the designation *Lyssavirus*.[27] During the 1970s and 1980s, placement within the taxonomic group was defined by serologic cross-reactivity of viral antigens (e.g., by complement fixation, immunofluorescence, neutralization tests, etc.) based on antigenic sites on the nucleoprotein (N) and glycoprotein (G) using monoclonal antibodies (MAbs).[28,29] More recently, sequence data became available, with a trend toward phylogenetic classification.[30–35] Application of MAb typing and gene sequencing to the study of lyssaviruses provided substantive evidence for considerable antigenic and genetic variation. Major virus species currently or putatively assigned to the *Lyssavirus* genus,[36] all isolated from mammals, include rabies virus, Lagos bat virus (LBV), Mokola virus (MOK), Duvenhage virus (DUV), European bat virus type 1 (EBV-1), European bat virus type 2 (EBV-2), and Australian bat virus (ABV). Several viruses, such as Obodhiang and Kotonkan, found only in Africa and originally isolated from mosquitoes or midges,[37] and Rochambeau virus,[38] isolated from mosquitoes in French Guiana, have been suggested by some for consideration in the genus, primarily based on serologic data alone, but are unlikely candidates. Other more likely *Lyssavirus* prospects, such as those isolated from bats, with shared antigenic and genetic properties, and known to produce encephalitis, await ultimate taxonomic assignment.[39]

Modern molecular methods have been particularly useful in determining the extent of natural variation among lyssaviruses isolated from wildlife reservoirs within restricted geographic areas or from separate continents over time.[40] In particular, distinctions between viruses isolated from bats and terrestrial carnivores became obvious.[41] Notwithstanding genetic variation and the general tendency or relatively rapid evolution of RNA viruses, striking global patterns have emerged that are highly suggestive of a rather conservative strategy presented by any particular variant.[35] Intragenotypic viral clusters are distinguishable, suggestive of historical, geographic, or host-species relationships. Combined with historical temporal and spatial disease surveillance data, antigenic characterization with MAbs and nucleotide sequence analysis can help to assign isolates to different animal rabies reservoirs. In addition, antigenic and molecular characterization is useful in investigating unusual or unexpected mortality from rabies, especially in domestic animals or humans with no obvious exposure history. The antigenic patterns or nucleotide sequences obtained can be compared with variants from known animal reservoirs. For example, analysis of recent human rabies cases from the United States implicate specific viral variants associated with insectivorous bats in the etiology of infection.[42]

Rabies is enzootic on all continents except Antarctica. Rabies virus is the prototype species of the *Lyssavirus* genus and can infect warm-blooded animals (including birds) under experimental conditions, but only mammals are significant natural hosts. Host range is broad, stretching from an exotic alphabet of species from armadillos to zebras, but most of these are epidemiologic dead ends, even if an episode is as dramatic as an infected pachyderm.[43] Major species responsible for transmission include dogs, foxes, jackals, coyotes, wolves, cats, raccoons, skunks, mongoose and their relatives, and bats.[44] Several countries, such as Japan and many islands, are reportedly "rabies free" either because of their isolation or due to considerable animal control efforts, but bats can reach even distant islands.[45]

The lyssaviruses DUV, LBV, and MOK are restricted to Africa. Although bats and small mammals such as shrews have been suggested as potential reservoirs,[46] relatively little is known about these African agents compared with rabies virus. Compared with other lyssaviruses, MOK appears to be the most disparate member recognized to date, with divergent amino acid changes in the antigenic sites mapped to the G protein, partially explaining the absence of cross-protection with vaccine.[47,48] In Europe, phylogenetic analysis of EBV suggests at least two genetically distinguishable lineages, possibly related to spatiotemporal introduction from different geographic locations, such as North Africa.[49] Bats, such as *Eptesicus serotinus, Myotis dasycneme,* and *M. daubentonii,* appear to be principal reservoirs for EBV. Australia was believed to be free of the disease until 1996,[50] when indigenous lyssaviruses were discovered among bats. These viruses appear to use either frugivorous Megachiroptera or insectivorous Microchiroptera as primary reservoirs and have caused at least two human deaths. The ultimate importance of the nonrabies lyssaviruses remains a matter of speculation. All mammals are likely susceptible to some degree, but experimental results suggest a rough hierarchy for species susceptibility. However, most experimental animal studies occurred before antigenic or genetic differences between lyssaviruses were appreciated. Wild canids are very susceptible to infection. Cats, important as vectors but not as reservoirs, and some wildlife species, such as raccoons, appear moderately susceptible to infection. The opossum (*Didelphis virginiana*) appears especially resistant.[51] Despite their varying ability to infect different cell cultures, no lyssaviruses have been isolated from cold-blooded vertebrates. Laboratory rodents, such as mice, have been used extensively for rabies diagnosis, vaccine testing, and pathogenesis studies, but laboratory rodents are epidemiologically insignificant as *Lyssavirus* vectors or reservoirs[52] compared with species among the Carnivora and Chiroptera.

An accurate calculation of the true incidence of human rabies from a global perspective is difficult due to the lack of reporting and accurate diagnosis in most developing countries but has been estimated at between 0.1 to 29 cases per 1 million inhabitants.[53] In developing countries, although most age ranges may be represented, most are young (<20 years), and more than 50 percent are male.[54] Clearly, human rabies may be prevented by avoiding exposure to rabid animals or by the application of prophylaxis after exposure occurs. Practical animal control efforts should be based on local rabies epidemiology. Most developed countries have eliminated canine rabies, and human fatalities are at or near zero, either imported or related to wildlife cases. Nevertheless, when exposures do occur, especially en masse, most tend to be associated with an infected domestic animal, even in the United States.[55]

In effect, *Lyssavirus* epidemiology is influenced in part by host species distribution, abundance, demographics, behavioral ecology, dispersal, and interactions with humans. Due to its severe consequences when ignored, rabies is a reportable disease in several, but not all, countries. Epidemiologic information on rabies usually originates from results of the examination of brain material submitted to public health or veterinary diagnostic laboratories when contact with wildlife or a domestic animal is suspected. The spatiotemporal distribution and relative intensity of rabies infection in various mammalian species thus often are described based on the passive monitoring of suspicious contact cases and frequently on a clinical basis only.

Rabies virus does not persist in the environment but rather is perpetuated in a variety of reservoirs. The dog is the principal host and major vector of rabies throughout the world.[56] International reporting of both human and animal rabies cases, suggested in the tens of thousands and tens of millions, respectively, grossly underestimates the magnitude of the problem. Predominant wild reservoirs include foxes in Arctic areas (*Alopex lagopus*), central and western Europe (*Vulpes vulpes*), and scattered foci elsewhere throughout the United States (e.g., *Urocyon cinereoargenteus*); the raccoon dog (*Nyctereutes procyanoides*) in Eurasia; jackals (*Canis* species) and other wild canids in Asia and Africa; skunks (*Mephitis mephitis, Spilogale putorius*) in North America; procyonids, such as the raccoon (*Procyon lotor*), in the eastern United States; and viverrids (e.g., the yellow mongoose, *Cynictis penicillata*) in Asia and Africa. The Indian mongoose (*Herpestes auropunctatus*) was introduced into several Caribbean islands during the nineteenth century and persists as a major agricultural and public health threat. Rabies detection in rodents and lagomorphs is uniformly rare. Bat rabies (due to true rabies virus, as opposed to ABV, DUV, EBV, LBV, etc.) predominates as a New World phenomenon, described primarily among the insectivorous species of the United States and Canada (some 40 species) and the three hematophagus vampire species (principally *Desmodus rotundus*) ranging from northern Mexico to Argentina. Renewed investigations suggest that other bat species also may be important throughout Latin America.

In contrast to parts of Europe and North America, where wildlife rabies predominates, in Asia, Africa, and much of Latin America, dogs continue to be the principal causative vectors to humans. Vaccination of a critical percentage of dogs, on the order of 40 to 70 percent, should be adequate to interrupt canine rabies transmission.[57] Realizing the importance of dogs as the primary reservoirs, the Pan American Health Organization began a program in 1983 to eliminate urban rabies from the principal cities of Latin America by the year 2000, and results to date have been very encouraging.[58] From the 1980s to the 1990s, the annual number of human rabies cases decreased from some 350 to less than 114; rabies-specific mortality declined from 1.3 to less than 0.2 deaths per 1 million exposures, and the proportion of 414 cities free of rabies increased from 75 percent to more than 80 percent. These results suggest that widespread vaccination of canine populations can reach sufficient levels for the herd immunity needed to prevent rabies epizootics and that elimination of canine rabies, at least in major urban areas, may be an achievable goal. Rabies transmission by hematophagous bats, unique to the Americas, is an emerging public health problem, in addition to being a historically important disease of livestock with widespread economic implications.

Properly applied, regional epidemiologic surveillance on animal rabies can reduce human morbidity (from inappropriate treatment) and mortality ascribed to lyssaviruses significantly by identifying typical versus unlikely reservoirs, developing treatment algorithms, assessing occupational groups at risk, and targeting veterinary efforts in animal control. Efforts in the United States illustrate the benefits of a systematic surveillance approach that defines rabies as single- or multiple-species assemblages.[59] For example, during 2001, 7437 cases (an increase of ~1 percent over 2000) were recorded. In contrast to widespread canine rabies of the 1940s, more than 90 percent of current cases are from wildlife. Most of the cases (37 percent) resulted from the continued spread of raccoon rabies due to progression of an outbreak initiated in the late 1970s when animals from an infected location in the southeastern United States were transported to the Virginias. Rabies cases increase after primary introduction, whereas the infection spreads successively within local populations.[60] Other major wildlife contributors included bats

(17 percent), skunks (31 percent), and foxes (6 percent). Cases of coyote rabies from an outbreak in southern Texas continued substantial decline. Domestic species included cats (4 percent), cattle (1 percent), and dogs (1 percent). Historically, Hawaii remained the only rabies-free U.S. state, never having reported a case of indigenously acquired rabies, due in part to its remote location.

Rabies is not considered a practical candidate for actual global disease eradication at this time because of the numerous wild reservoirs. However, the historical correlation between the reduction of canine rabies and decreased human fatalities has led to the successful application of herd health programs using vaccine-laden baits for wildlife, which ultimately may help to reduce the associated disease burden, if it can be accomplished over large areas with diverse hosts of high population density in a cost-effective manner.[61]

▶ CAUSATIVE AGENTS

Together with its taxonomic allies, rabies virus with its distinct bullet shape is in the family Rhabdoviridae and in the genus *Lyssavirus*. Both terms are of Greek derivation, meaning "rod" and "rage or frenzy," respectively.[62,63] At present, the genus *Lyssavirus* contains seven putative genotypes. Rabies virus is representative of genotype 1, whereas the other six genotypes are composed of: LBV (genotype 2), MOK (genotype 3), DUV (genotype 4), EBV-1 and EBV-2 (genotypes 5 and 6), and ABV (genotype 7). All of these, except genotype 2, have been associated with human disease (however, one has to realize that few diagnostic facilities exist in Africa with the laboratory ability to detect and differentiate non-rabies virus infections). Clinical manifestations in most *Lyssavirus* infections share several features of a classic rabies encephalitis.[64] Rabies virus and the other members of the family Rhabdoviridae, as well as several other RNA virus groups (the families Paramyxoviridae, Filoviridae, and Bornaviridae) that contain nonsegmented, negative-sense, single-strand RNA genomes, constitute the order Mononegavirales.

Rabies virus particles measure approximately 180 × 75 nm. Its genome consists of 11,932 or 11,928 nucleotides [based on an analysis of Pasteur virus (PV) and Street Alabama Dufferin (SAD)–B19 strains, respectively] and contains a leader sequence at the 3′ end, followed by five monocistronic genes that encode the nucleoprotein (N), phosphoprotein (P), matrix protein (M), glycoprotein (G), and RNA transcriptase (L).[62,63] At the core of this bullet-shaped virus is the ribonucleoprotein (RNP), which consists of helical RNA and the N, P, and L proteins. The M and G proteins are associated with a lipid bilayer envelope. The G protein forms approximately 400 trimeric spikes covering all but the flat end of the virion. The events during infection require transcription of these genomes to produce complementary messenger RNA (mRNA) molecules for synthesizing their corresponding proteins and a full-length positive-strand intermediate RNA. This antigenome RNA serves as the template for replication. Transcription and replication are ensured by the RNP complexes of the N, P, and L proteins. The classic neuronal inclusion, or Negri body, is an accumulation of intracellular matrix formed by an excess amount of RNA-protein complex.

▶ PATHOGENESIS

Rabies is the quintessential neurotropic virus infection. It is considered the most dramatic infection of the nervous system owing to its high fatality rate, unpredictable incubation period, and horrific clinical picture. Rabies virus may infect all mammalian species. However, species have different levels of susceptibility and variable transmission potentials.[65] Foxes and other wild canids are extremely susceptible to infection.[63] The pathogenesis of rabies virus infections can be considered according to "bite" or "nonbite" acquisition. However, it is the bite route that usually accounts for human disease. Sequential steps or cascades following peripheral inoculation of rabies virus include an eclipse phase, access to the peripheral nerve (with or without replication in peripheral tissues) with centripetal spread to the central nervous system (CNS), dissemination within and spread from the CNS to extraneural sites (particularly the salivary glands), and neuronal dysfunction and death.

Exposure

Human rabies cases are almost always attributable to a bite from a rabid animal. Animal bites were the cause of 99 percent of 3920 human rabies cases examined at Pasteur Institutes throughout the world in the first half of the twentieth century.[66] Virus does not enter intact skin. Although it is an almost universally fatal disease once signs develop, not all bites from rabid dogs result in death. Mortality after untreated bites by rabid dogs varies from 38 to 57 percent.[65,67] However, exposure to rabid animals of other species, such as wolves, may result in 80 percent or more mortality. Efficient transmission, therefore, depends in part on the degree of severity of the bites, the locations of the wound, the quantity of inoculum in the saliva, and the variant of the virus.

Bites at areas that contain a high density of nicotinic acetylcholine receptors (AchR), such as the head or face, particularly with bleeding, carry the highest risk and usually are associated with a shorter incubation period due to proximity to the CNS. Highest mortality tends to occur in persons bitten on the head and face (up to 80 percent or more), with intermediate mortality in those bitten on the hands or arms (15 to 40 percent) and least in those bitten on the trunk or legs (5 to 10 percent) or through clothing (<5 percent), when no specific prophylaxis was initiated.[68,69] Nevertheless, single bites at any location that are deep enough to reach the muscles should be treated with the same urgency.[70] The risk of rabies acquisition is at least 50 times higher with a bite than with scratches (5 to 80 percent versus 0.1 to 1.0 percent).[71] Most recent bat rabies–associated human deaths did not have a reported exposure source, but these cases are likely due to bat bites in which either the risk was not appreciated or the bites were not recognized by the patient owing partly to the unique ability of these agents to replicate in the nonneural tissues.[42,72,73]

Nonbite transmission includes inhalation from aerosolized virus in caves inhabited by millions of rabid bats and in laboratory accidents with aerosolized virus.[1,2] Transmission is also possible by handling and skinning of infected carcasses and through corneal transplantation. Other exposures, such as aerosols, licks, scratches, or other unusual events that lead to contamination of an open wound or mucous membrane, rarely cause rabies.[1,63] Although there is a potential risk from contact with patients, because secretions commonly contain viable virus,[74–76] there are no such documented cases.[65,77] Since secretions contain viable virus, masks should be worn when caring for these patients. Transplacental transmission has been reported very infrequently and has not been verified recently. The potential mechanism for such an unusual occurrence is not known. In contrast, infants born to mothers with rabies were found to be healthy.[78] Immediate rabies PEP and interferon were initiated at delivery. The importance of oral transmission of rabies infection remains uncertain, although this can occur under experimental conditions in animal models either by direct oral route or by gastric tube administration.[79] Rabies PEP was given to people who consumed nonpasteurized milk from a rabid cow without incident.[80]

Transit to the Central Nervous System (CNS)

Eclipse Phase Versus Direct Nerve Entry

Another characteristic of rabies is an extremely variable incubation period, which may range from less than 7 days to more than 6 years.[81–84] Persistence at the site of exposure may explain the long incubation period. Those who died in less than 1 week usually sustained a direct injury to a nerve or brachial plexus from dog bites.

Following a successful introduction into the wound, rabies virus may go directly into nerves. This ability was confirmed by inoculation of rabies virus into the anterior chamber of the eye in rats and in a mouse model by inoculation into the masseter muscle or the forelimb.[79,85–87] Alternatively, rabies virus may be localized within the muscle cells, at the neuromuscular junction, or in the skin at the site of exposure and undergo an "eclipse" phase. The eclipse phase during incubation specifically refers to the period after viral entry in the periphery and passage in the axoplasm when we are in the dark as to where virus may be or in what form, hence in eclipse or unable to be visualized. The eclipse phase ends when virus may be detected in the CNS, but in the more common scenario, this occurs with the onset of clinical disease. The role of rabies virus persistence in bone marrow cells to explain this eclipse phase is still intriguing but unproven.[88] The factors that control the length of this silent period are undefined.

In the case of canine rabies virus, the viral G protein (residues 174 to 202) may bind to the alpha subunit of the nicotinic AchR on the muscle and subsequently multiply in the muscle cells.[89–94] In one study in skunks, rabies virus antigen and genome could be demonstrated as long as 2 months after inoculation into muscle.[95] In the case of some bat lyssaviruses, the virus may bind to unknown receptors in the epidermis or dermis.[42,72] This silent phase of localization at exposure sites, in turn, provides an opportunity for host immune clearance and for PEP.[96]

Centripetal Spread to the CNS

After budding from the plasma membrane of muscle cells, virus is taken up into unmyelinated nerve endings at the neuromuscular junctions or at the muscle spindles. Rabies virus is transported to the CNS via retrograde fast axonal transport, which can be blocked by colchicine or vinblastine injection.[97] Studies in rhesus monkeys indicate that motor nerves are preferentially involved.[98] Rabies virus P protein (residues 138 to 172) interacts with dynein light chain 8 (LC 8), a component in actin- and microtubule-based transport, in this retrograde movement within the peripheral nerve and in the CNS.[99–101] The virus replicates again in the dorsal root ganglia and anterior horn cells.[102] At the dorsal root ganglia, viral replication may be recognized and attacked by immune effector cells, resulting in ganglioneuronitis and a clinical prodrome of neuropathic pain at the exposure site.[1,103] This local prodrome is found more frequently in bat-related than in dog-related cases (70 versus 30 percent).[81] Some bat rabies virus variants also may replicate more effectively in the skin than in the muscle.[72] These observations suggest a preferential sensory pathway in bat-related cases.

Travel from the peripheral nerves to the CNS occurs at a constant rate of 8 to 20 mm/day. However, the first development of the local prodrome, even with the absence of any other neurologic deficits, defines the patient's fate. Studies with the fixed-challenge virus standard strain of rabies virus in cocultures of chick spinal cord and muscles showed that the neuromuscular junction is the major site of entry into neurons.[94] Colocalization of virus and endosome tracers within the nerve terminals, which subsequently accumulate in axons and nerve cell bodies, indicates retrograde transport of endocytosed virus from motor-nerve terminals.

Although nicotinic AchR is an important rabies virus receptor for virus spread from the inoculation site to the CNS, it is unlikely to be the only receptor that mediates viral entry into neurons. Nicotinic AchR is not present on all types of neurons susceptible to rabies virus. Rabies virus also may use other central receptors, such as carbohydrates, phospholipids, gangliosides, the neural cell adhesion molecule (NCAM or CD56), and low-affinity nerve growth factor receptor p75 neurotrophin receptor (NTR) to gain entry into cells.[79]

Spread Within the CNS

Once the virus is in the neurons, rapid amplification and dissemination take place. Virus disseminates through plasma membrane budding and direct cell-to-cell transmission or by transsynaptic propagation, which occurs exclusively by retrograde axonal transport.[98,102] It is not known which tract is preferentially involved.[104] The G protein is required for attachment to neuronal receptors, as well as for transsynaptic spread.[62,105]

The hippocampus was once believed to be predominantly involved, suggesting that virus localization to this area may account for the altered behavior and rage reaction. Subsequent studies showed that infection involves the brain stem and thalamus most prominently both in animals and in humans.[106,107] In human rabies, rabies virus antigen is found predominantly in brain stem, thalamus, and spinal cord regardless of the clinical type if the survival period is less than 7 days.[107] Moreover, the hippocampus contains a minimal amount of rabies virus antigen.[106–108] Studies in skunks infected with skunk street rabies virus showed that the areas that contained heavy accumulations were the motor nucleus of the vagus nerve, midbrain raphe, hypoglottis, and red nuclei.[109] These street rabies virus–infected skunks manifested as furious rabies.

Spread from the CNS

An important component of disease is the centrifugal spread of virus back out of the CNS to peripheral sites.[63] Specifically, virus is transmitted to acinar cells of the salivary and submaxillary glands, resulting in salivary excretion of virus. Transport of virus back out of the CNS can lead to infection of head and neck tissues. The observation of virus infection at these sites has resulted in the recognition that biopsies of the nape of the neck are extremely helpful for diagnostic purposes.[96] Additionally, virus can be found in corneal cells, drawing the association between corneal smears and a rapid diagnosis of rabies infection, although this may not be as sensitive as biopsies of the nape of the neck.[110] Thus corneal transplants can be a source of infection for person-to-person transmission, as reported.[1,63] Virtually all organs can become involved following natural infection, including the heart, kidney, lung, and gastrointestinal tract.[96,111,112]

▶ PATHOPHYSIOLOGY

Lack of Correlation Between Clinical Severity and Pathology

The amount of rabies virus in the CNS does not appear to determine the clinical and functional severity of the disease. Access of the virus to the CNS does not necessarily lead to a rapid development of symptoms and death. High titers of virus in the brain and spinal cord can be found in animals long before clinical signs appear.[113] Rabies virus antigen has been demonstrated extensively in the frontal lobe of one paralytic rabies patient who had quadriplegia and respiratory failure requiring ventilatory support. He was euphoric but still fully conscious at the time of biopsy, which was performed 19 days after onset of the clinical illness.[110] The degree of muscarinic AchR functional modifications in the hippocampus of rabid dogs was not dependent on the amount of virus.[114]

Pathologic findings, although similar to those encountered with other encephalitides, are significantly less extensive. This is in drastic contrast to the striking clinical symptomatology of hydrophobia, frenzied activity, and bizarre behaviors. Perivascular cuffing, neuronophagia, neuronal necrosis, and parenchymal infiltrations are limited.[107,115] Moreover, virus localization may not solely explain limbic symptomatology or the diversity of clinical manifestations (furious and paralytic rabies).

Furious and Paralytic Rabies

Differential Response Versus Differential Infection

In human rabies, cerebral symptoms dominate the clinical picture in furious rabies, and peripheral nerve or anterior horn cell symptoms dominate the clinical presentation in paralytic rabies. There is no correlation between the two distinct clinical patterns and the site of the bite, species of responsible vector, presence or absence of a history of previous immunization, and the incubation period.[65,107,108,116] Almost all human rabies

cases in Thailand were associated with canine rabies virus of genotype 1. Similar regional CNS rabies antigen distribution, as well as similar magnetic resonance imaging (MRI) findings, could be found in both furious and paralytic rabies.[107,116] The brain stem and thalamus were predominantly involved. An MRI in a case of nonclassic rabies due to a bat bite revealed similar findings.[117] This suggests that functional changes and clinical manifestations (including mood and behavior, motor weakness, etc.) are due to a differential response of the various CNS regions.[108] Areas that contained a minimal amount of rabies virus antigen, such as the hippocampi, hypothalami, and subcortical white matter, also were abnormal on MRI in both clinical forms.[116]

Specific Rabies Virus Variants in Furious and Paralytic Rabies

Different rabies virus variants associated with particular vectors have been postulated to be responsible for these clinical manifestations. Differences in G protein may affect G protein–receptor interactions, such as nicotinic AchR at the bite site, the NCAM (CD56), and the p75 NTR, as well as glycolipid or ganglioside CNS receptors.[62] Minor variations on the G protein, such as an amino acid substitution of arginine at position 333, also can affect neuroinvasiveness and the use of different neuronal pathways and distribution in the CNS.[62] Furthermore, some bat lyssaviruses may bind to other unidentified receptors in the epidermis or dermis.[72] Patients with some acquired bat-related rabies viruses are reported to have clinical features substantially different from those of dog-related cases.[1] In addition, the rabies viral capsid P protein interacts with the microtubule dynein light chain in retrograde axonal transport.[62] Modifying the dynein light chain binding site can reduce the efficiency of the peripheral spread of certain rabies viruses.[101] Differences in genotypes or in associated structures required for binding and transport may affect rabies virus propagation and spread, thus resulting in variations in clinical manifestations (nonclassic rabies).[1]

Arguing against the concept of specific rabies virus variants in determining clinical manifestations, patients with classic rabies displayed a stereotypic clinical pattern and progression, unlike nonclassic rabies patients.[1] Although rabies acquired after exposure to a particular host, such as a vampire bat, generally is described as the paralytic form, a recent outbreak of rabies in Peru transmitted by vampire bats presented as the encephalitic form.[118,119] A single infected dog in Thailand transmitted the furious form of rabies to one patient and paralytic rabies to another.[110]

Comparison of a 1432-, a 1575-, and an 894-nucleotide region from the rabies virus N, G, and P protein genes of samples obtained from two furious and two paralytic rabies patients associated with canine rabies virus of genotype 1 showed only minor nucleotide differences.[120] Deduced amino acid patterns of N protein were identical among both human and canine samples that belonged to the same geographic location regardless of the clinical forms. All differences in the amino acid of G protein were not in an interactive region with receptors known to be responsible for virus pathogenicity, nor did they lie in an immunodominant G domain. Arginine-333 was present in all samples. None of the amino acid differences of P protein were within the putative interactive site with dynein. These findings support the concept that clinical manifestations are not explained solely by the infecting rabies virus variant.

Peripheral Nerve in Paralytic Rabies

The site of neural involvement responsible for weakness in paralytic rabies is not clearly defined. There have been no reliable electrophysiologic data defining whether the defect is in peripheral nerve or anterior horn cells. Nonetheless, a histopathologic study performed in 11 paralytic rabies patients suggested peripheral nerve demyelination as the prime pathologic change.[121] Such demyelination was absent in patients with encephalitic rabies.[103] In the 17 peripheral nerve specimens studied, there was mild to moderate loss of myelinated nerve fibers in 11 nerves. Segmental demyelination and remyelination were present in 16 teased nerve preparations. Axonal loss of a variable degree was present in only 4 cases, and Wallerian-like degeneration in teased single fibers was noted in 6 nerves. In 9 nerves, the primary abnormality was segmental demyelination and remyelination or myelinated nerve fiber loss either singly or in combination. In none of these cases was Wallerian-like degeneration seen as the only pathologic feature. All spinal nerves studies showed evidence of Wallerian-like degeneration as well as segmental demyelination.[121] Our recent study agrees with a previous pathology report[121] that peripheral nerve is the prime target.[116] There was an intense inflammation and demyelination in spinal nerve roots corresponding to enhancing nerve root lesions on MRI.[116] Inflammatory reactions were much more intense in the spinal cord in furious rabies patients. Only mild inflammation of the spinal nerve roots of all levels was seen.

Immunologic Parameters in Furious and Paralytic Rabies

The particular involvement of the peripheral nerves in paralytic rabies, plus unexplained aggression and extreme excitability in furious rabies (despite similar virus distributions in the CNS and similar MRI patterns in the brain) and the lack of specific virus variants, suggests a participation of host factors. The degree of functional impairment of muscarinic AchR in the brains of rabies virus–infected dogs does not correlate with virus distribution and virus load.[114] Patients with intact T-cell immunity to rabies virus, with a high concentration of serum interleukin 2 (IL-2) receptor and IL-6, die earlier and present with furious rabies, whereas those lacking such responses survive longer and present with paralytic rabies.[108,110,122] Lack of T-cell responses to virus in paralytic rabies is not explained by excessive cortisol production or by a panimmunosuppressive process. Cortisol concentrations, although significantly higher than normal, were similar among patients with furious and others with paralytic rabies. Reaction against myelin basic protein was found in both furious and paralytic rabies patients who died rapidly.[108,110,122] An immune phenomenon also may be responsible for nerve injury, although neutralizing antibody to rabies virus could not be demonstrated in the cerebrospinal fluid (CSF) of paralytic rabies patients.[116] This immune phenomenon can be further supported by a patient with furious rabies who developed paralysis of all limbs soon after intravenous administration of human rabies immune globulin (RIG).[123] An immune attack against virus in the axons has been suggested in one Chinese paralytic rabies patient.[124]

Hypothetical Mechanisms in Furious Rabies

Participation of host response to neuronal infection also may explain aggression, the rage reaction, and autonomic stimulation signs in furious rabies.[1] Rabies virus infection in the brain stem leads to the production of cytokines and proinflammatory molecules, such as interleukins 1 alpha/beta, 6, and 10; tumor necrosis factor alpha (TNF-α), interferons, nitric oxide, and chemokines (Fig. 11-1). These cytokines can modify the hippocampus and other limbic system functions, including electrical cortical activity, the hypothalamic-pituitary-adrenal axis, and serotonin metabolism.[81] In furious rabies, these locally produced cytokines may further activate the p55 TNF-α receptor, resulting in the recruitment of T and B cells.[125] This action may lead to the promotion of immune recognition against rabies virus at "immune privileged" sites and provoke another amplification of the cytokine cascade, intensifying the limbic symptom pattern. Delayed mortality was observed in mice deficient in the p55 TNF-α receptor as a result of an increase in interferon gamma and IL-10 and a reduction in inflammatory cells in the CNS.[125] Furthermore, if Vβ8 T cells are stimulated by rabies virus nucleocapsid antigen,[126] more cytokines are produced, thus exaggerating the functional disturbance in the limbic system even in the absence of virus in such structures. This process possibly explains the relative paucity of limbic dysfunction and the absence of cellular immune activity to rabies virus in patients with the paralytic form.

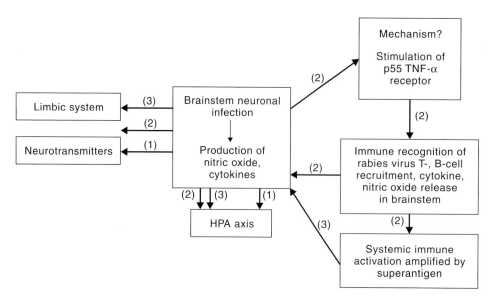

Figure 11-1. Hypothetical mechanisms in encephalitic rabies. Production of proinflammatory molecules results from rabies virus–infected neuronal processes in the brain stem. These substances, in turn, lead to functional modification of the limbic system and stimulation of the hypothalamic-pituitary-adrenal (HPA) axis (arrow 1). In furious rabies, the p55 TNF-α receptors also may be activated. Rabies virus antigen is thus recognized. Subsequently, recruitment of immune cells and intensification of limbic symptoms and HPA stimulation follow (arrow 2). Once Vβ8 T cells are stimulated by rabies virus nucleocapsid antigens (arrow 3), these cytokine cascades are reamplified, exaggerating the disturbance of the limbic and sympathetic nervous systems.
(Reprinted with permission from Human rabies: A disease of complex neuropathogenetic mechanisms and diagnostic challenge. Lancet Neurol 1:101, 2002, Fig. 4; used by permission of Elsevier.)

Neuronal Death, Vulnerability of Different Neuronal Type, and Neurodestructive Immunity

Programmed cell death during rabies virus infection had been proposed as a principal pathologic mechanism; however, recent studies suggest otherwise.[127] Apoptosis appears to be one of the most important defense mechanisms against rabies virus infection. Apoptosis leads to depolymerization of actin filaments, which would prevent transport of viral nucleocapsid protein and the neuronal spread of virus. The extent of apoptosis correlates with the amount of expression of rabies virus G protein in infected neurons.[128–130] Downregulation of G protein expression in neuronal cells contributes to pathogenesis by preventing apoptosis.[127] However, the process of cell death is also modulated by the types of the neurons infected and the quality of immune response to infecting virus, as well as its virulence.[131] There is a delay of apoptosis in spinal cord motoneurons after rabies virus infection compared with hippocampal cells.[132]

Nonfatal or abortive infection induced by the attenuated strain of Pasteur rabies virus is associated with paralysis.[130] This mechanism of viral clearance is mediated by local recruitment of T cells, as well as the development of apoptosis of infected neurons and surrounding cells. It is hoped that rabies virus clearance can be made possible by other nonlytic mechanisms than this neurodestructive immunity, as shown in the Sindbis virus model.[133]

Depletion of metabolic pools by excessive viral replication, which ultimately leads to downregulation of expression of the late response gene and cell death, is one likely explanation of the virulence of rabies virus.[127]

▶ CLINICAL FEATURES

Rabies continues to be underreported in most developing countries. One of the most important contributors to this is that diagnosis depends on symptomatology alone. Rabies can manifest variably, and once coma supervenes, there is no reliable sign.

Clinical features can be divided into five stages: incubation period, prodrome, acute neurologic phase, coma, and death or recovery.[1,65,134] During the acute neurologic phase, rabies can be distinguished clinically as classic (furious or paralytic forms) and nonclassic forms. Furious and paralytic forms also differ in the survival period (interval between onset of disease and death) and immunologic features (see "Pathophysiology" above).

Incubation Period

The incubation period of rabies is usually 1 to 2 months after exposure. However, patients have been reported who developed the first signs of rabies as early as 5 days after a severe dog bite injury to the brachial plexus with possible direct inoculation of the virus into the nerve.[81] On the other hand, unusually long periods of 27 months and 4 and 6 years have been reported.[1] These patients had Australian bat *Lyssavirus* infection and canine rabies variant of genotype 1. The incubation period of more than 1 year is considered exceptionally rare. The WHO recommends that rabies PEP should be given to an exposed person regardless of the time that has elapsed since exposure, but PEP usually is not administered after a time interval of longer than 1 year.[96] Absence of a history of exposure is not uncommon in dog rabies–endemic countries, where exposures frequently occur and tend to be neglected.[1] This is also true in cryptic bat rabies cases, whose exposure may be considered trivial.[135] Most deaths occur because individuals are unaware that they had been exposed and infected with rabies virus.[136]

Prodrome

Prodromal symptoms can be vague and nonspecific, such as fever, muscular aching, flulike symptoms, diarrhea, abdominal pain, etc. Only local symptoms at the bitten region in the form of burning, numbness, tingling, itching, or pruritus are regarded as reliable indicators of rabies.[1] This neuropathic pain is presumed to be due to ganglioneuronitis. As many as a third of patients with dog-related infections (equally common in furious and paralytic rabies) and three-quarters of those with bat-related disease may experience local symptoms.

The appearance of the local symptoms at the bitten region marks the end of the incubation period, and most patients die within the next 2 weeks. This local reaction is intense and progressive, starting at the bite site and spreading gradually to involve the whole limb in a nonradicular pattern or the ipsilateral side of the face. Rarely, these symptoms can occur at locations remote from the bite site. Prodromal symptoms usually last only a few hours or days.

Acute Neurologic Phase

During this phase, objective signs of nervous system dysfunction begin. Furious and paralytic forms of human rabies have been widely recognized, although the latter is not easily diagnosed. These patients display a stereotypic pattern of manifestations (see below).[1,65,81] Increasing awareness of atypical forms of rabies has been emphasized.[81,136] Both paralytic and atypical (or nonclassic) forms of rabies may pose diagnostic problems not only in clinical practice but also in disease surveillance. Underestimation of case numbers is undoubtedly a contributory factor to rabies being ranked low on the priority lists for disease-control programs.[137]

Classic Rabies

Classic rabies is almost always associated with true rabies virus (genotype 1), particularly the canine rabies virus variant. Mental status abnormalities can be seen in patients with furious rabies, as well as in some with paralytic forms, but to a much greater extent in the former group.

FURIOUS RABIES. Two-thirds of patients with classic rabies have a furious form, and the remainder present with paralysis. Most furious rabies patients die within 7 days (average 5 days) of onset, and the survival period is about 13 days in paralytic cases.[1,65,81]

The earliest feature is hyperactivity, aggravated by internal (fear, thirst, etc.) and external (light, noise, etc.) stimuli. Mentation is preserved, but attention span is shortened. Fever, already apparent during the prodrome, is fairly constant, persisting through the preterminal phase. Cranial nerve deficits are detected rarely. Focal neurologic deficits, such as hemiparesis and hemihypalgesia, are not present. Seizures and hallucinations are rare. There are three major cardinal signs of furious rabies:

Fluctuating consciousness. Mental status alternates between periods of progressively more severe agitation and periods of relative normality and depression (Fig. 11-2). The patient abruptly becomes confused and disoriented without any warning. This bizarre behavior lasts only for minutes and then abates. The patient then becomes lucid and may not recall these events. Confusion becomes severe and may evolve to wild agitation and aggressiveness. Between these episodes of agitation the patient is drowsy but arousable. The period of irritability is gradually succeeded by impaired consciousness and coma. Biting behavior and barking have never been observed (authors' experience). The electroencephalogram (EEG) is normal during the initial stage (Fig. 11-3). It will not be abnormal until the patient exhibits severe aggression, with the appearance of high-amplitude sharp and slow waves interspersed within the slow background (Fig. 11-4).

Phobic spasms. Aero- and hydrophobia are seen in all furious rabies patients at some stage. These spasms can be elicited by blowing or fanning air on the face or chest wall or merely by offering a drink or showing a cup of water. Aerophobia and hydrophobia may not coexist and are not necessarily associated with laryngeal spasms.

Figure 11-2. Fluctuation of consciousness in furious rabies. This is characterized by alternating periods of relative normality (*A*) and severe agitation (*B*).

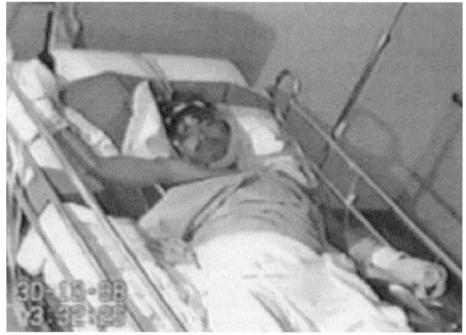

A

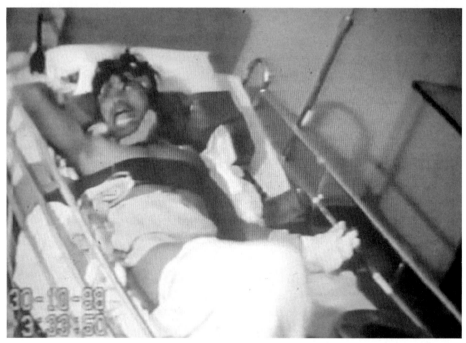

B

However, when these are present, the patient may spit saliva. These phobic spasms (or startle reactions) result from spasms of the accessory neck muscles and diaphragm followed by neck flexion (or rarely by neck extension). During the episode, the patient may have a fearful facial expression. These phobic spasms cannot be explained by a conditioned reflex because many patients have their first hydrophobic attack while bathing with no previous swallowing difficulties. Soft palate and pharyngeal sensations remain intact, but the gag reflex is hyperactive. Phobic spasms cannot be elicited once drowsiness and coma supervene. However, these are replaced by spontaneously occurring inspiratory spasms. Since inspiratory spasms are less intense and less frequent, they can escape notice. Opisthotonos, a characteristic sign of tetanus, is extremely rare.

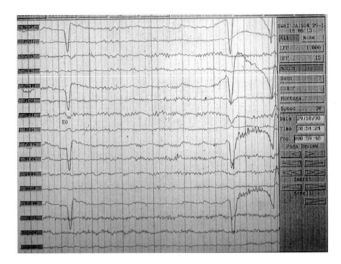

Figure 11-3. Electroencephalogram (EEG) in furious rabies displays a normal finding in the presence of fluctuating consciousness.

Autonomic dysfunction. Hypersalivation is a unique feature. Transient reactions can include fixed, dilated, or constricted pupils; anisocoria; localized (usually on the bitten region) or generalized piloerection; pulmonary edema (only in 3 among more than 170 patients in our experience); excessive sweating; priapism; and spontaneous ejaculations.

PARALYTIC RABIES. This form of rabies resembles the axonal form of Guillain-Barré syndrome (GBS), acute motor axonal neuropathy (AMAN).[124,138] The major cardinal signs appear late and are not prominent. Phobic spasms occur in only half the patients and are less ev-

ident because of weakness. Many, but not all, of the patients have weakness starting at the bitten limb. In patients with facial bites, weakness initially may involve facial and oculomotor muscles. Nevertheless, bilateral symmetric weakness of the legs develops in all patients regardless of the bite site. Bilateral weakness in an ascending fashion progressively involves all limbs and the pharyngeal, bulbar, and respiratory muscles. Facial diparesis is common (Fig. 11-5). Loss of deep tendon reflexes is found in all cases. Limb weakness is almost always proximal; however, this also can be seen in GBS. Sensory functions of all modalities are intact except, in some cases, at the bitten region. Persistent fever from the onset of weakness, intact sensory function, percussion myoedema, and bladder dysfunction may differentiate paralytic rabies from GBS.[134] Percussion myoedema is seen from the prodromal to the preterminal stage.[139] This is best elicited by percussion of the chest, deltoid, and thigh regions with a tendon hammer and consists of mounding of a part of the muscle at the percussion site, which then flattens and disappears over a few seconds. Patients with extreme cachectic conditions, hyponatremia, hypothyroidism, and renal failure may have myoedema signs. Myoedema during the late stage in rabies patients may be due in part to severe hyponatremia from the syndrome of inappropriate secretion of antidiuretic hormone.

Nonclassic Rabies
Patients with bat-related rabies have been reported to have clinical features substantially different from those with dog-related rabies.[1,81,113,117] Neuroimaging studies

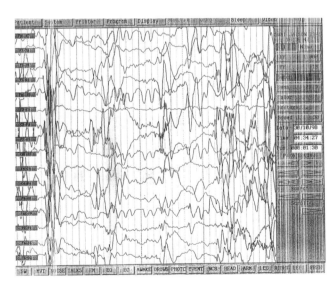

Figure 11-4. Paroxysmal bursts of high-amplitude sharp and slow waves appear only when the patient becomes severely agitated.

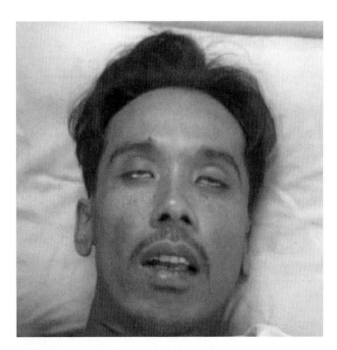

Figure 11-5. Facial diparesis in paralytic rabies.

in classic and nonclassic rabies patients appear remarkably similar.[116,117,140] Local neuropathic pain during the prodromal phase is more common in bat-related rabies. Moreover, there are reports of radicular pain, objective motor and sensory deficits, and choreiform movements of the bitten limb. Focal brain stem signs and myoclonus are observed frequently. Other patients have been described as having hemiparesis or hemisensory loss, ataxia, vertigo, or Horner's syndrome. Convulsive and nonconvulsive seizures and hallucinations are common. Phobic spasms were described in only one of six bat-related cases during 1997–2000.[1,74]

These atypical presentations have been observed in at least six patients with dog-related rabies since 1997 at Chulalongkorn University Hospital alone.[113] These included paraparesis, facial and bulbar weakness with preserved arm strength or bilateral arm weakness, repeated spontaneous ejaculations, ocular myoclonus, and hemichorea. One patient had nocturnal agitation but remained calm during the day. Phobic spasms or autonomic hyperactivity and hypersalivation were lacking.

Coma

Once a patient becomes comatose, it is extremely difficult to diagnose rabies. Although some suggest that the oculocephalic reflex (doll's-eye response) disappears early, this also happens in other viral encephalitis patients with brain stem involvement. Only inspiratory spasms can suggest the diagnosis of rabies at this stage. The EEG is nondiagnostic and similar to cases of metabolic encephalopathy (Fig. 11-6). Sinus tachycardia, disproportionate to fever, is usually seen even when hydration is adequate. This is followed by a nodal rhythm and, in some cases, by supraventricular and ventricular arrhythmias. Echocardiography shows reduction of the ejection fraction at the time of, or even before, hypotension. Viral involvement at the conduction pathways and myocardial involvement are the likely responsible mechanisms.[1] Coma precedes circulatory insufficiency, a prime cause of death, in almost all cases. Hematemesis is seen in 30 to 60 percent of patients 6 to 12 hours before death.

Recovery

Eight rabies survivors have been reported to date.[1,141] Most of them had atypical presentations.[108,113] The first patient (1972), who was exposed to a rabid bat, had unsteady gait, dysarthria, and hemiparesis. The second (1976), exposed to a rabid dog, had quadriparesis and generalized myoclonus at the early stage and later developed cerebellar signs, frontal lobe signs, and bibrachial weakness. The third patient (1977) had aerosol exposure to a highly concentrated fixed rabies virus strain. The five additional survivors include four Mexican children (between 1992 and 1995) and one Indian child (2002). Four patients were bitten by rabid dogs and one by a vampire bat. Each patient promptly received cell culture vaccine but not rabies immune globulin. All had significant sequelae. No spontaneous survivors have been reported to date.

▶ DIAGNOSIS

Antemortem Diagnosis

Clinical Features and Routine Laboratory Findings

Diagnosis on clinical grounds alone causes an imprecise assumption of low mortality from human rabies. Lack of a history of exposure is common in bat-related cases and is found in as many as 6 percent of dog-related cases.[113] Several patients with paralysis in Thailand had undergone plasma exchange because of a misdiagnosis of GBS. For a definitive diagnosis, all three cardinal signs of rabies should be present. Such a diagnosis is often not possible. Phobic spasms are evident at some stage. Many patients in developing countries seek medical attention late, and these signs cannot be demonstrated once the patients become comatose. In more developed countries, failure to diagnose rabies may be explained by a lack of medical familiarity even with typical clinical features of the disease. Moreover, clinical presentations may be variable in most cases associated with exposure to rabid bats or other wild animals[74] and even to rabid dogs.[81]

There are no characteristic findings in routine laboratory tests. The CSF examination is normal in most cases or shows only mild pleocytosis with lymphocytic predominance. The EEG shows no specific finding.

Neuroimaging

Computed tomographic (CT) scan of the brain is insufficient to detect abnormal parenchymal changes in

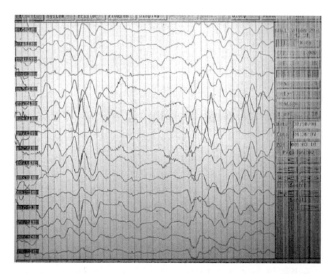

Figure 11-6. EEG during the comatose phase in rabies.

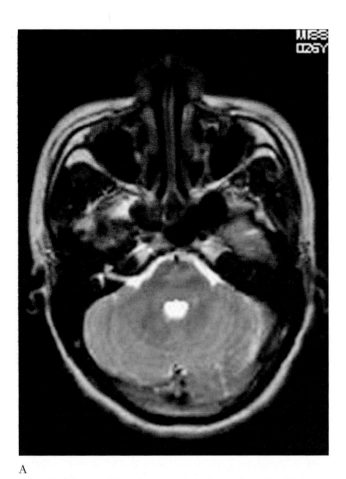

A

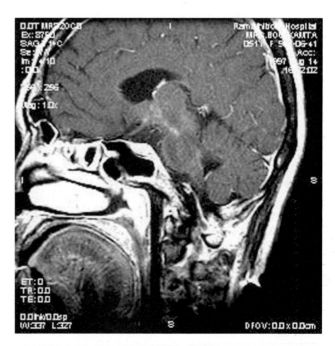

B

rabies. The MRI is more precise and can give specific findings suggestive of rabies.[116,117] A nonenhancing mild hyperintensity on T_2-weighted images in the brain stem, hippocampi, hypothalami, subcortical white matter, and deep and cortical gray matter can be demonstrated in noncomatose rabies patients[117] (Fig. 11-7). Enhancement with gadolinium can be seen only when the patient becomes comatose (Fig. 11-8). Human rabies of both forms demonstrate similar MRI abnormalities.

Similar abnormalities in the brain stem on MRI can be seen in Japanese encephalitis (JE); eastern equine encephalitis (EEE); rhombencephalitis from *Listeria monocytogenes*, herpes simplex virus (HSV), and adenovirus infections; acute hemorrhagic leukoencephalitis (AHL); acute disseminated encephalomyelitis (ADEM); and Behçet's disease.

The MRI findings in JE and EEE were similar to rabies in terms of localization but without enhancement. However, a much more prominent nonenhancing increased signal abnormality on T_2-weighted MRI images was found in the former with only a mild degree of cortical gray and white matter involvement.[142,143] Foci of hemorrhages are demonstrated frequently on MRI and CT scan in JE but are unusual in rabies.[116] The abnormality seen in adenovirus rhombencephalitis was composed of a more prominent moderate hyperintensity on T_2-weighted images involving the brain stem and cerebellum with patchy enhancement along the pe-

Figure 11-7. Axial (*A*) and coronal (*B*) T_2-weighted MRI of the brain in a patient with furious rabies demonstrating areas of increased signal intensity in the pons (*A*) and subcortical white matter and hippocampi (*B*). *(Courtesy of Dr. Jiraporn Laothamatas, Ramathibodi Hospital, Mahidol University, Bangkok, Thailand.)*

Figure 11-8. Postgadolinium sagittal T_1-weighted MRI of the brain in a comatose patient with paralytic rabies showing mild to moderate enhancement in the hypothalamus, midbrain, dorsal pons, and upper medulla. *(Courtesy of Dr. Jiraporn Laothamatas, Ramathibodi Hospital, Mahidol University, Bangkok, Thailand.)*

riphery of the involved areas.[144] The abnormality seen in AHL and ADEM consisted of bilateral symmetric abnormal hyperintensities on T_2-weighted images that selectively involved the white matter of supra- and infratentorial structures and spinal cord.[145] The MRI in Behçet's disease involved basal ganglia, thalamus, and the central part of the pons with the absence of a predominance of white matter lesions.[146]

Special Laboratory Tests

Serum and CSF can be tested for IgM and IgG rabies virus antibodies (in previously unvaccinated individuals), but these often are not positive when the patient first presents.[1,147] Furthermore, this may produce variable results among diagnostic laboratories.

Rabies virus antigen in the nerve plexus at the hair follicles can be demonstrated by the fluorescent-antibody (FA) technique on frozen sections of the skin from the nape of the neck. However, this may not always be practical because it requires a dedicated cryostat. Earlier studies suggested that the number of positive results tends to increase as the disease progresses, but these findings were not always confirmed.[75] Corneal and salivary impressions for detection of rabies virus antigen may yield conflicting results partly due to differences in technique and difficulty in interpretation.

Isolation of rabies virus in neuroblastoma cells from saliva specimens is sensitive and specific. Results are known within 48 hours; however, all samples tested must be maintained frozen after collection with no preservative. Patients who have serum rabies virus antibody tend to have negative results.[74]

Brain biopsy is not practical but is highly sensitive by the FA test. However, false-negative results can occur due to a relative paucity of virus antigen at the biopsy areas, usually in the frontotemporal region, during the first few days after clinical onset.[74,110] This can be overcome by rabies virus isolation or molecular detection.

Molecular technology can improve clinical diagnosis. Although molecular diagnostic facilities for rabies are limited in developing countries, these do exist in parts of India, the Philippines, Latin America, Sri Lanka, and Thailand. The best specimens include saliva, tear secretions, nuchal skin biopsy specimens, CSF, and urine. Performing reverse-transcription polymerase chain reaction (RT-PCR) or nucleic acid sequence–based amplification (NASBA) on several sequential samples is mandatory in patients suspected of rabies because not all samples are positive.[1,74,75,148,149] Secretion of virus is intermittent in saliva, urine, and even CSF. The CSF appears to be the least sensitive source for rabies virus RNA detection. Any PCR products will need to be sequenced for confirmation because of the occurrence of nonspecific bands. Rapid clinical and, where available, laboratory diagnosis is important to prevent potential exposure to the health care team and to reduce anxiety and treatment costs.

Postmortem Diagnosis

A definitive test for rabies requires an examination of brain tissue. Brain necropsy via the transorbital approach is an alternative whenever a full autopsy cannot be done. Brain examination should be performed in all patients with encephalitis or paralysis who progress to coma and death. The presence of inflammation and Negri bodies is not always indicative of rabies. Moreover, inclusion bodies may not always be present.[2] The direct FA test on brain tissue remains a gold standard in rabies diagnosis. Touch impressions of brain tissue are made on glass slides and fixed in cold acetone and subsequently stained with fluorescein isothiocyanate–labeled polyclonal or monoclonal antibodies against rabies virus antigens. Areas to be examined include brain stem, spinal cord, cerebellum, and hippocampus.[106,107]

Although the FA test on brain impressions is simple, many developing countries have limited facilities to do this. For example, in Thailand, where there are 33 FA diagnostic laboratories, the number of human and animal cases diagnosed by laboratory analysis remains low. Often without maintenance of the cold chain, transfer of the specimens for a FA test in many rural areas cannot be done easily within 24 hours, before the brain begins to decompose (Ministry of Public Health report, Thailand, September 2002). Although brain tissue samples can be stored frozen at the collection site and during transport, this is not always possible in remote areas where there is no or little electricity. Molecular assays may be useful, in such conditions, in confirming a diagnosis and in epidemiologic surveillance. Results may be reliable, even in decomposed brain samples.[150] Rabies virus RNA also can be recovered from brain tissues dried on filter paper and stored at room temperature after 222 days.[151]

▶ DIFFERENTIAL DIAGNOSIS

The differential diagnosis includes encephalitis caused by pathogens that may selectively involve midline structures or those which are associated with behavioral changes and includes arboviruses [JE, EEE, and West Nile (WNV) viruses], enterovirus 71 (EV-71), herpes simplex virus (HSV), and varicella-zoster virus (VZV) infections.[143,152–157] A combination of the clinical symptomatology, the presence of behavioral abnormalities from the onset, the rapidity of disease progression (from onset to coma), the presence or absence of brain stem signs, and MRI abnormalities may differentiate rabies from other pathogens (Fig. 11-9). Most rabies patients

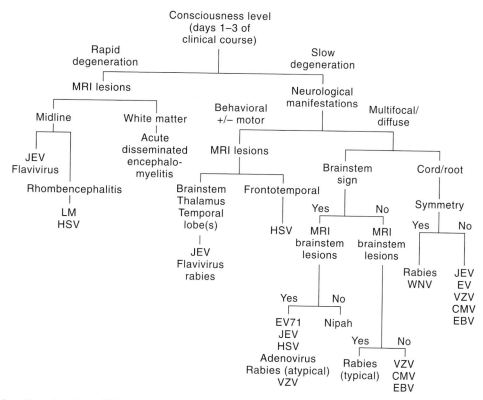

Figure 11-9. Algorithm for the differential diagnosis of rabies. The model considers the rapidity of disease progression, clinical manifestations, the presence or absence of brain stem signs on clinical examination and/or in MRIs, behavioral changes, MRI details, and the pattern of spinal cord/root involvement (see text for details). JEV = Japanese encephalitis virus; LM = *Listeria monocytogenes;* HSV = herpes simplex virus; EV = enterovirus; CMV = cytomegalovirus; EBV = Epstein-Barr virus; VZV = varicella zoster virus. *(Reprinted with permission from Rabies reexamined. Lancet Infect Dis 2:327, 2002, Fig. 11; used by permission of Elsevier.)*

remain alert and able to communicate during the first 3 days after clinical onset.

Patients with rabies and JE and HSV encephalitis may or may not have dramatic behavioral changes. An asymmetric MRI involvement with hyperintense lesions on T_2-weighted images in the frontotemporal region favors HSV encephalitis. Absence of enhancing lesions during the noncomatose phase and less intense signal in T_2-weighted images may separate rabies from other brain stem encephalitides due to EV-71, JE, and adenovirus infections. By comparison, HSV, VZV, and other herpesvirus infections are infrequently associated with brain stem lesions. Myoclonus and other brain stem signs, such as bilateral ptosis and nystagmus (similar to those in patients infected by bat rabies virus), have been found in Nipah virus encephalitis of acute, relapsed, and late-onset forms. However, the MRI usually shows multiple and widespread discrete hyperintense lesions, mainly in white matter, representing vasculitis in the acute form and confluent lesions involving primarily the cortical gray matter in late-onset or relapsed forms of Nipah virus encephalitis.[154,158] Diffuse flaccid paralysis was found in 10 percent of patients with WNV encephalitis. Asymmetric pure motor poliomyelitis-like

weakness can be seen in patients with JE and WNV infections. An asymmetric radiculomyelitis may be due to infection with cytomegalovirus (CMV), Epstein-Barr virus, and other herperviruses.

Acute hepatic porphyria with neuropsychiatric disturbances, such as psychosis, seizures, signs of autonomic dysfunctions, and ascending paralysis with bilateral facial weakness, may mimic rabies. Fluctuating consciousness is observed in both conditions, but phobic and inspiratory spasms are seen only in rabies. A family history, ingestion of porphyrinogenic agents, severe abdominal pain, and dark urine color after being exposed to sunlight or added with concentrated nitric acid with elevated urinary delta-aminolevulinic acid and porphobilinogen should establish the diagnosis. Other conditions mimicking rabies are substance abuse, alcohol withdrawal or delirium tremens, and acute serotonin syndrome from taking serotonin reuptake inhibitors. Tetanus resembles rabies only in the form of reflex spasms. Tetanus patients have a clear sensorium. Rabies patients do not have persistent rigidity or sustained contraction of the jaw, neck, back, and abdomen as seen in tetanus. Spasms in rabies predominantly affect accessory respiratory muscles and the diaphragm, whereas in tetanus spasms occur in axial muscles. Opisthotonos is rarely, if ever, present in rabies.

The axonal form of GBS, AMAN, shares many clinical features with paralytic rabies. Inspiratory spasms with abnormal behavior may appear late in the clinical course and may be masked by generalized paralysis and superimposed metabolic disturbances that can occur in both conditions. Nerve conduction studies cannot differentiate paralytic rabies from GBS.

In some parts of the world where nervous tissue (sheep, monkey, and mouse brain)–derived rabies vaccine is still widely used, neuroparalytic accidents must be included in the differential diagnosis. These developed in as many as 1 in 400 Semple vaccine–treated patients but less often in individuals who received mouse brain vaccine.[159–161] Delayed onset and a picture of chronic progressive encephalitis also have been observed. Phobic spasms, local prodromal symptoms, and fluctuating consciousness are not present in these postvaccination reactions.

▶ MANAGEMENT

Comfort care should be the management goal for the patient with rabies.[162] Previous attempts at treating symptomatic rabies patients have failed.[108,123] Invasive procedures and even respiratory support should be avoided in virtually every laboratory-proven case of rabies. Liberal use of barbiturates and intravenous morphine are best for relief of the terrifying attacks of anxiety, agitation, and respiratory spasms.

▶ PREVENTION

The WHO issued a current guideline for rabies pre- and postexposure prophylaxis (PEP) in humans in November 2002 (*www.who.int/emc.diseases/zoo/RabiesPET.pdf*). Due to reports of rabies prophylaxis failures,[1,163–165] this current guideline emphasizes the need to adhere strictly to its recommendations. Assessment of wounds or bite exposures helps define the risk and the need to use vaccine and RIG. Immediate washing and flushing with soap and water and disinfection with appropriate agents are as important as the use of vaccine and RIG. In less developed countries, where the use of commercial tissue-culture vaccines is not readily affordable, the practice of intradermal (ID) vaccination has been proven effective and economical. Therefore, the use of nerve-tissue vaccines, which carries serious side effects, should be abandoned by the year 2006.

General Considerations in Rabies PEP

Rabies PEP is a medical emergency and, as a general rule, should not be delayed or deferred. There are no contraindications if modern purified rabies biologicals are used. Pregnancy and infancy are never contraindications to rabies PEP. Persons who present for evaluation *even weeks or months after having been bitten* should be dealt with in the same manner as if the contact occurred recently.

Prophylaxis consists of vaccine regimens and routes of administration that have been proven to be safe and effective. Initiation of prophylaxis should *not await* the results of laboratory diagnosis or be delayed by dog observation when rabies is strongly suspected. Wounds should be washed and flushed with soap and water immediately or with water alone and disinfected with ethanol (700 ml/liter) or iodine (tincture or aqueous solution). Prophylaxis may be deferred if the species is unlikely to be infected with rabies and if results of laboratory diagnosis can be obtained in a timely manner, usually within 48 hours. Most dogs tend to shed virus concomitant with or shortly before the development of clinical signs. If the domestic dog or cat is unlikely to be rabid, it may be observed for 10 days. If the animal remains well, no prophylaxis is indicated. For example, the animal may be observed in cases where the bite is provoked and the animal is healthy, up to date on rabies vaccination, well maintained, etc. However, even vaccinated animals may become rabid. If the dog shows any sign of illness during the observation period, the patient should receive full rabies PEP urgently, and the animal's brain should be examined by a competent laboratory for a definitive rabies diagnosis.

Rabies PEP Modalities

Whether to use rabies immune globulin in addition to vaccine, vaccine alone, or none at all depends on the WHO category of exposure. These decisions may vary from country to country because epidemiologic circumstances vary. These broad categories are

Category III. Single or multiple transdermal bites, scratches, or contamination of mucous membrane with saliva (i.e., licks): Use RIG plus vaccine.

Category II. Minor scratches or abrasions without bleeding or licks on broken skin and nibbling of uncovered skin: Use vaccine alone.

Category I. Touching, feeding of animals, or licks on intact skin: No exposure; therefore, no PEP is required if the history is reliable.

Administration of Rabies Immune Globulin

Rabies immune globulin (RIG) must be infiltrated into the depth of the wound and around the wound. As much as anatomically feasible of the RIG should be infiltrated. Any remainder should be injected at an intramuscular site distant from that of vaccine inoculation, e.g., into the anterior thigh. The quantity used is 20 IU/kg of human RIG or 40 IU/kg of equine RIG. The total recommended dose should not be exceeded. If the calculated dose is insufficient to infiltrate all wounds, sterile saline may be used to dilute it two- to threefold to permit thorough infiltration. Suturing should be postponed to avoid further wound contamination with virus. If suturing is necessary, it should be ensured that RIG has been applied locally. Antimicrobial agents and tetanus toxoid may be required accordingly.

Rabies PEP: Vaccination

Tissue-culture rabies vaccine can be administered intramuscularly (IM) or ID where licensed or approved by the administrative authority. The efficacy and adverse events are comparable between these two regimens. However, the use of ID vaccination may decrease the cost by as much as 60 to 80 percent. Given that there has been no substantive data comparing one vaccine with the others in terms of vaccine immunogenicity and a change in the route of vaccine administration (e.g., from IM to ID), the routine interchangeability of modern rabies vaccines and routes is not recommended for liability concerns alone. However, when completion of PEP with the same rabies vaccine is not possible, the switch can be done, provided that it is with one of the WHO-recommended cell-culture vaccines.

Intramuscular Regimen

Vaccines should not be injected into the gluteal region. A classic five-dose IM or "Essen" regimen consists of one dose of vaccine on days 0, 3, 7, 14, and 28 in the deltoid region or in small children into the anterolateral area of the thigh muscle. As an alternative, the 2-1-1 regimen may be used. Two doses are given on day 0 in the deltoid muscle and right and left arms. In addition, one dose is given in the deltoid muscle on day 7 and one on day 21.

Intradermal Regimen

Since these regimens require considerably less vaccine than the IM regimens, this method is particularly appropriate where vaccine or funds are in short supply. The ID approach reduces the volume of vaccine required and hence vaccine cost by 60 to 80 percent.

The decision to implement an economical ID PEP scheme rests with government agencies that define rabies prevention and treatment policies in their own countries. When the ID route is used, attention must be given to staff training, conditions and duration of vaccine storage after reconstitution, use of an appropriate 1-ml syringe and short hypodermic needles, etc.

Vaccines suggested for use with the ID regimen are the HDCV Rabivac; the purified vero cell vaccines (PVRV) Verorab, Imovax, Rabies vero, and TRC Verorab;

and the purified chick embryo cell vaccine (PCECV) Rabipur. There are two methods of ID administration:

1. Eight-site ID method (8-0-4-0-1-1; 8 sites on day 0, 4 sites on day 7, 1 site on days 30 and 90) for use with HDCV (Rabivac) and PCECV (Rabipur). The volume per ID site for both vaccines is 0.1 ml. Although there has been no supporting scientific evidence, the eight-site regimen may be considered in emergency situations when no RIG is available. The RIG may be administered within 7 days after the first dose of vaccination.
2. Two-site ID method (2-2-2-0-1-1; 2 sites on days 0, 3, and 7; 1 site on days 30 and 90) for use with PVRV (Verorab, Imovax, Rabies vero, TRC Verorab) and PCECV (Rabipur). The volume per ID site is 0.1 ml for PVRV (Verorab, Imovax, Rabies vero, TRC Verorab) and 0.2 ml for PCECV (Rabipur) or, *as an option,* 0.1 ml for PCECV (Rabipur) may be considered for use by national health authorities. This does not apply to any other vaccine brand.

Rabies PEP Prophylaxis in Immunosuppressed Individuals

There is no reliable PEP method to ensure efficacy in immunosuppressed individuals. Therefore, the importance of wound treatment should be further stressed. RIG should be administered deeply into the wound for all exposures. Vaccine always should be administered, and no modification of the recommended number of doses is advisable. An infectious disease specialist with expert knowledge of rabies prevention should be consulted.

Rabies PEP in Previously Vaccinated Persons

Apart from local wound treatment, there is no need for RIG administration. Two boosters, either IM or ID, are required on days 0 and 3. However, full PEP should be given to persons who received pre- or postexposure prophylaxis with vaccine of unproven potency or who have not demonstrated acceptable rabies neutralizing antibody titer.

Preexposure Rabies Vaccination

Three doses of vaccine on days 0, 7, and 21 or 28 are recommended for persons at high risk of exposure to rabies virus (laboratory staff, veterinarians, animal handlers, and wildlife officers). Toddlers and children in highly endemic areas also may be considered for vaccine. A dose is either 1.0 or 0.5 ml (according to the vaccine type) standard IM or 0.1 ml ID (if antimalarial chemoprophylaxis is applied concurrently, IM injections are preferable to ID).

Persons working with rabies virus in diagnostic, research, and vaccine-production laboratories should have serum tested for neutralizing antibody every 6 months and have a booster when the titer falls below 0.5 IU/ml. People in other professions (such as veterinarians, animal handlers, and wildlife officers) who are at frequent risk of exposure to rabies should have serum testing every 2 years and receive a booster when the titer falls below 0.5 IU/ml.

▶ ACKNOWLEDGMENT

Dr. Hemachudha has been supported in part by grants from the Thai Red Cross Society, the Thailand Research Fund, and the General Prayudh Charumani, Cherdchai Wilailak, and the Phraya Athakraweesunthorn and Khunying Foundation.

REFERENCES

1. Hemachudha T, Laothamatas J, Rupprecht CE: Human rabies: A disease of complex neuropathogenetic mechanisms and diagnostic challenge. *Lancet Neurol* 1:101, 2002.
2. Rupprecht CE, Hanlon CA, Hemachudha T: Rabies re-examined. *Lancet Infect Dis* 2:327, 2002.
3. Steele J: History of rabies, in Baer G (ed): *The Natural History of Rabies,* 1st ed. New York: Academic Press, 1975, pp 1–29.
4. Wilkinson L: Understanding the nature of rabies: An historical perspective, in Campbell J, Charlton KM (eds): *Rabies.* Boston: Kluwer Academic, 1988, pp 1–23.
5. Wilkinson L: History, in Jackson A, Wunner WH (eds): *Rabies.* Amsterdam: Academic Press, 2002, pp 1–22.
6. Kaplan M, Koprowski H: Rabies. *Sci Am* 242:120, 1980.
7. Hurst E, Pawan JL: An outbreak of rabies in Trinidad. *Lancet* 2:622, 1931.
8. Baer G, Neville J, Turner GS: *Rabbis and Rabies.* Mexico City: Laboratorios Baer, 1996.
9. Zinke G: Neue Ansichten der Hundswuth, ihrer Ursachen und Folgen, nebst einer sichern Behandlungsart der von tollen Tieren gebissenen Menschen. *Gabler Jena* 16:212, 1804.
10. Negri A: Zur aetiologie der tollwuth: Die diagnose der tollwuth auf grund der neueren befunde. *Z Hug Infektkrankh* 44:519, 1903.
11. Goldwasser R, Kissling RE.: Fluorescent antibody staining of street and fixed rabies virus antigens. *Proc Soc Exp Biol Med* 98:219, 1958.
12. Debre P: *Louis Pasteur.* Baltimore: Johns Hopkins University Press, 1998.
13. Vodopija I, Clark HF: Human vaccination against rabies, in Baer G (ed): *The Natural History of Rabies.* Boca Raton, FL: CRC Press, 1991, pp 571–595.
14. Fermi C: Uber die Immunisierung gegen Wutkrankheit. *Z Hyg Infectionskrankh* 58:233, 1908.
15. Semple D: The preparation of a safe and efficient antirabic vaccine. *Sci Mem Med Sanit Dept India* 44, 1911.
16. Peck F, Powell HM, Culbertson CG: Duck-embryo rabies vaccine: Study of fixed virus vaccine grown in embryonated duck eggs and killed with beta-propriolactone. *JAMA* 162:1373, 1956.
17. Fuenzalida E, Palacios R, Borgono JM: Antibody response in man to vaccine made from infected suckling-mouse brain. *Bull WHO* 30:431, 1964.
18. Appelbaum E, Greenberg H, Nelson J: Neurologic complications following antirabies vaccine. *JAMA* 151:188, 1953.
19. Cabasso V: Local wound treatment and passive immunization, in Baer G (ed): *The Natural History of Rabies,* 2d ed. Boca Raton, FL: CRC Press, 1991, pp 551–570.
20. Baltazard M, Ghodssin M: Prevention of human rabies-treatment of persons bitten by rabid wolves. *Bull WHO* 10:797, 1954.
21. Habel K, Koprowski H: Laboratory data supporting the clinical trial of antirabies serum in person bitten by a rabid wolf. *Bull WHO* 13:773, 1955.
22. Kissling R: Growth of rabies virus in nonnervous tissue culture. *Proc Soc Trop Med Hyg* 98:223, 1958.
23. Fenje P: A rabies vaccine from hamster kidney tissue cultures: Preparation and evaluation in animals. *Can J Microbiol* 6:605, 1960.
24. Wiktor T, Fernandes MV, Koprowski H: Cultivation of rabies virus in human diploid cell strain WI-38. *J Immunol* 93:353, 1964.
25. Plotkin S, Rupprecht CE, Koprowski H: Rabies vaccine, in Plotkin S, Orenstein WA (eds.): *Vaccines,* 3d ed. Philadelphia: Saunders, 1999, pp 743–766.
26. Cleaveland S, Dye C: Maintenance of a microparasite infecting several host species: rabies in the Serengeti. *Parasitology* 111:S33, 1995.
27. Shope R: Rabies virus antigenic relationships, in Baer G (ed): *The Natural History of Rabies.* New York: Academic Press, 1975, pp 141–152.
28. Wiktor T, Koprowski H: Monoclonal antibodies against rabies virus produced by somatic cell hybridization: Detection of antigenic variants. *Proc Natl Acad Sci USA* 75:3938, 1978.
29. Rupprecht C, Dietzschold B, Wunner WH, et al: Antigenic relationship of lyssaviruses, in Baer G (ed): *The Natural History of Rabies,* 2d ed. Boca Raton, FL: CRC Press, 1991, pp 69–100.
30. Smith JS, Orciari LA, Yager PA, et al: Epidemiologic and historical relationships among 87 rabies virus isolates as determined by limited sequence analysis. *J Infect Dis* 166:296, 1992.
31. Bourhy H, Kissi B, Tordo N: Molecular diversity of the *Lyssavirus* genus. *Virology* 194:70, 1993.
32. Tordo N, Badrane H, Bourhy H, et al: Molecular epidemiology of lyssaviruses: Focus on the glycoprotein and pseudogenes. *Onderstepoort J Vet Res* 60:315, 1993.
33. Kissi B, Tordo N, Bourhy H: Genetic polymorphism in the rabies virus nucleoprotein gene. *Virology* 209:526, 1995.
34. Le Mercier P, Jacob Y, Tordo N: The complete Mokola virus genome sequence: structure of the RNA-dependent RNA polymerase. *J Gen Virol* 78:1571, 1997.

35. Smith J: Molecular epidemiology, in Jackson A, Wunner WH (eds): *Rabies*. Amsterdam: Academic Press, 2002, pp 79–111.

36. van Regenmortel M, Fauquet CM, Bishop DHL, et al: *Virus Taxonomy: Seventh Report of the International Committee on Taxonomy of Viruses*. New York: Academic Press, 1999.

37. Shope R, Murphy FA, Harrison AK, et al: Two African viruses serologically and morphologically related to rabies virus. *J Virol* 6:690, 1970.

38. Karabatsos N: *International Catalogue of Arboviruses*, 3d ed. San Antonio, TX: American Society of Tropical Medicine and Hygiene, 1985.

39. Arai Y, Kuzmin IV, Kameoka Y, et al: New *Lyssavirus* genotype from the lesser mouse-eared bat (*Myotis blythi*), Kyrghyzstan. *Emerg Infect Dis* 9:333, 2003.

40. Holmes EC, Woelk CH, Kassis R, Bourhy H: Genetic constraints and the adaptive evolution of rabies virus in nature. *Virology* 292:247, 2002.

41. Badrane H, Tordo N: Host switching in *Lyssavirus* history from the Chiroptera to the Carnivora orders. *J Virol* 75:8096, 2001.

42. Messenger SL, Smith JS, Orciari LA, et al: Emerging pattern of rabies deaths and increased viral infectivity. *Emerg Infect Dis* 9:151, 2003.

43. Wimalaratne O, Kodikara DS: First reported case of elephant rabies in Sri Lanka. *Vet Rec* 144:98, 1999.

44. Niezgoda M, Hanlon CA., Rupprecht CE: Animal rabies, in Jackson A, Wunner WH (eds): *Rabies*. Amsterdam: Academic Press, 2002, pp 163–218.

45. Constantine DG: Geographic translocation of bats: Known and potential problems. *Emerg Infect Dis* 9:17, 2003.

46. King AA, Meredith CD, Thomson GR: The biology of southern African *Lyssavirus* variants. *Curr Top Microbiol Immunol* 187:267, 1994.

47. Nel L, Jacobs J, Jaftha J, et al: New cases of Mokola virus infection in South Africa: A genotypic comparison of southern African virus isolates. *Virus Genes* 20:103, 2000.

48. Badrane H, Bahloul C, Perrin P, et al: Evidence of two *Lyssavirus* phylogroups with distinct pathogenicity and immunogenicity. *J Virol* 75:3268, 2001.

49. Armengual B, Whitby JE, King A, et al: Evolution of European bat lyssaviruses. *J Gen Virol* 78:2319, 1997.

50. Gould AR, Hyatt AD, Lunt R, et al: Characterisation of a novel *Lyssavirus* isolated from Pteropid bats in Australia. *Virus Res* 54:165, 1998.

51. Baer GM, Shaddock JH, Quirion R, et al: Rabies susceptibility and acetylcholine receptor. *Lancet* 335:664, 1990.

52. Childs JE, Colby L, Krebs JW, et al: Surveillance and spatiotemporal associations of rabies in rodents and lagomorphs in the United States, 1985–1994. *J Wildl Dis* 33:20, 1997.

53. Bogel K, Motschwiller E: Incidence of rabies and post-exposure treatment in developing countries. *Bull WHO* 64:883, 1986.

54. Singh J, Jain DC, Bhatia R, et al: Epidemiological characteristics of rabies in Delhi and surrounding areas, 1998. *Ind Pediatr* 38:1354, 2001.

55. Rotz LD, Hensley JA, Rupprecht CE, et al: Large-scale human exposures to rabid or presumed rabid animals in the United States: 22 cases (1990–1996). *J Am Vet Med Assoc* 212:1198, 1998.

56. Haupt W: Rabies: Risk of exposure and current trends in prevention of human cases. *Vaccine* 17:1742, 1999.

57. Coleman PG, Dye C: Immunization coverage required to prevent outbreaks of dog rabies. *Vaccine* 14:185, 1996.

58. PAHO: *Epidemiological Surveillance of Rabies in the Americas*. Washington: Pan American Health Organization, 2000.

59. Krebs JW, Noll HR, Rupprecht CE, et al: Rabies surveillance in the United States during 2001. *J Am Vet Med Assoc* 221:1690, 2002.

60. Childs JE, Curns AT, Dey ME, et al: Predicting the local dynamics of epizootic rabies among raccoons in the United States. *Proc Natl Acad Sci USA* 97:13666, 2000.

61. Foroutan P, Meltzer MI, Smith KA: Cost of distributing oral raccoon-variant rabies vaccine in Ohio: 1997–2000. *J Am Vet Med Assoc* 220:27, 2002.

62. Wunner W: Rabies virus, in Jackson A, Wunner WH (eds): *Rabies*. Amsterdam: Academic Press, 2002, pp 23–77.

63. Rupprecht C, Hemachudha T: Rabies, in Scheld M, Whitley RJ, Marra C (eds): *Infections of the Central Nervous System*, 3d ed, Philadelphia: Lippincott Williams and Wilkins, 2003.

64. Jackson A: Human disease, in Jackson A, Wunner WH (eds): *Rabies*. Amsterdam: Academic Press, 2002, pp 219–244.

65. Hemachudha T: Rabies, in Vinken P, Bruyn GW, Klawans HL (eds): *Handbook of Clinical Neurology,* revised series. Amsterdam: Elsevier Science, 1989, pp 383–404.

66. McKendrick A: A ninth analytical review of reports from Pasteur Institutes. *Bull WHO* 9:31, 1941.

67. Sitthi-Amorn C, Jiratanavattana V, Keoyoo J, et al: The diagnostic properties of laboratory tests for rabies. *Int J Epidemiol* 16:602, 1987.

68. Babes V: *Traite de la rage.* Paris: Bailliere, 1912.

69. Shah U, Jaswal GS: Victims of a rabid wolf bite in India: Effect of severity and location of bites on development of rabies. *J Infect Dis* 134:25, 1976.

70. World Health Organization: *WHO Recommendations on Rabies Post-Exposure Treatment and the Correct Technique of Intradermal Immunization Against Rabies* (WHO/EMC/ZOO/96.6), 1–24 ed. Geneva: World Health Organization, 1997.

71. Hattwick M: Human rabies. *Public Health Rev* 3:229, 1974.

72. Morimoto K, Patel M, Corisdeo S, et al: Characterization of a unique variant of bat rabies virus responsible for newly emerging human cases in North America. *Proc Natl Acad Sci USA* 93:5653, 1996.

73. Gibbons RV: Cryptogenic rabies, bats, and the question of aerosol transmission. *Ann Emerg Med* 39:528, 2002.

74. Noah DL, Drenzek CL, Smith JS, et al: Epidemiology of human rabies in the United States, 1980–1996. *Ann Intern Med* 128:922, 1998.

75. Crepin P, Audry L, Rotivel Y, et al: Intravitam diagnosis of human rabies by PCR using saliva and cerebrospinal fluid. *J Clin Microbiol* 36:1117, 1998.

76. Helmick C, Tauxe RV, Vernon AA.: Is there a risk to contacts of patients with rabies. *Rev Infect Dis* 9:511, 1987.

77. Fishbein DB, Robinson LE: Rabies. *New Engl J Med* 329:1632, 1993.

78. Lumbiganon P, Wasi C: Survival after rabies immunisation in newborn infant of affected mother. *Lancet* 336:319, 1990.

79. Jackson A: Pathogenesis, in Jackson A, Wunner WH (eds): *Rabies*. Amsterdam: Academic Press, 2002, pp 245–282.

80. Mass treatment of humans who drank unpasteurized milk from rabid cows—Massachusetts, 1996–1998. *MMWR* 48:228, 1999.

81. Hemachudha T, Phuapradit P: Rabies. *Curr Opin Neurol* 10:260, 1997.

82. Hanna JN, Carney IK, Smith GA, et al: Australian bat *Lyssavirus* infection: A second human case, with a long incubation period. *Med J Aust* 172:597, 2000.

83. Smith JS, Fishbein DB, Rupprecht CE, et al: Unexplained rabies in three immigrants in the United States: A virologic investigation. *New Engl J Med* 324:205, 1991.

84. Hemachudha T, Chutivongse S, Wilde H: Latent rabies. *New Engl J Med* 324:1890, 1991.

85. Kucera P, Dolivo M, Coulon P, et al: Pathways of the early propagation of virulent and avirulent rabies strains from the eye to the brain. *J Virol* 55:158, 1985.

86. Coulon P: Invasion of the peripheral nervous systems of adult mice by the CVS strain of rabies virus and its avirulent derivative Av01. *J Virol* 63:3550, 1989.

87. Shankar V, Dietzschold B, Koprowski H: Direct entry of rabies virus into the central nervous system without prior local replication. *J Virol* 65:2736, 1991.

88. Ray NB, Power C, Lynch WP, et al: Rabies viruses infect primary cultures of murine, feline, and human microglia and astrocytes. *Arch Virol* 142:1011, 1997.

89. Charlton KM: The pathogenesis of rabies and other lyssaviral infections: recent studies. *Curr Top Microbiol Immunol* 187:95, 1994.

90. Lentz TL, Burrage TG, Smith AL, et al: The acetylcholine receptor as a cellular receptor for rabies virus. *Yale J Biol Med* 56:315, 1983.

91. Lentz TL: Rabies virus binding to an acetylcholine receptor alpha-subunit peptide. *J Mol Recognit* 3:82, 1990.

92. Lentz TL: Structure-function relationships of curaremimetic neurotoxin loop 2 and of a structurally similar segment of rabies virus glycoprotein in their interaction with the nicotinic acetylcholine receptor. *Biochemistry* 30:10949, 1991.

93. Hanham CA, Zhao F, Tignor GH: Evidence from the anti-idiotypic network that the acetylcholine receptor is a rabies virus receptor. *J Virol* 67:530, 1993.

94. Lewis P, Fu Y, Lentz TL: Rabies virus entry at the neuromuscular junction in nerve-muscle cocultures. *Muscle Nerve* 23:720, 2000.

95. Charlton KM, Nadin-Davis S, Casey GA, et al: The long incubation period in rabies: Delayed progression of infection in muscle at the site of exposure. *Acta Neuropathol (Berl)* 94:73, 1997.

96. WHO Expert Committee on Rabies: *World Health Organization Technical Report Series* 824:1, 1992.

97. Tsiang H: Interaction of rabies virus and host cells, in Campbell J, Charlton KM (eds): Rabies. Boston: Kluwer Academic, 1988, pp 67–100.

98. Kelly RM, Strick PL: Rabies as a transneuronal tracer of circuits in the central nervous system. *J Neurosci Methods* 103:63, 2000.

99. Raux H, Flamand A, Blondel D: Interaction of the rabies virus P protein with the LC8 dynein light chain. *J Virol* 74:10212, 2000.

100. Jacob Y, Badrane H, Ceccaldi PE, et al: Cytoplasmic dynein LC8 interacts with *Lyssavirus* phosphoprotein. *J Virol* 74:10217, 2000.

101. Mebatsion T: Extensive attenuation of rabies virus by simultaneously modifying the dynein light chain binding site in the P protein and replacing Arg333 in the G protein. *J Virol* 75:11496, 2001.

102. Tsiang H: Pathophysiology of rabies virus infection of the nervous system. *Adv Virus Res* 42:375, 1993.

103. Tangchai P, Vejjajiva A: Pathology of the peripheral nervous system in human rabies: A study of nine autopsy cases. *Brain* 94:299, 1971.

104. Charlton KM, Casey GA, Wandeler AI, et al: Early events in rabies virus infection of the central nervous system in skunks (*Mephitis mephitis*). *Acta Neuropathol (Berl)* 91:89, 1996.

105. Etessami R, Conzelmann KK, Fadai-Ghotbi B, et al: Spread and pathogenic characteristics of a G-deficient rabies virus recombinant: An in vitro and in vivo study. *J Gen Virol* 81:2147, 2000.

106. Bingham J, van der Merwe M: Distribution of rabies antigen in infected brain material: Determining the reliability of different regions of the brain for the rabies fluorescent antibody test. *J Virol Methods* 101:85, 2002.

107. Tirawatnpong S, Hemachudha T, Manutsathit S, et al: Regional distribution of rabies viral antigen in central nervous system of human encephalitic and paralytic rabies. *J Neurol Sci* 92:91, 1989.

108. Hemachudha T: Human rabies: Clinical aspects, pathogenesis, and potential therapy. *Curr Top Microbiol Immunol* 187:121, 1994.

109. Smart NL, Charlton KM: The distribution of Challenge virus standard rabies virus versus skunk street rabies virus in the brains of experimentally infected rabid skunks. *Acta Neuropathol (Berl)* 84:501, 1992.

110. Hemachudha T, Phanuphak P, Sriwanthana B, et al: Immunologic study of human encephalitic and paralytic rabies: Preliminary report of 16 patients. *Am J Med* 84:673, 1988.

111. Jackson AC, Ye H, Phelan CC, et al: Extraneural organ involvement in human rabies. *Lab Invest* 79:945, 1999.

112. Jogai S, Radotra BD, Banerjee AK: Rabies viral antigen in extracranial organs: A postmortem study. *Neuropathol Appl Neurobiol* 28:334, 2002.

113. Hemachudha T, Mitrabhakdi E: Rabies, in Davis L,

Kennedy PGE (eds): *Infectious Diseases of the Nervous System*. Oxford, England: Butterworth-Heinemann, 2000, pp 401–444.

114. Dumrongphol H, Srikiatkhachorn A, Hemachudha T, et al: Alteration of muscarinic acetylcholine receptors in rabies virus–infected dog brains. *J Neurol Sci* 137:1, 1996.

115. Tangchai P, Yenbutr D, Vejjajiva A: Central nervous system lesions in human rabies. *J Med Assoc Thailand* 53:471, 1970.

116. Laothamatas J, Hemachudha T, Mitrabhakdi E, et al: Magnetic resonance imaging in human rabies. *Am J Neuroradiol* 24:1102, 2003.

117. Pleasure SJ, Fischbein NJ: Correlation of clinical and neuroimaging findings in a case of rabies encephalitis. *Arch Neurol* 57:1765, 2000.

118. Lopez A, Miranda P, Tejada E, et al: Outbreak of human rabies in the Peruvian jungle. *Lancet* 339:408, 1992.

119. Warner CK, Zaki SR, Shieh WJ, et al: Laboratory investigation of human deaths from vampire bat rabies in Peru. *Am J Trop Med Hyg* 60:502, 1999.

120. Hemachudha T, Wacharapluesadee S, Lumlertdaecha B, et al: Sequence analysis of rabies virus in humans exhibiting either furious or paralytic rabies. *J Infect Dis* 188:960, 2003.

121. Chopra J, Banerjee AK, Murphy JMK, et al: Paralytic rabies: A clinicopathological study. *Brain* 103:789, 1980.

122. Hemachudha T, Panpanich T, Phanuphak P, et al: Immune activation in human rabies. *Trans R Soc Trop Med Hyg* 87:106, 1993.

123. Hemachudha T, Sunsaneewitayakul B, Mitrabhakdi E, et al: Paralytic complications following intravenous rabies immune globulin treatment in a patient with furious rabies. *Int J Infect Dis* 7:76, 2003.

124. Sheikh K, Jackson AC, Ramos-Alvarez MR, et al: Paralytic rabies: Immune attack on nerve fibres containing axonally transported viral proteins (abstract). *Neurology* 501:183, 1998.

125. Camelo S, Lafage M, Galelli A, et al: Selective role for the p55 Kd TNF-alpha receptor in immune unresponsiveness induced by an acute viral encephalitis. *J Neuroimmunol* 113:95, 2001.

126. Lafon M, Lafage M, Martinez-Arends A, et al: Evidence for a viral superantigen in humans. *Nature* 358:507, 1992.

127. Dietzschold B, Morimoto K, Hooper DC: Mechanisms of virus-induced neuronal damage and the clearance of viruses from the CNS. *Curr Top Microbiol Immunol* 253:145, 2001.

128. Faber M, Pulmanausahakul R, Hodawadekar SS, et al: Overexpression of the rabies virus glycoprotein results in enhancement of apoptosis and antiviral immune response. *J Virol* 76:3374, 2002.

129. Yan X, Prosniak M, Curtis MT, et al: Silver-haired bat rabies virus variant does not induce apoptosis in the brain of experimentally infected mice. *J Neurovirol* 7:518, 2001.

130. Galelli A, Baloul L, Lafon M: Abortive rabies virus central nervous infection is controlled by T-lymphocyte local recruitment and induction of apoptosis. *J Neurovirol* 6:359, 2000.

131. Griffin D, Hardwick JM: Perspective: Virus infections and the death of neurons. *Trends Microbiol* 7:155, 1999.

132. Guigoni C, Coulon P: Rabies virus is not cytolytic for rat spinal motoneurons in vitro. *J Neurovirol* 8:306, 2002.

133. Binder G, Griffin DE: Interferon-gamma-mediated site-specific clearance of alphavirus from CNS neurons. *Science* 293:303, 2001.

134. Hemachudha T: Rabies, in Roos KL (ed): *Central Nervous System Infectious Diseases and Therapy*. New York: Marcel Dekker, 1997, pp 573–600.

135. Jackson AC, Fenton MB: Human rabies and bat bites. *Lancet* 357:1714, 2001.

136. Messenger SL, Smith JS, Rupprecht CE: Emerging epidemiology of bat-associated cryptic cases of rabies in humans in the United States. *Clin Infect Dis* 35:738, 2002.

137. Anonymous: Rabies: What can neurologists do? *Lancet Neurol* 1:73, 2002.

138. Seneviratne U: Guillain-Barré syndrome. *Postgrad Med J* 76:774, 2000.

139. Hemachudha T, Phanthumchinda K, Phanuphak P, et al: Myoedema as a clinical sign in paralytic rabies. *Lancet* 1:1210, 1987.

140. Brass D: *Rabies in Bats: Natural History and Public Health Implications*. Ridgefield, CT: Livia Press, 1994.

141. Madhusudana SN, Nagaraj D, Uday M, et al: Partial recovery from rabies in a six-year-old girl. *Int J Infect Dis* 6:85, 2002.

142. Kalita J, Misra UK: Comparison of CT scan and MRI findings in the diagnosis of Japanese encephalitis. *J Neurol Sci* 174:3, 2000.

143. Deresiewicz R, Thaler SJ, Hsu L, et al: Clinical and neuroradiographic manifestations of eastern equine encephalitis. *New Engl J Med* 336:1867, 1997.

144. Zagardo M, Shanholtz CB, Zoarski GH, et al: Rhombencephalitis caused by adenovirus: MR imaging appearance. *Am J Neuroradiol* 19:1901, 1998.

145. Vartanian T: Case records of the Massachusetts General Hospital. Weekly clinicopathological exercises. Case 1, 1999: A 53-year-old man with fever and rapid neurologic deterioration. *New Engl J Med* 340:127, 1999.

146. Falini A, Kesavadas C, Pontesilli S, et al: Differential diagnosis of posterior fossa multiple sclerosis: Neuroradiological aspects. *Neurol Sci* 22:S79, 2001.

147. Morrill P, Niezgoda M, Rupprecht CE: Use of serology in human rabies diagnosis (abstract 73). XII International Meeting on Research Advances and Rabies Control in the Americas, Oaxaca, Mexico, 2002.

148. Wacharapluesadee S, Hemachudha T: Nucleic acid sequence–based amplification in the rapid diagnosis of rabies. *Lancet* 358:892, 2001.

149. Wacharapluesadee S, Hemachudha T: Urine samples for rabies RNA detection in the diagnosis of rabies in humans. *Clin Infect Dis* 34:874, 2002.

150. Kamolvarin N, Tirawatnpong T, Rattanasiwamoke R, et al: Diagnosis of rabies by polymerase chain reaction with nested primers. *J Infect Dis* 167:207, 1993.

151. Wacharapluesadee S, Phumesin P, Lumlertdaecha B, et al: Diagnosis of rabies by use of brain tissue dried on filter paper. *Clin Infect Dis* 36:674, 2003.

152. Solomon T, Dung NM, Kneen R, et al: Japanese encephalitis. *J Neurol Neurosurg Psychiatry* 68:405, 2000.

153. Solomon T, Kneen R, Dung NM, et al: Poliomyelitis-like illness due to Japanese encephalitis virus. *Lancet* 351:1094, 1998.

154. Goh K, Tan CT, Chew NK, et al: Clinical features of Nipah virus encephalitis among pig farmers in Malaysia. *New Engl J Med* 342:1229, 2000.

155. Huang C, Liu CC, Chang YC, et al: Neurologic complications in children with enterovirus 71 infection. *New Engl J Med* 341:936, 1999.

156. Johnson RT: *Viral Infection of the Nervous System,* 2d ed. Philadelphia: Lippincott-Raven, 1998.

157. Kleinschmidt-DeMasters BK, Gilden DH: The expanding spectrum of herpesvirus infections of the nervous system. *Brain Pathol* 11:440, 2001.

158. Tan C, Goh KJ, Wong KT, et al: Relapsed and late-onset Nipah encephalitis. *Ann Neurol* 51:703, 2002.

159. Hemachudha T, Griffin DE, Giffels JJ, et al: Myelin basic protein as an encephalitogen in encephalomyelitis and polyneuritis following rabies vaccination. *New Engl J Med* 316:369, 1987.

160. Hemachudha T, Phanuphak P, Johnson RT, et al: Neurologic complications of Semple-type rabies vaccine: Clinical and immunologic studies. *Neurology* 37:550, 1987.

161. Piyasirisilp S, Schmeckpeper BJ, Chandanayingyong D, et al: Association of HLA and T-cell receptor gene polymorphisms with Semple rabies vaccine-induced autoimmune encephalomyelitis. *Ann Neurol* 45:595, 1999.

162. Jackson AC, Warrell MJ, Rupprecht CE, et al: Management of rabies in humans. *Clin Infect Dis* 36:60, 2003.

163. Hemachudha T, Mitrabhakdi E, Wilde H, et al: Additional reports of failure to respond to treatment after rabies exposure in Thailand. *Clin Infect Dis* 28:143, 1999.

164. Hemachudha T, Mitrabhakdi E, Wilde H, et al: Reply. *Clin Infect Dis* 29:1606, 1999.

165. Wilde H, Sirikawin S, Sabcharoen A, et al: Failure of postexposure treatment of rabies in children. *Clin Infect Dis* 22:228, 1996.

CHAPTER 12

Fungal Infections of the Central Nervous System

J. Andrew Alspaugh and John R. Perfect

► OVERVIEW

Fungi serve a primary role in nature in the decomposition and recycling of organic material. Many of these organisms also have been harnessed to provide additional benefit to humans, including the production of antibiotics, industrial biosynthetic processes, and the creation of various foods. Among the more than 100,000 species of fungi, only a few hundred cause human disease. Moreover, only a small percentage of these are encountered frequently by practicing physicians. However, human fungal pathogens cause significant morbidity and mortality. By many measures, the incidence of fungal diseases has increased dramatically over the

past three decades. Several factors have contributed to an increase in fungal diseases, including the movement of populations into endemic regions, such as the southwestern United States. However, the most significant factor for the rise in the incidence of human mycoses is the increased number of patients with varying defects of immunity. Antibacterial agents, cytotoxic chemotherapy, corticosteroids, organ transplantation, and human immunodeficiency virus (HIV) infection have each resulted in large numbers of compromised patients at risk for fungal disease. Also, seemingly immunocompetent individuals can acquire central nervous system (CNS) infections due to fungi such as *Cryptococcus neoformans*, *Coccidioides immitis*, and the dematiacious molds. As a result of these trends, CNS infections due to fungal pathogens are increasingly relevant in clinical practice.

The clinician faces several challenges in the diagnosis and management of fungal meningitis. CNS infections due to fungi present with varied clinical manifestations and rapidity of progression depending on the infecting organism, the CNS location of infection, and the immune state of the host. Also, traditional diagnostic methods, such as culture, may not be routinely positive. As more effective treatment options become available for these CNS infections, accurate and rapid diagnoses are imperative in these seriously ill patients. This chapter will review features in common to various types of fungal infections and focus on specific fungal species known to cause CNS disease.

▶ PATHOPHYSIOLOGY AND PATHOGENESIS

Fungal infections of the CNS most often are the result of hematogenous dissemination of fungi from primary infection elsewhere in the body. Most fungi enter the host by inhalation and establish a primary site of infection in the lungs. Among immunocompetent individuals, the initial infection is often unrecognized and resolves without the need for antifungal therapy. However, due to genetic factors or immunocompromising conditions, certain fungi are able to disseminate throughout the body and establish active sites of infection.

Candida species are notable exceptions to this. As resident colonizers of human mucosal surfaces, *Candida* species most often gain access to deeper tissues through alterations in the mucosa or skin due to wounds, intravenous catheters, or chemotherapy-induced mucositis. Immune defects, especially neutropenia or other granulocyte disorders, dramatically inhibit host clearance of *Candida* once it establishes infection in deep tissues.

Prolonged neutropenia is the major risk factor for the development of invasive aspergillosis. *Aspergillus* species are ubiquitous molds that are infrequent pathogens among immunocompetent individuals. However, *Aspergillus* species may gain access to compromised hosts through various routes, including the lungs, altered skin integrity, or mucosal lesions. Once disseminated, infections due to these molds are associated with a high mortality.

In addition to *Aspergillus* species, other nonpigmented molds also often enter the host through extrapulmonary routes. *Fusarium* species represent an increasing cause of systemic disease in neutropenic patients, and these molds may gain access to the bloodstream through paronychia or other sites of skin alteration. *Fusarium* and *Paecilomyces* species can establish primary infection at intravenous catheter sites.

In most cases, the fungal pathogen appears to seed the CNS hematogenously. However, fungal infections involving the cranial bones or sinuses can gain access to the subarachnoid space by direct extension, usually resulting in mass lesions or basilar meningitis.

Although any human fungal pathogen may, in theory, cause CNS disease in a suitably immunocompromised host, certain fungal species demonstrate a specific predilection for neural tissue and cause CNS disease as a major manifestation of their disease spectrum. Such fungi include *Cryptococcus neoformans*, *Coccidioides immitis*, and the pigmented molds (phaeohyphomycetes). Each has been implicated in causing meningitis in apparently immunocompetent hosts, and they thus may be considered primary CNS pathogens.

▶ CLINICAL FEATURES

Fungal infections of the CNS vary from rapidly progressive mold infections in neutropenic patients to indolent meningeal infections in immunocompetent hosts. However, most patients with fungal meningitis have a chronic meningitis syndrome, defined as meningitis that fails to improve or progress over 4 weeks of observation.[1] In fact, in this patient population, mycobacterial and fungal processes should be among the most likely infections considered. Most patients with fungal meningitis present initially with malaise or failure to thrive. Headache and fever are also observed commonly. As the disease progresses, lethargy, confusion, nausea, emesis, neck stiffness, and focal neurologic deficits may develop. Cranial nerve palsies, seizures, and symptoms of hydrocephalus often are present later in the course of the infection.

Given the nonspecific signs and symptoms associated with fungal meningitis, repeated clinical evaluations and cerebrospinal fluid (CSF) studies often are required before the diagnosis is evident. Symptoms may fluctuate over time, giving the temporary appearance of improvement, but without complete resolution. There are reports of cases of fungal meningitis that required several years for diagnosis. However, among immunosuppressed patients, the time course of the disease is more rapid, and the disease can progress quickly to permanent neurologic deficits and death. In cases of cryptococcal meningitis in patients with advanced HIV infection, the period of time from clinical presentation to death can be as short as a few days to weeks.[2]

▶ DIAGNOSIS

The diagnosis of fungal meningitis is considered most often in immunocompromised patients with CNS symptoms. In fact, the host is the most important factor when considering the likelihood of fungi as the cause of the

CNS infection. However, as in the case of *C. immitis,* immunocompetent individuals living in or visiting endemic areas are at risk for developing fungal meningitis.

Evaluation of the CSF yields important clues to the diagnosis of fungal meningitis. Lymphocytic pleocytosis is observed in most cases of fungal meningitis, with total cell counts in the range of 20 to 500 cells/mm^3. A predominance of neutrophils may be observed in meningitis due to *Blastomyces dermatitidis, Aspergillus* species, Zygomycetes, and *Scedosporium apiospermum.* There may be an eosinophilic pleocytosis in coccidioidal meningitis. In severely immunosuppressed patients with cryptococcal meningitis, a total CSF cell count less than 20 cells/mm^3 is well described and is associated with a poor prognosis. CSF protein concentrations are elevated in fungal meningitis. Importantly, decreased glucose concentrations in the CSF are observed frequently but not universally, and some noninfectious causes of chronic meningeal inflammation also can result in hypoglycorrhachia. In cryptococcal meningitis, the encapsulated yeast cell often can be directly visualized microscopically by counterstaining the CSF cell pellet with India ink. In other causes of fungal meningitis, it is uncommon to visualize fungi directly in the CSF. Culture of large volumes (15 to 30 ml) of CSF should be obtained, but the organism may fail to grow in culture, especially with the rapidity often demanded by the clinical deterioration of the patient. Therefore, biochemical identification of fungal components in the CSF complements culture data. Of these tests, the cryptococcal antigen test for capsular polysaccharide is the most reliable. Similar tests for *Histoplasma capsulatum* are available but less sensitive and specific. Identification of antibody response to specific fungal species can help in the diagnosis of meningitis due to *C. immitis* and *Sporothrix schenckii,* conditions in which the CSF culture is often negative. Other newer antigen assays and molecular microbiologic techniques for diagnosing fungal meningitis are being developed but are not standardized or routinely available.

Neurosurgical intervention is often required to make a timely diagnosis of fungal infections of the CNS. Meningeal biopsies or stereotactic biopsies of mass lesions may be the only means by which a diagnosis can be made. In CNS infections due to Zygomycetes and dematiacious molds, aggressive surgical therapy is the most important aspect of management.

▶ DIFFERENTIAL DIAGNOSIS

Clinical manifestations of fungal meningitis vary considerably. When they include headache, meningismus, and depressed levels of consciousness, they mimic meningeal inflammatory processes due to many conditions. The CSF profile of partially treated bacterial meningitis may be that of a lymphocytic pleocytosis

with an elevation in the protein concentration and a low glucose concentration, similar to many fungal causes of meningitis. *Mycobacterium tuberculosis* CNS disease commonly presents as a chronic basilar meningitis, frequently accompanied by cranial nerve palsies with similar CSF abnormalities to CNS mycoses. Parameningeal infections, viral meningitis, and syphilis also may have similar CSF abnormalities to fungal meningitis.

Noninfectious causes of chronic meningitis such as sarcoidosis, Behçet's disease, and carcinomatous meningitis have similar clinical symptoms to infectious etiologies and may even present with a CSF lymphocytic pleocytosis and hypoglycorrhachia. Idiopathic chronic meningitis is a poorly characterized entity and a diagnosis of exclusion. That this condition might represent several disease processes is supported by the fact that some of these patients respond to antituberculous therapy, whereas others respond to steroid treatment alone.[3,4] The varying treatments for infectious and noninfectious causes of chronic meningitis reinforce the recommendation to vigorously pursue effective diagnostic strategies in this condition.

▶ TREATMENT

Fungal meningitis always requires therapy. Conditions such as cryptococcal meningitis have been exceptionally well studied in clinical trials, and effective drug therapies are established and can result in complete cure. In contrast, meningitis due to *C. immitis* is potentially treatable but cannot be cured reliably with current therapeutic strategies. Fungal meningitis due to *Aspergillus* or Zygomycetes have very limited effective treatments. Pharmacologic and surgical options in fungal infections of the CNS are described below.

Amphotericin B

Amphotericin B has a broad antifungal spectrum of activity and was the first major advance in drug therapy of CNS fungal infections. It remains the primary treatment of most causes of fungal meningitis, especially among more seriously ill patients. In fact, this agent is the only acceptable treatment option in patients with CNS zygomycosis. Surprisingly, levels of amphotericin B in the CSF are often quite low or unmeasurable.[5,6] This observation may be explained by drug accumulation in the brain and meninges rather than in the CSF. In addition, amphotericin B has been demonstrated to possess an immunostimulatory activity that may enhance its antimicrobial effect.

To increase amphotericin B levels in the CSF, clinicians have administered amphotericin B intrathecally, either via a subcutaneous reservoir or by direct injection into the lumbar or cisternal space.[7–9] Intrathecal administration of amphotericin B at 0.25 to 0.5 mg/day has been used in the therapy of cryptococcal and coccidioidal meningitis. However, such approaches have not been studied in comparative trials and are associated with the potential for serious side effects such as arachnoiditis, cerebral vasculitis, and secondary bacterial superinfections.[9] Therefore, intrathecal amphotericin B is used only in rare instances, such as coccidioidal meningitis refractory to azole suppressive therapy, and then with great caution.

Lipid-associated formulations of amphotericin B are indicated primarily when nephrotoxicity or infusional side effects need to be minimized. These formulations appear to be reasonable, albeit expensive, alternatives to standard amphotericin B deoxycholate (Fungizone).[10] Anecdotal reports demonstrated efficacy of high-dose lipid-associated amphotericin B in zygomycosis involving the CNS.[11,12] An animal model of cryptococcal meningitis indicated that AmBisome was more effective than other formulations of amphotericin B in this experimental system. Given the ability to administer high drug doses, AmBisome was very effective in its ability to sterilize CSF in cryptococcal meningitis compared with amphotericin B deoxycholate.[10] However, no clinical comparative data have yet demonstrated that one formulation of amphotericin B is superior to others in the final outcome of curing the infection.

Flucytosine

The mechanisms by which flucytosine inhibits fungal cell growth are not completely understood. This compound likely competitively inhibits nucleoside entry into the cell. It is converted intracellularly into 5-fluorouracil, inhibiting DNA and RNA synthesis. Flucytosine is highly bioavailable, and CSF concentrations approach 85 percent of the serum levels. It possesses excellent activity against *Candida* species, *C. neoformans*, and dematiacious molds. However, the rapid development of resistance to this drug has been demonstrated both in vitro and in vivo, resulting in documented treatment failures when used as a single agent.[13,14] Clinically, this could be particularly problematic in CNS infections in which prolonged antimicrobial therapy may be required. Therefore, flucytosine should be used only in combination therapy with other antifungals. The addition of flucytosine to amphotericin B has been documented to improve survival and fungal clearance in cryptococcal meningitis and to reduce the incidence of relapsing disease.[15–17] This drug possesses excellent activity against many *Candida* species. It also has been demonstrated to reduce mortality when added to other antifungals in animal models of cerebral phaeohyphomycosis.[18]

Flucytosine is eliminated primarily unchanged in the urine. Therefore, renal insufficiency can result in drug accumulation and toxicity, especially hematologic side effects and hepatic injury. Drug levels should be monitored to ensure adequate dosing and to minimize side effects.

Azoles

Fluconazole

Fluconazole is a triazole antifungal with excellent CNS penetration.[19,20] It is an important treatment option in meningitis due to *C. neoformans*, *Candida* species, and *C. immitis*. This drug has both intravenous and oral forms and displays excellent oral bioavailability. It has few serious side effects and generally is well tolerated.

Fluconazole alone or in combination with flucytosine has been used in the primary management of cryptococcal meningitis, and although success rates are reasonable, its rapidity of activity is probably inferior to amphotericin-based regimens for the initial treatment of cryptococcal meningitis.[15] Although fluconazole is not recommended as first-line therapy for the initial treatment of cryptococcal infections, it plays a crucial role in subsequent maintenance therapy for this disease, especially in the lifelong secondary prophylaxis required in patients with acquired immunodeficiency syndrome (AIDS).[21] Furthermore, in developing countries in which intravenous therapy is not practical, oral fluconazole for the primary therapy of AIDS-associated cryptococcosis has been profoundly beneficial.[22] Fluconazole is also indicated in the lifelong secondary suppression required for coccidioidal meningitis. Prior to the use of fluconazole, intermittent intrathecal amphotericin B was the mainstay of therapy in this disease.

Itraconazole

Compared with fluconazole, itraconazole possesses increased antifungal potency against certain molds, especially *Aspergillus* species[23] and endemic dimorphic fungi such as *H. capsulatum*, *B. dermatitidis,* and *C. immitis.* However, its oral bioavailability and CSF penetration are limited.[24] This drug nonetheless has been used to successfully treat cryptococcal meningitis in patients with AIDS, perhaps due to its lipophilic nature allowing avid host cell binding and intracellular accumulation.[25,26] It is clearly less effective than fluconazole in the suppressive phase of CNS cryptococcosis,[17] perhaps due to inconsistent bioavailability of the oral regimen. Itraconazole does have an intravenous formulation that has not been studied extensively in the management of fungal meningitis. Therefore, for CNS mycoses, itraconazole most often is used only as a second-line agent in cryptococcal and coccidioidal meningitis in patients intolerant of fluconazole.

Voriconazole

Voriconazole is an expanded-spectrum triazole with excellent antifungal activity against a variety of yeasts and molds. Its CNS penetration exceeds that of itraconazole, and it is well-absorbed from the gastrointestinal tract. Importantly, this agent displays significant activity against *Aspergillus, Fusarium, Scedosporium,* and dematiacious mold species.[27,28] Historically, mold infections of the CNS have been exceptionally difficult to treat, even with amphotericin B.[29] Voriconazole has been used successfully to treat CNS aspergillosis and scedosporiosis.[28,30–32] As more clinical experience is accumulated with this agent, it is likely to become the drug of choice for the treatment of susceptible mold infections in the CNS. It remains uncertain whether this agent in combination with other antifungals will improve the outcome of CNS mold infections. Importantly, the zygomycete molds are not treated effectively by currently available azoles.

Ketoconazole

Prior to introduction of more effective antifungal therapy, ketoconazole was used extensively for the treatment of systemic mycoses due to endemic fungi and *Candida.*[33] Its CNS penetration, however, is poor. Despite accelerated dosing schedules, ketoconazole has been incompletely effective against cryptococcal and coccidioidal meningitis.[34,35] High drug doses also were associated with a significant incidence of side effects. Because of better azole options today, ketoconazole is not commonly used for CNS mycoses.

Miconazole

Miconazole is an imidazole used primarily for topical treatment of cutaneous infections due to dermatophytes and *Candida.* It is not absorbed from the gastrointestinal (GI) tract, and although there is an intravenous formulation of miconazole, it does not penetrate well into the CNS. Early studies demonstrated some activity against CNS mycoses when injected intrathecally,[36,37] but this drug is not currently used for invasive fungal infections.

Echinocandins

Caspofungin

Caspofungin is the first of several echinocandins that will become available in the near future. Caspofungin has excellent antifungal activity against several *Candida* species, and it also has activity against *Aspergillus* and other molds. There are no data on caspofungin use in *Candida* CNS infections, and current data indicate minimal CNS penetration for this drug. Therefore, caspofungin is unlikely to play a major role as monotherapy for fungal meningitis caused by molds, but it may potentiate the effect of other antifungals in combination therapy. Caspofungin has no significant clinical activity in *Cryptococcus* infections and will not be used in the treatment of this disease.

Role of Neurosurgery

Neurosurgical biopsies may be necessary to make a definitive diagnosis of fungal meningitis. Once the diagnosis is made, surgery plays a primary role in the treatment of CNS mycoses due to several molds, including the Zygomycetes and dematiacious molds. In fact, in retrospective studies of cerebral phaeohyphomycosis, complete surgical resection was the only intervention associated with improved survival.[38] Fungal mass lesions in the CNS greater than 3 cm and particularly mold infections should be considered for surgical debridement to allow for a complete cure. Clearly, the lesion needs to be surgically accessible. Also, complete resection is often not feasible, requiring debulking of the lesion followed by aggressive antifungal chemotherapy.

Hydrocephalus can complicate fungal meningitis, requiring neurosurgical shunt procedures. Once a patient is receiving antifungal therapy, placing a shunt when necessary does not compromise the management of fungal meningitis. A ventriculosotomy can be used during therapy and then be converted to a ventriculoperitoneal shunt.

▶ PREVENTION

Fungal CNS infections could, in theory, be prevented by multiple interventions, including vaccination strategies to prevent primary or reactivation fungal disease, elimination of latent fungi, immune reconstitution, or prevention of exposure of highly susceptible patient populations to primary infection. A vaccine was developed for *C. neoformans,* but it has never been validated in human trials.[39] Vaccines for endemic fungi, especially *C. immitis,* are being actively pursued.

The largest impact on reducing fungal infections in patients with AIDS has been the introduction of highly active antiretroviral therapy and subsequent immune reconstitution.[40] However, prior to the current era of combination antiretrovirals, the incidence of symptomatic cryptococcal disease in HIV-infected patients was significantly reduced in patients who had taken at least 1 year of fluconazole. This effect may be due to inhibition or killing of dormant fungi or by prevention of new primary infections.[41,42]

The use of antifungal therapy during periods of greatest immunosuppression has been studied widely among patients with bone marrow and solid-organ transplants to prevent symptomatic fungal disease.[43,44] Disinfection of patient areas in bone marrow transplant units reduces the mean air concentrations of various molds, including *Aspergillus* species, *F. solani,* dematiacious molds, and *Penicillium* species.[45] The impact that this latter intervention will have on the incidence of systemic fungal infections is not yet known.

▶ SPECIFIC FUNGAL INFECTIONS

Cryptococcus neoformans

The encapsulated yeast *C. neoformans* is the most common cause of fungal meningitis. Human disease due to *C. neoformans* was first described over 100 years ago (Busse, 1894). During the next two decades, meningoencephalitis became a prominent clinical manifestation of this disease. Due to the HIV epidemic, the incidence of *C. neoformans* disease has increased dramatically to the point that it is now one of the most common CNS microbial pathogens worldwide.

Epidemiology

There was an increase in the reported incidence of systemic mycoses, including cryptococcosis, in selected hospitals during the 1960s and 1970s.[46] Most explanations for this include the associated rise in immunosuppressed patient populations due to increased corticosteroid use, cytotoxic chemotherapy for malignancies, and more aggressive immunosuppression for organ transplantation. In the 1980s, a dramatic increase in the rates of cryptococcal disease was reported in the United States and certain African countries, directly attributable to the HIV epidemic. Prior to the introduction of highly active antiretroviral therapy (HAART), several U.S. cities reported rates of cryptococcal disease of 17 to 66 per 1000 patients with AIDS. In countries with a very high prevalence of HIV infection, 15 to 30 percent of patients diagnosed with AIDS-related opportunistic infections had cryptococcosis.

The more industrialized nations have witnessed a steady decrease in the incidence of cryptococcosis since introduction of combination therapy for HIV disease.[40–47] However, since most of the HIV-infected population worldwide does not have access to antiretroviral therapy, cryptococcal meningitis remains a serious opportunistic infection in untreated patients with AIDS.[2]

C. neoformans is a free-living fungus found throughout the world, often isolated from soil associated with decaying trees or avian excreta. Three varieties of this yeast have been described, each associated with unique environmental niches and clinical manifestations of disease. *C. neoformans* var. *grubii* (or serotype A) strains are isolated mostly from temperate climates, and they represent the most common clinical isolates, especially in people with AIDS. *C. neoformans* var. *neoformans* (serotype D) is reported primarily from Europe and some regions of the United States. The third variety, *C. neoformans* var. *gattii* (serotypes B and C), is isolated primarily from tropical and subtropical regions of Australia, Southeast Asia, Africa, and California in association with flowering trees such as eucalyptus species and firs. All varieties display a predilection for causing disease in the CNS, but the latter variety is more likely to cause disease in immunologically normal individuals and to manifest with cryptococcal abscesses (cryptococcomas) and hydrocephalus.

There is a strong association between HIV infection and cryptococcal disease due to strains of serotype A and D; however, the mechanism of this observation is incompletely understood. In regions of the world such as Central Africa, cryptococcosis prior to widespread HIV disease was due primarily to var. *gattii* strains. However, with the introduction of endemic HIV infection into these populations, disease due to *C. neoformans* var. *gattii* has practically vanished. Almost all cryptococcosis in these regions is now due to serotype A and D strains. In fact, this observation has provided indirect evidence for the timing of the introduction of HIV into these areas of the world.[48]

Pathogenesis

C. neoformans is introduced as a small yeast or spore into the host by inhalation. Once the infectious propagule has reached the lung, it germinates and establishes the primary site of infection. The resulting inflammatory response to the yeast cells often involves the lung and the regional lymph node, similar to a Ghon focus of primary pulmonary tuberculosis.[49] In most patients this inflammatory response completely limits spread of the organism from this site. However, fungal cells that are not killed by the host response can remain dormant for years, capable of reactivation when host immunity wanes. Primary pulmonary *C. neoformans* infections in immunologically normal individuals often are asymptomatic and self-limited, but clinically apparent pneumonia can occur, often resolving over weeks to months without specific therapy.[50] Immunosuppressed patients can develop progressive and diffuse pneumonia that requires antifungal therapy.

If the yeast cells are not contained by the host immune response, *C. neoformans* gains access to the blood through thoracic lymph channels. Disseminated disease has been described in a variety of organs and tissues. However, this fungus displays a remarkable tropism for the CNS. The specific mechanisms by which *C. neoformans* crosses the blood-brain barrier have not been defined, but the existence of a receptor on CNS cells for ligands on the yeast cells has been proposed.[51]

In order to survive in the host, *C. neoformans* induces the expression of phenotypes demonstrated to be required for pathogenesis. In response to physiologic concentrations of CO_2 and iron, *C. neoformans* cells produce a large polysaccharide capsule.[52,53] The capsule likely serves several functions, including inhibition of phagocytosis, activation of complement proteins, and direct inhibition of leukocytes. Genetic studies of capsular and hypocapsular mutant strains have demonstrated that the induction of this phenotype is required for pathogenesis in animal models of *C. neo-*

formans disease.[54,55] Additionally, a mutant clone isolated from a virulent clinical isolate was demonstrated to retain capsular polysaccharide but was unable to regulate capsule synthesis in response to CO_2. This strain was unable to survive in the subarachnoid space of rabbits, indicating that appropriate capsule regulation, and not merely the presence of capsule, is required to establish and maintain a CNS infection in the host.[52]

In addition to capsule, *C. neoformans* also induces the expression of a laccase enzyme in response to host physiologic conditions.[56] The activity of this enzyme is associated with melanin production by the yeast cell. The biosynthetic pathway of melanin in *C. neoformans* requires diphenolic substances such as dopamine, epinephrine, and norepinephrine. These compounds are found at higher concentrations in the CNS than elsewhere in the body, perhaps offering one mechanism for the neurotropism of this organism. Diphenolic compounds are not required for the growth of *C. neoformans*, but they do allow it to make melanin. *C. neoformans* has been demonstrated to make melanin in vivo, and mutant strains that are unable to produce melanin are avirulent in animal models. Melanin-deficient strains are also more susceptible to reactive nitrogen and oxygen compounds. Therefore, cryptococcal melanin may act as an antioxidant to protect this fungus from immune effector mechanisms involving oxidative and nitrosative damage.

Both cell-mediated and humoral immune responses are important aspects of the host defense in cryptococcal meningitis. A vigorous TH_1 immune response is important for the clearance of this infection. In humans and in animal models, CD4 lymphocyte depletion results in ineffective clearance of *C. neoformans* cells and allows dissemination from the initial site of infection.[57,58] Therefore, patients with AIDS or idiopathic CD4 lymphopenia have a dramatically increased risk of symptomatic cryptococcal disease. The genetic defects in cellular immunity in beige, nude, and SCID mice strain backgrounds result in increased susceptibility to *C. neoformans* infection.[59,60] Natural killer (NK) cells in animal models are required for effective clearance of a primary *C. neoformans* infection.[61] Also, the passive transfer of cytotoxic lymphocytes offers protection in experimental cryptococcosis.[62] Additionally, macrophage activation likely plays a central role in immunity to cryptococcosis. Activated macrophages are fungistatic for *C. neoformans* cells in vitro, and the appearance of activated macrophages in the CSF of infected rabbits correlates with clearance of these yeast cells from the CNS.[63]

Humoral aspects of immunity also help protect against *C. neoformans* infections. Alterations in the complement system have been demonstrated to predispose to the dissemination of *C. neoformans* cells from the lung to the CNS in experimental systems.[64] Both IgG

and C3b bind to capsular components and enhance phagocytosis. Passive administration of a monoclonal antibody directed against capsular components resulted both in prolongation of survival in a murine model of cryptococcosis and in decreased tissue burden of organisms.[65,66] However, immunization with polysaccharide capsule did not protect rabbits against *C. neoformans* cells injected intrathecally, even though these animals developed high titers of anticapsular antibodies.[67] Importantly, patients with primary disorders of antibody production do not develop cryptococcosis as frequently as patients with AIDS or CD4 lymphopenia. Therefore, humoral immunity is an important aspect of host resistance to *C. neoformans* infections but likely must act in concert with cellular immunity components for optimal host protection.

Clinical Manifestations

Most patients with cryptococcal meningitis have fever and headache, often lasting for more than 1 week. Cranial neuropathies are described frequently in later stages of disease as a result of basilar meningitis. Visual changes can be due to optic neuritis or impairment of ocular mobility. Initial presentations with subacute dementia are also reported. Although this disease was described classically to proceed in a subacute or chronic form, patients with advanced AIDS may present with a rapidly progressive neurologic syndrome. In fact, in developing nations with a high incidence of HIV disease, the median time between initial presentation and death due to cryptococcosis was 14 days, with only 22 percent of these patients surviving more than 30 days without treatment.[68]

Diagnosis

The laboratory diagnosis of cryptococcal meningitis is perhaps the most rapid and reliable among all the CNS mycoses. In contrast to other causes of fungal meningitis, encapsulated *C. neoformans* cells are visualized microscopically when the CSF cell pellet is counterstained with India ink in approximately 50 percent of all cases and in more than 80 percent of patients with AIDS-associated cryptococcal meningitis.[69,70] The organism can be cultured routinely from CSF. Additionally, the latex agglutination assay and the enzyme-linked immunosorbent assay (ELISA) for *C. neoformans* polysaccharide antigens in the CSF are sensitive and specific tests for cryptococcal meningitis.[71,72] The cryptococcal antigen test also can be performed on serum samples; if this test is positive, CNS disease must be assumed or ruled out by CSF examination. Although the antigen tests are excellent for diagnosing cryptococcal disease, their usefulness in subsequent monitoring of clinical progress is unclear because capsular components may be present after the infection is completely cured. Other CSF parameters, such as hypoglycorrhachia and pleocytosis, are also often present and may offer insight into prognosis.[73]

Treatment

Cryptococcal meningitis always should be treated. Although there have been reports of prolonged survival in patients with this disease prior to effective antifungal chemotherapy,[74] cryptococcal meningitis is eventually uniformly fatal. Current treatment options have been developed and studied in prospective and randomized trials.[15,16] The optimal treatment for cryptococcal meningitis entails three phases: induction, clearance, and maintenance. Initial induction therapy should result in rapid sterilization of the CSF. Amphotericin B (0.7 to 1 mg/kg daily) with flucytosine (100 mg/kg daily in four divided doses) has performed best in clinical trials as induction therapy[15,16,75] and should be continued for at least 2 weeks, until CSF cultures are negative.

After induction therapy, several options are available for complete clearance of the infection. Prolonged administration of amphotericin B for a total of 6 to 10 weeks has resulted in acceptable cure rates in immunocompetent patients. However, high-dose oral fluconazole (400 mg daily) for at least 10 weeks after induction therapy also may be used if negative CSF cultures can be documented. This latter option is attractive in order to minimize the length of intravenous therapy with its associated costs and adverse side effects. Maintenance-phase therapy for cryptococcosis is required indefinitely in all patients with AIDS. Most patients are maintained on lower dose oral fluconazole (100 to 200 mg daily), although itraconazole is an acceptable alternative in patients who do not tolerate fluconazole.[17] Intravenous or intrathecal amphotericin B currently is used only in unusual circumstances for secondary prophylaxis. In patients with AIDS who experience immune reconstitution with antiretroviral therapy, studies are attempting to determine whether secondary prophylaxis may be able to be discontinued if viral replication is completely inhibited. However, the details and long-term effects of this intervention have yet to be defined. Since the period of highest risk for relapsing disease is during the first few months after therapy is initiated, 6 to 12 months of fluconazole maintenance therapy in all patients with cryptococcal meningitis is recommended. This is especially important for patients who do not have HIV infection but do have other types of immunodeficiency states such as organ transplantation. However, cost issues and drug side effects must be carefully and individually considered.

Lipid formulations of amphotericin B have excellent activity against *C. neoformans*. AmBisome 4 mg/kg daily or ABLC 5 mg/kg daily can be substituted for amphotericin B deoxycholate in patients with cryptococcal meningitis with renal insufficiency.[10]

Fluconazole plays an important role in both the clearance and maintenance phases of cryptococcal disease, but it is inferior to amphotericin B–based regimens as initial induction therapy.[15] However, in regions of the world where resource limitation does not currently allow prolonged intravenous therapies, oral fluconazole monotherapy has resulted in dramatic improvements in mortality from cryptococcal meningitis.[22]

Coccidioides immitis

C. immitis is a primary human fungal pathogen endemic in desert regions of the southwestern United States and Mexico. Residents and visitors to these areas are frequently exposed to this fungus by the inhalation of infectious arthroconidia. Once inhaled, *C. immitis* conidia germinate in the lungs, most often resulting in an asymptomatic or self-limited respiratory infection known as *valley fever*. Infrequently, dissemination from the primary pulmonary focus of infection occurs. Among patients with disseminated disease, the CNS is involved in approximately one-third of cases. Certain ethnic groups, such as African-Americans and some populations from Southeast Asia, as well as patients with immunocompromising disorders, are at an increased risk for the developing disseminated disease and thus for coccidioidal meningitis. Without treatment, CNS infections due to *C. immitis* are most often fatal. Even when treated effectively, these infections require lifelong antifungal therapy to prevent recrudescent disease.

Clinical Manifestations

Coccidioidal meningitis most frequently manifests as headache, with or without accompanying signs of chronic basilar meningitis, such as cranial nerve palsies or alterations in consciousness. Less commonly, the CNS involvement presents as a meningoencephalitis, with focal neurologic defects resulting from parenchymal brain injury. Intracranial mass lesions, cerebral vasculitis, and communicating hydrocephalus resulting from coccidioidal infections also have been described uncommonly. Interestingly, *C. immitis* infection of facial skin may correlate with an increased relative risk of CNS involvement compared with skin involvement in other areas of the body.

Diagnosis

The diagnosis of coccidioidal meningitis requires a high index of suspicion among people with CNS disease living in endemic areas or among travelers to these areas. CSF findings typically demonstrate a lymphocytic pleocytosis, with white blood cell (WBC) counts ranging from 20 to 500 cells/ml; however, early disease can be accompanied by a predominance of neutrophils in the CSF. Interestingly, *C. immitis* can result in a CSF eosinophilia in approximately 70 percent of meningitis cases, an unusual finding in other types of fungal meningitis.[76] Spherules, the tissue form of *C. immitis*, are rarely visualized in the CSF.

Cultures of the CSF for the infecting organism are only positive in 25 percent of cases, making this diagnostic test quite limited in its utility. Complement-fixation tests and ELISA of CSF for anticoccidioidal antibodies may complement culture results and should be performed in patients with chronic meningitis and an appropriate exposure history. The detection of antibodies against the 33-kDa antigen from *C. immitis* spherules has a sensitivity of 72 percent and a specificity of 99 percent for *C. immitis* CNS infection.[77] Rarely, a parameningeal focus of *C. immitis* infection can result in a false-positive CSF antibody test.

Treatment

Previously, intravenous and intrathecal amphotericin B were moderately successful in the treatment of CNS disease due to *C. immitis*. However, introduction of the azoles has significantly improved the therapeutic options for coccidioidal meningitis. Recently, published treatment guidelines recommend high-dose fluconazole (400 to 800 mg daily) as initial induction therapy for coccidioidal meningitis.[78] The duration of this initial induction therapy is variable but, if successful, should be followed by lower doses of fluconazole indefinitely (200 to 400 mg daily). Among patients with coccidioidal meningitis who discontinued antifungal therapy, observational studies indicated that 78 percent experience relapsing disease. Thus CNS infection due to *C. immitis* is not routinely curable, and lifelong secondary prophylaxis in all patients is recommended.[79] The exceptional CSF penetration of fluconazole makes this antifungal agent the currently preferred azole for this condition, although itraconazole has been used with some success.

The newer triazoles, such as voriconazole and posaconazole, have excellent activity against *C. immitis* but have not been studied adequately in human trials to allow them to be considered as first-line therapy. Animal studies have demonstrated moderate activity of the echinocandin caspofungin against *C. immitis*,[80] but the limited CNS penetration of this drug and the lack of clinical data in CNS mycoses do not yet support a role for this class of drugs in coccidioidal meningitis.

Treatment failures are not uncommon and may require intrathecal administration of amphotericin B in addition to continued azole therapy. In fact, some clinicians advocate intrathecal amphotericin B in all initial regimens. However, the dose and frequency of intrathecal amphotericin B administration have not been well defined.[78] All patients who respond to induction therapy that includes an azole should be treated with this medication indefinitely to prevent relapsing disease. Rarely, patients require intermittent administration of intrathecal amphotericin B as secondary prophylaxis. Hydrocephalus can be observed as a late complication of coccidioidal meningitis, even with sterilization of the CSF. A ventriculostomy followed by a ventriculoperitoneal shunt may be required for treatment of this complication.

Histoplasma capsulatum

H. capsulatum has been isolated throughout the world, most often from soil associated with bird habitats. The most endemic areas of the world are the Mississippi/Ohio River valleys and regions of Central and South America. Humans in these endemic areas frequently are exposed to infectious propagules through inhalation into the lungs. Local outbreaks of symptomatic pulmonary infections due to *H. capsulatum* are often associated with construction, excavation, or other instances when large amounts of contaminated soil are aerosolized. Interestingly, pulmonary calcifications identified by chest radiographs previously were assumed to be synonymous with tuberculosis. However, in endemic areas, this finding is most frequently due to healed pulmonary histoplasmosis.[81]

Most cases of *H. capsulatum* pulmonary disease resolve without specific therapy. However, this fungus resides in mononuclear cells and can remain in a dormant state for many years. Symptomatic disseminated disease, during the primary or reactivated infection, is observed in patients with normal immune systems. However, populations with decreased cellular immunity are at a significantly increased risk for the development of extrapulmonary disease. CNS involvement occurs in 10 to 20 percent of patients with disseminated histoplasmosis.[82]

Clinical Manifestations

Disseminated histoplasmosis occurs most frequently in patients with profound defects in cellular immunity, such as late-stage HIV infection or organ transplantation.[83,84] Symptoms of this progressive infection result from end-organ involvement and often also include fever and malaise. Hepatosplenomegaly, cytopenias, lymphadenopathy, and mucosal ulcerations are among the most frequent findings.

CNS infection due to *H. capsulatum* presents most frequently as a chronic meningitis, with headache and possibly altered sensorium. This syndrome also can manifest with seizures, encephalitis, or mass lesions of the brain or spinal cord. Additionally, asymptomatic CNS involvement has been observed infrequently in patients with disseminated histoplasmosis.

Diagnosis

The limitations of laboratory testing in *H. capsulatum* meningitis underscore the importance of maintaining a high index of suspicion for disseminated histoplasmosis in immunocompromised patients from endemic regions. *H. capsulatum* may be cultured from blood and bone marrow in patients with disseminated histoplasmosis. The characteristic yeast form also can be observed in bone marrow biopsy specimens, buffy coat smears, and biopsies from involved organs. Identification of *H. capsulatum* antigens from serum and urine provides a sensitive and specific test for disseminated histoplasmosis in immunocompromised patients.

Radiologic studies may indicate the presence of a mass lesion in the brain or spinal cord due to *H. capsulatum*. However, there are no specific findings for this infection. In fact, focal CNS lesions due to *H. capsulatum* often have been mistaken for malignancies or abscesses.

The CSF from patients with *H. capsulatum* meningitis frequently demonstrates a mononuclear pleocytosis, increased total protein concentration, and a decreased glucose concentration.[85] Culture of the CSF for *H. capsulatum* is not a sensitive test in meningitis and is positive only in a minority of true cases of disease.[85,86] It is recommended that large volumes of CSF (15 to 20 ml) be obtained to improve the sensitivity of cultures. To complement fungal cultures, several investigators have proposed direct testing of the CSF for *H. capsulatum* antigens as well as antibodies against this fungus. Although there have been reports of cross-reactivity with *C. immitis* and *C. neoformans* in histoplasma serologic tests of CSF, such studies are often helpful in establishing a correct diagnosis.[86–88] Since meningitis often occurs as one component of a progressive systemic infection, tests for disseminated histoplasmosis also should be pursued to complement CNS-specific tests.[82]

Treatment

Patients with meningitis due to *H. capsulatum* should be treated with intravenous amphotericin B (0.7 to 1.0 mg/kg daily). Lipid-associated forms of amphotericin B have not demonstrated superiority to the standard drug formulation in this condition, but their use is recommended in patients with renal dysfunction or in combination with other nephrotoxic agents. Treatment generally continues to a target of approximately 30 mg/kg amphotericin B and should be guided by frequently repeated lumbar punctures to demonstrate microbiologic cure as well as resolution of CSF abnormalities.[82,85] Despite this aggressive therapy, relapses occur in as many of 50 percent of patients. In selected patients with progressive symptoms and focal CNS lesions, surgical resection may be warranted.[82]

Adjunctive therapy with ketoconazole and itraconazole has limited utility for meningitis due to the poor CSF penetration of these agents. However, use of these azoles may be warranted for long-term treatment of the disseminated infection. In contrast, fluconazole achieves excellent CNS levels, but the activity of this drug against *H. capsulatum* is limited. In fact, animal models of *Histoplasma* meningitis demonstrated antagonism when fluconazole and amphotericin B were used in combination compared with amphotericin B alone.[89,90] Newer triazoles, such as voriconazole and posaconazole, have CNS penetration and excellent activity against *H. capsulatum* but have untested benefit in this disease.

Blastomyces dermatitidis

B. dermatitidis is a free-living fungus isolated in many areas of the world. In the United States, *B. dermatitidis* is endemic in the Southeast as well as in states bordering the Great Lakes and the Mississippi, Ohio, and St. Lawrence rivers. Outdoor activities, especially associated with waterways, predispose to infection. Interestingly, dogs can become naturally infected in endemic areas. Humans become infected most frequently through the pulmonary route. Although most pulmonary infections resolve spontaneously, symptomatic primary lung infections frequently present as a chronic pneumonia that is unresponsive to empirical antibacterial therapy. Extrapulmonary disease, although uncommon, most often includes infection of the skin, bones, and genitourinary tract. CNS involvement in blastomycosis is uncommon, occurring primarily as a late manifestation of untreated disseminated disease.

Clinical Manifestations

CNS involvement by *B. dermatitidis* can present as a chronic meningitis with headache, lethargy, and meningismus. However, in contrast to *C. neoformans*, *B. dermatitidis* CNS infection more commonly results in abscess formation and mass lesions in the brain and spinal cord presenting with focal neurologic deficits, alterations of consciousness, and seizures. Meningitis often occurs in association with other signs of disseminated blastomycosis such as pneumonitis, genitourinary infection, and pyogranulomatous skin lesions. Systemic signs typically include fever and weight loss.

Diagnosis

Historically, the diagnosis of meningitis due to *B. dermatitidis* has been difficult. Examination of the CSF typically reveals an elevated opening pressure, elevated protein concentration, low glucose concentration, and a lymphocytic pleocytosis. However, neutrophils may predominate in the CSF early in the clinical course of *B. dermatitidis* meningitis.[91] Fungal forms are not typically visualized by direct examination of CSF, but cytology occasionally has been used to make this diagnosis.[92] Culture of the CSF is rarely positive for the causative fungus. Large-volume samples from lumbar punctures, as well as ventricular or cisternal punctures, have been advocated to improve the diagnostic yield of cultures when blastomycosis is strongly considered.[93,94] Stereotactic biopsies of mass lesions or meningeal biopsy may be required to make a definitive diagnosis.

Extraneural evidence of blastomycosis also should be pursued to complement the CSF examination. Thorough evaluations of the lungs should be done for infectious processes. Importantly, pulmonary blastomycosis rarely results in calcifications, in contrast to histoplasmosis and tuberculosis. The skin, joints, and genitourinary tract also should be assessed carefully for associated lesions.

Treatment

All patients with CNS blastomycosis should be treated with intravenous amphotericin B (0.7 to 1.0 mg/kg daily) to a target cumulative dose of at least 2 g.[95] Lipid formulations of amphotericin B have not been studied adequately in this syndrome, but they likely can be used in patients who are intolerant of standard amphotericin B preparations, who are being treated with other nephrotoxic agents, or who have preexisting renal dysfunction.

Itraconazole is currently recommended for the treatment of mild to moderate disseminated blastomycosis that does not involve the CNS. However, due to the poor CNS penetration of both itraconazole and ketoconazole, these agents should not be used for the primary treatment of *B. dermatitidis* meningitis. Fluconazole at high doses (400 to 800 mg daily) was demonstrated to be effective in non-life-threatening blastomycosis,[96] but patients with CNS blastomycosis were not included in this study. Its relatively limited activity against *B. dermatitidis* makes high-dose fluconazole (800 mg daily) a second-tier option for CNS blastomycosis and for use only in extraordinary circumstances.[97] Fluconazole may, however, be useful in consolidation therapy after initial amphotericin B therapy, but this has yet to be tested clinically. Newer azoles, such as voriconazole, are active against *B. dermatitidis* and have adequate CNS penetration. These agents have the potential to be primary therapies for CNS blastomycosis, but their clinical utility in this infection is currently untested.

Patients with certain immunodeficiency disorders, especially HIV infection, have high rates of relapse after therapy for blastomycosis.[97] These patients may benefit from long-term secondary prophylaxis after an aggressive primary treatment course. Azoles with good CNS penetration, such as fluconazole, may be useful in this role to prevent recurrent CNS blastomycosis.[95]

In addition to medical therapy, surgery may be required for diagnosis and management of patients with CNS blastomycosis, especially if mass lesions are present. Neurosurgical shunting also may be required for hydrocephalus complicating these infections. Rarely, osteomyelitis associated with *B. dermatitidis* CNS infections that does not respond to medical therapy also may require surgical debridement.[98]

Candida

Epidemiology

In contrast to many of the other human fungal pathogens, *Candida* species are often isolated as commensal microbial flora in immunocompetent individuals. In such patients, candidal disease primarily involves mucosal and skin infections without invasion of deeper structures or distant spread. However, *Candida* species also represent the most common causes of systemic mycoses, occurring mostly in patients with immunosuppression or alterations of the integument or mucosal surfaces. Although *Candida albicans* is the most common *Candida* species isolated from patients, other species such as *C. glabrata*, *C. tropicalis*, *C. parapsilosis*, and *C. lusitaniae* are increasingly identified pathogens and have been reported to cause CNS disease.[99–103]

Perhaps due to incomplete development of the blood-brain barrier or to the degree of fungemia, CNS infection resulting from candidemia is much more common in very young children than in adults. In a recent study from the Slovak Republic, 8 of 40 neonates with candidemia also were found to have concurrent candidal meningitis.[104] In some studies, *C. albicans* was the most common fungal isolate from the CSF of neonates and young children.[104,105] Most *Candida* isolates from CSF are obtained from premature neonates, children with chemotherapy-induced neutropenia, and as a result of neurosurgical procedures or head trauma.[106] One retrospective review of CNS fungal infections in Japanese patients reported *C. albicans* in 6 of 129 CSF cultures.[107]

Neutrophils are the primary immune effector cells responsible for preventing systemic infections with *Candida* species. Therefore, neutropenia is a major risk factor for candidal infections, including meningitis. Additionally, acquired and congenital neutrophil defects, such as myeloperoxidase deficiency and chronic granulomatous disease, also result in an increased risk for meningitis due to *Candida* species.[108,109] Any patient who spontaneously develops meningitis due to *Candida* probably should be evaluated for neutrophil disorders.

Patients with HIV infection also have been reported to develop *Candida* meningitis; however, most of these patients had additional risks for systemic mycoses such as neutropenia, trauma, or prior antibiotic use.[110,111] Chronic neutrophilic meningitis due to *C. albicans* has been described among intravenous drug users, with several weeks to months intervening between the onset of symptoms and diagnosis.[112]

Indwelling CNS devices such as ventriculostomy tubes or CNS shunts are also risk factors for the development of *Candida* meningitis.[113,114] Rare cases of *Candida* meningitis have resulted from direct extension from infected paranasal sinuses.[115] Importantly, candidemia in adult patients is rarely associated with meningitis. Therefore, routine lumbar punctures are not required in immunocompetent candidemic adults in the absence of CNS signs or symptoms.

Clinical Manifestations

The clinical presentation of meningitis due to *Candida* species varies from an acute and devastating CNS syndrome to a chronic and indolent meningitis. Most patients have headache and fever, and patients without HIV infection typically have meningismus.[111,116] Underlying immunodeficiency syndromes and risk factors for candidemia are typically present. In rare instances, often in patients with a preexisting anatomic defect, *Candida* infection may begin in the paranasal sinuses and spread contiguously into the subarachnoid space through adjacent bone.[115] Cases of vascular invasion and subarachnoid hemorrhage also have been attributed to *Candida* meningitis.[117]

Most neurosurgical patients who develop *Candida* meningitis have ventriculostomy tubes or ventricular shunts in place. In this patient population, antibiotic use and prior bacterial meningitis are also associated with the development of this infection.[113,118] Therefore, clinicians who care for patients with head trauma or neurosurgery should be vigilant for *Candida* superinfections in patients on antibacterial therapy, especially those with prior bacterial meningitis.

Diagnosis

The CSF of patients with *Candida* meningitis most often displays a mild pleocytosis and hypoglycorrhachia, often clinically indistinguishable from tuberculous or cryptococcal meningitis. CSF differential cell counts in this disease demonstrate either a mononuclear or a neutrophilic predominance.[116] Since many of the patients with candidemia are neutropenic, even the presence of nucleated cells in the CSF of patients with *Candida* meningitis may be quite variable.

Microbiologic staining and culture for *Candida* species in CSF reveal the organism in a minority of cases. Gram's stain correctly identified *Candida* in 17 percent of CSF samples, and cultures were positive in 44 percent of samples,[116] despite the fact that *Candida* species grow well on routine bacterial media. This observation may reflect a low burden or compartmentalization of organisms in the CNS, underscoring the importance of culturing large-volume CSF samples. Biochemical or molecular tests for fungal components or the identification of anti-*Candida* antibodies in the CSF may complement culture data. In fact, PCR-based studies have been used in the diagnosis and subsequent clinical monitoring of patients with *Candida* meningitis.[119,120] Such assays are being tested currently for more widespread use.

The clinical significance of a single positive culture for *Candida* from a CNS prosthetic device, such as a ventriculostomy tube, is unclear.[121] In the absence of other abnormal CSF parameters, repeat CSF sampling is likely required, often from a distant site such as a lumbar puncture. Without symptoms suggestive of CNS infection or an abnormal CSF profile, specific antifungal therapy may not be necessary, but the device likely should be removed.[105,122]

Treatment

Prospective comparisons of different treatment options in *Candida* meningitis have not been performed due to the relative rarity of this disease. However, several studies have indicated that aggressive antifungal therapy can reduce morbidity and mortality in this serious infection.[116,118,123] Of reported cases, most clinical experience has been with intravenous amphotericin B, which achieves rapid penetration into the CNS. The combination of amphotericin B and flucytosine resulted in excellent rates of cure, likely due to high achievable CNS levels of flucytosine and the synergistic activity in vitro of these two agents against *Candida* species.[124] Historically, most amphotericin B regimens have been used for 6 to 8 weeks, but shorter courses may be appropriate depending on the clinical response and whether combination therapies are used. Intraventricular amphotericin B has been used in apparent treatment failures, but this method of drug delivery was associated with significant drug toxicity.[113]

Liposomal amphotericin B (AmBisome) also has been used in instances of poor response to standard formulations of amphotericin B.[125,126] The combination of this drug with flucytosine is a reasonable option for treatment failures or relapses.

No human trials have compared fluconazole with amphotericin B in *Candida* meningitis. Despite excellent CSF penetration of fluconazole, animal studies suggest that amphotericin B may sterilize the CSF faster than fluconazole alone. Similar to its use in cryptococcal meningitis, fluconazole may play a role in the maintenance phase of treatment after initial intensive therapy with an amphotericin B–based regimen. Long-term secondary prophylaxis with fluconazole in HIV-infected patients with *Candida* meningitis also has been proposed.[111]

In patients with *Candida* meningitis due to ventriculostomies or CNS shunts, the device should be removed or replaced to allow for complete cure. Systemic antifungal therapy also is indicated.[113]

Aspergillus Species

Invasive aspergillosis occurs almost exclusively in profoundly immunosuppressed patients, especially those with prolonged neutropenia, graft-versus-host disease, and organ transplantation. This ubiquitous group of molds typically enters the host by inhalation into the lungs. Pulmonary macrophages are the primary effector cells that respond to and kill inhaled *Aspergillus* spores, but neutrophils are also important aspects of constitutive immunity against this group of fungi. Thus neutropenic patients and recipients of lung transplants are at a particularly increased risk of *Aspergillus* disease.[127,128] CNS aspergillosis has been described infrequently in patients with AIDS.[129]

Aspergillus fumigatus, A. terreus, and *A. flavus* are the most common *Aspergillus* species observed to cause CNS infections.[130–132] Most aspergillosis of the CNS results from local extension from the paranasal sinuses. However, hematogenous dissemination and direct inoculation by trauma, surgery, or lumbar puncture are mechanisms by which *Aspergillus* species also may gain access to the CNS.[132,133]

Clinical Manifestations

The most common clinical manifestations of *Aspergillus* infection of the CNS are infarctions and abscesses. Rare cases of meningitis have been reported, some as a result of direct invasion from infected vertebrae in chronic granulomatous disease of childhood.[134] A high index of suspicion for aspergillosis in immunosuppressed patients must be maintained due to the potential for rapid progression and due to the limited treatment options for late-stage disease.

Treatment

Surgical resection of mass lesions has resulted in long-term survival.[135] However, patients historically have fared poorly with antifungal therapy when immune restoration did not rapidly occur. Preliminary data with voriconazole in CNS aspergillosis have demonstrated significantly improved responses compared with historical treatment regimens.[27,136] Therefore, voriconazole may be considered first-line therapy for this disease.

Dematiacious (Pigmented) Molds

The dematiacious molds are a diverse group of environmental fungi having in common the ability to produce melanin in their cell walls. This dark pigment is made both in vitro and in vivo, and the brown coloration of the fungal elements often allows presumptive identification in histopathologic and cytologic materials. Melanin has been demonstrated experimentally to be required for virulence in dematiacious fungal pathogens. Disease due to these organisms is termed *phaeohyphomycosis,* encompassing superficial, cutaneous, subcutaneous, and disseminated infections. Epidemiologic studies have demonstrated an association between the development of phaeohyphomycosis and exposure to soil, especially with traumatic inoculation of organic material.

Several dozen species of pigmented molds have been described to cause phaeohyphomycosis.[137] However, similar to *C. neoformans,* certain species of the dematiacious molds appear to possess a neurotropism, with a disproportionate number of infections due to these species involving the CNS.[18] *Cladophialophora bantiana, Fonsacaea pedrosoi, Bipolaris spicifera,* and *Dactylaria gallopavum* are among the most common black molds to cause CNS infection in the United States. One species, *Dactylaria gallopavum,* is rarely identified as a pathogen in clinical practice, but even these limited reports frequently associate this species with CNS disease.[18] *Ramichloridium obovoideum* (*mackenziei*) is isolated primarily in patients in the Middle East, and this fungus also demonstrates a striking neurotropism.[138]

CNS disease due to these fungi is quite rare, most often presenting as brain abscesses and less commonly as meningitis.[139,140] Past reports of cerebral phaeohyphomycosis have presumed an anatomic origin of infection in the paranasal sinuses with local extension to the CNS. Hematogenous dissemination to the CNS and direct inoculation by penetrating trauma also have been described.[141–143] Recently, iatrogenic meningitis due to the dematiacious mold *Wangiella dermatitidis* was linked to contaminated steroid preparations used for epidural anesthesia.[144] Immunocompromised patients are likely at an increased risk for dissemination of phaeohyphomycosis.

The diagnosis of CNS phaeohyphomycosis requires culture or histopathologic confirmation from the CSF or from brain/meningeal biopsies. Due to the limited number of cases, treatment options have not been studied in clinical trials. However, in one retrospective review, complete neurosurgical excision of mass lesions was the only intervention associated with survival.[140] Antifungal therapy, in this series, did not affect clinical outcomes. However, given in vitro susceptibility data[145] and the high mortality of this disease, CNS phaeohyphomycosis should be treated with surgical intervention, when possible, as well as combination antifungal therapy with a polyene, flucytosine, and a newer extended-spectrum triazole such as voriconazole.

Hyaline (Nonpigmented) Molds

In contrast to dematiacious fungi, hyaline molds are environmental organisms that do not produce extensive melanin pigments. This grouping encompasses a variety of species, several of which are opportunistic human pathogens.

Fusarium species have long been recognized as common causes of mycotic keratitis. More recently, these species have been observed causing life-threatening infections in neutropenic patients, similar to *Aspergillus* species. In contrast to aspergillosis, *Fusarium* infections frequently involve metastatic foci of infection characterized by diffuse cutaneous lesions. Blood cultures in disseminated fusariosis are positive for the infecting mold in most cases. This is rarely the case in disease due to *Aspergillus*. *Fusarium* very infrequently involves the CNS.[146] Due to variable antifungal resistance patterns, therapy in all cases of fusariosis needs to be individualized. Clinical responses have been observed with triazoles, such as voriconazole, and amphotericin B, but susceptibility testing helps to guide therapy. Reversal of immunosuppression, when possible, is essential for optimal treatment of *Fusarium* infections. Other hyaline molds that primarily cause infection in profoundly immunosuppressed patients but which rarely invade the CNS include *Paecilomyces* and *Acremonium* species.

One hyaline mold that infects the CNS with some regularity is *Scedosporium apiospermum* (teleomorph, *Pseudallescheria boydii*). This environmental fungus is isolated worldwide from soil and water, and it is a common cause of mycetoma. Several cases of *S. apiospermum* meningitis have been described, especially in patients with neutropenia or other profound degrees of immunosuppression.[147,148] In these instances, corticosteroid therapy may predispose to CNS invasion by this mold. Interestingly, infection due to *S. apiospermum* is well described after near-drowning episodes in freshwater.[149] Access to the CNS during these events may occur by direct extension through the cribiform plate or secondary to fungal pneumonitis resulting from water aspiration. Due to polyene resistance, *S. apiospermum* infections historically have been quite difficult to treat. Triazoles such as voriconazole may become the primary therapy for CNS infections due to this fungus.

Sporothrix schenckii

In contrast to many other human fungal pathogens, *S. schenckii* generally does not enter the host through the respiratory tract. This environmental mold is introduced most often by direct inoculation. From the initial site of infection, *S. schenckii* spreads to distant regions by venous or lymphangitic channels.

CNS involvement by *S. schenckii* is very uncommon. Furthermore, diagnosis can be extremely difficult because traditional culture methods result in a very low yield of detection, and concurrent extrameningeal infection is evident in a minority of patients. Antibodies against *S. schenckii* in the CSF can be measured by latex agglutination methods or enzyme immunoassay, and these may be the methods of choice for diagnosis. Titers of greater than or equal to 1:8 displayed no cross-reactivity with other fungal pathogens.[150]

Penicillium marneffei

P. marneffei is an environmental fungus isolated in Southeast Asia and southern China. Although disease due to this fungus was very uncommon prior to the HIV era, it is now a common opportunistic infection in AIDS patients in endemic areas. The primary clinical manifestation of infection due to *P. marneffei* is a disseminated syndrome with fever and diffuse, umbilicated skin lesions. Additionally, many organs and tissues, including the meninges, have been reported to be involved in disseminated *P. marneffei* infection.[151] The worldwide significance of this fungus is underscored by case reports of patients with HIV infection who have developed disease due to *P. marneffei* after remote travel to endemic regions.[152,153] Therefore, clinicians in areas outside of Asia also should be familiar with this fungal pathogen.

Meningitis due to *P. marneffei* should be considered in patients with AIDS and a chronic meningitis who are either from or who have a travel history to an endemic area. Characteristic skin lesions or other organ involvement may be evident clinically as well. Most successful treatments of *P. marneffei* infections have included amphotericin B with or without flucytosine. This drug combination should be used in *P. marneffei* meningitis. Itraconazole has been used successfully in disseminated *P. marneffei* infections without CNS involvement.[154] This drug's poor CNS penetration limits its use in meningitis. Fluconazole failures have been described in this disease. Newer triazoles such as voriconazole are promising agents for CNS *P. marneffei* infections because early results in treating invasive infection are quite encouraging.[27]

Zygomycetes

The Zygomycetes are a broad class of molds that are commonly isolated from the environment. Many of the clinical manifestations of zygomycosis can be caused by any of the fungi in this group, and clinical distinction among the various species is rarely possible. Some of the more common Zygomycetes include *Rhizopus arrhizus*, *Mucor* species, *Rhizomucor*, *Apophysomyces elegans*, and *Cunninghamella bertholletiae*. The term *mucormycosis* also has been used to describe disease due to these environmental molds.

Most patients with zygomycosis have specific underlying conditions that suppress their immune system or otherwise predispose to these unusual infections. Such conditions include organ transplantation, hematologic malignancies, poorly controlled diabetes mellitus with frequent episodes of acidemia, intravenous drug abuse, and deferoxamine therapy. Among organ transplant patients, antirejection therapy with corticosteroids places patients at highest risk for zygomycosis.[155]

Involvement of the CNS by Zygomycetes most frequently occurs by direct extension from an initial infection in the nose and sinuses. This syndrome results in cerebral infarctions rather than meningitis. Rhinocerebral zygomycosis can proceed in a slow and indolent form, but a rapidly progressive form is also described and must be assumed in order to proceed quickly to potentially curative therapy. In both cases, nonspecific symptoms of sinus disease in a susceptible patient may be the only clinical manifestation of early, resectable disease. Later findings include palatal eschars, sanguineous nasal drainage, facial pain, and eventually, cranial neuropathies from extension into the cavernous sinus.

Cerebral zygomycosis complicating neurosurgical procedures, associated with intravenous drug abuse, and from hematologic dissemination have been described.[156] Such patients typically present with rapidly progressive neurologic deterioration. CSF findings are variable and nondiagnostic, and cultures of CSF rarely grow the causative organism. Radiologic imaging of the CNS and neurosurgical biopsies usually are required to make this diagnosis. Cerebral zygomycosis is fatal if not treated. Surgical removal of infected tissue is the cornerstone of effective therapy in this disease. Amphotericin B at the highest tolerated doses (1 to 1.5 mg/kg daily) is the only antifungal agent with reasonable activity against this group of molds. Reports indicate that lipid-associated amphotericin B preparations at high doses (3 to 5 mg/kg daily) may be effective alternatives in zygomycete infections of the CNS with decreased dose-limiting side effects compared with conventional amphotericin B.[11,12,157]

REFERENCES

1. Ellner JJ, Bennett JE: Chronic meningitis. *Medicine* 55:341, 1976.
2. Haki JG, Gangaidzo IT, Heyderman RS: Impact of HIV infection on meningitis in Harare, Zimbabwe: A prospective study of 406 predominantly adult patients. *AIDS* 14:1401, 2000.
3. Anderson NE, Willoughby EW: Chronic meningitis without predisposing illness: A review of 83 cases. *Q J Med* 63:283, 1987.
4. Smith JE, Aksamit AJ: Outcome of chronic idiopathic meningitis. *Mayo Clin Proc* 64:548, 1994.
5. Bindschadler DD, Bennett JE: A pharmacologic guide to the clinical use of amphotericin B. *J Infect Dis* 120:427, 1969.
6. Drutz DJ, Spickard A, Rogers DE, et al: Treatment of disseminated mycotic infections. *Am J Med* 45:405, 1968.
7. Polsky B, Depman MR, Gold JW, et al: Intraventricular therapy of cryptococcal meningitis via a subcutaneous reservoir. *Am J Med* 81:24, 1986.
8. Labadie EL, Hamilton RH: Survival improvement in coccidioidal meningitis by high-dose intrathecal amphotericin B. *Arch Intern Med* 146:2013, 1986.
9. Diamond RD, Bennett JE: A subcutaneous reservoir for intrathecal therapy of fungal meningitis. *New Engl J Med* 288:186, 1973.
10. Leenders AC, Reiss P, Portegies P, et al: Liposomal amphotericin B (Ambisome) compared with amphotericin B followed by oral fluconazole in the treatment of AIDS-associated cryptococcal meningitis. *AIDS* 11:1463, 1997.
11. Del Palacio A, Gomez-Hernando C, Revenga F, et al: Cutaneous *Alternaria alternata* infection successfully treated with itraconazole. *Clin Exp Dermatol* 21:241, 1996.
12. Strasser MD, Kennedy RJ, Adam RD: Rhinocerebral mucormycosis: Therapy with amphotericin B lipid complex. *Arch Intern Med* 156(3):337, 1996.
13. Bennett JE: Flucytosine. *Ann Intern Med* 86:319, 1977.
14. Utz JP, Shadomy S, McGehee RF: 5-Flucytosine: Experience in patients with pulmonary and other forms of cryptococcosis. *Am Rev Respir Dis* 99:975, 1969.
15. Saag MS, Powderly WG, Cloud GA, et al: Comparison of amphotericin B with fluconazole in the treatment of acute AIDS-associated cryptococcal meningitis. *New Engl J Med* 326:83, 1992.
16. van der Horst C, Saag MS, Cloud GA, et al: Treatment of cryptococcal meningitis associated with the acquired immunodeficiency syndrome. *New Engl J Med* 337:15, 1997.
17. Saag MS, Cloud GA, Graybill JR, et al: A comparison of itraconazole versus fluconazole as maintenance therapy for AIDS-associated cryptococcal meningitis. *Clin Infect Dis* 28:291, 1999.
18. Singh N, Chang FY, Gayowski T, et al: Infections due to dematiacious fungi in organ transplant recipients: Case report and review. *Clin Infect Dis* 24:369, 1997.
19. Foulds G, Brennan DR, Wajszczvk CP, et al: Fluconazole penetration into cerebrospinal fluid in humans. *J Clin Pharmacol* 28:363, 1988.
20. Arndt CA, Walsh T, McCully CL, et al: Fluconazole penetration into cerebrospinal fluid: Implications for treating fungal infections of the central nervous system. *J Infect Dis* 157:178, 1988.
21. Sugar AM, Saunders C: Oral fluconazole as suppressive therapy of disseminated cryptococcosis in patients with acquired immunodeficiency syndrome. *Am J Med* 85:481, 1988.
22. Laroche R, Dupont B, Touze JE, et al: Cryptococcal meningitis associated with acquired immunodeficiency syndrome (AIDS) in African patients: Treatment with fluconazole. *J Med Vet Mycol* 30:71, 1992.

23. Denning DW, Tucker RM, Hanson LH, et al: Treatment of invasive aspergillosis with itraconazole. *Am J Med* 86:791, 1989.

24. Perfect JR, Durack DT: Penetration of imidazoles and triazoles into cerebrospinal fluid of rabbits. *Antimicrob Agents Chemother* 16:81, 1985.

25. Denning DW, Tucker RM, Hanson LH, et al: Itraconazole therapy for cryptococcal meningitis and cryptococcosis. *Arch Intern Med* 149:2301, 1989.

26. Viviani MA, Tortorano AM, Giani PC, et al: Itraconazole for cryptococcal infection in the acquired immunodeficiency syndrome (letter). *Ann Intern Med* 106:166, 1987.

27. Perfect JR, Marr KA, Walsh TJ, et al: Voriconazole treatment for less common, emerging, or refractory fungal infections. *Clin Infect Dis* 36:1122, 2003.

28. Walsh TJ, Lutsar I, Driscoll T, et al: Voriconazole in the treatment of aspergillosis, scedosporiosis, and other invasive fungal infections in children. *Pediatr Infect Dis J* 21:240, 2002.

29. Denning DW, Stevens DA: Antifungal and surgical treatment of invasive aspergillosis: Review of 2121 published cases. *Rev Infect Dis* 12:1147, 1990.

30. Machetti M, Zotti M, Veroni L: Antigen detection in the diagnosis and management of a patient with probable cerebral aspergillosis treated with voriconazole. *Transpl Infect Dis* 2:140, 2000.

31. Schwartz S, Milatovic D, Thiel E: Successful treatment of cerebral aspergillosis with a novel triazole (voriconazole) in a patient with acute leukemia. *Br J Haematol* 97:663, 1997.

32. Nesky MA, McDougal EC, Peacock JE Jr: *Pseudoallescheria boydii* brain abscess successfully treated with voriconazole and surgical drainage: Case report and literature review of central nervous system pseudoallescheriasis. *Clin Infect Dis* 31:673, 2000.

33. Dismukes WE, Cloud G, Bowles C: Treatment of blastomycosis and histoplasmosis with ketoconazole: Results of a prospective, randomized clinical trial. *Ann Intern Med* 103:861, 1985.

34. Perfect JR, Durack DT, Hamilton JD, et al: Failure of ketoconazole in cryptococcal meningitis. *JAMA* 247:3349, 1982.

35. Craven PC, Graybill JR, Jorgensen JH, et al: High-dose ketoconazole for treatment of fungal infections of the central nervous system. *Ann Intern Med* 98:160, 1983.

36. Graybill JR, Levine HB: Successful treatment of cryptococcal meningitis with intraventricular miconazole. *Ann Intern Med* 138:814, 1978.

37. Sung JP, Campbell GD, Grendahl JG: Miconazole therapy for fungal meningitis. *Arch Intern Med* 35:443, 1978.

38. Dixon DM, Walsh TJ, Merz WG, et al: Infections due to *Xylohypha bantiana* (*Cladosporium trichoides*). *Rev Infect Dis* 11(4):515, 1989.

39. Devi SJ, Scheerson R, Egan W, et al: *Cryptococcus neoformans* serotype A glucuronoxylomannan protein conjugate vaccines: Synthesis, characterization, and immunogenicity. *Infect Immun* 59:3700, 1991.

40. Mirza S, Phelan M, Rimland D, et al: The changing epidemiology of cryptococcosis: An update from population-based active surveillance in two large metropolitan areas, 1992–2000. *Clin Infect Dis* 36:789, 2002.

41. Nightingale SD, Cal SX, Peterson DM, et al: Primary prophylaxis with fluconazole against systemic fungal infections in HIV-positive patients. *AIDS* 6:191, 1992.

42. Powderly WG, Finkelstein DM, Feinberg J, et al: A randomized trial comparing fluconazole with clotrimazole troches for the prevention of fungal infections in patients with advanced human immunodeficiency virus infection. *New Engl J Med* 332:700, 1995.

43. Behre G, Schwartz S, Lenz K: Aerosol amphotericin B inhalations for prevention of invasive pulmonary aspergillosis in neutropenic cancer patients. *Ann Hematol* 71:287, 1995.

44. Hertenstein B, Stefanic M, Novotny J, et al: Low incidence of invasive fungal infections after bone-marrow transplantation in patients receiving amphotericin-B inhalations during neutropenia. *Ann Hematol* 68:21, 1994.

45. Anaissie E, Stratton S, Dignani M, et al: Cleaning patient shower facilities: A novel approach to reducing patient exposure to aerosolized aspergillus species and other opportunistic molds. *Clin Infect Dis* 38(8):E86, 2002.

46. Fraser DW, Ward JI, Ajello L, et al: Aspergillosis and systemic mycosis. *JAMA* 242:1631, 1979.

47. van Elden LJ, Walenkamp AM, Lipovsky MM: Declining number of patients with cryptococcosis in the Netherlands in the era of highly active antiretroviral therapy. *AIDS* 14:2787, 2000.

48. Molez J: The historical question of acquired immunodeficiency syndrome in the 1960s in the Congo River basin area in relation to cryptococcal meningitis. *Am J Trop Med Hyg* 58:273, 2001.

49. Baker RD: The primary pulmonary lymph node complex of cryptococcosis. *Am J Clin Pathol* 65:83, 1976.

50. Warr W, Bates JH, Stone A: The spectrum of pulmonary cryptococcosis. *Ann Intern Med* 69:1109, 1968.

51. Merkel GJ, Scofield BA: Conditions affecting the adherence of *Cryptococcus neoformans* to rat glial and lung cells in vitro. *J Med Vet Mycol* 31:55, 1993.

52. Granger DL, Perfect JR, Durack DT: Virulence of *Cryptococcus neoformans:* Regulation of capsule synthesis by carbon dioxide. *J Clin Invest* 76:508, 1985.

53. Vartivarian SE, Anaissie EJ, Cowart RE, et al: Regulation of cryptococcal capsular polysaccharide by iron. *J Infect Dis* 167:186, 1993.

54. Kwon-Chung KJ, Lehman D, Good C, et al: Genetic evidence for role of extracellular proteinase in virulence of *Candida albicans*. *Infect Immun* 49:571, 1985.

55. Chang YC, Kwon-Chung KJ: Complementation of a capsule-deficiency mutation of *Cryptococcus neoformans* restores its virulence. *Mol Cell Biol* 14:4912, 1994.

56. Williamson PW. Biochemical and molecular identification of the diphenol oxidase of *Cryptococcus neoformans:* Identification as a laccase. *J Bacteriol* 176:676, 1994.

57. Mody CH, Lipscomb MF, Street NE, et al: Depletion of

CD4+ (L3T4+) lymphocytes in vivo impairs murine host defenses to *Cryptococcus neoformans. J Immunol* 144:1472, 1990.

58. Hill JO: CD4+ T cells cause multinucleated giant cells to form around *Cryptococcus neoformans* and confine the yeast within the primary site of infection in the respiratory tract. *J Exp Med* 175:1685, 1992.

59. Marquis G, Montplaisir S, Pelletier M: Genetic resistance to murine cryptococcosis: The beige mutation (Chediak-Higashi syndrome) in mice. *Infect Immun* 47:288, 1985.

60. Cauley LK, Murphy JW: Response of congenital athymic (nude) and phenotypically normal mice to *Cryptococcus neoformans* infection. *Infect Immun* 23:644, 1979.

61. Hidore MR, Murphy JW: Correlation of natural killer cell activity and clearance of *Cryptococcus neoformans* from mice after adoptive transfer of splenic nylon wool-nonadherent cells. *Infect Immun* 51:547, 1986.

62. Lim TS, Murphy JW: Transfer of immunity to cryptococcosis by T-enriched splenic lymphocytes from *Cryptococcus neoformans*–sensitized mice. *Infect Immun* 30:5, 1980.

63. Perfect JR, Hobbs MM, Granger DL, et al: Cerebrospinal fluid macrophage response to experimental cryptococcal meningitis: Relationship between in vivo and in vitro measurements of cytotoxicity. *Infect Immun* 56:849, 1988.

64. Diamond RD, May JE, Kane MA: The role of the classical and alternative complement pathways in host defense against *Cryptococcus neoformans* infection. *J Immunol* 112:2260, 1974.

65. Dromer F, Charreire J, Contrepois A, et al: Protection of mice against experimental cryptococcosis by anti-*Cryptococcus neoformans* monoclonal antibody. *Infect Immun* 55:749, 1987.

66. Mukherjee J, Pirofski LA, Scharff MD, et al: Antibody-mediated protection in mice with lethal intracerebral *Cryptococcus neoformans* infection. *Proc Natl Acad Sci USA* 90:3636, 1993.

67. Perfect JR, Lang DR, Durack DT: Influence of agglutinating antibody in experimental cryptococcal meningitis. *Br J Exp Pathol* 62:595, 1981.

68. Heyderman RS, Gangaidzo IT, Hakim JG, et al: Cryptococcal meningitis in human immunodeficiency virus–infected patients in Harare, Zimbabwe. *Clin Infect Dis* 26:284, 203.

69. Kovacs JA, Kovacs AA, Polis M, et al: Cryptococcosis in the acquired immunodeficiency syndrome. *Ann Intern Med* 103:533, 1985.

70. Eng RH, Bishburg E, Smith SM: Cryptococcal infections in patients with acquired immune deficiency syndrome. *Am J Med* 81:19, 1986.

71. Goodman JS, Kaufman L, Loening MG: Diagnosis of cryptococcal meningitis: Detection of cryptococcal antigen. *New Engl J Med* 285:434, 1971.

72. Snow RM, Dismukes WE: Cryptococcal meningitis: Diagnostic value of cryptococcal antigen in cerebrospinal fluid. *Arch Intern Med* 135:1155, 1975.

73. Diamond RD, Bennett JE: Prognostic factors in crypto-

coccal meningitis: A study of 111 cases. *Ann Intern Med* 80:176, 1974.

74. Beeson PB: Cryptococcal meningitis of nearly sixteen years' duration. *Arch Intern Med* 89:797, 1952.

75. Bennett JE, Dismukes W, Duma RJ, et al: A comparison of amphotericin B alone and combined with flucytosine in the treatment of cryptococcal meningitis. *New Engl J Med* 301:126, 1979.

76. Ragland AS, Arusa E, Ismail Y, et al: Eosinophilic pleocytosis in coccidioidal meningitis: frequency and significance. *Am J Med* 195:254, 1993.

77. Galgiani JN, Peng T, Lewis ML, et al: Cerebrospinal fluid antibodies detected by ELISA against a 33-kDa antigen from spherules of *Coccidioides immitis* in patients with coccidioidal meningitis. The National Institute of Allergy and Infectious Diseases Mycoses Study Group. *J Infect Dis* 173:499, 1996.

78. Galgiani JN, Ampel NM, Catanzaro A: Practice guidelines for the treatment of coccidioidomycosis. *Clin Infect Dis* 30:658, 2000.

79. Dewsnup DH, Galgiani JN, Graybill JR, et al: Is it ever safe to stop azole therapy for *Coccidioides immitis* meningitis? *Ann Intern Med* 124:305, 1996.

80. Gonzales G, Tijerina R, Najvar L, et al: Correlation between antifungal susceptibilities of *Coccidioides immitis* in vitro and antifungal treatment with caspofungin in a mouse model. *Antimicrob Agents Chemother* 45:1854, 2001.

81. Goodwin RA Jr, Shapiro JL, Thurman GH, et al: Disseminated histoplasmosis: Clinical and pathologic correlations. *Medicine* 59:1, 1980.

82. Wheat LJ, Batteiger BE, Sathapatayavongs B: *Histoplasma capsulatum* infections of the central nervous system. *Medicine* 69:244, 1990.

83. Anaissie E, Fainstein V, Samo T, et al: Central nervous system histoplasmosis: An unappreciated complication of the acquired immunodeficiency syndrome. *Am J Med* 84:215, 1988.

84. Wheat LJ, Smith EJ, Sathapatayavongs B, et al: Histoplasmosis in renal allograft recipients: Two large urban outbreaks. *Arch Intern Med* 143:703, 1983.

85. Livramento JA, Machado LR, Nobrega JPS, et al: Histoplasmosis of the central nervous system: study of cerebrospinal fluid in eight patients. *Arq Neuropsiquiatr* 51:80, 1993.

86. Wheat LJ, Kohler RB, Tewari RP, et al: Significance of *Histoplasma* antigen in the cerebrospinal fluid of patients with meningitis. *Arch Intern Med* 149:302, 1989.

87. Wheat LJ, French M, Batteiger B, et al: Cerebrospinal fluid *Histoplasma* antibodies in central nervous system histoplasmosis. *Arch Intern Med* 145:1237, 1985.

88. Plouffe JF, Fass RJ: Histoplasma meningitis: Diagnostic value of cerebrospinal fluid serology. *Ann Intern Med* 92:189, 1980.

89. Haynes R, Connolly P, Durkin M, et al: Antifungal therapy for central nervous system histoplasmosis, using a newly developed intracranial model of infection. *J Infect Dis* 185:1830, 2001.

90. LeMonte AM, Washum KE, Smedema ML, et al: Amphotericin B combined with itraconazole or flucona-

zole for treatment of histoplasmosis. *J Infect Dis* 182:545, 2000.

91. Harley WB, Lomis M, Haas DW: Marked polymorphonuclear pleocytosis due to blastomycotic meningitis: A case report and review. *Clin Infect Dis* 18:816, 1994.

92. Mendel E, Milefchik EN, Amadi J, et al: Coccidioidomycosis brain abscess: Case report. *J Neurosurg* 81:614, 1994.

93. Gonyea EF: The spectrum of primary blastomycotic meningitis: A review of central nervous system blastomycosis. *Ann Neurol* 3:26, 1978.

94. Kravitz GR, Davies SF, Eckman MR, et al: Chronic blastomycotic meningitis. *Am J Med* 71:501, 1981.

95. Chapman SW, Lin AC, Hendricks A: Endemic blastomycosis in Mississippi: Epidemiological and clinical studies. *Semin Respir Infect* 12:219, 1997.

96. Pappas PG, Bradsher RW, Kauffman CA: Treatment of blastomycosis with higher-dose fluconazole. *Clin Infect Dis* 25:200, 1997.

97. Pappas PG, Threlkeld MG, Bedsole GD, et al: Blastomycosis in immunocompromised patients. *Medicine* 72:311, 1993.

98. Ward BA, Parent A, Raila F: Indications for the surgical management of central nervous system blastomycosis. *Surg Neurol* 43:379, 1995.

99. Heing E, Djaldetti M, Pinkhas J, et al: *Candida tropicalis* meningitis in Hodgkin's disease. *JAMA* 199:214, 1967.

100. Flynn PM, Mariana NM, Rivera GK, et al: *Candida tropicalis* infections in children with aspergillus leukemia. *Leuk Lymphoma* 10:369, 1993.

101. Faix RG: *Candida parapsilosis* meningitis in a premature infant. *Pediatr Infect Dis J* 2:462, 1983.

102. Leggiadro RJ, Collins T: *Candida lusitaniae* meningitis. *Pediatr Infect Dis J* 7:368, 1988.

103. Sanchez PJ, Cooper BH: *Candida lusitania:* Sepsis and meningitis in a neonate. *Pediatr Infect Dis J* 6:758, 1987.

104. Huttova M, Hartmanova I, Kralinsky K, et al: *Candida fungemia* in neonates treated with fluconazole: Report of forty cases, including eight with meningitis. *Pediatr Infect Dis J* 17:1012, 1998.

105. Arisoy ES, Arisoy AE, Dunne WM Jr: Clinical significance of fungi isolated from cerebral fluid in children. *Pediatr Infect Dis J* 13:127, 1994.

106. Huttova M, Kralinsky K, Horn J, et al: Prospective study of nosocomial fungal meningitis in children: Report of 10 cases. *Scand J Infect Dis* 30:485, 1998.

107. Mori T, Ebe T: Analysis of cases of central nervous system fungal infections reported in Japan between January 1979 and June 1989. *Intern Med* 31:174, 1992.

108. Ludviksson BR, Thoraparensen O, Gudnason T, et al: *Candida albicans* meningitis in a child with myeloperoxidase deficiency. *Pediatr Infect Dis J* 12:162, 1993.

109. Oleske J, Minnefor A, Cooper R, et al: Immune deficiency syndrome in children. *JAMA* 249:2345, 1983.

110. Rodriquez-Arrondo F, Aquirrebengoa K, De Arce A, et al: Candidal meningitis in HIV-infected patients: Treatment with fluconazole. *Scand J Infect Dis* 30:417, 1998.

111. Casado JL, Quereda C, Oliva J, et al: Candidal meningitis in HIV-infected patients: Analysis of 14 cases. *Clin Infect Dis* 25:673, 1997.

112. del Pozo MM, Bermejo F, Molina JA, et al: Chronic neutrophilic meningitis caused by *Candida albicans.* *Neurologia* 13:362, 1998.

113. Sanchez-Portocarrero J, Martin-Rabadan P, Saldana CJ, et al: *Candida* cerebrospinal fluid shunt infection: Report of two new cases and review of the literature. *Diagn Microbiol Infect Dis* 20:33, 1994.

114. Poon WS, Ng S, Wai S: CSF antibiotic prophylaxis for neurosurgical patients with ventriculostomy: A randomized study. *Acta Neurochir Suppl* 71:146, 1998.

115. Kaji M, Shoji H, Oizumi K: Intractable meningitis and intracranial abscess following sinusitis due to *Candida* species. *Kurume Med J* 45:279, 1998.

116. Voice RA, Bradley SF, Sangeorzan JA, et al: Chronic candidal meningitis: An uncommon manifestation of candidiasis. *Clin Infect Dis* 19:60, 1994.

117. Kupsky RR, Kupsky WJ, Haas JE: Arteritis and fatal subarachnoid hemorrhage complicating occult *Candida* meningitis: Unusual presentation in pediatric acquired immunodeficiency syndrome. *Arch Pathol Lab Med* 122:1030, 1998.

118. Nguyen MH, Yu VL: Meningitis caused by *Candida* species: An emerging problem in neurosurgical patients. *Clin Infect Dis* 21:323, 1995.

119. Ralph ED, Hussain Z: Chronic meningitis caused by *Candida albicans* in a liver transplant recipient: Usefulness of the polymerase chain reaction for diagnosis and for monitoring treatment. *Clin Infect Dis* 23:191, 1996.

120. Tsuge I, Makimura K, Natsume J, et al: Successful polymerase chain reaction–based diagnosis of fungal meningitis in a patient with chronic granulomatous disease. *Acta Paediatr Jpn* 40:356, 1998.

121. Geers TA, Gordon SM: Clinical significance of *Candida* species isolated from cerebrospinal fluid following neurosurgery. *Clin Infect Dis* 28:1139, 1999.

122. Martino P, Girmenia C, Venditti M, et al: *Candida* colonization and systemic infection in neutropenia patients: A retrospective study (abstract). *Cancer* 64:2030, 1989.

123. Walsh TJ, Hiemenz JW, Seibel N, et al: Amphotericin B lipid complex for invasive fungal infections: Analysis of safety and efficacy in 556 cases. *Clin Infect Dis* 26:1383, 1998.

124. Smego RA, Perfect JR, Durack DT: Combined therapy with amphotericin B and 5-fluorocytosine for *Candida* meningitis. *Rev Infect Dis* 6:791, 1984.

125. Jarlov JO, Born P, Bruun B: *Candida albicans* meningitis in a 27 weeks' premature infant treated with liposomal amphotericin-B. *Scand J Infect Dis* 27:419, 1995.

126. Houmeau L, Monfort-Gouraud M, Boccara JF, et al: *Candida* meningitis, in a premature infant, treated with liposomal amphotericin B and flucytosine. *Arch Fr Pediatr* 50:227, 1993.

127. Gerson SL, Talbot GH, Hurwitz S, et al: Prolonged granulocytopenia: The major risk factor for invasive pulmonary aspergillus in patients with acute leukemia. *Ann Intern Med* 100:345, 1984.

128. Kanj SS, Welty-Wolf K, Madden J: Fungal infections in

lung and heart-lung transplant recipients. *Medicine* 75:142, 1996.

129. Carrazana EJ, Rossitch E Jr, Morris J: Isolated central nervous system aspergillosis in the acquired immunodeficiency syndrome. *Clin Neurol Neurosurg* 93:227, 1991.

130. Iyer S, Dodge P, Adams RD: Two cases of aspergillus infection of the central nervous system. *J Neurol Neurosurg Psychiatry* 15:152, 1952.

131. Gordon MA, Holzman RS, Senter H, et al: Aspergillus orzyme meningitis. *JAMA* 235:2122, 1976.

132. Mukoyama M, Gimple K, Poser CM: Aspergillosis of the central nervous system: Report of a brain abscess due to *A. fumigatus* and review of the literature. *Neurology* 19:967, 1969.

133. Guisan von M: Sclerosing posttraumatic meningeal aspergillosis. *Schweiz Arch Neurol Psychiatr* 90:235, 1962.

134. Cohen MS, Isturiz RE, Malech HL, et al: Fungal infection in chronic granulomatous disease. *Am J Med* 71:59, 1981.

135. Goodman ML, Coffey RJ: Stereotaxic drainage of *Aspergillus* brain abscess with long-term survival: Case report and review. *Neurosurgery* 24:96, 1989.

136. Denning DW, Ribaud P, Milpied N, et al: Efficacy and safety of voriconazole in the treatment of acute invasive aspergillosis. *Clin Infect Dis* 34:563, 2002.

137. Perfect JR, Schell WA: The newer fungal opportunists are coming. *Clin Infect Dis* 22:112, 1996.

138. Sutton DA, Slifkin M, Yakulis R, et al: U.S. case report of cerebral phaeohyphomycosis caused by *Ramichloridium obovoideum* (*R. mackenziei*): Criteria for identification, therapy, and review of other known dematiacious neurotropic taxa. *J Clin Microbiol* 36:708, 1998.

139. Bennett JE, Bonner H, Jennings AE, et al: Chronic meningitis caused by *Cladosporium trichoides. Am J Clin Pathol* 59:398, 1973.

140. Perfect JR, Rude T, Penning L, et al: Cloning of a *Cryptococcus neoformans* mannitol dehydrogenase gene. XI Congress of the International Society for Human and Animal Mycoses, Montreal, CA, 1991 (abstract no 1.45).

141. Fletcher H, Williams NP, Nicholson A, et al: Systemic phaeohyphomycosis in pregnancy and the puerperium. *West Ind Med J* 49:79, 2000.

142. Walz R, Bianchin M, Chaves ML, et al: Cerebral phaeohyphomycosis caused by *Cladophialophora bantiana* in a Brazilian drug abuser. *J Med Vet Mycol* 35:427, 1997.

143. Biggs PJ, Allen RL, Powers JM, et al: Phaeohyphomy-cosis complicating compound skull fracture. *Surg Neurol* 25:393, 1986.

144. *Exophiala* infection from contaminated injectable steroids prepared by a compounding pharmacy. *MMWR* 51, 2002.

145. Dixon D, Polak A: In vitro and in vivo drug studies with three agents of central nervous system phaeohyphomycosis. *Chemotherapy* 33:129, 1987.

146. Steinberg GK, Britt RH, Enzmann DR: Fusarium brain abscess. Case report. *J Neurosurg* 58:598, 1983.

147. Yoo D, Lee WHS, Kwon-Chung KJ: Brain abscess due to *Pseudallescheria boydii* associated with primary non-Hodgkin's lymphoma of the central nervous system: A case report and literature review. *Rev Infect Dis* 7:272, 1985.

148. Selby R: Pachymeningitis secondary to *Allescheria boydii:* Case report. *J Neurosurg* 36:225, 1972.

149. Dworzack DL, Clark RB, Padgett PJ: New causes of pneumonia, meningitis, and disseminated infections associated with immersion. Infect Control Hosp, *Epidemiology* 1:615, 1987.

150. Scott EN, Kaufman L, Brown AC, et al: Serologic studies in the diagnosis and management of meningitis due to *Sporothrix schenckii. New Engl J* Med 317:935, 1987.

151. Kozel TR, Pfrommer GST, Guerlain AS, et al: Role of the capsule in phagocytosis of *Cryptococcus neoformans. Rev Infect Dis* 10:S436, 1988.

152. Jones PD, See J: *Penicillium marneffei* in patients with human immunodeficiency virus: Late presentation in an area of nonendemicity. *Clin Infect Dis* 15:744, 1992.

153. Sekhon AS, Stein L, Garg AK, et al: Pulmonary penicillosis *marneffei:* Report of the first imported case in Canada. *Mycopathologia* 128:3, 1994.

154. Supparatpinyo K, Chiewchanvit S, Hirunsri P, et al: *Penicillium marneffei* infection in patients infected with human immunodeficiency virus. *Clin Infect Dis* 14:871, 1992.

155. Singh N, Gayowski T, Singh J, et al: Invasive gastrointestinal zygomycosis in a liver transplant recipient: Case report and review of zygomycosis in solid-organ transplant recipients. *Clin Infect Dis* 20:617, 1995.

156. Hopkins RJRM, Fiore A, Goldblum SE: Cerebral mucormycosis associated with intravenous drug use: Three case reports and review. *Clin Infect Dis* 21:1133, 1994.

157. Larkin J, Montero JA: Efficacy and safety of amphotericin B lipid complex for zygomycosis. *Infections in Medicine* 20(4):201, 2003.

CHAPTER 13

CNS Tuberculosis and Mycobacteriosis

Juan C. Garcia-Monco

Mycobacterial infections in humans represent a growing international health problem. Tuberculosis (TB) is the leading infectious cause of death in the world today. The mycobacteria that cause human disease belong to two groups: *Mycobacterium tuberculosis* complex and nontuberculous mycobacteria (NTM) or atypical mycobacteria. *M. tuberculosis* causes the vast majority of central nervous system (CNS) infections.

▶ CNS TUBERCULOSIS

Recent estimates from the World Health Organization (WHO) indicate that the global burden of tuberculosis is enormous mainly because of a high incidence of disease in Southeast Asia, sub-Saharan Africa, and eastern Europe and because of high rates of *M. tuberculosis* and human immunodeficiency virus (HIV) coinfection in some African countries.[1] In the United States, after decades of steadily declining rates of infection there was a resurgence of tuberculosis in the mid-1980s. The highest incidence was reached in 1992, followed by a steady decrease in the cure rate. In 2000, 16,377 cases (5.8 cases per 100,000 population) were reported to the Centers for Disease Control and Prevention (CDC), which represented a 45 percent decrease from the peak rate and was the lowest in U.S. history. Despite this, the number of cases among foreign-born persons per 100,000 population continues to rise (7270 cases in 1992 and 7554 cases in 2000), with a case rate that remains seven times higher than that among people born in the United States.[2] The acquired immune deficiency syndrome (AIDS) epidemic accounts for a large number of tuberculosis cases, in addition to immigration and urban crowding. This, combined with an increase in drug-resistant *M. tuberculosis* strains, makes this disease a global public health priority.

Etiologic Agent

Tuberculosis is caused by mycobacteria belonging to the *Mycobacterium tuberculosis* complex, which consists of *M. tuberculosis, M. bovi,* and *M. africanum. M. tuberculosis* is the main pathogen in human disease, and the term *tuberculosis* should be reserved exclusively for infection or disease caused by this organism. The other two species rarely cause human diseases. *M. bovis* is transmitted by ingestion of unpasteurized milk, and the distribution of *M. africanum* is largely restricted to central and west Africa. Infection by these organisms should be referred to as *mycobacteriosis due to M. bovis or M. africanum,* avoiding the term *atypical tuberculosis. M. tuberculosis* is an obligate aerobic bacillus whose entire genome has been sequenced,[3] providing a wealth of information that may result in much needed improvement in treatment, diagnosis, and prevention. More important, the main biologic characteristics of this bacillus (Table 13-1) underscore the basis for many of the difficult challenges presented by CNS tuberculosis.

Pathogenesis

The mycobacteria are primarily soil or environmental organisms. However, *M. tuberculosis* has become so adapted to the human body that it has no natural reservoirs in nature other than infected/diseased persons. The principal mode of contagion is by inhalation of aerosolized droplet nuclei. These nuclei contain few bacilli, and it is estimated that only 1 to 10 organisms are needed to cause infection.[4] The severity of disease in the infecting individual is important in determining

▶ **TABLE 13-1.** BIOLOGIC CHARACTERISTICS OF *MYCOBACTERIUM TUBERCULOSIS*

Gram-positive bacterium

Aerobic, nonmotile, and non-spore-forming bacillus

Very slow growth in vivo and under laboratory culture conditions

Generation time (cell division) is about 22–24 hours

Slow growth contributes to the chronic course of infection and to the need for lengthy antibiotic therapy

Has a circular chromosome with 4.4 million base pairs and about 4000 genes

Genome has a very rich G+C content (66%)

Cell wall contains rich and unusual lipids, glycolipids, and sugars

These lipids form a hydrophobic layer external to the cell wall that interferes with antibiotic penetration

Bacillus is naturally resistant to many antibiotics and has specific antibiotic resistance genes

Genome has many insertional sequences that could have a role in molecular diagnostics

Genome does not disclose the presence of acquired pathogenicity islands of different nucleotide composition

Genome is stable

SOURCE: Adapted from Cole,[3] with permission.

the risk of contagion; nodular lesions produce less bacilli than cavitary lesions.[5] Mycobacteria reach the alveoli, where they multiply in alveolar spaces or in macrophages. Within 2 to 4 weeks, many bacilli are killed, but some survive, and a silent hematogenous dissemination to extrapulmonary sites, including the CNS, can occur. A magnetic resonance imaging (MRI) study disclosed the presence of asymptomatic CNS granulomas in patients with miliary tuberculosis.[6] Ten percent of immunocompetent patients with tuberculosis will develop CNS disease.[7] Extrapulmonary tuberculosis, including CNS involvement, is considered an AIDS-defining condition. In the United States, 5 to 9 percent of AIDS patients have pulmonary or extrapulmonary tuberculosis. HIV serology should be obtained in patients with tuberculosis.[8]

Tubercles consisting of mononuclear cells surrounding a necrotic (caseous) center can be formed in the lungs as well as in secondary sites. Protein-purified derivative (PPD) reactivity develops and, together with radiologic evidence of the small tubercles, sometimes provides the only indication of infection. The complex cellular immune response in tuberculosis largely influences the development of active disease, although the factors that determine the degree of immune protection are not completely understood.[9,10] In some individuals (immune dysfunction plays a role here), further attempts by the mononuclear cells to control the infection result in expansion of the caseous lesions with central necrosis, liquefaction, and viable bacilli. If these lesions expand and break into the bronchi, a cavity can result, and the patient may release bacilli by coughing. If this progression occurs in the CNS from an initial or secondary tubercle, tuberculous meningitis or parenchymal disease (tuberculomas or, less frequently, abscesses) can develop. The inciting CNS tubercle has been called a *Rich focus,* which is thought to develop early in the infection during dissemination from the primary focus.[11] The location of the expanding tubercle determines the type of CNS involvement. Tubercles rupturing into the subarachnoid space cause meningitis. Those deeper in the brain or spinal cord parenchyma cause tuberculomas or abscesses.

Several important pathologic findings are strikingly apparent in tuberculous meningitis. A diffuse exudate composed of neutrophils, mononuclear cells, erythrocytes, and variable numbers of bacilli within a loose fibrin network occupies the subarachnoid space, particularly in the basilar cisterns and choroid plexus. As the disease evolves, lymphocytes and connective tissue elements predominate. Small and medium-sized arteries (but other vessels as well) adjacent to and traversing the exudate become inflamed with subsequent subendothelial cell thickening. This vasculitis can lead to focal brain or spinal cord ischemic disease as a result of vessel occlusion. Hydrocephalus, often of the communicating type and more prominent in children than in adults, results from blockage of the flow and resorption of cerebrospinal fluid (CSF) secondary to the inflammatory exudate. Damage to the brain parenchyma adjacent to areas of exudate (*border-zone encephalitis*) can occur and lead to sequelae even after appropriate therapy. A leukoencephalopathy adjacent or distant to sites of prominent exudate has been reported. All these pathophysiologic changes have been known for many years.[7,12–14]

Clinical Features

Tuberculous meningitis (TBM) is the most frequent and severe manifestation of CNS involvement in tuberculosis.[15] Tuberculoma and abscess formation, as well as spinal cord involvement, also can occur. The different clinical manifestations of TBM, tuberculomas, abscesses, and spinal cord involvement will be discussed separately. The characteristics pertaining to HIV-infected patients are included.

Tuberculous Meningitis

The main characteristics of tuberculous meningitis reported in the literature are listed in Tables 13-2 and 13-3 and separated into three categories to allow for a comparison between adults,[16–30] children,[31–44] and HIV-infected patients.[26,45–48] The British Medical Research Council devised a staging system to assess the severity of tuberculous meningitis and consists of three stages.[49] In stage 1, patients are fully conscious and rational and do not have any neurologic signs. In stage 2, patients are confused but not comatose or have neurologic signs of localization such as hemiparesis or a single cranial nerve palsy. In stage 3, patients are comatose or stuporous or have multiple cranial nerve palsies or complete hemiplegia or paraplegia.

Typically, there is a prodromal period of 2 to 4 weeks (it may range from a few days to several months) during which nonspecific symptoms, including fatigue, malaise, myalgia, and fever, are present. Not infrequently, in the first stage of meningitis, children have infection of the upper respiratory tract. Meningitis should be considered when the concurrent fever and irritability or lethargy seem out of proportion to the obvious infection or when general symptoms persist after improvement in the local manifestations.[31] Chest x-ray abnormalities, a history of close contact with an individual with tuberculosis, and tuberculin skin test positivity are present more frequently in children than in adults, likely reflecting the shorter period between contact and the development of meningitis in children. In adults, meningitis develops long after primary infection.

In adults, the most prominent clinical features of tuberculous meningitis are fever, headache, and vomiting with a variable degree of mental status abnormalities and meningismus and evidence of hydrocephalus on neuroimaging. Malaise, anorexia, and fatigue are also present in 50 percent of patients. Cranial nerve palsies occur in approximately one-fourth of patients, involving mainly the sixth and, less frequently, the third, fourth, seventh, and eighth cranial nerves. Other cranial nerves are affected only rarely, and occasionally there is bilateral involvement. Hemiparesis, pap-

► **TABLE 13-2.** TUBERCULOUS MENINGITIS: ASSOCIATED DATA

	Adults*	Children†	HIV-Infected Individuals‡
Mean duration of illness prior to admission (range)	2 weeks (1 day–9 months)	2 weeks (3 days–3 months)	2 weeks (1 day–3 months)
Mean frequency of close contact with tuberculosis (range)	28% (2–50%)	56% (45–70%)	NA
Prior history of tuberculosis	23% (5–45%)	NA	NA
Abnormal chest x-ray (range)	45% (25–55%)	61% (35–75%)	59% (55–65%)
Positive tuberculin skin test (range)	51% (40–70%)	72% (50–95%)	29%
Patients with hyponatremia (plasma sodium level < 135 meq/dl) (range)	46% (25–75%)	44% (25–65%)	NA
Mortality	27% (7–45%)	19% (3–40%)	25% (20–30%)

Note: NA = data not available or incomplete.
*Data pooled from references 16 to 22 and 24 to 30.
†Data pooled from references 31 to 44.
‡Data pooled from references 26 and 45 to 47.

▶ **TABLE 13-3.** SIGNS AND SYMPTOMS IN PATIENTS WITH TUBERCULOUS MENINGITIS

	Adults*		Children†		HIV-Infected Individuals‡	
	Mean (%)	Range (%)	Mean (%)	Range (%)	Mean (%)	Range (%)
Fever	72	55–85	76	45–95	82	75–90
Headache	67	45–85	34	20–40	79	60–100
Meningismus	67	55–90	62	25–75	65	NA
Abnormal mental status§	59	30–80	42	25–75	36	25–45
Hydrocephalus (CT scan)	52	40–65	85	75–100	42	NA
Vomiting	43	30–70	58	30–70	27	NA
Malaise-anorexia	41	45–65	52	30–70	27	NA
Cranial nerve palsies	24	20–40	29	10–45	NA	NA
Papilledema	15	5–30	9	9	NA	NA
Hemiparesis/hemiplegia	12	5–20	24	5–40	NA	NA
Seizures	11	7–10	25	10–55	3	NA

Note: NA = data not available or incomplete.
*Data pooled from references 16 to 30, 33, 35, 43, and 44.
†Data pooled from references 31 to 44.
‡Data pooled from references 26, 45 to 48, and 212.
§Includes any degree of drowsiness, lethargy, stupor, coma, and behavioral changes.

illedema, and seizures occur in 10 to 15 percent of the patients. Funduscopic evidence of choroidal tubercles, an almost confirmatory finding of tuberculosis, is found in only a minority (<10 percent) of patients, most frequently in association with miliary tuberculosis.[50] Children present with some differences in the clinical picture compared with adults, although the main features, such as fever, meningismus, vomiting, and altered sensorium or behavioral changes, are present in the vast majority. As compared with adults, a significantly smaller percentage of children complain of headache, which is absent in children under age 3 for obvious reasons. Hydrocephalus is present more frequently in children than adults, and several series have reported a 100 percent occurrence.[35] Children also may present with abdominal pain and constipation. In one series, constipation was present in 37 percent of patients.[19] This may have been underestimated in other series. The rest of the clinical manifestations do not differ very much between the pediatric and adult age groups.

The clinical features and CSF profiles of tuberculous meningitis are not modified by HIV infection.[26,30,51] This is in contrast with cryptococcal meningitis, which has a different clinical presentation in HIV-infected patients compared with non-HIV-infected individuals.[45] In terms of extraneurologic localization of tuberculosis, there was no significant differences in a group of 48 patients admitted to the intensive care unit (ICU) between HIV-infected and non-HIV-patients, except for the presence of tuberculous lymph nodes in 50 percent of HIV-infected patients as compared with 3 percent of HIV-negative patients.[30] Some studies have reported a

greater frequency of tuberculous intracerebral mass lesions in HIV-positive patients, mainly among intravenous drug users.[48,51] HIV-infected patients show a lower percentage of tuberculin skin test positivity (see Table 13-2), undoubtedly reflecting their cell-mediated immune deficiency. Tuberculin skin tests are positive in approximately one-third of patients, particularly in the early stages of HIV infection, whereas anergy develops with more advanced immunosuppression.

CSF Findings (Table 13-4)

Characteristically, the CSF has a lymphocytic pleocytosis with an average cell count around 200 cell/μl, increased protein concentration (around 200 mg/dl), and low glucose concentration. In 20 to 25 percent of non-HIV-infected patients, a neutrophilic predominance is present. Usually, there is a shift to a lymphocytic predominance over the ensuing 24 to 48 hours,[30] although occasionally neutrophils persist, resulting in the so-called persistent neutrophilic meningitis, a syndrome of varied etiology in which TB has to be carefully excluded.[52] This syndrome also occurs in HIV-infected patients, where it is more common when meningitis is caused by multidrug-resistant mycobacteria.[45] It also has been described in immunocompromised non-HIV-infected patients with tuberculous meningitis.[53]

On the other hand, an initial mononuclear pleocytosis may briefly change in the direction of a polymorphonuclear predominance when therapy is initiated, and this may be associated with clinical deterioration. This therapeutic paradox has been regarded by some authors as virtually pathognomonic of tuberculous

▶ **TABLE 13-4.** CSF PROFILE IN PATIENTS WITH TUBERCULOUS MENINGITIS

	Adults*	Children†	HIV-Infected Individuals‡
Mean cell count (range)	223 cells/μl (0–4000)	200 cells/μl (5–950)	230 cells/μl
Mean percentage of patients with neutrophilic pleocytosis (>50% neutrophils) (range)	27% (15–55)	21% (15–30)	42% (30–55)
Percentage of CSF with normal cell count	6% (5–15)	3% (1–5)	11%
Mean protein level in mg/dl (range)	224 mg/dl (20–1000)	219 mg/dl (50–1300)	125 (50–200)
Percentage of CSF with normal protein concentration	6% (0–15)	16% (10–30)	43%
Percentage of patients with decreased glucose concentration (<45 mg/dl or 40% of serum glucose)	72% (50–85)	77% (65–85)	69 (50–85)
Positive smear	25% (5–85)	3% (0–6)	NA
Positive culture	61% (40–85)	58% (35–85)	23%

Note: NA = not available.
*Data pooled from references 16 to 30.
†Data pooled from references 31 to 44.
‡Data pooled from references 26, 45 to 48, and 212.

meningitis.[32] It manifests clinically within a few days after the commencement of antituberculous therapy with the patient's rapid deterioration into coma or even death. This syndrome is thought to represent an uncommon hypersensitivity reaction to the massive release of tuberculoproteins into the subarachnoid space.[7,54]

Some studies have found that mean protein concentrations were higher in patients with stage 3 disease than in those with stage 1 or 2 disease.[36] Normal protein concentrations are seen in 5 to 15 percent of patients and normal glucose concentrations in less than a third.

HIV-infected patients have a neutrophilic predominance more frequently (around 40 percent) than non-HIV-infected patients and less increased protein concentrations, the latter being normal in up to 40 percent of patients. Their CSF is acellular in up to 16 percent of patients as compared with 3 to 6 percent in non-HIV-infected patients. Acellular CSF samples may show pleocytosis if a spinal tap is repeated 24 to 48 hours later.[24]

Over time, CSF glucose concentrations normalize first, followed by the cell count and the protein concentration.[17,30] In one series, the most rapid return to normal of the CSF glucose concentration was 19 days, the slowest 11 weeks.[30] Mycobacterial stain of CSF samples is positive in 5 to 25 percent of patients and culture in 60 percent of patients. A combination of both microscopic examination and culture of several samples of CSF (sometimes up to four are necessary) provides the highest yield. Positive direct examinations of ventricular CSF samples from patients whose direct examinations of CSF from lumbar punctures were negative

have been reported.[30] This difference could be related to the larger volume of CSF obtained from ventricular drainage than from lumbar punctures. Adenosine deamine levels are usually increased in the CSF and can help in the diagnosis (see "Diagnosis" below).

Neuroimaging

Enhancement of the basal cisterns, either on contrast-enhanced computed tomographic (CT) scan or on post-gadolinium MRI is often striking, corresponding to the thick exudate that is observed pathologically.[55–57] The interpeduncular fossa, the ambiens cistern, and the chiasmatic region are the sites of predilection.[58,59] Meningeal enhancement is more common in HIV-infected patients. In one study, meningeal enhancement was present in 23 percent of HIV-positive patients but only in 6 percent of HIV-negative individuals.[26] Hydrocephalus is observed on CT scan and MRI usually as the result of tuberculous meningitis (communicating type), although obstructive hydrocephalus may occur due to a focal parenchymal lesion and the associated mass effect.[60–62] Some cases of so-called hypertrophic pachymeningitis have been associated with TB, either intracranial or cervical, but this association needs to be better defined, since most cases reported to date have been idiopathic.[63,64]

Complications

During the course of tuberculous meningitis, several complications can develop and should be monitored closely because they contribute to outcome.[60] Ischemic infarctions occur during the course of tuberculous meningitis in 25 to 40 percent of patients.[14,40,65] The inflammatory exudate involves the adventitia and progresses to affect the entire vessel wall, leading to panarteritis with secondary thrombosis and occlusion involving mainly the small and medium-sized arteries at the base of the brain. The anterior circulation is involved most frequently, whereas the vertebrobasilar system is affected less frequently. In one series, 25 percent of patients developed unilateral choreoathetoid movements due to contralateral caudate nucleus infarction.[14] Other movements disorders such as myoclonus, tremor, and dystonia also have been described.[66] Angiographic findings in tuberculous meningitis consist mainly of a triad that includes narrowing of the arteries at the base of the brain, narrowed or occluded small and medium-sized arteries, and hydrocephalus.[14,67]

As described earlier, hydrocephalus that eventually may require a shunting procedure is quite common in tuberculous meningitis, particularly in children. Also frequent is the development of a variable degree of hyponatremia or true SIADH that contributes to a further deterioration in the level of consciousness and can be attributed mistakenly to the infection itself. The serum sodium concentration should be corrected carefully so as to avoid a too rapid restoration of natremia with the risk of pontine myelinolysis. Syringomyelia also can develop as a complication of tuberculous meningitis, usually occurring several years after the initial infection, although a few acute cases have been reported.[68–71] Inflammatory edema and spinal cord ischemia appear to be the underlying mechanisms in early cases, whereas chronic arachnoiditis is the underlying mechanism in late-onset cases.

Diagnosis

The laboratory is of moderate assistance in the diagnosis of tuberculous meningitis. Approximately 10^4 organisms are required for reliable detection of bacilli using acid-fast stains (Ziehl-Neelsen, Kinyoun, and auramine-rhodamine stains), and for this reason, these techniques are seldom of diagnostic value in the CSF. Cultures of CSF, when positive, can take 4 to 8 weeks for a full and unequivocal identification. The frequency of positive CSF cultures in clinically diagnosed patients with tuberculous meningitis has a wide range of 25 to 85 percent (see Table 13-4) and an average of approximately 50 percent. Given that the patient with untreated tuberculous meningitis can have a rapid deterioration within the same period of time that it takes for cultures to grow, empirical therapy is mandatory. Therefore, the decision to treat patients where there is a high index of suspicion of tuberculous meningitis is made by the clinician without adequate laboratory support. Despite the low productivity of CSF cultures, it is highly recommended that they always be attempted not only for confirmation of the clinical and other laboratory diagnoses but also for drug sensitivity studies of the isolated strains. It is important to remember that both microscopic analysis and cultures should be attempted with as much CSF volume and with as many serial CSF samples as possible. Newer culture media—either radiometric, such as BACTEC, or nonradiometric systems—represent an improvement in that they may give positive results in 7 to 10 days.[72]

Serologic assays for TB have been notoriously lacking in the laboratory arsenal for this infection. A review of this topic is outside of the scope of this chapter because the host response in TB is very complex, but there are excellent recent reviews.[10,73–76] Although newer techniques using recombinant antigens for serology may become available in the future, the measurement of levels of antibodies to *M. tuberculosis* is not in routine use at present. Recent studies have shown promising results in detecting antibodies to this organism in cases of meningitis and pulmonary involvement.[77–79]

Determination of adenosine deaminase (ADA) in CSF, an enzyme associated with disorders that induce cell-mediated responses, is useful for the diagnosis of tuberculous meningitis.[80–85] However, high ADA levels also can be seen in other CNS disorders, e.g., lymphoma with meningeal involvement,[81] such other infectious disorders as neurobrucellosis,[84] subarachnoid hemorrhage,[86] or sarcoidosis.[87] False-negative results occur occasionally.[88,89] Several studies have reported a sensitivity and specificity of approximately 90 percent or even higher using a cut-off value between 5 and 10 IU/liter. Patients with tuberculous meningitis and AIDS do not differ greatly in CSF ADA values from non-HIV-infected individuals.[26,84,90] One study found a correlation between the CSF ADA levels and the CSF cell count, the percentage of lymphocytes, and the protein concentration.[91] ADA values may increase during the first 1 to 2 weeks of therapy and then decrease progressively.[80]

The unique features of tuberculous meningitis with its paucity of organisms, the poor yield of present laboratory techniques for the detection of bacilli, and the availability of a completely sequenced genome of *M. tuberculosis* provide reasons to be enthusiastic about the use of the polymerase chain reaction (PCR) as an important tool for the laboratory diagnosis of this disease. A large body of literature already exists on the use and parameters for the amplification of mycobacterial DNA in CSF. This literature is derived from studies that provide measurements of sensitivity and specificity for CSF PCR in tuberculous meningitis. In general, the use of primers derived from the insertional sequence *IS*6110, which is an element repeated many times in the genome of members of the *M. tuberculosis* complex, has yielded amplifications of high sensitivity. Other primers have been used as well with similar results. The sensitivity of the PCR in CSF has been variable, ranging from 54 to 100 percent, and the specificity has ranged between 94 and 100 percent.[92–105] As with other uses of this technique for the detection of microorganisms, its full use for the diagnosis of tuberculous meningitis is limited by the lack of standardization.[106] Nonetheless, a review of the existing literature shows convincing evidence that PCR is more sensitive than microscopic examination and cultures of CSF. A nucleic acid amplification assay intended for use on respiratory specimens, the Gen-Probe Amplified *Mycobacterium tuberculosis* Direct Test, also has been shown to provide a rapid (within 24 hours) and accurate diagnosis of tuberculous meningitis and intracranial tuberculoma.[107–109] In some studies, the evolution of a positive to a negative PCR before and after treatment suggests a role for this technique in deciding on treatment efficacy.

Therapy

The prognosis of tuberculous meningitis, an almost uniformly fatal condition at the beginning of the century, greatly improved after the introduction of streptomycin in the 1940s and of isoniazid in the 1950s. Since then, much debate has existed as to which regimens are ideal. Antituberculous drugs have been divided by general consensus into first-line (e.g., isoniazid, rifampin, ethambutol, pyrazinamide, and streptomycin) and second-line drugs (e.g., *para*-aminosalicylic acid, ethionamide, cycloserine, and some aminoglycosides and quinolones).[110] The search for new drugs, however, is imperative.[111] Guidelines for therapy of TB have been established by the American Thoracic Society, the CDC,[112] and the Infectious Disease Society of America.[8] The treatment of tuberculous meningitis, like that of other forms of TB, is aimed at killing both intracellular and extracellular organisms and must make use of several drugs. Although the number of organisms present in tuberculous meningitis is considerably lower than in other forms of TB and seemingly could represent an advantage, the treatment of tuberculous meningitis is hindered by the difficulty of antituberculous drug penetration into the CNS (Table 13-5). Isoniazid and pyrazinamide are bactericidal and penetrate both inflamed and uninflamed meninges, easily achieving therapeutic CSF concentrations. The CSF concentrations of oral rifampin and ethambutol and of intramuscular streptomycin are only marginally above the minimal inhibitory concentration (MIC) for *M. tuberculosis*. These drugs do not penetrate uninflamed meninges.[110]

Given a reasonable suspicion of tuberculous meningitis and the fact that antituberculous therapy is not particularly toxic in the short term, broad empirical antituberculous treatment should be initiated as early as possible to reduce morbidity and mortality.[113,114] At present, much of the decision as to which regimen should be employed depends on whether there is evidence of drug resistance. Cases of multidrug-resistant tuberculosis (i.e., resistance to at least isoniazid and rifampin) present a difficult treatment problem where therapy should be individualized and based on susceptibility studies.[115,116] The importance of antituberculous multidrug therapy, particularly in the initial phases of treatment to prevent the appearance of drug resistance, cannot be overemphasized. In this regard, the patient's compliance is crucial not only to cure the infection but also to avoid resistance. At present, drug resistance does not seem to represent a serious threat for tuberculous meningitis because there has been only the occasional single case report of multidrug-resistant meningitis,[33,117–121] although this aspect requires utmost vigilance. Intrathecal therapy with amikacin and levofloxacin was successful in an HIV-infected patient with multidrug-resistant tuberculous meningitis.[122] Whenever drug resistance is unlikely, a regimen with three drugs (e.g., isoniazid, rifampin, and pyrazinamide, all daily) for 2 months and two drugs (e.g., isoniazid and rifampin, daily or twice a week) for 10 months is recommended.[112,116] If the local incidence of drug resistance to *M. tuberculosis* is greater than 4 percent or is unknown, a fourth drug (e.g., streptomycin or ethambutol) should be added for 2 months, followed by isoniazid and rifampin to complete 12 months of therapy. If cultures remain positive for extended periods or signs or symptoms respond slowly, therapy should be extended to 18 months or 6 months after cultures are negative.[123] If resistance to one of these drugs is present, susceptibility studies will mandate the drug(s) to use. Ethambutol should be considered, particularly if the patient is over 50 years of age or has renal disease. Occasionally, five to six drugs are needed simultaneously in resistant cases, their choice being determined by sensitivity studies.

Liver enzymes should be monitored throughout therapy. In the event of significant elevations of alanine aminotransferase (>5 times normal), isoniazid and rifampin usually are stopped, and ethambutol and streptomycin are started and continued until enzymes return to normal, at which time isoniazid may be resumed with biweekly determinations of liver enzymes. In most cases the isoniazid, ethambutol, pyrazinamide, and streptomycin combination will be well tolerated. During pregnancy, streptomycin (which can cause congenital deafness) and pyrazinamide (with which there is not enough experience) should be avoided, and the preferred regimen is isoniazid, ethambutol, and rifampin. Shorter regimens could suffice, although there have been few controlled trials of treatment in patients with extrapulmonary disease. A study reported that the 6-month therapeutic regimen resulted in a morbidity-mortality ratio similar to that found in the longer-course therapies.[124] Chemotherapy with isoniazid and rifampin for 9 months

▶ **TABLE 13-5.** CHARACTERISTICS OF THE FIRST-LINE ANTITUBERCULOUS DRUGS

Drug	Bactericidal or Bacteriostatic	Penetration into the CSF with Normal Meninges*	Penetration into the CSF with Inflamed Meninges	Daily Dose (Route)	Special Remarks
Isoniazid	Bactericidal (against intra- and extracellular organisms)	+ (20% of plasma levels)	+++ (90% of plasma levels)	A: 300 mg/d (PO, IM) Ch: 10 mg/kg	Monitor for liver toxicity Add pyridoxine to avoid peripheral neuropathy
Rifampin	Bactericidal (against intra- and extracellular organisms)	No	+ (up to 10% of plasma levels)	A: 600 mg/d (PO, IV) Ch: 10–20 mg/kg	Monitor for liver toxicity Interacts with protease inhibitors for HIV infection
Ethambutol	Bacteriostatic	No	++ (10–50% of plasma levels)	15–25 mg/kg/d	Monitor for optic neuritis
Pyrazinamide	Bactericidal (against intracellular organisms at high concentrations)	+++ (similar to plasma levels)	+++ (similar to plasma levels)	A: 20–35 mg/kg (PO) Ch: 20–30 mg/kg	Monitor for liver toxicity
Streptomycin	Bacteriostatic (against extracellular organisms)	No	++ (25% of plasma levels)	A: 15 mg/kg (IM) Ch: 20–30 mg/kg	Monitor for vestibular and auditory toxicity

*Maximal penetration is represented by three crosses. A = adults; Ch = children; IM = intramuscular.

also has proven successful in 95 percent of patients, equivalent to conventional therapy with two to three drugs for 18 to 24 months.[125] A schedule that uses isoniazid, streptomycin, and pyrazinamide daily for 2 months and then two to three times per week for 7 months has an advantage of reduced cost, fewer doses, and ease of supervision when needed. A recent prospective study concluded that young children with tuberculous meningitis can be treated safely for 6 months with high doses of antituberculous agents (e.g., isoniazid, rifampin, ethionamide, and pyrazinamide) without overt hepatotoxicity and with a low risk of relapse.[126]

There is uncertainty regarding the role of corticosteroids as adjunctive therapy for tuberculous meningitis.[114,127,128] Two criticisms of the use of corticosteroids are interference with the interpretation of CSF studies and with penetration of antituberculous drugs into the CSF. The first criticism has not been supported by clinical experience. Through extensive follow-up of sequential CSF samples, in a retrospective series of 58 patients with tuberculous meningitis, low CSF glucose concentrations and positive smears persisted despite the use of corticosteroids.[25] The penetration of drugs into the CSF is not significantly affected by corticosteroid therapy.[129] Corticosteroid therapy probably improves neurologic outcomes of and decreases mortality resulting from tuberculous meningitis of moderate severity.[130] A recent study showed that corticosteroids significantly improved the survival rate and intellectual outcome of children with tuberculous meningitis, with enhanced resolution of the basal exudate and tuberculomas by steroids, as shown by serial CT scanning. Corticosteroids did not affect the intracranial pressure or the incidence of basal ganglia infarction significantly.[131] Therefore, their use seems warranted because the benefits probably exceed the risks.

Surgery is sometimes required to alleviate hydrocephalus not responsive to medical therapy, including steroids and/or diuretics (e.g., furosemide and acetazolamide). Usually ventriculoatrial or ventriculoperitoneal shunting is done, in general with favorable results.[132–135]

Vaccination with the bacille Calmette-Guérin (BCG) is administered routinely to newborns in developing countries where the prevalence rate of TB is high, as well as in some lower-incidence countries.[136] The reported efficacy of the BCG vaccine in preventing tuberculous meningitis ranges from 60 to 80 percent and from 84 to 100 percent in preventing TB-related death.[137–139] Although the duration of protection generally has been found to be limited, recent follow-up of a trial in newborns showed that the efficacy against both death and disease due to TB persisted for 20 years.[140] It also has been suggested that vaccination with BCG is effective in reducing the incidence of TB among health care workers.[141]

However, when the findings from all well-designed, prospective trials are combined, including data from trials that have involved older subjects, the relative risk of disease is in the range of 0.20 to 1.56, with an average efficacy of 50 percent,[142,143] which is substantially lower than that for mycobacteria-naive newborn populations. There are inadequate data to determine whether childhood BCG immunization provides protection against HIV-associated bacteremic or pulmonary TB.[144] As with most other vaccines, BCG has been shown to prevent disease, not infection.[145] Development of a more effective, better standardized, affordable vaccine with durable activity and fewer side effects is a major priority, including attenuated or enhanced whole-cell live, whole-cell inactivated, subunit, DNA, and prime-boost vaccines.[146]

Prognosis

All authors have emphasized the prognostic importance of the level of consciousness at hospital admission and the timing of initiation of therapy. Patients initially classified as stage 3 at admission and those in whom therapy is delayed are known to have a poor prognosis.[19,36,37,49] Also, patients under the age of 3 or over age 65, as well as those with associated miliary TB, have a poorer outcome.[32,36,67,147] In a study on adults admitted to the ICU with tuberculous meningitis, three variables correlated with outcome: time to onset of treatment of 3 days or more, coma, and a simplified acute physiology score of greater than 11.[30] Delays in treatment may be due to lack of suspicion of tuberculous meningitis, lack of characteristic CSF abnormalities, absence of meningeal signs, and no evidence of prior exposure to TB.[18,19,36]

HIV Infection and CNS Tuberculosis

Coinfection with HIV and TB has important implications because the prognosis of TB is poorer in these individuals due to their immunosuppressed state. Perform HIV testing on all patients with TB.[8] There is mounting evidence that the host immune response to *M. tuberculosis* enhances HIV replication and may accelerate the natural progression of HIV infection. Recently, the CDC recommendations for the diagnosis, treatment, and prevention of TB among adults and children coinfected with HIV in the United States have been updated.[148] In treating HIV-infected individuals, several factors should be considered. First, they usually have difficulty in controlling the infection due to the associated immunodeficiency. Second, rifamycins (e.g., rifampin, rifabutin, and rifapentine) interact with protease inhibitors, resulting in decreased activity of these drugs due to induction of cytochrome CYP450 by rifamycins (all protease inhibitors are metabolized by CYP450). For this reason, rifabutin—which has substantially less activity as an inducer of cytochrome enzymes—is used instead of rifampin in HIV-infected individuals, at a dose of 150 mg daily. Conversely, if protease inhibitors, particularly ritonavir or saquinavir, which are potent CYP450 inhibitors, are administered with rifabutin, blood concentrations of the latter increase markedly, and rifabutin toxicity increases as well.[148] Rifabutin is efficacious in nonresistant TB and is also active against *M. avium*; its role in multiresistant cases is less clear.[149] Third, HIV-infected patients can have malabsorption of antituberculous drugs[150] and are particularly prone to adverse drug reactions,[151] which makes drug monitoring particularly important. Ideally, the management of TB among HIV-infected patients taking antiretroviral drugs should include directly observed therapy.[148] Paradoxical reactions may occur during the course of TB treatment when antiretroviral therapy restores immune function.[152] It is also important to remember that HIV-infected patients have an increased prevalence of infections caused by atypical nontuberculous mycobacteria (see below). Aside from classic regimens of long duration (see above), a 6-month (isoniazid, rifabutin, and pyrazinamide for 2 months and isoniazid and rifabutin for 4 additional months) and a 9-month schedule (isoniazid, streptomycin, and pyrazinamide daily for 2 months and then two to three times per week for 7 months) are accepted regimens for HIV-infected patients.[148]

Parenchymal CNS Disease: Tuberculomas and Abscesses

Parenchymal CNS lesions may occur in patients with TB in the form of tuberculomas or abscesses. The differential characteristics of both entities are summarized in Table 13-6. Tuberculous granulomas (tuberculomas) are composed of a central zone of solid caseation necrosis that is surrounded by a capsule of collagenous tissue, epithelioid cells, multinucleated giant cells, and mononuclear inflammatory cells.[153–157] They contain a few bacilli in the necrotic center. Outside the capsule

there is parenchymal edema and astrocytic proliferation. They can be found in the cerebrum, cerebellum, subarachnoid space, subdural space, or epidural space. Tuberculomas are most commonly infratentorial in children, whereas in adults they tend to be supratentorial.[158] They may coexist with meningitis in 10 percent of patients[157,159,160] and are multiple in up to one-third of patients.[159,161,162] Clinical findings suggestive of TB are frequently subtle or absent. Extraneural disease or a past history of TB is present in fewer than 50 percent of patients.[157,159] The common presenting signs and symptoms are headache, intracranial hypertension, seizures, and papilledema.[157,163–165] The clinical course is subacute or chronic, usually weeks or months. The tuberculin skin test is positive in up to 85 percent of patients,[153,166,167] and chest x-rays suggest pulmonary TB in 30 to 80 percent of patients.[156,157] CSF findings are unremarkable or show a mild nonspecific increased protein concentration, and bacteriology is usually negative.[157] The diagnosis is made on the basis of neuroimaging findings, PPD test results, and response to antituberculous therapy. Parenchymal disease by neuroimaging most often involves the corticomedullary junction and periventricular regions, as expected with a hematogenously disseminated infection. On CT scan, tuberculomas appear as solid-enhancing, ring-enhancing, or mixed lesions; on occasion, there is a central calcification surrounded by a hypodense area with peripheral ring enhancement (target sign),[59] a pattern highly suggestive, although not pathognomonic, of TB. On MRI, tuberculomas appear as isointense to gray matter on T_1-weighted images and may have a slightly hyperintense rim.[168] Noncaseating lesions are bright on T_2-weighted images with nodular enhancement. Caseating tuberculomas vary from isointense to hypointense on T_2-weighted images and also exhibit rim enhancement.[59,168–170] They may demonstrate a variable degree of mass effect and perilesional edema, which usually are more prominent in the early stages.[168] Tuberculomas demonstrate no abnormalities on diffusion-weighted MRI with normal ADC values.[171]

▶ **TABLE 13-6.** DIFFERENTIAL DIAGNOSIS BETWEEN TUBERCULOMAS AND TUBERCULOUS ABSCESSES

	Tuberculoma	**Abscess**
Frequency	Relatively common	Rare
Lesion number	Multiple in one-third of cases	Single
Pathology	Solid caseation with few bacilli; lymphocytic infiltration	Liquefaction (pus) with many bacilli Neutrophilic infiltration
Course	Subacute–chronic	Acute
Location	Variable	Supratentorial
Neuroimaging	Solid, ring-, or mixed-enhancing lesions	Hypodense (CT scan), edema, mass effect, and peripheral enhancement of capsule

The differential diagnosis includes neoplasms and other granulomatous processes such as sarcoidosis and parasitic diseases such as cysticercosis and toxoplasmosis. Magnetization transfer imaging analysis has proved helpful in differentiating tuberculomas and pyogenic abscess from brain tumors.[172] With therapy, tuberculomas usually decrease in size to complete resolution within 3 months, although it may take longer (even to years), sometimes leaving a residual calcification.[153,165,167,170,173] Therefore, medical therapy alone is indicated initially, and surgery is indicated in the presence of intolerably increased intracranial pressure and in medical failure.[153,156,157] Mortality with current chemotherapeutic regimens is less than 10 percent. Prior to the availability of antituberculous drugs, mortality after decompression and excision was 35 to 85 percent.[159] Some patients develop intracranial tuberculomas or present a paradoxical enlargement of preexisting ones during the first weeks or months of treatment for tuberculous meningitis.[174] In a series of intracranial tuberculomas during therapy ($N = 24$), they generally appeared within 3 months of the start of therapy. Paradoxical deterioration in HIV-negative patients frequently is accompanied by an increase in peripheral blood lymphocyte count and an exaggerated tuberculin skin reaction.[175] Steroids seem to improve the general outcome, and dexamethasone is recommended for 4 to 8 weeks.[176] A recent review of the literature shows that surgery was done in approximately 60 percent of these patients.[176]

When the caseous core of a tuberculoma liquefies, a tuberculous abscess will result. Tuberculous abscesses are usually larger and less frequent than tuberculomas, may be multiloculated, and often have greater mass effect and edema. In contrast to the solid caseation and few organisms seen in tuberculomas, the abscess is formed by pus, where many bacilli can be found.[177] Its wall is devoid of the granulomatous reaction that surrounds the tuberculoma, with its appearance resembling that of a typical pyogenic abscess. A tuberculous abscess has a more accelerated clinical course than a tuberculoma, usually presenting acutely with fever, headache, and neurologic focal signs, often in the third and fourth decades, and is most commonly supratentorial.[178,179] However, a clear distinction between tuberculomas and abscesses is not always easy.[177] On CT scan, abscesses are hypodense, with surrounding edema and mass effect, and show peripheral enhancement, usually thin and uniform, although less often thick and irregular. On MRI, there is a central area of hyperintensity on T_2-weighted images.[59,169,170] This pattern is not specific; thus tuberculous abscesses are difficult to differentiate from toxoplasmic, fungal, or pyogenic abscesses or even from lymphoma in AIDS patients.[59,180] Localized areas of cerebritis with gyriform enhancement are observed less frequently.[62] Appropriate therapy includes antituberculous chemotherapy and surgical excision or aspiration where indicated. Ofloxacin was successful in a patient with intracranial tuberculomas in whom first-line therapy failed.[181] Parenchymal disease is more common in HIV-infected patients[26,51] and has been reported in 15 to 44 percent of AIDS patients with CNS TB.[169]

Spinal Cord Involvement

The spinal cord, as well as the nerve roots (radiculomyelitis) and spine, may be involved in TB. Spinal meningitis most frequently accompanies intracranial disease, although it may occur alone.[182–184] Pathologically, spinal tuberculous meningitis is characterized by a gross granulomatous exudate that fills the subarachnoid space and extends over several segments. Vasculitis involving arteries and veins can result in ischemic spinal cord infarction.[185] Clinically, tuberculous myelitis or radiculomyelitis usually presents as an acute or subacute (in fewer cases it runs a chronic course) transverse myelitis with variable degrees of radicular pain. Radiculomyelitis also occurs in HIV-positive patients.[186] CSF analysis reveals an increased protein concentration with a lymphocytic pleocytosis; low glucose concentrations are seen in one-third of patients.[182,184] The thoracic cord is affected most commonly, followed by the lumbar and the cervical regions. MRI shows contrast-enhancing tissue that surrounds the spinal cord and the roots and obliterates the subarachnoid space with focal or diffuse increased intramedullary signal on T_2-weighted images and variable degrees of edema and mass effect. Postcontrast T_1-weighted images may reveal leptomeningeal enhancement (Fig. 13-1). The nerve roots may be clumped and show contrast enhancement depending on the degree of involvement.[58,187,188] Corticosteroids seem to improve the prognosis.[189] Rarely, tuberculomas occur in the spinal cord either as intramedullary lesions or located in the dural space.[190–195] A combination of microsurgical resection and antituberculous chemotherapy is the best choice of treatment for intramedullary tuberculomas.[195] Also, infrequent cases of intramedullary tuberculous abscesses have been reported.[196]

Tuberculous spondylitis most often involves the thoracolumbar region, with L1 being the most commonly affected level and the cervical and sacral spine being involved only rarely.[59] The infection initially occurs in the anterior part of the vertebral body, usually involving more than one vertebral level, and disseminates to the disk and eventually extends along the anterior or posterior longitudinal ligaments or through the endplate. Vertebral collapse may occur, resulting in kyphosis. On occasion, infection of disks located at sites distant from the initial focus occurs, leaving intervening parts unaffected. In the lumbar region, tuberculous spondylitis may result in a psoas abscess that often cal-

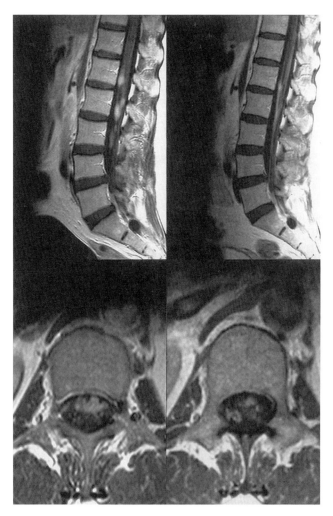

Figure 13-1. Spinal leptomeningeal tuberculosis. Serial T$_1$-weighted postgadolinium sagittal and coronal MRIs demonstrating nodular leptomeningeal enhancement of the conus medullaris and cauda equina on admission (*left*) and after 1 month of antituberculous therapy (*right*) without steroids. Notice the decrease in contrast enhancement after empirical antituberculous therapy.

cifies. Neuroimaging discloses bone destruction and fragmentation with involvement of the disk space and calcified paravertebral mass. MRI is the neuroimaging procedure of choice, with an accuracy of 94 percent in the detection of vertebral osteomyelitis.[197] MRI reveals hypointense T$_1$-weighted areas in the vertebral bodies alternating with areas of hyperintense T$_2$-weighted signal in the disk space and paravertebral soft tissue. Postgadolinium images show enhancement of infected bone and disk. Psoas abscess calcification can accompany spondylitis and is a finding very suggestive of TB. It is best detected by CT scan. It usually runs a subacute or chronic course with back pain, fever, and variable neurologic deficits. Spondylitis also can be associated with an epidural abscess, resulting in different combinations of local and radicular pain, limb motor and sensory loss, and sphincter disturbances. Eventually, complete spinal cord compression with paraplegia, the most dreaded complication, may supervene. Epidural deposits are best shown by MRI, which reveals a soft tissue mass that is iso- to hypointense compared with spinal cord on T$_1$-weighted images, hyperintense on proton-density and T$_2$-weighted images, and with variable degrees of contrast enhancement.[59] Spinal cord disease is treated with prolonged antimicrobial therapy and systemic steroids, with the prognosis being better in patients with recent-onset disease and those in whom prompt treatment is established. Surgery should be considered on an individualized basis depending on the extent and nature of the lesion and on the presence and degree of neurologic deficit.

► CNS INFECTION BY NONTUBERCULOUS OR ATYPICAL MYCOBACTERIA

Nontuberculous mycobacteria (NTM), or atypical mycobacteria, are categorized into different groups based on characteristic colony morphology, growth rate, and pigmentation (the Runyon system of classification), although this classification system is being replaced by more efficient and rapid systems of molecular diagnosis. Growth rates in culture remain a practical means for grouping species and classify NTM into slow (>7 days), rapid (within 7 days), and intermediate (usually 7 to 10 days) growing mycobacteria. The slow-growth group includes the *M. avium* complex (MAC), consisting of *M. avium* and *M. intracellulare* (also known as MAI), *M. kansasii*, *M. scrofulaceum*, *M. xenopi*, and *M. genavense*, among others. Mycobacteria that grow at the intermediate rate include *M. gordonae* and *M. marinum*. Among the rapidly growing organisms are the *M. fortuitum* complex (*M. fortuitum* group and *M. chelonei/abscessus* group). MAC is responsible for most of the infections caused by NTM.[198] Currently, approximately 50 species of NTM are considered to be potential pathogens. The rate of isolation of NTM is increasing and has surpassed that for *M. tuberculosis* in some areas. NTM are ubiquitous in the environment, including soil, water, and animals.[198] Most infections, including those which are hospital-acquired, result from inhalation or direct inoculation from environmental sources. Ingestion may be the source of infection for children with NTM cervical adenopathy and for patients with AIDS, whose disseminated infection may begin in the gastrointestinal tract. Because person-to-person transmission is extremely rare, infected patients do not require isolation.

NTM usually infect immunosuppressed individuals, primarily those with AIDS and very low CD4 counts (<50 cells/μl), in whom prophylaxis with clarithromycin (500 mg twice daily) or azithromycin (1200 mg once weekly) is recommended. NTM produce a broad spectrum of disease, including chronic pulmonary disease in adults, lymphadenitis (mainly cervical) in children, skin and soft tissue disease, skeletal infection, catheter-related infections, and disseminated infection.[198] CNS infection is rare and occurs in the setting of disseminated disease. The definitive diagnosis is made by culture of samples depending on the organ involved and, in cases of systemic infection, by blood cultures because there may be a high degree of mycobacteremia. The diagnosis is also established if transbronchial, percutaneous, or open-lung biopsy tissue reveals mycobacterial histopathologic changes and yields the organism. Radiometric culture systems, DNA probes, and PCR assays have increased the speed and accuracy of laboratory diagnosis of pulmonary and extrapulmonary infections.[199,200] Specific skin test antigens for NTM are not available. Since NTM are ubiquitous bacteria, their isolation from a clinical sample may represent a contamination. Thus it is very important to consider the clinical features when evaluating a positive culture. In contrast, isolation from a sterile fluid such as CSF usually represents a genuine infection of the nervous system.

CNS infection by NTM is infrequent and usually consists of meningitis or meningoencephalitis.[201] *M. avium* is the most common etiologic agent of this group, especially in AIDS patients. Most patients have evidence of extensive disseminated disease. *M. kansasii* meningitis is similar to that of tuberculous meningitis but with a somber prognosis. *M. fortuitum* meningitis is related to prior CNS surgery and trauma and frequently associated with abscess and foreign bodies. Prognosis in these patients can be more favorable if the concomitant abscess can be drained successfully or the foreign body removed. Overall prognosis for NTM meningitis is poor, with a mortality rate close to 70 percent.[201–203] CSF examination in NTM meningitis shows mild lymphocytic pleocytosis, with glucose and protein concentrations close to normal.[201] Less frequently, these infections result in mass lesions[204] or rhombencephalitis.[205] A case of chronic meningitis with a brain abscess in an immunocompetent patients also has been described.[206] In a patient with Hodgkin's disease, the histopathologic examination of the brain showed a perivascular infiltrate of lymphocytes and macrophages containing acid-fast resistant bacilli.[207] In a series of CSF cultures from 2083 AIDS patients with concomitant neurologic manifestations, *M. tuberculosis* was the most commonly isolated microorganism (4.2 percent), followed by NTM (0.7 percent). Of 130 positive cultures, 89 (68.5 percent) were *M. tuberculosis* and 15 (11 percent) an NTM.[208] In another series, *M. avium* was isolated from CSF in 11 of a total of 1273 (0.63 percent) AIDS patients.[209] A

potential role has been suggested for bacteria of the MAC infection in contributing to AIDS peripheral neuropathy as a consequence of macrophage activation resulting in an increased macrophage-derived toxin production.[210] Therapy for disseminated NTM infections requires consultation with an expert and has been revised by the American Thoracic Society,[211] although approaches to neurologic infection are unclear due to their rarity. Decisions must weigh all potential drug toxicities and interactions as well as the results of susceptibility testing. Regimens usually include a macrolide (clarithromycin 500 mg twice daily or azithromycin 600 mg daily), ethambutol (15 mg/kg daily), and an additional third drug (rifampin 600 mg daily or rifabutin 150 to 300 mg daily or ciprofloxacin). Optimal duration of therapy is unclear; immunocompetent patients probably should be treated for 18 to 24 months and AIDS patients for life.[212]

REFERENCES

1. Dye C, Scheele S, Dolin P, et al: Consensus statement: Global burden of tuberculosis: Estimated incidence, prevalence, and mortality by country. WHO Global Surveillance and Monitoring Project. *JAMA* 282(7):677, 1999.
2. Centers for Disease Control and Prevention: Tuberculosis morbidity among U.S.-born and foreign-born populations—United States, 2000. *MMWR* 51:1014, 2002.
3. Cole ST, Brosch R, Parkhill J, et al: Deciphering the biology of *Mycobacterium tuberculosis* from the complete genome sequence. *Nature* 393(6685):537, 1998.
4. Canetti G: Present aspects of bacterial resistance in tuberculosis. *Am Rev Respir Dis* 92(5):687, 1965.
5. Bloom BR, Murray CJ: Tuberculosis: Commentary on a reemergent killer. *Science* 257(5073):1055, 1992.
6. Gupta RK, Kohli A, Gaur V, et al: MRI of the brain in patients with miliary pulmonary tuberculosis without symptoms or signs of central nervous system involvement. *Neuroradiology* 39(10):699, 1997.
7. Udani PM, Parekh UC, Dastur DK: Neurological and related syndromes in CNS tuberculosis: Clinical features and pathogenesis. *J Neurol Sci* 14(3):341, 1971.
8. Horsburgh CR Jr, Feldman S, Ridzon R: Practice guidelines for the treatment of tuberculosis. *Clin Infect Dis* 31(3):633, 2000.
9. Dunlap NE, Briles DE: Immunology of tuberculosis. *Med Clin North Am* 77(6):1235, 1993.
10. Orme IM: Immunity to mycobacteria. *Curr Opin Immunol* 5(4):497, 1993.
11. Rich AR, MacCordick HA: The pathogenesis of tuberculosis. *Bull Johns Hopkins Hosp* 52:5, 1933.
12. Tandon PN, Rao MA, Pathak SN, et al: Radioisotope scanning of cerebrospinal fluid pathways. *Ind J Med Res* 62(2):281, 1974.
13. Winkelman NW, Moore MT: Meningeal blood vessels in tuberculous meningitis. *Am Rev Tuberc* 42:315, 1940.
14. Leiguarda R, Berthier M, Starkstein S, et al: Ischemic

infarction in 25 children with tuberculous meningitis. *Stroke* 19(2):200, 1988.

15. Garcia-Monco JC: Central nervous system tuberculosis. *Neurol Clin* 17(4):737, 1999.

16. Hinman AR: Tuberculous meningitis at Cleveland Metropolitan General Hospital 1959 to 1963. *Am Rev Respir Dis* 95(4):670, 1967.

17. Barret-Connor E: Tuberculous meningitis in adults. *South Med J* 60:1060, 1967.

18. Haas EJ, Madhavan T, Quinn EL, et al: Tuberculous meningitis in an urban general hospital. *Arch Intern Med* 137(11):1518, 1977.

19. Kennedy DH, Fallon RJ: Tuberculous meningitis. *JAMA* 241(3):264, 1979.

20. Klein NC, Damsker B, Hirschman SZ: Mycobacterial meningitis: Retrospective analysis from 1970 to 1983. *Am J Med* 79(1):29, 1985.

21. Kilpatrick ME, Girgis NI, Yassin MW, et al: Tuberculous meningitis: Clinical and laboratory review of 100 patients. *J Hyg (Lond)* 96(2):231, 1986.

22. Clark WC, Metcalf JC Jr, Muhlbauer MS, et al: *Mycobacterium tuberculosis* meningitis: A report of twelve cases and a literature review. *Neurosurgery* 18(5):604, 1986.

23. Traub M, Colchester AC, Kingsley DP, et al: Tuberculosis of the central nervous system. *Q J Med* 53(209):81, 1984.

24. Ogawa SK, Smith MA, Brennessel DJ, et al: Tuberculous meningitis in an urban medical center. *Medicine* 66(4):317, 1987.

25. Kent SJ, Crowe SM, Yung A, et al: Tuberculous meningitis: A 30-year review. *Clin Infect Dis* 17(6):987, 1993.

26. Berenguer J, Moreno S, Laguna F, et al: Tuberculous meningitis in patients infected with the human immunodeficiency virus. *New Engl J Med* 326(10):668, 1992.

27. Davis LE, Rastogi KR, Lambert LC, et al: Tuberculous meningitis in the southwest United States: A community-based study. *Neurology* 43(9):1775, 1993.

28. Girgis NI, Sultan Y, Farid Z, et al: Tuberculosis meningitis, Abbassia Fever Hospital–Naval Medical Research Unit No. 3, Cairo, Egypt, from 1976 to 1996. *Am J Trop Med Hyg* 58(1):28, 1998.

29. Hosoglu S, Ayaz C, Geyik MF, et al: Tuberculous meningitis in adults: An eleven-year review. *Int J Tuberc Lung Dis* 2(7):553, 1998.

30. Verdon R, Chevret S, Laissy JP, et al: Tuberculous meningitis in adults: Review of 48 cases. *Clin Infect Dis* 22(6):982, 1996.

31. Lincoln EM, Sordillo SVR, Davis PA: Tuberculous meningitis in children: A review of 167 untreated and 74 treated patients with special reference to early diagnosis. *J Pediatr* 57:807, 1960.

32. Smith AL: Tuberculous meningitis in childhood. *Med J Aust* 1(3):57, 1975.

33. Steiner P, Portugaleza C: Tuberculous meningitis in children: A review of 25 cases observed between the years 1965 and 1970 at the Kings County Medical Center of Brooklyn with special reference to the problem of infection with primary drug-resistant strains of *M. tuberculosis*. *Am Rev Respir Dis* 7(1):22, 1973.

34. Sumaya CV, Simek M, Smith MH, et al: Tuberculous

meningitis in children during the isoniazid era. *J Pediatr* 87(1):43, 1975.

35. Waecker NJ Jr, Connor JD: Central nervous system tuberculosis in children: A review of 30 cases. *Pediatr Infect Dis J* 9(8):539, 1990.

36. Delage G, Dusseault M: Tuberculous meningitis in children: A retrospective study of 79 patients, with an analysis of prognostic factors. *Can Med Assoc J* 120(3):305, 1979.

37. Idriss ZH, Sinno AA, Kronfol NM: Tuberculous meningitis in childhood: Forty-three cases. *Am J Dis Child* 130(4):364, 1976.

38. Naughten E, Weindling AM, Newton R, et al: Tuberculous meningitis in children: Recent experience in two English centres. *Lancet* 2(8253):973, 1981.

39. Cassleman ES, Hasso AN, Ashwal S, et al: Computed tomography of tuberculous meningitis in infants and children. *J Comput Assist Tomogr* 4(2):211, 1980.

40. Bhargava S, Gupta AK, Tandon PN: Tuberculous meningitis: A CT study. *Br J Radiol* 55(651):189, 1982.

41. Bullock MR, Welchman JM: Diagnostic and prognostic features of tuberculous meningitis on CT scanning. *J Neurol Neurosurg Psychiatry* 45(12):1098, 1982.

42. Naheedy MH, Azar-Kia B, Fine M: Radiologic evaluation of tuberculous meningitis. *Invest Radiol* 18(3):224, 1983.

43. Witrak BJ, Ellis GT: Intracranial tuberculosis: manifestations on computerized tomography. *South Med J* 78(4):386, 1985.

44. Yaramis A, Gurkan F, Elevli M, et al: Central nervous system tuberculosis in children: A review of 214 cases. *Pediatrics* 102(5):E49, 1998.

45. Sanchez-Portocarrero J, Perez-Cecilia E, Jimenez-Escrig A, et al: Tuberculous meningitis: Clinical characteristics and comparison with cryptococcal meningitis in patients with human immunodeficiency virus infection. *Arch Neurol* 53(7):671, 1996.

46. Yechoor VK, Shandera WX, Rodriguez P, et al: Tuberculous meningitis among adults with and without HIV infection: Experience in an urban public hospital. *Arch Intern Med* 156(15):1710, 1996.

47. Fischl MA, Pitchenik AE, Spira TJ: Tuberculous brain abscess and *Toxoplasma* encephalitis in a patient with the acquired immunodeficiency syndrome. *JAMA* 253(23):3428, 1985.

48. Bishburg E, Sunderam G, Reichman LB, et al: Central nervous system tuberculosis with the acquired immunodeficiency syndrome and its related complex. *Ann Intern Med* 105(2):210, 1986.

49. Council. BMR: Streptomycin treatment of tuberculous meningitis. *Lancet* 1:582, 1948.

50. Illingworth RS: The early diagnosis of tuberculous meningitis. *Br Med J* 1:479, 1950.

51. Dube MP, Holtom PD, Larsen RA: Tuberculous meningitis in patients with and without human immunodeficiency virus infection. *Am J Med* 93(5):520, 1992.

52. Peacock JE Jr: Persistent neutrophilic meningitis. *Infect Dis Clin North Am* 4(4):747, 1990.

53. Mizutani T, Kurosawa N, Matsuno Y, et al: Atypical manifestations of tuberculous meningitis. *Eur Neurol* 33(2):159, 1993.

54. O'Toole RD, Thornton GF, Mukherjee MK, et al: Dexamethasone in tuberculous meningitis: Relationship of cerebrospinal fluid effects to therapeutic efficacy. *Ann Intern Med* 70(1):39, 1969.

55. Ozates M, Kemaloglu S, Gurkan F, et al: CT of the brain in tuberculous meningitis: A review of 289 patients. *Acta Radiol* 41(1):13, 2000.

56. Engin G, Acunas B, Acunas G, et al: Imaging of extrapulmonary tuberculosis. *Radiographics* 20(2):471, 2000.

57. Boukobza M, Tamer I, Guichard JP, et al: Tuberculosis of the central nervous system: MRI features and clinical course in 12 cases. *J Neuroradiol* 26(3):172, 1999.

58. Gupta RK, Gupta S, Kumar S, et al: MRI in intraspinal tuberculosis. *Neuroradiology* 36(1):39, 1994.

59. Whiteman ML: Neuroimaging of central nervous system tuberculosis in HIV-infected patients. *Neuroimaging Clin North Am* 7(2):199, 1997.

60. Visudhiphan P, Chiemchanya S: Tuberculous meningitis in children: Treatment with isoniazid and rifampicin for twelve months. *J Pediatr* 114(5):875, 1989.

61. Kilani B, Ammari L, Tiouiri H, et al: Neuroradiologic manifestations of central nervous system tuberculosis in 122 adults. *Rev Med Intern* 24(2):86, 2003.

62. Villoria MF, de la Torre J, Fortea F, et al: Intracranial tuberculosis in AIDS: CT and MRI findings. *Neuroradiology* 34(1):11, 1992.

63. Parney IF, Johnson ES, Allen PB: "Idiopathic" cranial hypertrophic pachymeningitis responsive to antituberculous therapy: Case report. *Neurosurgery* 41(4):965, 1997.

64. Goyal M, Sharma A, Mishra NK, et al: Imaging appearance of pachymeningeal tuberculosis. *AJR* 169(5):1421, 1997.

65. Dastur DK, Lalitha VS, Udani PM, et al: The brain and meninges in tuberculous meningitis: Gross pathology in 100 cases and pathogenesis. *Neurol India* 18(2):86, 1970.

66. Alarcon F, Duenas G, Cevallos N, et al: Movement disorders in 30 patients with tuberculous meningitis. *Mov Disord* 15(3):561, 2000.

67. Lehrer H: The angiographic triad in tuberculous meningitis: A radiographic and clinicopathologic correlation. *Radiology* 87(5):829, 1966.

68. Fehlings MG, Bernstein M: Syringomyelia as a complication of tuberculous meningitis. *Can J Neurol Sci* 19(1):84, 1992.

69. Daif AK, al Rajeh S, Ogunniyi A, et al: Syringomyelia developing as an acute complication of tuberculous meningitis. *Can J Neurol Sci* 24(1):73, 1997.

70. Caplan LR, Norohna AB, Amico LL: Syringomyelia and arachnoiditis. *J Neurol Neurosurg Psychiatry* 53(2):106, 1990.

71. Schon F, Bowler JV: Syringomyelia and syringobulbia following tuberculous meningitis. *J Neurol* 237(2):122, 1990.

72. Watterson SA, Drobniewski FA: Modern laboratory diagnosis of mycobacterial infections. *J Clin Pathol* 53(10):727, 2000.

73. Orme IM, Andersen P, Boom WH: T-cell response to *Mycobacterium tuberculosis. J Infect Dis* 167(6):1481, 1993.

74. Fenton MJ, Vermeulen MW: Immunopathology of tuberculosis: Roles of macrophages and monocytes. *Infect Immun* 64(3):683, 1996.

75. Bloom BR, Flynn J, McDonough K, et al: Experimental approaches to mechanisms of protection and pathogenesis in *M. tuberculosis* infection. *Immunobiology* 191(4–5):526, 1994.

76. Rook GA, Hernandez-Pando R: The pathogenesis of tuberculosis. *Annu Rev Microbiol* 50:259, 1996.

77. Kameswaran M, Shetty K, Ray MK, et al: Evaluation of an in-house-developed radioassay kit for antibody detection in cases of pulmonary tuberculosis and tuberculous meningitis. *Clin Diagn Lab Immunol* 9(5):987, 2002.

78. Katti MK, Acharya MT: Immunodiagnosis of tuberculous meningitis: Detection of antibody reactivity to antigens of *Mycobacterium tuberculosis* and *Cysticercus cellulosae* in cerebrospinal fluid tuberculous meningitis patients by ELISA. *J Immunoassay Immunochem* 22(4):401, 2001.

79. Katti MK: Assessment of antibody responses to antigens of *Mycobacterium tuberculosis* and *Cysticercus cellulosae* in cerebrospinal fluid of chronic meningitis patients for definitive diagnosis as TBM/NCC by passive hemagglutination and immunoblot assays. *FEMS Immunol Med Microbiol* 33(1):57, 2002.

80. Ribera E, Martinez-Vazquez JM, Ocana I, et al: Activity of adenosine deaminase in cerebrospinal fluid for the diagnosis and follow-up of tuberculous meningitis in adults. *J Infect Dis* 155(4):603, 1987.

81. Pettersson T, Klockars M, Weber TH, et al: Diagnostic value of cerebrospinal fluid adenosine deaminase determination. *Scand J Infect Dis* 23(1):97, 1991.

82. Malan C, Donald PR, Golden M, et al: Adenosine deaminase levels in cerebrospinal fluid in the diagnosis of tuberculous meningitis. *J Trop Med Hyg* 87(1):33, 1984.

83. Mishra OP, Loiwal V, Ali Z, et al: Cerebrospinal fluid adenosine deaminase activity for the diagnosis of tuberculous meningitis in children. *J Trop Pediatr* 42(3):129, 1996.

84. Lopez-Cortes LF, Cruz-Ruiz M, Gomez-Mateos J, et al: Adenosine deaminase activity in the CSF of patients with aseptic meningitis: Utility in the diagnosis of tuberculous meningitis or neurobrucellosis. *Clin Infect Dis* 20(3):525, 1995.

85. Burnat P, Perrier F, Perrier E, et al: Value of determining the activity of adenosine deaminase in tuberculous meningitis. *Presse Med* 18(21):1077, 1989.

86. Egido JA, Gonzales JL, Cubo E: False positive of ADA determination in cerebrospinal fluid. *Acta Neurol (Napoli)* 16(5–6):288, 1994.

87. Garcia-Monco C, Berciano J: Sarcoid meningitis, high adenosine deaminase levels in CSF and results of cranial irradiation. *J Neurol Neurosurg Psychiatry* 51(12):1594, 1988.

88. More J, Matas E, Garau J: Determination of adenosine deaminase in tuberculous meningitis: Initial false-negative reactions exist in adults. *Med Clin (Barc)* 90(14):595, 1988.

89. Fernandez Carril JM, Guijarro Castro IC, Munoz Lasa S,

et al: Adenosine deaminase: False negatives in tuber-culous meningitis. *Neurologia* 7(7):202, 1992.

90. Ena J, Crespo MJ, Valls V, et al: Adenosine deaminase activity in cerebrospinal fluid: A useful test for meningeal tuberculosis, even in patients with AIDS. *J Infect Dis* 158(4):896, 1988.

91. Misra UK, Kalita J, Srivastava M, et al: Prognosis of tu-berculous meningitis: A multivariate analysis. *J Neurol Sci* 137(1):57, 1996.

92. Bonington A, Strang JI, Klapper PE, et al: Use of Roche AMPLICOR *Mycobacterium tuberculosis* PCR in early diagnosis of tuberculous meningitis. *J Clin Micro-biol* 36(5):1251, 1998.

93. Monno L, Angarano G, Romanelli C, et al: Polymerase chain reaction for noninvasive diagnosis of brain mass lesions caused by *Mycobacterium tuberculosis:* Report of five cases in human immunodeficiency virus-posi-tive subjects. *Tuberc Lung Dis* 77(3):280, 1996.

94. Miorner H, Sjobring U, Nayak P, et al: Diagnosis of tu-berculous meningitis: A comparative analysis of 3 im-munoassays, an immune complex assay and the poly-merase chain reaction. *Tuberc Lung Dis* 76(5):381, 1995.

95. Nguyen LN, Kox LF, Pham LD, et al: The potential contribution of the polymerase chain reaction to the diagnosis of tuberculous meningitis. *Arch Neurol* 53(8):771, 1996.

96. Scarpellini P, Racca S, Cinque P, et al: Nested poly-merase chain reaction for diagnosis and monitoring treatment response in AIDS patients with tuberculous meningitis. *AIDS* 9(8):895, 1995.

97. Seth P, Ahuja GK, Bhanu NV, et al: Evaluation of polymerase chain reaction for rapid diagnosis of clini-cally suspected tuberculous meningitis. *Tuberc Lung Dis* 77(4):353, 1996.

98. Lin JJ, Harn HJ: Application of the polymerase chain reaction to monitor *Mycobacterium tuberculosis* DNA in the CSF of patients with tuberculous meningitis after antibiotic treatment. *J Neurol Neurosurg Psychiatry* 59(2):175, 1995.

99. Lin JJ, Harn HJ, Hsu YD, et al: Rapid diagnosis of tu-berculous meningitis by polymerase chain reaction as-say of cerebrospinal fluid. *J Neurol* 242(3):147, 1995.

100. Kox LF, Kuijper S, Kolk AH: Early diagnosis of tuber-culous meningitis by polymerase chain reaction. *Neu-rology* 45(12):2228, 1995.

101. Folgueira L, Delgado R, Palenque E, et al: Polymerase chain reaction for rapid diagnosis of tuberculous meningitis in AIDS patients. *Neurology* 44(7):1336, 1994.

102. Liu PY, Shi ZY, Lau YJ, et al: Rapid diagnosis of tuber-culous meningitis by a simplified nested amplification protocol. *Neurology* 44(6):1161, 1994.

103. Donald PR, Victor TC, Jordaan AM, et al: Polymerase chain reaction in the diagnosis of tuberculous meningi-tis. *Scand J Infect Dis* 25(5):613, 1993.

104. Kaneko K, Onodera O, Miyatake T, et al: Rapid diag-nosis of tuberculous meningitis by polymerase chain reaction (PCR). *Neurology* 40(10):1617, 1990.

105. Shankar P, Manjunath N, Mohan KK, et al: Rapid diag-

nosis of tuberculous meningitis by polymerase chain reaction. *Lancet* 337(8732):5, 1991.

106. Noordhoek GT, Kolk AH, Bjune G, et al: Sensitivity and specificity of PCR for detection of *Mycobacterium tuberculosis:* A blind comparison study among seven laboratories. *J Clin Microbiol* 32(2):277, 1994.

107. Chedore P, Jamieson FB: Rapid molecular diagnosis of tuberculous meningitis using the Gen-Probe Amplified *Mycobacterium tuberculosis* Direct Test in a large Canadian public health laboratory. *Int J Tuberc Lung Dis* 6(10):913, 2002.

108. O'Sullivan CE, Miller DR, Schneider PS, et al: Evalua-tion of Gen-Probe Amplified *Mycobacterium tuberculo-sis* Direct Test by using respiratory and nonrespiratory specimens in a tertiary care center laboratory. *J Clin Microbiol* 40(5):1723, 2002.

109. Woods GL: Molecular techniques in mycobacterial de-tection. *Arch Pathol Lab Med* 125(1):122, 2001.

110. Mandell GL, Petri WA: Drugs used in the chemother-apy of tuberculosis, *Mycobacterium avium* complex disease, and leprosy, in Hardman JE, Limbird LE, Moli-noff PB, Ruddon RW, Gilman AG (eds): *Goodman and Gilman's The Pharmacological Basis of Therapeu-tics*, 9th ed. New York: McGraw-Hill, 1996, pp 1155–1174.

111. O'Brien RJ, Nunn PP: The need for new drugs against tuberculosis: Obstacles, opportunities, and next steps. *Am J Respir Crit Care Med* 163(5):1055, 2001.

112. Bass JB Jr, Farer LS, Hopewell PC, et al: Treatment of tuberculosis and tuberculosis infection in adults and children. American Thoracic Society and The Centers for Disease Control and Prevention. *Am J Respir Crit Care Med* 149(5):1359, 1994.

113. Humphries M: The management of tuberculous menin-gitis. *Thorax* 47(8):577, 1992.

114. Kendig EL Jr: Steroids for meningitis: Tuberculous and bacterial. *Pediatr Infect Dis J* 8(8):541, 1989.

115. Iseman MD, Cohn DL, Sbarbaro JA: Directly observed treatment of tuberculosis: We can't afford not to try it. *New Engl J Med* 328(8):576, 1993.

116. Small PM, Fujiwara PI: Management of tuberculosis in the United States. *New Engl J Med* 345(3):189, 2001.

117. Jereb JA, Klevens RM, Privett TD, et al: Tuberculosis in health care workers at a hospital with an outbreak of multidrug-resistant *Mycobacterium tuberculosis*. *Arch Intern Med* 155(8):854, 1995.

118. Fortun J, Gomez-Mampaso E, Navas E, et al: Tubercu-lous meningitis caused by resistant microorganisms: Therapeutic failure in two patients with HIV infection and disseminated tuberculosis. *Enferm Infect Microbiol Clin* 12(3):150, 1994.

119. Horn DL, Hewlett D Jr, Peterson S, et al: RISE-resistant tuberculous meningitis in AIDS patient. *Lancet* 341(8838):177, 1993.

120. Steiner P, Rao M, Victoria MS, et al: A continuing study of primary drug-resistant tuberculosis among children observed at the Kings County Hospital Med-ical Center between the years 1961 and 1980. *Am Rev Respir Dis* 128(3):425, 1983.

121. Watt G, Selkon JB, Bautista S, et al: Drug resistant tu-

berculous meningitis in the Philippines: Report of a case. *Tubercle* 70(2):139, 1989.

122. Berning SE, Cherry TA, Iseman MD: Novel treatment of meningitis caused by multidrug-resistant *Mycobacterium tuberculosis* with intrathecal levofloxacin and amikacin: Case report. *Clin Infect Dis* 32(4):643, 2001.

123. Holdiness MR: Management of tuberculosis meningitis. *Drugs* 39(2):224, 1990.

124. Alarcon F, Escalante L, Perez Y, et al: Tuberculous meningitis. Short course of chemotherapy. *Arch Neurol* 47(12):1313, 1990.

125. Dutt AK, Moers D, Stead WW: Short-course chemotherapy for extrapulmonary tuberculosis: Nine years' experience. *Ann Intern Med* 104(1):7, 1986.

126. Donald PR, Schoeman JF, Van Zyl LE, et al: Intensive short course chemotherapy in the management of tuberculous meningitis. *Int J Tuberc Lung Dis* 2(9):704, 1998.

127. Girgis NI, Farid Z, Kilpatrick ME, et al: Dexamethasone adjunctive treatment for tuberculous meningitis. *Pediatr Infect Dis J* 10(3):179, 1991.

128. Leonard JM, Des Prez RM: Tuberculous meningitis. *Infect Dis Clin North Am* 4(4):769, 1990.

129. Kaojarern S, Supmonchai K, Phuapradit P, et al: Effect of steroids on cerebrospinal fluid penetration of antituberculous drugs in tuberculous meningitis. *Clin Pharmacol Ther* 49(1):6, 1991.

130. Dooley DP, Carpenter JL, Rademacher S: Adjunctive corticosteroid therapy for tuberculosis: A critical reappraisal of the literature. *Clin Infect Dis* 25(4):872, 1997.

131. Schoeman JF, Van Zyl LE, Laubscher JA, et al: Effect of corticosteroids on intracranial pressure, computed tomographic findings, and clinical outcome in young children with tuberculous meningitis. *Pediatrics* 99(2):226, 1997.

132. Gropper MR, Schulder M, Sharan AD, et al: Central nervous system tuberculosis: Medical management and surgical indications. *Surg Neurol* 44(4):378; discussion 384, 1995.

133. Chitale VR, Kasaliwal GT: Our experience of ventriculoatrial shunt using Upadhyaya valve in cases of hydrocephalus associated with tuberculous meningitis. *Prog Pediatr Surg* 15:223, 1982.

134. Murray HW, Brandstetter RD, Lavyne MH: Ventriculoatrial shunting for hydrocephalus complicating tuberculous meningitis. *Am J Med* 70(4):895, 1981.

135. Singhal BS, Bhagwati SN, Syed AH, et al: Raised intracranial pressure in tuberculous meningitis. *Neurol India* 23(1):32, 1975.

136. Romanus V, Svensson A, Hallander HO: The impact of changing BCG coverage on tuberculosis incidence in Swedish-born children between 1969 and 1989. *Tuberc Lung Dis* 73(3):150, 1992.

137. Guerin N, Levy-Bruhl D: Update on the BGC vaccine: Indications for use in Europe and in developing countries. *Med Trop (Mars)* 56(2):173, 1996.

138. Thilothammal N, Krishnamurthy PV, Runyan DK, et al: Does BCG vaccine prevent tuberculous meningitis? *Arch Dis Child* 74(2):144, 1996.

139. Rodrigues LC, Diwan VK, Wheeler JG: Protective effect of BCG against tuberculous meningitis and miliary tuberculosis: A meta-analysis. *Int J Epidemiol* 22(6):1154, 1993.

140. Aronson N, Santosham M, Howard R, et al: The long term efficacy of BCG vaccine. In *Programs and Abstracts of the 39th Interscience Conference on Antimicrobial Agents and Chemotherapy, 1999.* San Francisco: American Society for Microbiology, 1999, p 381.

141. Brewer TF, Colditz GA: Bacille Calmette-Guérin vaccination for the prevention of tuberculosis in health care workers. *Clin Infect Dis* 20(1):136, 1995.

142. Colditz GA, Berkey CS, Mosteller F, et al: The efficacy of bacillus Calmette-Guérin vaccination of newborns and infants in the prevention of tuberculosis: Meta-analyses of the published literature. *Pediatrics* 96:29, 1995.

143. Colditz GA, Brewer TF, Berkey CS, et al: Efficacy of BCG vaccine in the prevention of tuberculosis. Meta-analysis of the published literature. *JAMA* 271(9):698, 1994.

144. von Reyn CF: The significance of bacteremic tuberculosis among persons with HIV infection in developing countries. *AIDS* 13(16):2193, 1999.

145. Letvin NL, Bloom BR, Hoffman SL: Prospects for vaccines to protect against AIDS, tuberculosis, and malaria. *JAMA* 285(5):606, 2001.

146. von Reyn CF, Vuola JM: New vaccines for the prevention of tuberculosis. *Clin Infect Dis* 35(4):465, 2002.

147. Lincoln EM, Gilbert LA: Disease in children due to mycobacteria other than *Mycobacterium tuberculosis. Am Rev Respir Dis* 105(5):683, 1972.

148. Anonymous: Prevention and treatment of tuberculosis among patients infected with human immunodeficiency virus: Principles of therapy and revised recommendations. Centers for Disease Control and Prevention. *MMWR* 47(RR-20):1, 1998.

149. Wallace RJ: Antimycobacterial agents, in Mandell GI, Bennet JE, Dolin R (eds): *Principles and Practice of Infectious Diseases.* Philadelphia: Churchill-Livingstone, 2000, pp 436–448.

150. Gordon SM, Horsburgh CR Jr, Peloquin CA, et al: Low serum levels of oral antimycobacterial agents in patients with disseminated *Mycobacterium avium* complex disease. *J Infect Dis* 168(6):1559, 1993.

151. Pozniak AL, MacLeod GA, Mahari M, et al: The influence of HIV status on single and multiple drug reactions to antituberculous therapy in Africa. *AIDS* 6(8):809, 1992.

152. Rao GP, Nadh BR, Hemaratnan A, et al: Paradoxical progression of tuberculous lesions during chemotherapy of central nervous system tuberculosis. *J Neurosurg* 83:359, 1995.

153. Bagga A, Kalra V, Ghai OP: Intracranial tuberculoma: Evaluation and treatment. *Clin Pediatr (Phila)* 27(10):487, 1988.

154. Dastur HM: A tuberculoma review with some personal experiences: I. Brain. *Neurol India* 20(3):111, 1972.

155. Haskett JR Jr, Branch CE Jr, Buscemi JH: Brain stem tuberculoma: Value of sequential computed tomography. *Ann Neurol* 6(3):275, 1979.

156. Loizou LA, Anderson M: Intracranial tuberculomas: Correlation of computerized tomography with clinicopathological findings. *Q J Med* 51(201):104, 1982.

157. Mayers MM, Kaufman DM, Miller MH: Recent cases of intracranial tuberculomas. *Neurology* 28(3):256, 1978.

158. Dastur DK, Lalitha VS, Prabhakar V: Pathological analysis of intracranial space-occupying lesions in 1000 cases including children: 1. Age, sex, and pattern and the tuberculomas. *J Neurol Sci* 6(3):575, 1968.

159. Arseni C: Two hundred and one cases of intracranial tuberculoma treated surgically. *J Neurol Neurosurg Psychiatry* 21:308, 1958.

160. Anderson JM, Macmillan JJ: Intracranial tuberculoma: An increasing problem in Britain. *J Neurol Neurosurg Psychiatry* 38(2):194, 1975.

161. Jinkins JR: Computed tomography of intracranial tuberculosis. *Neuroradiology* 33(2):126, 1991.

162. Sibley WA: Intracranial tuberculomas: A review of clinical features and treatment. *Neurology* 6:157, 1956.

163. Maurice-Williams RS: Tuberculomas of the brain in Britain. *Postgrad Med J* 48(565):678, 1972.

164. Peatfield RC, Shawdon HH: Five cases of intracranial tuberculoma followed by serial computerised tomography. *J Neurol Neurosurg Psychiatry* 42(4):373, 1979.

165. DeAngelis LM: Intracranial tuberculoma: Case report and review of the literature. *Neurology* 31(9):1133, 1981.

166. Meyers BR: Tuberculous meningitis. *Med Clin North Am* 66(3):755, 1982.

167. Harder E, Al-Kawi MZ, Carney P: Intracranial tuberculoma: Conservative management. *Am J Med* 74(4):570, 1983.

168. Gupta RK, Jena A, Singh AK, et al: Role of magnetic resonance (MR) in the diagnosis and management of intracranial tuberculomas. *Clin Radiol* 41(2):120, 1990.

169. Whiteman M, Espinoza L, Post MJ, et al: Central nervous system tuberculosis in HIV-infected patients: Clinical and radiographic findings. *AJNR* 16(6):1319, 1995.

170. Garcia-Monco JC, Gomez Beldarrain M, Fernandez Canton G, et al: Resolution of a brainstem abscess through antituberculous therapy. *Neurology* 49(1):265, 1997.

171. Basoglu OK, Savas R, Kitis O: Conventional and diffusion-weighted MR imaging of intracranial tuberculomas: A case report. *Acta Radiol* 43(6):560, 2002.

172. Pui MH, Ahmad MN: Magnetization transfer imaging diagnosis of intracranial tuberculomas. *Neuroradiology* 44(3):210, 2002.

173. Choudhury AR: Nonsurgical treatment of tuberculomas of the brain. *Br J Neurosurg* 3(6):643, 1989.

174. Afghani B, Lieberman JM: Paradoxical enlargement or development of intracranial tuberculomas during therapy: Case report and review. *Clin Infect Dis* 19(6):1092, 1994.

175. Cheng VC, Ho PL, Lee RA, et al: Clinical spectrum of paradoxical deterioration during antituberculosis therapy in non-HIV-infected patients. *Eur J Clin Microbiol Infect Dis* 21(11):803, 2002.

176. Hejazi N, Hassler W: Multiple intracranial tuberculomas with atypical response to tuberculostatic chemotherapy: Literature review and a case report. *Acta Neurochir (Wien)* 139(3):194, 1997.

177. Tyson G, Newman P, Strachan WE: Tuberculous brain abscess. *Surg Neurol* 10(5):323, 1978.

178. Whitener DR: Tuberculous brain abscess: Report of a case and review of the literature. *Arch Neurol* 35(3):148, 1978.

179. Kumar R, Pandey CK, Bose N, et al: Tuberculous brain abscess: Clinical presentation, pathophysiology, and treatment (in children). *Childs Nerv Syst* 18(3–4):118, 2002.

180. Reichenthal E, Cohen ML, Schujman CB, et al: Tuberculous brain abscess and its appearance on computerized tomography: Case report. *J Neurosurg* 56(4):597, 1982.

181. Sermet-Gaudelus I, Stambouli F, Abadie V, et al: Rapid improvement of intracranial tuberculomas after addition of ofloxacin to first-line antituberculosis treatment. *Eur J Clin Microbiol Infect Dis* 18(10):726, 1999.

182. Wadia NH, Dastur DK: Spinal meningitides with radiculomyelopathy: 1. Clinical and radiological features. *J Neurol Sci* 8(2):239, 1969.

183. Nussbaum ES, Rockswold GL, Bergman TA, et al: Spinal tuberculosis: A diagnostic and management challenge. *J Neurosurg* 83(2):243, 1995.

184. Dastur HM: A tuberculoma review with some personal experiences: II. Spinal cord and its coverings. *Neurol India* 20(3):127, 1972.

185. Kocen RS, Parsons M: Neurological complications of tuberculosis: Some unusual manifestations. *Q J Med* 39(153):17, 1970.

186. Hernandez-Albujar S, Arribas JR, Royo A, et al: Tuberculous radiculomyelitis complicating tuberculous meningitis: Case report and review. *Clin Infect Dis* 30(6):915, 2000.

187. Freilich D, Swash M: Diagnosis and management of tuberculous paraplegia with special reference to tuberculous radiculomyelitis. *J Neurol Neurosurg Psychiatry* 42(1):12, 1979.

188. Kumar A, Montanera W, Willinsky R, et al: MR features of tuberculous arachnoiditis. *J Comput Assist Tomogr* 17(1):127, 1993.

189. De La Blanchardiere A, Stern JB, Molina JM, et al: Spinal tuberculous arachnoiditis. *Presse Med* 25(29):1333, 1996.

190. Gokalp HZ, Ozkal E: Intradural tuberculomas of the spinal cord: Report of two cases. *J Neurosurg* 55(2):289, 1981.

191. MacDonnell AH, Baird RW, Bronze MS: Intramedullary tuberculomas of the spinal cord: Case report and review. *Rev Infect Dis* 12(3):432, 1990.

192. Rhoton EL, Ballinger WE Jr, Quisling R, et al: Intramedullary spinal tuberculoma. *Neurosurgery* 22(4):733, 1988.

193. Tacconi L, Arulampalam T, Johnston FG, et al: Intramedullary spinal cord abscess: Case report. *Neurosurgery* 37(4):817, 1995.

194. Garg M, Singh S: Intramedullary spinal tuberculoma. *Br J Neurosurg* 16(1):75, 2002.

195. Kayaoglu CR, Tuzun Y, Boga Z, et al: Intramedullary

spinal tuberculoma: A case report. *Spine* 25(17):2265, 2000.

196. Hanci M, Sarioglu AC, Uzan M, et al: Intramedullary tuberculous abscess: A case report. *Spine* 21(6):766, 1996.

197. Modic MT, Feiglin DH, Piraino DW, et al: Vertebral osteomyelitis: Assessment using MR. *Radiology* 157(1):157, 1985.

198. Brown BA, Wallace RJ Jr: Infections due to nontuberculous mycobacteria, in Mandell GI, Bennet JE, Dolin R (eds): *Principles and Practice of Infectious Disease.* Philadelphia: Churchill-Livingstone, 2000, pp 2630–2636.

199. Cook VJ, Turenne CY, Wolfe J, et al: Conventional methods versus 16S ribosomal DNA sequencing for identification of nontuberculous mycobacteria: Cost analysis. *J Clin Microbiol* 41(3):1010, 2003.

200. Brown-Elliott BA, Griffith DE, Wallace RJ Jr: Diagnosis of nontuberculous mycobacterial infections. *Clin Lab Med* 22(4):911, 2002.

201. Flor A, Capdevila JA, Martin N, et al: Nontuberculous mycobacterial meningitis: Report of two cases and review. *Clin Infect Dis* 23(6):1266, 1996.

202. Jacob CN, Henein SS, Heurich AE, et al: Nontuberculous mycobacterial infection of the central nervous system in patients with AIDS. *South Med J* 86(6):638, 1993.

203. Weiss IK, Krogstad PA, Botero C, et al: Fatal *Mycobacterium avium* meningitis after misidentification of *M. tuberculosis.* *Lancet* 345(8955):991, 1995.

204. Berman SM, Kim RC, Haghighat D, et al: *Mycobacterium genavense* infection presenting as a solitary brain mass in a patient with AIDS: Case report and review. *Clin Infect Dis* 19(6):1152, 1994.

205. Duong M, Piroth L, Chavanet P, et al: A case of rhombencephalitis with isolation of cytomegalovirus and *Mycobacterium avium* complex in a woman with AIDS. *AIDS* 8(9):1356, 1994.

206. Uldry PA, Bogousslavsky J, Regli F, et al: Chronic *Mycobacterium avium* complex infection of the central nervous system in a nonimmunosuppressed woman. *Eur Neurol* 32(5):285, 1992.

207. Gyure KA, Prayson RA, Estes ML, et al: Symptomatic *Mycobacterium avium* complex infection of the central nervous system: A case report and review of the literature. *Arch Pathol Lab Med* 119(9):836, 1995.

208. Landgraf IM, Palaci M, Vieira MF, et al: Bacterial agents isolated from cerebrospinal fluid of patients with acquired immunodeficiency syndrome (AIDS) and neurological complications. *Rev Inst Med Trop Sao Paulo* 36(6):491, 1994.

209. Hadad DJ, Petry TC, Maresca AF, et al: *Mycobacterium avium* complex (MAC): An unusual potential pathogen in cerebrospinal fluid of AIDS patients. *Rev Inst Med Trop Sao Paulo* 37(2):93, 1995.

210. Norton GR, Sweeney J, Marriott D, et al: Association between HIV distal symmetric polyneuropathy and *Mycobacterium avium* complex infection. *J Neurol Neurosurg Psychiatry* 61(6):606, 1996.

211. Diagnosis and treatment of disease caused by nontuberculous mycobacteria: American Thoracic Society statement. *Am J Respir Crit Care Med* 156(2 pt 2):S1, 1997.

212. Sanchez-Portocarrero J, Perez-Cecilia E, Romero-Vivas J: Infection of the central nervous system by *Mycobacterium tuberculosis* in patients infected with human immunodeficiency virus (the new neurotuberculosis). *Infection* 27(6):313, 1999.

CHAPTER 14
Neurosyphilis

Edward W. Hook, III, and David H. Chansolme

Throughout the twentieth century and continuing to the present, efforts to diagnose and manage syphilis, including neurosyphilis, have challenged clinicians, biomedical scientists, public health officials, and medical ethicists. As numerous questions have been addressed, others have arisen. Syphilis remains difficult to recognize, diagnose, and treat. Syphilis is now far less common than it was previously. Likewise, the prevalence of clinical neurosyphilis has decreased substantially, perhaps even to a greater degree than the incidence of syphilis itself. Nonetheless, since the emergence of human immunodeficiency virus (HIV) in the 1980s, potential interactions of syphilis and HIV have raised questions regarding how to best manage both diseases. For HIV-infected persons in particular, the diverse array of neurologic disorders that may occur, combined with the strong associations between HIV and syphilis and the myriad potential presentations of neurosyphilis, has proven particularly challenging.

The term *neurosyphilis* encompasses a spectrum of clinical syndromes including aseptic meningitis, meningovascular disease, tabes dorsalis, general paresis, gummatous neurosyphilis, and asymptomatic central nervous system (CNS) infection, all of which can present independent of one another or with considerable overlap. Although often misconceived of as a late manifestation of untreated syphilis, CNS involvement with *Treponema pallidum* occurs throughout the natural course of infection and may become apparent at any stage of untreated infection, as well as being a presenting manifestation of treatment failure. Because of this variability, neurosyphilis must be considered in the differential diagnosis of disorders varying from psychiatric complaints to focal neurologic or ophthalmologic disease and a wide range of presentations in between.

▶ HISTORY OF NEUROSYPHILIS

The origins of syphilis have been debated for many years, but it is believed that syphilis was transported to Europe from the New World by European sailors.[1,2] At that time, it seemed to be an aggressive disease with prominent cutaneous manifestations. Little neurosyphilis was reported.[1] Manifestations of CNS syphilis did not begin to be described extensively until the eighteenth century when the mental hospitals of Europe were crowded with syphilitic patients.[2] Some authors have estimated that by the beginning of the twentieth century, as many as 20 percent of all patients in mental hospitals were afflicted with neurosyphilis.[3] As Merritt and colleagues[1] noted, "paretic neurosyphilis is the combined result of 'syphilization' and civilization."

Another distinguishing feature of syphilis in the nineteenth and early twentieth centuries is that unlike today, syphilis was not limited to persons living on the margins of society. Indeed, many of history's most notable figures are believed or, in some cases, proven to have contracted syphilis and suffered the effects of neurosyphilis. The last days of Guy de Maupassant were spent in the throes of general paresis, replete with violent behavior, severe depression, hallucinations, and somatic disturbances.[4] Lord Randolph Churchill (the father of Sir Winston Churchill) died with all the signs and symptoms of tabes dorsalis and general paresis.[5] Others, such as Friedrich Nietzsche, Baudelaire, and Paul Gauguin, were all purported to have succumbed to neurosyphilis. Sir Oscar Wilde died penniless under a pseudonym in a Paris hotel, ravaged by neurosyphilis.[6]

Similarly, syphilis has been a prominent topic for biomedical research, and many treatments have been used in an effort to cure syphilis and neurosyphilis. Toxic mercurial compounds were used from the 1500s into the early twentieth century. In the last 100 years, two Nobel Prizes were awarded for contributions to the therapy of this disorder. In 1910, Paul Ehrlich developed arsphenamine (Salvarsan) as an alternative to mercury therapy, for which he received a Nobel Prize. Salvarsan was quickly incorporated into treatment regimens, but its administration and utility for long-term treatment were limited by local pain and thrombophlebitis. Other intravenous arsenical compounds were less irritating but still had toxic effects and, on the whole, were not particularly well tolerated. Nonetheless, the advantages of these compounds over earlier therapies contributed to a commitment to arsenical therapy (often used in combination with bismuth subsalicylate), which persisted as the cornerstone of syphilis therapy until penicillin became widely available.[7]

The second Nobel Prize directly related to advances in syphilotherapy was awarded to Wagner von Jauregg, a Viennese psychiatrist who introduced fever therapy into the armamentarium of therapy for neurosyphilis in 1917. Building on observations that people living in areas where febrile illnesses were common (malaria, typhoid, etc.) appeared less likely to develop neurosyphilis despite the high prevalence of early syphilis, Dr. von Jauregg began taking blood from patients with malaria and injecting it into paretics.[2] The fever would be allowed to relapse for 10 to 12 episodes, and then quinine would be given to arrest the malaria.[8] Earlier studies had shown the mortality rate of general paresis in the 1920s to be around 40 percent in many European hospitals. In malaria-treated patients, the case-fatality rate declined to about 10 percent.[8] This work earned Dr. von Jauregg a Nobel Prize in 1927.

Penicillin was first used to treat primary syphilis in 1943. It began to be used in neurosyphilis in 1944 and shortly thereafter was adopted as the treatment of choice, although early confusion regarding dosage, untoward reactions, and clinical efficacy delayed universal acceptance.[7] Ultimately, however, the ease of administration, the shorter courses of therapy, and the reduction in treatment-associated complications made penicillin the treatment of choice for neurosyphilis for more than 60 years. Many other antibiotics have been examined as possible alternatives, but none has shown the dependability of penicillin.

During the twentieth century, syphilis research increased, as did public health efforts to control the disease. Development of serologic tests, which could be used for diagnosis and to follow response to therapy, helped to define both the prevalence of syphilis and its manifestations. The famous Oslo study outlined the natural history of syphilis in a way no previous endeavor had done. The infamous Tuskegee study followed a cohort of men with latent syphilis in the absence of therapy even after the widespread availability of penicillin. The abuses of trust and the clear conflicts of interest inherent in the Tuskegee study were the foundation for many of the legal, ethical, and institutional changes integrated into the medical research system. Subsequently, large multicenter trials helped to define recommended regimens for syphilis treatment. Entering the twenty-first century, syphilis remains an important topic of biomedical research, as well as occupying an important place in the differential diagnosis of a number of clinical syndromes.

▶ SPECTRUM OF DISEASE

Without therapy, syphilis reliably progresses through a series of clinical stages. These stages have been divided broadly into early (those in the first few years of infection) and late (more long-standing) syphilis. Early syphilis is further divided into primary syphilis, characterized by the presence of a chancre; secondary syphilis, which may be manifest by the presence of a rash, generalized lymphadenopathy, and other more general clinical manifestations; and early latent syphilis, in which the clinical signs and symptoms of early syphilis have resolved, and the only readily apparent indication of infection is a reactive serologic test. Latent syphilis may persist for years or decades without therapy. Years later, tertiary syphilis may develop in up to one-third of untreated persons and manifest as gummatous, cardiovascular, or late neurologic syphilis. Although often misconceptualized as a late manifestation of syphilis, the CNS actually is involved throughout the course of syphilis. Laboratory evidence of treponemal CNS invasion is present in many patients with primary syphilis even before development of reactive serologic tests (see below.)

The signs and symptoms of syphilis can vary dramatically from person to person and case to case, and so syphilis often has been called the "great imitator." After sexual exposure to *T. pallidum*, an incubation period averaging about 3 weeks typically is followed by the development of an ulcerative lesion at the site of inoculation known as a *chancre*. The appearance of the chancre heralds the onset of primary syphilis and often coincides with regional lymphadenopathy. The classic chancre is painless with an indurated, raised border around a central, clean-based ulcer. Spirochetes often are demonstrable by dark-field microscopy. Untreated, chancres may persist for 3 to 6 weeks and will resolve without any scar or other persistent abnormality. Most untreated patients will progress to secondary syphilis while the chancre is resolving or soon thereafter.

Secondary syphilis coincides with development of mild generalized symptoms, which include low-grade fever, headache, malaise, arthralgias or myalgias, and clinical involvement of a number of organs. A macular rash involving the palms and soles is the classic manifestation of secondary syphilis; however, the rash of secondary syphilis is highly variable and may present as a more generalized macular rash, as pustules mimicking pityriasis rosea, or as a rash resembling any of a number of other dermatologic conditions. Other clinical findings include generalized lymphadenopathy, mucosal lesions, renal involvement, hepatitis, and neurologic involvement. Untreated, the secondary stage typically will last from 2 to 8 weeks, after which, as for primary syphilis, the signs and symptoms will resolve, and the disease will enter a clinically quiescent or latent stage.

In latent syphilis, clinical signs and symptoms are absent, but serologic evidence of infection is present. At this time, examination of cerebrospinal fluid (CSF) and serum may provide evidence of an ongoing disease. For management purposes, latent syphilis is further subdivided into the early latent stage (as determined by being detected within 1 year of acquisition of infection or being diagnosed within 1 year of the resolution of signs of primary or secondary syphilis), when the patient is at greatest risk for relapse of secondary syphilis and is most infectious to sexual partners, and the late latent stage, when sexual transmission of infection to others almost never occurs. During early latent syphilis, as many as 25 percent of untreated

patients may experience recurrence of clinical signs. About one-third of untreated latent syphilis patients will progress to late (tertiary) syphilis.[1,9,10]

Late, or tertiary, syphilis can affect any organ in the body. The cardiovascular system and the CNS are involved most commonly. Included in the broader category of tertiary syphilis are disease processes such as aortitis, iritis, and "late benign" or gummatous syphilis, which can vary in presentation and may be present independently of each other or in combination. Gummas are inflammatory mass lesions that can involve a variety of organs but seem to show a predilection for soft tissues, mucocutaneous tissue, and bone. These lesions are thought to represent an intense host response to a small number of treponemes, affect patients primarily through mass effect, and respond readily to penicillin therapy.[10]

Neurosyphilis has been further subdivided into four distinct disease manifestations that span the natural history of untreated infection: syphilitic meningitis, meningovascular syphilis, parenchymatous syphilis, and gummatous disease. With the possible exception of gummatous neurosyphilis, clinical neurosyphilis syndromes are preceded by asymptomatic CNS involvement in which only CSF abnormalities are present. Successful treatment of asymptomatic CNS involvement will prevent progression to clinical neurosyphilis. Syphilitic meningitis is an aseptic meningitis syndrome most often seen early during the course of syphilis and responds well to therapy. Meningovascular syphilis may present with focal neurologic deficits corresponding to areas of ischemia due to syphilitic vasculitis involving small and medium-sized CNS arteries and is seen several years after primary infection but not as late as parenchymatous disease. Therapy frequently halts disease progression, and some measure of clinical improvement is seen as well. Parenchymatous syphilis is comprised mostly of patients with general paresis, tabes dorsalis, or a combination of the two, but some patients with cranial nerve findings and ocular disease are included in this category as well. Disease onset usually is seen many years after the primary infection, and clinical deficits may not improve following treatment due to the irreversible nature of the pathology involved. Gummatous neurosyphilis is rare but can occur in late syphilis, presenting with findings due to space-occupying lesions in the CNS parenchyma. Penicillin can improve the clinical picture and resolve many of the symptoms associated with this disorder. Patients often present with overlapping symptoms, indicating a mixed syndrome.[1,9–11]

▶ EPIDEMIOLOGY

Prior to the availability of modern antibiotic therapy, syphilis was widespread and common throughout all

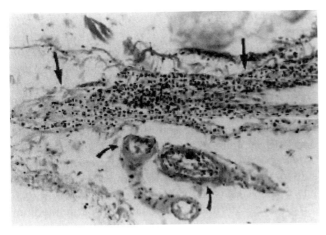

Figure 14–2. Microscopic findings of syphilitic meningitis. There is a lymphoplasmacytic infiltrate with thickened meninges *(straight arrows)* with involvement of the perivascular structures *(curved arrows)*. *(Used with permission from Brightbill TC, et al: Neurosyphilis in HIV-positive and HIV-negative patients: Neuroimaging findings. AJNR 16:708, 1995.)*

cytes (Fig. 14-2). This can cause further destruction of the meningeal space and rarely leads to a fibrosing arachnoiditis.[32] More recently, efforts to study the CNS immune response also have shown increasing levels of IgG (both total and *T. pallidum*–specific) in the CSF in syphilitic CNS involvement.[33–35] In early syphilis with CNS involvement, appropriate therapy may halt this antibody response and also may lead to a restitution of the blood-brain barrier. In later neurosyphilitic syndromes, the levels of IgG do not seem to decline following therapy as reliably, and abnormalities persist for longer periods.[34] The humoral response to syphilis appears to predominate in the first several weeks of infection but quickly transitions into a T-cell-predominant cellular immune response. Evidence of developing cell-mediated immunity, expressed as increasing CSF interferon and interleukin levels with time, has been demonstrated in a monkey model.[36] The role of T-helper-stimulated macrophages also appears crucial with regard to spirochetal eradication.[31] Demonstration of the importance of a T-helper cellular response in clearance of CSF treponemes provides an explanation for the apparent increased risk for neurosyphilis among persons whose T-cell response has been compromised by infection with HIV. Neurosyphilis appears more likely to develop in HIV-infected patients with low CD4 counts, the impaired immunity presumably delaying clearance of spirochetes from the CSF as well.[31] Although clinical manifestations of neurosyphilis may vary, the basic pathologic process involved in these syndromes may be similar across the spectrum of disease.

▶ CLINICAL FEATURES

The clinical manifestations of neurosyphilis can vary greatly with regard to signs, symptoms, time course, epidemiologic factors, and diagnostic parameters. As noted previously, there are five general categories into which neurosyphilis traditionally has been divided: asymptomatic CNS involvement, syphilitic meningitis, meningovascular syphilis, parenchymatous neurosyphilis (including general paresis and tabes dorsalis), and gummatous neurosyphilis (Fig. 14-3). These syn-

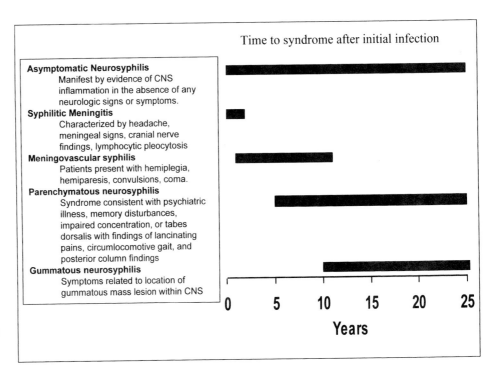

Figure 14–3. Signs and symptoms associated with the neurosyphilis syndromes and the time course for these syndromes.

Time to syndrome after initial infection

Asymptomatic Neurosyphilis
Manifest by evidence of CNS inflammation in the absence of any neurologic signs or symptoms.
Syphilitic Meningitis
Characterized by headache, meningeal signs, cranial nerve findings, lymphocytic pleocytosis
Meningovascular syphilis
Patients present with hemiplegia, hemiparesis, convulsions, coma.
Parenchymatous neurosyphilis
Syndrome consistent with psychiatric illness, memory disturbances, impaired concentration, or tabes dorsalis with findings of lancinating pains, circumlocomotive gait, and posterior column findings
Gummatous neurosyphilis
Symptoms related to location of gummatous mass lesion within CNS

Years

dromes may present independently of one another, with considerable overlap with other neurosyphilis syndromes and even coexisting with other CNS disorders.[37]

Most descriptions of clinical presentations of neurosyphilis were recorded prior to the availability of modern antibiotic therapy, before the HIV epidemic, and before modern descriptions of many other CNS diseases that may have been misdiagnosed as neurosyphilis in the past.[9] Each of these potential confounders of neurosyphilis diagnoses may have contributed to changes in the clinical spectrum and distribution of neurosyphilis syndromes during the antibiotic era. Whereas dementia and personality changes attributed to parenchymatous neurosyphilis were the most frequently encountered manifestations in the preantibiotic era, focal neurologic findings, seizure activity, and neuroophthalmologic findings appear to predominate now, although the former syndromes are still seen occasionally.[32,38] Another possible contributor to this shift is the widespread use of antibiotics for disorders other than syphilis and the potential for them to modify the course of disease through partial treatment of occult syphilis.[32]

Despite progress following the discovery and widespread use of penicillin, treatment of syphilis (or neurosyphilis) does not always result in complete resolution of clinical manifestations. While clearly more effective than its predecessors (mercury, arsenicals, etc.), penicillin therapy at any stage of syphilis may not totally prevent development of later complications of infection, including neurosyphilis.

Asymptomatic CNS Infection

Studies conducted in the preantibiotic era described a high prevalence of abnormal CSF findings in syphilis patients without clinical neurologic abnormalities by history or physical examination.[20] These abnormalities included abnormal CSF cell counts, protein concentrations, and serologic tests, as well as the presence of *T. pallidum*.[20] Further studies in the preantibiotic era showed that the presence of CSF abnormalities predicted increased risk for progression to clinical neurosyphilis, and as a result, LP became a routine part of syphilis management, being used to determine the length of syphilis treatment.[20] As penicillin became the therapy of choice for syphilis, despite studies confirming the high prevalence of CSF abnormalities in early syphilis patients, LP was relegated to evaluation of patients with late syphilis or for diagnosis of suspected clinical neurosyphilis.

At present, the clinical significance of CSF abnormalities in otherwise asymptomatic early syphilis patients is a topic of continuing debate. Over half of patients with early (primary, secondary, and early latent) syphilis have abnormal CSF findings (leukocytosis, elevated protein concentrations, or reactive serologic tests).[1,22] However, because these abnormalities do not clearly predict treatment failure or future clinical deficits, at present LP is not recommended routinely for patients with early syphilis. In contrast, for patients with late latent or latent syphilis of unknown duration, LP to rule out asymptomatic neurosyphilis is recommended, particularly if those patients have relatively high nontreponemal tests or are HIV-infected. Evaluation of the CSF in late syphilis in one series revealed abnormal CSF values in 32 percent of patients manifest by either elevated protein concentrations, elevated CSF white blood cell (WBC) counts, or reactive CSF Venereal Diseases Research Laboratory (VDRL) tests.[39] Earlier studies had shown only about 11 percent of these patients to have an abnormal CSF formula.[1] Patients coinfected with syphilis and HIV were more likely to have an abnormal CSF formula despite the absence of neurologic symptoms.[40] The relevance of these findings in relation to the prognosis of syphilis for individual patients, the subsequent risk of developing clinically apparent neurosyphilis, and the potential impact on response to traditional therapeutic interventions is less clear. The absence of longitudinal data in patients with asymptomatic CNS infection will ensure that this continues to be debated. Whether or not other tests used to detect the presence of spirochetes in the CNS will shed any light on this controversial area remains to be seen (see below).

Syphilitic Meningitis

In a subset of syphilis patients, meningeal inflammation is pronounced. Syphilitic meningitis is most common in secondary syphilis and usually is seen during the first 2 years of infection.[9] In the preantibiotic era, Merritt and colleagues[1] reported the frequency of syphilitic meningitis to be 0.3 to 2.4 percent, making it one of the less common neurosyphilitic syndromes; however, this relatively low prevalence may reflect the authors' high threshold (in terms of signs and symptoms) for making the diagnosis (see below). Musher and colleagues[25] reported that 23 of 40 cases of neurosyphilis were syphilitic meningitis, and others have described rates of 10 to 25 percent.[21] There has been speculation that syphilitic meningitis may be more common in persons with concomitant HIV infection.[22,25]

The largest series of patients with syphilitic meningitis was reported by Merritt and Moore,[41] who described 80 patients seen at Boston area hospitals in the 1920s. Among their patients, the most common symptoms were headache, nausea, vomiting, neck stiffness, and a variety of cranial nerve findings, as well as occasionally altered mental status or seizures. Almost all patients had meningeal signs (e.g., meningismus, Kernig's sign) and papilledema on physical examination.[41] Sixty-four percent of cases occurred in the first year of infection, and over 71 percent were noted in the first 2 years. A more recent series in San Francisco found 19 patients with syphilitic meningitis, all with HIV or AIDS, and appears to confirm earlier descriptions. Symptoms encountered in the San Francisco patients included headache (18 of 19), fever (4 of 19), cranial nerve deficits (5 of 19), and meningismus (4 of 19).[22] Involvement of nearly every cranial nerve has been described in the literature as a part of syphilitic meningitis.[1,11,41] The cranial nerves most commonly involved are cranial nerves VII and VIII and less commonly the oculomotor nerve (cranial nerve III). Most cranial nerve deficits resolve following therapy, although persistent visual disturbance and hearing deficits occur.[1]

The CSF formula in patients with acute syphilitic meningitis is typical of other aseptic meningitides. The CSF white blood cell (WBC) count is usually greater than 10/mm³ with a mononuclear predominance, the CSF protein concentration is elevated (88 percent in Merritt and Moore's series), and the glucose concentration can be normal or slightly decreased in up to 50 percent of cases.[1,9,11,22] CSF serological tests (Wasserman tests in the preantibiotic era, VDRL tests more recently) frequently are abnormal in patients with syphilitic meningitis. In Merritt and Moore's series, 86 percent of patients had positive CSF serologic tests. Radiologic studies have not been used routinely in the diagnosis of syphilitic meningitis, although there are case reports of meningeal enhancement seen by computed tomographic (CT) scanning and magnetic resonance imaging (MRI)[42–44] (Fig. 14-4).

The differential diagnosis of syphilitic meningitis should include other causes of aseptic meningitis. In syphilis patients with HIV coinfection, cryptococcal and tuberculous meningitis should be considered. Viral meningitis also may present with similar signs and symptoms.

Syphilitic meningitis responds well to therapy; unlike neurosyphilis occurring later in disease, clinical improvement approaches 100 percent.[9] Many of the earlier studies reported improvement even in the absence of therapy.[1] However, in some patients, focal cranial nerve deficits may persist despite appropriate high-dose penicillin therapy—most notably optic atrophy and deafness.[9,11]

Meningovascular Syphilis

Meningovascular syphilis refers to the neurosyphilis syndrome characterized most prominently by focal neurologic findings resembling cerebrovascular events due to hypertension or atheroembolic disease. Merritt and colleagues[1] stated that about 3 percent of syphilitics will develop meningovascular syphilis during the course of illness. More recent studies have found meningovascular syphilis to comprise up to 30 percent of all cases of

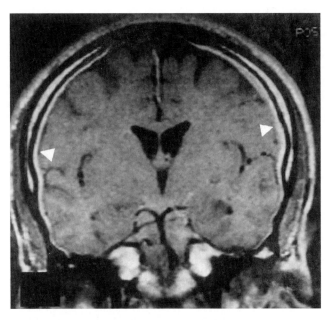

Figure 14–4. Contrast-enhanced image showing high-signal CSF outlining the basilar and posterior cerebral arteries and enhancement (*arrowheads*) of the meninges overlying the cerebral hemispheres in a patient with syphilitic meningitis. *(Used with permission from Good CD: Contrast enhancement of the cerebrospinal fluid on MRI in two cases of spirochaetal meningitis. Neuroradiology 42:449, 2000.)*

neurosyphilis. Flood and colleagues[22] found that 8 of 117 (7 percent) neurosyphilitics presented with meningovascular syphilis, while an earlier series[32] from the same area reported 13 percent of neurosyphilis to be meningovascular syphilis. Musher and colleagues[25] found that 11 of 40 (28 percent) patients presented with focal signs and symptoms consistent with meningovascular syphilis in a review of cases from 1971 to 1990.

Meningovascular syphilis typically presents within the first 10 years of syphilis infection and appears to peak around 7 years after primary infection, although there is substantial variation; syndromes consistent with meningovascular syphilis have been reported as early as 4 months after primary infection.[1,9,27,45]

Meningovascular syphilis is characterized by focal deficits corresponding to the area of ischemia in the distribution of the affected blood flow. Patients also may present with signs and symptoms of syphilitic meningitis, i.e., headache, neck stiffness, dizziness, and impaired cognitive ability. In about one-quarter of cases, patients will describe transient premonitory symptoms, including focal neurologic deficits, headache, and dizziness, prior to the sudden onset of a lasting neurologic event. Hemiplegia or hemiparesis was seen in 83 percent of patients.[1] Other presenting findings include convulsions (14 percent), coma (12 percent), cranial nerve deficits, and cerebellar findings including ataxia.[1] Although evidence of syphilitic vasculitis can be demonstrated to affect multiple CNS vessels by angiography, only 5 of 42 (12 percent) patients in the series of Merritt and colleagues[1] had clinical evidence of more than one affected vessel. Most patients (about two-thirds) present with symptoms attributable to cerebral ischemia in the distribution of the middle cerebral artery, with the basilar artery being the next most commonly involved.[1]

The clinical findings of meningovascular syphilis may resemble those due to hypertensive or arteriosclerotic CNS disease; however, persons with meningovascular syphilis tend to be younger. Seventy-four percent of the patients reported by Merritt and colleagues[1] were under the age of 50. Although routine screening for syphilis is not recommended for all patients who present with focal neurologic deficits, serologic testing for syphilis in patients without other identifiable risk factors for acute cerebrovascular events is appropriate.[46] Importantly, patients with meningovascular syphilis tend to have a less severe course of illness than their counterparts with disease due to arteriosclerosis and overall have a better prognosis.[1] Reasons suggested for these differences include the involvement of smaller-caliber vessels by syphilis, the younger age of the cohort with syphilis, and the indolent process of vascular fibrosis leading to obliterative endarteritis, which facilitates the development of collateral flow and the potential for "rescue" perfusion to the affected tissues in the event of an acute occlusion.[1,9]

A vascular syndrome analogous to meningovascular syphilis also can affect the spinal cord and cause signs and symptoms that reflect the segment of the spinal cord involved.[1] Alterations in bowel or bladder function, upper motor neuron signs, and sensory disturbances all have been described in patients with this syndrome, corresponding to the vessel affected and/or the segment of spinal cord involved. These patients do not fare as well as patients with cerebral/cerebellar disease, and the deficits are less likely to resolve following therapy. Only 8 of 25 (32 percent) patients in the series by Merritt and colleagues[1] showed improvement with therapy, although there have been case reports of reversal of clinical disease in the antibiotic era.[47]

CSF abnormalities are common in patients with meningovascular syphilis.[11] The inflammatory process that causes the clinical pathology also appears to involve the vessels that supply the leptomeninges. In 8 patients described by Flood and colleagues,[22] all had a CSF WBC count of 33/mm^3 or greater, predominantly lymphocytes. CSF protein concentrations also were elevated in these patients, and 5 of 8 (63 percent) patients had CSF VDRL titers of 1:4 or greater.[22] Cerebral angiography by conventional means or magnetic resonance angiography (MRA) may show concentric narrowing of involved vessels, and neuroimaging by CT scan or MRI demonstrates changes in the parenchyma consistent with ischemia.[11,44]

Parenchymatous Neurosyphilis

Parenchymatous neurosyphilis (general paresis and tabes dorsalis) is the latest of the neurosyphilis syndromes to appear in persons with untreated syphilis. Whereas the pathologic process in the neurosyphilis syndromes previously discussed results primarily from vascular inflammation, in parenchymatous neurosyphilis syndromes, progressive destruction of neurons occurs. The clinical presentations of parenchymatous neurosyphilis varies based on the affected anatomy and may resemble a number of other illnesses.[1] Although the pathologic process involved is similar, the presentation of general paresis and tabes dorsalis is distinct with regard to onset, symptomatology, physical examination findings, and prognosis. Whereas patients with tabes dorsalis present with a specific symptom complex due to involvement of the dorsal columns in the spinal cord, patients with general paresis can present in a variety of ways depending on which area of the cerebral cortex is most involved. Many patients present with elements of both disorders, so-called taboparesis.[11,48]

General paresis is one of the best-described forms of neurosyphilis and in the preantibiotic era was the second-most commonly encountered form of symptomatic neurosyphilis, comprising 12 percent of all neurosyphilis cases.[1] As mentioned earlier, more recent studies suggest that the proportion of neurosyphilis that fits into this category has declined.[22,32,38] General paresis classically is described to occur most often 10 to 20 years after primary infection but can occur anytime in the course of late syphilis.[9] Men are affected four to seven times more often than women, and it appears to strike most commonly between the ages of 35 to 50 years, although this certainly can vary based on the time of initial infection and has been shown to be higher in some more recent studies.[1,11,22]

A number of monikers have been attached to this syndrome, including *dementia paralytica* and *general paralysis of the insane*. Both these terms are reflective of the signs and symptoms that accompany this disease process, primarily dementing in nature and reflecting a disturbance of cognition and thought. Paresis is insidious in onset; often the duration of symptoms can be established only retrospectively because early disease may be difficult to recognize.[11] The earliest symptoms include irritability, personality changes, forgetfulness, sleep disturbances, and easy fatigability. Physical symptoms of weight loss and headache also may be encountered.[1] Focal neurologic deficits per se may be absent at this stage, and the physical examination can be entirely normal. As the disease progresses, cognition and judgment become increasingly affected, and delusional symptoms may appear. Classically, grandiose delusions and euphoria are present, although this occurs in a minority of paretic neurosyphilitics. More commonly, deterioration in personal appearance, intellectual performance, and judgment is accompanied by emotional lability, confusion, and frank psychosis.[1] Physical examination findings at this time may include tremors, expressionless facies, speech and handwriting impairment, and pupillary abnormalities, including but not limited to the Argyll-Robertson pupil.[1,11] If the disease process is allowed to continue untreated, these symptoms recede, and the predominant characteristic becomes dementia. Seizures may be seen during this later period as well and may herald the terminal phase of the disease, in which the patient becomes bedridden and neurologically incompetent with loss of voluntary motor power and sphincter control.[1] Physical examination in these later stages of the disease may reveal a slouching posture and a generalized hypotonia with an inability to perform even the most basic activities.[1] The entire course of general paresis may take as little as a few months or as long as 3 to 4 years and can be arrested with appropriate therapy.

Gross pathology of paretic brains reveals generalized cortical atrophy, most pronounced in the frontal lobes, with a diminishing involvement in the more posterior structures of the cerebrum. Microscopic examination of affected parenchyma demonstrates a paucity of neurons, marked gliosis, and proliferation of astrocytes.[1] Using special stains, spirochetes can be found in the tissue in 25 to 40 percent of specimens.[9] Accompanying this cortical process, meningeal inflammation by lymphocytes and plasma cells in a distribution similar to the cortical process is also pronounced.[1,9] This is reflected in the CSF, which is abnormal in the vast majority of patients with untreated general paresis.[1,11] Findings include an elevated CSF WBC count and protein concentrations and reactive serologic tests, although any one specimen may not have all these abnormalities. More recently, of five patients with paretic neurosyphilis reported by Flood and colleagues,[22] one patient had a CSF WBC count of less than $5/mm^3$, and other reports[11,38] suggest that up to 10 percent of patients with paresis will not have an elevated CSF WBC count. It has been postulated that as more people receive antibiotics for a variety of infectious disorders (not necessarily syphilis) with activity against *T. pallidum*, partially treated neurosyphilis may develop, thus making the diagnosis of neurosyphilis more difficult to establish because CNS inflammation may be attenuated and classic CSF findings may be absent.[32]

The differential diagnosis of general paresis includes a number of psychiatric disorders in addition to organic disease. Microvascular dementia, Alzheimer's disease, schizoaffective disorders, personality disorders, and frank psychosis all may present with similar symp-

toms. Viral encephalitis also may present with cognitive dysfunction and have a similar CSF formula, although the time course of viral encephalitis typically is more rapid. In addition, mycobacterial and fungal meningitides may have similar signs and symptoms and should be ruled out in the evaluation of these patients.

In tabes dorsalis, neuronal destruction primarily involves the posterior columns of the spinal cord. Tabes dorsalis is thought to affect men more often than women, with peak incidence occurring 10 to 20 years following acquisition of infection.[1,11] The course of untreated tabes dorsalis, however, is considerably longer than general paresis, sometimes exceeding 20 years. In the preantibiotic era, Merritt and colleagues[1] reported that tabes dorsalis was the most commonly recognized form of neurosyphilis, comprising 30 percent of almost 700 cases. At present, with the rising proportion of meningeal and meningovascular varieties of neurosyphilis, the incidence of tabes dorsalis has declined substantially both absolutely and as a percentage of neurosyphilis syndromes.[22,32,38]

Merritt and colleagues[1] reported that 75 percent of patients with tabetic neurosyphilis experienced recurrent, lancinating pain episodes that best characterize this disorder—sharp, fleeting pains that are found most often in the legs but also can affect the back, arms, and face. The pain can be mild or incapacitating, and the duration of pain episodes may last only a few minutes or several days. Likewise, pain-free intervals can vary from minutes to months and may migrate from one location to another.[1,9,11] Ataxia, due to impaired position and vibration sensation, is another common symptom of tabes dorsalis and is most evident in the lower extremities. Patients compensate for these deficiencies by adopting the characteristic tabetic broad-based gait, leaning backwards and lifting and throwing the legs forward in a circumlocomotive manner.[1,11] Classically, the triad of symptoms attributed to tabes dorsalis includes lancinating pain, ataxia, and bladder dysfunction. As the destructive process continues, bladder hypotonia develops and may be seen in up to a third of patients, resulting in overflow incontinence.[1,11] Tabes dorsalis also may present as abdominal pain or discomfort and colonic distension. These less common symptoms, called *visceral crises,* include abdominal pain, particularly epigastric pain, as the predominant symptom without accompanying signs or symptoms of a surgical abdomen.[1,9] Sexual dysfunction and impotence also may be seen in both men and women and is accompanied by anesthesia of the involved organs.[1] Up to 20 percent of patients complain of visual symptoms that may begin with a decrease in vision in one eye and then the other and lead to blindness within 7 to 8 years.[1] Unlike paresis, which will progress continuously if untreated, in the preantibiotic era tabes was diagnosed during its active phase but then would evolve to the "burned-out phase," reflecting arrest of the primary pathologic process. The patient was left with residual symptoms and signs attributable to destruction of spinal cord neurons during the active phase.[1] Because of this propensity for the destructive process to spontaneously abort, tabes dorsalis has been said rarely to be the cause of death in tabetic neurosyphilitics.[1,11]

Physical examination in patients with tabes dorsalis reveals a number of characteristic findings. A Romberg's sign is encountered in over 50 percent of patients, and impaired vibratory sense, pain sensation, and position sense can be detected on neurologic examination.[1] The reflexes are diminished, with the absence of an ankle jerk being most common and involvement of the biceps and triceps reflexes being less common. Musculoskeletal examination may reveal Charcot joints due to the inadvertent repeated trauma sustained by tabetic patients with loss of proprioception and pain sensation.[1] Pupillary involvement also is seen at some point during the course of disease in over 90 percent of tabetic patients. Classically, the Argyll-Robertson pupil, in which the pupils constrict with accommodation but do not react to direct illumination, has been described in tabetics, but other pupillary abnormalities also have been described in equal numbers.[1]

Examination of the CSF in patients with tabes dorsalis may not aid in the diagnosis of this disorder because it is frequently devoid of evidence of inflammation and serologic markers of syphilis. Merritt and colleagues[1] reported that half the patients with tabes dorsalis had a CSF WBC count of less than 5/mm³, 47 percent had a normal protein concentration, and over 25 percent had a nonreactive CSF Wasserman test.

Pathologic examination of the spinal cord reveals atrophic posterior columns and posterior nerve roots.[1] Early tabes dorsalis is accompanied by an inflammation of the meninges, with cellular inflammation similar to that seen in the meninges of paretic patients. Microscopic examination reveals astrocyte proliferation and gliosis, as well as a decreased number of neurons, but only rarely can spirochetes be demonstrated in the affected tissue.[1,9]

Gummatous Neurosyphilis

The least common form of neurosyphilis is gummatous neurosyphilis. The clinical manifestations of CNS gummas are due to mass effect rather than direct neuronal destruction by syphilis. As a result, there may be focal neurologic deficits as well as seizures and altered mental status.[9,30,49,50] CNS gummas can arise from the meningeal surfaces and extend directly into the brain or, more rarely, may arise in the brain parenchyma without associated meningeal involvement.[30] CSF examination may be normal.[9] Special stains (immunofluorescence or silver stains) of biopsy specimens may reveal spirochetes. More recently, polymerase chain reaction (PCR) techniques also have been used to demonstrate *T. pallidum* in gummatous tissues.[49,51]

▶ DIAGNOSIS

Unlike most bacteria causing CNS infection, culture of *T. pallidum* is impractical, and as a result, the diagnosis of CNS syphilis relies on markers of infection, including cell count, protein concentration, and serologic testing. No single laboratory test has proven optimal for neurosyphilis diagnosis, but in most instances the combination of historical and physical findings, along with the composite results of laboratory tests, gives the clinician reasonable confidence in the presence or absence of neurosyphilis.

Routine CSF studies of patients with suspected neurosyphilis, including a cell count with differential and protein and glucose concentrations and serologic tests, provide important clues for neurosyphilis diagnosis. In active neurosyphilis, an elevated CSF WBC count with a lymphocytic pleocytosis is the most common abnormality, although a normal CSF WBC count also may be seen in some cases, particularly in late disease. For instance, over 50 percent of all tabetic patients have normal CSF WBC counts (<5/mm³), whereas almost 100 percent of patients with syphilitic meningitis will have CSF WBC counts greater than 10/mm³ and rarely as high as 2000 cells/mm³. More recently, of 117 patients with HIV and neurosyphilis, 76 of 117 (65 percent) had CSF WBC counts of greater than 5 cells/mm³.[22] In other studies, 18 of 21 neurosyphilis patients with a reactive CSF-VDRL test had CSF mononuclear cell counts of greater than 5 cells/mm³.[33]

Although less specific than the cell count, most patients with neurosyphilis also have an elevated CSF protein concentration (>45 mg/dl).[1,52] The CSF glucose concentration has been found to be a less reliable marker of syphilitic activity in the CNS and is of little utility in diagnosis or in assessing response to therapy.

While CSF pleocytosis and an elevated protein concentration are nonspecific abnormalities, CSF serologic testing improves diagnostic accuracy. In the preantibiotic era, the Wasserman test, a precursor of the present-day VDRL test and rapid plasma reagin (RPR) test, was used as the preferred serologic test for syphilis and neurosyphilis diagnosis. Although a positive Wasserman test was felt to be diagnostic of neurosyphilis, up to 30 percent of patients with neurosyphilis syndromes in the prepenicillin era did not have reactive CSF serologic tests.[1] While relatively insensitive, the specificity of the CSF VDRL is high; in the absence of blood contamination from a traumatic LP, the frequency of biologic false-positive CSF VDRL tests is very low and has been reported only in the context of case reports. At present, the CSF VDRL is used rather than the Wasserman test and has been reported to have a sensitivity for neurosyphilis of between 10 and 30 percent.[53] Negative CSF VDRL results do not rule out a diagnosis of neurosyphilis.[54] The RPR test, which is currently more widely used for nontreponemal serologic syphilis testing, has not been well studied using CSF and is not recommended for this purpose.

In an effort to improve the sensitivity of CSF serologic testing for neurosyphilis diagnosis, treponemal serologic tests for neurosyphilis have been studied. The fluorescent treponemal antibody (FTA) test, used with or without an absorption step, and the *T. pallidum* hemagglutination assay (TPHA) have been used most commonly. A number of studies have found these treponemal assays to be more sensitive than the CSF VDRL. Luger and colleagues[52] found the TPHA index to have a sensitivity of 98.3 percent compared with 91.7 percent for CSF VDRL in an Austrian study. Tomberlin and colleagues[35] found positive TPHA indices in patients with negative CSF VDRL reactivity, although the reverse also could be found. Unfortunately, the specificity of CSF treponemal tests for syphilis appears to be low, with reactive tests being relatively common in syphilis patients with no other data to suggest CNS involvement. Hooshmand and colleagues[48] demonstrated a positive FTA-abs in the CSF of 156 of 156 patients with neurosyphilis, thus demonstrating a high positive predictive value for the diagnosis of neurosyphilis with this treponemal test. While a negative CSF treponemal test almost certainly rules out a neurosyphilis diagnosis, a positive test is not necessarily diagnostic of neurosyphilis.

The difficulties associated with CSF serologic testing for suspected neurosyphilis have prompted some investigators to attempt to improve the diagnostic accuracy using an antibody index to quantify the ratio of *T. pallidum*–specific antibody in the CSF to that in the serum, sometimes also in comparison with CSF and serum total IgG and/or albumin levels, reasoning that patients with neurosyphilis are more likely to have elevated antibody indices.[33–35,54–55] As with other tests, the antibody indices can be elevated in the absence of any other CSF abnormalities. To date, none of these tests has been demonstrated clearly to have the combination of sensitivity and specificity required to improve the diagnosis of neurosyphilis.

For demonstration of *T. pallidum* in CSF, dark-field microscopy is insensitive. Investigators studying syphilis pathogenesis have used the rabbit inoculation test (RIT) and, more recently, polymerase chain reaction (PCR) to demonstrate the presence of *T. pallidum* in CSF from syphilis patients. In the RIT, clinical specimens (i.e., CSF) are injected into rabbit testes, and the animals are monitored both serologically and through microscopic evaluation of testicular aspirates for evidence of infection. This method of diagnosis is time-consuming (it may take 4 to 8 weeks to become positive) and labor-intensive and is not feasible in clinical practice. More recently, PCR techniques have been found to be much faster and as—or perhaps more—sensitive than RIT for *T. pallidum* detection in CSF specimens. While these methods have been used to demonstrate *T. pallidum* in CSF from patients with early (primary, secondary, or early latent) syphilis, PCR is negative in over 50 percent of patients with syphilitic involvement of the CNS.

PCR is appealing for the diagnosis of neurosyphilis because the *T. pallidum* assays can detect a single whole organism down to 10^{-2} *T. pallidum* RNA equivalents in CSF.[56] Several studies have shown PCR to have comparable sensitivity and specificity to RIT with a much shorter turnaround time and a decreased cost.[51] In their report of the most recent large multicenter study of early syphilis treatment, Rolfs and colleagues[40] found that 32 of 131 CSF specimens were positive for *T. pallidum* by PCR, but this did not correlate with CSF WBC counts, protein concentrations, or CSF VDRL reactivity. Thus exactly what the presence of *T. pallidum* in the CSF means is still not exactly clear; as with RIT, PCR can detect microorganisms in the absence of abnormal CSF WBC counts, protein concentrations, or CSF VDRL reactivity, a fact that further complicates interpretation of positive PCR results.[40]

At present, with the exception of syphilis patients who have concomitant HIV infection, LP is recommended primarily for evaluation of patients with latent syphilis or possible treatment failure. While many patients with early syphilis will have one or more abnormal CSF test results, the clinical significance of these findings for treatment outcome is unclear. Up to 50 percent of patients with early syphilis have reactive CSF VDRL tests, and up to 70 percent of secondary syphilis patients will have at least one abnormal value.[18,33,45] While the small proportion of syphilis patients who fail therapy may have abnormal CSF findings before treatment, the vast majority of those with CSF abnormalities respond to therapy in a fashion similar to patients without CSF abnormalities. Thus the significance of the high prevalence of CSF abnormalities in early syphilis patients remains unclear and the subject of debate.

Current CDC sexually transmitted diseases treatment guidelines advocate LP for syphilis patients who meet the following criteria: (1) having any neurologic or ophthalmologic signs and symptoms (irrespective of clinical stage of infection), (2) having evidence of tertiary syphilis in other organ systems, (3) having failed treatment, (4) having HIV infection and late latent syphilis or syphilis of unknown duration, or (5) patients in whom an examination of the CSF is otherwise deemed necessary[57] (Table 14-1). These recommendations are based on data from the preantibiotic era, when patients with varying degrees of CSF abnormalities were at a higher risk for progression to clinical neurosyphilis.[20] There also has been evidence of neurosyphilis in patients with latent syphilis and nonspecific

► **TABLE 14-1.** INDICATIONS FOR LUMBAR PUNCTURE IN PATIENTS WITH SYPHILIS

---

1. Any neurologic or ophthalmologic signs and symptoms irrespective of clinical stage of infection
2. Evidence of tertiary syphilis in other organ systems
3. Treatment failure
4. HIV infection and late latent syphilis or syphilis of unknown duration
5. Any patient in whom an examination of the CSF is otherwise deemed necessary.

Source: From Centers for Disease Control and Prevention: Sexually transmitted diseases treatment guidelines 2002. MMWR 51(RR-6):22, 2002.

treponemal test titers of more than 1:32, and many experts recommend LP in this patient population as well.[57,58]

► THERAPY

For neurosyphilis treatment, the goals of therapy vary based on the clinical syndrome. With the early neurosyphilis syndromes, such as syphilitic meningitis, the goal of therapy is to cure or accelerate resolution of symptoms and return the patient to his or her previous state of health. With later-stage neurosyphilis, such as meningovascular syphilis or general paresis, treatment may arrest the progression of disease and prevent further neurologic deterioration, but reversal of clinical deficits is uncommon. In contrast, for asymptomatic neurosyphilis patients, the goal of therapy is to prevent development of clinical neurosyphilis. As mentioned earlier, for asymptomatic neurosyphilis, there is debate about how to best accomplish this goal or what proportion of affected persons will benefit from intensive therapy. Thus the goals of therapy for neurosyphilis have been a "moving target" and certainly will continue to evolve.

Few diseases have had their impact on society as profoundly altered by the advent of penicillin as syphilis. Previous therapeutic regimens included heavy metals, fever therapy, and other agents. The demonstration of penicillin's efficacy stimulated dramatic changes in neurosyphilis management. Unlike therapy for nearly all other bacterial infections, penicillin continues to be the treatment of choice for neurosyphilis today. Treatment failures do still occur in a minority of patients (particularly since the advent of HIV infection), and some syphilologists whose clinical experiences include use of both penicillin and heavy metal therapy, malaria therapy, and other compounds have argued that the major advantage of penicillin is not the rate of success but rather the relative ease of therapy.[9] Treatment regimens in the preantibiotic era for neurosyphilis could be expected to last months to years and were fraught

with complications. The advent of penicillin markedly changed the landscape of syphilis therapy in terms of ease of administration, tolerability, and the proportion of patients completing a full course of therapy.[9] A number of reports have documented the failure of stage-appropriate penicillin therapy to prevent or effectively cure neurosyphilis.[11,18,22–24,26–29,59–61] Many of these studies also have shown appropriate declines in serologic markers of syphilis infection in the short term with recrudescent disease at a much later date.[28] A growing body of evidence has shown HIV infection to be a risk factor for relapse and has led to some debate as to the most appropriate therapy for various stages of syphilis in patients who are infected with both HIV and syphilis.[27,28,62]

Penicillin has been the preferred therapy for syphilis for over 60 years. Although penicillin resistance has developed in a wide variety of bacteria and has become a dilemma in the management of other diseases, there are no data to indicate that penicillin resistance has developed in *T. pallidum*. While referred to inclusively as "penicillin therapy," over the years a number of compounds have been formulated in an effort to enhance delivery, half-life, and tolerability of penicillin. Among the formulations used in various studies are aqueous penicillin G, procaine penicillin, procaine penicillin in aluminum monostearate (PAM), benzathine penicillin, benethamine penicillin, and penicillin in beeswax, as well as related drugs such as ampicillin and amoxicillin. Animal studies suggest that a serum penicillin level of 0.018 μg/ml is treponemicidal, and in some studies, these CSF penicillin concentrations have been used as a surrogate for clinical efficacy.[63] In contrast, others have suggested that the slow multiplication time of *T. pallidum* permits subtreponemicidal serum or CSF levels for extended periods of time to be effective for neurosyphilis therapy when provided in a longer course of therapy.[64,65] Other recent studies have suggested that the serum level of penicillin is not a reliable indicator of CSF penicillin levels, and therefore, more frequent dosing schedules with higher doses of penicillin may be required to achieve desirable levels in the CSF.[64–67] Mohr and colleagues[67] demonstrated that 12 of 13 patients treated with 3.6 million units of intramuscular benzathine penicillin G weekly for 4 weeks did not have detectable levels of penicillin in the CSF.[67] Conversely, Scheroth and colleagues[64] showed CSF penicillin levels of 0.10 μg/ml or greater in 8 of 8 patients treated with 10.5 to 13.5 million units of intravenous aqueous penicillin G per day given at 4-hour intervals.[64]

In the late 1940s, Dr. Richard Hahn and colleagues[68,69] studied the probability of progression to clinical neurosyphilis in 765 patients with asymptomatic neurosyphilis and syphilis of greater than 2 years' duration. Patients were given varying amounts of penicillin throughout the study period and were followed for up to 8 years after completion of therapy. Only the group of patients who received less than 2.4 million units of penicillin progressed to neurosyphilis more frequently than those who received higher amounts of penicillin, and those who received 2.4 to 4.8 million units or 4.8 to 9 million units of penicillin did just as well as the group receiving more than 9 million units. Similar proportions of patients in the 2.4 to 4.8 million unit and in the 4.8 to 9.0 million unit groups had resolution of CSF abnormalities after treatment.[68,69] Currently, the CDC recommends 18 to 24 million units of aqueous penicillin G per day given in divided doses for 10 to 14 days[57] (Table 14-2). This recommendation appears to be based in large part on the body of data documenting treponemicidal levels of penicillin in the CSF with high-dose penicillin therapy.[11,63,64,66,67] Studies evaluating various penicillin compounds given with probenecid have found CSF levels of penicillin comparable with those attained with high-dose penicillin therapy. As a result, the CDC also recommends an alternate regimen of procaine penicillin 2.4 million units intramuscularly with probenecid 500 mg orally four times a day for 10 to 14 days.[57]

For patients unable to tolerate penicillin, alternate medications in small numbers of patients have been studied for neurosyphilis treatment. Despite the risk of cross-reactivity for penicillin-allergic patients, ceftriaxone is probably the most commonly used alternative. It has been studied prospectively and retrospectively in HIV patients with neurosyphilis with results comparable with those receiving penicillin. Marra and colleagues[70] studied 30 HIV-infected patients in a prospective, randomized trial and found that ceftriaxone therapy lead to resolution of CSF abnormalities at a rate similar to that in patients randomized to penicillin G treatment. Other studies have shown similar results. Dowell and colleagues[71] examined the results of 43 patients with latent syphilis or asymptomatic neurosyphilis treated with varying dosages of ceftriaxone as compared with 13 patients with latent syphilis treated with three doses of benzathine penicillin and found similar rates of treatment success, serologic relapse, and progression to clinical neurosyphilis. Formal studies in HIV-nega-

tive neurosyphilis patients have not been done, and the efficacy of this regimen in that setting has not been described. However, in a recent survey of infectious disease specialists, 20 percent of those surveyed reported using ceftriaxone as an alternative therapy for various stages of syphilis, with six failures noted.[72]

Tetracycline derivatives also have been studied as a possible alternative to penicillin because of their excellent penetration into the CSF and evidence of activity against *T. pallidum*. Minocycline has shown some efficacy in HIV-negative patients with neurosyphilis when given over a 9-month period.[73] Doxycycline has been shown to achieve high CSF levels and is suggested for patients intolerant of penicillin; however, long-term follow-up and the lack of evidence regarding treponemicidal activity have been cited as potential concerns.[74] At present, penicillin is the preferred regimen for therapy, and an effort to desensitize patients with allergies to penicillin should be made prior to use of alternate therapies.

As a rule, the "earlier" neurosyphilis syndromes (i.e., syphilitic meningitis, iritis) respond better to high-dose penicillin therapy than syndromes occurring after longer time intervals from primary infection. Symptoms of syphilitic meningitis, i.e., neck stiffness and headache, resolve quickly and completely with appropriate treatment.[32] Likewise, most patients with meningovascular syphilis will improve with therapy. Patients with meningovascular syphilis are younger than the nonsyphilitic group with cerebrovascular disease and thus have a greater capacity for improvement. Second, the pathologic process is related to inflammation rather than atherosclerosis; although endothelial damage is present in both cases, the inflammation associated with infection responds quickly to penicillin. Third, there is more collateral flow to ischemic regions of the brain in patients with meningovascular syphilis because of the caliber of vessels (i.e., smaller) involved in the endarteritis.[9] However, effective treatment can only be instituted with prompt recognition of this syndrome.

Treatment of general paresis and tabes dorsalis does not appear to be as effective as for other neurosyphilis syndromes. As noted earlier, the pathologic process involves destruction of the CNS parenchyma. In one study, 39 percent of patients treated for general paresis with penicillin or heavy metal therapy went on to develop new neurologic symptoms after completion of therapy irrespective of antibiotic therapy.[75] In this series, seizures and strokes were the most frequently encountered new symptoms indicating progression of disease. Neurologic deterioration despite adequate therapy may reflect a progression of parenchymal destruction due to nonsyphilitic causes or healing of "scars" induced by *T. pallidum*.[76]

Penicillin also has proven to be effective in improving the CSF abnormalities associated with neurosyphilis. The early work of Hahn and colleagues dem-

▶ **TABLE 14-2.** 2002 CDC RECOMMENDATIONS FOR NEUROSYPHILIS TREATMENT

---

1. Aqueous crystalline penicillin G 18–24 million units per day administered as 3–4 million units IV every 4 hours or continuous infusion for 10–14 days
2. Procaine penicillin 2.4 million units IM once daily
   plus
   Probenecid 500 mg orally four times a day for 10–14 days

Source: From Centers for Disease Control and Prevention: Sexually transmitted diseases treatment guidelines 2002. MMWR 51(RR-6):23, 2002.

onstrated the efficacy of penicillin in patients with latent and asymptomatic neurosyphilis. At the time of enrollment, 60 percent of patients had CSF WBC counts of $11/mm^3$ or higher. Repeat LPs revealed that pleocytosis fell to 12.2 percent at 6 months and 6 percent at 1 year regardless of the amount of penicillin given.[69] A more recent study in HIV-positive patients with neurosyphilis demonstrated a marked improvement in the CSF WBC count after a course of intravenous penicillin therapy, but CSF VDRL tests were slower to resolve.[22] A study comparing HIV-positive with HIV-negative patients with neurosyphilis treated with high-dose penicillin therapy showed that those with concomitant HIV infection were somewhat slower to resolve their CSF abnormalities irrespective of neurologic abnormalities, stage of syphilis, or treatment regimen.[15] The authors suggested that the immune dysfunction in HIV-positive patients may contribute to delayed normalization of CSF parameters. However, the clinical relevance of these differences in resolution of abnormalities is not clear; cure rates in both HIV-positive and HIV-negative individuals are similar.[15,61]

The relationship between CSF VDRL reactivity and seroreactivity also was addressed by Hahn and colleagues in their study of patients with asymptomatic neurosyphilis. It was noted that serologic response to therapy (or lack thereof) did not reflect the resolution of the CSF abnormalities to therapy and was not useful as a surrogate marker of resolution of neurosyphilis in adequately treated patients.[69] The CDC currently recommends reexamining the CSF at 6-month intervals to monitor response to therapy and to consider retreatment if improvement is not noted at 6 months or if the CSF WBC count is not normal after 2 years.[57]

► HIV AND NEUROSYPHILIS

In the past 20 years, the interrelationship between syphilis and HIV infection has been the subject of much study. Factors associated with risk for both diseases are similar, and concomitant infection is common.[12,77,78] Many experts believe that HIV coinfection in syphilis patients may modify the natural history of syphilis, risk for neurosyphilis, and response to recommended therapy. Patients with early syphilis and HIV infection are more likely to present with secondary syphilis, and those with secondary syphilis and HIV are more likely to have coexisting chancres at the time of diagnosis.[79] In addition, there are many instances of treatment failure in patients with concomitant syphilis and HIV infection, including neurosyphilis. There are a number of case reports from the literature describing patients who have received therapy for early syphilis, late syphilis, and neurosyphilis who have gone on (or relapsed) to develop neurosyphilis.[25,27,61,80,81] In a study by Malone and colleagues,[28] 10 of 56 (17.9 percent) dually infected patients experienced either a clinical or serologic relapse, including 2 of 11 patients with primary or secondary syphilis treated appropriately with intramuscular penicillin.[28] However, in the only prospectively conducted, randomized study to compare outcomes of early syphilis treatment in patients with and without HIV infection, there were no significant differences in serologic response to therapy at 6, 9, or 12 months of follow-up, and none of the patients developed symptomatic neurosyphilis.[40] Similarly, neurologic symptoms in early syphilis were noted to occur with similar frequency in both groups of patients and were related more closely to the stage of disease (i.e., secondary syphilis) than to the presence or absence of HIV infection.[45] Marra and colleagues[15,31,82] demonstrated delayed healing of syphilitic lesions in a monkey model of HIV, and it has been shown the T-cell response to *T. pallidum* infection is essential for clearance of the microorganism. However, in one of the only studies in the HIV era documenting both pre- and posttherapy CSF findings in patients with early syphilis, no difference was seen in the rate of detection of *T. pallidum* from the CSF at follow-up examinations based on HIV status[40] (Table 14-3). The follow-up period was short (12 months), and other studies have shown higher sero-

► **TABLE 14-3.** RESULTS OF CEREBROSPINAL FLUID OF PATIENTS WITH EARLY SYPHILIS WHO UNDERWENT LUMBAR PUNCTURE ACCORDING TO HIV STATUS AT ENROLLMENT

Laboratory Test	HIV-Infected	Not HIV-Infected
White cells	20/46 (43%)	22/99 (22%) p < 0.01
Reactive VDRL test	7/45 (16%)	7/99 (7%)
Protein	17/47 (36%)	25/102 (25%)
Any of the above tests	28/46 (61%)	39/97 (40%) p < 0.05
*T. pallidum**	11/43 (26%)	21/88 (24%)

*As detected by PCR, RIT, or both.
Source: Used with permission from Rolfs et al: A randomized trial of enhanced therapy for early syphilis in patients with and without human immunodeficiency virus infection. New Engl J Med 337:307, 1997.

logic and CSF relapse rates after therapy.[28] Whether or not these findings are applicable to patients treated for late syphilis with standard regimens is less clear.

A growing body of evidence indicates patients identified with neurosyphilis and HIV infection and treated appropriately with high-dose penicillin may relapse more frequently than the HIV-negative cohort. A small study by Gordon and colleagues[61] demonstrated either no improvement or clinical failure in 3 of 7 patients treated for neurosyphilis with high-dose intravenous penicillin. In another study, Marra and colleagues demonstrated reduction of CSF VDRL titers in only 5 of 14 HIV-infected patients treated for neurosyphilis with either intravenous penicillin or ceftriaxone for an appropriate period of time.[70]

These data magnify the need for vigilance on the part of the clinician when treating patients infected with both HIV and neurosyphilis. Close follow-up with frequent monitoring for symptoms and periodic reevaluation of the CSF should be undertaken in an effort to identify relapsing neurosyphilis and to institute prompt therapy in this setting.

REFERENCES

1. Merritt HH, Adams RD, Solomon HC: *Neurosyphilis.* New York: Oxford University Press, 1946.
2. Jacobowsky B: General paresis and civilization. *Acta Psychiatr Scand* 41(3):267, 1965.
3. Braslow JT: Punishment or therapy: Patients, doctors, and somatic remedies in the early twentieth century. *Psychiatr Clin North Am* 17(3):493, 1994.
4. Critchley M: Four illustrious neuroleptics. *Proc R Soc Med* 62(7):669, 1969.
5. Greenblatt RB: The humiliating demise of Lord Randolph Churchill, 1849–1895. *Postgrad Med* 75(1):31, 1984.
6. Cawthorne T: The fatal illness of Oscar Wilde. *Ann Otol Rhinol Laryngol* 75(3):657, 1966.
7. Benedek TG, Erlen J: The scientific environment of the Tuskegee study of syphilis, 1920–1960. *Perspect Biol Med* 43:1, 1999.
8. Chernin E: The malariatherapy of neurosyphilis. *J Parasitol* 70(5):611, 1984.
9. Hook EW: Syphilis, in Scheld WM, Whitley RJ, Durack DT (eds): *Infections of the Central Nervous System,* 2d ed. Philadelphia: Lippincott-Raven Publishers, 1997, p 669.
10. Tramont EC: Syphilis, in Mandell GL, Bennett Ge, and Dolin R (eds): *Mandell, Douglas, and Bennett's Principles and Practice of Infectious Diseases,* 5th ed. Philadelphia: Churchill Livingstone, 2000, pp 2474–2490.
11. Simon RP: Neurosyphilis. *Arch Neurol* 42:606,1985.
12. Nakashima AK, Rolfs RT, Flock ML, et al: Epidemiology of syphilis in the United States, 1941–1993. *Sex Transm Dis* 23(1):16, 1996.
13. Centers for Disease Control and Prevention: Sexually transmitted disease surveillance 2001 supplement,

14. Syphilis surveillance report. Atlanta: U.S. Department of Health and Human Services, Centers for Disease Control and Prevention. February 2003.
14. Centers for Disease Control and Prevention: Sexually transmitted disease surveillance 2002 supplement, Syphilis surveillance report. Atlanta: U.S. Department of Health and Human Services, Centers for Disease Control and Prevention. January 2004.
15. Marra CM, Longstregth WT, Maxwell CL, et al: Resolution of serum and cerebrospinal fluid abnormalities after treatment of neurosyphilis. *Sex Transm Dis* 23(3):184, 1996.
16. Rolfs RT, Goldberg M, Sharrar RG: Risk factors for syphilis: Cocaine use and prostitution. *Am J Public Health* 80(7):853, 1990.
17. Clark EG, Danbolt N: The Oslo study of the natural course of untreated syphilis: An epidemiologic investigation based on a restudy of the Boeck-Bruusgaard material. *Med Clin North Am* 48:613, 1964.
18. Hook EW, Marra CM: Acquired syphilis in adults. *New Engl J Med* 326(16):1060, 1992.
19. Rockwell DH, Yobs AR, Moore MB: The Tuskegee study of untreated syphilis. *Arch Intern Med* 114:792, 1964.
20. Moore JE, Hopkins HH: Asymptomatic neurosyphilis: VI. The prognosis of early and late asymptomatic neurosyphilis. *JAMA* 95:1637, 1930.
21. Katz DA, Berger JR: Neurosyphilis in acquired immunodeficiency syndrome. *Arch Neurol* 46:895, 1989.
22. Flood JM, Weinstock HS, Guroy ME, et al: Neurosyphilis during the AIDS epidemic, San Francisco 1985–1992. *J Infect Dis* 177:931, 1998.
23. Berry CD, Hooton TM, Collier AC, et al: Neurologic relapse after benzathine penicillin therapy for secondary syphilis in a patient with HIV infection. *New Engl J Med* 316(25):1587, 1987.
24. Moskovitz BL, Klimek JJ, Goldman RL, et al: Meningovascular syphilis after "appropriate" treatment of primary syphilis. *Arch Intern Med* 142:139, 1982.
25. Musher DM, Hamill RJ, Baughn RE: Effect of human immunodeficiency virus infection on the course of syphilis and on the response to treatment. *Ann Intern Med* 113:872, 1990.
26. Dibbern DA, Ray SC: Recrudescence of treated neurosyphilis in a patient with human immunodeficiency virus. *Mayo Clin Proc* 74:53, 1999.
27. Johns DR, Tierney M, Felsenstein D: Alteration in the natural history of neurosyphilis by concurrent infection with the human immunodeficiency virus. *New Engl J Med* 316(25):1569, 1987.
28. Malone JL, Wallace MR, Hendrick BB, et al: Syphilis and neurosyphilis in a human immunodeficiency virus type-1 seropositive population: Evidence for frequent serologic relapse after treatment. *Am J Med* 99:55, 1995.
29. Lukehart SA, Hook EW, Baker-Zander MS, et al: Invasion of the central nervous system by *Treponema pallidum*: Implications for diagnosis and treatment. *Ann Intern Med* 109:855, 1988.
30. Stokes JH, Beerman H, Ingraham NR: *Modern Clinical Syphilology,* 3rd ed. Philadelphia: Saunders, 1944.
31. Arroll TW, Centurion-Lara A, Lukehart SA, et al: T-cell

responses to *Treponema pallidum* subsp. *pallidum* antigens during the course of experimental syphilis infection. *Infect Immun* 67(9):4757, 1999.

32. Hotson JR: Modern neurosyphilis: A partly treated chronic meningitis. *West J Med* 135:191, 1981.

33. van Eijk RVW, Wolters EC, Tutuarima JA, et al: Effect of early and late syphilis on central nervous system: Cerebrospinal fluid changes and neurological deficit. *Genitourinary Med* 63:77, 1987.

34. Prange HW, Moskophidis M, Schipper HI, et al: Relationship between neurological features and intrathecal synthesis of IgG antibodies to *Treponema pallidum* in untreated and treated human neurosyphilis. *J Neurol* 230:241, 1983.

35. Tomberlin MG, Holtom PD, Owens JL, et al: Evaluation of neurosyphilis in HIV-infected individuals. *Clin Infect Dis* 18:288, 1994.

36. Marra CM, Castro CD, Kuller L, et al: Mechanisms of clearance of *Treponema pallidum* from the CSF in a nonhuman primate model. *Neurology* 51:957, 1998.

37. Mantadakis E, Samonis G: Common symptoms—different diseases: Coexistence of neurosyphilis and non-Hodgkin's lymphoma. *Infection* 30(1):43, 2002.

38. Burke JM, Schaberg DR: Neurosyphilis in the antibiotic era. *Neurology* 35:1368, 1985.

39. Graman PS, Trupei MA, Reichman RC: Evaluation of cerebrospinal fluid in asymptomatic late syphilis. *Sex Transm Dis* 14(4):205, 1987.

40. Rolfs RT, Joesoef MR, Hendershot EF, et al for the Syphilis and HIV Study Group: A randomized trial of enhanced therapy for early syphilis in patients with and without HIV infection. *New Engl J Med* 337(5):307, 1997.

41. Merritt HH, Moore M: Acute syphilitic meningitis. *Medicine* 14:119, 1935.

42. Smith MM, Anderson JC: Neurosyphilis as a cause of facial and vestibulocochlear nerve dysfunction: MR imaging features. *AJNR* 21:1673, 2000.

43. Good CD, Jäger HR: Contrast enhancement of the cerebrospinal fluid on MRI in two cases of spirochaetal meningitis. *Neuroradiology* 42:448, 2000.

44. Brightbill TC, Ihmeidan IH, Post MJD, et al: Neurosyphilis in HIV-positive and HIV-negative patients: Neuroimaging findings. *AJNR* 16(4):703, 1995.

45. Rompalo AM, Joesoef MR, O'Donnell JA, et al for the Syphilis and HIV Study Group: Clinical manifestations of early syphilis by HIV status and gender. *Sex Transm Dis* 28(3):158, 2001.

46. Kelley RE, Bell L, Kelley SE, et al: Syphilis detection in cerebrovascular disease. *Stroke* 20(2):230, 1989.

47. Berger JR: Spinal cord syphilis associated with human immunodeficiency virus infection: A treatable myelopathy. *Am J Med* 92:101, 1992.

48. Hooshmand H, Escobar MR, Kopf SW: Neurosyphilis: A study of 241 patients. *JAMA* 219(6):726, 1972.

49. Horowitz HW, Marius PV, Wicher V, et al: Cerebral syphilitic gumma confirmed by the polymerase chain reaction in a man with human immunodeficiency virus infection. *New Engl J Med* 331:1488, 1994.

50. Roeske LC, Kennedy PR: Syphilitic gummas in a patient with HIV infection. *New Engl J Med* 335(15):1123, 1996.

51. Liu H, Rodes B, Chen C-Y, et al: New tests for syphilis: rational design of a PCR method for detection of *Treponema pallidum* in clinical specimens using unique regions of the DNA polymerase I gene. *J Clin Microbiol* 39(5):1941, 2001.

52. Luger AF, Schmidt BL, Kaulich M: Significance of laboratory findings for the diagnosis of neurosyphilis. *Int J STD AIDS* 11:224, 2000.

53. Davis LE, Schmitt JW: Clinical significance of cerebrospinal fluid tests for neurosyphilis. *Ann Neurol* 25:50, 1989.

54. MacLean S, Luger A: Finding neurosyphilis without the VDRL test. *Sex Transm Dis* 23(5):392, 1996.

55. Luger A, Schmidt BL, Steyrer K, et al: Diagnosis of neurosyphilis by examination of the cerebrospinal fluid. *Br J Vener Dis* 57:232, 1981.

56. Centurion-Lara A, Castro C, Shaffer JM, et al: Detection of *Treponema pallidum* by a sensitive reverse transcriptase PCR. *J Clin Microbiol* 35(6):1348, 1997.

57. Centers for Disease Control and Prevention: Sexually transmitted diseases treatment guidelines 2002. *MMWR* 51(RR-6), 2002.

58. Marra CM, Maxwell CL, Smith SL, et al: Cerebrospinal fluid abnormalities in patients with syphilis: Association with clinical and laboratory features. *J Infect Dis* 189(3):369, 2004.

59. Giles AJH: Tabes dorsalis progressing to general paresis after 20 years despite routing penicillin therapy. *Br J Vener Dis* 56:368, 1980.

60. Whiteside DM: Persistence of neurosyphilis despite multiple treatment regimens. *Am J Med* 87:225, 1989.

61. Gordon SM, Eaton ME, George R, et al: The response of symptomatic neurosyphilis to high-dose intravenous penicillin G in patients with human immunodeficiency virus infection. *New Engl J Med* 331(22):1469, 1994.

62. Hook EW: Syphilis and HIV infection. *J Infect Dis* 160(3):530, 1989.

63. Dunlop EMC, Al-Eigaly SS, Houang ET: Penicillin levels in blood and CSF achieved by treatment of syphilis. *JAMA* 241(23):2538, 1979.

64. Schoth PEM, Wolters EC: Penicillin concentrations in serum and CSF during high-dose intravenous treatment for neurosyphilis. *Neurology* 37:1214, 1987.

65. Eagle H: Speculations as to the therapeutic significance of the penicillin blood level. *Ann Intern Med* 28:260, 1948.

66. Polnikorn N, Witoonpanich R, Vorachit M, et al: Penicillin concentrations in cerebrospinal fluid after different treatment regimens for syphilis. *Br J Vener Dis* 56:363, 1980.

67. Mohr JA, Griffiths W, Jackson R, et al: Neurosyphilis and penicillin levels in cerebrospinal fluid. *JAMA* 236(19):2208, 1976.

68. Hahn RD, Cutler JC, Curtis AC, et al: Penicillin treatment of asymptomatic central nervous system syphilis: I. Probability of progression to symptomatic neurosyphilis. *Arch Dermatol* 74:355, 1956.

69. Hahn RD, Cutler JC, Curtis AC, et al: Penicillin treatment of asymptomatic central nervous system syphilis: II. Results of therapy as measured by laboratory findings. *Arch Dermatol* 74:367, 1956.

70. Marra CM, Boutin P, McArthur JC, et al: ACTG145 team:

A pilot study evaluating ceftriaxone and penicillin G as treatment agents for neurosyphilis in human immunodeficiency virus-infected individuals. *Clin Infect Dis* 30:540-544, 2000.

71. Dowell ME, Ross PG, Musher DM, et al: Response of latent syphilis or neurosyphilis to ceftriaxone therapy in persons infected with human immunodeficiency virus. *Am J Med* 93:481, 1992.

72. Augenbraun M, Workowski K: Ceftriaxone therapy for syphilis: Report from the emerging infections network. *Clin Infect Dis* 29(5):1337, 1999.

73. De Maria A, Solaro C, Abbruzzese M, et al: Minocycline for symptomatic neurosyphilis in patients allergic to penicillin. *New Engl J Med* 337(18):1322, 1997.

74. Yim CW, Flynn NM, Fitzgerald FT: Penetration of oral doxycycline into the cerebrospinal fluid of patients with latent or neurosyphilis. *Antimicrob Agents Chemother* 28(2):347, 1985.

75. Wilner E, Brody JA: Prognosis of general paresis after treatment. *Lancet* 2:1370, 1968.

76. Jordan KG: Modern neurosyphilis: A critical analysis. *West J Med* 149:47, 1988.

77. Hook EW: Management of syphilis in human immunodeficiency virus-infected patients. *Am J Med* 93:477, 1992.

78. Blocker ME, Levine WC, St. Louis ME: HIV prevalence in patients with syphilis, United States. *Sex Transm Dis* 27(1):53, 2000.

79. Hook EW: Editorial response: Diagnosing neurosyphilis *Clin Infect Dis* 18:295, 1994.

80. Fox PA, Hawkins DA, Dawson S: Dementia following an acute presentation of meningovascular syphilis in an HIV-1-positive patient. *AIDS* 14(13):2062, 2000.

81. Berger JR: Neurosyphilis in human immunodeficiency virus type 1–seropositive individuals: A prospective study. *Arch Neurol* 48:700, 1991.

82. Marra CM, Handsfield HH, Kuller L, et al: Alterations in the course of experimental syphilis associated with concurrent simian immunodeficiency virus infection. *J Infect Dis* 165:1020, 1992.

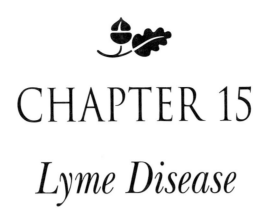

CHAPTER 15

Lyme Disease

John J. Halperin

▶ OVERVIEW

Although the term *Lyme disease* was coined in the 1970s,[1] this infectious disease's most important clinical manifestations were well known through much of the twentieth century. The characteristic rash, erythema migrans (EM), a typically painless erythroderm that expands slowly to many centimeters in diameter, was well described by Afzelius in 1910 (Fig. 15-1). In 1922, two French clinicians, Garin and Bujadoux, elegantly described the syndrome of tick bite–associated lymphocytic meningitis with painful radiculoneuritis, a disorder they even postulated was due to a spirochetal infection. In the early 1940s, the German neurologist Bannwarth recognized that this neurologic syndrome was common and often was associated with "rheumatism." In the 1950s it was demonstrated that the disorder could be treated successfully with antibiotics.

Curiously, clinical phenomena typical of this infection were not recognized in North America until many years later. It has been suggested that the causative organism was first introduced in the United States early in the twentieth century when a small herd of deer was brought to Shelter Island, New York. Per-

haps the causative organism then went through many cycles of unobserved amplification among the unique vectors and permissive hosts in this environment until sufficient numbers of humans finally invaded the rather rural environs in which the infection survived, permitting the occurrence and recognition of human illness.

By the mid-1950s, cases of recurrent nontraumatic knee arthritis, dubbed *Montauk knee,* were well recognized among practitioners in eastern Long Island, New York. The characteristic rash, erythema migrans, was first reported in the United States in 1970 in a patient infected in Minnesota. Then, in the mid-1970s, a group of parents in Old Lyme, Connecticut, recognized that an inordinate number of the children in that small area were being diagnosed as having juvenile rheumatoid arthritis. In a series of elegant epidemiologic studies, Steere and colleagues established that this rheumatologic disorder was actually due to an infection transmitted by bites of hard-shelled *Ixodes* ticks, associated with the same rash, erythema migrans, and the same neurologic disorders[2] long described in Europe. Finally, in the early 1980s, a series of reports from the United States and then Scandinavia identified the tick-borne spirochete, which was named *Borrelia burgdor-*

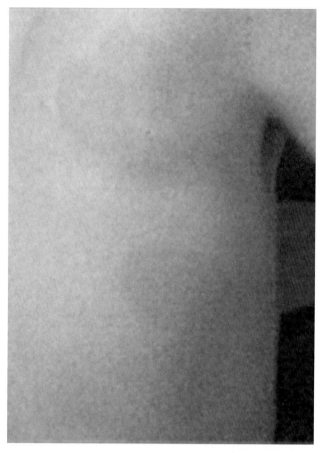

Figure 15.1. Multifocal erythema migrans, demonstrating the multicentric nature of the rash. Each focus develops from a separate nidus of disseminated infection.

feri, responsible for this group of previously only clinically defined syndromes. This, in turn, permitted the development of serologic and microbiologic tests to better refine our understanding of the spectrum of human disease caused by this infection. Despite some years of either misinterpretation or misapplication of such testing, as well as its intrinsic limitations, the characteristics of this multisystem infectious disease now gradually have become better defined.

▶ EPIDEMIOLOGY

Lyme disease, despite its mystique and mythology, is simply an infectious disease—one with a particular predilection to affect joints, the nervous system, and skin. The causative organism, the spirochete *B. burgdorferi,* can be transmitted only by hard-shelled *Ixodes* ticks—*I. scapularis* in most of the United States, predominantly *I. ricinus* in Europe, and other related species in other parts of the world. This tick family prefers temperate, moist environments. Hence, in the United States, 95 percent of all cases occur either along the East Coast, between the District of Columbia and New Hampshire, or in Wisconsin and Minnesota. In Europe, it occurs throughout Scandinavia and in areas of Austria, France, Germany, and central Europe where the climate is similar.

Even though *Ixodes* ticks may be present elsewhere, the infection must first be introduced into the local ecosystem, where it must take root and be perpetuated. The tick goes through a complex 2-year life cycle that is essential to propagating the infection. Since transovarial infection probably does not occur, the larval nymph can become infected only when it takes its first blood meal, typically on a small host, such as a field mouse. Only if this host is spirochetemic can the tick itself become infected. Once fed, the tick larva matures into a nymph and eventually takes its second blood meal—which may be on an inopportunely located human.

To facilitate unobserved attachment and continued feeding (a full meal typically requires that the tick remain in place for a number of days), the tick injects local anesthetics and anticoagulants both at the onset and during feeding. Blood entering the tick gut triggers the local proliferation of spirochetes, which then migrate through the tick, eventually to be injected into the host later in the feeding. This cycle probably requires at least 24 hours of feeding. If the duration of tick attachment is less than this, the likelihood of this second host becoming infected is extremely low. Following this meal, the nymphal tick will mature into an adult, which may in turn feed on one last host, often a larger animal such as a bear, deer, sheep, or human, potentially infecting it. Since this constitutes the tick's last supper, control strategies aimed just at deer (the most common host for adult ticks in the northeastern United States) may not be wholly successful. The deer's role in the tick life cycle is primarily permissive, allowing the tick to overwinter and lay its eggs. However, whether or not the deer is infected is irrelevant—ticks feeding on it will never feed again. In temperate climates, this entire three-stage, three-meal life cycle typically requires 2 years. At the end, the adult tick dies—in the case of the female, after laying her eggs. Importantly, ticks generally are inactive—and consequently, do not feed—in cold weather. Thus new-onset infection in winter is extremely unlikely.

As a result of these geographic and temporal considerations, acute Lyme disease occurs only in specific locales and at specific times of the year. In a patient who has never been outside an urban center or who develops symptoms in January, the likelihood of the illness being attributable to acute Lyme disease is extremely small, any laboratory results notwithstanding.

▶ PATHOPHYSIOLOGY AND PATHOGENESIS

Originally characterized as a single organism, molecular analysis of *B. burgdorferi* has now resulted in the spirochete being subclassified into three distinct strains.[3] In the United States, only one strain occurs naturally, and it has been named *B. burgdorferi sensu stricto*. In Europe, two strains predominate; *B. garinii*, responsible for many of the neurologic manifestations, and *B. afzelii*, particularly likely to cause an unusual cutaneous manifestation, acrodermatitis atrophicans, which occurs rarely, if ever, in the United States. *B. burgdorferi sensu stricto* occurs in Europe as well. Much has been said about differences in clinical manifestations of this infection among European versus American patients. Specifically, nervous system involvement is said to be much more common in European patients, and arthritis is more prevalent among Americans. To what extent this reflects bacterial strain differences, differing biases of ascertainment, or other factors remains to be determined.[4] Although a great deal has been learned about the biology of the responsible microorganism, the precise reasons for specific organotropisms remain unclear.

Once inoculated into the host's skin by the tick, spirochetes migrate centrifugally—the leading edge of the EM typically contains large numbers of spirochetes. Bacteria, particularly *B. burgdorferi sensu stricto,* also can disseminate hematogenously. In the United States, patients quite frequently develop multifocal EM—each focus representing a separate nidus of hematogenously disseminated infection. Disseminated bacteria also can lodge in other organs. There is good evidence that the central nervous system is commonly seeded quite early in infection.[5,6] It appears that much like syphilis, this infection then may subside spontaneously or persist, causing subsequent neurologic disease that may be brief and self-limited, or progressive. Some studies have suggested that *B. burgdorferi* may have a particular affinity for oligodendroglia or for the gangliosides they produce.[7] The significance of these observations remains to be clarified, but this could provide an explanation for the apparent predilection for cerebral white matter.

▶ CLINICAL FEATURES

Lyme disease affects the nervous system in very specific ways (Table 15-1). Although the literature is replete with suggestions that it can mimic virtually any known neurobehavioral disorder, such is not the case. The literature also suggests that the manifestations of this disease differ in Europe and the United States, which is thought to be related to strain differences. This also may be more apparent than real. Certainly in both, the most typical form of neuroborreliosis is the classic triad of cranial neuropathy (particularly facial nerve palsy), lymphocytic meningitis, and painful radiculoneuritis (known in Europe as the syndrome of Garin-Bujadoux-Bannwarth).

To understand nervous system involvement more clearly, it is helpful to go beyond such syndromic descriptions and attempt to group disorders based on their underlying pathophysiology. Disorders first can be divided into those affecting the peripheral versus the central nervous system (CNS). The latter, in turn, can be divided into those affecting the CNS parenchyma and the CNS milieu—either the subarachnoid space or the overall homeostatic environment in which the brain functions.

It is simplest to begin with the peripheral nervous system (PNS).[8] PNS disorders can be conceptualized as those primarily affecting myelin (e.g., the Guillain-Barré syndrome), those affecting axons (such as many toxic neuropathies), and those affecting nerves in a multifocal fashion (a mononeuropathy multiplex such as occurs in diabetes, vasculitis, or leprosy). Case reports have attributed virtually every conceivable clinical phe-

▶ **TABLE 15-1.** NEUROLOGIC MANIFESTATIONS, THEIR PATHOPHYSIOLOGY, AND CLINICAL PICTURE

Peripheral Nervous System		Central Nervous System	
Mechanism	Clinical	Mechanism	Clinical
		Meningeal infection	Meningitis
		Toxic/metabolic encephalopathy	"Lyme encephalopathy"
Mononeuropathy multiplex	Cranial neuropathy	Multifocal encephalomyelitis	"MS-like" (but monophasic)
	Radiculopathy		Transverse myelitis
	Brachial plexopathy		
	Lumbosacral plexopathy		
	Mononeuropathy multiplex		
	Confluent mononeuropathy multiplex-acute or indolent		

nomenon to Lyme disease. However, some of these (acute inflammatory demyelinating polyneuropathy) have been seen so infrequently as to quite likely be chance associations.

Most systematic studies have demonstrated multifocal involvement of peripheral nerve, primarily with axonal damage. Careful analysis of the available neurophysiologic data suggests that all patients, in fact, have a mononeuropathy multiplex—either manifest as a confluent form, mimicking a diffuse axonopathy, or as a more classic focal syndrome of a monoradiculopathy, plexopathy, or cranial nerve palsy. The limited neuropathologic data available have demonstrated perivascular inflammatory changes with no evidence of primary demyelination, a pattern entirely consistent with a mononeuropathy multiplex. In the only good animal model of nervous system Lyme disease, the rhesus macaque monkey, virtually all infected animals develop a typical mononeuropathy multiplex, evident clinically, neurophysiologically, and histopathologically.

Clinically, PNS neuroborreliosis can be manifest in any of a number of ways. Probably the best known is a cranial neuropathy, of which the overwhelming majority involve the facial nerve. Lyme disease, along with Guillain-Barré syndrome and sarcoidosis, is one of the few disorders likely to feature bilateral facial nerve involvement, which occurs in one of every four or five individuals with Lyme disease–associated facial nerve palsy. Interestingly, even though the majority of patients with Lyme disease–associated facial nerve palsy have a concomitant meningitis, clinical observations suggest that even in this setting the nerve is damaged peripherally as part of a mononeuropathy multiplex and not as it crosses through the purulent exudate in the subarachnoid space.[9] The other fairly frequent but often missed PNS manifestation is a painful radiculopathy that can be indistinguishable clinically from a mechanical one. Patients present with quite severe dermatomal pain and corresponding sensory, motor, and reflex changes. Signs of a myelopathy at the same segmental level may be present. Lyme disease should be suspected if a radiculopathy occurs in the summer or autumn months in Lyme disease–endemic areas, particularly in the absence of an antecedent injury and if imaging studies do not demonstrate a herniated disk or other abnormality. Cerebrospinal fluid (CSF) often shows inflammatory changes. Involvement of thoracic roots may present with atypical chest or abdominal pain that is often misdiagnosed as a visceral process.

Lyme disease may present with brachial or lumbosacral plexopathies or more typical mononeuropathies. Patients with long-standing and indolent disease may develop a more slowly evolving and symmetric "stocking glove" neuropathy that suggests neurophysiologically a confluent mononeuropathy multiplex. Although a few case reports of myositis have

been published, and creatine kinase elevations are observed in some patients, muscle involvement probably is rarely clinically significant.

CNS disease similarly can be conceptualized based on thematic rather than structural anatomy. Approximately 10 percent of infected, untreated patients will develop a lymphocytic meningitis.[10] CSF abnormalities resemble those found in viral infections, typically with fewer than 100 to 200 lymphocytes/mm^3, mildly elevated protein, and normal glucose concentrations. Symptoms vary from minimal to marked, with some patients having typical photosensitivity, severe headache, neck stiffness, and so on, whereas others with the same CSF white blood cell count are asymptomatic.

Parenchymal brain involvement occurs quite rarely. It has been estimated that approximately 0.1 percent of untreated patients will develop white matter inflammation, with clinical manifestations determined by the site of the lesions. Whether this is similar to immune-mediated acute demyelinating encephalomyelitis or is a multifocal white matter infection (as suggested by the demonstrated affinity of *B. burgdorferi* for oligodendroglia) remains unclear. However, anecdotally, long-term improvement appears more likely to occur following antimicrobial rather than immunosuppressive therapy. It is worth noting the parallelism between this multifocal inflammatory process observed (rarely) in the brain and the far more frequently observed but conceptually analogous multifocal inflammatory process in the PNS.

Perhaps the most frequently discussed and widely misperceived clinical phenomenon is the entity that has been termed *Lyme encephalopathy*.[11] This disorder was recognized initially in patients who had Lyme arthritis. These individuals had significant systemic inflammatory disease, presumably with a high concentration of circulating cytokines and other neuroimmune modulators. They complained of difficulty with memory, concentration, and cognitive processing. These abnormalities could be confirmed on formal mental status testing. This is probably analogous to the frequently observed cognitive dysfunction in individuals with other immune activated states such as sepsis, lupus, or other diseases.

Two crucial elements of this disorder are often ignored. First, many patients with depression or other psychiatric disorders describe similar symptoms. Essential in diagnosing any encephalopathy is confirming the patient's described difficulty with objective testing, with either a mini–mental status examination or more formal and detailed neuropsychologic testing, and demonstrating the existence of a causative, underlying medical illness. The other essential but often forgotten consideration is that encephalopathies generally are due to systemic factors and not to irreversible damage to the brain. Although a few of the patients originally described as having Lyme encephalopathy actually had evidence of active CNS inflammation with abnormal brain magnetic resonance imaging (MRI) and CSF, this is probably only a small minority of such patients, a group that can be identified readily with these two procedures. Many patients in whom the diagnosis of Lyme encephalopathy is considered are mistakenly but understandably terrified that they have a chronic brain infection that ultimately will destroy all cognitive function—a prospect that may induce severe anxiety or depression, even if none existed originally. Reports have described associations between innumerable other neuropsychiatric disorders and Lyme disease. In some, the evidence in support of Lyme disease has been stronger than in others. The few controlled studies that have been performed suggest that the incidence of neuropsychiatric symptoms is no greater in patients with Lyme disease than in those with other systemic inflammatory disorders. What does appear clear from the available published data is that even in the unlikely event that these associations are biologically real, they do not reflect CNS infection. This is an important consideration in designing therapeutic strategies.

▶ DIAGNOSIS ✓

Unlike in other bacterial infections, culturing readily available patient samples has not been very productive. Although the pathognomonic skin lesion, erythema migrans, often contains innumerable spirochetes, culture of joint fluid, CSF, or peripheral nerve is rarely informative. This probably reflects a variety of factors, not the least of which is the rather small number of organisms present in these tissues and fluids. Even using polymerase chain reaction (PCR)–based techniques to amplify samples, the sensitivity of organism-specific assays remains remarkably low. Tests to detect bacterial antigens, although informative in other illnesses, has been disappointing in Lyme disease. The often-touted Lyme urine antigen test (LUAT) has been shown to have results no different from chance.[12] Several authors have described detecting Lyme antigens and antibodies in immune complexes. This has been neither widely replicated nor generally available. As a result, diagnosis has

rested largely on serologic testing. These techniques have been heavily criticized for their shortcomings, even though many of these are no different in Lyme disease than in any other illness. Although there continues to be legitimate debate about technical aspects of these assays, including which *B. burgdorferi* strains to use, the benefit of using specified antigens versus whole-organism sonicates, criteria for defining positivity, and so on, most of the issues relate to test misapplication and misinterpretation.

In most infections, it is considered understandable that antibodies are undetectable very early in infection, before the immune system has mounted a measurable response. In Lyme disease, this insensitivity in the first few weeks is considered a peculiar shortcoming. In most illnesses, serologic testing is used to demonstrate an evolving antibody titer, typically looking for a significant rise in antibody concentration between acute and convalescent samples. In Lyme disease it has been commonplace to look at a single value and use it to determine the presence of acute, active disease. In all other (bacterial) serologic testing it is generally accepted that a single test demonstrating the presence of IgG antibody may reflect active infection or remote exposure or even irrelevant cross-reactivity and is not definitive evidence of infection.

Two particular problems occur in serologic testing for Lyme disease. First, many of the antigens detected in standard Lyme enzyme-linked immunosorbent assays (ELISAs) are common to other spirochetal organisms (such as oral treponemes), resulting in significant cross-reactivity and many false-positive results. This has been addressed by using Western blots (Table 15-2), a technique used to demonstrate the specific antigens to which the patient's antibodies react. Western blot criteria have been developed for use primarily in patients in whom the ELISA is positive or borderline. Since these criteria were developed primarily in seropositive patients, the validity of extrapolation to seronegative individuals is at best questionable. It is important to emphasize, though, that these criteria were developed to improve specificity, not sensitivity; in fact, sensitivity is somewhat limited.[13] Two-thirds of patients with acute disease do not have detectable IgM antibodies, and IgG

▶ **TABLE 15-2.** WESTERN BLOT CRITERIA FOR THE DIAGNOSIS OF LYME DISEASE, PRIMARILY IN SEROPOSITIVE PATIENTS

	IgM (Acute Disease)	IgG (Established Disease)
Bands (kDa)	23, 39, 41	18, 23, 28, 30, 39, 41, 45, 60, 66, 93
Criterion	2 of 3	5 of 10
Sensitivity	32%	83%
Specificity	100%	95%

SOURCE: *Used with permission from ref. 13.*

antibodies are absent in one in six with established infection. Thus neither a negative serologic result in a patient with classic EM nor a positive serology but negative Western blot in a patient from a Lyme disease–endemic area with facial palsy should be interpreted as negating the diagnosis of Lyme disease. Both patients should be treated. In contrast, a patient with a negative ELISA who comes from a nonendemic area and has only nonspecific symptoms, even the presence of multiple IgG bands, should not be given antimicrobial therapy for possible Lyme disease. In fact, a consideration of the positive and negative predictive values of serologic tests leads to the conclusion that in patients from nonendemic areas with nonspecific symptoms, the likelihood of a false-positive result so exceeds the chance of a true positive that even obtaining the test should be discouraged. The other unusual limitation of serologic testing is that in some individuals treated with noncurative doses of antibiotics early in infection, spirochetes may persist (perhaps in immunologically protected sites), but the humoral response may be permanently abrogated. This uncommon but interesting observation has led to widespread speculation about seronegative Lyme disease—something that probably does occur, albeit rarely.

An additional diagnostic option is available for patients with suspected CNS infection. As in patients with other CNS infections, localization of microorganisms in the CNS can trigger a local autonomous immune response, with trapping of targeted B cells within the CNS and local production of specific antibody. Assessment of this intrathecal antibody production requires simultaneous measurement of CSF and serum specific antibodies, correcting for any overall immune stimulation by normalizing for CSF immunoglobulin concentration, and comparing the patient's CSF and serum Lyme disease ELISA values, a ratio that conceptually should exceed 1.0 in individuals with intrathecal antibody production. This approach has several intrinsic limitations. First, in patients with treated CNS infection, apparent intrathecal antibody production may persist for 10 years or more. However, evidence of active inflammation, such as increased white blood cell counts or protein concentration, would resolve. More important conceptually, in the absence of any other absolutely diagnostic criterion for CNS infection, the sensitivity of this (or any) approach is undefinable, with estimates ranging from 95+ percent in the European literature to 90 percent in U.S. patients with meningitis to 50 percent in patients thought to have more indolent CNS disease.[14]

▶ DIFFERENTIAL DIAGNOSIS

As suggested by the preceding discussion, the differential diagnosis can be broad, depending on clinical presentation. First and foremost, though, in considering the possibility of Lyme disease is the epidemiologic possibility of exposure. Absent any potential exposure in Lyme disease–endemic areas, the likelihood of this infection is very remote. From a laboratory point of view, other spirochetal infections (syphilis, relapsing fevers) can give false-positive Lyme disease ELISAs. Fortunately, there is very little geographic overlap between the relapsing fevers and Lyme disease. Although Lyme disease can cause a false-positive FTA (which detects specific spirochetal antigens that are common to both organisms), it should not cause a positive RPR (which actually detects anticardiolipin antibodies typically produced in syphilis). Although other infections and inflammatory states (subacute bacterial endocarditis, lupus) can cause a false-positive ELISA, Western blots typically readily identify such nonspecific false-positive results.

Other forms of basilar meningitis should be considered in the differential diagnosis of disorders causing multiple cranial neuropathies, including sarcoidosis; fungal, syphilitic, or HIV infection; and cancer. In patients with radiculopathies, mechanical and neoplastic processes should be considered. The differential diagnosis of peripheral neuropathies is vast, but in light of the typical mononeuropathy multiplex–like pattern, vasculitic and vasculopathic processes in particular must be considered.

On those rare occasions when parenchymal brain or spinal cord inflammation occurs, a first episode of demyelinating disease must be considered. In this specific circumstance, since CSF immunoglobulin will be elevated in either Lyme disease or a first episode of demyelinating disease, CSF serologic testing should be virtually 100 percent diagnostic. If CSF IgG is elevated because of the presence of organism-specific antigens in the CNS, intrathecal production of antibodies targeted against those antigens should be detected. In Lyme disease, antibodies against *B. burgdorferi* should be evident. On the other hand, if CSF IgG is elevated because of a first episode of multiple sclerosis, antibody directed against *B. burgdorferi* should be no more evident than any other antibodies.

▶ TREATMENT

Despite frequently expressed concerns that Lyme disease is "never cured, just controlled," this is in fact a bacterial infection that is very sensitive to appropriate antimicrobial therapy[15] (Table 15-3). In patients with early disease, a 2- to 3-week course of amoxicillin, doxycycline, or cefuroxime is curative in over 90 percent of patients. Recent studies indicate that adding a dose of ceftriaxone or extending treatment beyond 10 days confers no additional benefit to the already excellent prog-

▶ **TABLE 15-3.** RECOMMENDED TREATMENT REGIMENS

Indication	Medication, Dose	Duration
Early disease	Doxycycline 100 mg PO bid	2–4 weeks
	Amoxicillin 500 mg PO tid	2–4 weeks
	Cefuroxime axetil 500 mg PO bid	3 weeks
CNS/Late disease	Ceftriaxone 2 g IV qd	14–28 days
	Cefotaxime 2 g IV q8h	14–28 days
	Penicillin 20–24 mU/d IV (q4h dosing)	14–28 days
Selected circumstances	Doxycycline 100–200 mg PO bid	30 days

NOTE: Doxycycline or other tetracyclines should not be used in pregnancy or in children under age 8.
SOURCE: *Used with permission from ref. 15.*

nosis.[16] Even in patients with Lyme arthritis, initial treatment with oral agents is recommended because the response is quite good. Parenteral antimicrobial therapy is recommended whenever there is evidence of CNS invasion despite the suggestion in the European literature that oral treatment is sufficient for Lyme meningitis and even facial palsy.

Definitive treatment of neuroborreliosis is typically with ceftriaxone or cefotaxime. Although studies show no advantage of treatment for more than 2 weeks, most recommendations list 2- to 4-week courses based on anecdotal experience, with evidence of occasional treatment failures with 2-week courses. Assessing treatment success can be difficult. There should be no specific expectation that antibody titers will fall rapidly, although this may occur, particularly in early disease. In CNS disease, follow-up lumbar punctures can be informative, as in neurosyphilis, where a decline or normalization in the cell count and protein concentration typically occurs. However, generally, treatment efficacy must be judged clinically with at least stabilization and hopefully improvement in symptoms and their objective correlates. Although there are practitioners who recommend extremely protracted courses of treatment, not only is there no evidence to support this approach, but there are now at least two studies demonstrating no additional benefit from protracted therapy.[17]

▶ COMPLICATIONS

Acute infection can be associated with a number of serious complications. Heart block can occur and may require a temporary pacemaker. Although rare cases of heart failure have been linked to *B. burgdorferi* infection, the causal link is controversial. In patients who develop frank arthritis, some (probably HLA determined) may progress to a destructive and persistent arthritis that may not resolve no matter how much antimicrobial therapy is given. When the nervous system

is involved, residual neurologic deficits may occur. For example, patients with facial nerve paralysis may have a persistent deficit, although this appears to occur even more rarely than in patients with idiopathic Bell's palsy. In patients with other forms of PNS involvement, recovery typically occurs, although, as with any nerve injury, this is a long, slow process. Similarly, in rare patients with demonstrable parenchymal CNS inflammation who develop clinical deficits, some residua may remain. However, much as in patients with other small and nonprogressive CNS lesions, slow improvement may occur over time. Although a prolonged chronic fatigue–like state (post-Lyme disease syndrome) has been described following successful treatment of Lyme disease, neither the biology of this disorder, its relationship to *B. burgdorferi* infection, nor its optimal treatment are understood. However, it is now clear that prolonged antimicrobial therapy has no significant impact on the further evolution of this syndrome.[18]

▶ PREVENTION

Lyme disease occurs because humans invade areas inhabited by infected ticks and their hosts. Ticks must be attached for at least 24 and probably 48 hours before there is a significant risk of infection. Thus this disease can be prevented by (1) avoiding high-risk habitats, (2) limiting the risk of tick bites when in such habitats by applying tick repellants to clothes and minimizing the amount of exposed skin or at least increasing the likelihood of noticing ticks by wearing light-colored clothing, or (3) doing a "tick check" at the end of each day when at risk of tick exposure to remove feeding ticks before they have the opportunity to infect the host. Ticks are best removed by grasping with forceps inserted between the skin and the tick mouth and then retracting slowly. There is no role for prophylactic antibiotics after tick bites.

► SUMMARY

Lyme disease, the multisystem infectious disease caused by the tick-borne spirochete *B. burgdorferi*, is preventable by avoiding the typical habitats of infected ticks or by removing ticks before they have been able to feed for an extended period of time. If infection occurs, the nervous system is commonly involved, most commonly evidenced by facial nerve palsy, lymphocytic meningitis, mononeuropathy multiplex, or rarely, multifocal involvement of the brain and spinal cord. Treatment with antibiotics almost invariably is successful; long-term neurologic sequelae are rare.

REFERENCES

1. Steere AC, Malawista SE, Hardin JA, et al: Erythema chronicum migrans and Lyme arthritis: The enlarging clinical spectrum. *Ann Intern Med* 86:685, 1977.
2. Reik L, Steere AC, Bartenhagen NH, et al: Neurologic abnormalities of Lyme disease. *Medicine* 58:281, 1979.
3. Busch U, Hizo-Teufe C, Boehmer R, et al: Three species of *Borrelia burgdorferi sensu lato* (*B. burgdorferi sensu stricto, B afzelii,* and *B. garinii*) identified from cerebrospinal fluid isolates by pulsed-field gel electrophoresis and PCR. *J Clin Microbiol* 34:1072, 1996.
4. Halperin JJ: Clinical features, diagnosis and therapy of neuroborreliosis, in *Vector Borne and Zoonotic Diseases* 2:241, 2002.
5. Luft BJ, Steinman CR, Neimark HC, et al: Invasion of the central nervous system by *Borrelia burgdorferi* in acute disseminated infection. *JAMA* 267:1364, 1992.
6. Logigian EL, Steere AC: Invasion of the central nervous system by *Borrelia burgdorferi* in acute disseminated infection. *JAMA* 267:1364, 1992.
7. Garcia-Monco JC Benach JL: Lyme neuroborreliosis. *Ann Neurol* 37:691, 1995.
8. Halperin JJ: Lyme disease and the peripheral nervous system. *Muscle Nerve* (in press).
9. Halperin JJ: Facial nerve palsy associated with Lyme disease. *Muscle Nerve* 28:133, 2003.
10. Pachner AR, Steere AC: The triad of neurologic manifestations of Lyme disease. *Neurology* 35:47, 1985.
11. Halperin JJ, Krupp LB, Golightly MG, et al: Lyme borreliosis–associated encephalopathy. *Neurology* 40:1340, 1990.
12. Klempner MS, Schmid CH, Hu L, et al: Intralaboratory reliability of serologic and urine testing for Lyme disease. *Am J Med* 110:217, 2001.
13. Dressler F, Whalen JA, Reinhardt BN, et al: Western blotting in the serodiagnosis of Lyme disease. *J Infect Dis* 167:392, 1993.
14. Steere AC, Berardi VP, Weeks KE, et al: Evaluation of the intrathecal antibody response to *Borrelia burgdorferi* as a diagnostic test for Lyme neuroborreliosis. *J Infect Dis* 161:1203, 1990.
15. Wormser GP, Nadelman RB, Dattwyler RJ, et al: Practice guidelines for the treatment of Lyme disease. The Infectious Diseases Society of America. *Clin Infect Dis* 31(suppl 1):1, 2000.
16. Wormser GP, Ramanathan R, Nowakowski J, et al: Duration of antibiotic therapy for early Lyme disease. *Ann Intern Med* 138:697, 2003.
17. Klempner M, Hu L, Evans J, et al: Two controlled trials of antibiotic treatment in patients with persistent symptoms and a history of Lyme disease. *New Engl J Med* 345:85, 2001.
18. Krupp LB, Grimson R: A randomized, double-masked clinical trial studying the treatment of post-Lyme disease. *Neurology* 58:A405, 2002.

CHAPTER 16

Helminthic Infections

Oscar H. Del Brutto

Helminths are common parasites of humans and contribute extensively to morbidity and mortality in developing countries. In recent years, increased tourism, refugee movements, and migration of people from endemic areas to industrialized nations have caused a spread of helminthic diseases to areas where these infections no longer should be considered exotic or rare.[1] Helminths are classified as flatworms and roundworms (nematodes). The former are further classified as cestodes (tapeworms) and trematodes (flukes). These highly structured parasites require two or more hosts to complete their complex life cycles. Humans may be either intermediate or definitive hosts of helminths.[2] The unpredictable nature of the immunologic reaction of the host against helminthic infections, as well as the myriad pathologic lesions that these parasites cause in hu-

mans, makes these infections highly pleomorphic. About 20 of the helminths that infect humans may invade the central nervous system (CNS) causing meningitis, encephalitis, space-occupying brain lesions, stroke, and myelopathy (Table 16-1).

▶ CESTODE INFECTIONS

Coenurosis

Coenurosis is caused by *Coenurus cerebralis*, the larval stage of *Taenia multiceps*, the dog tapeworm. Canids are definitive hosts of this cestode, and sheep are intermediate hosts. Humans who ingest dog feces contaminated with eggs of *T. multiceps* also may become

▶ **TABLE 16-1.** HELMINTHIC INFECTIONS OF THE CENTRAL NERVOUS SYSTEM

Agent	Disease	Main Pathologic Features
Angiostrongylus cantonensis	Angiostrongyliasis	Eosinophilic meningitis
Ascaris lumbricoides	Ascariasis	Thalamic granulomas, obstruction of CSF shunt devices
Ascaris zuum	Ascariasis	Acute encephalitis
Baylisascaris procyonis	Baylisascariasis	Eosinophilic meningoencephalitis
Coenurus cerebralis	Coenurosis	Parenchymal cysts, arachnoiditis, hydrocephalus, cerebral infarctions
Cysticercus (*Taenia solium*)	Neurocysticercosis	Parenchymal, subarachnoid, ventricular, and spinal cysts; arachnoiditis; hydrocephalus; angiitis; encephalitis
Dracunculus medinensis	Dracontiasis	Extradural spinal abscess
Echinococcus granulosus	Cystic hydatid disease	Parenchymal, subarachnoid, epidural, ventricular, orbital, and spinal cysts; cerebral infarctions
Echinococcus multilocularis	Alveolar hydatid disease	Parenchymal cysts
Gnathostoma spinigerum	Gnathostomiasis	Eosinophilic meningitis, encephalitis, intracranial hemorrhages
Helicephalobus deletrix	Micronemiasis	Meningoencephalitis
Lagochilascaris minor	Lagochilascariasis	Intracranial hemorrhages
Loa loa	Loiasis	Encephalitis
Paragonimus spp.	Paragonimiasis	Parenchymal granulomas, arachnoiditis, intracranial hemorrhages
Schistosoma spp.	Schistosomiasis	Parenchymal granulomas, arachnoiditis, granulomas of conus medullaris and cauda equina, spinal cord infarctions
Spirometra mansoni	Sparganosis	Parenchymal granulomas, arachnoiditis, intracranial hemorrhages
Strongyloids stercoralis	Strongyloidiasis	Meningitis, brain abscess, cerebral infarctions, pyogenic meningitis
Toxocara spp.	Visceral larva migrans	Parenchymal granulomas, diffuse brain swelling, cerebral infarctions
Trichinella spiralis	Trichinosis	Parenchymal granulomas, arachnoiditis, cerebral infarctions

intermediate hosts.[3] After being ingested, eggs hatch into oncospheres in the intestine. Oncospheres enter the bloodstream and are carried to the tissues where the larvae develop. Target organs of *C. cerebralis* are the eye and the CNS.

Epidemiology

Human coenurosis is rare. Cases have been recognized from sheep-raising areas of the United States and Europe, as well as from Canada, South America, and Africa.[4–7]

Pathophysiology and Pathogenesis

C. cerebralis is a vesicle that includes a cloudy fluid and one larva with multiple scolices.[3] Vesicles may be found in subcutaneous tissues, skeletal muscles, orbits, and the CNS.[8–10] In the latter, cysts usually are located

in the subarachnoid space at the base of the skull, where they induce arachnoiditis with obstruction of the flow of cerebrospinal fluid (CSF). The blood vessels in the circle of Willis are affected by this process of arachnoiditis and develop inflammatory changes in their walls that may cause arterial narrowing or occlusion.[11] Cystic lesions also may be located within the brain parenchyma, where they elicit a focal inflammatory reaction around the cysts.[9]

Clinical Features

Patients with subarachnoid coenurosis and hydrocephalus usually present with increased intracranial pressure of subacute onset and a slowly progressive course. Focal neurologic signs and seizures may result from parenchymal brain cysts or a stroke may be caused by inflammatory occlusion of leptomeningeal blood vessels.[9,11]

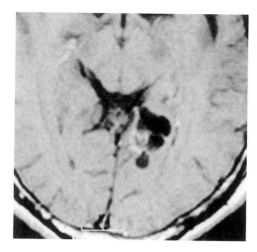

Figure 16-1. Contrast-enhanced T₁-weighted MRI of a patient with cerebral coenurosis showing a multilobulate hypointense lesion in the quadrigeminal ambiens cistern.

Diagnosis

Cytochemical analysis of CSF may show a mild lymphocytic pleocytosis with a low glucose concentration. Computed tomographic (CT) scan and magnetic resonance imaging (MRI) may demonstrate hydrocephalus or cystic or ring-enhancing lesions located in the brain parenchyma or in the basal subarachnoid cisterns (Fig 16-1). Intracranial calcifications, reflecting dead parasites, are common in patients with cerebral coenurosis.[9] There are no serologic tests for coenurosis.

Differential Diagnosis

It is impossible to differentiate coenurosis from cysticercosis on clinical and neuroimaging grounds. Microscopic examination of the lesion allows for a correct diagnosis because the larvae of *C. cerebralis* have multiple scolices and that of *Taenia solium* have only one scolex.

Treatment

Therapy includes shunt placement for the relief of hydrocephalus and surgical resection of brain lesions.[12] Corticosteroids may be used to ameliorate the inflammatory reaction induced by the presence of the parasites in the brain parenchyma or the subarachnoid space. There have been no trials of antiparasitic agents for this infection, and a single patient with intraocular coenurosis treated with praziquantel was left with visual loss due to the inflammatory reaction from the death of the parasite in the eye.[10]

Prevention

Disease in humans may be prevented by promoting hygienic practices to reduce contact with the feces of dogs.

Treatment of dogs with praziquantel or niclosamide destroys adult parasites and reduces environmental contamination with eggs.[3]

Cysticercosis

Cysticercosis occurs when humans become the intermediate hosts of *Taenia solium*, the pork tapeworm. Humans are definitive hosts of this parasite, and both humans and pork may be intermediate hosts.[13] The two main sources from which humans acquire cysticercosis are ingestion of food contaminated with *T. solium* eggs and the fecal-oral route in individuals harboring the adult parasite in the intestine. While the former was considered the most common form of transmission, recent studies have shown clustering of patients with cysticercosis around taeniasic individuals, changing previous concepts that the environment was the main source of human contamination with *T. solium* eggs.[14,15] Cysticerci may lodge in subcutaneous tissues, skeletal muscles, the eye, and the CNS.

Epidemiology

Cysticercosis constitutes a threat to millions of people all over the world. The disease is endemic in Latin America, sub-Saharan Africa, and some regions of Asia, including the Indian subcontinent, Indonesia, and China.[16–18] In the United States, massive immigration of people from endemic areas has caused a recent increase in the prevalence of this parasitic disease, particularly in Texas and California.[19,20] In endemic areas, cysticercosis accounts for 10 to 12 percent of all admissions to neurologic hospitals. This disease is the most common cause of acquired epilepsy in developing countries, where the prevalence of epilepsy is almost twice the prevalence in Western countries.[21]

Pathophysiology and Pathogenesis

Cysticerci are vesicles containing an invaginated scolex that has a structure similar to the adult *T. solium*. Within the CNS, cysticerci may be located in brain parenchyma, the ventricular system, the subarachnoid space, and the spinal cord. Parenchymal cysts are small and tend to lodge in the cerebral cortex or the basal ganglia (Fig. 16-2A). Subarachnoid cysts are located most often in the Sylvian fissure or in the cisterns at the base of the brain and may attain a large size because their growth is not limited by the brain parenchyma (see Fig. 16-2B). Ventricular cysticerci may be attached to the choroid plexus or may be freely floating in the ventricular cavities. Spinal cysticerci may be found in both the cord parenchyma and the subarachnoid space.[22]

After entering the CNS, cysticerci are in a vesicular stage in which the parasites elicit few inflammatory changes in the surrounding tissues. Cysticerci may remain in this stage for years or undergo a process of de-

Figure 16-2. Macroscopic appearance of parenchymal brain cysticerci (*A*) and subarachnoid racemose cysticercus located in the Sylvian fissure (*B*). Parenchymal brain cysts are small, and the scolex is seen as a small dot inside the vesicle. In contrast, racemose cysts are composed of several membranes attached to each other, and the scolex is not identified.

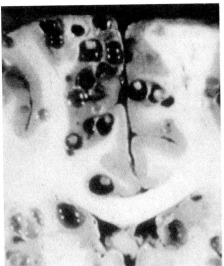 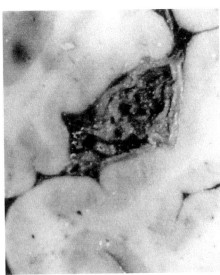

generation and death as a result of the host's immune response. The three stages of involution through which cysticerci pass during this process are the colloidal, granular, and calcified stages.[23] The inflammatory reaction around cysticerci induces pathologic changes in the CNS. Within the brain parenchyma, the inflammatory reaction is usually associated with edema and reactive gliosis. In the subarachnoid space, there is thickening of the leptomeninges with entrapment of cranial nerves and blood vessels at the base of the skull.[22,24] Luschka and Magendie's foramina may be occluded by the thickened leptomeninges with the subsequent development of hydrocephalus. Ventricular cysticerci also elicit a local inflammatory reaction if they are attached to the choroid plexus or the ventricular wall. In such cases, ependymal cells proliferate and may block the transit of CSF at the level of the cerebral aqueduct or Monro's foramina; this process of granular ependymitis causes obstructive hydrocephalus. Cysticerci located in the spinal subarachnoid space may induce inflammatory and demyelinating changes in ventral and dorsal roots of peripheral nerves in a similar way to that which occurs in cranial nerves.

Clinical Features

Cysticercosis is pleomorphic due to marked differences in the number and location of lesions within the CNS, as well as to differences in the degree of the host's immune response to the parasites. Seizures are the most common symptom and usually represent the primary or sole manifestation of the disease.[25] A number of focal signs with a subacute onset and progressive course (pyramidal tract signs, sensory deficits, involuntary movements) have been described in patients with neurocysticercosis. Focal signs also may occur abruptly in patients who develop a cerebral infarction due to cys-

ticercotic angiitis.[24] Patients may present with increased intracranial pressure associated with seizures or dementia; hydrocephalus is the most common cause of this syndrome.[26] Intracranial hypertension also may occur when ventricular cysts cause obstructive hydrocephalus and in cases of cysticercotic encephalitis. The latter is a particularly severe form of the disease that results from a massive cysticercotic infection of the brain parenchyma inducing an intense immune response from the host.[27] Manifestations of spinal cysticercosis include root pain, weakness, and sensory deficits that vary according to the level of the lesion.[13]

Diagnosis

The diagnosis of neurocysticercosis is possible in most cases after proper interpretation of clinical data together with neuroimaging findings and results of immunologic tests.[28] Neuroimaging studies usually provide objective evidence about the location of lesions and the degree of the host inflammatory response against the parasites. These include cystic lesions imaging the scolex, parenchymal brain calcifications, ring-enhancing lesions, abnormal enhancement of the leptomeninges, hydrocephalus, and cerebral infarctions (Fig. 16-3). Cytochemical analysis of CSF is normal in most patients with parenchymal brain cysticercosis. However, in those with the subarachnoid or ventricular forms of the disease, the CSF has a lymphocytic pleocytosis and increased protein concentration with a normal glucose concentration. From the many serologic tests developed for the diagnosis of cysticercosis, the recommended test is the immunoblot performed on serum.[29] However, false-positive results occur in patients who have cysticerci outside the CNS, and false-negative results are common in patients with a single intracranial cyst or with inactive (calcified) lesions.[30,31]

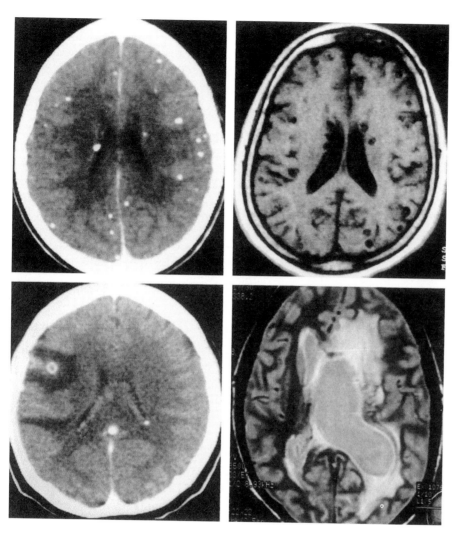

Figure 16-3. Neuroimaging findings in neurocysticercosis, including parenchymal brain calcifications (*A*), multiple vesicular cysts (*B*), single enhancing colloidal cyst (*C*), and large ventricular cyst (*D*).

Differential Diagnosis

Cysticercosis may mimic almost any other neurologic disease.[13] The main diagnostic problems occur in patients with ring-enhancing lesions because pyogenic brain abscesses, tuberculomas, mycotic granulomas, toxoplasmosis, and brain tumors may produce similar findings on neuroimaging studies. In such cases, the shape and size of the lesions (which in cysticercosis are usually round and measure less than 20 mm in diameter), as well as the absence of fever and signs of meningeal irritation (very rare in cysticercosis), together with data provided by serologic testing, x-ray films of the chest, and CSF analysis (glucose concentrations are usually normal in cysticercosis), usually permit an accurate diagnosis.

Treatment

Characterization of the disease in terms of viability and location of lesions, as well as the severity of the host's immune response, is important before planning therapy.[32] In most cases, management of these patients includes the use of both symptomatic drugs and cystici-

dal agents. Surgical procedures are needed in some patients.

CALCIFICATIONS

Calcifications do not need specific therapy. While treatment with antiepileptic drugs is recommended when parenchymal brain calcifications are associated with seizures, the optimal length of therapy in such cases remains undefined. Some studies have shown that the risk of seizure recurrence after antiepileptic drug withdrawal is high.[33] Moreover, neuroimaging studies performed immediately after seizure relapse have shown focal edema and abnormal contrast material uptake around previously inert calcifications.[34,35] These changes suggest that parenchymal brain calcifications represent epileptogenic foci susceptible to reactivation when the inhibitory influence of antiepileptic drugs is withdrawn.

CYSTIC LESIONS

Praziquantel and albendazole provide clinical improvement and resolution of lesions in most patients with parenchymal brain or subarachnoid cysticerci.[36] From the first controlled trials of therapy, it was demonstrated that vesicular cysts remain unchanged for several years; in contrast, praziquantel destroyed more than 60 percent of parenchymal brain cysts.[37,38] Praziquantel reaches its highest plasma concentration 1 to 3 hours after administration. The drug is metabolized in the liver; therefore, simultaneous use of drugs that induce the cytochrome P450 microsomal system decrease praziquantel plasma levels.[39] Recommended dosages of praziquantel have ranged from 10 to 100 mg/kg for periods of 3 to 21 days. It has been suggested recently that if intracranial cysts are exposed to a high concentration of praziquantel maintained for up to 6 hours by giving three doses of 25 to 33 mg/kg at 2-hour intervals, this might be sufficient to destroy the parasites.[40–42]

Albendazole is another cysticidal drug. It is not metabolized by the liver, and its plasma levels do not depend on the activity of the cytochrome P450 microsomal system. In a preliminary study, albendazole was administered at daily doses of 15 mg/kg for 30 days, resulting in an 86 percent reduction in the number of cysts.[43] Subsequent studies showed that a 1-week course of therapy is as effective as the 1-month course.[44] There is recent evidence, however, that patients with large subarachnoid cysts may require longer courses of albendazole.[45] Corticosteroid administration is mandatory when treating these patients to ameliorate the inflammatory reaction within the subarachnoid space, which may cause occlusion of leptomeningeal blood vessels.[46] A few controlled trials have compared the efficacy of albendazole with that of praziquantel. Albendazole was found to be more effective than praziquantel in these trials, destroying 80 to 90 percent of parenchymal brain cysts, compared with 60 to 70 percent for praziquantel.[47–49] However, there is still insufficient data to conclude that albendazole is definitively superior to praziquantel.

Praziquantel and albendazole should not be used in patients with cysticercotic encephalitis because these drugs may exacerbate the inflammatory response within the brain parenchyma that occurs in this form of the disease.[27] Corticosteroids and osmotic diuretics are recommended for initial therapy in these patients to reduce the severity of brain edema and to preserve visual function. In addition, ventricular cysticerci should not be treated with cysticidal drugs but removed by endoscopic aspiration to avoid the adverse reaction related to death of the parasite within the ventricular cavities.[50]

HYDROCEPHALUS

Patients with hydrocephalus due to cysticercosis usually require a ventricular shunt before other therapeutic measures.[32] Despite therapy, most of these patients have a protracted course and a poor prognosis. The main problem is the high frequency of shunt dysfunc-

tion because mortality has been related to the number of surgical interventions to change the shunt.[51] A recent study demonstrated that continued administration of prednisone significantly reduced the risk of shunt dysfunction.[52]

Prevention

Cysticercosis is closely linked to poverty and ignorance, and its eradication will be possible only with socioeconomic development. To be effective, control programs should be directed at all the steps in the cycle of transmission of *T. solium*, including human carriers of the adult tapeworm, infected pigs, and eggs in the environment. Targets of control to be considered in eradication programs include education, mass chemotherapy, improved husbandry, routine pork inspection, freezing of pork before public distribution, and improved sanitation.[53,54]

Echinococcosis (Hydatidosis Disease)

Echinococcosis (hydatidosis) is caused by infection with the larval forms of the canine tapeworm *Echinococcus* spp. Canids are definitive hosts of these parasites, and sheep or rodents may be intermediate hosts. Humans also may become intermediate hosts by ingesting water or food contaminated with dog feces containing eggs of these tapeworms.[55] After entering the body, eggs transform into cysts that grow in different organs, including lungs, kidneys, heart, liver, and CNS. In the latter, cysts may grow from direct implantation of oncospheres or from metastatic dissemination of a previously developed visceral cyst. Less than 5 percent of patients with echinococcosis have cerebral involvement. CNS hydatidosis is more common in children than in other age groups.[56]

Epidemiology

E. granulosus is the most common and widespread *Echinococcus* spp. and has been reported from Australia and from European and Asian countries bordering the Mediterranean, as well as from North and South America. In contrast, *E. multilocularis* is geographically restricted to the Arctic and to northern regions of Canada, Europe, and countries of the former Soviet Union.[57]

Pathophysiology and Pathogenesis

The two main forms of echinococcosis are cystic hydatid disease, caused by *E. granulosus*, and alveolar hydatid disease, caused by *E. multilocularis*. *E. granulosus* cysts are spherical and well demarcated from the surrounding tissue, which does not show marked inflammatory changes.[58] These cysts may achieve a size of 10 cm or more in diameter. While in most cases *E. granulosus* cysts are single, formation of daughter vesicles may give the lesion a multiloculated appearance.[59] Within the CNS, cysts may be located in brain parenchyma, the ventricular system, the subarachnoid space, the epidural space, and the spinal canal at both epidural and subarachnoid spaces. Intracranial and spinal epidural cysts are associated with vertebral bone erosion.[60,61] In contrast, *E. multilocularis* cysts are small, group in clusters, elicit a severe inflammatory reaction from the host, and tend to metastize both locally and distantly. Within the CNS, they usually are located within brain parenchyma.[62–64]

Hydatid disease of the heart may cause a cerebral infarction that usually is located in the territory of the middle cerebral artery. In some cases, hydatid cysts subsequently grow within the necrotic brain tissue, suggesting that the infarction is caused by embolic occlusion of the intracranial artery with fragments of a cyst previously broken within cardiac cavities.[65]

Clinical Features

Cerebral involvement in patients with cystic hydatid disease is manifest by seizures or increased intracranial pressure of subacute onset and progressive course.[66] Focal neurologic deficits are common and result from cysts strategically located in the thalamus, the internal capsule, or the brain stem or are due to a cerebral infarction from cardiogenic brain embolism of cystic membranes.[66–71] Cranial nerve palsies, mainly ophthalmoplegia, are frequent in patients with parasellar extradural cysts due to involvement of the lateral wall of the cavernous sinus.[72] Cerebral alveolar hydatid disease also presents with intracranial hypertension, seizures, and focal neurologic deficits. However, the clinical course is usually more rapid and more severe than in cystic hydatid disease.[62–64] Spinal cord involvement, associated with root pain and motor or sensory deficits below the level of the lesion, is more common in patients with cystic hydatid disease but may be observed in both forms of hydatid diseases.[61,73,74] Orbital involvement in patients with cystic hydatid disease is characterized by proptosis and ophthalmoplegia.[75]

Diagnosis

Cystic hydatid disease is usually seen on CT scan or MRI as a single, large, and nonenhancing cystic lesion, that is well demarcated from the surrounding brain parenchyma (Fig. 16-4). Some lesions may show calcifications.[76] Cystic lesions located in the subarachnoid space may be multiple and confluent. Epidural cysts have a biconvex shape or a multilocular appearance and may be associated with bone erosion.[61] Alveolar hydatid disease causes different neuroimaging findings because the lesions are multiple, surrounded by edema, and show ringlike enhancement.[62] Alveolar hydatidosis of the spinal canal may be visualized by MRI, although the findings are nonspecific; CT scan is better than MRI

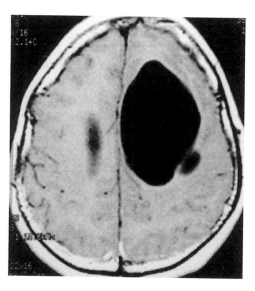

Figure 16-4. T$_1$-weighted MRI of a patient with a cystic hydatid disease of the brain. Lesion is cystic and well demarcated from the surrounding brain parenchyma. A small daughter vesicle is noted in the vicinity of the cyst.

to demonstrate bone erosion in vertebral bodies. Immunologic diagnosis of echinococcosis is not accurate due to cross-reaction with other parasitic diseases and false-negative results in patients with intact cystic hydatid lesions.[57]

Differential Diagnosis

As with other parasitic diseases of the CNS, the clinical manifestations of hydatidosis are nonspecific and similar to those caused by primary or metastatic brain tumors, neurocysticercosis, tuberculomas, toxoplasmosis, or mycotic granulomas.[66] Neuroimaging studies facilitate the diagnosis in cases of cystic hydatid disease but are nonspecific in patients with alveolar hydatidosis. In the latter, accurate diagnosis is only possible after surgical resection and microscopic examination of the lesion.

Treatment

The therapy of CNS hydatidosis is divided into cystic hydatid disease of the brain, cystic hydatid disease of the spine, and alveolar hydatid disease.

CYSTIC HYDATID DISEASE OF THE BRAIN

Hydatid cysts traditionally have been removed by surgery.[77] However, accidental rupture of the cyst may cause an allergic reaction or recurrent hydatid disease due to spillage of the cyst's contents.[69,78] Albendazole has been used with success in patients with hepatic, pulmonary, or renal cystic hydatid disease.[79] Albendazole has been given at doses ranging from 10 to 15 mg/kg per day for several 1-month cycles with therapy-free intervals of 14 days between cycles. However, experience with albendazole therapy for cerebral cystic hydatid disease is scarce. In most patients, albendazole has been given before surgery to avoid the complications of transoperative rupture of cysts or postoperatively to treat recurrent hydatid disease.[69,80] It also has been suggested that chemotherapy alone may destroy cerebral cysts, obviating the need for surgery.[81] Some patients experience clinical deterioration during albendazole therapy due to the development of an intense inflammatory reaction surrounding the dying cyst.[82]

CYSTIC HYDATID DISEASE OF THE SPINE

Treatment of patients with spinal hydatid disease includes a combination of decompressive laminectomy, removal of cysts, excision of involved bone, and stabilization of the spine.[61,74] However, resection of spinal hydatid cysts is more difficult than that of cerebral cysts, and most lesions rupture during surgery.[69] Albendazole, in similar doses to that used for patients with intracranial cystic hydatid disease, is recommended to reduce the risk of recurrent hydatid disease after surgery.[83,84]

ALVEOLAR HYDATID DISEASE OF THE BRAIN

Surgical removal of alveolar cysts usually requires resection of adjacent tissue, and this may cause neurologic deficits if the lesion is located in an eloquent cerebral area.[64,69] Albendazole administration should follow or even precede the surgical procedure or may be used as primary therapy for patients with inoperable alveolar hydatid disease.[85] The drug is given in similar doses to that described for cystic hydatid disease. Using this approach, 90 percent of lesions regress or remain static, and only 10 percent continue to grow.[86] A single patient with inoperable alveolar hydatid disease of the CNS was treated successfully with gamma knife radiosurgery and albendazole.[87]

Prevention

Echinococcosis may be prevented by reducing human contact with dog feces.[88] Periodic treatment of dogs with praziquantel and housing of stray dogs also decrease environmental contamination with eggs and reduce human infection.

Sparganosis

Sparganosis is caused by infection with the migrating second-stage plerocercoid larva of *Spirometra mansoni*. Dogs and cats are definitive hosts of this cestode, cyclops are first intermediate hosts, and frogs and snakes are second intermediate hosts.[89] Humans acquire the disease by drinking water contaminated with cyclops harboring the larva (sparganum), by eating infected frog or snake meat, or by applying the flesh of a frog as a poultice to the eye. Once in the human body, the sparganum migrates to subcutaneous tissue or skeletal mus-

cles, where it produces slowly growing nodules.[90] In some cases, the larvae migrate through the foramina of the skull base to invade the CNS.

Epidemiology

Sparganosis is a rare disease that occurs in Southeast Asia (China, Japan, Korea), the Indian subcontinent, and the Americas (Brazil, Mexico, Venezuela, and the United States).[91–94] Less than 100 cases with cerebral involvement have been reported.

Pathophysiology and Pathogenesis

The sparganum is a ribbon-shaped motile worm measuring several centimeters long. It has a protruding head with a central groove called a *bothrium*.[89] Sparganum may be located in the subarachnoid space, the brain parenchyma, or the spinal cord.[92,95] The brain parenchyma around the lesion shows an inflammatory infiltrate and reactive gliosis. Hemorrhages are common along the tracks of migration of these larvae.[96–98]

Clinical Features

Cerebral sparganosis may present with seizures, headache, or focal neurologic signs of subacute onset that vary according to the location of the parasite, as well as to the degree of the host's inflammatory reaction.[92,99] Symptoms may occur suddenly in patients with sparganosis-induced hemorrhagic stroke.[98,100] Spinal cord sparganosis begins with root pain followed by progressive motor deficits and sensory disturbances below the level of the lesion.[95,96]

Diagnosis

Neuroimaging abnormalities in cerebral sparganosis usually are confined to one hemisphere and include multiple areas of low density within the subcortical white matter, ventricular enlargement, calcifications, and enhancing nodules.[99,101,102] Lesions may change in location on sequential scans due to migration of the larvae. Cerebral hemorrhages also may be detected by CT scan or MRI.[97,100] In patients with intramedullary sparganosis, neuroimaging studies may reveal spinal cord enlargement and obliteration of spinal subarachnoid spaces at the level of the lesion.[95,96] The diagnostic accuracy of serologic diagnosis has not been established.[103]

Differential Diagnosis

Clinical manifestations of sparganosis resemble those caused by brain tumors or other focal infections of the brain and spinal cord. In most cases, diagnosis is possible after surgical resection of the lesion and microscopic identification of the larvae.[91,104]

Treatment

Surgical resection of the parasite is the treatment of choice because no specific medical therapy exists for

CNS sparganosis. A handful of patients have been treated with praziquantel without success because the drug does not destroy living sparganum.[92]

Prevention

Control measures include proper cooking of frog or snake meat before consumption and avoidance of the ancient use of the flesh of frogs as a poultice to the eye.

▶ NEMATODE INFECTIONS

Angiostrongyliasis

Angiostrongyliasis is caused by infection with *Angiostrongylus cantonensis*, the rat lungworm. The life cycle of this parasite involves rats as definitive hosts and snails or slugs as intermediate hosts.[105] Humans are accidental hosts and become infected by eating raw snails or vegetables contaminated with rat feces. After ingestion, motile larvae of the parasite cross the intestinal wall and migrate to the tissues of the host, including the CNS.

Epidemiology

Angiostrongyliasis is endemic to some regions of Southeast Asia, particularly in Japan and Thailand.[106,107] With increased travel and massive immigration of people from endemic areas, this parasitic disease will be recognized more frequently in developed countries.

Pathophysiology and Pathogenesis

Most neuropathologic findings in *A. cantonensis* infections are related to congestion and inflammation of leptomeninges due to immunologic damage.[108] Necropsy studies have shown necrotic tracts in the brain parenchyma caused by migration of the larvae.[109] This suggests that mechanical injury directly induced by movement of the parasite is important in the pathogenesis of the neurologic complications of the disease.

Clinical Features

A. cantonensis is the most common etiologic agent of eosinophilic meningitis, a self-limited syndrome characterized by headache, neck stiffness, and cranial nerve palsies.[106,110] However, angiostrongyliasis also may present as a more severe disease, with seizures, intracranial hypertension, or deterioration of consciousness due to diffuse cerebral involvement or hydrocephalus.[111–113] Sudden blindness due to retinal detachment may occur if *A. cantonensis* migrates through the eye.[114]

Diagnosis

CSF analysis in patients with *A. cantonensis* meningitis usually reveals a severe pleocytosis with 20 to 70 per-

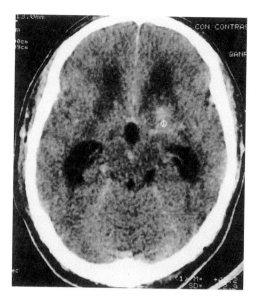

Figure 16-5. Contrast-enhanced CT scan in a patient with eosinophilic meningitis. Findings include acute hydrocephalus and abnormal enhancement of leptomeninges.

cent eosinophils and a mild increase in protein concentration. Glucose concentrations are normal.[106,110] Neuroimaging studies may show abnormal enhancement of leptomeninges at the base of the skull, periventricular edema, and hydrocephalus (Fig 16-5). Detection of specific antibodies to *A. cantonensis* has been reported by the use of ELISA and immunoblot; however, the diagnostic accuracy of these tests is largely unknown.[107]

Differential Diagnosis

Many infectious and noninfectious conditions may cause meningitis with increased eosinophils in the CSF. Therefore, accurate diagnosis of eosinophilic meningitis caused by this tissue nematode requires identification of the larvae in tissues.[106]

Treatment

Most patients with CNS angiostrongyliasis improve with the use of analgesics and antiemetics. CSF drainage through serial lumbar punctures is effective for headache relief in patients who do not respond to conservative therapy.[105] While the use of corticosteroids in patients with *A. cantonensis*–related eosinophilic meningitis has been controversial, a recent double-blind, placebo-controlled study confirmed the value of a 2-week course of prednisolone at doses of 60 mg daily in this condition.[115] The role of antiparasitic drugs for therapy of eosinophilic meningitis has not been defined, and it has been suggested that antiparasitic drugs should not be used in patients with CNS involvement because destruction of the larvae may increase cerebral edema and induce further clinical deterioration.[105]

Prevention

A. cantonensis meningitis can be prevented by properly cooking snails and other mollusks and by washing vegetables before consumption.[105] Measures to reduce the population of rats in endemic areas also will help to control disease transmission.

Gnathostomiasis

Gnathostomiasis is caused by the tissue nematode *Gnathostoma spinigerum*. This parasite has a complex life cycle involving more than two hosts. Dogs and cats are definitive hosts, cyclops are the first intermediate hosts, and many animal species are the second intermediate hosts.[116] Humans become infected by eating undercooked fish or poultry contaminated with the larvae of this parasite. After ingestion, these highly motile larvae cross the intestinal wall and migrate to subcutaneous tissues, skeletal muscles, the eye, and the CNS.

Epidemiology

Gnathostomiasis is common in countries of Southeast Asia, particularly Thailand, where it accounts for a large number of cases of nonaneurysmal subarachnoid hemorrhage.[116–118] The disease is also common in South America; however, there are marked geographic differences in the severity of disease expression because South American cases do not present with neurologic disorders but only with subcutaneous involvement.

Pathophysiology and Pathogenesis

G. spinigerum induces tissue damage by mechanical injury because the hooks and spines of this parasite leave hemorrhagic tracts as it passes through the CNS.[107] It is not uncommon to see large parenchymal brain hemorrhages extending from the frontal lobe to the brain stem caused by migration of the parasite.[119]

Clinical Features

Neurologic manifestations of gnathostomiasis are severe and include radicular pain, transverse myelitis, meningitis, encephalitis, and intracranial hemorrhages.[117–123] Blindness may occur as a result of migration of *G. spinigerum* through the eye.[124,125]

Diagnosis

Neuroimaging studies may show hemorrhagic tracts in the brain parenchyma or subarachnoid hemorrhage.[118] These are nonspecific findings, and the diagnosis usually rests on identification of the larvae in tissues. The diagnostic accuracy of detection of specific antibodies to *G. spinigerum* in serum is unknown.

Differential Diagnosis

Gnathostomiasis should be included in the differential diagnosis of patients with intracranial hemorrhage from areas where the disease is endemic. A history of vanishing, painful subcutaneous nodules may suggest the correct diagnosis.

Treatment

Therapy of *G. spinigerum* infections of the CNS includes the use of high doses of intravenous dexamethasone and osmotic diuretics to reduce the intracranial hypertension that usually accompanies this condition. Although albendazole is highly effective for the subcutaneous form of the disease, its role in the therapy of the neurologic complications of gnathostomiasis is not known.

Prevention

Gnathostomiasis can be prevented by properly cooking freshwater fish, poultry, and other reservoir animals before consumption.[116] The common practice of eating raw fish should be discouraged in endemic areas of Asia and South America.

Strongyloidiasis

Strongyloidiasis is caused by the intestinal nematode *Strongyloides stercoralis*. Larvae of this parasite are found in the soil and enter the human body through the skin, mature in the lungs, and migrate to the intestine, where they mature into adult worms. Autoinfection is possible because eggs may transform into infective larvae in the intestine. The larvae also may enter the body through the perianal skin.[126] Under normal conditions, strongyloidiasis is a benign condition. However, disseminated disease may occur when the host's immune system fails to control the normal cycle of autoinfection (hyperinfection syndrome). The hyperinfection syndrome is common in patients with acquired immune deficiency syndrome (AIDS), HTLV-I-related tropical spastic paraparesis, and hematologic malignancies.[127–131]

Epidemiology

S. stercoralis is worldwide in distribution. Infections predominate in tropical areas of Central and South American, the Caribbean, Africa, and Asia.[132]

Pathophysiology and Pathogenesis

CNS involvement is common during the course of disseminated disease. It may occur as a result of direct larval invasion or may be secondary to recurrent bacteremia associated with migrating larvae.[133–135] Larval invasion of the CNS may cause arachnoiditis and parenchymal brain granulomas or abscesses.[136–138] Cerebral infarctions occur as a result of plugging of intracranial arteries by larvae.[139]

Clinical Features

Strongyloidiasis of the CNS may present with an acute meningeal syndrome characterized by fever, headache, and neck stiffness.[133,134] Brain abscesses and granulomas present with seizures, focal neurologic deficits, or intracranial hypertension.[138] Small cerebral infarctions may be associated with hemiparesis or sensory deficits.[139] The hyperinfection syndrome usually occurs with an underlying disease; as such, neurologic manifestations of strongyloidiasis are associated with symptoms of pulmonary, cardiac, or gastrointestinal involvement.[127–131]

Diagnosis

Examination of the CSF may demonstrate a neutrophilic pleocytosis with an increased protein concentration and a normal glucose concentration.[140] Gram's stain is needed to rule out pyogenic meningitis. Neuroimaging studies may reveal ring-enhancing lesions or small cortical infarctions.[138] Definitive diagnosis depends on identification of the larvae in CSF, sputum, stool, or tissue specimens (Fig. 16-6). The specificity of serologic tests for the diagnosis of this condition is decreased by the high rate of false-positive results due to cross-reaction with other parasitic infections.[141,142]

Differential Diagnosis

Accurate diagnosis of strongyloidiasis usually requires a high index of suspicion because clinical manifestations and neuroimaging findings are nonspecific and may be caused by a number of infectious and noninfectious diseases of the CNS.

Treatment

The hyperinfection syndrome is treated with thiabendazole at a dose of 50 mg/kg per day for 5 to 14 days

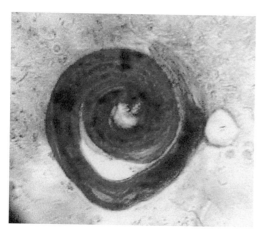

Figure 16-6. Larvae of *S. stercoralis* obtained from the sputum of a patient with the hyperinfection syndrome. *(Courtesy of Dr. José Navarrete, Guayaquil-Ecuador.)*

or with ivermectin at a dose of 200 μg/kg per day for 10 to 14 days.[127,143,144] Patients with disseminated strongyloidiasis who have superimposed bacterial infections of the CNS should be managed by the general rules of therapy for pyogenic meningitis. Corticosteroids should be withdrawn once the hyperinfection syndrome is diagnosed.[133]

Prevention

It is important to detect and treat *S. stercoralis* infection in immunocompromised patients before the hyperinfection syndrome occurs. Regimens used to treat such infections include thiabendazole (50 mg/kg per day for 3 days), albendazole (400 mg/d for 3 days), or ivermectin (200 μg/kg per day for 2 days).[145,146]

Toxocariosis

Toxocariosis is caused by tissue nematodes of the genus *Toxocara* (*T. canis, T. cati*). Dogs and cats are definitive hosts of these parasites. Humans acquire the infection by ingesting soil contaminated with dog or cat feces containing *Toxocara* eggs.[147] The infection is more common among pet owners, mentally retarded children, and people with poor hygiene.[148–150] After ingestion, the eggs mature into larvae that cross the intestinal wall and migrate to the tissues of the host to produce one of two clinical diseases, visceral larva migrans or ocular larva migrans.[151]

Epidemiology

Toxocariosis is worldwide in distribution; its prevalence, however, is difficult to assess due to the high rate of asymptomatic infections.[147,152]

Pathophysiology and Pathogenesis

Tissue damage in toxocariosis is due to the migration of larvae, which leave necrotic tracks, or to the inflammatory response of the host around dead larvae.[151] In ocular larva migrans, eye invasion of the parasite may cause retinal detachment, uveitis, endophthalmitis, and subretinal granulomas.[153–155] In visceral larva migrans, target organs are the liver, lungs, and CNS. In the latter, pathologic lesions include brain swelling, parenchymal brain or spinal cord granulomas, and cerebral infarctions due to occlusion of intracranial arteries.[151]

Clinical Features

Ocular larva migrans is usually associated with unilateral diminution of visual acuity.[153,154] Visceral larva migrans with CNS involvement may present with seizures only, with a rapidly progressive encephalopathy, or with a transverse myelopathy when the spinal cord is affected.[156–158] Some epidemiologic studies have suggested a possible relationship between epilepsy and

Toxocara infection.[159,160] This may represent only chance association due to the high prevalence of toxocariosis in some areas.

Diagnosis

Funduscopic examination reveals the parasite in ocular larva migrans. CT scan and MRI are useful to visualize intracranial granulomas and spinal cord lesions in patients with toxocariosis of the CNS. Intracranial granulomas appear as multiple, nodular-enhancing lesions located in the subcortical white matter of cerebral hemispheres.[156] Spinal cord lesions present with cord swelling and large high-signal areas on T_2-weighted images.[158] Accurate diagnosis of toxocariosis is possible in most cases by detection of specific antibodies by ELISA or immunoblot.[161,162]

Differential Diagnosis

Toxocariosis should be included in the differential diagnosis of patients with a history of pica or pet owners presenting with sudden unilateral blindness, acute encephalopathy, or myelopathy.[151]

Treatment

Diethylcarbamazine at a dose of 6 mg/kg per day for 10 days or albendazole at a dose of 10 to 15 mg/kg per day for 5 days is effective for toxocaral infections. Patients with ocular and brain lesions usually require the simultaneous administration of corticosteroids to reduce the risk of tissue damage as a result of death of the parasite.[151,156,163]

Prevention

Control of stray dogs, periodic treatment of domestic dogs and cats with antiparasitic drugs, and education of the population are important preventive measures to reduce the risk of *Toxocara* infection.[152]

Trichinosis

Trichinosis (trichinellosis) is a zoonosis caused by the tissue nematode *Trichinella spiralis*. Humans are infected by ingesting the undercooked meat of pigs, horses, bears, and other animals contaminated with larvae of the parasite.[164] Once ingested, larvae cross the intestinal wall, enter the bloodstream, and encyst in the tissues of the host.

Epidemiology

Trichinosis is worldwide in distribution and has been reported from the United States, Central and South America, eastern Europe, Asia, and Africa. It may be endemic or present as outbreaks related to the eating habits of a particular population.[164,165]

Pathophysiology and Pathogenesis

T. spiralis encysts in skeletal muscles, causing swelling and degeneration of muscle fibers.[165] Trichinosis may cause pathologic lesions in the CNS, including granuloma formation, arachnoiditis, and cerebral infarction.[166–168] Trichinosis-related stroke may be secondary to occlusion of intracranial blood vessels due to migrating larval emboli or may be caused by an eosinophilic-induced vascular damage.[169]

Clinical Features

Encystment of larvae in muscle is associated with fever, periorbital edema, diplopia, and generalized weakness and myalgias.[170] Myocardial involvement may present with arrhythmias. Acute meningoencephalitis, stroke, and cranial or peripheral neuropathies are the most common neurologic complications of trichinosis.[166–172] Stroke subtypes in trichinosis include hemorrhagic infarction due to venous thrombosis and subcortical infarction caused by small-artery disease.[166,169]

Diagnosis

Patients with myositis usually develop peripheral blood eosinophilia and increased serum creatine phosphokinase and lactic dehydrogenase concentrations. In patients with CNS involvement, CSF analysis reveals an eosinophilic pleocytosis with an increased protein concentration and a normal glucose concentration. Neuroimaging studies reveal hemorrhagic infarctions due to venous thrombosis or multiple subcortical infarctions.[167–169,173] Diagnosis is confirmed by the finding of specific antibodies in serum by ELISA or by the identification of the parasite in muscles.[165,174]

Differential Diagnosis

Muscle involvement due to trichinosis may be confused with viral or immune-related myositis, and clinical and neuroimaging manifestations of neurotrichinosis may be caused by a wide range of infectious or noninfectious conditions affecting the CNS. The occurrence of other cases of trichinosis in the community is helpful in diagnosis.

Treatment

The role of antiparasitic therapy in striated muscle trichinosis has been controversial.[164] However, mebendazole at doses of 400 mg daily for 10 days appears to be the drug of choice for this condition.[175] In patients with cerebral trichinosis, corticosteroids are recommended to suppress the eosinophilic-induced vascular damage and to reduce the inflammatory reaction to migrating larvae in the brain.[169] There is no solid evidence favoring the use of antiparasitic drugs in cerebral trichinosis.

Prevention

Cooking meat or pork before human consumption will destroy encysted larvae and reduce the risk of human infection.[164] Routine inspection of meat at slaughter before distribution also has helped to eradicate the disease in many countries.

► UNCOMMON NEMATODE INFECTIONS OF THE CNS

Ascarioid Infections

A number of nematodes of the family Ascarididae may infect humans. The most important parasites in this family are *Ascaris lumbricoides, A. suum, Baylisascaris procyonis,* and *Lagochilascaris minor. A. lumbricoides* is a common intestinal nematode, but there are only two well-documented cases of CNS infection by *A. lumbricoides*; in one of these patients, a larva was located in the center of a thalamic granuloma, and in the other, an adult worm was found in the third ventricle.[176] CNS infection by *A. suum* is also rare, and only one case of acute encephalopathy caused by this nematode has been described.[177] In contrast, infections with *L. minor* and *B. procyonis* are recognized with increasing frequency, and the latter has become an emerging infectious disease in the United States and Canada owing to the high population of raccoons (its animal reservoir) in these countries.[178–183] Both conditions, lagochilascariasis and baylisascariasis, may present as an acute and severe eosinophilic meningoencephalitis associated with foci of hemorrhagic necrosis in the brain parenchyma.[182–184] Diagnosis of these conditions is difficult on clinical grounds and should be confirmed by the detection of specific antibodies in serum by ELISA or immunoblot.[183] There is no specific therapy for these disorders.

Dracontiasis

The nematode *Dracunculus medinensis* (guinea worm) causes dracontiasis (dracunculiasis), a common disease in India, Africa, and the Middle East.[185] Humans acquire the infection by drinking water contaminated with infected copepods. After being ingested, the larvae cross the intestine and lodge in the retroperitoneum, where they mature and migrate down to the legs to protrude through painful skin ulcers. Rare patients with dracontiasis develop extradural abscesses that compress the spinal cord.[186–188] Such abscesses usually are located at the thoracic levels and present with paraplegia associated with loss of sensory modalities below the level of the lesion. Histologic examination has shown the parasites surrounded by granulomatous tissue typical of a foreign-body reaction.[188] Therapy requires surgical excision of the abscess to decompress the spinal cord.

Loiasis

Loiasis is caused by the filarial nematode *Loa loa* and transmitted from human to human by the bite of red flies of the genus *Chrysops*. It is geographically restricted to tropical Africa.[189] The disease is characterized by transient subcutaneous nodules called *calabar swellings*. In addition, loiasis may be associated with visceral involvement, including an acute encephalitis characterized by seizures, clouded consciousness, and focal neurologic signs.[190,191] Most reported cases of encephalitis have occurred after diethylcarbazine or ivermectin treatment of lymphatic filariasis or onchocerciasis (in patients who also had been infected with *Loa loa*), suggesting that such therapy may exacerbate a previously asymptomatic infection by unmasking the parasites to the host's immune system.[192]

Micronemiasis

Micronemiasis is caused by *Helicephalobus deletrix,* a saprophagous nematode that is found in manure and decaying organic material. Only a few cases of human infection with this parasite have been reported, all from North America.[193–195] Patients have developed an acute and fatal meningoencephalitis. Autopsy studies have shown a dense purulent exudate with thickening of the leptomeninges with multiple larvae and eggs of *H. deletrix* in and around intracranial vessels, as well as in the brain parenchyma. There is no known therapy for this condition.

► TREMATODE INFECTIONS

Paragonimiasis

Paragonimiasis is caused by lung flukes of the genus *Paragonimus,* including *P. westermani, P. skrjabini, P. mexicanus, P. skrjabini,* and *P. africanus*. Humans acquire the infection by ingesting flukes' metacercariae in raw or undercooked crabs or crayfish.[196] After ingestion, metacercariae liberate larvae that enter the peritoneal cavity and migrate to the lungs, where they mature into worms. Erratic migration of worms through the jugular veins and carotid arteries causes involvement of the CNS.[130]

Epidemiology

Paragonimiasis is worldwide in distribution; however, there is a geographic variability in the prevalence and distribution of the different *Paragonimus* spp. Most of the cases of cerebral paragonimiasis have been caused by *P. westermani,* a parasite endemic in Asia and the South Pacific islands.[198] Sporadic cases of cerebral paragonimiasis resulting from *P. skrjabini, P. miyazakii,* and *P. mexicanus* have been reported from Japan, China, and Central America.

Pathophysiology and Pathogenesis

The migration of worms within the CNS and the host's inflammatory reaction to them may cause several pathologic lesions, including hemorrhagic tracks in the brain parenchyma, cystic lesions, granulomatous reactions, diffuse arachnoiditis, obstructive hydrocephalus, and spinal cord lesions located in both the subdural and epidural spaces.[197–200]

Clinical Features

Clinical manifestations depend on the location of lesions within the CNS and the severity of the host's inflammatory reaction. Arachnoiditis presents as a meningeal syndrome with headache, fever, neck stiffness, cranial nerve palsies, and focal neurologic signs due to cerebral infarction caused by endarteritis.[198,199] Parenchymal brain granulomas may cause seizures, focal signs, or intracranial hypertension.[197,198] Paragonimiasis of the spinal cord is characterized by radicular pain, weakness, and sensory disturbances.[201]

Diagnosis

There is a CSF pleocytosis with an increased protein concentration and a normal glucose concentration in patients with *Paragonimus*-induced meningitis. CT scan and MRI in patients with parenchymal brain involvement show calcifications, cysts, or ring-enhancing lesions that usually are located in the occipital and temporal lobes, closely related to each other, giving the appearance of "soap bubbles."[202–207] Intracranial hemorrhages may be seen in some cases. The diagnosis is confirmed by the presence of specific antibodies in blood and CSF by ELISA or immunoblot, by the demonstration of *Paragonimus* eggs in sputum, or by the finding of adult worms in tissue samples.[196]

Differential Diagnosis

Many other infectious and noninfectious disorders of the CNS may mimic paragonimiasis. Neuroimaging studies showing confluent lesions are highly suggestive of paragonimiasis, but alveolar hydatidosis, tuberculosis, and cysticercosis may have similar findings on MRI.

Treatment

The therapy of cerebral paragonimiasis includes a combination of symptomatic and antiparasitic agents and surgery.[198] There is little experience with the use of antiparasitic drugs in cerebral paragonimiasis. An old study suggested that bithionol may be effective when used early in the disease.[208] Praziquantel, given at doses of 75 mg/kg per day for 2 days, also has been used with success in a few patients with cerebral paragonimiasis.[198] Corticosteroids and antiepileptic agents usually are recommended to treat seizures and to reduce the inflammatory reaction induced by the host's immune system. Surgical resection of intracranial lesions also has a role in the management of cerebral paragonimiasis, but the large size and multiplicity of lesions make their radical resection difficult without damaging the surrounding brain parenchyma.[197,198] For cystic lesions located in the spinal subdural and epidural spaces, surgical removal of the cysts with decompression of the spinal cord is recommended.[201]

Prevention

Preventive measures should focus on avoidance of dietary habits that include eating raw or undercooked crab or crayfish, particularly in endemic areas of Asia.[196]

Schistosomiasis

Schistosomiasis is caused by flukes of the genus *Schistosoma* (*S. japonicum, S. mansoni,* and *S. haematobium*). These parasites enter the human body through the skin after aquatic exposure to their larvae.[209] Then the larvae migrate, mature, and settle in the mesenteric or bladder veins. Ectopic migration of worms or embolic deposition of eggs within the spinal cord or cerebral vasculature causes neuroschistosomiasis. *S. japonicum* usually infects the brain, and the other two species more often infect the spinal cord than the brain.[210]

Epidemiology

Schistosoma spp. are common parasites of humans, affecting more than 200 million people worldwide. *S. haematobium* is endemic in the Arab peninsula, as well as in some African countries. *S. japonicum* is prevalent in Southeast Asia. *S. mansoni* is distributed widely and is found in Africa, the Middle East, South America, and some islands of the Caribbean basin.[209]

Pathophysiology and Pathogenesis

All *Schistosoma* spp. induce an intense inflammatory reaction in the host's tissues. Cerebral schistosomiasis caused by either *S. japonicum, S. haematobium,* or *S. mansoni* is associated with diffuse arachnoiditis, parenchymal brain granulomas, and intracranial hemorrhages due to segmental damage of small blood vessels.[211,212] In addition, *S. mansoni* and *S. haematobium* may cause inflammatory necrosis of the spinal cord, occlusion of the anterior spinal artery, and granuloma formation at the level of the conus medullaris or the cauda equina.[213]

Clinical Features

Neurologic complications of schistosomiasis differ according to the offending agent. *S. japonicum* infections may cause acute meningoencephalitis with fever, seizures, neck stiffness, and decreased level of consciousness. Chronic disease is associated with seizures, focal neurologic signs, and intracranial hypertension. These manifestations are related to the development of parenchymal brain granulomas or intracranial hemorrhages.[210] In contrast, *S. mansoni and S. haematobium* infections usually cause acute transverse myelitis, due to necrosis of the lower spinal cord, that is characterized by flaccid paraplegia, sphincter dysfunction, and

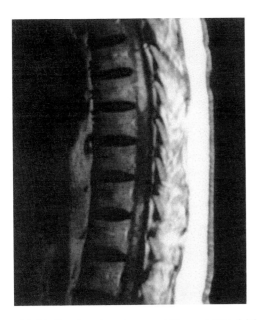

Figure 16-7. Contrast-enhanced T_1-weighted MRI showing patchy areas of abnormal enhancement of the spinal cord in a patient with *S. mansoni* schistosomiasis. *(Courtesy of Dr. Francisco J. Carod, Brasilia, Brazil.)*

sensory loss.[214] Granulomatous masses involving the conus medullaris and cauda equina cause saddle anesthesia, sphincter dysfunction, and weakness.[213] Occlusion of the anterior spinal artery by parasites may cause acute paraplegia due to necrosis of the spinal cord.[215]

Diagnosis

Cytochemical analysis of the CSF in neuroschistosomiasis usually demonstrates a mononuclear pleocytosis with an increased protein concentration and a normal glucose concentration.[213] Neuroimaging studies show single or multiple enhancing lesions in the brain parenchyma in cerebral schistosomiasis and enlargement or abnormal enhancement of the spinal cord in spinal schistosomiasis[216–218] (Fig. 16-7). Most patients with spinal cord schistosomiasis have a positive ELISA for the detection of schistosomal antibodies in the CSF; however, this test lacks specificity. The demonstration of schistosomal eggs in stool or urine is helpful when positive, but their absence does not exclude the diagnosis.[209,210]

Differential Diagnosis

Cerebral schistosomiasis should be included in the differential diagnosis of acute meningitis or parenchymal brain granulomas in areas where the disease is endemic, particularly Asia, where *S. japonicum* is endemic. Spinal cord schistosomiasis should be considered in African or South American patients presenting with acute transverse myelitis affecting the lower spinal cord, particularly when neuroimaging studies show abnormal en-

hancement or segmental enlargement at the level of the conus medullaris.[214]

Treatment

For a rational management of neuroschistosomiasis, infections due to *S. japonicum* should be differentiated from those due to *S. mansoni* and *S. haematobium.*

S. JAPONICUM NEUROSCHISTOSOMIASIS

Praziquantel at a dose of 30 to 60 mg/kg for 1 day is the drug of choice for systemic *S. japonicum* schistosomiasis.[219] However, experience with this drug for the therapy of cerebral involvement is limited.[220] *S. japonicum* neuroschistosomiasis should be treated with corticosteroids to reduce the inflammatory reaction in the CNS that may cause further tissue damage.

S. MANSONI AND *S.* HAEMATOBIUM NEUROSCHISTOSOMIASIS

Therapy for *S. mansoni* and *S. haematobium* spinal cord disease usually requires antischistosomal drugs, corticosteroids, and laminectomy.[210,213,221] Praziquantel, at a dose of 40 mg/kg per day for 1 or 2 days, is effective for both *S. mansoni* and *S. haematobium* infections, and oxamniquine, at a dose of 15 to 30 mg/kg per day for 1 or 2 days, is also effective for infections caused by *S. mansoni.*[222–224] Therapy for cerebral *S. mansoni* and *S. haematobium* infections is less clear. Some patients have improved after surgical resection of the brain lesion or after therapy with either praziquantel, oxamniquine, or praziquantel plus corticosteroids.[221,225–227]

Prevention

Eradication of schistosomiasis will be possible only when control programs are directed at all the steps in the cycle of transmission of these parasites. These steps include mass human chemotherapy, snail control, reduction of water contact and contamination, improved sanitation, and vaccination.[209]

REFERENCES

1. Nishimura K, Hung TP: Current views on geographic distribution and modes of infection of neurohelminthic diseases. *J Neurol Sci* 145:5, 1997.
2. Strickland GT: Helminthic infections: General principles. In Strickland GT (ed): *Hunter's Tropical Medicine and Emerging Infectious Diseases,* 8th ed. Philadelphia: Saunders, 2000, p 713.
3. Diaz FJ, Gilman RH: Coenurosis. In Strickland GT (ed): *Hunter's Tropical Medicine and Emerging Infectious Diseases,* 8th ed. Philadelphia: Saunders, 2000, p 877.
4. Bertrand I, Callot J, Terrase J, et al: A proos d'un noveau cas de cénurose cérébrale. *Press Med* 64:333, 1956.

5. Templeton AC: Human coenurus infection: A report of 14 cases from Uganda. *Trans R Soc Trop Med Hyg* 62:251, 1968.

6. Benger A, Rennie RP, Roberts JT, et al: Human coenurus infection in Canada. *Am J Trop Med Hyg* 30:638, 1981.

7. Ing MB, Schantz PM, Turner JA: Human coenurosis in North America: Case report and review. *Clin Infect Dis* 27:519, 1998.

8. Kurtycz DF, Alt B, Mack E: Incidental coenurosis: Larval cestode presenting as an axillary mass. *Am J Clin Pathol* 80:735, 1983.

9. Pau A, Turtas S, Brambilla M, et al: Computed tomography and magnetic resonance imaging of cerebral coenurosis. *Surg Neurol* 27:548, 1987.

10. Ibechukwu BI, Onwukeme KE: Intraocular coenurosis: A case report. *Br J Ophthalmol* 75:430, 1991.

11. Hermos JA, Healy GR, Schultz MC, et al: Fatal human coenurosis. *JAMA* 213:1461, 1970.

12. Pau A, Perria C, Turtas S, et al: Long-term follow-up of the surgical treatment of intracranial coenurosis. *Br J Neurosurg* 4:39, 1990.

13. Del Brutto OH, Sotelo J, Román GC: *Neurocysticercosis: A Clinical Handbook.* Lisse, Netherlands, Swets & Zeitlinger, 1998.

14. Sarti E, Schantz PM, Lara-Aguilera R, et al: Epidemiological investigation of *Taenia solium* taeniosis and cysticercosis in a rural village of Michoacán state, México. *Trans R Soc Trop Med Hyg* 88:49, 1994.

15. Gilman RH, Del Brutto OH, Garcia HH, et al: Prevalence of taeniosis among patients with neurocysticercosis is related to severity of infection. *Neurology* 55:1062, 2000.

16. García HH, Del Brutto OH: *Taenia solium* cysticercosis. *Infect Dis Clin North Am* 14:97, 2000.

17. Preux PM, Melaku Z, Druet-Cabanac M, et al: Cysticercosis and neurocysticercosis in Africa: Current status. *Neurol Infect Epidemiol* 1:63, 1996.

18. Wadia NH: Neurocysticercosis. In Shakir RA, Newman PK, Poser CM (eds): *Tropical Neurology.* London: Saunders, 1996, p 248.

19. White AC Jr: Neurocysticercosis: Update on epidemiology, pathogenesis, diagnosis, and management. *Annu Rev Med* 51:187, 2000.

20. Ong S, Talan DA, Moran GJ, et al: Neurocysticercosis in radiographically imaged seizure patients in U.S. emergency departments. *Emerg Infect Dis* 8:608, 2002.

21. Commission on Tropical Diseases of the International League Against Epilepsy: Relationship between epilepsy and tropical diseases. *Epilepsia* 35:89, 1994.

22. Pitella JEH: Neurocysticercosis. *Brain Pathol* 7:681, 1997.

23. Escobar A: The pathology of neurocysticercosis. In Palacios E, Rodriguez-Carbajal J, Taveras JM (eds): *Cysticercosis of the Central Nervous System.* Springfield, IL: Charles C Thomas, 1983, p 27.

24. Cantu C, Barinagarrementeria F: Cerebrovascular complications of neurocysticercosis: Clinical and neuroimaging spectrum. *Arch Neurol* 53:233, 1996.

25. Del Brutto OH, Santibañez R, Noboa CA, et al: Epilepsy due to neurocysticercosis: Analysis of 203 patients. *Neurology* 42:389, 1992.

26. Sotelo J, Del Brutto OH: Review of neurocysticercosis. *Neurosurg Focus* 12:1, 2002.

27. Rangel R, Torres B, Del Brutto O, et al: Cysticercotic encephalitis: A severe form in young females. *Am J Trop Med Hyg* 36:387, 1987.

28. Del Brutto OH, Rajshekhar V, White AC Jr, et al: Proposed diagnostic criteria for neurocysticercosis. *Neurology* 57:177, 2001.

29. Richards F, Schantz PM: Laboratory diagnosis of cysticercosis. *Clin Lab Med* 11:1011, 1991.

30. Garcia HH, Gilman RH, Catacora M, et al: Serologic evolution of neurocysticercosis patients after antiparasitic therapy. *J Infect Dis* 175:486, 1997.

31. Rajshekhar V, Oommen A: Serological studies using ELISA and EITB in patients with solitary cysticercus granuloma and seizures. *Neurol Infect Epidemiol* 2:177, 1997.

32. Garcia HH, Evans CAW, Nash TE, et al: Current consensus guidelines for treatment of neurocysticercosis. *Clin Microbiol Rev* 15:747, 2002.

33. Del Brutto OH: Prognostic factors for seizure recurrence after withdrawal of antiepileptic drugs in patients with neurocysticercosis. *Neurology* 44:1706, 1994.

34. Nash TE, Pretell J, Garcia HH: Calcified cysticerci provoke perilesional edema and seizures. *Clin Infect Dis* 33:1649, 2001.

35. Antoniuk SA, Bruck I, Dos Santos LHC, et al: Seizures associated with calcifications and edema in neurocysticercosis. *Pediatr Neurol* 25:309, 2001.

36. Del Brutto OH: Medical treatment of cysticercosis—effective. *Arch Neurol* 52:102, 1995.

37. Sotelo J, Escobedo F, Rodriguez-Carbajal J, et al: Therapy of parenchymal brain cysticercosis with praziquantel. *New Engl J Med* 301:1001, 1984.

38. Sotelo J, Torres B, Rubio-Donnadieu F, et al: Praziquantel in the treatment of neurocysticercosis: A long-term follow-up. *Neurology* 35:752, 1985.

39. Jung H, Vazquez ML, Sanchez M, et al: Clinical pharmacokinetics of praziquantel. *Proc West Pharmacol Soc* 34:335, 1991.

40. Corona T, Lugo R, Medina R, et al: Single-day praziquantel therapy for neurocysticercosis. *New Engl J Med* 334:125, 1996.

41. Del Brutto OH, Campos X, Sánchez J, et al: Single-day praziquantel versus 1-week albendazole for neurocysticercosis. *Neurology* 52:1079, 1999.

42. López-Gómez M, Castro N, Jung H, et al: Optimization of the single-day praziquantel therapy for neurocysticercosis. *Neurology* 57:1929, 2001.

43. Escobedo F, Penagos P, Rodriguez J, et al: Albendazole therapy for neurocysticercosis. *Arch Intern Med* 147:738, 1987.

44. Garcia HH, Gilman RH, Horton J, et al: Albendazole therapy for neurocysticercosis: A prospective, double-blind trial comparing 7 versus 14 days of treatment. *Neurology* 48:1421, 1997.

45. Proaño JV, Madrazo I, Avelar F, et al: Medical treatment for neurocysticercosis characterized by giant subarachnoid cysts. *New Engl J Med* 345:879, 2001.

46. Del Brutto OH, Sotelo J, Aguirre R, et al: Albendazole therapy for giant subarachnoid cysticerci. *Arch Neurol* 49:535, 1992.

47. Sotelo J, Del Brutto OH, Penagos P, et al: Comparison of therapeutic regimen of anticysticercal drugs for parenchymal brain cysticercosis. *J Neurol* 237:69, 1990.

48. Takayanagui OM, Jardim E: Therapy for neurocysticercosis: Comparison between albendazole and praziquantel. *Arch Neurol* 49:290, 1992.

49. Cruz M, Cruz I, Horton J: Albendazole versus praziquantel in the treatment of cerebral cysticercosis: Clinical evaluation. *Trans R Soc Trop Med Hyg* 85:244, 1991.

50. Bergsneider M, Holly LT, Lee JH, et al: Endoscopic management of cysticercal cysts within the lateral and third ventricles. *J Neurosurg* 92:14, 2000.

51. Sotelo J, Marin C: Hydrocephalus secondary to cysticercotic arachnoiditis: A long-term follow-up review of 92 cases. *J Neurosurg* 66:686, 1987.

52. Roman RAS, Soto-Hernández JL, Sotelo J: Effects of prednisone on ventriculoperitoneal shunt function in hydrocephalus secondary to cysticercosis: A preliminary study. *J Neurosurg* 84:629, 1996.

53. Bern C, Garcia HH, Evans C, et al: Magnitude of the disease burden from neurocysticercosis in a developing country. *Clin Infect Dis* 29:1203, 1999.

54. Roman GC, Sotelo J, Del Brutto OH, et al: A proposal to declare neurocysticercosis an international reportable disease. *Bull WHO* 78:399, 2000.

55. Schantz PM: Echinococcosis. In Guerrant RL, Walker DH, Weller PF (eds): *Tropical Infectious Diseases: Principles, Pathogens, and Practice.* New York: Churchill Livingstone, 1999, p 1005.

56. Onal C, Unal F, Barlas O, et al: Long-term follow-up and results of thirty pediatric intracranial hydatid cysts: Half a century of experience at the department of neurosurgery of the school of medicine at the university of Istanbul (1952–2001). *Pediatr Neurosurg* 35:72, 2001.

57. Moro PL, Gonzalez AE, Gilman RH: Cystic hydatid disease. In Strickland GT (ed): *Hunter's Tropical Medicine and Emerging Infectious Diseases,* 8th ed. Philadelphia: Saunders, 2000, p 866.

58. Taratuto AL, Venturiello SM: Echinococcosis. *Brain Pathol* 7:673, 1997.

59. Fabiani A, Trebini F, Torta R: Brain hydatidosis: Report of two cases. *J Neurol Neurosurg Psychiatry* 43:91, 1980.

60. Ciurea AV, Valisescu G, Nuteanu L, et al: Cerebral hydatid disease in children: Experience of 27 cases. *Childs Nerv Syst* 11:679, 1995.

61. Karadereler S, Orakdogen M, Kilic K, et al: Primary spinal extradural cyst in a child: Case report and review of the literature. *Eur Spine J* 11:500, 2002.

62. Tunaci M, Tunaci A, Engin G, et al: MRI of cerebral alveolar echinococcosis. *Neuroradiology* 41;844, 1999.

63. Piotin M, Cattin F, Kantelip B, et al: Disseminated intracerebral alveolar echinococcosis: CT and MRI. *Neuroradiology* 39:431, 1997.

64. Aydin Y, Barlas O, Yolas C, et al: Alveolar hydatid disease of the brain: Report of four cases. *J Neurosurg* 65:115, 1986.

65. Benomar A, Yahyaoui M, Birouk N, et al: Middle cerebral artery occlusion due to hydatid cyst of myocardial and intraventricular cavity cardiac origin: Two cases. *Stroke* 25:886, 1994.

66. Turgut M: Hydatidosis of central nervous system and its coverings in the pediatric and adolescent age groups in Turkey during the last century: A critical review of 137 cases. *Childs Nerv Syst* 18:670, 2002.

67. Khaldi M, Mohamed S, Kallel J, et al: Brain hydatidosis: Report on 117 cases. *Childs Nerv Syst* 16:765, 2000.

68. Turgut M, Bavulkem K: Cerebrovascular occlusive disease: hydatidosis. *Childs Nerv Syst* 14:697, 1998.

69. Altinors N, Bavbek M, Caner HH, et al: Central nervous system hydatidosis in Turkey: A cooperative study and literature survey analysis of 458 cases. *J Neurosurg* 93:1, 2000.

70. Abbassioun K, Amirjamshidi A, Moinipoor MT: Hydatid cyst of the pons. *Surg Neurol* 26:297, 1986.

71. Ersahin Y, Mutluer S, Dermirtas E, et al: A case of thalamic hydatid cyst. *Clin Neurol Neurosurg* 97:321, 1995.

72. Guo HR, Lu YJ, Bao YH, et al: Parasellar epidural hydatid cysts. *Neurosurgery* 32:662, 1993.

73. Bhojraj SY, Shetty NR: Primary hydatid disease of the spine: An unusual cause of progressive paraplegia. Case report and review of the literature. *J Neurosurg* 91(suppl 2):216, 1999.

74. Islekel S, Zileli M, Ersahin T: Intradural sinal hydatid cysts. *Eur Spine J* 7:162, 1998.

75. Ergun R, Okten AI, Yuksel M, et al: Orbital hydatid cysts: report of four cases. *Neurosurg Rev* 20:33, 1997.

76. Micheli F, Lehkuniec E, Giannaula R, et al: Calcified cerebral hydatid cyst. *Eur Neurol* 27:1, 1987.

77. Arana-Iñiguez R, San Julián J: Hydatid cysts of the brain. *J Neurosurg* 12:323, 1955.

78. Sandhu P, Saggar K, Sodhi KS: Multiple hydatid cysts after brain surgery. *J Neurol Neurosurg Psychiatry* 68:97, 2000.

79. Horton RJ: Albendazole in treatment of human cystic echinococcosis: 12 years of experience. *Acta Trop* 64:79, 1997.

80. Aydin MD, Ozkan U, Altinors N: Quadruplets hydatid cysts in brain ventricles: a case report. *Clin Neurol Neurosurg* 104:300, 2002.

81. Singounas EG, Leventis AS, Sakas DE, et al: Successful treatment of intracranial hydatid cysts with albendazole: Case report and review of literature. *Neurosurgery* 31:571, 1992.

82. Hagemann G, Gottstein B, White OW: Isolated *Echinococcus granulosus* hydatid cyst in the CNS with severe reaction to treatment. *Neurology* 52:1100, 1999.

83. Baykaner MK, Dogulu F, Ozturk G, et al: A viable residual spinal hydatid cyst cured with albendazole: Case report. *J Neurosurg* 93(suppl 1):142, 2000.

84. García-Vicuña R, Carvajal I, Ortiz-García A, et al: Primary solitary echinococcosis in cervical spine: Postsurgical successful outcome after long-term albendazole treatment. *Spine* 25:520, 2000.

85. Todorov T, Vutova K, Mechlov G, et al: Experience in the chemotherapy of severe, inoperable echinococcosis in man. *Infection* 20:19, 1992.

86. Gilman RH, Lee BH: Alveolar hydatid disease. In Strickland GT (ed): *Hunter's Tropical Medicine and Emerging Infectious Diseases,* 8th ed. Philadelphia: Saunders, 2000, p 872.

87. Schmid M, Pendl G, Samonigg H, et al: Gamma-knife

radiosurgery and albendazole for cerebral alveolar hydatid disease. *Clin Infect Dis* 26:1379, 1998.

88. Campos-Bueno A, Loez-Abente G, Andres-Cercadillo AM: Risk factors for *Echinococcus granulosus* infection: A case-control study. *Am J Trop Med Hyg* 62:329, 2000.

89. Diaz FJ, Gilman RH: Sparganosis. In Strickland GT (ed): *Hunter's Tropical Medicine and Emerging Infectious Diseases*, 8th ed. Philadelphia: Saunders, 2000, p 876.

90. Chae SW, Choi JH, Lee HM: Sparganosis presenting as a lateral neck mass. *Head Neck* 25:74, 2003.

91. Holodniy M, Almenoff J, Loutit J, et al: Cerebral sparganosis: Case report and review. *Rev Infect Dis* 13:155, 1991.

92. Kim DG, Paek SH, Chang KH, et al: Cerebral sparganosis: Clinical manifestations, treatment, and outcome. *J Neurosurg* 85:1066, 1996.

93. Landero A, Hernandez F, Abasolo MA, et al: Cerebral sparganosis caused by *Spirometra mansonoides:* Case report. *J Neurosurg* 75:472, 1991.

94. Boero AM, Garaguso PP, Navarre J: A case of cerebral sparganosis in South America. *Arq Neuropsiquiatr* 49:111;1991.

95. Cho YD, Huh JD, Hwang YS, et al: Sparganosis in the spinal canal with partial block: An uncommon infection. *Neuroradiology* 34:241, 1992.

96. Kudesia S, Indira DB, Sarala D, et al: Sparganosis of the brain and spinal cord: Unusual tapeworm infestation (report of two cases). *Clin Neurol Neurosurg* 100:148, 1998.

97. Jeong SC, Bae JC, Hwang SH, et al: Cerebral sparganosis with intracerebral hemorrhage: A case report. *Neurology* 50:503, 1998.

98. Chamadol W, Tangdumrongkul S, Thanaphaisal C, et al: Intracerebral hematoma caused by sparganum: A case report. *J Med Assos Thai* 75:602, 1992.

99. Chang KH, Chi JG, Cho SY, et al: Cerebral sparganosis: Analysis of 34 cases with emphasis on CT features. *Neuroradiology* 34:1, 1992.

100. Wong CW, Ho YS: Intraventricular hemorrhage and hydrocephalus caused by intraventricular parasitic granuloma suggesting cerebral sparganosis. *Acta Neurochirur (Wien)* 29:205, 1994.

101. Moon WK, Chang KH, Cho SY, et al: Cerebral sparganosis: MR imaging versus CT features. *Radiology* 188:751, 1993.

102. Kim CY, Cho BK, Kim IO, et al: Cerebral sparganosis in a child. *Pediatr Neurosurg* 26:103, 1997.

103. Nishiyama T, Ide T, Hilmes SR, et al: Immunodiagnosis of human sparganosis *mansoni* by microchemiluminescence enzyme-linked immunosorbent assay. *Trans R Soc Trop Med Hyg* 88:663, 1994.

104. Tsai MD, Chang CN, Ho YS, et al: Cerebral sparganosis diagnosed and treated with stereotactic techniques: Report of two cases. *J Neurosurg* 78:129, 1993.

105. Bunnag T: Angiostrongyliasis. In Strickland GT (ed): *Hunter's Tropical Medicine and Emerging Infectious Diseases*, 8th ed. Philadelphia: Saunders, 2000, p 793.

106. Weller PF, Liu LX: Eosinophilic meningitis. *Semin Neurol* 13:161, 1993.

107. Schmutzhard E, Boongird P, Veijjajiva A: Eosinophilic meningitis and radiculomyelitis in Thailand caused by CNS invasion of *Gnathostoma spinigerum* and *Angiostrongylus cantonensis*. *J Neurol Neurosurg Psychiatry* 51:80-87, 1988.

108. Koo J, Pien F, Kliks MM: Angiostrongyliasis (parastrongylus) eosinophilic meningitis. *Rev Infect Dis* 10:1155, 1988.

109. Punyagupta S, Bunnag T, Juttijudata P, et al.: Eosinophilic meningitis in Thailand: Epidemiologic studies of 484 typical cases and the role of *Angiostrongylus cantonensis*. *Am J Trop Med Hyg* 19:950, 1970.

110. Kuberski T, Wallace GD: Clinical manifestations of eosinophilic meningitis caused by *Angiostrongylus cantonensis*. *Neurology* 29:1566, 1979.

111. Pien FD, Pien BC: Angiostrongylus cantonensis eosinophilic meningitis. *Int J Infect Dis* 3:161, 1999.

112. Witoonpanich R, Chuahirun S, Soranastaporn S, et al: Eosinophilic myelomeningoencephalitis caused by *Angiostrongylus cantonensis*: A report of three cases. *Southeast Asian J Trop Med Public Health* 22:262, 1991.

113. Noskin GA, McMenamin MB, Grohmann SM: Eosinophilic meningitis due to *Angiostrongylus cantonensis*. *Neurology* 42:1423, 1992.

114. Toma H, Matsumura S, Oshiro C, et al: Ocular angiostrongyliasis without meningitis symptoms in Okinawa, Japan. *J Parasitol* 88:211, 2002.

115. Chotmongkol V, Sawanyawisuth K, Thavornpitak Y: Corticosteroid treatment of eosinophilic meningitis. *Clin Infect Dis* 31:660, 2000.

116. Bunnag T: Gnathostomiasis. In Strickland GT (ed): *Hunter's Tropical Medicine and Emerging Infectious Diseases*, 8th ed. Philadelphia: Saunders, 2000, p 790.

117. Rusnak JM, Lucey DR: Clinical gnathostomiasis: Case report and review of the English-language literature. *Clin Infect Dis* 16:33, 1993.

118. Visudhipan P, Chiemchanya S, Somburanasin R, et al: Causes of spontaneous subarachnoid hemorrhage in Thai infants and children: A study of 56 patients. *J Neurosurg* 53:185, 1980.

119. Chitanondh H, Rosen L: Fatal eosinophilic encephalomyelitis caused by the nematode *Gnathostoma spinigerum*. *Am J Trop Med Hyg* 16:638, 1967.

120. Chandenier J, Husson J, Canaple S, et al: Medullary gnathostomiasis in a white patient: Use of immunodiagnosis and magnetic resonance imaging. *Clin Infect Dis* 32:E154, 2001.

121. Booongird P, Phuappradit P, Siridej N, et al: Neurological manifestations of gnathostomiasis. *J Neurol Sci* 31:279, 1977.

122. Kawamura J, Kohri Y, Oka N: Eosinophilic meningoradiculomyelitis caused by *Gnathostoma spinigerum*: A case report. *Arch Neurol* 40:583, 1983.

123. Punyagupta S, Bunnag T, Juttijudata P: Eosinophilic meningitis in Thailand: Clinical and epidemiological characteristics of 162 patients with myeloencephalitis probably caused by *Gnathostoma spinigerum*. *J Neurol Sci* 96:241, 1990.

124. Baquera-Heredia J, Cruz-Reyes A, Flores-Gaxiola A, et al: Case report: Ocular gnathostomiasis in northwestern Mexico. *Am J Trop Med Hyg* 66:572, 2002.

125. Biswas J, Gopal L, Sharma T, et al: Intraocular *Gnathostoma spinigerum:* Clinicopathologic study of two cases with review of literature. *Retina* 14:438, 1994.

126. Genta RM: Strongyloidiasis. In Guerrant RL, Walker DH, Weller PF (eds): *Tropical Infectious Diseases: Principles, Pathogens, and Practice.* New York: Churchill Livingstone, 1999, p 975.

127. Tabacof J, Feher O, Katz A, et al: *Strongyloides* hyperinfection in two patients with lymphoma, purulent meningitis, and sepsis. *Cancer* 68:1821, 1991.

128. Morgello S, Soifer FM, Lin CS, et al.: Central nervous system *Strongyloides stercoralis* in acquired immunodeficiency syndrome: A report of two cases and review of the literature. *Acta Neuropathol (Berl)* 186:285, 1993.

129. Cahill KM, Shevchuk M: Fulminant, systemic strongyloidiasis in AIDS. *Ann Trop Med Parasitol* 90:313, 1996.

130. Greaff-Texeira C, Leite CS, Sperhacke CL, et al: Prospective study of strongyloidiosis in patients with hematologic malignancies. *Rev Soc Bras Med Trop* 30:355, 1997.

131. Gotuzzo E, Terashima A, Alvarez H, et al: *Strongyloides stercoralis* hyperinfection associated with human T cell lymphotropic virus type 1 infection in Perú. *Am J Trop Med Hyg* 60:146, 1999.

132. Gilman RH: Intestinal nematodes that migrate through skin and lungs. In Strickland GT (ed): *Hunter's Tropical Medicine and Emerging Infectious Diseases,* 8th ed. Philadelphia: Saunders, 2000, p 730.

133. Cappello M, Hotez PJ: Disseminated strongyloidiasis. *Semin Neurol* 13:169, 1993.

134. Smallman LA, Young JA, Shortland-Webb WR, et al: *Strongyloides stercoralis* hyperinfestation syndrome with *Escherichia coli* meningitis: Report of two cases. *J Clin Pathol* 39:366, 1986.

135. Thompson AJ, Brown MM, Ridley A: *Escherichia coli* meningitis and disseminated strongyloidiasis. *J Neurol Neurosurg Psychiatry* 51:1596, 1988.

136. Owor R, Wamukota WM: A fatal case of strongyloidiasis with *Strongyloides* larvae in the meninges. *Trans R Soc Trop Med Hyg* 70:497, 1977.

137. Vishwanath S, Baker RA, Mansheim BJ: *Strongyloides* infection and meningitis in an immunocompromised host. *Am J Trop Med Hyg* 33:857, 1982.

138. Masdeu JC, Tantulavanich S, Gorelick PP, et al: Brain abscess caused by *Strongyloides stercoralis. Arch Neurol* 39:62, 1982.

139. Neefe LI, Pinilla O, Garagusi VF, et al: Disseminated strongyloidiasis with cerebral involvement: A complication of corticosteroid therapy. *Am J Med* 55:832, 1973.

140. Takayanagui OM, Lofrano MM, Araújo MBM, et al: Detection of *Strongyloides stercoralis* in the cerebrospinal fluid of a patient with acquired immunodeficiency syndrome. *Neurology* 45:193, 1995.

141. Sato Y, Kobayashi J, Shiroma Y: Serodiagnosis of strongyloidiasis: The application and significance. *Rev Inst Med Trop Sao Paolo* 37:35, 1995.

142. Siddiqui AA, Berk SL: Diagnosis of *Strongyloides stercoralis* infection. *Clin Infect Dis* 33:1040, 2001.

143. Belani A, Leptrone D, Shands JW Jr: *Strongyloides* meningitis. *South Med J* 80:916, 1987.

144. Chiodini PL, Reid AJ, Wiselka MJ, et al: Parenteral ivermectin in *Strongyloides* hyperinfection. *Lancet* 355:43, 2000.

145. Schaffel R, Nucci M, Portugal R, et al: Thiabendazole for the treatment of strongyloidiasis in patients with hematologic malignancies. *Clin Infect Dis* 31:821, 2000.

146. Zaha O, Hirata T, Kinjo F, et al: Strongyloidiasis: Progress in diagnosis and treatment. *Intern Med* 39:695, 2000.

147. Schantz PM: Toxocariasis. In Strickland GT (ed): *Hunter's Tropical Medicine and Emerging Infectious Diseases,* 8th ed. Philadelphia: Saunders, 2000, p 787.

148. Marmor M, Glickman L, Shofer F, et al: *Toxocara canis* infection of children: Epidemiologic and neuropsychologic findings. *Am J Public Health* 77:554, 1987.

149. Baboolal S, Rawlins SC: Seroprevalence of toxocariasis in schoolchildren in Trinidad. *Trans R Soc Trop Med Hyg* 96:139, 2002.

150. Mizgajska H: Eggs of *Toxocara* spp. in the environment and their public health implications. *J Helminthol* 75:147, 2001.

151. Hotez PJ: Visceral and ocular larva migrans. *Semin Neurol* 13:175, 1993.

152. Giacometti A, Cirioni O, Fortuna M, et al: Environmental and serologic evidence for the presence of toxocariasis in the urban area of Ancona, Italy. *Eur J Epidemiol* 16:1023, 2000.

153. Mirdha BR, Khokar SK: Ocular toxocariasis in a North Indian population. *J Trop Pediatr* 48:328, 2002.

154. Sabrosa NA, de Souza EC: Nematode infections of the eye: Toxocariasis and diffuse unilateral subacute neuroretinitis. *Curr Opin Ophthalmol* 12:450, 2001.

155. Molk R: Ocular toxocariasis: A review of the literature. *Ann Ophthalmol* 15:216, 1983.

156. Ruttinger P, Hadidi H: MRI in cerebral toxocaral disease. *J Neurol Neurosurg Psychiatry* 54:361, 1991.

157. Sommer C, Ringelstein EB, Biniek R, et al: Adult *Toxocara canis* encephalitis. *J Neurol Neurosurg Psychiatry* 57:229, 1994.

158. Duprez TP, Bigaignon G, Delgrange E, et al: MRI of cervical cord lesions and their resolution in *Toxocara canis* myelopathy. *Neuroradiology* 38:792, 1996.

159. Arpino C, Gattinara GC, Piergili D, et al: *Toxocara* infection and epilepsy in children: A case-control study. *Epilepsia* 31:33, 1990.

160. Nicoletti A, Bartolino A, Reggio A, et al: Epilepsy, cysticercosis, and toxocariasis: A population-based case-control study in rural Bolivia. *Neurology* 58:1256, 2002.

161. Magnaval JF, Malard L, Morassin B, et al: Immunodiagnosis of ocular toxocariasis using Western blot for the detection of specific anti-*Toxocara* IgG and CAP for the measurement of specific anti-*Toxocara* IgE. *J Helminthol* 76:335, 2002.

162. Matos MFC, Militao DNA, Brum MAR, et al: Presence of anti-*Toxocara* antibodies in children selected at hospital universitario, Campo Grande, MS, Brazil. *Rev Inst Med Trop Sao Paulo* 39:49, 1997.

163. Barisani-Asenbauer T, Maca SM, Hauff W, et al: Treatment of ocular toxocariasis with albendazole. *J Ocular Pharmacol Ther* 17:287, 2001.

164. Murrell KD: Trichinosis. In Strickland GT (ed):

Hunter's Tropical Medicine and Emerging Infectious Diseases, 8th ed. Philadelphia: Saunders, 2000, p 780.

165. Taratuto AL, Venturiello SM: Trichinosis. *Brain Pathol* 7:663, 1997.

166. Gay T, Pankey GA, Beckman EN, et al: Fatal CNS trichinosis. *JAMA* 247:1024, 1982.

167. Ellrodt A, Halfon P, Le Bras P, et al: Multifocal central nervous system lesions in three patients with trichinosis. *Arch Neurol* 44:432, 1987.

168. Mawhorter SD, Kazura JW: Trichinosis of the central nervous system. *Semin Neurol* 13:148, 1993.

169. Fourestie V, Douceron H, Brugieres P, et al: Neurotrichinosis: A cerebrovascular disease associated with myocardial injury and hypereosinophilia. *Brain* 116:603, 1993.

170. Davis MJ, Cilo M, Plaitakis A, et al: Trichinosis: Severe myopathic involvement with recovery. *Neurology* 26:37, 1976.

171. Clausen MR, Meyer CN, Krantz T, et al: *Trichinella* infection and clinical disease. *Q J Med* 89:631, 1996.

172. Lopez-Lozano JJ, Garcia-Merino JA, Liaño H: Bilateral facial palsy secondary to trichinosis. *Acta Neurol Scand* 78:194, 1988.

173. Feydy A, Touze E, Miaux Y, et al: MRI in a case of neurotrichinosis. *Neuroradiology* 38(suppl 1):S80, 1996.

174. Harms G, Binz P, Feldmier H, et al: Trichinosis: A prospective controlled study of patients ten years after acute infection. *Clin Infect Dis* 17:637, 1993.

175. Watt G, Sairson S, Jongsakul K, et al: Blinded, placebo-controlled trial of antiparasitic drugs for trichinosis. *J Infect Dis* 182:371, 2000.

176. Thompson AF: Other helminthic infections (*Echinococcus,* ascariasis, and hookworm). In Vinken PJ, Bruyn GW (eds): *Handbook of Clinical Neurology,* Vol 35. Amsterdam: North Holland, 1978, p 343.

177. Inatomi Y, Murakami T, Tokunaga M, et al: Encephalopathy caused by visceral larva migrans due to *Ascaris suum. J Neurol Sci* 164:195, 1999.

178. Gavin PJ, Kazacos KR, Tan TQ, et al: Neural larva migrans caused by the raccoon roundworm *Baylisascaris procyonis. Pediatr Infect Dis J* 21:971, 2002.

179. Sorvillo F, Ash LR, Berlin OG, et al: *Baylisascaris procyonis*: An emerging helminthic zoonosis. *Emerg Infect Dis* 8:355, 2002.

180. Rowley HA, Uht RM, Kazacos KR, et al: Radiologic-pathologic findings in raccoon roundworm (*Baylisascaris procyonis*) encephalitis. *AJNR* 21:415, 2000.

181. Park SY, Glaser C, Murray WJ, et al: Raccoon roundworm (*Baylisascaris procyonis*) encephalitis: Case report and field investigation. *Pediatrics* 106:E56, 2000.

182. Moertel CL, Kazacos KR, Butterfield JH, et al: Eosinophil-associated inflammation and elaboration of eosinophil-derive proteins in two children with raccoon roundworm (*Baylisascaris procyonis*) encephalitis. *Pediatrics* 108:E93, 2001.

183. Cunningham CK, Kazacos KR, McMillan JA, et al: Diagnosis and management of *Baylisascaris procyonis* infection in an infant with nonfatal meningoencephalitis. *Clin Infect Dis* 18:868, 1994.

184. Rosemberg S, Lopes MB, Masuda Z, et al: Fatal encephalopathy due to *Lagochilascaris minor* infection. *Am J Trop Med Hyg* 35:575, 1986.

185. Hours M, Cairneross S: Long-term disability due to guinea worm disease. *Trans R Soc Trop Med Hyg* 88:559, 1994.

186. Mitra AK, Haddock RW: Paraplegia due to Guinea worm infection. *Trans R Soc Trop Med Hyg* 64:102, 1970.

187. Legmann P, Chiras J, Launay M, et al: Epidural dracunculiasis: A rare cause of spinal cord compression. *Neuroradiology* 20:43, 1980.

188. Reddy CRRM, Valli VV: Extradural Guinea worm abscess. *Am J Trop Med Hyg* 16:23, 1967.

189. Walker-Deemin A, Kombila M, Mouray H, et al: Detection of circulating antigens in Gabonese patients with *Loa loa* filariasis. *Trop Med Int Health* 1:772, 1996.

190. Carme B, Boulesteix J, Boutes H, et al: Five cases of encephalitis during treatment of loiasis with diethylcarbamazine. *Am J Trop Med Hyg* 44:684, 1991.

191. Vitris M, Nkam M, Binam F, et al: Meningoencephalite filarienne: Discussion a propos dún cas. *Med Trop Mars* 49:293, 1989.

192. Gardon J, Gardon-Wendel M, Ngangue D, et al: Serious reaction after mass treatment of onchocerciasis with ivermectin in an area endemic for *Loa loa* infection. *Lancet* 350:18, 1997.

193. Hoogstraten J, Young WG: Meningoencephalomyelitis due to the sacrophagous nematode *Micronema deletrix. Can J Neurol Sci* 2:121, 1975.

194. Shadduck IA, Ubelaker J, Telford VO: *Micronema deletrix* meningoencephalitis in an adult man. *Am J Clin Pathol* 72:640, 1979.

195. Gardiner CH, Koh DS, Cardella TA: *Micronema* in man: Third fatal infection. *Am J Trop Med Hyg* 30:586, 1981.

196. Bunnag D, Cross JH, Bunnag T: Lung fluke infections: Paragoniamiasis. In Strickland GT (ed): *Hunter's Tropical Medicine and Emerging Infectious Diseases,* 8th ed. Philadelphia: Saunders, 2000, p 847.

197. Kusner DJ, King CH: Cerebral paragonimiasis. *Semin Neurol* 13:201, 1993.

198. Hung TP, Chen ER: Paragonimiasis of the central nervous system. *Neurol Infect Epidemiol* 1:11, 1996.

199. Kim SK: Cerebral paragonimiasis: A report of 47 cases. *Arch Neurol* 1:30, 1959.

200. Madrigal RB, Rodriguez-Ortiz B, Solano GV, et al: Cerebral hemorrhagic lesions produced by *Paragonimus mexicanus. Am J Trop Med Hyg* 31:522, 1982.

201. Oh SJ: Spinal paragonimiasis. *J Neurol Sci* 6:125, 1968.

202. Yoshida M, Moritaka K, Kuga S, et al: CT findings of cerebral paragonimiasis in the chronic stage. *J Comput Assist Tomogr* 6:195, 1982.

203. Udaka F, Okuda B, Okada M, et al: CT findings of cerebral paragonimiasis in the chronic stage. *Neuroradiology* 30:31, 1988.

204. Li HZ, Xie FW, Sun SC: CT findings in "fresh" cerebral paragonimiasis. *Neurol Surg* 20:91, 1992.

205. Cha SH, Chang KH, Cho SY, et al: Cerebral paragonimiasis in early active stage: CT and MR features. *AJR* 162:141, 1994.

206. Im JG, Chang KH, Reeder MM: Current diagnostic imaging of pulmonary and cerebral paragonimiasis, with pathological correlation. *Semin Roentgenol* 32:301, 1997.

207. Kang SY, Kim TK, Kim TY, et al: A case of chronic cerebral aragonimiasis *westermani. Korean J Parasitol* 38:167, 2000.

208. Oh SJ: Bithionol treatment in cerebral paragonimiasis. *Am J Trop Med Hyg* 16:585, 1967.

209. Strickland GT, Ramirez BL: Schistosomiasis. In Strickland GT (ed): *Hunter's Tropical Medicine and Emerging Infectious Diseases,* 8th ed. Philadelphia: Saunders, 2000, p 804.

210. Liu LX: Spinal and cerebral schistosomiasis. *Semin Neurol* 13:189, 1993.

211. Pittella JEH: Neuroschistosomiasis. *Brain Pathol* 7:649, 1997.

212. Pittella JE, Gusmao SN, Carvalho GT, et al: Tumoral form of cerebral schistosomiasis *mansoni:* A report of four cases and a review of the literature. *Clin Neurol Neurosurg* 98:15, 1996.

213. Scrimgeour EM, Gajdusek DC: Involvement of the central nervous system in *Schistosoma mansoni* and *S. haematobium* infection: A review. *Brain* 198:1023, 1985.

214. Bennett G, Provenzale JM: Schistosomal myelitis: Findings at MR imaging. *Eur J Radiol* 27:268, 1998.

215. Siddorn JA: Schistosomiasis and anterior spinal artery occlusion. *Am J Trop Med Hyg* 27:532, 1978.

216. Schils J, Hermanus N, Durant-Flament J, et al: Cerebral schistosomiasis. *AJNR* 6:840, 1985.

217. Preidler KW, Riepl T, Szolar D, et al: Cerebral schistosomiasis: MR and CT appearance. *AJNR* 17:1598, 1996.

218. Junker J, Eckardt L, Husstedt I: Cervical intramedullar schistosomiasis as a rare cause of acute tetraparesis. *Clin Neurol Neurosurg* 103:39, 2001.

219. King CH, Mahmoud AAF: Drugs five years later: Praziquantel. *Ann Intern Med* 110:290, 1989.

220. Watt G, Long GW, Ranoa CP, et al: Praziquantel in treatment of cerebral schistosomiasis. *Lancet* 2:529, 1986.

221. Fowler R, Lee C, Keystone JS: The role of corticosteroids in the treatment of cerebral schistosomiasis caused by *Schistosoma mansoni:* Case report and discussion. *Am J Trop Med Hyg* 61:47, 1999.

222. Cosnett JE, van Dellen JR: Schistosomiasis (bilharzia) of the spinal cord: Case reports and clinical profile. *Q J Med* 61:1131, 1986.

223. Efthimiou J, Denning D: Spinal cord disease due to *Schistosoma mansoni* successfully treated with oxamniquine. *Br Med J* 288:1343, 1984.

224. Haribhai HC, Bhigjee AL, Bill PLA, et al: Spinal cord schistosomiasis: A clinical, laboratory and radiological study, with a note on therapeutic aspects. *Brain* 114:709, 1991.

225. Bambirra EA, de Souza Andrade E, Cesarino I, et al: The tumoral form of schistosomiasis: Report of a case with cerebellar involvement. *Am J Trop Med Hyg* 33:76, 1984.

226. Pollner JH, Schwartz A, Kobrine A, et al: Cerebral schistosomiasis caused by *Schistosoma haematobium:* Case report. *Clin Infect Dis* 18:354, 1994.

227. Mackenzie IR, Guha A: Manson's schistosomiasis presenting as a brain tumor: Case report. *J Neurosurg* 89:1052, 1998.

CHAPTER 17
Protozoal Infections

Erich Schmutzhard

► OVERVIEW

Protozoa are a polyphyletic collection of extremely diverse and diversely organized single-celled organisms of the kingdom Eukaryota.[1,2] The smallest protozoa have a size of less than 1 μm; the largest, of more than 150 μm. There is a cell membrane in the trophozoite stage of protozoa. Trophozoites are capable of ingestion of nutrients, growth, multiplication, and movement. However, they do not possess a cell wall sensu stricto. It is only the rigid wall of the cysts and other permanent stages in which this membrane can be correctly termed a wall.[3] More than 40,000 species have been described; the estimation of the total number reaches beyond 100,000.[1–3]

Around 70 protozoal species exist in humans, half of them being of theoretically pathogenic importance.[4] Some of the protozoal species are intracellular parasites (e.g., plasmodia, *Toxoplasma* spp.), whereas others are extracellular parasites (e.g., *Trypanosoma* spp., *Entamoeba* spp.). Although the protozoa are an extremely heterogeneous group of organisms—some of them very primitive, others highly developed—and although the relationship of specific groups of protozoa to each other is not understood at all, the term *protozoa* is still used, mainly for practical reasons.[5]

Detailed knowledge of the epidemiology, geographic and seasonal distribution, mode of transmission, and in particular, predisposing factors of protozoal infections of the central nervous system (CNS) is necessary for timely diagnosis and antiparasitic chemotherapy.[6–8] Protozoal infections of the CNS include extremely diverse diseases, such as cerebral malaria, sleeping sickness, Chagas disease, indirect CNS complications of babesiosis (due to hypotension and multiorgan dysfunction), and infections by free-living amebae that cause a granulomatous encephalitis. Additionally, *Entamoeba histolytica* and *Toxoplasma gondii* produce multiple brain abscesses. Table 17-1 lists the classification of protozoa causing CNS disease.[9,10] Table 17-2 classifies the human parasitic protozoa into six groups.[12,13]

▶ **TABLE 17-1.** CLASSIFICATION OF PROTOZOA CAUSING CNS DISEASE

Flagellates (locomotion by flagella)
    Phylum: Kinetoplasta
        Species: *Trypanosoma* spp.
    Of uncertain taxonomic position: *Naegleria* spp.
Amebae (locomotion by pseudopodia)
    Phylum: Rhizopoda
        Species: *Entamoeba histolytica, Acanthamoeba* spp.
Sporozoa (no locomotory organelles)
    Phylum: Apicomplexa (=Sporozoa)
        Class: Coccidia
            Species: *Toxoplasma gondii*
        Class: Haemosporidea
            Species: *Plasmodium falciparum*
        Class: Piroplasmea
            Species: *Babesia* spp.

SOURCES: Based on Cox[10] and Schmutzhard.[9]

Sir Ronald Ross, a Nobel laureate for the elucidation of the life cycle of plasmodia, the causative agent of malaria, wrote in his autobiography in 1923 that he hoped the great malaria problem would be solved within due short time.[11] This disease, as with most other protozoal diseases, is very far from being eradicated. With growing expansion of tropical and subtropical terrain endemic to protozoal parasitoses, together with the continuing emergence of parasite resistance to many of the chemotherapeutic agents and the need for highly toxic therapies for some of the protozoal diseases, e.g., sleeping sickness, the global health problems presented by protozoal infections are probably greater today than they were in Ross' lifetime. Furthermore, as with all other parasitic infections and infestations (e.g., helminthic), satisfactory vaccines are far away.[7]

Trypanosoma species, both African and South American, present major health problems in respect to both timely diagnosis and efficacious chemotherapy. Similarly, little is known about the best possible diagnostic procedures and chemotherapies for *Acanthamoeba* spp. and *Babesia* spp., protozoa that rarely cause disease in the CNS but may cause life-threatening disease in immunocompromised patients. With the exception of *Plasmodium falciparum*, the causative agent of cerebral malaria, *T. gondii* is best known due to the experience with this infection in immunocompromised adults. Since the recognition of its potentially fatal effect in the embryo/fetus, and since introduction of the respective prophylactic prenatal screenings, this protozoon may be the only one that is assumed to be coming under control.

This chapter highlights protozoa that have the capacity to damage the CNS either by direct invasion or by indirect mechanisms. The life-threatening course of cerebral malaria (*P. falciparum*) is caused by a number of indirect mechanisms. In sleeping sickness (African trypanosomiasis), the chronic encephalitis is caused by *Trypanosoma brucei gambiense* and *rhodesiense*. Both direct and indirect effects are seen in *T. cruzi* infection (South American trypanosomiasis, Chagas disease). Free-living amebae (*Naegleria* spp. and *Acanthamoeba* spp.) cause a granulomatous encephalitis by direct invasion of the CNS; *E. histolytica* causes abscess formation. Table 17-3 summarizes the CNS disease, geographic distribution, predisposing factors, and mode of transmission of the protozoal pathogens. These will be described in detail separately.

▶ **CEREBRAL MALARIA**

History/Overview

Malaria is the most important protozoal disease of humans; more than 10 percent of the world's population is infected, and up to 3 million people die each year. Most deaths are due to multiorgan dysfunction, cerebral malaria being the most life-threatening complication.

Periodic fever (malaria) was described more than 3000 years ago in early East Asian and Indian writings. In the fourth century B.C. an association between exposure to swamps and periodic fever (*malaria* = "bad air") had been recognized and led to the drainage of swamps to control this disease.[7,11] In the seventeenth century the bark of the South American *Cinchona* tree was in widespread use for periodic fever. Quinine, its active alkaloid, is still in use for severe malaria.[15] The modern drugs artemisinine and related substances are an extract of *Artemisia annua*, a plant that has been in use in traditional Chinese herbal medicine (as *Quinghaosu*) for more than 2000 years to contain fever.[16] In 1879, malaria was reported to be caused by a bacterial organism, *Bacillus malariae*; however, only a few years later the causative organism of malaria was identified as a parasite.[17] In 1897, Ronald Ross suggested that the pathogenic agent of malaria was transmitted by a mosquito.[18] In 1880, Laveran observed moving bodies (most likely gametocytes exflagellating) in the fresh blood of a patient with high fever, and he correctly suggested that these "germs," which were parasites of the red blood cells, were the cause of malaria.[19] He and Ross received the Nobel prize for their respective discoveries.

Until the nineteenth century, malaria was found in northern Europe, North America, and Russia, transmission in southern Europe and other Mediterranean countries being intense.[11] Nowadays, malaria, in particular *P. falciparum* malaria, the only form of the disease afflicting the CNS, is seen in both tropical and subtropical countries.[20] In holoendemic areas, cerebral malaria is seen mainly in children[17,21,22] and pregnant women,[23,24] whereas in nonimmune individuals (e.g.,

▶ **TABLE 17-2.** MODERN/RECENT CLASSIFICATION OF PROTOZOA CAUSING CNS DISEASE

Phylum	Class	Order	Family	Species Causing Disease	Species Causing CNS Disease
Metamonada	Diplomonadea	Diplomonadida	Diplomonadidae	*Giardia lamblia*	Indirect: encephalopathy in tropical sprue
Axostylata	Parabasalea	Trichomonadida	Trichomonadidae	*Trichomonas* spp.	
Heterolobosa	Schizopyrenidea	Schizopyrenida	Vahlkampfiidae	*Naegleria fowleri*	*N. fowleri*
Euglenozoa					
Subphylum: Kinetoplasta	Trypanosomatidea	Trypanosomatida	Trypanosomatidae	*Trypanosoma* spp.	*T. cruzi* *T. brucei rhodesiense* *T. brucei gambiense*
Alveolata					
Subphylum: Apicomplexa	Coccidea	Adeleida Eimeriida	Cryptosporidiidae	*Cryptosporidium* spp.	
			Sarcocystidae	*Sarcocystis* *Toxoplasma gondii* *Isosopora belli*	*T. gondii*
	Haematozoa	Haemosporida Piroplasmida	Eimeriidae Plasmodiidae Babesiidae	*Plasmodium* spp. *Babesia* spp.	*P. falciparum* *Babesia* spp.
Subphylum: Ciliophora	Litostomatea	Trichostomatida	Balantidiidae	*Balantidium coli*	—
Amoebozoa					
Subphylum: Lobosea		Amoebida Acanthopodida	Entamoebidae Acanthamoebidae	*Entamoeba histolytica* *Acanthamoeba* spp.	*E. histolytica* *Acanthamoeba* spp.

SOURCE: Based on Aspoeck et al.[4]

▶ **TABLE 17-3.** EPIDEMIOLOGY OF PROTOZOA CAUSING CNS DISEASE

Pathogen	CNS Disease	Geographic Distribution	Predisposing Factor	Mode of Transmission
P. falciparum	Cerebral malaria (multiorgan malaria)	Tropical areas	—	Vector: *Anopheles* mosquitoes Very rare: blood transfusion
Babesia spp.	Hypoxic encephalopathy	Temperate climate zones	Postsplenectomy	Vector: ticks Very rare: blood transfusion
Acanthamoeba spp. Balamuthia mandrillaris	Granulomatous encephalitis	Worldwide	Rarely: immunosuppressive therapy, AIDS	Contact lens, swimming in freshwater pools Inhalation
Naegleria spp.	Fulminant purulent meningoencephalitis	Worldwide	—	Swimming in freshwater pools
Entamoeba histolytica	Brain abscess	Tropical and subtropical areas	Intestinal amebiasis and amebic liver abscess	Fecal-oral
Trypanosoma brucei gambiense or rhodesiense	Chronic meningoencephalitis	Africa	—	Tsetse fly
Trypanosoma cruzi	Acute meningitis, cerebrovascular-embolic disease	South America (Central America and southern states of U.S.)	—	Reduviid bugs
Toxoplasma gondii	Encephalopathy (congenital) Encephalitis, focal granulomatous intracerebral lesion	Worldwide	Intrauterine infection Posttransplantation HIV infection	Congenital, foodborne

European and American travelers to tropical areas), cerebral malaria is seen more frequently in the elderly.[20,25–27] Four species of the genus *Plasmodium* may infect humans. Only *P. falciparum* causes cerebral malaria or multiorgan malaria. Almost all deaths are caused by *P. falciparum*. The three benign malarias are caused by *P. vivax*, *P. ovale*, and *P. malariae*. Only single case reports attribute a fatal cerebral course of disease to *P. vivax*. The possibility of a double infection, from which only one *Plasmodium* species, e.g., *P. vivax*, is identified, needs to be considered in such cases.[17] Within the past decades, growing concern has resulted from the emergence of resistant strains of *P. falciparum*. Mefloquin and haloflantrin were introduced in the late 1980s and early 1990s after recognition of the seriousness of chloroquin resistance and development of resistance against the combination-drug Fansidar (pyrimethamin and sulfamethoxazole). At this time, the rapid development of resistance to these drugs, as well as atovaquone, a naphthaquinone compound, raised the possibility that humans may become infected by untreatable strains of *P. falciparum*. Nevertheless, in recent years, new combination drugs and new compounds have been tested and seem to alleviate the fear of an omniresistant *P. falciparum* strain killing people by the thousands. In addition to the development of new antimalarial compounds, further progress in decreasing the morbidity and mortality of multiorgan malaria/cerebral malaria caused by *P. falciparum* can only be achieved by early diagnosis and timely initiation of all therapeutic strategies available, including intensive care monitoring and neurocritical care management.[28]

Epidemiology

Malaria is found throughout the tropical countries. *P. falciparum* causes disease in Africa, Papua New Guinea, and Haiti. In other tropical areas, South America, and the Indian subcontinent, *P. vivax* is more common. In East Asia and Oceania, both *P. vivax* and *P. falciparum* are similarly prevalent. This distribution explains why almost all severe patients diagnosed with multiorgan malaria/cerebral malaria in Europe have a history of recent travel to African countries.[17]

The pathogenetic agents of all forms of malaria are transmitted by anopheline mosquitoes. Transmission does not occur below 16°C and at altitudes higher than 2000 m above sea level. An ambient/average temperature between 20 and 30°C and high humidity are optimal for transmission. It is only female mosquitoes that bite humans, human blood being essential for maturation of their eggs. There must be a human reservoir of viable sexual forms (gametocytes) to allow transmission. In areas of high transmission rates it is mainly infants and young children who develop severe malaria,

older children and adults developing some sort of immunity (semi-immunity). The endemicity of malaria is defined in terms of the frequency of splenomegaly in children younger than age 9. Hypoendemic areas have a splenomegaly rate of less than 10 percent in children; mesoendemic areas have a splenomegaly rate of 10 to 50 percent in children; hyperendemic areas have a rate between 50 and 75 percent (the adult splenomegaly rate is usually also high); and holoendemic areas have a rate of more than 75 percent (and a low adult splenomegaly rate).[17] It is mainly tropical Africa and coastal New Guinea where most of the hyper- and holoendemic areas are located. In these areas, cerebral malaria/multiorgan malaria is seen exclusively in children younger than age 5. Eventually, if the child survives, a state of premonition (semi-immunity) is achieved. In semi-immune patients, an infection with *P. falciparum* causes little or no longer life-threatening disease. However, in pregnancy, particularly in primigravidae, as well as in persons having left the holoendemic area for more than 1 year, this state of semi-immunity is severely altered, rendering these patients likely to develop a more severe form of *P. falciparum* infection, even a cerebral malaria.[23] In mesoendemic areas, the development of semi-immunity may take longer; cerebral malaria is also seen in older children (<10 years of age). In hypoendemic and nonendemic areas, cerebral malaria may be seen in all ages; imported malaria, however, is more likely to have a life-threatening course in elderly individuals.[25–27] The incubation period of *P. falciparum* ranges from 10 to 16 days, with single reports as short as 8 to 9 days and as long as 3 months or more.

For detailed information about preerythrocytic development, asexual blood-stage development, and sexual-stage development within humans and development in mosquitoes, the reader is referred to textbooks of parasitology or tropical medicine, respectively (e.g., refs. 7 and 8). Detailed epidemiologic studies support the hypothesis that certain genetically determined red cell abnormalities confer protection against malaria, in particular, against a severe course of disease. This is certainly true for sickle-cell trait[17,29] and Melanesian ovalocystosis.[30] Thalassaemias and glucose-6-phosphate dehydrogenase (G6PD) deficiency are also—although to a lesser extent—protective against malaria, reducing the risk of severe malaria by more than 50 percent.[31,32] Certain human leukocyte antigens (HLAs) are seen frequently in various African areas. Some of them also may confer protection against severe malaria.[33,34] In recent years, a large number of genetic polymorphisms have been detected both in patients being highly susceptible to severe *P. falciparum* malaria and also in those who seem to be protected from its severe form. It is mainly the tumor necrosis factor (TNF) promotor polymorphisms that seem to be associated with severe malaria in African children, but also the polymorphism in the inducible nitric oxide synthesis gene promotor region and polymorphism in CD36 and intercellular adhesion molecule (ICAM-1) receptors (essential receptors for *P. falciparum* cytoadherence) may predispose to a more severe course. On the other hand, some authors report that these polymorphisms protect against cerebral malaria.[17,35–38] Rarely, plasmodia may be transmitted by blood transfusion.[17]

Pathophysiology and Pathogenesis

Four plasmodial species may cause the clinical syndrome of malaria. However, only *P. falciparum* causes multiorgan dysfunction, in particular cerebral dysfunction, i.e., cerebral malaria. Only a very few single case reports have described *P. vivax* as the causative agent of cerebral involvement.[39] It is the asexual blood-stage development (schizogony) that causes the signs and symptoms of multiorgan malaria. After the preerythrocytic life cycle, the asexual erythrocytic life cycle commences. The erythrocytic life cycle takes approximately 48 hours (range 42 to 54 hours). Many parasitized erythrocytes rupture simultaneously, releasing parasites in their merozoitic form into the bloodstream. Parasite debris and malarial pigment cause fever peaks and destruction of erythrocytes, leading to hemolytic anemia.[17] Parasitemia upregulates TNF-α, cytokines, and adhesion molecules.[17,40–49] The parasitized erythrocytes have knob-like protrusions, which are essential for erythrocytic adhesion to the vascular endothelium lining the capillaries and venules. Parasitic development within the parasitized erythrocytes usually takes 13 to 16 hours. These parasitized erythrocytes are the nucleus for rosette formation,[17] adding to capillary blockage induced by the upregulated adhesion molecules ("sticking and rolling"). Adhesion molecules lead to loosening of tight junctions of the endothelial cell lining, perivascular hemorrhage, and finally, edema formation.[50]

The pathogenesis of the impairment of consciousness in patients with multiorgan malaria, in particular, cerebral malaria, is manyfold. The upregulated cytokines [in particular interleukin 1 (IL-1), IL-6, and IL-10] and adhesion molecules (e.g., ICAM-1; the average serum values of ICAM-1 are significantly higher in patients with cerebral malaria than in those with non-cerebral severe malaria) lead to reduced cerebral microcirculation,[51–56] cerebral anaerobic glycolysis, increased cerebral rate of lactate metabolism, increased lactate levels in brain tissue and cerebrospinal fluid (CSF),[57] and a disturbed/impaired blood-brain barrier, as shown by the accumulation of endostatin/collagen XVIII in brains of patients who died with cerebral malaria.[50] In addition to red blood cells and leukocytes, platelets also have been shown to accumulate in brain microvessels in severe cerebral malaria in children.[58]

Besides these "mechanical factors," increased cytokines play an instrumental role in the increase in nitric oxide.[59–62] Recently, it has been shown that inducible nitric oxide synthase expression is increased in brain tissue in patients with fatal cerebral malaria.[60] Neurotransmission is inhibited in patients with cerebral malaria.[57]

The key pathogenetic pathways responsible for impairment of consciousness in cerebral malaria are impairment of microcirculation, impairment of the blood-brain barrier, and local synthesis of nitric oxide. In addition to all these pathogenetic mechanisms, cerebral malaria as a part of multiorgan dysfunction is frequently accompanied by thrombocytopenia and signs of coagulopathy.[17] Although disseminated intravascular coagulation (DIC) as an integral part of the pathogenesis of cerebral malaria has not yet been confirmed by prospective studies, it is fully accepted that in patients with cerebral malaria a severe coagulopathy, going beyond the effects of thrombocytopenia, is observed regularly. It has been shown that the activation of the coagulation cascade is directly proportional to disease severity. Recent studies have shown that patients with severe malaria, in particular, cerebral malaria, show—during the initial phase of the life-threatening disease—a marked reduction of antithrombin III, protein S, and in particular, protein C.[63] Table 17-4 summarizes the pathophysiologic and pathogenetic processes of cerebral malaria.

In cerebral malaria, the microvasculature of the brain is packed with erythrocytes containing mainly mature forms of *P. falciparum* but also macrophages and microglial cells.[64] Sequestration is seen overwhelmingly in the brain but also in the heart, intestine, lungs, and kidney. The brain is usually (mildly) swollen and has multiple petechial hemorrhages[8,17] mainly within the white matter, sometimes confluent and forming sizable hemorrhages. Both lacunae and larger brain infarctions may be seen. A high percentage of the capillaries and venules are packed with parasitized erythrocytes, frequently outnumbering the parasitized erythrocytes seen in peripheral blood smears. This sequestration is more prominent in the white matter; the accumulation of glial cells (macrophages) surrounding hemorrhagic foci is termed *Duercks's granuloma*.[64] Knoblike surface projections lead to attachment of infected red blood cells to the vascular endothelium, as easily visualized by electron microscopy.[17] Recently, platelet aggregation and accumulation have been shown to be more prominent in cerebral blood vessels than in other blood vessels.[58]

Clinical Features

The incubation period of *P. falciparum* ranges from 9 days to more than 3 months, usually being between 10 and 16 days. However, it may be prolonged by inef-

▶ **TABLE 17-4.** PATHOPHYSIOLOGIC PROCESSES IN CEREBRAL MALARIA

Upregulation of TNF-α and cytokines

Upregulation of adhesion molecules

Dysproportionate upregulation of sICAM-1 in cerebral malaria

Sequestration and cytoadherence leading to disturbance of microcirculation

Rosetting and aggregation, adding to disturbance of microcirculation

Loss of deformability of erythrocytes, adding to disturbance of microcirculation

Loosening of endothelial tight junctions, leading to destruction of blood-brain barrier and increasing permeability

Platelet accumulation in brain microvessels, adding to impairment of microcirculation

Increase of nitric oxide and inhibition of neurotransmission

Increase in cerebral anaerobic glycolysis and increase in brain tissue (and CSF) lactate

Extracerebral organ dysfunction, adding to impairment of cerebral metabolism
  Renal failure
  Pulmonary edema
  Anemia
  Electrolyte changes
  Coagulopathy
  Thrombocytopenia
  Finally, systemic inflammatory response syndrome (SIRS) and sepsis syndrome, resembling septic shock syndrome at the end stage of multiorgan dysfunction
  Gastrointestinal dysfunction, increasing the risk of secondary gram-negative infection/sepsis syndrome
  Possibly: acidosis and hypoglycemia

fective antimalarial chemoprophylaxis or insufficient treatment. Semi-immunity reduces/impairs effective multiplication of parasites, thus prolonging the incubation period. Furthermore, semi-immunity effectively inhibits the development of severe malarial signs and symptoms. Thus cerebral malaria is seen on a regular basis only in children in holo- and hyperendemic areas.[65] In contrast, cerebral malaria is seen more frequently in the elderly in nonendemic or hypoendemic

areas, a fact that applies fully to imported cases of severe *P. falciparum* malaria.[25,26]

In 1990, the World Health Organization (WHO) defined cerebral malaria as unarousable coma, *P. falciparum* in a blood smear or bone marrow smear, and exclusion of other causes of the encephalopathy.[17] This WHO definition was changed in 2000.[66] The WHO recommendation now adds to its former definition the following parameters: impairment of consciousness less marked than unarousable coma, prostration, and hyperparasitemia (>4 percent; in hyper- or holoendemic areas, 20 percent or more). In adults the Glasgow coma scale[67] (Table 17-5) and in children the Blantyre scale[68] (Table 17-6) are recommended to assess impairment of consciousness.

Frequently, a matter of discussion has been the assessment of convulsions as a feature of severe malaria, i.e., cerebral malaria.[69–71] The following issues have to be addressed carefully when assessing the causative relationship between convulsions and the diagnosis of cerebral malaria: Generalized tonic/clonic seizures are seen frequently in children, in particular, infants, with cerebral malaria. The presence of a prolonged postictal impairment of consciousness has to be interpreted as being in favor of the diagnosis of cerebral malaria. Persistent postictal impairment of consciousness has to be differentiated from a nonconvulsive status epilepticus. A tonic/clonic status epilepticus may be the main presenting feature of cerebral malaria.[72] Both repeated generalized tonic/clonic seizures and primarily focal beginning and secondarily generalizing tonic/clonic seizures are associated with a higher incidence of neurologic long-term sequelae.[73]

Since the development of cerebral malaria depends on both the parasite density and the duration of parasitemia, the earliest possible recognition of a patient being at risk for cerebral malaria is essential.[74] The multiorgan dysfunction score (MODS) has been tested recently in a pilot study to assess the risk for the development of multiorgan malaria. This multiorgan dysfunction score[75] has been validated with the clinical course, the baseline TNF-α concentrations, the duration of symptoms after admission, and parasite count. Besides a positive correlation with all these aspects, MODS also has shown a positive correlation with parasite clearance time and fever clearance time. All these correla-

▶ **TABLE 17-5.** GLASGOW COMA SCALE (GCS)

Eye opening	4 spontaneous	3 to speech	2 to pain	1 none		
Best verbal response	5 oriented	4 confused conversation	3 inappropriate words	2 incomprehensible sounds		1 none
Best motor response (upper limbs)	6 obeying	5 localizing	4 withdrawal	3 flexor response	2 extensor response	1 none

SOURCE: Used with permission from ref. 67.

▶ **TABLE 17-6.** BLANTYRE COMA SCALE FOR CHILDREN

	Score*
Best motor response	
Localizes painful stimulus†	2
Withdraws limb from pain‡	1
Nonspecific or absent response	0
Verbal response	
Appropriate cry	2
Moan or inappropriate cry	1
None	0
Eye movements	
Directed (e.g., follows mother's face)	1
No directed	0

*Total score can range from 0 to 5; 2 or less indicates unarousable coma.
†Painful stimulus: rub knuckles on patient's sternum.
‡Painful stimulus: firm pressure on thumbnail bed with horizontal pencil.
SOURCE: *Used with permission from ref. 68.*

tions remained significant even after controlling for the initial level of parasitemia.[75]

Diagnosis of Cerebral Malaria

According to the WHO recommendations, every patient coming from a possibly endemic malarial area presenting with fever must be evaluated for plasmodial infection. Thus every patient with respective travel or exposure history presenting with impairment of consciousness, prostration, and/or convulsions, as well as impairment or dysfunction of other organ systems, needs a careful diagnostic workup with respect to *P. falciparum* malaria. The gold standard is the microscopic examination of both thick and thin blood films, i.e., the presence of intraerythrocytic ringforms or, rarely, gametozytes in Giemsa stain (Figs. 17-1 and 17-2). Bone marrow smears also may be positive but do not increase the diagnostic yield. The visualization of parasitic DNA by means of staining the blood film with fluorescent dyes (e.g., Acridine orange) or the presence of monoclonal antibodies against *P. falciparum* histidinde-rich protein 2 are two additional diagnostic procedures that have been in testing but have not replaced the microscopic examination of blood smear by means of Giemsa stain.[6,8,17] Typically, the CSF is normal, in particular, cell count and glucose concentration (also CSF/serum glucose ratio); however, CSF lactate may be increased. The CSF protein concentration may be normal, but mildly to moderately increased protein concentrations may be seen. In children, the opening pressure is usually elevated, depending on the stage of disease.

Neuroimaging may visualize brain edema and multifocal areas of hemorrhage.[76,77] Transcranial doppler

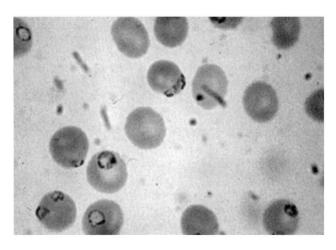

Figure 17-1. Thin blood film (Giemsa stain): *Plasmodium falciparum,* ring forms.

sonography, measuring blood flow velocity in the large basal intracranial arteries, is usually normal; however, perfusion single photon emission computerized tomography (SPECT) and tissue oxygen measurement (by means of near-infrared spectroscopy) may show impairment.[56] Electrophysiologic methods do not add to the diagnostic accuracy.[73,78] However, they may be indicated in the final stage of disease in assessing imminent or definite brain death and in patients with prolonged seizures or nonconvulsive status epilepticus.[72]

In cerebral malaria, which is usually part of a multiorgan disease, close monitoring of all organ functions is mandatory, in particular, circulation; cardiac, renal, and hepatic function; and the coagulation system. Impairment of pulmonary function, typically an adult respiratory distress syndrome (ARDS), is seen 3 to 5 days after the clinical signs and symptoms of severe malaria have started. In patients developing recurrence of fever on days 3 to 5, the possibility of sepsis due to translocation of intestinal gram-negative bacteria has to be recognized at the earliest possible stage.[6,8,17] Regular blood

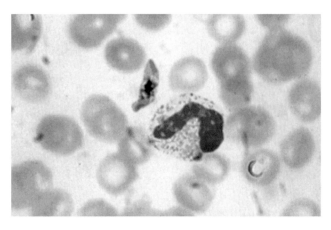

Figure 17-2. Thin blood film (Giemsa stain): *Plasmodium falciparum,* gametocyte.

cultures are recommended. Every patient showing signs and symptoms of multiorgan dysfunction needs close observation. If cerebral dysfunction is the leading feature, timely transfer to a well-equipped neurointensive care unit is recommended. Determinations of blood glucose concentration, red blood cell count, and platelet count are mandatory on a regular basis (initially up to four times daily). Persistent fever or recurring fever may indicate a failure of antimalarial drug but also may indicate development of secondary gram-negative sepsis. In order to diagnose such a gram-negative bacteremia/sepsis, measurement of acute-phase proteins (e.g., C-reactive protein, fibrinogen levels, procalcitonin) is recommended during the initial phase of disease (<5 days). Blood smears have to be taken on a regular basis (at least every 12 hours) to assess parasite clearance. Parasite clearance time, duration of coma, and fever clearance time are all important clinical parameters.[6,8,17]

Differential Diagnosis

Table 17-7 lists the diseases in the differential diagnosis of cerebral malaria.[6,8,17] Taking the best and most thorough history is essential in directing the differential diagnostic evaluation. All these diseases require immediate diagnostic and therapeutic management steps.

▶ **TABLE 17-7.** DIFFERENTIAL DIAGNOSIS OF CEREBRAL MALARIA

Bacterial meningitis
Meningoencephalitis
Encephalitis
Sinus venous thrombosis
Sepsis syndrome
Babesiosis
Rickettsiosis
Salmonellosis
T. b. rhodesiense meningoencephalitis
Malignant neuroleptic syndrome
Heat stroke
Metabolic encephalopathy

Therapy

Antimalarial chemotherapy (schizontocidal therapy) (Table 17-8) and adjunctive therapeutic management strategies (Table 17-9) are the two mainstays of therapy in cerebral malaria.[6,8,9,17,79,80]

▶ **TABLE 17-8.** ANTIPROTOZOAL CHEMOTHERAPY IN CEREBRAL MALARIA

Drug	ICU	Rural Hospital	Duration of Therapy
Quinine*	Loading dose: 20 mg salt/kg bw infused over 4 hours Maintenance dose: 10 mg salt/kg bw infused over >2 hours and at 8-hour intervals	20 mg salt/kg bw diluted 1:2 with sterile water IM Maintenance dose: 10 mg salt/kg bw IM 8 hourly	7 days
Quinidine (quinidine gluconate)*	Loading dose: 10 mg base/kg bw infused within 1–2 hours Maintenance dose: 10 mg base/kg bw infused over >4 hours and at 8-hour intervals *or* 0.02 mg base/kg bw per minute Electrocardiographic monitoring recommended	—	7 days
Artemisinin derivatives		See: ICU	
Artemether	Loading dose: 3.2 mg/kg bw IM Maintenance dose: 1.6 mg/kg bw at 12- to 24-hour intervals	*or* Artemisinin suppositories 10 mg/kg bw at hours 0 and 4, followed by 7 mg/kg bw at 24, 36, 48, and 60 hours	5 days
Artesunate†	Loading dose: 2 mg/kg bw IV Maintenance dose: 1 mg/kg bw IV at 12 hours; then 1 mg/kg bw daily IV	Loading dose: 3.2 mg/kg bw IM Maintenance dose: 1.6 mg/kg bw IM every 12/24 hours	5 days

*Infusions are either 0.9% normal saline or 5% glucose
†It is currently dispensed as dry artesunic acid, which is made up for injection with 5% sodium bicarbonate solution.[66]

▶ **TABLE 17-9.** ADJUNCTIVE THERAPY STRATEGIES IN CEREBRAL MALARIA

Admission to intensive care unit

Closest possible monitoring of airway, breathing, and circulation

Stabilization of vital functions (ABCs)

Early intubation and fluid resuscitation

Close monitoring of pulmonary function

If necessary, invasive ventilation strategies (increase of PEEP, oxygen content, etc.)

Early sedation when necessary (impairment of consciousness, reduction of gag reflex)

Early enteral nutrition

Close observation/monitoring of intestinal function (peristalsis?)

In case of epileptic seizures, sedation with benzodiazepines (e.g., Midazolam), propofol, or barbiturates

Avoid prophylactic application of anticonvulsants

Close monitoring of blood gases, biochemistry (glucose, electrolytes), red blood cell count, platelets, lactate

Correction of lactatic acidosis

In case of clinical and neuroimaging signs of raised intracranial pressure:
   Elevation of the upper trunk (30°)
   Cautious hyperventilation (PCO_2 32–35 mmHg)
   Give mannitol (dosage, e.g., 100 ml, 20%) only if serum osmolality can be monitored
   If necessary and possible (caveat: coagulopathy!), ICP monitoring

If possible, plasma concentration of L-arginine (the substrate of NO synthesis)

In case of severe initial protein C deficiency, consider use of recombinant protein C

If extremely high parasitemia (>20%), consider carefully weighed exchange blood transfusion

There is no scientific support to give corticosteroids or desferrioxamin

Schizontocidal Therapy

Cinchona alkaloids still constitute the major therapeutic antimalarial strategy. Artemisinine derivatives, however, are used increasingly.[81] Several prospective, randomized studies have proven the efficacy of artemisinine derivatives in treating patients with severe malaria, in particular, cerebral malaria. Table 17-8 lists the antiprotozoal chemotherapeutic agents for cerebral malaria.[81–89] Intramuscular artemether and intravenous quinine were compared in a prospective study in the treatment of Sudanese children with severe *P. falciparum* malaria, including cerebral malaria. In comatose patients with a Blantyre scale of less than 2 (severe cerebral malaria), the time of recovery from coma was significantly shorter in the artemether-treated group than

▶ **TABLE 17-10.** ALGORITHM FOR THE TREATMENT OF RECRUDESCENT *P. FALCIPARUM* MALARIA

Quinine → quinine + tetracycline

Quinine + tetracycline → artesunate

Artesunate → mefloquine + artesunate

Reconsider analgesia + sedation

in the quinine-treated group.[89] Both drugs were equally safe. The rectal application of artemesinine derivatives has been proposed in moderately to severely sick children with malaria[90–93]; however, the absorption of rectally administered drugs may be reduced in severe multiorgan-diseased malarial children. Table 17-10 is an algorithm for the treatment of recrudescent *P. falciparum* malaria, and Table 17-11 lists the adverse effects of antimalarial drugs currently in use for the treatment of cerebral malaria.[6–9,94–96]

Adjunctive Therapeutic Strategies

Table 17-9 lists the adjunctive therapeutic strategies in cerebral malaria.[97–103] Routine phenobarbital has been found to be associated with fewer convulsions but possibly more deaths.[104] Rectal administration of diazepam did not terminate all convulsions; plasma drug concentrations were more variable.[105] Thus the selection of antiepileptic drugs and mode of application has to be decided on an individual basis.[104,105]

A patient with severe cerebral malaria with clinical and/or laboratory signs and symptoms of multiorgan dysfunction needs—very similar to a patient with a septic syndrome or septic shock syndrome—full-scale intensive care management.[6–9,79,106,107] The first, foremost, and most important therapeutic strategy for a patient with multiorgan malaria (septic shock syndrome) is sedation and analgesia to allow for artificial ventilation and fluid resuscitation.[108] In the early stage of multiorgan malaria, there is no restriction to fluid administration. In the case of severe multiorgan dysfunction (septic shock syndrome), which is defined by the absence of an appropriate response to vasopressors, the only way to maintain organ perfusion, in particular, cerebral perfusion, is to administer intravenous fluids without restriction.[109] There is no upper limit of intravenous volume administration. Not only is central venous pressure monitoring required, but even better, the best possible monitoring of the circulation is by pulmonary catheter and/or the modern strategy of thermodilution in order to assess cardiac output and cardiocirculatory and cardiorespiratory condition.[110–112] There is little experience with these invasive techniques in patients with multiorgan malaria. Patients with multiorgan malaria, in particular, cerebral malaria, resemble in many respects pa-

▶ **TABLE 17-11.** ADVERSE EFFECTS OF ANTIMALARIAL DRUGS

Antimalarial	Adverse Effects	Frequency
Quinine	Cinchonism (tinnitus, high-tone hearing impairment, nausea, vomiting)	Frequent
	Prolongation of repolarization in cardiac muscle (also in skeletal muscle); prolongation of the QT interval on ECG	Rare
	Iatrogenic dysrhythmias	Extremely rare
	Exacerbation of orthostatic hypotension	Frequent
	Blindness (retinal ganglion cell toxicity)	Rare
	Deafness	Rare
	Stimulatory effect on the pancreatic beta cells, causing hyperinsulinemic hypoglycemia	Frequent
	Allergic reactions (e.g., immune thrombocytopenia)	Rare
	Black water fever	Possible
	In case of intramuscular administration: Local pains Abscess	If given undiluted, frequent
Quinidine	Myocardial conduction and repolarization abnormalities (prolongation of the QRS complex and QT interval)	Frequent (more frequent than in quinine)
	Hypotension	Frequent (more frequent than in quinine)
	Stimulatory effect on the pancreatic beta cells, hypoglycemia, deafness	Frequent Rare (less frequent than in quinine)
Mefloquine	Nausea, vomiting	Frequent
	Dizziness	Frequent
	Dysphoria	Frequent
	"Encephalopathy" (acute brain syndrome): psychotic reaction, convulsions	1:200 to 1:1500 (when used in therapeutic dosage) 1:15,000 (when used as a prophylactic)
Halofantrine	Slowing of atrioventricular conduction (dose-related prolongation of QT interval)	Frequent (in particular when treatment with mefloquine preceded)
	Ventricular tachyarrhythmias resulting in sudden death	Rare
	Diarrhea	Frequent (associated with high doses)
Pyrimethamine	Megaloblastic anemia	
	Neutropenia	
	Thrombocytopenia (when folate deficiency preexisting)	Rare
	Allergic reactions	Most likely due to combination with long-acting sulfonamides
Sulfonamides	Allergic reactions (severe skin reaction, hepatopathy)	
	Toxic epidermal microlysis, Lyell syndrome, Stevens-Johnson syndrome	1:30,000
	Blood dyscrasias	Rarely
	Methemoglobinemia	Rather frequent
Proguanil (Chlorproguanil)	Mouth ulcers	Occasional
	Hair loss	Very rare
	Pancytopenia (in patients with renal failure)	Very rare
Qinghaosu derivatives (artemisinine, artemether, artesunate)	No documented toxicity in therapeutic doses Possible side effects (animal studies): Depression of reticulocyte counts, neurotoxicity, cardiac toxicity, and gut toxicity—only in case of high doses	

tients with septic shock syndrome, and they should be managed accordingly. The same applies to the use of low-dose hydrocortisone, which has been shown to be of some benefit in septic shock syndrome,[113] but this contradicts the 20-year-old study on dexamethasone in cerebral malaria, which suggested dexamethasone was deleterious.[114]

Complications

Table 17-12 lists the neurologic and nonneurologic complications seen in patients with cerebral/multiorgan malaria.[6–9,21,115–129]

Prognosis

Cerebral malaria still carries mortality rates of up to 30 percent.[7,8,21,65,115–118] Poor prognosis is associated with very young age in holoendemic areas[115,116] and old age in nonendemic areas,[25–27,77] multiorgan dysfunction, severe anemia, high-grade parasitemia, low blood glucose levels, low plasma bicarbonate, and metabolic acidosis.[130] Up to 10 percent of patients surviving cerebral malaria have long-term neurologic sequelae of seizures and focal neurologic deficits mainly consisting of speech and language problems.[7,8,21,117,128] Children with cerebral malaria suffer more frequently from difficulties with comprehension, failure to conceive the content of words and the function of words, and syntax errors.[128,129] Previously, low plasma glucose levels and high TNF-α levels were reported to be associated with increased mortality. Recently, neither was found to be associated with long-term neurologic sequelae or increased mortality; however, low plasma bicarbonate concentrations and metabolic acidosis were found to be associated with poor neurologic outcome.[130]

The initial neurologic presentation, in particular, the duration of impairment of consciousness, has the strongest predictive value for mortality and long-term morbidity. It is the timing of the diagnosis and the initiation of specific antimalarial chemotherapy, as well as the timely initiation of intensive care monitoring and management, that are the most important factors for mortality and long-term morbidity. The prevention and therapy of complications, in particular, gram-negative sepsis, are mandatory in order to reduce morbidity and mortality. Highly sophisticated laboratory examinations also may be helpful in prognosis; i.e., low plasma concentrations of L-arginine (the substrate for nitric oxide synthesis) have been associated with poor outcome.[131]

The postmalarial neurologic syndrome (PMNS) is rare and has been reported primarily in children in the Indian subcontinent. Symptoms include psychosis, rigors, tremor, and mainly cerebellar ataxia.[127,132] The pathophysiology of PMNS is not understood.[133] Genetic studies have indicated a weak but significant association of certain polymorphisms to the susceptibility and clinical course of cerebral malaria.[134,135] Certain polymorphisms have been found (e.g., CD36 polymorphism) to be associated with protection from cerebral malaria.[35] Other polymorphisms, in particular, in IL-1β and IL-1 receptor antagonist genesis, have been shown to play a possible role in the clinical outcome of malaria (IL-1β exon 5 allele 2).[136]

Prevention

Exposition prophylaxis and chemoprophylaxis are the most powerful tools to prevent cerebral malaria. Although exposition prophylaxis, e.g., by means of impregnated bed nets, may be a tool to reduce the likelihood of acquiring cerebral malaria in African children, the use of exposition preventive measures, e.g., bed nets, repellents, etc., is more applicable for European or North American travelers to endemic areas than to the local African or New Guinean population. Chemoprophylaxis is almost impossible in the local, endogenous population of holo- and hyperendemic areas. Persons at risk for developing severe malaria (e.g., pregnant women, in particular, primigravidae) and nonimmune individuals (e.g., travelers to holoendemic areas, including semi-immune persons having left the holoendemic area for more than 1 year, thus losing their semi-immunity within this time) should adhere to the respective chemoprophylactic recommendations from WHO, the Centers for Disease Control and Prevention (CDC), or national tropical medicine societies. Detailed information is provided in the respective publications, which are updated on an annual basis.[6–8] The most powerful tool to prevent multiorgan malaria/cerebral malaria is timely diagnosis and appropriate and timely initiation of antimalarial (schizontocidal) chemotherapy. The second most important step is early recognition of the development of multiorgan malaria/cerebral malaria and the earliest possible transfer to an intensive care unit.

▶ **TABLE 17-12.** NEUROLOGIC COMPLICATIONS/LONG-TERM SEQUELAE OF CEREBRAL MALARIA

Neurologic complications
  Seizures
  Focal neurologic deficits
  Raised intracranial pressure
  Neuropsychological defects
Nonneurologic complications:
  All complications seen in sepsis syndrome and septic shock syndrome (organ failure, coagulopathy, hemorrhages, gastric ulcers, aspiration pneumonia, nosocomial infections, etc.)

► BABESIOSIS

History/Overview

Babesiosis is a malaria-like illness that was shown to be transmitted by arthropods in 1888. However, it was not until 1957 that the first human case was documented. Since then, not more than a hundred human cases have been diagnosed, mainly in Europe, the United States, and very recently, Canada. Humans represent dead-end hosts for all *Babesia* spp. Most human cases of babesiosis are due to *B. bovis, B. divergens,* or *B. microti*; others, such as *B. caucasica, B. canis,* and a new *Babesia* (WA 1), have been reported as single cases within the last decade.[137,138] Very rarely, human infection may occur via blood transfusion or intrauterine infection.[139] It is the ecology and biology of the vector tick that defines the pattern of risk for the human population.

Epidemiology

Human infection occurs after the bite of a tick, blood transfusion, or transplacentally/perinatally.[137,139] In Europe, most cases have been due to *B. divergens* and, rarely, *B. microti* and *B. canis*. The vector of *B. divergens* is the common European hard tick, *Ixodes rhizinus*, and *B. microti* has been shown to be transmitted by *I. trianguliceps*. Fatal *B. divergens* infection usually is associated with an asplenic state. In North America, almost all cases of human babesiosis have been due to *B. microti*; most reports have come from northeastern United States, a few from Wisconsin, sporadic cases from California and Georgia, and very recently, some from Canada. In North America, the vector of *B. microti* is *I. dammini*; the reservoir animals are both mice (*Peromyscus leucopus*) and deer (*Odocoileus virginianus*).[138–143] *I. dammini* is also the vector for *Borrelia burgdorferi*, the causative agent of Lyme disease. Coinfection with *B. burgdorferi* and *B. microti* has been reported.[144] *B. microti* infects both healthy individuals and splenectomized patients, in the latter usually causing a more severe, potentially life-threatening disease. In addition to splenectomy, autoimmune disease, cytostatic therapy in cancer patients, and old age have been reported to be risk factors. In human immunodeficiency virus (HIV)–positive patients, severe and persistent disease has occurred.[145,146]

Pathogenesis and Pathophysiology

Sporozoites of *Babesia* spp. are injected into the bloodstream by a tick bite. No tissue stage has ever been demonstrated for *B. bovis* or *B. divergens*. Sporozoites of *B. microti* first enter lymphocytes and undergo merogony, and the daughter parasites then may enter the erythrocytes. This part of the life cycle has been shown

in the small mammal hosts of *B. microti*; however, up to now there is no published report of this preerythrocytic stage in human *B. microti* infections.[137]

Babesia spp. multiply in erythrocytes by budding, releasing daughter parasites that reinvade erythrocytes, and then intraerythrocytic asexual multiplication continues. Recently, the formation of intraerythrocytic gametocytes, which are thought to undergo further development in the tick vector, has been reported.[147] After the formation of zygotes, the parasite develops further outside the intestine of the transmitting vector, *Ixodes* spp., finally invading the salivary glands. Sporozoites are injected via the tick saliva at the next blood meal. Transovarial transmission of *B. bovis* and transstadial transmission to nymph and adult stages of all *Babesia* spp. can take place.[5,137,147]

Babesia organisms are hematozoa of the order Piroplasmida. The molecular basis for their attachment to and invasion of erythrocytes is unknown. *B. microti* in erythrocytes resembles the ring stages of *P. falciparum*. The absence of pigment distinguishes *B. microti* from plasmodia and may be helpful diagnostically.[10,13] Splenectomized patients experience an intense parasitemia and develop a severe anemia, hemoglobinemia, and hemoglobinuria, followed by renal and hepatic failure and hypotension. It is at this stage that the patient also develops metabolic and hypoxic encephalopathy.[145] Macrophage-derived TNF-α has been postulated to play a role in pathogenesis. Formation of immune complexes and activation of the clotting and complement systems also may contribute to the pathogenesis of multiorgan dysfunction in severe *Babesia* infections (in particular, *B. divergens* in splenectomized patients).[148–151] T cells are regarded as vital for developing resistance to *Babesia* infections. Nonspecific responses via natural killer cells and macrophages are important for resistance to babesial infections.[148,151]

Clinical Features

Most human infections by *B. microti* are subclinical. In patients requiring hospitalization, DIC, ARDS, and renal and cardiac failure have been reported, typically associated with the presence of severe anemia. The incubation period of *B. microti* ranges from 1 to 3 weeks (in tick-transmitted infections it may reach 6 weeks, whereas in posttransfusion infections up to 9 weeks has been reported). The illness usually begins with anorexia, nonperiodic fever, sweating, and generalized myalgias.[6,137] A patient with *B. bovis* or *B. divergens* infection usually presents—after an incubation period of 1 to 4 weeks—with high fever, prostration, severe anemia and hemoglobinuria, severe myalgias, and gastrointestinal symptoms. Due to the fulminant nature of *B. bovis/divergens* infection, frequently the diagnosis is only confirmed after the patient has died.[6,137]

Diagnosis

The neurologic features are a result of the secondary effects of the *Babesia* infection, due to both hypotension and anemia, as well as multiorgan dysfunction.[6] The definitive diagnosis is based on demonstration of intraerythrocytic parasites on blood film examination. The size of the parasites varies; they may be rather pleomorphic, *B. divergens* usually being smaller than *B. bovis*, both being pear-shaped, oval, or round. In fulminant cases, *B. divergens* may show ring forms. Up to eight parasites may be seen in a single red cell. Up to 70 percent of erythrocytes have been parasitized in a fatal case. *B. bovi* and *B. divergens* are smaller than malaria parasites, they do not form schizonts, and no pigment can be shown.

B. microti is similar in size to *B. bovis* (2 by 1.5 μm) and presents in various forms (ring, rod-shaped, ameboid). In patients with very high parasitemias, even extracellular merozoites may be found.[5] Patients with *B. bovis/divergens* infection usually have a severe anemia, a leukocytosis, signs of hemolysis (hyperbilirubinemia), and early indications of renal failure. Hemoglobinuria is typical.[137] In *B. microti* infection, there is a mild to moderate hemolytic anemia, thrombocytopenia (mild), and increased bilirubin levels. An indirect fluorescent antibody test is available for *B. bovis* and *B. microti*. The usual diagnostic tool is the microscopic examination of thick and thin blood smears stained with Giemsa. Repeated smears may be needed. DNA amplification techniques (polymerase chain reaction) are a useful diagnostic tool in patients with low-level or transient parasitemia. Polymerase chain reaction (PCR) also may be used to monitor the treatment response.[152,153] *B. microti* recovered from humans may be isolated in hamsters, and *B. divergens* has been passaged successfully to gerbils and to a splenectomized calf. However, animal inoculation is not in use for routine diagnosis in individual cases.[152]

Differential Diagnosis

B. bovi/divergens may be mistaken for *P. falciparum* malaria, in particular, when intraerythrocytic parasites are seen in the blood film. Acute viral hepatitis or acute leptospirosis has to be considered. Since *B. microti* is transmitted by the same ticks as *B. burgdorferi*, the causative agent of Lyme borreliosis, this disease may be mistaken in patients having been to Lyme borreliosis–endemic areas.[6,137,155]

Treatment

B. bovi/divergens infection in splenectomized individuals is usually a fulminant illness that is fatal. There are no prospective, randomized, controlled therapy trials. Based on single case reports and small series, exchange blood transfusion plus intravenous clindamycin and intravenous (possibly also oral) quinine is recommended for the treatment of severe, life-threatening *B. bovi/divergens* infection.[137,156,157] Quinine plus pyrimethamine has proven ineffective.[137] In *B. microti* infections, a combination of atovaquone (750 mg bid) plus azithromycin 500 mg (on day 1) followed by 250 mg daily thereafter for a total of 7 days has been recommended. This combination of atovaquone plus azithromycin is as effective as clindamycin (600 mg tid) plus quinine (650 mg tid) for 7 days. Atovaquone and azithromycin ought to be recommended as the therapy of first choice. Most recently, an increase in the dosage of azithromycin (600 mg/d) has been recommended in combination with atovaquone (for dosage, see above).[158]

Whole-blood exchange transfusion has produced a rapid and substantial fall in parasitemia, and its use as an adjunctive therapy should be considered in every patient with high parasitemia and severe clinical signs and symptoms.[156,157] It is mainly the multiorgan dysfunction that may respond to this adjunctive therapy. Diminacene (Berenil) has been recommended; however, this therapy has been associated with an inflammatory polyradiculoneuropathy.[137]

Complications

Multiorgan dysfunction and severe anemia are directly associated with different degrees of encephalopathy. Hemoglobinuria may lead to aggravation of kidney failure.[6,137]

Prevention

Prevention of all types of human babesiosis depends directly on avoidance of tick bites and prompt removal of ticks. In endemic areas, awareness of the possibility of tick-transmitted and transfusion-transmitted *Babesia* infection should be maintained at a level high enough that both the exclusion from blood donation and the possibility of occurrence of this potentially life-threatening disease in persons at risk, e.g., splenectomized humans, are considered routinely. In *B. bovis* and *B. divergens* infections, the course is usually fulminant and rapidly fatal, in particular, in untreated, splenectomized patients.[159]

▶ INFECTIONS OF THE CNS BY FREE-LIVING AMEBAE

History/Overview

Free-living amebae, e.g., *Naegleria fowleri*, *Acanthamoeba* spp., and *Balamuthia mandrillaris*, are found commonly in lakes, swimming pools, tap water, and heating or air-conditioning units. The term *free-living amebae* was coined originally to differentiate these amebae from parasitic amebae, i.e., amebae causing disease in humans. However, it has been clearly established that some of these free-living amebae cause disease of the CNS in humans. The term *free-living amebae* includes a wide variety of organisms that are not or are only distantly related.[160,161] However, it is the consensus that the term *free-living amebae* should be retained unchanged because it allows the grouping of organisms of similar and comparable human pathologic relevance. Nevertheless, it should be repeated that the term *free-living amebae* does not hold any significance with respect to systematic grouping.[160]

The first case of a primary amebic meningoencephalitis caused by *Naegleria* spp. was reported in a severely malnourished patient in 1948.[162] The first case of *Acanthamoeba* spp. primary granulomatous encephalitis was reported in the early 1970s.[163] This organism usually produces infections in various tissues in severely immunocompromised patients. Recently, *B. mandrillaris* has been described as causing a similar granulomatous encephalitic disease.[164]

A new facet of the medical importance of these organisms is that free-living amebae, particularly in their extremely resistant cystic form, may harbor opportunistic bacteria; hence these ameba may act as vectors. This is very important and of medical relevance in immunocompromised individuals. *Acanthamoeba* spp. may act as vectors for *Legionella pneumophilia*, *Listeria monocytogenes*, *Chlamydia pneumoniae*, a wide variety of opportunistic mycobacteria, *Pseudomonas aeruginosa*, etc. *Naegleria fowleri* and *Hartmanella* spp. act as vectors for *L. pneumophilia*, *Vibrio cholerae*, and *Pseudomonas* and *Bacillus* spp. *Legionella* spp., *Listeria* spp., *C. pneumoniae*, and *V. cholerae* may even proliferate within the amebic host, whereas others use the amebic host simply as a mean of persistence. Most recently, *Acanthamoeba* spp. have been incriminated as a vector for mycobacteria and hepatitis viruses.[160,165]

Primary Amebic Meningoencephalitis (PAM)

Epidemiology

N. fowleri has been reported living in warm freshwater worldwide. The feeding, growing, and multiplying form is called a *trophozoite* and is found on surfaces of vegetation and within the mud. The biflagellate form with the capacity to move rapidly is found in the surface layers of water, whereas the normal cyst prefers the same habitat as the trophozoite. Both the trophozoite and the flagellate forms are infectious to humans; infection takes place via nasal epithelium when contaminated water (during swimming, diving, etc.) enters the nasal cavity. So far, around 200 cases have been reported from all over the world.[160] In the 10-year period from 1989 to 1998 in the United States, 22 cases of PAM due to *N. fowleri* have been reported, all fatal.[165] *N. fowleri* has been shown to be responsible for 0.3 percent of all cases of illnesses associated with recreational water; however, it is responsible for almost all fatal diseases associated with recreational water.[165]

Pathophysiology and Pathogenesis

Both trophozoite and flagellate forms are able to penetrate the epithelium and then pass along the olfactory nerve branches, finally reaching the meninges, where they multiply in the perivascular Virchow Robin species.[165–167] A possible route of infection via the intestinal tract has been discussed recently.[168] The trophozoites penetrate the brain, "ingesting" cerebral tissue, adding to the clinical signs and symptoms of meningitis progressing to cerebritis, and sometimes causing focal neurologic signs and symptoms.[165,169] The severe purulent meningitis quickly progresses to diffuse brain edema, abnormalities of cerebral perfusion, and finally, death.[170,171] The microscopic pathologic finding is that of a typical purulent meningitis and cortical cerebritis. The cerebral hemispheres are grossly edematous with numerous, frequently focal cortical hemorrhages, rarely involving the white matter.[170]

N. fowleri destroys nerve cells by trogocytosis (ingestion of the cytoplasm through a feeding cup) and contact-dependent lysis by altering the permeability of the target cell by lytic proteins. The integrity of the blood-brain barrier is damaged by the cellular influx due to the acute inflammatory reaction and, in particular, the direct invasion of amebae into the blood-brain barrier and brain tissue. *Naegleria* harbors an agent that is capable of causing cytopathic changes in cultured vertebrate cells named *N. ameba cytopathic agent* (NACA), which is a protein of 35 kDa. Invading trophozoites are killed by complement in the bloodstream, a fact that probably explains the usual restriction of the fulminant disease to the CNS.[172,173]

Diffuse brain edema, hydrocephalus (pyozephalus), and secondary vascular perfusion abnormalities due to both vascular occlusion and increased intracranial pressure (ICP) lead to uncontrollable ICP, diffuse cerebral ischemia, and hypoxic brain damage.[170,171] The trophozoites of *N. fowleri* dissolve brain tissue by means of lysosomal hydrolyases and phospholipases. It is both the high speed of locomotion and the capacity of naegleriae to intrude into the intercellular space that are responsible for the fulminant course of disease. Moreover, *N. fowleri* still proliferates even if the body temperature surpasses 40°C, a biologic property that contributes to the fulminant course of disease.[160,165] A very high percentage of the general population has antibodies against *Naegleria;* however, it is highly unlikely that these antibodies provide a protective immunity.[160]

Clinical Features

The signs and symptoms of a PAM very closely resemble those of a severe purulent bacterial meningitis. Incubation period is usually less than 7 days and frequently 2 to 3 days. In a few cases, sore throat and rhinitis have been reported as a prodromal feature. Within a very short time, the disease progresses from headache and slight pyrexia to intense headache, vomiting, and stiff neck. Within hours, the patient develops qualitative and finally quantitative impairment of consciousness. The duration of illness is usually less than 7 days until death.[159,163,172,173]

Diagnosis

The CSF is turbid and frequently slightly hemorrhagic, with a markedly increased cell count, mainly polymorphonuclear cells. The presence of erythrocytes in the CSF has been suggested as being characteristic of PAM; however, red blood cells can be due to accidental contamination of the CSF during the lumbar puncture (a traumatic tap), decreasing the specificity of the presence of red blood cells. CSF protein concentration is generally extremely high, whereas the CSF glucose concentration is typically decreased.[174,175]

An immediate wet microscopic examination of the CSF is recommended in all suspected cases of PAM; although trophozoites may be mistaken for highly active mononuclear or other white cells, careful observation should allow the appropriate diagnosis. Naegleriae move actively at a rate of up to three body lengths per minute with progressive movement and the characteristic explosive protrusion of a pseudopodium. Warming the wet preparation enhances and stimulates the movement of naegleriae. In addition to wet microscopy, cytospine films stained with Romanovsky stain or Acridine orange stain should be done. Giemsa stain or Calcofluor white stain is useful in demonstrating naegleriae in CSF.[160,165] In contrast to *Acanthamoeba* spp., in *N. fowleri*–associated PAM there are never cysts in the CSF. *N. fowleri* can be distinguished easily from other, nonhuman pathogenic *Naegleria* spp. by its capacity to grow even at 45°C. To confirm the diagnosis, cultures of the CSF sample on 1.5% nonnutrient agar coated with washed *E. coli* bacteria and maintained in a moist box at 37°C overnight should be examined. Cell cultures used in virus isolation techniques also provide the appropriate growth substrate for *N. fowleri*. It is important, however, to make sure that no antifungal agents are incorporated in the culture medium.[177] *N. fowleri*–specific monoclonal antibodies and PCR techniques for the identification of *N. fowleri* have been described.[160,176–178,180]

Differential Diagnosis

The main differential diagnosis of a PAM is acute purulent (bacterial) meningitis. Viral meningoencephalitis, tuberculous meningitis, and malignant carcinomatous meningitis are easily differentiated by means of cytologic examination of the CSF.[6,165,170,171]

Treatment

There are no prospective, randomized studies on the antiprotozoal therapy of *N. fowleri* meningoencephalitis. However, in vitro and animal studies have shown a potential synergism of amphotericin B with tetracycline, miconazole, and rifamycin.[181,182] In particular, the combination of amphotericin B with miconazole is supported by in vitro studies carried out on the strain of *N. fowleri* isolated from the CSF of a patient in California because synergism was seen with amphotericin B. There is a clear synergism between rifampicin and amphotericin B, whereas rifampicin and miconazole may be mildly antagonistic.[183–185] Recently, qinghaosu and its derivatives have been proposed with partial in vitro success.[186,187]

Because of the typically fulminant course of this disease, an extremely high level of suspicion is necessary to allow timely initiation of therapy, which is recommended to consist of amphotericin B (AmB; 0.5 to 1.5 mg/kg daily). In a patient with a ventriculostomy, the administration of intraventricular AmB 0.05 mg initially and increasing to 0.1 mg daily should be considered. Rifampicin may be given intravenously or orally (600 mg/d). Intravenous miconazole (350 mg/m² of body surface) can be considered. Miconazole may be given intrathecally at a dosage of 10 mg daily every other day.[9,165] Whether a patient needs external ventricular drainage, dexamethasone, or anticonvulsive therapy depends on the specific course of the patient's disease.[165]

Prevention

N. fowleri is sensitive to disinfectants, particularly chlorine. This may be important for public baths and swimming pools but is not applicable to lakes and ponds. However, since a local infection of the upper respiratory tract is thought to promote the invasion of *Naegleria* through the nasal mucosa, persons with such an infection are strongly discouraged from immersing the head into potentially dangerous waters, particularly when the ambient and water temperatures are high. *N. fowleri* is usually not isolated from water at temperatures below 35°C. Both cysts and trophozoites are killed only by temperatures above 60°C. Ozonation has been tested with some success in eliminating *N. fowleri* from baths and pools. However, *Naegleria* is a much more serious problem for natural waters than for artificial pools, which can be maintained properly to prevent the growth of these organisms.[192–194]

Granulomatous Amebic Encephalitis

Epidemiology

Human pathogenic *Acanthamoeba* spp. and *B. mandrillaris* have a cosmopolitan distribution, although most cases of granulomatous amebic encephalitis (GAE) have been reported from the United States. Predisposing factors are various forms of immunosuppression, organ transplantation, HIV infection, splenectomy, corticosteroid therapy and chemotherapy, chronic alcoholism, malignant disease, diabetes mellitus, and chronic kidney and liver diseases.[160,165] Two hundred cases of GAE have been reported from all over the world.[158,188–191] Recently in AIDS patients, the leptomyxid ameba, *B. mandrillaris*, has been shown to cause a granulomatous encephalitis.[192–194]

Pathophysiology and Pathogenesis

A wide variety of *Acanthamoeba* species (e.g., *A. castellani*, *A. culbertsoni*, *A. polyphaga*, *A. astronyxis*, *A. hatchetti*, and *A. rhysodes*) and the only known species of *Balamuthia* (*B. mandrillaris*) have been reported as the causative agents of GAE.[160] Although no patient in a series of 15 cases of GAE[189] had any recent history of swimming or water sports, infection presumably takes place by contact with contaminated water or by inhalation of amebic cysts. Lesions within the skin, the mucosa of the respiratory tract, or the olfactory neuroepithelium may enhance the invasion of *Acanthamoeba*. An inflammatory primary focus frequently is identified from which hematogeneous spread with final invasion of the CNS (and other organs) takes place.[160] The spread of the amebae within the brain tissue is centrifugally; they usually invade central areas of brain tissue and finally advance to the cortical areas.

Trophozoites invade the CNS by hematogenous dissemination, leading to microthrombosis in periventricular capillaries.[192] Various enzymatic reactions, mainly using hydrolases, phospholipases, and cysteinproteinases, allow the spread of the acanthamoebae into the surrounding brain tissue.[165,169] Thermotolerance of *Acanthamoeba* plays an important role in the pathogenesis of GAE. Similar to naegleriae, acanthamoebae probably injure cells by the mechanism of trogocytosis and by means of contact-mediated lysis of cellular components due to secreted enzymes (hydrolases, etc.; see above).[160,172,173] The granulomatous cellular response adds to the pathology. In the healthy person, the development of antibodies and cell-mediated immunity usually protects the infected person from invasion of amebae into the brain. Very recently, a few single cases of GAE due to *B. mandrillaris* have been reported in immunocompetent children.[188,190,195]

Clinical Features

GAE manifests with multiple necrotizing lesions within the brain. All areas of the brain, mainly both cerebral hemispheres but also the cerebellum and brain stem, may be involved. The signs and symptoms are initially highly nonspecific, mimicking chronic inflammatory diseases of the CNS (e.g., mycoses, tuberculosis, autoimmune diseases, malignant diseases, and even vas-

culitis). In *B. mandriallaris* infection, frequently an initial lesion of the skin may be seen, sometimes in the nasal pyramid, ulcerating and persisting for weeks or months. Due to vasculitic lesions, the initial diagnosis may be stroke.[195] Headache, focal neurologic lesions, seizures, and finally, impairment of consciousness progressing to coma are seen developing over days, weeks, or even months.[9,160,165,171,175,189]

Diagnosis

Since both the clinical features and the CSF findings are highly nonspecific in GAE, direct proof of the pathogenetic agent is the gold standard of diagnosis. The CSF cell count may be increased with a predominance of lymphocytes. The CSF glucose and protein concentrations are usually normal.[160,165,192,196,197] In a few cases in AIDS patients, amebic trophozoites were identified in the CSF.[198] Serologic testing would be ideal in view of the chronic nature of the infection. A complement fixation test with *A. culbertsoni* antigen has been reported in a patient with fatal cerebrovascular disease in whom postmortem histologic examination demonstrated amebae similar to *Acanthamoeba*.[165] PCR techniques are still experimental but may be a useful diagnostic test in the future.[199,200] Cerebral biopsy is thought to be the gold standard in granulomatous inflammatory intraparenchymal brain lesions.[9,160,165] *Acanthamoeba*-specific monoclonal antibodies are likely to prove valuable in diagnosing GAE. Biopsy material quickly incubated at 37°C (for up to a week under humid conditions) should be cultured (see "Primary Amoebic Meningoencephalitis (PAM)" above].[171] Both naegleriae and acanthamoebae can be isolated in cell cultures, and attempts at culturing the CSF can be successful. It should be noted, however, that *B. mandrillaris* does not grow on nonnutrient agar media coated with *Escherichia coli* (as recommended for naegleriae or acanthamoebae).[160,171]

Neuroimaging will show nonspecific multiple granulomatous enhancing lesions with the typical centrifugal progression (starting from periventricular areas and finally reaching the cortical regions). Initially, the lesions are seen frequently in the cerebral hemispheres, eventually also involving the cerebellar hemispheres and brain stem structures. Hydrocephalus may develop.[195,201]

Differential Diagnosis

Any kind of granuloma-forming, space-occupying disease (inflammatory, infectious, malignant, etc.) may be mistaken for GAE.[9]

Treatment

In mice, *Acanthamoeba* infections have been treated successfully with rifampicin and paromomycin. Solitary *Acanthamoeba* brain lesions may be excised. Combination therapy with fluconazole and sulfadiazine has been reported recently in an AIDS patient with GAE.[194]

No prospective studies exist with respect to antiamebic therapy; a multidrug regimen usually is recommended. This may contain AmB, intravenous pentamidine, oral fluconazole, ketoconazole, miconazole, sulfadiazine, and/or rifampicin.[195–202] Improvement of the immunologic deficiency by treating both the underlying disease and by means of immunomodulation has to be discussed in every single case.[9,160,165] Since the diagnosis of GAE is very difficult, in many cases the disease ends fatally.

Complications

Depending on the anatomic location, any kind of granuloma may cause focal neurologic deficits, impairment of CSF circulation, or epileptic seizures.

Prevention

Since *Acanthamoeba* cysts occur in tap water and in the air, there is no way to prevent infection with these agents, particularly since the occurrence of GAE is not linked with any kind of risky, improper, or negligent behavior or exposure.[160]

Amebic Brain Abscess

History/Overview

Invasive amebiasis due to infection by the parasitic protozoon *E. histolytica* is responsible for 70,000 deaths per year worldwide.[203] The pathogenic agent, *E. histolytica*, was first described in 1875 in the autopsy of a patient with fatal dysentery. Only a few years later, in 1890, William Osler reported the first case of dysentery complicated by fatal hepatic abscess.[160] Cerebral involvement has been documented in 1.2 to 2.5 percent of patients who had amebiasis at autopsy, amebic liver abscess usually being a prerequisite.[204,205]

Epidemiology

E. histolytica has a worldwide distribution and is endemic in most countries with low socioeconomic conditions. By now it is accepted that pathogenic and nonpathogenic strains of *Entamoeba* exist, the nonpathogenic *E. dispar* being the more prevalent species (with a ratio of 10:1).[160] Up to 10 percent of patients infected with the pathogenic *E. histolytica* develop invasive disease. It is estimated that up to 50 million people (worldwide) are infected with *E. histolytica*, the global mortality reaching up to 70,000 deaths per year.[203,204] The infection occurs via the fecal-oral route, contaminated food and drinks being the main source of infection. In rare instances, infection occurs by sexual transmission. Severe infections occur in very young children, pregnant women, the malnourished, and individuals taking corticosteroids. Patients with AIDS do not have an increased risk of severe or invasive infection, respectively.[206]

Approximately 40 different species have been described as parasites of vertebrates, rarely also as parasites of invertebrates.[204] In endemic areas, up to 90 percent of the population carries *E. histolytica* or *E. dispar*, in northern and western countries these parasites can be found rather frequently.[165] In North America, 4 percent of the population carries *Entamoeba coli*, another 4 percent *Endolimax nana*, 1.5 percent *E. hartmanni*, 0.6 percent *Jodamoeba buetschlii*, and 0.9 percent the potentially invasive *E. histolytica*.[204] With the exception of *E. gingivalis*, all intestinal amebae usually live in the colon, where they survive primarily on bacteria. The cystic form, however, is highly resistant and may survive in a humid habitat for months. Cysts can survive underneath the fingernails for up to 45 minutes. Cysts of *E. histolytica* are the typical infective stage.

Pathophysiology and Pathogenesis

The trophozoites of *E. histolytica* have a size of 10 to 20 μm, usually containing vacuoles that are full of bacteria. The mature cysts have a diameter of 10 to 16 μm and have four nuclei. *E. histolytica* is highly pathogenic and is the only cause of amebic dysentery, amebic liver abscess, and all other extraintestinal manifestations, including intracerebral abscesses.[160,204] The ingested cyst is infectious for humans (it is only the cyst). Within the intestine, the cyst releases motile trophozoites that multiply in the colon, feeding on bacteria, epithelial cells, and erythrocytes.

E. histolytica is a parasite of humans, but its full life cycle has also been demonstrated in monkeys; thus these animals possibly constitute a reservoir. The invasive manifestations, such as liver abscess and intracerebral abscess, which carry the highest mortality rate, have been found not only in tropical areas but also in subtropical and temperate climatic regions, wherever hygiene is poor.[203,204] The invasiveness of *E. histolytica* is determined by the capacity of its trophozoitic form to attach itself by means of lectine to the epithelial cells and to invade the epithelial lining of the intestine. As soon as *E. histolytica* has contact with these cells, a rapid cytolytic process begins, leading to swelling of cells, formation of vacuoles, and finally, cell lysis. *E. histolytica* proteins have been named *amebic pores* in analogy to the reaction that is induced by the enzyme perforin of cytotoxic T cells. Besides these amebic pores and lectine, it is mainly cystein proteinases that constitute the main factor of invasiveness of *E. histolytica*. An additional virulence factor may be the capacity to modulate the immune response of the host, which leads to chemotaxis of neutrophils and macrophages, which, however, are not able to contain the infectious focus.[160,204]

Amebae probably spread from the intestine to the liver through the portal circulation. In severe cases, amebic trophozoites can be found in the "abscess walls" of liver abscesses and virtually in every organ of the body, including the brain, finally leading to space-occupying brain abscesses. Cerebral involvement has been documented in up to 2.5 percent of patients who had amebiasis at autopsy but in less than 0.1 percent of patients in large clinical series of amebic dysentery. Rupture of an intracranial abscess manifests by the acute onset of signs and symptoms and results in a fulminant, fatal course of disease.[160,204,205]

Diagnosis

The detection of the parasite (amebic trophozoites having phagocytosed erythrocytes) in the feces or in a rectal/colonic biopsy is the gold standard for the diagnosis of amebic dysentery.[204] Since cerebral amebic abscesses usually accompany abscesses in other locations, in particular, liver abscesses, the aspiration of a liver abscess can be considered to make the diagnosis. Amebic trophozoites are sparse in necrotic material from the center of the abscess and are more abundant on the marginal walls; therefore, the aspirate should be collected in several different containers because the trophozoites are found more commonly in the last portions of the aspirated material.[207] The demonstration of trophozoites is extremely difficult because they may be trapped in debris and do not show their typical pseudopodic motility. For this reason, the diagnosis of extraintestinal amebiasis, in particular, cerebral amebic abscess, depends heavily on immunologic tests to detect specific antibodies against *E. histolytica*, enzyme-linked immunosorbent assay (ELISA) being the most commonly used technique.[208,209]

Other methods to detect antiamebic antibodies include the immunofluorescent antibody test, the indirect hemagglutination assay (IHA), radioimmunoassay, and countercurrent immunoelectropheresis. These immunologic tests are particularly useful in nonendemic areas, whereas in highly endemic areas in the population at risk (lower social levels) high titers of antiamebic antibodies are seen frequently in the majority of tested persons.[160] In invasive *E. histolytica* disease, antibody response is present in up to 95 percent, particularly if more than one technique is employed. Serologic responses measured by agar gel diffusion, countercurrent immunoelectropheresis, and ELISA may persist for more than 3 years, and IHA may remain positive for more than 10 years after parasitologic cure.[160]

In every patient with suspected cerebral amebic abscess, usually visualized by neuroimaging methods (cCT, MRT), a thorough radiologic examination of chest, lungs, and abdomen/liver (sonography and/or computed tomography) is mandatory.[205] Single abscesses frequently present with less acute symptoms, whereas patients presenting acutely tend to have multiple lesions. In most instances, aspiration of an intracranial/cerebral amebic abscess is not indicated because intraaspiration rupture may lead to a deleterious spread of the infection. A concomitant liver abscess only should be aspirated unless there is a clear indication to aspirate the cerebral abscess. Such indications[204,207] are to rule out a pyogenic abscess, particularly with multiple lesions; as an adjunct to medical therapy (no response after 72 hours of pharmacologic therapy); if rupture is believed to be imminent; and an abscess in the left liver lobe, where the risk of rupture is increased. Patients with an extraintestinal amebiasis, particularly with multiple brain and liver abscesses, usually present in critical condition with high fever and high leukocytosis in the peripheral blood.

Differential Diagnosis

Any kind of primary or secondary intracranial abscess or other space-occupying lesion (e.g., metastasis) constitutes the differential diagnosis of intracranial amebic brain abscess. The combination of a liver abscess with a brain abscess is highly suggestive of amebic origin; however, apurulent gallbladder disease leading to anaerobic septicemia similarly may present with both abdominal and intracranial abscess formation. Thus the main differential diagnostic considerations are pyogenic liver abscess, inflammatory gallbladder disease, and sepsis syndrome.[6]

Treatment

Two classes of drugs are used in the treatment of *E. histolytica* infections. Luminal amebicides, such as diloxanide furoate and iodoquinol, act on organisms in the intestinal lumen and are not effective against tissue organisms.[160,204] Tissue amebicides are metronidazole, dehydroemetine, and chloroquine. They are highly effective in the treatment of invasive amebiasis, including amebic brain abscess. Metronidazole in a dose of 750 mg tid for 10 days (in children, 35 to 50 mg/kg of body weight per day divided into the three doses for 10 days) followed by diloxanide furoate (500 mg tid for 10 days; pediatric dosage: 20 mg/kg of body weight divided into three doses for 10 days) is the drug regimen of first choice in extraintestinal amebiasis, including amebic brain abscess. An alternative is tinidazole (2 g/d for 5 days; pediatric dosage: 50 mg/kg of body weight per day for 5 days) followed by diloxanide furoate (for dosage, see above). Paromomycin or iodoquinol may be used as an alternative to diloxanide furoate. Third choice is dehydroemetine in a dosage of 1 to 1.5 mg/kg of body weight per day (maximum: 90 mg/d) intravenously for 5 days, with a pediatric dosage of 1 mg/kg of body weight per day for 10 days (maximum), followed by diloxanide furoate (for dosage, see above). A combination of metronidazole and chloroquine may be considered in patients with severe and multiple extraintestinal amebic abscesses.[203]

Complications

The typical complications of amebic brain abscess correspond to those of other space-occupying inflammatory intracranial lesions; rupture of an amebic brain abscess leads to a fulminant cerebritis and meningitis with a usually fatal course.

Prevention

Improving the standard of living and the establishment of adequate sanitary conditions in countries where the disease is prevalent are the best possible means to control invasive amebiasis, including amebic brain abscesses. On an individual level, early detection and treatment of invasive amebiasis are essential. Since metronidazole and tinidazole have little effect on the intestinal cysts, reinfection and recurrence of the extraintestinal manifestation may occur; for this reason, the appropriate therapy of extraintestinal amebiasis has to be followed by luminal agents such as diloxanide furoate, paromomycin, or iodoquinol (in the latter, myelooptic neuropathy has been reported after long-term use).[160,204] Individual chemoprophylaxis for travelers is not indicated; however, close observation of hygiene for food and drinking water is essential. The probability of acquiring the infection (for travelers) has been shown to be very low (0.3 percent) of all travelers' diarrheas.[210]

► NEUROLOGIC MANIFESTATIONS OF CHAGAS DISEASE (AMERICAN TRYPANOSOMIASIS)

History/Overview

When working as a malaria control officer in the Brazilian state of Minas, Gerais Carlos Chagas found, in 1907, protozoan flagellates in the feces of large blood-sucking insects, the triatomine bugs, that attacked inhabitants of poor-quality housing. Oswaldo Cruz exposed marmosets to these infected triatomine bugs and developed a circulating trypanosome that was named *Trypanosoma cruzi*. Chagas found the same organisms circulating in the blood of patients, mainly children, with an acute febrile illness. All the major features of the *T. cruzi* life cycle and the discovery of natural reservoir hosts (e.g., armadillos) have to be attributed to Carlos Chagas. However, in 1912, the mechanism of transmission was proven to be by contamination with infected bug feces. It took years/decades until the widespread distribution and public health significance of this protozoal parasite were recognized.[211]

Serologic surveys throughout the Americas led to a prevalence estimate of up to 90 million people, up to 10 percent being expected to die in the acute phase of infection. Up to 30 percent of those surviving the acute phase may enter the chronic state of disease, with the chagasic heart disease/cardiomyopathy and, more rarely, denervation of the esophagus, stomach, and large intestine.[212] An infected individual retains a low-level infection for life, although not all will develop a chronic Chagas disease state. An immunocompromised state (e.g., HIV infection or organ transplantation) can reactivate the acute infection.[213–215]

Epidemiology

T. cruzi infection is seen solely in the Americas, extending from South Argentina into the southern states of the United States.[216–218] The natural habitat of triatomine bugs is the nests or resting sites of mammals and birds. Five species of triatomine bugs are known to be vectors of *T. cruzi*: *Triatoma infestans*, *T. timidiata*, *T. brasiliensis*, *Panstrongylus megistus*, and *Rodninus prolixus*.[212,219–222] Theoretically, all mammalian species are considered to be susceptible to *T. cruzi*, thus serving as reservoir hosts, armadillos and the common opossum being the main species. In recent years it has been confirmed that *T. cruzi* is much more heterogeneous than previously thought. Isoenzyme electrophoresis originally classified *T. cruzi* into principal zymodemes (Z1–Z3).[221–223] There is consensus, however, at the present time that at least two major subspecific divisions exist within this species, simply named *T. cruzi I* and *T. cruzi II*, although this may constitute an oversimplified division.

Pathophysiology and Pathogenesis

T. cruzi is a single-celled protozoal parasite of the family Trypanosomatidae. *T. cruzi* divides intracellularly in nonphagocytic and phagocytic cells as well. In mammals, *T. cruzi* is predominantly an intracellular parasite, thus influencing the pathogenesis of the disease and the immune response to infection. In the vector, this parasite multiplies only within the intestinal tract and does not enter the hemocele. In the rectum of the triatomine bug, the trypanosomas transform to infective trypomastigotes. Every time the triatome bug takes a blood meal, feces and urine are released containing metacyclic trypomastigotes. Infection in humans is established when *T. cruzi* crosses mucous membranes such as the conjunctiva, nasal, or oral mucosa or through lesioned skin, e.g., a bite wound. The intact skin, however, is an impenetrable barrier. As soon as the feces is dried up, the metacyclic trypomastigotes lose their infectivity. The triatomine bugs acquire infection by feeding on the blood of an infected mammal. So far no transovarial transmission of *T. cruzi* has been reported. Having entered the host, *T. cruzi* penetrates nonphagocytic cells, e.g., muscle cells, but also phagocytic cells. Within these cells, *T. cruzi* transforms to the amastigote stage, which multiplies by binary fission, forming a pseudocyst. After 5 days, the amastigotes are transformed to trypomastigotes, which are finally released when the pseudocyst ruptures. Multiplication usually takes place at the initial site of infection, causing a cutaneous or ocular lesion, and from there, systemic spread of the organism sets in. Pseudocysts are seen most frequently in heart muscle, skeletal muscle, and smooth muscle of the alimentary tract. Parasitemia is usually transient in the acute phase of infection, although very low numbers of circulating trypomastigotes may remain for life, thus making the host a lifelong potential source of infection to triatomine bugs. Besides the triatomine bug acting as an "indirect" vector, transmission by blood transfusion also has been reported, as well as congenital transmission. When eating food contaminated by triatomine feces, an oral transmission of *T. cruzi* is possible, as is milk transmission from mother to child.[211,212,224]

Pseudocysts may be widespread. In addition to cardiac, skeletal muscle, and reticuloendothelial cells, they may be found in perivascular spaces or even in glial and neuronal cells, representing the histopathologic picture of acute meningoencephalitis.[225] In chronic Chagas disease, the pathogenetic basis of the neurogenic "signs and symptoms" is the rupture of pseudocysts with antigenic stimulation of surrounding uninfected cells, focal immunologic destruction of unaffected cells including ganglion cells, further loss of ganglion cells with age and dysfunction, and enlargement of the affected organs when the loss of ganglion cells crosses a critical threshold. In addition to their neurogenically caused megacolon, megaesophagus, etc., these patients suffer from cardiomegaly with impairment of the conduction system, eventually leading to cardiogenic embolism, including cerebral embolism. The inflammatory response in the tissues may lead to acute myocarditis, similarly leading to cardiogenic embolism, as well as to acute meningitis and meningoencephalitis. The inflammation within the tissues usually subsides after the acute phase of infection, but it may show a renewed inflammatory response leading to progressive myocarditis and secondary cerebral emboli.[226–229] Hence the pathogenetic and pathophysiologic mechanisms in South American trypanosomiasis are twofold: (1) the acute myocarditis and acute meningoencephalitis that are seen during the acute stage of disease and (2) the chronic myocarditis with a risk of secondary cardiogenic embolism, this mechanism being one of the most important reasons for stroke (juvenile) in South America.[226]

Clinical Features

Romana's sign, a very well known clinical entity (unilateral conjunctivitis and periophthalmic edematous swelling), is highly suggestive of acute *T. cruzi* infection in endemic areas. Local lymphadenopathy is followed by generalized signs and symptoms of myalgia,

fever, headache, vomiting, diarrhea, and anorexia. Electrocardiographic (ECG) changes indicate acute myocarditis that may be fatal. Meningoencephalitis is seen rarely in adults; however, in children, in particular, in congenital infections, meningoencephalitis is more common, with a poor prognosis. The acute meningoencephalitis is not distinguishable clinically from other causes of meningoencephalitis. The incubation period may be as short as 2 weeks and as long as several months.[211] In immunocompromised patients, a meningoencephalitis and an ocular myositis have been described.[230–232]

Symptomatic (but also nonsymptomatic) acute *T. cruzi* infection is usually followed by a variable long phase without clinical signs of an infection. This indeterminate phase may last for life; in up to 30 percent of patients, however, after years or decades ECG abnormalities develop and typically include conduction disturbances such as right bundle-branch block and left anterior hemiblock. Any other kind of arrhythmia may be seen. Cardiomegaly with major parts of the myocardium being silent may ensue. Both the acute cardiac arrhythmias and the silent areas within the myocardium may be responsible for cardiogenic embolism leading to an acute stroke syndrome.[226] Regurgitation and dysphagia are early signs of megaesophagus (achalasia) due to neurogenic dysfunction (on the ganglion level) of the entire intestine.[212]

Diagnosis

The typical sequence of clinical signs and symptoms (see above) is highly suggestive of acute Chagas disease in a known endemic area. Similarly, the development of cardiomegaly and/or neurogenic megacolon, megaesophagus, etc. is equally highly suggestive of Chagas disease (chronic syndrome).[212] In the acute stage it is essential to investigate not only for the presence of a supporting history (exposure to triatomine bugs, blood transfusion, intake of contaminated food) but also for the presence of trypanosomes in peripheral blood and tissue.[233] In some acute cases, microscopy of thick blood films, microscopy of the puffy-coat layer after hematocritic centrifugation, or searching for trypomastigotes in centrifuged serum after blood coagulation may be helpful. In rare instances, direct microscopy of unstained wet blood films may be positive.[234] Serology, including the indirect hemagglutination test (IHAT), the indirect immunofluorescent antibody test (IFAT), and ELISA, should be positive if Chagas disease is present.[235]

After the acute-phase infection, the parasitemia subsides to very low levels; in an immunocompromised patient, however, the parasitemia may recur, which may be visualized in a thick blood film.[230] In the chronic phase, the only possibly effective parasitologic techniques are xenodiagnosis and blood culture. In xenodiagnosis, triatomine bugs from laboratory colonies feed on the patients and are allowed to take a blood meal. Some 3 weeks later the intestinal tract of each triatomine bug (up to 20 bugs may be necessary) is removed and examined microscopically for the presence of epimastigotes.[212] Using a blood agar base with physiologic saline overlay, cultures may be as sensitive as xenodiagnosis; however, contamination of the culture medium may interfere with the accuracy of diagnosis.[236] Xenodiagnosis is believed to be more robust than blood culture, both yielding similar positive results. PCR methods to detect parasite DNA have been tested; they are not yet sufficiently practical to replace parasitologic diagnostic procedures.[236–240]

Differential Diagnosis

Any form of acute meningoencephalitis, particularly viral meningoencephalitis, and even cerebral malaria may be mistaken for the acute stage of neurologic Chagas disease. Similarly, any kind of myocardial disease leading to cardiogenic embolism has to be considered in the differential diagnosis of secondary chagasic cerebral embolism.[6,212,226]

Therapy

Only two effective antiparasitic drugs are available for the treatment of *T. cruzi* infection. The synthetic nitrofuran nifurtimox is given in a dose of 8 to 10 mg/kg of body weight (in three divided doses) for a total of 3 months. A double dose may be necessary for children.[212,241] The reader is referred to a textbook of tropical medicine for detailed information about the many potential side effects that may interfere with compliance. The nitroimidazole benzonidazole is given in a dose of 5 to 7 mg/kg of body weight (in two divided daily doses) for 2 months; for children, a dosage of 10 mg/kg of body weight per day is recommended. Similarly, nifurtimox has many potential side effects. All acute cases, including trypanosomal meningoencephalitis, should be treated with benzonidazole as the drug of first choice. Early initiation of treatment is necessary to avoid potentially life-threatening complications (myocarditis or meningoencephalitis). Whether antiparasitic chemotherapy is necessary in chronic Chagas disease is controversial.[242] Cardiogenic embolism at this stage of disease is treated as any other type of (juvenile) embolic stroke.[226] Surgery constitutes a vital part of the best possible management of a megacolon, megaesophagus (achalasia), etc. For detailed information, the respective textbooks of surgery in tropical medicine are recommended. Most recently, adjunctive therapies have been discussed,[243] and several drugs have been found to influence positively—on an experimen-

tal level—acute Chagas disease (i.e., the antifungal ravuconazole).[244,245] In rare instances, spontaneous cure has been reported.[246]

Prevention

Chagas disease is a disease of poverty. Methods for controlling both triatomine bugs and transmission by blood transfusion, albeit having been proven highly effective, still are not available to all those in need.[247] Effective control would depend on improved housing, insecticide spraying, health education, and community participation. Serologic testing constitutes an integral part of monitoring the success of vector control. A joint prevention program has led to an 85 percent reduction of domestic transmission of *T. cruzi* in large areas of Brazil, and Chile and Uruguay have been rid of domestic transmission.[248]

▶ SLEEPING SICKNESS (HUMAN AFRICAN TRYPANOSOMIASIS)

History/Overview

In 1803, T. M. Winterbottom reported a febrile illness associated with cervical lymphadenopathy and lethargy. Almost 100 years later (1902), *Trypanosoma* spp. were demonstrated to be responsible for this condition, which was named *trypanosome fever of West Africa*. During the same time in eastern Africa (northern shores of Lake Victoria), an epidemic outbreak of "negro-lethargy" had been reported. With painstaking work, D. Bruce and D. Nabarro demonstrated *Trypanosoma* spp. in both CSF and blood of several patients with this disease. More than 50 years earlier (1847), David Livingstone had proposed that the tsetse fly was responsible for the transmission of "nagana," a disease that affected cattle in central Africa. It took many more years before Bruce and Nabarro demonstrated that *T. gambiense* was transmissible to monkeys via the bite of infected tsetse flies (*Glossina palpalis*). It took another 8 years until *T. rhodesiense* was discovered in Malawi and Zimbabwe. *T. rhodesiense* is transmitted to humans by the bite of *G. morsitans*. It is now known that human African trypanosomiasis is caused by protozoan parasites *T. brucei gambiense* in western and partially central Africa and *T. brucei rhodesiense* in eastern (southeastern) Africa.[249] Large-scale control and intervention programs led to a rapid decrease in the incidence and prevalence of this disease by the end of the 1960s; however, several major outbreaks have been reported from the Congo, Angola, Sudan, and Uganda throughout the past two decades, with incidence rates reaching more than 100,000 and prevalence figures going beyond 500,000.[250–252]

Epidemiology

Sleeping sickness is only found where *Glossina* spp. (tsetse flies) are endemic, i.e., from 14°N in western Africa (10°N in eastern Africa) reaching southward to 20°S (northern Botswana and Namibia). Climatic factors and typical vegetations determine the distribution of *Glossina* spp. Two groups of tsetse flies transmit sleeping sickness, the *G. palpalis* group transmitting *T. brucei gambiense* and the *G. morsitans* group transmitting *T. brucei rhodesiense*. In Uganda, *G. fuscipes* is responsible for the transmission of *T. brucei rhodesiense*. Sleeping sickness is endemic to more than 35 countries, with a prevalence of 500,000 patients and at least 50,000 new cases per year. It is believed that these figures are grossly underestimated, realistic estimates reaching figures as high as 500,000 new cases per year.[250,251,253–258] This estimate would correspond with the number of deaths, which the 2000 *World Health Report* estimated as 66,000 per year.[259] The economic and social impact of sleeping sickness is enormous, although this aspect has not been studied in detail. The *World Health Report* (2000) calculated the disability of adjusted life-years (DALYs) as being more than 2×10^6 (combining healthy life-years lost through premature death with those lost due to disability). After malaria and lymphatic filariosis, African sleeping sickness is the third most important parasitic disease in the world.[259] Single cases are imported to Europe or North America.[260]

T. brucei gambiense is endemic throughout western and central Africa and frequently is associated with foci of infection. Its transmission usually occurs near riverine vegetation, water collection points, forests, villages, and nearby rivers or lakes. The most intense transmission seems to occur at the end of the dry season when contact between humans and *G. palpalis* is most frequent. Once infected, a tsetse fly can transmit trypanosomes each time it bites. All isolates of *T. brucei gambiense* from humans in western and central Africa are comprised of six zymodemes.[261–264] Classic *T. brucei gambiense* of humans is not normally associated with endemicity in animals; thus animal reservoirs are highly unlikely, although early experimental studies have demonstrated that a wide range of domestic animals theoretically is capable of being infected with isolates of *T. brucei gambiense* from humans. Isoenzyme and DNA analysis forms a strong base for future detailed epidemiologic studies in this respect.

T. brucei rhodesiense is the causative agent of the more acute form of sleeping sickness seen primarily in eastern Africa from Uganda and Kenya (in the north) to Botswana in the south. Recent biochemical and molecular studies have identified two main strain groups of *T. brucei rhodesiens*; the Zambesi strain (from Zambia and Malawi), which is less virulent than the Usoga group (near the northern distribution areas).[252,265] It is mainly the *G. morsitans* group that is the vector. *G. morsitans* species prefer feeding on bovines and are not as strongly attracted to humans as the *G. palpalis* group. *G. morsitans* mainly feeds on humans when other hosts are not readily available. People whose activities or occupations bring them into close and frequent contact with the environment of *G. morsitans* are at particular risk of contracting East African trypanosomiasis (*T. brucei rhodesiense*). These groups include fishermen, honey gatherers, game wardens, hunters, and firewood collectors. In essence, *T. brucei rhodesiense* is a zoonosis with known reservoir hosts: domestic animals (cattle, sheep, goats) and a wide variety of game animals, including carnivores. Particular zymodemes of *T. brucei rhodesiense* are associated with particular mammalian hosts. In the mid-1980s in Busoga, Uganda, during an epidemic of *T. brucei rhodesiense* infection, there were 8000 cases per year. This epidemic is believed to have been caused by changes in agriculture. Political and economic constraints led to abandonment of cotton and coffee production, allowing certain weeds (e.g., *Lantana camara*) to grow abundantly. These weeds provided the perfect habitat for *G. fuscipes*, thus setting the stage for the epidemic. Cattle also were hosts in this epidemic.[266,267] Both *T. brucei* subspecies are transmitted to mammalian hosts by the bite of various tsetse flies (*Glossina* spp.) that transmit the infective metacyclic stage from the salivary gland into the bite wound after a complex developmental cycle within the fly.

Pathophysiology and Pathogenesis

Sleeping sickness produces multiple pathologic changes involving many organs. The disease is progressive, and its anatomic, histologic, physiologic, biochemical, and immunologic changes have been described extensively in textbooks of tropical medicine.[249] Briefly, after inoculation of the *T. brucei* subspecies into the human, a local inflammatory response with edema and mononuclear cell infiltration occurs at the site of infection; i.e., a trypanosomal chancre evolves. From there the trypanosomes spread via the lymphatic system into the lymphatic glands and to the bloodstream. Lymphadenopathy ensues, and trypanosomes can be found in lymph gland aspirates. The main feature of lymph node pathology is a vasculitis. General proliferation of the reticuloendothelial system follows, and focal necrosis with endothelial macrophages is seen. *T. brucei rhodesiense* may cause a pancarditis involving all layers of the heart. In experimental monkey infections, myocarditis and endocarditis have been observed regularly. Glomerulonephritis and pulmonary involvement (through intravascular proliferation, obstruction of capillaries with fibrosis, and collapse of the alveoli) follows. Involvement of the bone marrow results in anemia.[249,250]

After the trypanosomes invade the CNS, typical pathologic lesions are seen: progressive chronic leptomeningitis, involving mainly the Virchow Robin spaces as well as the vertex, followed by congestion and edema formation within the brain tissue.[6,249,268] Frequently, the ventricles are dilated, and perivascular cuffing (round cell infiltration) is seen throughout the parenchyma and meninges.[268] The invading cells are glia cells, lymphocytes, and plasma cells (so-called morula cells). Trypanosomes can be found within the brain, mainly in the frontal lobe and the brain stem. Finally, neural damage and demyelination set in. The organisms may invade the CSF via the choroidal plexus. Ventricular CSF more often than lumbar CSF yields the organisms.[269] Patients with sleeping sickness have a markedly altered plasma albumin-globulin ratio, IgM being increased in the early and first parasitemia. IgG production frequently is selectively suppressed. The CNS disease is associated with perivascular hemorrhages and petechiae due to vascular injury and coagulopathy with increased fibrinolysis and thrombocytopenia. The coagulopathy is most prominent in acute *T. brucei rhodesiense* disease.[249,250]

A major aspect in the pathogenesis of CNS trypansomiasis is the extremely complex and complicated immunopathology.[270,271] The major surface protein of bloodstream trypanosomes is the variant surface glycoprotein (VSG). This has the capacity to protect invariant constituents of the outer membrane from the patient's immune system. Each trypanosome genotype contains up to 1000 different *VSG* genes. At any given time, only one single *VSG* gene is actively transcribed at a telomeric expression site. Thus the antigenic conversion happening by duplicative transposition (gene conversion), by nonduplicative transposition (reciprocal recombination), and by in situ telomeric activation occurs in a spontaneous nonprogrammed nonforeseeable manner. The primary component of the antibody response to VSG is a T-cell-independent IgM response, the VSG coat (on intact trypanosomes) acting as a T-cell-independent antigen, whereas nonvariant "buried" T-cell epitopes are presented to T cells only after phagocytosis of the trypanosomes. This T-cell-mediated response is crucial for the typical cytokine response profile.[270,271,273–277] The successive peaks of recurring parasitemias are triggered by trypanosomes expressing immunologically different VSGs. The immune responses to a *Trypanosoma* infection are twofold: a nonspecific polyclonal activation of B cells and a generalized suppression of some humoral and cellular immune functions. In the CNS, autoantibodies against nervous tissue elements such as myelin basic protein, gangliosides, etc. have been reported.[277] There is evidence for the syn-

thesis of nitric oxide by activated macrophages, a fact that may be involved significantly in immunosuppression, as typically seen in patients with African trypanosomiasis.[278] For detailed description of the complex activation of the cytokine network during African trypanosomiasis, the reader is referred to specific textbooks on tropical medicine and to the excellent review by Rhind and Shek.[279]

Clinical Features

T. brucei gambiense and *T. brucei rhodesiense* differ in biology, vector epidemiology, clinical signs and symptoms, and treatment. The sequence of clinical stages, however, is similar in both *T. brucei gambiense* and *T. brucei rhodesiense*, although the time course differs considerably. After a variable incubation period, the patient develops a local chancre, which is followed by the hemolymphatic stage and finally the chronic meningoencephalitic stage of disease. The clinical signs and symptoms of *T. brucei gambiense* and *T. brucei rhodesiense* infection are described separately, the former usually running a chronic course of disease and the latter typically being a much more acute infection with CNS involvement developing after only a few weeks.[249,250]

First Stage of T. brucei gambiense (Hemolymphatic Stage)

The incubation period is usually less than 3 weeks, and then a chancre develops at the site of inoculation. The disease progresses with highly nonspecific signs; irregular fever, varying in cycles of hours to days, reflects the immune response to the ever-changing VSGs.[270,271] Typically, lymphadenopathy, headache, myalgia, and general malaise occur in various degrees of intensity during these cycles of irregular fever. In almost 90 percent of patients, the lymphadenopathy is most prominent on the nuchal/posterior cervical region (Winterbottom's sign). This phase may last for months. Finally, fever bouts become less frequent (now parasites are more difficult to find in the blood). There may be signs of endocrine dysfunction, such as amenorrhea, impotence, and anemia. Pruritis and facial edema are observed frequently. Typical clinical findings of *T. brucei gambiense* sleeping sickness are listed in Table 17-13. These data are compiled from a prospective, controlled clinical trial on sleeping sickness treatment with melarsoprol in Angola.[280]

First Stage of T. brucei rhodesiense (Hemolymphatic Stage)

In *T. brucei rhodesiense* infection, the inoculation chancre (trypanosomal chancre), which is frequently invisible, develops within 1 to 2 weeks after the tsetse fly bite. This chancre may be circumscribed, up to 5 cm in diameter, and disappears within 3 weeks. Typically,

▶ **TABLE 17-13.** SIGNS AND SYMPTOMS OF *T. B. GAMBIENSE* SLEEPING SICKNESS

	n/N*	Percent
Lymphadenopathy	425	85.0
Headache	349	69.8
General motor weakness	256	51.2
Menstruation absent†	66/214	30.8
Diurnal somnolence	143	28.6
Nocturnal insomnia	143	28.6
Aggressiveness	116	23.2
Tremors	95	19.0
Pruritus	87	17.4
Disturbed appetite	51	10.2
Unusual behavior	48	9.6
Fever (temp. >37.5°C)	47	9.4
Hepatomegaly	35	7.0
Abnormal movements‡	29	5.8
Splenomegaly	25	5.0
Epileptiform attacks§	14	2.8
Impaired speech	7	1.4
Inability to walk unaided	6	1.2

*If not indicated, *N* is 500.
†Considers only women who have not yet reached menopause.
‡Preventing the patient from performing daily tasks.
§History reported by patient.
SOURCE: *Used with permission from ref. 280.*

regional lymphadenopathy is present, and fever and parasitemia appear at this time. Generally, the parasites are much easier to visualize in the blood than in the *T. brucei gambiense* form of disease. In contrast, cervical lymphadenopathy (Winterbottom's sign) is less common in *T. brucei rhodesiense* disease; however, generalized lymphadenopathy is typical. Ophthalmic involvement includes keratitis and conjunctivitis.

Second Stage (Meningoencephalitic Stage)

CNS invasion by the trypanosomes marks the beginning of the meningoencephalitic stage of disease. Typically, trypanosomes cross the blood-brain barrier at the level of the choroid plexus, thalamus, and pineal and hypophyseal regions. This preference may explain, at least in part, the initial and principal neurologic signs and symptoms. Whereas the interval between the start of the infection and the meningoencephalitic stage in *T. brucei gambiense* infection may range from months to 2 years (even longer periods have been observed), the interval between the start of the infection and the meningoencephalitic stage in *T. brucei rhodesiense* infection is in the range of weeks to a few months. The duration of the meningoencephalitic stage ranges from months to 1 year in *T. brucei gambiense* infection. A patient with the meningoencephalitic stage of *T. bru-*

cei rhodesiense infection usually dies within 6 to 9 months. Headache is one of the major and initial features of this stage, frequently being unresponsive to analgesics. Motor function becomes progressively impaired due to abnormal movements, tremor, motor weakness (pareses), and rarely, ataxia (see Table 17-13). Speech becomes dysphasic. The abnormal movements and tremor may resemble Parkinson's syndrome. At this stage the patient shows aggressiveness, unusual behavior, and finally, dementia.[281] The diurnal somnolence seen in more than a quarter of patients is usually accompanied by nocturnal insomnia.[282] Finally, the patient becomes comatose. Aspiration pneumonia is frequently the eventual and immediate cause of death. It is generally accepted that sleeping sickness is ultimately fatal in all untreated patients.[6,249,250,280] In the second stage of *T. brucei rhodesiense* infection, severe myocardial and pericardial involvement may be the prominent clinical feature, even before clearcut signs and symptoms of CNS involvement have developed.[250]

Diagnosis

The direct detection of trypanosomes in the blood is diagnostic. The direct detection of the parasites in blood is the most difficult in *T. brucei gambiense* infection.[249,250,283–285] Serologic methods, usually employing the card agglutination test for trypanosomiasis (CATT), confirms the diagnosis. Recently, alternative serologic tests such as the card indirect antigen test for trypanosomiasis (CIAAT), the rapid latex agglutination test, the immunofluorescence (IF) test, the indirect hemagglutination assay (IHA), and ELISA, as well as different PCR methods, have been developed.[286–296] In the case of a positive blood slide result or positive serologic result, a lumbar puncture is done to allow stage determination.[249,250] Trypanosomes must be searched for in the CSF but also in blood and lymph node and/or bone marrow aspirates and even ascites fluid.[250,297,298] Several techniques are in use to detect trypanosomes in blood: blood films for direct detection of trypanosomes (Fig. 17-3) and concentration methods, such as the microhematocrit centrifugation technique (m-HCT), the miniature anion-exchange centrifugation technique (m-AECT), and the quantitative puffy-coat (QPC) technique.[297,298] For analysis of the lymph node aspirate, a wet preparation of the fluid obtained from enlarged lymph nodes is examined directly. Such a biologic material may be inoculated in vivo in guinea pigs, suckling rats, or mice. In vivo culture systems can be used for isolating trypanosomes from infected patients.[250]

Since melarsoprol is the only drug available for second-stage disease in *T. brucei rhodesiense* infection and carries a high risk of potentially life-threatening side effects, the exact and correct determination of the stage of disease is crucial before initiating antiparasitic che-

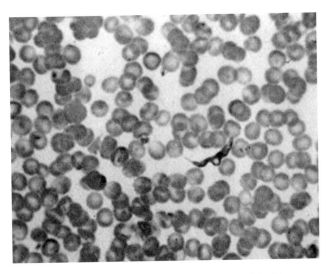

Figure 17-3. Thin blood film (Giemsa stain): *Trypanosoma brucei rhodesiense.*

motherapy. Examination of the CSF is the only way to determine the stage of disease. Parasites can be seen during white cell counting, but concentration techniques (e.g., double centrifugation) enhance the ability to visualize the parasite directly. Clearcut criteria for second-stage infection are detection of trypanosomes in the CSF and a raised leukocyte count of more than 5 cells/μm.[250,299] An increased CSF protein concentration is also a useful criterion for staging but has less of a predictive value compared with the white blood cell count. In the near future, a latex agglutination field test for the quantification of IgM in CSF may become useful for determination of the stage of infection.[300,301] Most recently, new diagnostic techniques have been described: a PCR for detecting *T. brucei rhodesiense* using a primer derived from the serum resistance-associated gene showing a very high specificity and sensitivity[302] and a novel *T. brucei* isolation method with the use of Kit for in vitro isolation (KIVI) based on rodent inoculations and allowing for *T. brucei* genotype selection.[303]

Differential Diagnoses

In first stage African trypanosomiasis, any cause of protracted or recurrent febrile illness (e.g., malaria, typhus, typhoid fever, relapsing fever, etc.) should be considered. Any infectious and noninfectious cause of lymphadenopathy also may be included in the differential diagnosis. In second-stage disease, any form of subacute or chronic meningitis/meningoencephalitis (e.g., tuberculosis, cryptococcosis, syphilis, etc.) may have similar signs and symptoms,[6] even masquerading as pulmonary infectious diseases.[304]

Treatment

The chemotherapeutic management of *T. brucei gambiense* and *T. brucei rhodesiense* infections is listed in Table 17-14.[6,9,249,250,305–309] Apart from the capacity of the drug to penetrate the blood-brain barrier, the following factors are important with respect to planning drug therapy: geographic origin; suspected subspecies; economic constraints, including the duration of therapy; and hospital stay.[310] There are four drugs available for the treatment of African trypanosomiasis; however, only melarsoprol and eflornithine penetrate the blood-brain barrier. Alternative chemotherapeutic agents should be chosen only if there is a relapse, treatment failure, or life-threatening side effects. If after two courses of melarsoprol the patient still has signs and symptoms of meningoencephalitis, the only alternative is nitrofurazone or nifurtimox. New regimens of suramin and melarsoprol have been proposed, during which simultaneous administration of these drugs is recommended to alleviate side effects and enhance efficacy.[309–311] Most recently, and for the first time in the past 20 years since the introduction of eflornithine,[303,308] new trypanocidal compounds have been developed. Megazol,[312] a pentamidine analogue, can be administered orally.[313] There are dicationic compounds related to pentamidine,[314] aromatic diamidines and dimidazolines,[315] conformationally restricted pentamidine congeners,[316] and melarsoprol metabolites, e.g., melarsen oxide.[317]

After "successful therapy," every patient with a meningoencephalitic stage of African trypanosomiasis needs follow-up lumbar puncture after 3, 6, 12, 18, and 24 months. The side effects and toxic reactions of the trypanocidal drugs are listed in Table 17-15.[6,9,249,250] It is mainly the risk of polyneuropathy and the potentially life-threatening encephalopathy that require extreme caution when using the trivalent arsenic melarsoprol.[6,249,250] Up to 10 percent of melarsoprol-treated patients develop a potentially life-threatening encephalopathy that affects mainly the white matter and the brain stem, leading to severe hemorrhagic abnormalities. The subcurative dosage[318] and the speed of drug application[319] have been incriminated in the development of the encephalopathy. Upregulation of TNF-α, interleukins, and a macrophage inflammatory protein (MIP-1) have been reported in a mouse model.[320,321] Up to 5 percent of patients with melarsoprol encephalopathy die from it. Corticosteroids may reduce the incidence of this complication. In addition, the severe diarrhea associated with melarsoprol and with nifurtimox therapy may limit the use of these drugs and also may cause a life-threatening disturbance of water and electrolyte metabolism, finally leading to death in the typical sleeping sickness with limited resources. The same applies to nephrotoxicity.[249,250]

► **TABLE 17-14.** ANTIMICROBIAL CHEMOTHERAPY IN AFRICAN TRYPANOSOMIASIS

Indication (Pathogenic Agent)	Drug	Dose	Duration

1. *T. brucei gambiense* hemolymphatic stage	Eflornithine	Adults:
		100 mg/kg bw IV qid
		  followed by
		75 mg/kg bw PO qid
		Children:
		150 mg/kg bw IV qid
		  followed by
		75 mg/kg bw PO qid
			2 weeks
			
			4 weeks
			
			2 weeks
			
			4 weeks

2. *T. b. gambiense* meningoencephalitic stage; see 1.			
3. *T. b. gambiense* hemolymphatic stage (alternative therapy)	Pentamidine (base)	4 mg/kg bw IM daily	10 days

4. *T. b. gambiense* hemolymphatic stage (in case of pentamidine resistance)	Suramine	Test dosage: 4 mg/kg bw IV
		  (in 10% solution)
		10 mg/kg bw IV
		20 mg/kg bw IV
		(Max. single dose: 100 mg)
			On day 1
			
			On day 3
			On days 5, 11, 17,
			  23, and 29

5. *T. b. gambiense* meningoencephalitic stage (alternative therapy)	Preceding 3 or 4 followed by Melarosprol	1.8 mg/kg bw IV 2.1 mg/kg bw IV 2.4 mg/kg bw IV 2.7 mg/kg bw IV 3.0 mg/kg bw IV 3.3 mg/kg bw IV 3.6 mg/kg bw IV	On day 1 On day 2 On day 3 On day 10 On day 11 On day 12 On days 19, 20, and 21
6. *T. b. rhodesiense* hemolymphatic stage	See 4		
7. *T. b. rhodesiense* meningoencephalitic stage	Combination of 4 and 5		
8. Relapse of meningoencephalitis (*T. b. gambiense* or *rhodesiense*)	Repeat 5		
9. In case of Melarsoprol resistance	Nifurtimox	Adults: 2–2.5 mg/kg bw PO qid 11–16 years: 3–4 mg/kg bw PO qid <11 years: 4–5 mg/kg bw PO qid Experimental in adults: Up to 7.5 mg/kg bw PO every 6 months	 3 months 3 months 3 months 1 month

SOURCE: Adapted from ref. 6.

Adjunctive Therapies

Prophylactic steroid therapy (e.g., 40 mg prednisolone daily) is recommended to prevent the occurrence of life-threatening encephalopathy from melarsoprol therapy.[320] In an animal model, the concomitant use of aza-thioprine therapy has reduced both the frequency and the severity of the arsenic encephalopathy.[322] Great care has to be taken to maintain sufficient nutrition, to prevent aspiration and treat aspiration pneumonia, to recognize psychotic attacks as being part of the disease or therapy, to treat seizures and their complications, and

▶ **TABLE 17-15.** SIDE EFFECTS/ADVERSE EVENTS OF TRYPANOSOMAL CHEMOTHERAPY

Medication	Clinical Entity	Frequency*
Eflornithine	Reversible bone marrow depression	Up to 50%
	Epileptic seizures	Only in case of high dosage
Suramin	Idiosyncrasy (hypotension, shock)	++
	Fever	++
	Arthralgia	++
	Pruritus	++
	Nephrotoxicity	++
	Polyneuropathy	+
Pentamidine	Sterile abscess (if given IM)	+
	Hypotension	++
	Hypoglycemia	++
	Nephrotoxicity	(+)
	Hepatotoxicity	(+)
	Bone marrow depression	(+)
Melarsoprol	Diarrhea	+++
	Life-threatening water and electrolyte disturbances	+
	Exfoliative dermatitis	(+)
	Hepatitis	+
	Polyneuropathy	++ (10%)
	Encephalopathy	++ (10%)
Nifurtimox	Anorexia	++
	Weight loss	++
	Diarrhea	+
	Exanthema	+
	Psychotic reactions	+
	Polyneuropathy	+

*+++ = very frequent; ++ = frequent; + = rare; (+) = single case report.

to regulate the disorganized sleep-wake rhythm with sleep medication where indicated. Careful monitoring for any complications of the disease and the therapy is necessary.

Complications

Both the complications of the disease and trypanocidal chemotherapeutics may be life-threatening. Neurologic complications include acute psychotic attacks, epileptic seizures, and cardioembolic cerebral ischemia as a complication of myocarditis (*T. brucei rhodesiense*). A relapse of the meningoencephalitis may occur despite adequate chemotherapy in up to 10 percent of second-stage trypanosomiasis patients and is seen more frequently in men than in women.[323] In addition to these neurologic complications of *T. brucei rhodesiense* infections, an acute myocarditis has the potential of a fatal course. Acute cardiac failure and malignant cardiac arrhythmias are the most frequent and most dangerous cardiac complications.[324] A pseudobulbar paralysis or direct involvement of the brain stem may aggravate the risk of aspiration and aspiration pneumonia, adding to loss of weight (in addition to the inherent anorexia), marasmus, and cachexia.[249,250] Patients with systemic African trypanosomiasis, particularly second-stage try-

panosomiasis, frequently show signs of humoral and cellular immunodeficiency. This immunosuppression may lead to superimposed infectious complications. Patients with systemic African trypanosomiasis do not react appropriately with antibody production in response to immunization (e.g. tetanus, cholera, salmonellosis).[249,250]

Prognosis

Without trypanocidal chemotherapy, both African trypanosomiases are fatal, although single case reports of patients with chronic parasitemia without signs and symptoms of disease and spontaneous cures have been reported. Despite appropriate trypanocidal chemotherapy, 10 percent of patients with trypanosomal meningoencephalitis develop a relapse.[325] The course and duration of *T. brucei gambiense* infection usually are protracted and may last up to 6 years. In contrast to this, a *T. brucei rhodesiense* infection usually runs an acute/subacute course very rarely exceeding 6 to 9 months. Patients with *T. brucei gambiense* infection typically die from the meningoencephalitis. Patients with *T. brucei rhodesiense* infection frequently die from complications of myocarditis or pancarditis.[249,250] Despite appropriate chemotherapy, there is a 10 to 12 percent mortality rate from *T. brucei rhodesiense* infection. Detailed follow-up examinations with neurologic, neuropsychological, and psychiatric long-term sequelae are lacking. Nevertheless, it must be assumed that both psychological and psychiatric long-term sequelae, as well as focal neurologic deficits and seizures as the consequence of meningoencephalitis, constitute an enormous potential for long-term morbidity. The extent to which the severe arsenic encephalopathy or polyneuropathy contributes to overall long-term sequelae has not been determined.

Prevention

Exposition prophylaxis is the mainstay and most important means to prevent African trypanosomiasis. Tsetse flies are exophageous and highly active during the daytime. For this reason, it is wise to avoid endemic areas; if this is not possible, appropriate clothing (long sleeves, etc.) should be worn and repellents used during the time spent in the endemic area.

In western Africa, chemoprophylaxis with pentamidine (4 mg/kg of body weight intramuscularly in a single dose) exists. However, this is only applicable for short-term travel to endemic areas (maximum 2 to 4 months). The prophylactic administration of suramine (20 mg/kg of body weight intravenously in a single dose) is less reliable and provides protection for a maximum of 2 months.[249,250] Individual chemoprophylaxis is discouraged because this may contribute to development of resistance, a fact that is extremely delicate in view of the scarcity and paucity of trypanocidal drugs. In a few instances, the surprising development of a second stage, i.e., meningoencephalitis, without the typical trypanosomal chancre and without the signs and symptoms of the hemolymphatic stage has been reported in patients taking chemoprophylactic therapy (most likely due to subcurative levels of pentamidine or suramine).[250] This may complicate or even hamper timely diagnosis and treatment.

No immunoprophylaxis (neither active nor passive) exists, although promising targets for the development of a parasite-specific broad-spectrum vaccine may have been identified.[326] With respect to control and eradication programs of African trypanosomiasis, the reader is referred to specialized tropical medicine literature.[327] Identification of animal reservoirs[328,329] and their appropriate management are crucial mainstays of all control programs.[330]

▶ TOXOPLASMOSIS

History/Overview

T. gondii, one of the most frequent parasites of humans, is usually harmless for the immunocompetent person.

However, in the immunocompromised patient—in former years mainly in those with HIV infection and in recent years more frequently in organ recipients than in AIDS patients—this protozoon may cause serious and life-threatening disease particularly of the CNS and the eye. Furthermore, in the fetus whose mother was infected for the first time during her pregnancy, toxoplasmosis may cause severe disease. Surveillance programs during pregnancy, including serologic examinations and adequate chemotherapy, have been successful in preventing intrauterine infection.[331,332] In 1908, the organism was first described in a North African rodent, but it took another 15 years for an association to be made with human disease, when parasitic cysts were found in the retina of a child with hydrocephalus and microophthalmia. In 1937, the significance of congenital toxoplasmosis was demonstrated, and in 1940, a postnatal infection was discovered and described by Pinkerton and Weinmann.[333] In 1948, Sabin and Feldmann developed the first reliable serologic assay, the so-called dye test.[334] Elucidation of the prevalence and clinical spectrum of the infection was then possible.[331,332]

Epidemiology

The prevalence of antibodies against *T. gondii* is proportional to the age of the population, clearly indicating that infection is acquired throughout life.[331] Although there are marked geographic variations, most likely due to different climates, cat contact, and diet (eating uncooked or raw meat),[335,336] *T. gondii* is prevalent throughout the entire world. In rural African countries, seroprevalence rates of up to 60 percent have been found.[337] In many northern and western countries, the prevalence of *T. gondii* disease has declined over the past few decades, most likely due to the practice of deep freezing meat and intensive farming techniques separating cats from livestock.[331] *T. gondii* is the causative agent of CNS toxoplasmosis. It is a coccidian parasite with a sexual cycle in the intestinal epithelium of the definitive host (e.g., cats) and an asexual cycle in secondary hosts, e.g., rodents, birds, and mammals, including humans.[331,332,335,338]

Pathophysiology and Pathogenesis

T. gondii is the only species of the genus *Toxoplasma*. In the late 1960s, the full life cycle of *T. gondii* was elucidated.[335] The characteristic form of *T. gondii* is the crescent-shaped trophozoite (6 μm in length). The sexual and asexual multiplication (gamogony and schizogony) of *T. gondii* occurs within the enterocytes of the definitive host, i.e., cats and other felides.[331,332] Finally, the sporogony leads to the formation of cysts that are excreted in the feces of the felide. In the felide, even an asexual multiplication by endodyogeny with formation of pseudocysts and cysts—after generalized tissue infection—may take place.[332] The oocysts sporulate within a few days and form the infectious sporocysts, which may remain viable for more than 1 year in moist and humid surroundings (soil, etc.). These oocysts are ingested by secondary hosts (natural intermediate host, e.g., mice or other preys of cats), in which asexual multiplication by endodyogony with formation of pseudocysts and cysts (after generalized tissue infection) takes place. These secondary/natural intermediate hosts do not excrete *T. gondii* but are important for maintaining the "wild" life cycle of *T. gondii* (being the favorite prey of cats). Cat feces may contaminate salads and vegetables that may be ingested by food animals such as sheep, pigs, etc.[331,332] Thus infection of humans can take place via three routes: ingestion of sporocysts in cat feces–contaminated soil or in unwashed salads and raw vegetables, ingestion of tissue cysts in raw or undercooked meat (lamb meat or pork), and theoretically, via organ transplantation.

Up to a third of the normal population carries within their brain or their musculature, cysts of *T. gondii*. Such cysts vary in size; they may be as small as 5 μm or as large as up to 300 μm. They are an infected cell of the definitive host into which the protozoon has intruded and multiplied, finally containing hundreds (possibly thousands) of bradyzoites. It is the membrane of the original host cell that delineates this cyst from the surrounding tissue, thus explaining the fact that the organism does not activate any immunologic or other defense mechanisms. As long as the host's immune system is intact, such cysts, even in the CNS (as seen in 30 to 50 percent of healthy persons in central Europe), are not harmful.[331] Every carrier of such cysts has immunity against *T. gondii*. It is this immunity that has an important advantage to females of childbearing age because this immunity protects the fetus from a diaplacentar infection in case of a reinfection during pregnancy. However, in immunosuppressed organ transplant recipients or HIV-infected individuals, these cysts may rupture and result in severe CNS disease.[332,338–344] An immunosuppressed pregnant woman loses the protection against *T. gondii* cysts, which may result in infection of the fetus.[329]

If tissue cysts or sporocysts are ingested by humans, the bradyzoites are released from the cysts within the intestine, enter epithelial cells of the intestine, and undergo an asexual multiplication. The bradyzoites now multiply with "high speed," with binary fission taking place within a few hours; this stage is named the *tachyzoite stage*.[331] In humans there is never sexual multiplication; thus oocyst formation will never occur. For this reason, humans never excrete oocysts in their feces. However, the tachyzoites invade the blood vessels and are distributed in various organs, including musculature and brain, where they multiply asexually, finally forming tissue pseudocysts (cells containing the parasitophorous vacuole).[336] Within days and after several multiplication cycles, the host's immune system enforces the transformation of the tachyzoites into bradyzoites, which leads to cyst formation. Periodic excystation may occur, controlled by mechanisms that are not yet established. Possibly cell-mediated immune mechanisms play an important role, e.g., activated macrophages and T cells, interferon-γ, and various cytokines inducing an effective immune response. Specific antibodies—in the presence of complement—eliminate extracellular parasites.[331]

Pathology

In the immunocompetent adult, lymphadenopathy, characterized by follicular hyperplasia and infiltration with mononuclear cells, is seen after primary infection with *T. gondii*.[331] In the immunosuppressed patient, in association with either primary infection or reactivation of latent infection, there are areas of central necrosis with surrounding astrocytosis in brain parenchyma. Pseudocysts are seen at the necrotic margins of the infected areas. In addition to these pseudocysts and areas of necrosis, thromboses of capillaries, venuoles, and arterioles are seen.[345,346] Congenital toxoplasmosis frequently is localized to the CNS but also may be a generalized disease. Within the cerebral tissue, encephalitic changes, infarctions, and necrosis are seen within the cortex, periventricular areas, and basal ganglia. Focal calcifications and glial nodules may be seen, as well as zones of necrosis. In addition to the pathologic changes within brain tissue, obstruction of the aqueduct of Sylvius results in hydrocephalus.[347] Frequently, in congenital toxoplasmosis there is infection of ocular tissue, destruction of the retina, proliferation of pigment, and occasionally, parasites at the lesion margins.[348]

Clinical Features

The clinical manifestations of *Toxoplasma* infection result in three different groups of infected persons: postnatal toxoplasmosis in the immunocompetent, postnatal toxoplasmosis in the immunosuppressed, and prenatal *T. gondii* infection (in primarily infected pregnant women).

Infection of the Immunocompetent Patient[349]

Most immunocompetent individuals infected by *T. gondii* do not show any signs and symptoms, the acute infection passing unnoticed. Patients who develop a discernible illness present with painless lymphadenopathy (Piringer-Kuchinka), sometimes accompanied by slight fever. Rarely, lymphadenopathy is accompanied by malaise and myalgias. The duration of the illness usually does not exceed weeks to a few months. The differential diagnosis is cytomegalovirus infection, Epstein-Barr virus infection, and lymphoma. Very rarely, a pericarditis can be the presenting clinical feature in the immunocompetent patient with acute *T. gondii* infection. Regularly, no CNS or peripheral nervous system (PNS) symptoms are present.

Postnatal Toxoplasmosis/Congenital T. gondii Infection[331,332,350,351]

The incidence and presentation of acute toxoplasmosis in the pregnant woman does not differ from those seen in the general population; this means that many infections may be asymptomatic unless close serologic surveillance during pregnancy is done. If a pregnant woman has been infected—for the first time in her life—with *T. gondii*, the tachyzoites spread throughout the entire body, including the placenta, and may lead to diaplacentar infection of the embryo or fetus, respectively. During the early phase of pregnancy (first trimester), the likelihood that maternal infection leads to infection of the embryo is very low, the probability rising continuously and reaching more than 80 percent immediately before birth.[331] The severity of disease, however, is indirectly proportional to the gestational age. If in the early embryonal period a diaplacentar infection takes place, in most cases the embryo dies. It is accepted that the majority of such early infections go unnoticed because an abortion occurs before the woman realizes that she is pregnant or the causal connection between infection and spontaneous abortion is not recognized. If the diaplacentar infection is contracted in the last trimenon, the newborn may seem healthy. However, a prenatal infection with *T. gondii* may lead to clinical manifestations during the first years of life, e.g., retinochoroiditis or even cerebral involvement. The features of congenital toxoplasmosis not necessarily already present at birth include hydrocephalus, mental retardation, and intracerebral calcifications. Myositis, myocarditis, hepatitis, and pneumonia may be present.[349,350] Some children born with congenital infection may develop ocular disease, e.g., chorioretinitis, in later life, even up to 20 years after birth, irrespective of the clinical status at birth.[351]

Postnatal Infection in the Immunosuppressed

Prior to the introduction of effective antiviral therapy, toxoplasmosis was the most common cause of focal brain lesions and one of the most frequent opportunistic infections in patients with HIV infection/AIDS.[352–354] Since introduction of highly active antiretroviral therapy, cerebral toxoplasmosis is not seen as frequently in HIV-infected individuals. Now toxoplasmosis represents a life-threatening complication in organ transplant recipients.[355] Cerebral toxoplasmosis in association with solid-organ transplantation is seen only in a seronegative organ recipient who has been given an organ containing viable cysts of *T. gondii*, i.e., from a seropositive donor. Since the frequency of such infections is higher in patients having received organs in which pseudocysts or cysts are common, such as the heart, toxoplasmosis is seen most frequently after heart transplantation. The disseminated disease, which is usually seen 1 or 2 months after transplantation, is heralded by fever, signs of respiratory failure, and finally, deterioration of consciousness due to acute meningoencephalitis. In patients with bone marrow transplantation, cerebral toxoplasmosis may occur and is usually due to reactivation of the recipient's previously latent chronic infection.[342] Fever, pulmonary dysfunction, and focal or generalized CNS signs and symptoms usually occur between 15 and 150 days after transplantation.[355]

In HIV-infected individuals, most cases result from reactivation of a chronic, previously unnoticed infection; in particular, when the individual's T-cell immune function has been grossly impaired. The main features of cerebral toxoplasmosis in an AIDS patient are persistent headache; focal neurologic signs and symptoms; focal, sometimes also generalized, epileptic seizures; deterioration of mental status; and finally, impairment of consciousness.[338,356] Movement disorders[357] and spinal involvement have been reported occasionally.[358] Retinochorioiditis and pulmonary disease have been described accompanying CNS toxoplasmosis.[338]

Diagnosis

The diagnosis of a *T. gondii* infection is impeded in a twofold way: many *T. gondii* infections do not lead to clinical signs and symptoms, and the pathogenic agent is usually not excreted from the human host. *T. gondii* cysts are harbored by the infected patient within muscular or cerebral tissue; these cysts remain there without eliciting focal lesions, focal inflammation, or clinical signs and symptoms. This means that direct proof of the invasive nature of *T. gondii* would necessitate a biopsy.[332,359] To determine if an intrauterine infection has occurred in a pregnant woman, examination of the amniotic fluid by amniocentesis for the pathogenic agent can be done.[332,360] This is done by microscopic examination of the amniotic fluid (after centrifugation). This has a relatively low yield. PCR or the mouse inoculation test has a much higher probability of a positive result.[360,361]

The main diagnostic procedure in CNS toxoplasmosis is serologic proof of infection. Today the most frequently used tests are the indirect immunofluorescence test, various enzyme immune tests to detect all classes of antibodies (IgG, IgM, and IgA), the Western blot (immunoblot), and the test of avidity. The presence of specific IgG antibodies indicates prior exposure to the parasites and the potential for reactivation in the immunosuppressed state. Specific IgM, IgA, or low-avidity IgG is associated with a more recent infection of an immunocompetent individual.[331,359,362] The Sabin Feldmann dye test is still the gold standard in the serodiagnosis of *Toxoplasma* infection.[331] In the immunocompromised patient, neuroimaging is the most important technique to visualize lesions of cerebral toxoplasmosis.[363] Histologic examination may be helpful. The sensitivity of the biopsy is improved if immunohistochemical studies are used.[359,364]

In the immunocompromised patient in whom serologic responses may be altered, thus not allowing for routine serodiagnosis, detection of antigen using ELISA and agglutination systems can confirm the diagnosis. PCR in CSF or, even better, in biopsied material represents a considerable advance as compared with the just-mentioned antigen-detection methods (ELISA, agglutination systems).[365,366] Cell-mediated immunity can be measured by in vitro tests and by a skin test, but this has not found wide use in general clinical practice.[331] If in the immunocompromised patient typical neuroimaging abnormalities are found, and if biopsy is not possible or not advisable, a therapeutic trial of antiparasitic drugs may be used to confirm the diagnosis of cerebral toxoplasmosis *ex iuvantibus*. This method, of course, should be employed only in profoundly immunosuppressed patients in whom any invasive method cannot be performed.

Differential Diagnosis

In the immunocompetent patient, a lymphadenopathy of any other origin (including other parasites, lymphoma, cytomegalovirus, HIV, or Epstein-Barr virus infection) may be mistaken for toxoplasmosis. The same applies to the rare case of a toxoplasmic pericarditis.[359] Similarly, in congenital/postnatal infection, any other form of intrauterine infection (such as rubella, lues, etc.) may be mistaken. In the immunocompromised individual, the differential diagnosis includes bacterial brain abscesses, metastases, cryptococcal infection, and CNS tuberculosis, as well as intracranial lymphoma. The rare event of acute toxoplasmic encephalitis may be mistaken for bacterial cerebritis or viral encephalitis.[364]

Treatment

Encysted forms (cysts, pseudocysts) are not treatable by any of the antiparasitic drugs in use for toxoplasmosis. Therefore, complete eradication of the parasite can never be achieved, and treatment is directed against the tachyzoite form.[331] The following antiparasitic agents are available: spiramycin, pyrimethamine, sulfonamide, clindamycin, azithromycin, and/or the combination drug trimethoprim-sulfamethoxazole.[9,331,332] Spiramycin is a protein synthesis inhibitor with few side effects; its diaplacentar passage, however, is rather limited.

Pyrimethamine and the sulfonamides are folic acid antagonists with possibly severe side effects (bone marrow suppression). Folinic acid is necessary as adjunctive therapy to counteract these side effects.

In animal studies, pyrimethamine has been shown to be teratogenic. Both pyrimethamine and sulfonamides penetrate the placental barrier easily. Clindamycin has the capacity to penetrate the choroidea readily but passes through the blood-brain barrier less easily. However, the combination of this drug with pyrimethamine and sulfonamides (e.g., in AIDS patients) allows for reduction of the dosage of pyrimethamine and sulfonamides, thus reducing the severity and frequency of severe side effects.[9]

Therapy of the Immunocompetent Patient

Anti-toxoplasma chemotherapy is usually not indicated in an immunocompetent patient with a first episode of toxoplasmosis. If, however, for whatever reason therapy is considered (in an unusually severe or protracted course of disease, lymphadenitis), sulfadiazine (2 g/d) in combination with pyrimethamine (25 mg/d) is given orally. Folinic acid (15 mg twice weekly) is given to counteract bone marrow toxicity. As an alternative, azithromycin (3 mg/kg of body weight daily for 10 days) may be used.[331,332]

Therapy of the Pregnant Woman

The macrolide antibiotic spiramycin is given in a dose of 3 g/day during confinement—as a prophylactic measure—to possibly reduce the risk of diaplacentar passage of the parasite. If amniocentesis (or ultrasound) has confirmed fetal infection, antiparasitic therapy is indicated to prevent or at least reduce the severity of prenatal/congenital toxoplasmosis. Sulfadiazine (50 to 100 mg/kg daily) in combination with pyrimethamine (0.5 to 1.0 mg/kg of body weight daily) is given for 3 weeks, followed by another 3 weeks of therapy with spiramycin (3 g/d). These alternating therapeutic cycles are to be repeated until delivery. Pyrimethamine toxicity is counteracted by giving vitamin supplements, in particular, folinic acid. Reduction of the dose of pyrimethamine is necessary if hematologic monitoring shows bone marrow suppression.[6,9,331,332,367]

Therapy of Congenital Infection

Every newborn/infant that has been shown either prenatally or postnatally to have been infected prenatally has to be given specific anti-toxoplasma chemotherapy for the first 12 months of life irrespective of the severity of disease. This therapy consists of alternating 3-week courses of the combination sulfadiazine (for dosage, see above) plus pyrimethamine and spiramycin (100 mg/kg daily). Folinic acid supplementation is self-evident. In case of ventricular dilatation, corticosteroids may be considered, although no prospective studies exist.[6,9,331,332]

Therapy of the Immunosuppressed Individual

An immunosuppressed patient with cerebral toxoplasmosis is treated with sulfadiazine (4 to 8 g/d) plus pyrimethamine (50 to 75 mg/d) with vitamin supplementation (folinic acid 15 mg) for at least 6 weeks. Clindamycin (2.4 to 4.8 g/d) can be the substitution drug if bone marrow suppression precludes further pyrimethamine therapy or if sulfonamide toxicity (renal toxicity) develops. Maintenance therapy with reduced pyrimethamine and sulfadiazine combination is necessary, in particular, if the immunosuppressed patient has a CD4 count of less than 100/μl. Seronegative transplant recipients of a seropositive solid organ (in particular, heart and liver) should be given pyrimethamine prophylaxis (25 mg/d) plus folinic acid (10 mg/d) for a duration of 6 weeks after transplantation to prevent primary infection. If the period of immunosuppression is envisioned to be prolonged, even in organ transplant recipients, maintenance therapy (pyrimethamine 25 to 50 mg/d + sulfadiazine 50 mg/d + folinic acid 10 mg/d) may be required.[6,9,331,332,367]

Complications

Cerebral toxoplasmosis is frequently accompanied by focal or generalized tonic/clonic epileptic seizures. An acute toxoplasmic encephalitis may lead to increased ICP. Both clinical entities must be recognized early in order to administer appropriate anticonvulsive and/or anti-ICP therapy. Care has to be taken in heart transplant recipients with the anticonvulsive drug diphenylhydantoin. Alternative antiepileptic drugs for intravenous treatment may be valproic acid or benzodiazepines. An acute phase of raised ICP is treated with intravenous mannitol and/or intravenous dexamethasone.[6,9]

Prevention/Prophylaxis

Health education is the mainstay to prevent infection during pregnancy. Women who are seronegative after conception should be informed of how to reduce the risk of acquiring toxoplasmosis during pregnancy (avoid raw or undercooked food, contaminated vegetables and fruits, etc.). If these women have to handle cat litter or have to do gardening, gloves should be worn. Similar advice should be given to HIV-infected individuals.[331,368] Presently, there is no vaccine suitable for humans, although a non-cyst-forming strain of *T. gondii* has been used to prevent toxoplasmosis in sheep.[369] Only the first/primary infection by *T. gondii* during pregnancy is dangerous for the unborn. Infection with *T. gondii* prior to the pregnancy leads to immunity that protects the unborn from a diaplacentar infection.[331,368]

Sequential serologic testing of the serum of pregnant initially seronegative women can detect early enough a primary infection acquired during pregnancy.[362]

Immediate initiation of antiparasitic chemotherapy either may prevent diaplacentar infection or may successfully treat the unborn in case of intrauterine infection. Exposition prophylaxis is highly efficacious but cannot fully exclude infection.[331] The first serologic examination of the pregnant women should be done as early as possible during pregnancy. If the pregnant woman is seronegative, follow-up serology should be done every 2 months. If in the first serologic screening the pregnant woman is seropositive, it has to be elucidated if the infection has taken place prior to or during the early phase of pregnancy; IgM antibodies and the avidity tests allow for discriminating recent from long-standing infection. If there is any doubt, a follow-up serology should be done within 2 to 3 weeks. Within the first 15 weeks of pregnancy, spiramycin can be given; beyond week 15, pyrimethamine plus sulfadiazine can be used. Before initiating antiparasitic chemotherapy, amniocentesis should be done to examine the amniotic fluid by PCR.[331] The "preventive" therapy of newborns that have no clinical signs and symptoms of *T. gondii* infection at birth but are likely to have been infected during pregnancy was described earlier.

► LEISHMANIASIS

In patients with HIV infection, *Leishmania* antigens have been detected in the CNS.[370] Usually, *L. donovani* is responsible for visceral leishmaniasis, a potentially fatal disease, in particular, in HIV patients. *L. amazonensis* is one of the etiologic agents of human tegumentary leishmaniases. In *BALB/c* and Swiss mice that have been infected subcutaneously with amastigotes of *L. amazonensis*, histologic examination showed that two-thirds of the infected mice had signs of inflammation and hyperemia of the meninges.[371] Parasitized macrophages were detected within the cerebral parenchyma, as well as mast cells, lymphocytes, and polymorphonuclear cells. Furthermore, necrosis in the cerebral parenchyma was observed. This experiment, published very recently,[371] shows that in *BALB/c* and Swiss mice, *L. amazonensis* is able to penetrate the blood-brain barrier and to cause significant inflammatory changes in the CNS. Whether this experimental finding can be extrapolated to potential human pathology is still a matter of discussion.[371] However—and possibly in favor of this—*L. infantum* has been detected in the choroid plexus,[372] and anti-*Leishmania* antibodies have been found in the cerebrospinal fluid of dogs.[373] Secondary CNS complications of visceral leishmaniasis (kala azar) may be seen due to either severe anemia, hypokalemia, or thrombocytopenia. The associated alterations of the plasmatic (hepatic) coagulation factors may be a possible source of intracranial hemorrhages.[374]

Treatment

The state-of-the-art treatment of systemic leishmaniasis is a short-term, high-dose course of liposomal AmB (AmBisome, 3 to 4 mg/kg of body weight for 5 days and one such repeat dose on day 10).[375] The oral alkyl phospholipid compound Miltefosine has been evaluated in several phase II studies with a 100 percent cure rate at a dose of 100 mg/day over 4 weeks.[376]

REFERENCES

1. Doolittle WE: Phylogenetic classification and the universal tree. *Science* 284:2124, 1999.
2. Baldauf SL, Roger AJ, Wenk-Siefert I, Doolittle WF: A kingdom-level phylogeny of eukaryotes based on combined protein data. *Science* 290:972, 2000.
3. De Meeus T, Renaud F: Parasites within the new phylogeny of eukaryotes. *Trends Parasitol* 18:247, 2002.
4. Aspoeck H: Protozoen als Erreger von Krankheiten des Menschen: Uebersicht und aktuelle Probleme in Mitteleuropa. *Kataloge Ooe Landesmuseums* 71:219, 1994.
5. Baker JR: Parasitic protozoa. In Cook GC, Zumla A (eds): *Mansons's Tropical Diseases*, 21st ed. London: Saunders, 2003:1629.
6. Schmutzhard E: Entzuendliche Erkrankungen des Nervensystems, 1. Aufl. Stuttgart: Thieme, 2000.
7. Cook GC, Zumla A: *Manson's Tropical Diseases*, 21st ed. London: Saunders, 2003.
8. Lang W, Loescher TH: Tropenmedizin in Klinik und Praxis, 3. Aufl. Stuttgart: Thieme, 2000.
9. Schmutzhard E: Protozoal infections. In Noseworthy JH (ed): *Neurological Therapeutics, Principles and Practice*, 1st ed. London: Martin Dunitz, 2003:1003.
10. Cox FE: Systematics of parasitic protozoa. In Kreier JP, Baker JR (eds): *Parasitic Protozoa*, 2d ed, Vol 1. San Diego: Academic Press, 1991, p 55.
11. Bruce Chwatt LJ: History of malaria from prehistory to eradication. In Wernsdorfer WH, McGregor I (eds): *Malaria: Principles and Practice of Malariology*. Edinburgh: Churchill Livingstone, 1988, p 1.
12. Cavalier-Smith T: A revised six-kingdom system of life. *Biol Rev Camb Philos Soc* 73:203, 1988.
13. Walochnik J, Aspoeck H: Die Protozoen des Menschen im phylogenetischen System. In Aspoeck H (ed): *Amoeben Bandwuermer, Zecken*, 1. Aufl. Linz: Kataloge des OOe Landesmuseums, Biologiezentrum OOe, 2002, p 115.
14. Breman JG: The ears of the hippopotamus: Manifestations, determinants, and estimates of the malaria burden. *Am J Trop Med Hyg* 64:1, 2001.
15. Duran-Reynolds MG: *The Fever Bark Tree*. New York: Doubleday, 1946.
16. Rediscovering wormwood, qinghaousu, for malaria (editorial). *Lancet* 339:649, 1993.
17. White NJ. Malaria. In Cook GC, Zumla A (eds): *Mansons's Tropical Diseases*, 21st ed. London: Saunders, 2003, p 1205.
18. Ross R: On some peculiar pigmented cells found in two mosquitoes fed on malarial blood. *Br Med J* 2:1786, 1897.
19. Laveran CLA: Note sur un nouveau parasite trouvé dans le sang de plusieurs malades atteints de fièvre palustre. *Bull Acad Med* 9:1235, 1880.
20. Jelinek T, Schulte C, Behrens R, et al: Imported *falciparum* malaria in Europe: Sentinel surveillance data from the European network on surveillance of imported infectious diseases. *Clin Infect Dis* 34:572, 2002.
21. Schmutzhard E, Gerstenbrand F: Cerebral malaria in Tanzania: Its epidemiology, clinical symptoms and neurological long term sequelae in the patients of 66 cases. *Trans R Soc Trop Med Hyg* 78:351, 1984.
22. Wolf-Gould C, Osei L, Commey JO: Pediatric cerebral malaria in Accra, Ghana. *J Trop Pediatr* 38:290, 1991.
23. Olsen BE, Hinderaker SG, Bergsjo P, et al: Causes and characteristics of maternal deaths in rural northern Tanzania. *Acta Obstet Gynaecol Scand* 81:1101, 2002.
24. Etard JF, Kodio B, Ronsmans C: Seasonal variation in direct obstetric mortality in rural Senegal: Role of malaria. *Am J Trop Med Hyg* 68:503, 2003.
25. Stich A, Zwicker M, Steffen T, et al: Old age as risk factor for complications of malaria in non-immune travellers. *Dtsch Med Wochenschr* 128:309, 2003.
26. Muehlberger N, Jelinek T, Behrens RH, et al: Age as a risk factor for severe manifestations and fatal outcome of *falciparum* malaria in European patients: Observations from Trop Net Europ and SIMPID Surveillance Data. *Clin Infect Dis* 36:990, 2003.
27. Stoppacher R, Adams SP: Malaria deaths in the United States: Case report and review of deaths, 1979–1998. *J Forens Sci* 48:404, 2003.
28. Gupta D, Chugh K, Sachdev A, et al: ICU management of severe malaria. *Ind J Pediatr* 68:1057, 2001.
29. Abdulhadi NH: Protection against severe clinical manifestations of *Plasmodium falciparum* malaria among sickle cell trait subjects is due to modification of the release of cytokines and/or cytoadherence of infected erythrocytes to the host vascular beds. *Med Hypoth* 60:912, 2003.
30. Pasvol G: Ovalocytosis in Papua New Guinea. *Trends Parasitol* 18:150, 2002.
31. Smith TG, Ayi K, Serghides L, et al: Innate immunity to malaria caused by *Plasmodium falciparum*. *Clin Invest Med* 25:262, 2002.
32. Chotivanich K, Udomsangpetch R, Pattanapanyasat K, et al: Hemoglobin E: A balanced polymorphism protective against high parasitemias and thus severe *P. falciparum* malaria. *Blood* 100:1110, 2002.
33. Weatherall DJ, Clegg JB: Genetic variability in response to infection: Malaria and after. *Genes Immun* 3:331, 2002.
34. Hill S, Elvin J, Willis AC, et al: Molecular analysis of an malaria. *Nature* 352:595, 1991.
35. Omi K, Ohashi J, Ptarapotikul J, et al: CD36 polymorphism is associated with protection from cerebral malaria. *Am J Hum Genet* 72:364, 2003.

36. Morahan G, Boutlis CS, Huang D, et al: A promoter polymorphism in the gene encoding interleukin-12 p40 (IL12β) is associated with mortality from cerebral malaria and with reduced nitric oxide production. *Genes Immun* 3:414, 2002.

37. Hobbs MR, Udhayakumar V, Levesque MC, et al: A new *NOS2* promoter polymorphism associated with increased nitric oxide production and protection from severe malaria in Tanzanian and Kenyan children. *Lancet* 360:1468, 2002.

38. Omi K, Ohashi J, Patarapotikul J, et al: Fcγ receptor IIA and IIIB polymorphisms are associated with susceptibility to cerebral malaria. *Parasitol Int* 51:361, 2002.

39. Beg MA, Khan R, Baig SM, et al: Cerebral involvement in benign tertian malaria. *Am J Trop Med Hyg* 67:230, 2002.

40. Heddini A: Malaria pathogenesis: A jigsaw with an increasing number of pieces. *Int J Parasitol* 32:1587, 2002.

41. Artavanis-Tsakonas K, Tongren JE, Riley EM: The war between the malaria parasite and the immune system: Immunity, immunoregulation and immunopathology. *Clin Exp Immunol* 133:145, 2003.

42. Kristensson K, Mhlanga JD, Bentivoglio M: Parasites and the brain: Neuroinvasion, immunopathogenesis and neuronal dysfunctions. *Curr Top Microbiol Immunol* 265:227, 2002.

43. Malaguarnera L, Musumeci S: The immune response to *Plasmodium falciparum* malaria. *Lancet Infect Dis* 2:472, 2002.

44. Beeson JG, Brown GV: Pathogenesis of *Plasmodium falciparum* malaria: The roles of parasite adhesion and antigenic variation. *Cell Mol Life Sci* 59:258, 2002.

45. Odeh M: The role of tumour necrosis factor-α in the pathogenesis of complicated falciparum malaria. *Cytokine* 14:11, 2001.

46. Engwerda CR, Mynott TL, Sawhney S, et al: Locally up-regulated lymphotoxin α not systemic tumor necrosis factor α is the principal mediator of murine cerebral malaria. *J Exp Med* 195:137, 2002.

47. Ubalee R, Suzuki F, Kikuchi M, et al: Strong association of a tumor necrosis factor-α promoter allele with cerebral malaria in Myanmar. *Tissue Antigens* 58:407, 2001.

48. Chang WL, LI J, Sun G, et al: P-selectin contributes to severe experimental malaria but is not required for leukocyte adhesion to brain microvasculature. *Infect Immun* 71:1911, 2003.

49. Bauer PR, Van Der Heyde HC, Sun G, et al: Regulation of endothelial cell adhesion molecule expression in an experimental model of cerebral malaria. *Microcirculation* 9:463, 2002.

50. Deininger MH, Fimmen B, Kremsner PG, et al: Accumulation of endostatin/collagen XVIII in brains of patients who died with cerebral malaria. *J Neuroimmunol* 131:216, 2002.

51. Hearn J, Rayment N, Landon DN, et al: Immunopathology of cerebral malaria: Morphological evidence of parasite sequestration in murine brain microvasculature. *Infect Immun* 68:5364, 2000.

52. Day NP, Hien TT, Schollaardt T, et al: The prognostic and pathologic role of pro- and antiinflammatory cytokines in severe malaria. *J Infect Dis* 180:1288, 1999.

53. Gosi P, Khusmith S, Looareesuwan S, et al: Complicated malaria is associated with differential elevations in serum levels of interleukins 10, 12 and 15. *Southeast Asian J Trop Med Public Health* 30:412, 1999.

54. Maneerat V, Pongponrain E, Viriyavejakul P, et al: Cytokines associated with pathology in the brain tissue of fatal malaria. *Southeast Asian J Trop Med Public Health* 30:64354, 1999.

55. Mori O, Ohaki Y, Oguro T, et al: Adhesion molecule detection in a case of early cerebral malaria: Immunohistochemical and electron microscopic findings. *Hum Pathol* 31:1175, 2003.

56. Kampfl A, Pfausler B, Haring HP, et al: Impaired microcirculation and tissue oxygenation in human cerebral malaria: A single photon emission computed tomographic and near-infrared spectroscopy study. *Am J Trop Med Hyg* 56:585, 1997.

57. Medana IM, Hien TT, Day NP, et al. The clinical significance of cerebrospinal fluid levels of kynurenine pathway metabolites and lactate in severe malaria. *Infect Dis* 185:650, 2002.

58. Grau GE, Mackenzie CD, Carr RA, et al: Platelet accumulation in brain microvessels in fatal pediatric cerebral malaria. *J Infect Dis* 187:461, 2003.

59. Brunet LR: Nitric oxide in parasitic infections. *Int Immunopharmacol* 1:1457, 2001.

60. Maneerat V, Virivavejakui P, Punpoowong B, et al: Inducible nitric oxide synthase expression is increased in the brain in fatal cerebral malaria. *Histopathology* 37:269, 2000.

61. Fritsche G, Larcher C, Schennach H, et al: Regulatory interactions between iron and nitric oxide metabolism for immune defense against *Plasmodium falciparum* infection. *J Infect Dis* 183:1388, 2001.

62. Clark IA, Awburn MM, Whitteh RO, et al: Tissue distribution of migration inhibitory factor and inducible nitric oxide synthase in *falciparum* malaria and sepsis in African children. *Malar J* 2:6, 2003.

63. Vogetseder A, Ospelt C, Reindl M, et al: Time course of coagulation parameters, cytokines and adhesion molecules in *Plasmodium falciparum* malaria (abstract 7). Kongress für Infektionskrankheiten und Tropenmedizin, Berlin, February 26–28, 2003.

64. Deininger MH, Kremsner PG, Meyermann R, et al: Macrophages/microglial cells in patients with cerebral malaria. *Eur Cytokine Network* 13:173, 2002.

65. Makani J, Matuja W, Liyombo E, et al: Admission diagnosis of cerebral malaria in adults in an endemic area of Tanzania: Implications and clinical description. *Q J Med* 96:355, 2003.

66. World Health Organization: Severe *falciparum* malaria. *Trans R Soc Trop Med Hyg* 1:812, 2000.

67. Teasdale G, Jennett B: Assessment and prognosis of coma after head injury. *Acta Neurochir* 43:45, 1976.

68. Newton CR, Chokwe T, Schellenberg JA, et al: Coma scales for children with severe *falciparum* malaria. *Trans R Soc Trop Med Hyg* 91:161, 1997.

69. Waruiru CM, Newton CR, Forster D, et al: Epileptic

seizures and malaria in Kenyan children. *Trans R Soc Trop Med Hyg* 90:152, 1996.

70. Versteeg AC, Carter JA, Dzombo J, et al: Seizure disorders among relatives of Kenyan children with severe *falciparum* malaria. *Trop Med Int Health* 8:12, 2003.

71. Crawley J, Kokwaro G, Ouma D, et al: Chloroquine is not a risk factor for seizures in childhood cerebral malaria. *Trop Med Int Health* 5:860, 2000.

72. Crawly J, Smith S, Kirkham F, et al: Seizures and status epilepticus in childhood cerebral malaria. *Q J Med* 89:591, 1996.

73. Crawley J, Smith S, Muthinji P, et al: Electroencephalographic and clinical features of cerebral malaria. *Arch Dis Child* 84:247, 2001.

74. Moore DA, Jennings RM, Doherty TF, et al: Assessing the severity of malaria. *Br Med J* 326:808, 2003.

75. Helbok R, Dent W, Nacher M, et al: Use of the multi-organ dysfunction score: A tool to discriminate different levels of severity in uncomplicated *Plasmodium falciparum* malaria. *Am J Trop Med Hyg* 68:372, 2003.

76. Patankar TF, Karnad DR, Shetty PG, et al: Adult cerebral malaria: Prognostic importance of imaging findings and correlation with postmortem findings. *Radiology* 224:811, 2002.

77. Roze E, Thiebaut MM, Mazevet D, et al: Neurologic sequelae after severe falciparum malaria in adult travelers. *Eur Neurol* 46:192, 2001.

78. Thornton C, Heyerman RS, Thorniley M, et al: Auditory- and somatosensory-evoked potentials in cerebral malaria and anaesthesia: A comparison. *Eur J Anaesthesiol* 19:717, 2002.

79. Wilairatana P, Looareesuwan S: Guideline in management of severe malaria. *J Ind Med Assoc* 98:628, 2000.

80. Mturi N, Musumba CO, Wamola BM, et al: Cerebral malaria: Optimising management. *CNS Drugs* 17:153, 2003.

81. Assimadi JK, Gbadoe AD, Agbodjan-Djossou O, et al: Treatment of cerebral malaria in African children by intravenous quinine: Comparison of a loading dose to a regimen without a loading dose. *Arch Pediatr* 9:587, 2002.

82. Abdin MZ, Israr M, Rehman RU, et al: Artemisinin, a novel antimalarial drug: Biochemical and molecular approaches for enhanced production. *Planta Med* 69:289, 2003.

83. Artemeter-Quinine Meta-analysis Study Group: A meta-analysis using individual patient data of trials comparing artemether with quinine in the treatment of severe *falciparum* malaria. *Trans R Soc Trop Med Hyg* 95:637, 2001.

84. Thumba PE, Bhat GJ, Mabeza GF, et al: A randomized controlled trial of artemotil (β-arteether) in Zambian children with cerebral malaria. *Am J Trop Med Hyg* 62:524, 2000.

85. Moyou-Somo R, Tietche F, Ondoa M, et al: Clinical trial of β-arteether versus quinine for the treatment of cerebral malaria in children in Yaounde, Cameroon. *Am J Trop Med Hyg* 64:229, 2001.

86. Faiz MA, Rahman E, Hossain MA, et al: A randomized, controlled trial comparing artemether and quinine in the treatment of cerebral malaria in Bangladesh. *Ind J Malariol* 38:9, 2001.

87. Satti GM, Elhassan SH, Ibrahim SA: The efficacy of artemether versus quinine in the treatment of cerebral malaria. *J Egypt Soc Parasitol* 32:611, 2002.

88. Goka BQ, Adabayeri V, Ofori-Adjei E, et al: Comparison of chloroquine with artesunate in the treatment of cerebral malaria in Ghanaian children. *J Trop Pediatr* 47:165, 2001.

89. Adam I, Idris HM, Mohamed-Ali AA, et al: Comparison of intramuscular artemether and intravenous quinine in the treatment Sudanese children with severe *falciparum* malaria. *East Afr Med J* 79:621, 2002.

90. Esamai F, Ayuo P, Owino-ONgor W, et al: Rectal dihydroartemisinin versus intravenous quinine in the treatment of severe malaria: A randomised clinical trial. *East Afr Med J* 77:273, 2000.

91. Awad MI, Alkadru AM, Behrens RH, et al: Descriptive study on the efficacy and safety of artesunate suppository in combination with other antimalarials in the treatment of severe malaria in Sudan. *Am J Trop Med Hyg* 68:153, 2003.

92. Karunjaeewa HA, Kemiki A, Alpers MP, et al: Safety and therapeutic efficacy of artesunate suppositories for treatment malaria in children in Papua New Guinea. *Pediatr Infect Dis J* 22:251, 2003.

93. Assimadi JK, Gbadoe AD, Agbodjan-Djossou O, et al: Diluted injectable quinine in the intramuscular and intrarectal route: Comparative efficacy and tolerance in malaria treatment for children. *Med Trop* 62:158, 2002.

94. Wooltorton E: Mefloquine: Contraindicated in patients with mood, psychotic or seizure disorders *Can Med Assoc J* 167:1147, 2002.

95. Genovese RF, Newman DB, Brewer TG: Behavioral and neural toxicity of the artemisinin antimalarial arteether but not artesunate and artelinate in rats. *Pharmacol Biochem Behav* 67:37, 2002.

96. Phillips-Howard PA, ter Kuile FO: CNS adverse events associated with antimalarial agents: Fact of fiction? *Drug Saf* 12:370, 1995.

97. Esamai F, Mining S, Forsberg P, et al: A comparison of brain, core and skin temperature in children with complicated and uncomplicated malaria. *J Trop Pediatr* 47:170, 2001.

98. Agbolosu NB, Cuevas LE, Milligan P, et al: Efficacy of tepid sponging versus paracetamol in reducing temperature in febrile children. *Ann Trop Paediatr* 17:283, 1997.

99. Biemba G, Dolmans D, Thuma PE, et al: Severe anaemia in Zambian children with *Plasmodium falciparum* malaria. *Trop Med Int Health* 5:9, 2000.

100. Burchard GD, Kroger J, Knobloch J, et al: Exchange blood transfusion in severe *falciparum* malaria: retrospective evaluation of 61 patients treated with, compared to 63 patients treated without, exchange transfusion. *Trop Med Int Health* 2:733, 1997.

101. Morch K, Feruglio SL, Ormassen V, et al: Severe *falciparum* malaria treated with exchange transfusion. *Tidsskr Nor Laegeforen* 122:999, 2002.

102. Tomlinson RJ, Morrice J: Does intravenous mannitol improve outcome in cerebral malaria. *Arch Dis Child* 88:640, 2003.

103. Crawley J, Waruiru C, Mithwani S, et al: Effect of phenobarbital on seizure frequency and mortality in child-

hood cerebral malaria: A randomised, controlled intervention study. *Lancet* 355:701, 2000.

104. Meremikwu M, Marson AG: Routine anticonvulsants for treating cerebral malaria. *Chocrane Database Syst Rev* CD002152, 2002.

105. Ogutu BR, Newton CR, Crawley J, et al: Pharmacokinetics and anticonvulsant effects of diazepam in children with severe *falciparum* malaria and convulsions. *Br J Clin Pharmacol* 53:49, 2002.

106. Hay F, Treluyer JM, Orbach D, et al: Severe malaria in children in intensive care: National survey 1990–1995. *Arch Pediatr* 7:1163, 2000.

107. Sowunmi A: Clinical study of cerebral malaria in African children. *Afr J Med Sci* 26:9, 1997.

108. Vincent JL, Abraham E, Annane D, et al: Reducing mortality in sepsis: new directions. *Crit Care* 3:51, 2000.

109. Wijdicks EJ: *The Clinical Practice of Critical Care Neurology,* 2d ed. Oxford, England: Oxford University Press, 2003.

110. Gerhardt UM, Scholler C, Bocker D, et al: Noninvasive estimation of cardiac output in critical care patients. *Clin Monit Comput* 16:263, 2002.

111. Sun Q, Rogiers P, Pauweis D, et al: Comparison of continuous thermodilution and bolus cardiac output measurement in septic shock. *Intensive Care Med* 28:1276, 2002.

112. Sakka SG, Reinhard K, Wegscheider K, et al: Comparison of cardiac output and circulatory blood volumes by transpulmonary thermodye dilution and transcutaneous indocyanine green measurement in critically ill patients. *Chest* 121:559, 2002.

113. Manglik S, Flores E, Lubarski L, et al: Glucocorticoid insufficiency in patients who present to the hospital with severe sepsis: A prospective clinical trial. *Crit Care Med* 31:1668, 2003.

114. Warell DA, Looareesuwan S, Warrell MJ, et al: Dexamethasone proves deleterious in cerebral malaria: A double-blind trial in 100 comatose patients. *New Engl J Med* 306:313, 1982.

115. Waller D, Krishna S, Crawley J, et al: The clinical features and outcome of severe malaria in Gambian children. *Clin Infect Dis* 21:577, 1995.

116. Jaffar S, Van Hensbroek MR, Palmer A, et al: Predictors of a fatal outcome following childhood cerebral malaria. *Am J Trop Med Hyg* 57:20, 1997.

117. Brewster DR, Kwiatkowski D, White NJ: Neurological sequelae of cerebral malaria in children. *Lancet* 336:1039, 1990.

118. Newton CR, Hien TT, Withe N: Cerebral malaria. *J Neurol Neurosurg Psychiatry* 69:433, 2000.

119. Koch J, Strik WK, Becker T, et al: Acute organic psychosis after malaria tropica. *Nervenarzt* 67:72, 1996.

120. Müller O, Traore C, Becher H, et al: Malaria morbidity, treatment-seeking behaviour, and mortality in a cohort of young children in rural Burkina Faso. *Trop Med Int Health* 8:290, 2003.

121. Hamann G, Schimrigk: Neurologic complications of malaria infection. *Fortschr Neurol Psychiatry* 61:46, 1993.

122. Saavedra-Lozano J, Booth TN, Weprin BE, et al: Isolated cerebellar edema and obstructive hydrocephalus in a child with cerebral malaria. *Pediatr Infect Dis* 20:908, 2001.

123. Schemann JF, Doumbo O, Malvy D: Ocular lesions associated with malaria children in Mali. *Am J Trop Med Hyg* 67:61, 2002.

124. Kochar DK, Joshi A, Vallabh B, et al: Effect of arteether on electrocardiogram in the patients of *falciparum* malaria: A preliminary study. *Ind J Malriol* 36:61, 1999.

125. Gupta GB, Varma S: Effect of intravenous quinine on capillary glucose levels in malaria. *J Assoc Phys Ind* 49:426, 2001.

126. Lochhead J, Movaffaghy A, Falsini B, et al: The effect of quinine on the electroretinograms of children with pediatric cerebral malaria. *J Infect Dis* 187:1342, 2003.

127. Senanayake N, Roman GC: Neurological complications of malaria. *Southeast Asian J Trop Med Public Health* 23:672, 1992.

128. Carter JA, Murira GM, Ross AJ, et al. Speech and language sequelae of severe malaria in Kenyan children. *Brain Inj* 17:217, 2003.

129. Boivin MJ: Effects of early cerebral malaria on cognitive ability in Senegalese children. *J Dev Behav Pediatr* 23:353, 2002.

130. Oguche S, Omokhodion SI, Adeyemo A, et al: Low plasma bicarbonate predicts poor outcome of cerebral malaria in Nigerian children. *West Afr J Med* 21:22276, 2002.

131. Lopansri BK, Anstey NM, Weinberg JB, et al: Low plasma arginine concentrations in children with cerebral malaria and decreased nitric oxide production. *Lancet* 361:676, 2003.

132. Senanayake N, de Silva HJ: Delayed cerebellar ataxia complicating *falciparum* malaria: A clinical study of 74 patients. *J Neurol* 24:456, 1994.

133. de Silva HJ, Senanayake N: Absence of anti-Purkinje cell antibodies in patients with cerebellar ataxia following *falciparum* malaria. *Southeast Asian J Trop Med Public Health* 25:707, 1994.

134. Burgner D, Usen S, Rockett K, et al: Nucleotide and haplotypic diversity of the *NOS2A* promoter region and its relationship to cerebral malaria. *Hum Genet* 112:379, 2003.

135. Burgner D, Levin M: Genetic susceptibility to infectious diseases. *Pediatr Infect Dis* 22:1, 2003.

136. Gyan B, Goka B, Cvetkovic JT, et al: Polymorphisms in interleukin-1β and interleukin-1 receptor antagonist genesis and malaria in Ghanaian children. *Scand J Immunol* 56:619, 2002.

137. Chiodini PL: Babesiosis. In Cook GC, Zumla A (eds): *Manson's Tropical Diseases,* 21st ed. London: Saunders, 2003, p 1297.

138. Persing DH, Mathiesen D, Marshall WF, et al: Detection of *Babesia microti* by polymerase chain reaction. *J Clin Microbiol* 30:2097, 1992.

139. Kain KC, Jassoum SB, Fong IW, et al: Transfusion-transmitted babesiosis in Ontario: First reported case in Canada. *Can Med Assoc J* 164:1721, 2001.

140. Herwaldt B, Persing DH, Precigout EA, et al: A fatal case of babeosis in Missouri: Identification of another piroplasm that infects humans. *Ann Intern Med* 124:643, 1996.

141. Meldrum SC, Birkhead GS, White DJ, et al: Human babesiosis in New York State: An epidemiological description of 136 cases. *Clin Infect Dis* 15:1019, 2000.

142. Uhnoo I, Cars O, Christensson D, et al: First documented case of human babesiosis in Sweden. *Scand J Infect Dis* 24:541, 1992.

143. Shi CM, Liu LP, Chung WC, et al: Human babesiosis in Taiwan: Asymptomatic infection with a *Babesia microti*–like organism in a Taiwanese woman. *J Clin Microbiol* 35:450, 1992.

144. Krause PJ, Telford SR III, Spielman A, et al: Concurrent Lyme disease and babesiosis: Evidence for increased severity and duration of illness. *JAMA* 275:1657, 1996.

145. Ong K, Stavropoulos C, Inada Y: Babesiosis, asplenia and AIDS. *Lancet* 360:112, 1990.

146. Falagas ME, Klempner MS: Babesiosis in patients with AIDS: A chronic infection presenting as fever of unknown origin. *Clin Infect Dis* 22:809, 1996.

147. Schuster FL: Cultivation of *Babesia* and *Babesia*-like blood parasites: Agents of an emerging zoonotic disease. *Clin Microbiol Rev* 15:365, 2002.

148. Shoda LK, Palmer GH, Florin-Christensen J, et al: *Babesia bovis*–stimulated macrophages express interleukin-1β, interleukin-12, tumor necrosis factor alpha, and nitric oxide and inhibit parasite replication in vitro. *Infect Immun* 68:5139, 2000.

149. Shoda LK, Kegerreis KA, Suarez CE: DNA from protozoan parasites *Babesia bovis, Trypanosoma cruzi,* and *T. brucei* is mitogenic for B lymphocytes and stimulates macrophage expression of interleukin-12, tumor necrosis factor alpha, and nitric oxide. *Infect Immun* 69:2162, 2001.

150. Goff WL, Johnson WC, Tuo W, et al: Age-related innate immune response in calves to *Babesia bovis* involves IL-12 induction and IL-10 modulation. *Ann NY Acad Sci* 969:164, 2002.

151. Goff WL, Johnson WC, Parish SM, et al: IL-4 and IL-10 inhibition of IFN-α and TNF-α–dependent nitric oxide production from bovine mononuclear phagocytes exposed to *Babesia bovis* merozoites. *Vet Immunol Immunopathol* 84:237, 2002.

152. Homer MJ, Aguilar-Delfin I, Telford S, et al: Babesiosis. *Clin Microbiol Rev* 13:451, 2000.

153. Krause PJ, Telford SR, Ryan R, et al: Diagnosis of babesiosis: Evaluation of a serologic test for the detection of *Babesia microti* antibody. *J Infect Dis* 169:923, 1994.

154. Krause PJ, Telford S, Spielman A, et al: Comparison of PCR with blood smear and inoculation of small animals for diagnosis of *Babesia microti* parasitemia. *J Clin Microbiol* 34:2791, 1996.

155. Schetters TP, Eling WM: Can *Babesia* infections be used as a model for cerebral malaria? *Parasitol Today* 15:492, 1999.

156. Dorman SE, Cannon ME, Telford SR, et al: Fulminant babesiosis treated with clindamycin, quinine, and whole-blood exchange transfusion. *Transfusion* 40:375, 2000.

157. Denes E, Roges JP, Darde ML, et al: Management of *Babesia divergens* babesiosis without a complete course of quinine treatment. *Eur J Clin Microbiol Infect Dis* 18:672, 1999.

158. Krause PJ, Telford SR, Sikand VK, et al: Atovaquone and azithromycin for the treatment of babesiosis. *New Engl J Med* 343:1454, 2000.

159. Krause PJ, Spielman A, Telford SR, et al: Persistent parasitemia after acute babesiosis. *New Engl J Med* 339:160, 1998.

160. Walochnik J, Aspoeck H: Amoeben und Amoebosen: gefaehrliche biologische und medzinische Sammelsurien. In Aspoeck H (ed): *Amoeben, Bandwuermer, Zecken,* 1. Aufl. Linz: Kataloge OOe Landesmuseums, Biologiezentrum OOe, 2002, p 229.

161. Warhurst DC: Pathogenic free-living amebae. *Parasitol Today* 1:24, 1985.

162. Derrick EH: A fatal case of generalized amebiasis due to a protozoon closely resembling if not identical to *Jodamoeba buetschlii. Trans R Soc Trop Med Hyg* 42:191, 1948.

163. Jaeger BV, Stamm WP: Brain abscesses caused by free living ameba probably of the genus *Hartmannella* in a patient with Hodgkin's disease. *Lancet* 2:1343, 1972.

164. Visvesvara GS, Martinez AJ, Schuster FL, et al: *Leptomyxid ameba,* a new agent of amebic meningoencephalitis in humans and animals. *J Clin Microbiol* 28:2750, 1990.

165. Warhurst DC: Potentially pathogenic free-living amebae. In Cook GC, Zumla A (eds): *Manson's Tropical Diseases,* 21st ed. London: Saunders, 2003, p 1411.

166. Kuhlencord A, Mergerian H, Bommer W: Studies on the pathogenesis of *Acanthamoeba*-associated meningoencephalitis. *Zentralbl Bakteriol* 271:256, 1989.

167. Ockert G: Review article: Occurrence, parasitism and pathogenetic potency of free-living ameba. *Appl Parasitol* 34:77, 1993.

168. Sadaka HA, Emam EE: Is the intestinal tract a portal of entry for *Acanthamoeba* infection? *J Egypt Soc Parasitol* 31:781, 2001.

169. Jarolim KL, McCosh JK, Howard MJ, et al: A light microscopy study of the migration of *Naegleria fowleri* from the nasal submucosa to the central nervous system during the early stage of primary amebic meningoencephalitis in mice. *J Parasitol* 86:50, 2000.

170. Scaglia M: Human pathology caused by free-living ameba. *Ann Ist Super Sanita* 33:551, 1997.

171. Martinez AJ, Visvesvara GS: Free-living, amphizoic and opportunistic amebas. *Brain Pathol* 7:583, 1987.

172. Marciano-Cabral F, Toney DM: Modulation of biological functions of *Naegleria fowleri* amebae by growth medium. *J Eukaryot Microbiol* 41:38, 1994.

173. Marciano-Cabral F, Zoghby KL, Braley SG: Cytopathic action of *Naegleria fowleri* amebae on rat neuroblastoma target cells. *J Protozool* 37:138, 1990.

174. Viriyavejakul P, Rochanwutanon M, Sirinavin S: *Naegleria* meningomyeloencephalitis. *Southeast Asian J Trop Med Public Health* 28:237, 1997.

175. Campos P, Cabrera J, Gotuzzo E, et al: Neurological involvement in free living amebiasis. *Rev Neurol* 29:316, 1999.

176. Pelandakis M, Pernin P: Use of multiplex PCR and PCR restriction enzyme analysis for detection and ex-

ploration of the variability in the free-living ameba *Naegleria* in the environment. *Appl Environ Microbiol* 68:2061, 2002.

177. Reveiller FL, Cabanes PA, Marciano-Cabral F: Development of a nested PCR assay to detect the pathogenic free-living ameba *Naegleria fowleri. Parasitol Res* 88:443, 2002.

178. Behets J, Seghi F, Declerck P, et al: Detection of *Naegleria* spp and *Naegleria fowleri:* A comparison of flagellation tests, ELISA and PCR. *Water Sci Technol* 17:117, 2003.

179. Schuster FL: Cultivation of pathogenic and opportunistic free-living amebas. *Clin Microbiol Rev* 15:342, 2002.

180. Visvesvara GS, Peralta MJ, Brandt FH, et al: Production of monoclonal antibodies to *Naegleria fowleri,* agent of primary amebic meningoencephalitis. *J Clin Microbiol* 25:1629, 1987.

181. Thong YH, Rowan-Kelly B, Shepherd C, et al: Growth inhibition of *Naegleria fowleri* by tetracycline, rifamycin, and miconazole. *Lancet* 22:876, 1977.

182. Lee KK, Karr SL, Wong MM, et al: In vitro susceptibilities of *Naegleria fowleri* strain HB-1 to selected antimicrobial agents, singly and in combination. *Antimicrob Agents Chemother* 16:217, 1979.

183. Jain R, Prabhakar S, Modi M, et al: *Naegleria* meningitis: A rare survival. *Neurol Ind* 50:470, 2002.

184. Hannisch W, Hallagan LF: Primary amebic meningoencephalitis: A review of the clinical literature. *Southeast Asian J Trop Med Public Health* 8:211, 1977.

185. Tieweharoen S, Junnu V, Chinabut P: In vitro effect of antifungal drugs on pathogenic *Naegleria* spp. *Southeast Asian J Trop Med Public Health* 33:38, 2002.

186. Gupta S, Dutta GP, Vishwakarma RA: Effect of α,β-arteether against primary amebic meningoencephalitis in Swiss mice. *Ind J Exp Biol* 36:824, 1998.

187. Cooke DW, Lallinger GJ, Durack DT: In vitro sensitivity of *Naegleria fowleri* to qinghaosu and dihydroqinghaosu. *J Parasitol* 73:411, 1987.

188. Kodet R, Nohyukova E, Tichy M, et al: Amebic encephalitis caused by *Balamuthia mandrillaris* in a Czech child: Description of the first case from Europe. *Pathol Res Pract* 194:423, 1998.

189. Martinez AJ: Infection of the central nervous system with *Acanthamoeba. Rev Infect Dis* 13(suppl 5):S399, 1991.

190. Shirabe T, Monobe Y, Visvesvara GS: An autopsy case of amebic meningoencephalitis: The first Japanese case caused by *Balamuthia mandrillaris. Neuropathology* 22:213, 2002.

191. Reed RP, Cooke-Yarhorough CM, Jaquiery AL, et al: Fatal granulomatous amebic encephalitis caused by *Balamuthia mandrillaris. Med J Aust* 21:82, 1997.

192. Recavarren-Arce S, Velarde C, Gotuzzo E, et al: Ameba angeitic lesions of the central nervous system in *Balamuthia mandrillaris* amebiasis. *Hum Pathol* 30:268, 1990.

193. Anzil AP, Rao C, Wrzolek MA, et al: Amebic meningoencephalitis in a patient with AIDS caused by a newly recognized opportunistic pathogen, *Leptomyxid ameba. Arch Pathol Lab Med* 115:21, 1991.

194. Seijo-Martinez M, Gonzalez-Mediero G, Santiago P, et al: Granulomatous amebic encephalitis in a patients with AIDS: Isolation of *Acanthamoeba* spp. group II from brain tissue and successful treatment with sulfadiazine and fluconazole. *J Clin Microbiol* 38:3892, 2000.

195. Duke BJ, Tyson RW, De Biasi R, et al: *Balamuthia mandrillaris* meningoencephalitis presenting with acute hydrocephalus. *Pediatr Neurosurg* 26:107, 1997.

196. Deol J, Robledo L, Meza A, et al: Encephalitis due to a free-living ameba (*Balamuthia mandrillaris*): Case report with literature review. *Surg Neurol* 53:611, 2000.

197. Katz JD, Ropper AH, Adelman L, et al: A case of *Balamuthia mandrillaris* meningoencephalitis. *Arch Neurol* 57:1210, 2000.

198. Hawley HP, Czachor JS, Malhotra V, et al. *Acanthamoeba* encephalitis in patients with AIDS. *AIDS Reader* 7:137, 1997.

199. Vodkin M, Howe DK, Visvesvara G, et al: Identification of *Acanthamoeba* at the generic and specific levels using the polymerase chain reaction. *J Protozool* 39:378, 1992.

200. Stothard DR, Hay J, Schroeder JM, et al: Fluorescent oligonucleotide probes for clinical and environmental detection of *Acanthamoeba* and the T4 185 rRNA gene sequence type. *J Clin Micriobiol* 37:2687, 1999.

201. Healy JF: *Balamuthia* amebic encephalitis: Radiographic and pathologic findings. *Am J Neuroradiol* 23:468, 2002.

202. Stater CA, Sickel JZ, Visvesvara GS, et al: Brief report: Successful treatment of disseminated *Acanthamoeba* infection in an immunocompromised patient. *New Engl J Med* 331:85, 1994.

203. Walsh JA: Problems in recognition and diagnosis of amebiasis: Estimation of the global magnitude of morbidity and mortality. *Rev Infect Dis* 8:226, 1986.

204. Farthing MJG, Cevallos AM, Kelly P: Intestinal protozoa. In Cook GC, Zumla A (eds): *Mansons's Tropical Diseases,* 21st ed. London: Saunders, 2003, p 1373.

205. Schmutzhard E, Mayr U, Rumpl E, et al: Secondary cerebral amebiasis due to infection with *Entamoeba histolytica:* A case report with computed tomographic findings. *Eur Neurol* 25:161, 1986.

206. Lowther SA, Dworkin MS, Hanson DL: *Entamoeba histolytica/Entamoeba dispar* infections in human immunodeficiency virus–infected patients in the United States. *Clin Infect Dis* 30:959, 2000.

207. Freeman O, Akamaguna A, Jarikre LN: Amebic liver abscess: The effect of aspiration on the resolution or healing time. *Ann Trop Med Parasitol* 84:281, 1990.

208. Espinosa-Cantellano MA, Martinez-Palomo A: Pathogenesis of intestinal amebiasis: From molecules to disease. *Clin Microbiol Rev* 13:318, 2000.

209. Eckert J: Parasitologie. In Kayser FH, Bienz KA, Eckert J, Zinkernagel RM (eds): *Medizinische Mikrobiologie,* 10. Aufl. Stuttgart: Thieme, 2001, p 479.

210. Weinke T, Friedrich-Janicke B, Hopp P, et al: Prevalence and clinical importance of *Entamoeba histolytica* in two high-risk groups: Travelers returning from the tropics and male homosexuals. *J Infect Dis* 161:1029, 1990.

211. Miles MA: New world trypanosomiasis. In Cox FEG (ed): *The Wellcome Trust Illustrated History of Tropical Diseases.* London: Wellcome Trust; 1996, p 192.

212. Miles MA. American trypanosomiasis (Chagas disease). In Cook GC, Zumla A (eds): *Mansons's Tropical Diseases,* 21st ed. London: Saunders, 2003, p 1325.

213. de Oliveira Santos E, dos Reis Caneia J, Gomes Monaco HC, et al: Reactivation of Chagas' disease leading to the diagnosis of acquired immunodeficiency syndrome. *Braz J Infect Dis* 6:317, 2002.

214. Sutmoller F, Penna TL, de Soza CT, et al: Human immunodeficiency virus incidence and risk behaviour in the Projeto Rio: Results of the first 5 years of the Rio de Janeiro open cohort of homosexual and bisexual men. *Int J Infect Dis* 6:259, 2002.

215. Ferreira MS, Borges AS: Some aspects of protozoan infections in immunocompromised patients, a review. *Mem Inst Oswaldo Cruz* 97:443, 2002.

216. Bosseno MF, Barnabe C, Magallon G, et al: Predominance of *Trypanosoma cruzi* lineage I in Mexico. *J Clin Microbiol* 40:627, 2002.

217. Beard CB, Pye G, Steurer FJ, et al: Chagas disease in a domestic transmission cycle, southern Texas, USA. *Emerg Infect Dis* 96:103, 2003.

218. Guzman-Bracho C. Epidemiology of Chagas disease in Mexico: An update. *Trends Parasitol* 17:372, 2001.

219. Ramirez LE, Lages-Silva E, Alvarenga-Franco F, et al: High prevalence of *Trypanosoma rangeli* and *Trypanosoma cruzi* in opossums and triatomids in a formerly endemic area of Chagas disease in southeast Brazil. *Acta Trop* 84:189, 2002.

220. Dumonteil E, Gourbiere S, Barrera-Perez M, et al: Geographic distribution of *Triatoma dimidiata* and transmission dynamics of *Trypanosoma cruzi* in the Yucatan peninsula of Mexico. *Am J Trop Med Hyg* 67:176, 2002.

221. Garzon EA, Barnabe C, Cordova X, et al: *Trypanosoma cruzi* isoenzyme variability Ecuador: First observation of zymodemie III genotypes in chronic chagasic patients. *Trans R Soc Trop Med Hyg* 96:378, 2002.

222. Santoz SS, Cupolillo E, Jungqueria A, et al: The genetic diversity of Brazilian *Trypanosoma cruzi* isolates and the phylogenetic positioning of zymodeme 3 based on the internal transcribed spacer the ribosomal gene. *Ann Trop Med Parasitol* 96:755, 2002.

223. Mendonca MB, Nehme NS, Santos SS, et al: Two main clusters within *Trypanosoma cruzi* zymodeme 3 are defined by distinct regions of the ribosomal RNA cistron. *Parasitology* 124:177, 2002.

224. Gurtler RE, Segura EL, Cohen JE: Congenital transmission of *Trypanosoma cruzi* infection in Argentina. *Emerg Infect Dis* 9:29, 2003.

225. Pan American Health Organization: *Chagas' Disease and the Nervous System* (Scientific Publication No 547). Washington: PAHO, 1994.

226. Carod-Artal FJ, Vargas AP, Melo M, et al: American trypanosomiasis (Chagas disease): An unrecognised cause of stroke. *J Neurol Neurosurg Psychiatry* 74:516, 2003.

227. Girones N, Fresno M: Etiology of Chagas disease myocarditis: Autoimmunity, parasite persistence, or both? *Trends Parasitol* 19:19, 2003.

228. Mortara RA, da Silva S, Patricio FR, et al: Imaging *Trypanosoma cruzi* within tissue from chagasic patients using confocal microscopy with monoclonal antibodies. *Parasitol Res* 85:800, 1999.

229. Gomes JA, Bahia-Oliveira LM, Rocha MO, et al: Evidence that development of severe cardiomyopathy in human Chagas' disease is due to a Th1-specific immune response. *Infect Immun* 71:118, 2003.

230. Corti M: AIDS and Chagas' disease. *AIDS Patient Care* 14:581, 2000.

231. Lages-Silva E, Ramirez LE, Silva-Vergara MI, et al: Chagasic meningoencephalitis in a patient with acquired immunodeficiency syndrome: Diagnosis, follow-up, and genetic characterization of *Trypanosoma cruzi.* *Clin Infect Dis* 34:118, 2002.

232. dos Santos Sde S, Almeida GM, Monteiro ML, et al: Ocular myositis and diffuse meningoencephalitis from *Trypanosoma cruzi* in an AIDS patient. *Trans R Soc Trop Med Hyg* 93:535, 1999.

233. Elias FE, Vigliano CA, Laguens RP, et al: Analysis of the presence of *Trypanosoma cruzi* in the heart tissue of three patients with chronic Chagas heart disease. *Am J Trop Med Hyg* 68:242, 2003.

234. Miles MA. New world trypanosomiasis. In Cox FEG, Kreier JP, Wakelin D (eds): *Topley & Wilson's Microbiology and Microbial Infections,* Vol 5. London: Arnold, 1997, p 283.

235. Umezawa ES, Bastos SF, Coura JR, et al: An improved serodiagnostic test for Chagas' disease employing a mixture of *Trypanosoma cruzi* recombinant antigens. *Transfusion* 43: 91, 2003.

236. Portela-Lindoso AA, Shikanai-Yasuda MA: Chronic Chagas' disease: from xenodiagnosis and hemoculture to polymerase chain reaction. *Rev Saude Publica* 37: 107, 2003.

237. Virreira M, Torrico F, Truyens C, et al: Comparison of polymerase chain reaction methods for reliable and easy detection of congenital *Trypanosoma cruzi* infection. *Am J Trop Med Hyg* 68:574, 2003.

238. Vera-Cruz JM, Magallon-Gastelum E, Grijalva G, et al: Molecular diagnosis of Chagas' disease and use of an animal model to study parasite tropism. *Parasitol Res* 89:480, 2003.

239. Marcon GE, Andrade PD, de Albuquerque DM, et al: Use of a nested polymerase chain reaction (N-PCR) to detect *Trypanosoma cruzi* in blood samples from chronic chagasic patients and patients with doubtful serologies. *Diagn Microbiol Infect Dis* 43:39, 2002.

240. Guhl F, Jaramillo C, Carrranza JC, et al: Molecular characterization and diagnosis of *Trypanosoma cruzi* and *T. rangeli.* *Arch Med Res* 33:362, 2002.

241. Kirchhoff LV: Changing epidemiology and approaches to therapy for Chagas disease. *Curr Infect Dis Rep* 5:59, 2003.

242. Villar JC, Marin-Neto JA, Ebrahim S, et al: Trypanocidal drugs for chronic asymptomatic *Trypanosoma cruzi* infection. *Cochrane Database Syst Rev* 1:CD003463, 2002.

243. Leon JS, Wang K, Engman DM: Captopril ameliorates myocarditis in acute experimental Chagas disease. *Circulation* 107:2264, 2003.

244. Urbina JA, Payares G, Sanoja C, et al: Parasitological cure of acute and chronic experimental Chagas disease using the long-acting experimental triazole TAK-187:

Activity against drug-resistant *Trypanosoma cruzi* strains. *Int J Antimicrob Agents* 21:39, 2003.

245. Urbina JA, Payares G, Sanoja C, et al: In vitro and in vivo activities of ravuconazole on *Trypanosoma cruzi,* the causative agent of Chagas disease. *Int J Antimicrob Agents* 21:27, 2003.

246. Francolino SS, Antunes AF, Talice R, et al: New evidence of spontaneous cure in human Chagas' disease. *Rev Soc Bras Med Trop* 36:103, 2003.

247. Dias JC, Silveira AC, Schofield CJ: The impact of Chagas disease control in Latin America: A review. *Mem Inst Oswaldo Cruz* 97:603, 2002.

248. WHO Expert Committee: *Control of Chagas Disease* (World Health Organ Technical Report Series 905). Geneva: WHO, 2002, p 1.

249. Burri C, Brun R: Human African trypanosomiasis. In Cook GC, Zumla A (eds): *Mansons's Tropical Diseases,* 21st ed. London: Saunders, 2003, p 1303.

250. Dumas M: Sleeping sickness, a reemerging sickness. *Bull Acad Natl Med* 184:1867, 2000.

251. Welburn SC, Odiit M: Recent development in human African trypansomiasis. *Curr Opin Infect Dis* 15:477, 2002.

252. Hutchinson OC, Fevre EM, Carrington M, et al: Lessons learned from the emergence of a new *Trypanosoma brucei rhodesiense* sleeping sickness focus in Uganda. *Lancet Infect Dis* 3:42, 2003.

253. Abaru DE: Sleeping sickness in Busoga, Uganda, 1976–1983. *Trop Med Parasitol* 36:72, 1985.

254. Molyneux DH: Vector-borne parasitic diseases: An overview of recent changes. *Int J Parasitol* 28:927, 1998.

255. Hide G: History of sleeping sickness in East Africa. *Clin Microbiol Rev* 12:112, 1999.

256. Enyaru JC, Odiit M, Winyi-Kaboyo R, et al: Evidence for the occurrence of *Trypanosoma brucei rhodesiense* sleeping sickness outside the traditional focus in southeastern Uganda. *Ann Trop Med Parasitol* 93: 817, 1999.

257. Legros D, Gaelle O, Gastellu-Etchegorry M, et al: Treatment of human African trypanosomiasis: Present situation and needs for research and development. *Lancet Infect Dis* 2:437, 2002.

258. WHO: *Control and Surveillance of African Trypanosomiasis* (reprint of a WHO expert committee. World Health Organization Technical Report Series 881). Geneva: WHO, 1998.

259. WHO: *Health Systems: Improving Performance* (World Health Report 2000). Geneva: WHO, 2000.

260. Oscherwitz SL: East African trypanosomiasis. *J Travel Med* 10:141, 2003.

261. Penchenier L, Mathieu-Daude F, Brengues C, et al: Population structure of *Trypanosoma brucei* S.L. in Cote d'Ivoire assayed by multilocus enzyme electrophoresis: Epidemiological and taxonomical considerations. *J Parasitol* 83:14, 1997.

262. Stevens JR, Lanham SM, Allingham R, et al: A simplified method for identifying subspecies and strain groups in Trypanaozoon by isoenzymes. *Ann Trop Med Parasitol* 86:9, 1992.

263. Jamonneau V, Barnabe C, Koffi M, et al: Identification of *Trypansoma brucei* circulating in a sleeping sickness focus in Cote d'Ivoire: Assessment of genotype selection by the isolation method. *Infect Genet Evol* 3:143, 2003.

264. Smith DH, Bailey JW: Human African trypanosomiasis in southeastern Uganda: Clinical diversity and isoenzyme profiles. *Ann Trop Med Parasitol* 91:851, 1997.

265. Truc P, Cuny G: Distribution and spread of human African trypanosomiasis: Value of genetic identification of the trypanosomes. *Med Trop* 61:433, 2001.

266. Okoth JO: Peridomestic breeding sites of *Glossina fuscipes* newts in Busoga, Uganda, and epidemiological implications for trypansomiasis. *Acta Trop* 43:283, 1986.

267. Mbulamberi DB: Possible causes leading to an epidemic outbreak of sleeping sickness: Facts and hypotheses. *Ann Soc Belg Med Trop* 69:173, 1989.

268. Enanga B, Burchmore RJ, Stewart ML, et al: Sleeping sickness and the brain. *Cell Mol Life Sci* 59:845, 2002.

269. Kristensson K, Bentivoglio M: Pathology of African trypanosomiasis. In Dumas M, Bouteille B, Buguet A (eds): *Progress in Human African Trypanosomiasis, Sleeping Sickness,* Part 5. Berlin: Springer, 1999, p 157.

270. Hunter C, Kennedy P: Immunopathology in central nervous system human African trypanosomiasis. *J Neuroimmunol* 36:91, 1992.

271. Sternberg JM: Immunobiology of African trypanosomiasis. *Chem Immunol* 70:186, 1998.

272. Sharafeldin A, Hamadien M, Diab A, et al: Cytokine profiles in the central nervous system and the spleen during the early course of experimental African trypanosomiasis. *Scand J Immunol* 50:256, 1999.

273. Sharafeldin A, Eltayeb R, Pashenkov M, et al: Chemokines are produced in the brain early during the course of experimental African trypanosomiasis. *J Neuroimmunol* 103:165, 2000.

274. Bakhiet M, Hamadien M, Tjernlund A, et al: African trypanosomes activate human fetal brain cells to proliferation and TFN-γ production. *Neuroreport* 21:53, 2002.

275. Shi M, Pau W, Tabel H: Experimental African trypanosomiasis: IFN-γ mediates early mortality. *Eur J Immunol* 33:108, 2003.

276. Lejon V, Lardon J, Kenis G, et al: Interleukin 6 (IL-6), IL-8 and IL-10 in serum and CSF of *Trypansoma brucei gambiense* sleeping sickness patients before and after treatment. *Trans R Soc Trop Med Hyg* 96:329, 2002.

277. Hunter CA, Jennings FW, Tierney JF, et al: Correlation of autoantibody titres with central nervous system pathology in experimental African trypanosomiasis. *J Neuroimmunol* 41:143, 1992.

278. Girard M, Ayed Z, Preux PM, et al: In vitro induction of nitric oxide synthase in astrocytes and microglia by *Trypansoma brucei. Parasite Immunol* 22:7, 2000.

279. Rhind SG, Shek PN: Cytokines in the pathogenesis of human African trypanosomiasis: Antagonistic roles of TNF alpha and IL-10. In Dumas M, Bouteille B, Buguet A (eds): *Progress in Human African Trypanosomiasis, Sleeping Sickness.* Berlin: Springer, 1999, p 119.

280. Burri C, Nkunku S, Merolle A, et al: Efficacy of a new

concise treatment schedule for melarsoprol in treatment of sleeping sickness caused by *Trypanosoma brucei gambiense:* A randomised trial. *Lancet* 355:1419, 2002.

281. Bedat-Millet AL, Charpentier S, Monge-Strauss MF, et al: Forme psychiatrique de trypanosomiase africaine: illustration des difficultés diagnostiques et apport de l'imagerie par résonance magnétique. *Rev Neurol* 156:5, 2000.

282. Lundkvist GB, Hill RH, Kristensson K: Disruption of circadian rhythms in synaptic activity of the suprachiasmatic nuclei by African trypanosomes and cytokines. *Neurobiol Dis* 11:20, 2002.

283. Woo PT: The haematocrit centrifuge for the detection of trypanosomes in blood. *Can J Zool* 47:921, 1996.

284. Lumsden WGR, Kimber CE, Evans DA, et al: *Trypansoma brucei:* Miniature anion exchange centrifugation for detection of low parasitemia: adaptation for field use. *Trans R Soc Trop Med Hyg* 73:314, 1979.

285. Bailey JW, Smith DH: The use of the acridine orange QBC technique in the diagnosis of African trypanosomiasis. *Trans R Soc Trop Med Hyg* 86:630, 1992.

286. Magnus E, Vervoort T, Van Meirvenne N: A card agglutination test with stained trypanosomes (CATT) for the serological diagnosis of *Trypansoma brucei gambiense* trypanosomiasis. *Ann Soc Belg Med Trop* 58:169, 1978.

287. Pansaerts R, Van Meirvenne N, Magnus E, et al: Increased sensitivity of the card agglutination test CATT/*Trypansoma brucei gambiense* by inhibition of complement. *Acta Trop* 70:349, 1998.

288. Nantulya VM: TrypTect CIATT: A card indirect agglutination trypanosomiasis test for diagnosis of *Trypanosoma brucei gambiense* and *Trypansoma brucei rhodesiense* infections. *Trans R Soc Trop Med Hyg* 91:551, 1997.

289. Buscher E, Lejon V, Magnus E, et al: Improved latex agglutination test for detection of antibodies in serum and cerebrospinal fluid of *Trypansoma brucei gambiense*–infected patients. *Acta Trop* 73: 11, 1999.

290. Truc P, Lejon V, Magnus E, et al: Evaluation of the micro-CATT, CATT/*Trypansoma brucei gambiense,* LATEX/*Trypansoma brucei gambiense* methods for serodiagnosis and surveillance of human African trypanosomiasis in west and central Africa. *Bull WHO* 80:882, 2002.

291. Penchenier L, Grebaut P, Njokou F, et al: Evaluation of LATEX/*Trypansoma brucei gambiense* for mass screening of *Trypanosoma brucei gambiense* sleeping sickness in central Africa. *Acta Trop* 85:31, 2003.

292. Kabiri M, Franco JR, Simarro PP, et al: Detection of *Trypanosoma brucei gambiense* in sleeping sickness suspects by PCR amplification of expression-site associated genes 6 and 7. *Trop Med Int Health* 4:658, 1999.

293. Penchenier L, Simo G, Grebaut P, et al: Diagnosis of human trypanosomiasis due to *Trypanosoma brucei gambiense* in central Africa, by the polymerase chain reaction. *Trans R Soc Trop Med Hyg* 94:392, 2000.

294. Kyambadde JW, Enyaru JC, Matovu E, et al: Detection of trypanosomes in suspected sleeping sickness patients in Uganda using the polymerase chain reaction. *Bull WHO* 78:119, 2000.

295. Solano P, Jamonneau V, N'Guessan P, et al: Comparison of different DNA preparation protocols for PCR diagnosis of human African trypanosomiasis in Cote d'Ivoire. *Acta Trop* 82:349, 2002.

296. Radwanska M, Claes F, Magez S, et al: Novel primer sequences for polymerase chain reaction–based detection of *Trypanosoma brucei gambiense*. *Am J Trop Med Hyg* 67:289, 2002.

297. Louis FJ, Buscher P, Lejon V: Diagnosis of human African trypanosomiasis in 2001. *Med Trop* 61:340, 2001.

298. Lejon V, Buscher P: Diagnosis of sleeping sickness stage: Towards a new approach. *Bull Soc Pathol Exot* 95:338, 2002.

299. Lejon V, Buscher P: Stage determination and follow-up in sleeping sickness. *Med Trop* 61:355, 2001.

300. Lejon V, Legros D, Richer M, et al: IgM quantification in the cerebrospinal fluid of sleeping sickness patients by latex card agglutination test. *Trop Med Int Health* 7:685, 2002.

301. Lejon V, Reiber H, Legros D, et al: Intrathecal immune response pattern for improved diagnosis of central nervous system involvement in trypanosomiasis. *J Infect Dis* 187:1475, 2003.

302. Radwanska M, Chamekh M, Vanhamme L, et al: The serum resistance-associated gene as a diagnostic tool for the detection of *Trypanosoma brucei rhodesiense*. *Am J Trop Med Hyg* 67:684, 2002.

303. Jamonneau V, Barnabe C, Koffi M, et al: Identification of *Trypanosoma brucei* circulating in a sleeping sickness focus in Cote d'Ivoire: Assessment of genotype selection by the isolation method. *Infect Genet Evol* 3:143, 2003.

304. Mbala L, Ngita F, Tsita J, Matumueni P, et al: Cerebrospinal trypanosomiasis masquerading as pulmonary infectious disease in a 1-year-old boy. *Ann Trop Pediatr* 20:293, 2000.

305. Barret MP: Problems for the chemotherapy of human African trypansomiasis. *Curr Opin Infect Dis* 13:647, 2000.

306. Kennedy PG, Murray M, Jennings F, et al: Sleeping sickness: new drugs from old? *Lancet* 359:1695, 2002.

307. Burchmore RJ, Ogbunude PO, Enanga B, et al: Chemotherapy of human African trypanosomiasis. *Curr Pharm Des* 8:256, 2002.

308. Burri C, Brun R: Eflornithine for the treatment of human African trypanosomiasis. *Parasitol Res* 90(supp 1):S49, 2003.

309. Jennings FW, Rodgers J, Bradley B, et al: Human African trypanosomiasis: Potential therapeutic benefits of an alternative suramin and melarsoprol regimen. *Parasitol Int* 51:381, 2002.

310. Masiga DK, Barrett MP: Sleeping sickness. *Africa Health* 22:5, 2000.

311. Dumas M, Bouteille B: *Progress in Human African Trypanosomiasis, Sleeping Sickness.* Berlin: Springer, 1999.

312. Chauviere G, Bouteille B, Enanga B, et al: Synthesis and biological activity of nitro heterocycles analogous

to megazol, a trypanocidal lead. *J Med Chem* 30:427, 2003.

313. Bouteille B, Onkem O, Bisser S, et al: Treatment perspectives for human African trypanosomiasis. *Fundam Clin Pharmacol* 17:171, 2003.

314. Donkor IO, Assefa H, Rattendi D, et al: Trypanocidal activity of dicationic compounds related to pentamidine. *Eur J Med Chem* 36:531, 2001.

315. Donkor IO, Clark AM: In vitro antimicrobial activity of aromatic diamidines and diimidazolines related to pentamidine. *Eur J Med Chem* 34:639, 1999.

316. Donkor IO, Huang TL, Tao B, et al: Trypanocidal activity of conformationally restricted pentamidine congeners. *J Med Chem* 46:1041, 2003.

317. Keiser J, Ericsson O, Burri C: Investigations of the metabolites of the trypanocidal drug melarsoprol. *Clin Pharmacol Ther* 67:478, 2000.

318. Hunter CA, Jennings FW, Adams JH, et al: Subcurative chemotherapy and fatal post-treatment reactive encephalopathies in African trypanosomiasis. *Lancet* 25:250, 1992.

319. Jennings FW, Hunter CA, Kennedy PG, et al: Chemotherapy of *Trypansoma brucei* infection of the central nervous system: Use of a rapid chemotherapeutic regimen and the development of post-treatment encephalopathies. *Trans R Soc Trop Med Hyg* 87:224, 1993.

320. Kennedy PG: The pathogenesis and modulation of the post-treatment reactive encephalopathy in a mouse model of human African trypanosomiasis. *J Neuoimmunol* 100:36, 1999.

321. Eckersall PD, Gow JW, McComb C, et al: Cytokines and the acute phase response in post-treatment reactive encephalopathy *Trypanosoma brucei*–infected mice. *Parasitol Int* 50:15, 2001.

322. Hunter CA, Jennings FW, Kennedy PG, et al: The use of azathioprine to ameliorate post-treatment encephalopathy associated with African trypanosomiasis. *Neuropathol Appl Neurobiol* 18:619, 1992.

323. Pepin J, Mpia B, Hoasche M: *Trypanosoma brucei gambiense* African trypanosomiasis: Differences between men and women in severity of disease and response to treatment. *Trans R Soc Trop Med Hyg* 96:421, 2002.

324. Koten JW, De Raadt P: Myocarditis in *Trypanosoma rhodesiense* infections. *Trans R Soc Trop Med Hyg* 63:485, 1969.

325. Brun R, Schumacher R, Schmid C, et al: The phenomenon of treatment failures in human African trypanosomiasis. *Trop Med Int Health* 6:906, 2001.

326. Lubega GW, Byarugaba DK, Prichard RK: Immunization with a tubulin-rich preparation from *Trypanosoma brucei* confers broad protection against African trypanosomosis. *Exp Parasitol* 102:9, 2002.

327. Rogers DJ, Randolph SE: A response to the aim of eradicating tsetse from Africa. *Trends Parasitol* 18:534, 2002.

328. Welburn SC, Picozzi K, Fevre EM, et al: Identification of human-infective trypanosomes in animal reservoir of sleeping sickness in Uganda by means of serum-resistance-associated (*SRA*) gene. *Lancet* 358:2017, 2001.

329. Fevre EM, Coleman PG, Odiit M, et al: The origins of a new *Trypanosoma brucei rhodesiense* sleeping sickness outbreak in eastern Uganda. *Lancet* 25:625, 2001.

330. Wendo C: Uganda revises cattle treatment of protect humans from sleeping sickness. *Lancet* 359:239, 2002.

331. Aspoeck H, Auer H, Walochnik J: Harmlose Unpaesslichkeit fuer gesunde-lebensbedrohliche Krankheit für Ungeborene und AIDS Patienten. In Aspoeck H (ed): *Amoeben, Bandwuermer, Zecken,* 1 Aufl. Linz: Kataloge des OOe Landesmuseums, Biologiezentrum OOe, 2002, p 179.

332. Holliman RE: Toxoplasmosis: Parasitic protozoa. In Cook GC, Zumla A (eds): *Mansons's Tropical Diseases,* 21st ed. London: Saunders, 2003, p 1365.

333. Pinkerton H, Weinman D: Toxoplasma infection in man. *Arch Pathol* 30:374, 1940.

334. Sabin AB, Feldman HA: Dyes as microchemical indicators of a new immunity phenomenon affecting a protozoan parasite. *Science* 108:660, 1948.

335. Hutchison WM, Dunachie JF, Work K, et al: The life cycle of the coccidian parasite *Toxoplasma gondii* in the domestic cat. *Trans R Soc Trop Med Hyg* 65:380, 1971.

336. Dubey JP, Beattle PB: *Toxoplasmosis of Animals and Man.* Boca Raton, FL: CRC Press, 1988, p 1.

337. Schmutzhard E, Fuchs D, Hengster P, et al: Retroviral infections (HIV-1, HIV-2, and HTLV-I) in rural northwestern Tanzania: Clinical findings, epidemiology, and association with infections common in Africa. *Am J Epidemiol* 130:309, 1989.

338. Gagne SS: Toxoplasmosis. *Prim Care Update Obstet Gynecol* 8:122, 2001.

339. Mimadi A, DeSimone JA, Pomerantz RJ: Central nervous system infections in individuals with HIV-1-infection. *J Neurovirol* 8:158, 2002.

340. Happe S, Fischer A, Heese Ch, et al: HIV-associated cerebral toxoplasmosis: Review and retrospective analysis of 36 patients. *Nervenarzt* 73:1174, 2002.

341. Singh N, Husain S: Infections of the central nervous system transplant recipients. *Transpl Infect Dis* 2:101, 2000.

342. Roemer E, Blau IW, Basar N, et al: Toxoplasmosis, a severe complication in allogeneic hematopoietic stem cell transplantation: Successful treatment strategies during a 5-year single-center experience. *Clin Infect Dis* 32:E1-8, 2001.

343. Gonzalez MI, Caballerio D, Lopez C, et al: Cerebral toxoplasmosis and Guillain-Barré syndrome after allogeneic peripheral stem cell transplantation. *Transpl Infect Dis* 2:145, 2000.

344. Pruitt AA: Nervous system infections in patients with cancer. *Neurol Clin* 21:193, 2003.

345. Jellinger KA, Setinek U, Drlicek M, et al: Neuropathology and general autopsy findings in AIDS during the last 15 years. *Acta Neuropathol* 100:213, 2002.

346. Martinez AJ: The neuropathology of organ transplantation: comparison and contrast in 500 patients. *Pathol Res Pract* 194:473, 1998.

347. Naessens A, Jenum PA, Pollak A, et al: Diagnosis of congenital toxoplasmosis in the neonatal period: A multicenter evaluation. *J Pediatr* 135:714, 1999.

348. Holland GN, Lewis KG, O'Connor GR: Ocular toxoplasmosis: A 50th anniversary tribute to the contributions of Helenor Campell Wilder Forerster. *Arch Ophthalmol* 120:1081, 2002.

349. Kean BH: Clinical toxoplasmosis: 50 years. *Trans R Soc Trop Med Hyg* 66:549, 1972.

350. Carter AO, Frank JW: Congenital toxoplasmosis: Epidemiological features and control. *Can Med Assoc J* 135:618, 1986.

351. Koppe JH, Loewer Steger DH, de Roever-Bonnet H: Results of 20 year follow-up of congenital toxoplasmosis. *Lancet* 1:254, 1986

352. Holliman RE: Toxoplasmosis and the acquired immune deficiency syndrome. *J Infect* 16:121, 1988.

353. Chaddha DS, Kalra SP, Singh AP, et al: Toxoplasmic encephalitis in acquired immunodeficiency syndrome. *J Assoc Phys Ind* 47:680, 1999.

354. Skiest DJ: Focal neurological disease in patients with acquired immunodeficiency syndrome. *Clin Infect Dis* 34:103, 2002.

355. Wreghitt TG, Hakim M, Gray JJ, et al: Toxoplasmosis in heart and heart and lung transplant recipients. *J Clin Pathol* 42:194, 1987.

356. Nakazaki S, Saeki N, Itoh S, et al: Toxoplasmic encephalitis in patients with acquired immunodeficiency syndrome: Four case reports. *Neurol Med Chir* 40:120, 2000.

357. Pezzini A, Zavarise P, Palvarini L, et al: Holmes' tremor following midbrain *Toxoplasma* abscess: Clinical features a treatment of a case. *Parkinsonism Relat Disord* 8:177, 2002.

358. Straathof CS, Kortbeek LM, Roerdink H, et al: A solitary spinal cord *Toxoplasma* lesion after peripheral stem-cell transplantation. *J Neurol* 248:814, 2001.

359. Hill D, Dubey JP: *Toxoplasma gondii:* Transmission, diagnosis and prevention. *Clin Microbiol Infect* 8:634, 2002.

360. Gross U, Pelloux H: Diagnosis in the pregnant woman. In Ambroise-Thomas P, Petersen E (eds): *Congenital Toxoplasmosis: Scientific Background, Clinical Management and Control.* Berlin: Springer-Verlag, 2000, p 121.

361. Forestier F, Hohfeld R, Soley Y, et al: Prenatal diagnosis of congenital toxoplasmosis by PCR: Extended experience. *Prenat Diagn* 18:405, 1990.

362. Auer H, Vander Mose A, Picher O, et al: Clinical and diagnostic relevance of the *Toxoplasma* IgG avidity test in the serological surveillance of pregnant women in Austria. *Parastiol Res* 86:965, 2002.

363. Vastava PB, Pradhan S, Jha S, et al: MRI features of *Toxoplasma* encephalitis in the immunocompetent host: A report of two cases. *Neuroradiolgy* 44: 834, 2002.

364. Chunha BA: Central nervous system infections in the compromised host: a diagnostic approach. *Infect Dis Clin North Am* 15:567, 2001.

365. Julander I, Martin C, Lappalainen M, et al: Polymerase chain reaction for diagnostic of cerebral toxoplasmosis in cerebrospinal fluid in HIV-positive patients. *Scand J Infect Dis* 33:538, 2001.

366. da Silva AV, Langoni H: The detection of *Toxoplasma gondii* by comparing cytology, histopathology, bioassay in mice, and the polymerase chain reaction (PCR). *Vet Parasitol* 97:191, 2001.

367. McCabe RE, Oser S: Current recommendations and future prospects in the treatment of toxoplasmosis. *Drugs* 38:973, 1989.

368. Carter AO, Gelmon SB, Wells GA, et al: The effectiveness of a prenatal education programme for the prevention of congenital toxoplasmosis. *Epidemiol Infect* 103:39, 1989.

369. Buston D, Innes EA: A commercial vaccine for ovine toxoplasmosis. *Parasitology* 110:811, 1955

370. Ramos Santos C, Hernandez-Montes O, Sanchez-Tejeda G, et al: Visceral leishmaniosis caused by *Leishmania (L.) mexicana* in a Mexican patient with human immunodeficiency virus infection. *Mem Inst Oswaldo Cruz* 95:733, 2000.

371. Abreu-Silva Al, Calabrese KS, Tedesco C, et al: Central nervous system involvement in experimental infection with *Leishmania (L.) amazonensis. Am J Trop Med Hyg* 68:661, 2003.

372. Nieto CG, Vinuelas J, Bianco A, et al: Detection of *Leishmania infantum amastigotes* in canine choroid plexus. *Vet Rec* 139:346, 1966.

373. Garcia-Alonso M, Nieto CG, Blanco A, et al: Presence of antibodies in the aqueous humour and cerebrospinal fluid during *Leishmania* infections in dogs: Pathologic features at the central nervous system. *Parasite Immunol* 18:539, 1996.

374. Dedet JP, Pratlong F: Leishmaniasis. In Cook GC, Zumla A (eds): *Manson's Tropical Diseases,* 21st ed. London: Saunders, 2003, p 1339.

375. Berman J, Badaro R, Thakur C, et al: Efficacy and safety of liposomal amphotericin B (AmBisome) for visceral leishmaniasis in endemic developing countries. *Bull WHO* 76:25, 1998.

376. Sundar S, Makharia A, More D, et al: Short course of oral miltefosine for treatment of visceral leishmaniasis. *Clin Infect Dis* 31:110, 2000.

CHAPTER 18

Prion Encephalopathies

Erik Johnson and James A. Mastrianni

The prion diseases are unique infectious diseases that also behave as typical neurodegenerative diseases. As such, they may occur spontaneously or sporadically, present as familial disease due to a germline mutation, or result from exposure to the infectious agent. The nature of the pathogenic agent of these diseases also sets them apart from other infectious diseases. This unconventional agent has been termed a *prion* to denote its *pro*teinaceous *in*fectious nature. The prion is composed largely, if not entirely, of a host-encoded protein that undergoes misfolding to an aberrant three-dimensional structure and appears to transfer this altered conformation to normally folded host-encoded prion protein without the need for nucleic acid. Study of the prion and how it causes disease has yielded insight into a number of previously poorly understood neurodegenerative diseases and has challenged fundamental biologic tenets on how information can be encoded within the cell.

The characterization of human prion disease began in the 1950s with work by Carleton Gajdusek on a strange disease, called *kuru,* endemic to the Fore tribe living in the Papua New Guinea highlands. Persons afflicted with the disease were largely women and children, who developed a severe progressive ataxia and dementia that led rapidly to death.[1–3] Gajdusek concluded that the disease was spread by horizontal transmission from the deceased relatives during cannibalistic rituals. Women and children were most affected, presumably from greater contact with the brain during the preparation and ceremony of the feast. Pathologic examination of the brains of afflicted individuals revealed extensive vacuolation (spongiform change) and deposition of amyloid plaques. Transmission of disease to chimpanzees by inoculation of brain material from kuru patients was reported in 1966.[4] Two years later, Creutzfeldt-Jakob disease (CJD), another obscure human neurologic disease with undetermined etiology but similar neuropathology to kuru, was also transmitted to chimpanzees.[5] Because of the unique spongy degeneration of the brain observed in CJD and kuru patients, these diseases were labeled *transmissible spongiform encephalopathies* (TSEs).

Although the etiologic agent of the TSEs was not identified, it was hypothesized to be a "slow virus" based on the long incubation times required for expression of disease.[6,7] This slow virus was indeed unconventional because it provoked no immune response in the host and was resistant to formalin, ultraviolet (UV) light, and ionizing radiation treatments that normally destroy viruses.[8–11] A significant protein content of the infectious agent was recognized early on, but Stanley Prusiner pursued this finding to show eventually that a single protein was consistently present in the infectious fraction, dubbed the *prion protein,* and that surprisingly this protein was encoded by a normal chromosomal gene of the host.[10–16] Sequencing of the prion protein gene (*PRNP*) was pivotal to understanding prion disease because it showed that mutations in the gene could give rise to CJD, as well as two other diseases not previously considered to be prion diseases, Gerstmann Sträussler Scheinker disease (GSS) and fatal familial insomnia (FFI).[17–19] Linkage of germline mutations in *PRNP* with prion disease confirmed the multiple modes of expression of this family of diseases: spontaneous, genetic, and infectious.

Prion diseases also occur in animals as a result of natural disease or by exposure to prions. A major focus of prion research is to determine the potential for transmission of animal-borne prion disease to humans. The apparent ability of some prions to cross the species barrier has garnered much public attention.[20] Transgenic animal studies have shown that the species barrier to infection seems to depend largely on the degree of amino acid sequence homology between the infectious prion and the host prion protein.[21–23] However, this species barrier is not absolute, as demonstrated by the recent identification of a new prion disease in humans linked to the consumption of beef products contaminated with bovine prions from bovine spongiform encephalopathy (BSE). An emerging natural prion disease of deer and elk, known as *chronic wasting disease* (CWD), is currently raising more concern about the species barrier as it relates to the safety of humans.

▶ EPIDEMIOLOGY

The worldwide yearly incidence of sporadic prion disease is 1 case per 1 million population and 1 case per 100 million population for genetic disease. No obvious gender bias has been noted.[24] A higher incidence of prion disease within certain countries and cultures was thought initially to be due to dietary habits but later was linked to causal genetic mutations.[18,25–27] Sporadic CJD (sCJD) accounts for about 85 percent of all cases of prion disease.[28] Onset is typically in the seventh decade, but patients aged 17 to 90 have been reported.[24] Because progression of disease to death is typically under 6 months, the annual incidence is roughly equal to the annual mortality rate. Environmental exposure and geographic location are not risk factors for sCJD.[29,30] Importantly, patient-to-patient spread does not occur.[24] About 15 percent of prion disease cases are autosomal dominantly inherited. In contrast to sporadic disease, familial cases of prion disease, on average, present earlier in life (prior to age 55) and have a more protracted disease course (1 to 5 years). In rare cases, patients have survived for over 20 years after the onset of disease.[31] The rate and character of progression of familial prion disease depend heavily on the associated mutation.

The relatively small number of acquired prion diseases are due either to ingestion or iatrogenic administration of prions. With the recognition of the link to kuru, cannibalism largely has been eliminated as a cause of the acquired form of disease. In recent years, however, a source of orally consumed prions has been the cow. Since 1995, at least 150 cases of CJD have been documented, mostly in the United Kingdom (U.K.) and Europe, as a result of BSE. In 1995, the first cases of what is now termed *variant CJD* (vCJD) were reported in teenagers.[32,33] In addition to epidemiologic evidence,[20] experimental evidence also supports a causal link between BSE and vCJD.[34–37] Why younger individuals are at higher risk is not known, but it may relate in part to the types of food consumed and their relative quantities. While it is unlikely that significant quantities of brain material were introduced into human food, mechanically rendered meats that went into foodstuffs such as hamburgers and sausages were likely contaminated with spinal cord material known to contain high titers of prions. Whether vCJD will evolve into a true epidemic is not currently known, the answer depending heavily on the range of its incubation period. The minimum incubation time appears to be 6 to 12 years, which is comparable with other forms of peripheral exposure, such as human growth hormone (hGH) and kuru.[20] In 1997, Cousens and colleagues applied a mathematical model to data from initial vCJD cases and estimated the potential number of future cases to be anywhere from a few hundred to over 80,000.[38] Fortunately, the incidence of new cases has been small and holding steady over the last few years. The likely cause of vCJD is sobering because it appears that bovine prions were able to cross the species barrier to infect humans. The potential for prion disease to occur in the wild is also of great concern. This has come to recent attention following the recognition of CWD in deer and elk in the western and central United States.[39] Although the source and transmission of prion disease in these animal populations are not known, the potential health threats to hunters and those who consume game meats has led to the culling and monitoring of certain deer populations in an effort to prevent the spread of prion disease in these and other animal populations. BSE was declared eliminated in the United Kingdom by the Ministry of Agriculture Fisheries and Food (MAFF) in December of 1999, and cases of vCJD currently seem to be leveling off. However, CWD provides an instructive example that prion disease can occur on a large scale in other animal populations and that vigilant monitoring of animals and the animal food supply for the presence of prion disease is prudent. In support of this, a single cow was identified with BSE in Canada in May 2003, and another in the U.S. in December 2003.

No studies have shown an increased occupational risk of contracting prion disease. However, prudence would argue for careful handling of tissue specimens by neurosurgeons, pathologists, and histologic technicians from suspected cases of prion disease in animals and humans.[40] Prions reportedly have been identified in the urine of patients suffering from prion disease,[41] but this finding has not been replicated by others.

The Polymorphic Codon 129 of *PRNP*

Although autosomal dominant mutations of *PRNP* are directly associated with familial prion disease, polymorphisms of the gene also play an important role in disease susceptibility and phenotype. The amino acid at position 129 in the prion protein (PrP) is predominately methionine (allelic frequency of 0.66.) in Caucasians, although valine encoding is prevalent (allelic frequency of 0.34).[42] The genotype distribution is 12 percent VV, 51 percent MV, and 37 percent MM. Interestingly, Met homozygosity is greatly overrepresented in sCJD cases, with some series identifying almost 90 percent of sCJD patients as 129MM.[43–46] In addition, all vCJD cases to date have been 129MM.[47,48] Taken together, these data suggest that homozygosity at residue 129 might predict disease; however, it is important to note that the allelic distribution within the Japanese population is Met (0.96):Val (0.04) with no obvious increase in CJD prevalence.[49] Thus homozygosity at codon 129 is a predisposing factor but not sufficient by itself for developing prion disease. Epidemiologic studies examining the nature of codon 129 in 25 cases of iatrogenic CJD (iCJD) found that 43 percent of the patients were 129VV and 57 percent were 129MM,[50] further supporting this notion.

In addition to imparting risk for disease, codon 129 also influences the phenotype of disease. Patients with sCJD who are 129MM typically have a rapid disease progression with dementia as the identifying feature, whereas patients who are 129VV or 129MV generally have a slower disease course with prominent ataxia.[51] In familial cases, the effect of the polymorphism at codon 129 is most striking when combined with a dominant mutation at codon 178 that causes a change in coding from aspartate (D) to asparagine (N). When 129M is allelic with the D178N mutation, the clinicopathologic phenotype of FFI results. If combined with Val, fCJD is the observed phenotype.[52] Homozygosity at codon 129 also can influence the phenotype of familial diseases. Coupling between F198S, a 144-base-pair insert mutation, and homozygosity at codon 129 seems to lower the age of onset and decrease the duration of GSS induced by these mutations.[53] Thus it appears that the residue at position 129 in PrP plays an important role in the expression of prion disease and the ability of prions to propagate. In addition to susceptibility polymorphisms, recent evidence suggests that another polymorphism at position 219 may protect against CJD.[54] Whereas 12 percent of the Japanese population carries a lysine (K) substitution at codon 219, no CJD patient has yet to be reported with that substitution, implying a protective feature. This has been further suggested in cell culture[55] and transgenic animal studies,[56] whereby expression of PrP carrying K at codon 219 acts to inhibit conversion of nonmutated PrP.

► PATHOPHYSIOLOGY AND PATHOGENESIS

Our understanding of the etiology of prion disease has undergone a major revolution within the past 20 years, and while the exact nature of the infectious agent in prion disease remains to be characterized fully, it has become clear that it is composed mainly, if not exclusively, of the host-encoded PrP. How a protein can apparently replicate itself and carry strain-specific information (see sections on strains below) has presented challenges to the "protein only" hypothesis, yet the details of how this may occur are currently being addressed. While the specifics of how prions replicate are still debated, an overwhelming amount of data have supported the prion concept as the best explanation for these diseases.

The Prion Concept

Early work to define the infectious agent of prion disease showed that it was highly resistant to treatments that normally degrade nucleic acid, such as ionizing and UV irradiation, but it was partially susceptible to prolonged treatment with proteases.[10–13] A relatively protease-resistant polypeptide of 27 to 30 kDa was consistently present in brain homogenate from animals with prion disease. Purification and N-terminal sequencing of this 27- to 30-kDa protein fraction identified its main component to be a chromosomally encoded host protein, dubbed *PrP*.[14–16] It has since been shown that the seminal event in the pathogenesis of prion disease seems to be a tertiary structural conversion of PrP from a mostly α-helical to significantly β-sheet conformation. The two isoforms have been labeled PrP^c and PrP^{Sc}, for the normal *cellular* α-helical protein and the pathogenic *scrapie* β-sheet protein, respectively. Both are 33 to 35 kDa in molecular weight and have no obvious covalent posttranslational modifications. However, PrP^c is soluble in nondenaturing detergents and susceptible to proteolytic digestion, whereas PrP^{Sc} is insoluble and largely resistant to proteolytic degradation. High-resolution nuclear magnetic resonance (NMR) and x-ray structures have been solved for PrP^c and show the protein to be composed of three well-ordered α helices and an unorthodox β sheet, with the N-terminus being largely disordered.[57,58] The insolubility of PrP^{Sc} has hampered attempts to obtain high-resolution structural information on the protein, but spectroscopic structural studies have shown it to be composed of at least 40 percent β sheet.[59] How PrP^c converts into PrP^{Sc} is not understood, and answering this question is currently a major research goal. It should be mentioned that PrP^c and PrP^{Sc} may each exist in multiple conformations (see section on strains below), and therefore, the terms *PrP^c* and *PrP^{Sc}* should be considered to denote functional rather than specific structural states.

De novo generation of PrP^{Sc} can occur via a familial or somatic mutation that increases the probability that PrP^c will convert to PrP^{Sc} or through a stochastic conformational change from PrP^c to PrP^{Sc}. Once PrP^{Sc} has been generated, its replication is thought to occur by protein-protein interaction, whereby PrP^{Sc} provides a structural template to convert more PrP^c into PrP^{Sc}. The strongest support for this mechanism comes from the finding that transgenic mice in which the *PRNP* gene has been ablated (PrP knockouts) are resistant to prions.[60–62] Furthermore, transgenic mice that express a chimeric PrP transgene constructed of both human and mouse segments (MHu2M-PrP^c) produce chimeric PrP^{Sc} (MHu2M-PrP^{Sc}) after inoculation of HuPrP^{Sc} from humans with prion disease, clearly demonstrating that HuPrP^{Sc} converts nonpathogenic host PrP^c (MHu2M-PrP^c) into pathogenic (MHu2M-PrP^{Sc}) PrP^{Sc} rather than self-replicating in the host.[63] However, attempts to convert PrP^c into PrP^{Sc} in vitro have been unsuccessful to date; while some properties of PrP^{Sc}, such as insolubility and protease resistance, have been reproduced in the test tube, infectivity has not. This result, along with other studies with transgenic mice, has pointed to the possibility of another cellular factor, perhaps an additional protein, that is necessary for the conversion reaction to occur.[63–65] This factor has not been isolated.

A direct protein-protein interaction between PrP^c and PrP^{Sc} is also supported by the existence of a species barrier. Transmission of prion disease from Syrian hamsters (SHa) to mice is highly inefficient, but mice expressing a SHa PrP transgene (SHaPrP) are susceptible to infection with SHa PrP^{Sc}.[21] Furthermore, transmission of human prion disease to mice was only efficient when the central segment of the mouse protein was replaced by a human sequence.[22,66] These and other studies have shown that sequence homology between infectious PrP^{Sc} and host PrP^c is an important determinant for the ability of PrP^{Sc} to convert PrP^c.

The minimum number of PrP^{Sc} molecules required to cause disease is not known. However, once an "infectious unit" is generated, a cascade of events occurs that eventually leads to cell death. Whether PrP^{Sc} is directly responsible for cell death is not yet known. Other possible causes have been proposed, including apoptosis, oxidative damage, and an astrocytic response that releases toxic levels of cytokines.[67–69] Once disease progression begins, it is irreversible and eventually leads to death of the host.

The Prion Protein

PrP is a 253-amino-acid protein encoded by the *PRNP* gene located on the short arm of chromosome 20.[70] Differential splicing of the *PRNP* transcript does not occur. The protein has two N-linked glycosylation sites at residues 181 and 197 and one disulfide bond, and it is attached to the cell membrane via a glycophosphatidylinositol (GPI) anchor.[71] PrP is constitutively expressed in the adult, and its expression is regulated during development. Highest expression is seen in neurons, but the protein is also expressed to a lesser degree in peripheral tissues, notably lung, heart, white blood cells, and platelets.[23,72,73] Immunocytology has localized PrP to the neuromuscular junction, which may explain why mice engineered to greatly overexpress PrP develop a spontaneous hind limb paralysis due to a demyelinating neuropathy and necrotizing myopathy.[74,75] The absence of PrP^{Sc} in these mice has raised the possibility that PrP^{Sc} is not responsible for cell death in prion disease, although PrP^c mRNA has not been shown to be upregulated during disease development in animals.[16,76] Peripheral and central anterograde neuronal transport also has been noted, which may have implications for the route of infection in acquired prion diseases.[76,77]

The function of PrP has remained enigmatic. Various reports have suggested a role in copper transport, synaptic function, and signal transduction, yet the original PrP knockout mice showed no obvious defects even though the protein sequence is highly conserved among species.[60,78–82] Subsequent PrP knockout mice generated in other laboratories showed a mild phenotype of altered circadian rhythm and ataxia, perhaps due to the interruption of a gene located next to the *PRNP* locus that codes for a protein with 25 percent homology to PrP named *doppel* (Dpl).[83–85] Dpl mRNA has been shown to be upregulated in mice that develop the ataxic phenotype but not in the normal PrP knockout mice.[85] Dpl has a similar tertiary structure to PrP, but whether it provides functional redundancy for PrP remains to be answered. To date, no studies have shown an increase in Dpl expression in human prion disease, and no mutations in Dpl have yet been linked to prion disease.[86,87]

Prion Strains

While the existence of prion strains in animals has been known for quite some time, only recently has the strain phenomenon been correlated with conformational differences in PrP^Sc. As an example, two types of transmissible mink encephalopathy (TME) strains passaged in hamsters, designated *HYPER* and *DROWSY,* show remarkably different behavioral phenotypes, pathologic profiles, and incubation periods, and the corresponding PrP^Sc molecules show different electrophoretic mobilities, suggesting a conformational difference between them.[88,89] BSE also shows a characteristic electrophoretic signature when passaged into hosts of different species, such as hamster, macaque, and mouse.[34–36,90,91] Other animal prion strains have been investigated, and several subconformations of PrP^Sc have been reported that correlate with strain.[92] This phenomenon is recapitulated in human prion disease. The five subtypes of human prion disease (CJD, vCJD, GSS, FI, and kuru) show unique PrP^Sc molecules by gel electrophoresis, and the differences in electrophoretic mobility in some are reproduced after passage to experimental animals. The unique forms also correlate with the observed phenotypes in the experimental host.[93,94] The *protein signature* can aid in the diagnosis of prion disease and has lent support to the theory that BSE is responsible for vCJD in the United Kingdom. How different PrP^Sc conformers can lead to such disparate clinical and pathologic profiles in prion disease is not well understood and has been interpreted by some as evidence that nucleic acid is involved in the generation of strain diversity.[95,96] The glycosylation pattern of PrP also may be important in explaining distinct prion strains. Transgenic animals in which one or both glycosylation sites are disrupted show different patterns of PrP^Sc distribution in the brain after inoculation with similar PrP^Sc isolates, implicating a dependence on glycosylation for trafficking of PrP^Sc.[97] Full structural characterization of these different PrP^Sc conformations awaits high-resolution structural information on PrP^Sc, and further work is needed to address how different PrP^Sc conformations can influence expression of prion disease.

► PHENOTYPES OF PRION DISEASE

Human prion disease shows a remarkable variation in clinical features resulting from a single etiologic factor. Long before PrP was identified as the central feature of these diseases, specific names were given to different phenotypes based on their clinical profiles. However, because clinical features vary so widely, disease classification now also rests on the presence of specific neuropathologic features. This has led to the classification of prion disease into five major categories: kuru, Creutzfeldt-Jakob disease (CJD), variant CJD (vCJD), Gerstmann-Sträussler-Scheinker disease (GSS), and fatal insomnia (FI) (Table 18-1). While these defined categories encompass most cases of prion disease, some patients present with overlapping clinical and/or pathologic features, and therefore, it may be more useful to think about prion disease classified into acquired, sporadic, and inherited subtypes. Since sCJD is by far the most common prion disease, most of this discussion will address the clinical features of this disease. Attention also will be given to the acquired prion diseases: kuru, iCJD, and vCJD. Familial forms will be mentioned for completeness, but detailed reviews of clinical features associated with specific mutations in familial forms of prion disease (fCJD, GSS, and FFI) can be found elsewhere.[98]

Sporadic CJD (sCJD)

The relentless and rapid progression of multifocal neurologic deficits distinguishes sCJD from many other neurologic diseases. The classic triad of sCJD includes progressive dementia, ataxia, and myoclonus. About 70 percent of patients present with cognitive decline alone or with ataxia, whereas about 15 to 20 percent present exclusively with ataxia, although nearly all patients eventually will develop frank dementia at some point during the disease course.[99] The cognitive decline may be heralded by complaints of concentration problems and difficulty performing mental calculations or maintaining train of thought, progressing to specific impairments of immediate and/or delayed recall, aphasia, constructional apraxias, and any other cortically based function. At initial evaluation, memory testing may show impairment of short- and long-term memory, difficulty with expressive and/or receptive language (dysphasia), problems with calculations (dyscalculia), difficulty carrying out a complex motor movement (dyspraxia), or loss of the ability to write (dysgraphia). Often the earliest problem noted is most obviously and severely affected by the time other features of disease begin to appear. In about 25 percent of patients a prodromal period characterized by vague complaints of fatigue, vertigo, headache, sleep disturbance, and anxiety may be apparent prior to the onset of clinically obvious disease.[100] Behavioral and personality changes, anorexia, and depression also can occur. Most cases of CJD develop subacutely over the course of several weeks, although about 10 percent of cases will have a more abrupt onset that suggests encephalitis, stroke, or acute inflammatory disease of the brain.

▶ **TABLE 18-1.** PHENOTYPES OF HUMAN PRION DISEASE

Disease	Occurrence	Age at Onset (Range)	Time to Death (Mos.)	Clinical Phenotype	Pathologic Phenotype
Kuru	Cannibalism	~40 years (29–60)	3–12	Gait ataxia, myoclonus, dementia	Presence of kuru-type plaques
CJD	Sporadic	~60 years (17–83)	<12 (typically 4–6)	Early dementia, then gait ataxia, and myoclonus	Extensive vacuolation (spongiosis) and gliosis
	Iatrogenic	Depends on age at "infection"	<12	Variable, often ataxia, then dementia	Extensive vacuolation (spongiosis) and gliosis
	Genetic	<55 years (20s–80s*)	>12 and <72	Early dementia, then gait ataxia, and myoclonus	Extensive vacuolation (spongiosis) and gliosis
GSS	Genetic	<60 years (20s to 80s)	12–60	Early ataxia and dysarthria, late dementia	PrP-amyloid plaques, gliosis, less vacuolation than CJD
FI	Sporadic (sFI)	~45 years	12–16	Refractory insomnia, autonomic dysfunction, then ataxia, and late dementia	Thalamic and olivary nucleus neuronal loss and gliosis, minimal spongiform pathology
	Genetic (FFI)	~45 years	12–16		
vCJD	Beef consumption?	~30 years (18–53)	12–18	Psychiatric (depression, apathy) or pain syndrome, then gait dysfunction, late dementia	Presence of florid-type PrP-amyloid plaques

*Typically less than 50 years, although some mutations may present later in life.

Soon after the cognitive problems appear, gait or truncal ataxia becomes prominent, although appendicular ataxia may appear simultaneously or follow shortly. Other signs of cerebellar involvement include vertigo, nystagmus, ocular dysmetria, intention tremor, and dysarthria. Worsening ataxia is evidenced by an increased frequency of falls, eventually necessitating the use of a wheelchair. Incoordination of swallowing, manifested initially as coughing during eating or drinking, is a consequence of ataxia. This increases the risk for aspiration pneumonia, a common cause of death in these patients. Pyramidal and extrapyramidal features may be present at onset in about 1 to 2 percent of patients, yet develop eventually in approximately 50 percent of patients during the course of the disease. In addition to dementia and motor signs, diffuse or focal weakness, peripheral neuropathy, choreiform movements, hallucinations, cortical blindness, primary language disturbance, supranuclear ophthalmoplegia, and alien hand syndrome, among others, have been observed at onset.[100–102] The extremely wide variation in clinical signs presumably reflects the fact that CJD can initiate from almost any cortical region, from which it then spreads throughout the brain.

Myoclonus, another cardinal feature of sCJD, develops in over 75 percent of patients, typically appearing during the middle to late stages of the disease. This appears as a spontaneous or stimulus-induced irregular multifocal jerking of large muscle groups. Startle myoclonus may appear early and be induced by a loud noise, such as from clapping the hands. In some cases this response may be so prominent that simply walking into the room, initiating speech during a quiet period, or turning on the light in a dark room may provoke the response. Even when warned of the stimulus, the patient is unable to suppress the startle response. In the final stage of disease, the patient is usually bedridden, akinetic, and mute. Sleep-wake cycles may be evident, and myoclonus may persist. Total disease duration averages 4 to 5 months, with 70 percent of patients dying within 6 months. Less typical cases extend for over a year. The cause of death may be due to aspiration pneumonia, starvation because of inability to eat, or sepsis.

True variants of CJD that defy the typical clinical pattern and course of the disease occur in less than 20 percent of patients. In some cases the phenotype is sufficiently unique and reproducible to have been labeled a syndrome. The Heidenhaim variant, described in 1929, is a syndrome in which the rapid dementia is associated with cortical blindness and extensive involvement of the occipital lobes.[103] An ataxic variant, as noted earlier, has been described in which cerebellar ataxia predominates and dementia is a late feature in the disease.[99,104] A panencephalopathic form, reported almost exclusively in Japan, shows extensive degeneration of the cerebral white matter and vacuolation of the gray matter. A variant that shows dementia along with lower

▶ **TABLE 18-2.** WHO CRITERIA FOR THE DIAGNOSIS OF sCJD

Definite CJD
1. Diagnosed by standard neuropathologic techniques and/or
2. Immunocytochemically and/or Western blot confirmed protease-resistant PrP and/or
3. Presence of scrapie-associated fibrils

Probable CJD
1. Progressive dementia *and*
2. At least two of the following four clinical features:
   a. myoclonus
   b. visual or cerebellar disturbance
   c. pyramidal/extrapyramidal signs
   d. akinetic mutism
   and
3. Periodic discharges on the EEG *and/or* a positive 14-3-3 CSF assay and a clinical duration to death <2 years
4. Routine investigations should not suggest an alternative diagnosis

Possible CJD:
1. Progressive dementia *and*
2. At least two of the following four clinical features:
   a. myoclonus
   b. visual or cerebellar disturbance
   c. pyramidal/extrapyramidal signs
   d. akinetic mutism
   and
2. No EEG available or atypical EEG and
3. Duration <2 years

motor neuron signs has been reported, but whether this "amyotrophic variant" is true prion disease has been questioned on the basis of conflicting reports of transmissibility.[105–108]

Diagnostic Evaluation of CJD

The World Health Organization (WHO) has proposed criteria for the diagnosis of "definite," "probable," and "possible" cases of CJD (Table 18-2). Estimates for the sensitivity and specificity of these criteria in defining "probable" CJD have been reported recently to be approximately 65 to 95 percent, respectively, whereas inclusion of the "possible" CJD category changes these figures to 91 and 28 percent, respectively. Inclusion of the criteria for possible CJD therefore increases the sensitivity but reduces specificity.[109] Overall, it was estimated that 12 percent of CJD was missed by these criteria, indicating that better diagnostic methods are needed.

Studies

Typical diagnostic tools include the electroencephalogram (EEG), magnetic resonance imaging (MRI), and cerebrospinal fluid (CSF) analysis. While best studied in sCJD, these tools are variably helpful in other forms of prion disease. These tools are discussed below and presented concisely in Table 18-3.

▶ **TABLE 18-3.** COMPARISON OF DIAGNOSTIC TESTING OF PRION DISEASE SUBTYPES

Phenotype	EEG	Neuroimaging	CSF Studies	Biopsy*
sCJD	~70% of cases have PSWCs	Nonspecific atrophy Increased signal in basal ganglia or cortex with DWI	14-3-3 positive in most cases of highly probable CJD, although not diagnostic on its own. May need to repeat to increase sensitivity Mild, nonspecific protein elevation common in all PrD	Frontal cortex shows spongiform change* Negative in tonsils and lymphoid organs
fCJD	Mutation-dependent: V210I, and E200K carriers, generally positive, most others negative	Similar to sCJD but variable— depends on mutation	Less consistent results with fCJD, some positive, most not	Mutation-dependent, but most will have positive spongiform change by frontal cortex biopsy Studies of lymphoid tissues lacking
iCJD	Slow waves	Insufficient data	Insufficient data	—
GSS	Typically, no PSWCs	Nonspecific, ?cerebellar atrophy Insufficient data on DWI	14-3-3 typically negative	May show regional pathology, cerebellar > frontal plaque path
FI	Slow waves	PET useful, thalamic hypometabolism	Insufficient data	Minimal pathology at cortex; may therefore be unhelpful
vCJD	Slow waves	Hyperintensity of pulvinar with proton-weighted MRI and DWI	<50% 14-3-3 positive	Tonsils and lymph nodes may contain protease-resistant PrP Cerebral cortex shows florid plaque pathology

*Biopsy often reserved for younger patients and those with atypical presentations.
DWI = diffusion-weighted MRI

The EEG usually shows bilateral periodic sharp wave complexes (PSWCs) of 0.5 to 2.0 Hz against a slow wave background at some point during the disease. A characteristic EEG is shown in Figure 18-1A; however, it should be noted that findings on the EEG are variable, and PSWCs also can be found in other diseases. When present with the clinical triad, PSWCs predict sCJD with about 90 percent certainty.[100,110,111] Serial monitoring of the EEG may be necessary to observe PSWCs because they are often absent in the early or late stages of the disease. The absence of PSWCs does not rule out prion disease because many atypical cases do not show EEG abnormalities.

Until recently, neuroimaging studies generally have been negative in sCJD. Generalized atrophy may be observed by MRI, but the MRI has been used primarily to rule out other diseases, such as central nervous system (CNS) vasculitis and infiltrating brain tumors. With the advent of diffusion-weighted imaging, however, MRI is proving to be a useful study for establishing the diagnosis of prion disease. Some series have estimated that up to 90 percent of patients with CJD show increased signal in either the basal ganglia or the cortical ribbon by diffusion-weighted MRI (DWI); however, the specificity of this finding for CJD is not yet clear (Fig. 18-1C). In the rare panencephalopathic form of sCJD, extensive degeneration of the cerebral white matter is apparent on MRI and may appear similar to leukodystrophy. Positron-emission tomographic (PET) scans generally show nonspecific cortical hypometabolism, which helps to exclude other dementias that show characteristic patterns on PET scans.

A specific serologic or CSF test for prion disease does not exist. Routine biochemical and hematologic tests usually are normal. Liver function tests may be slightly abnormal in some patients, but this is likely a consequence of medication or the general state of health of the patient rather than the disease process itself.[112] Mild protein elevation in CSF may be seen in fewer than 50 percent of patients, but it rarely exceeds 1.0 g/liter.[112] An inflammatory response is characteristically absent in prion disease, and therefore, the presence of inflammatory cells in CSF immediately should trigger a search for another disease. The identification of PrP^{Sc} in CSF would provide a definitive diagnosis of prion disease, but PrP^{Sc} has so far been undetectable in CSF by western blot even though prion disease can be transmitted through inoculation of CSF from affected individuals into healthy experimental animals.[5,113] Other proteins released into the CSF in prion disease are specific to neurons, such as 14-3-3 and neuron-specific enolase, and have been suggested to be sensitive and specific markers for prion disease.[114–120] The presence of these proteins in the CSF of prion disease patients reflects the rapid rate of neuron death and release of intracellular contents. There is currently significant debate

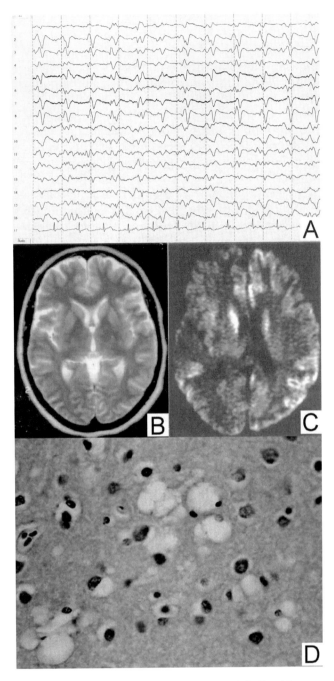

Figure 18-1. *A.* Typical EEG pattern of CJD with periodic sharp wave complexes (PSWCs) of 0.5 to 2.0 Hz. *B.* T$_2$-weighted MRI of patient with CJD demonstrating mild hyperintensity of the caudate and putamen seen in a minority of patients. *C.* Diffusion-weighted MRI demonstrating hyperintensity of the cortical ribbon (especially left parietal) and basal ganglia seen in a majority of patients. *D.* Characteristic spongiform change in the neuropil of a CJD brain.

regarding the usefulness of 14-3-3. Although it is widely used, recent reports suggest a sensitivity of less than 60 percent.[121,122]

The only definitive diagnostic test for sCJD and any other prion disease is brain biopsy. This test is considered primarily in younger individuals or patients with atypical presentations, where a differentiation cannot be made between prion disease and a potentially treatable condition, such as CNS vasculitis. If evidence of prion disease is found on pathologic examination of biopsy tissue, a definitive diagnosis of prion disease can be made; however, failure to find evidence of prion disease does not exclude prion disease due to the variability of cortical lesion sites and the potential for sampling error. The decision to perform a brain biopsy obviously should weigh the potential risks to the patient, such as brain abscess formation or hemorrhage. This decision also involves the neurosurgical team because preparation of the operating room for a CJD patient is not a minor procedure. The neuropathology of sCJD is defined by the presence of intracellular vacuoles that, when viewed by light microscopy, convey a picture of "spongy" degeneration (Fig. 18-1D). The vacuoles represent focal swellings of axonal and dendritic processes, with loss of synaptic organelles and accumulation of abnormal membranes apparent by electron microscopy.[123–125] Vacuoles are located between nerve cell bodies and usually range in size from 5 to 25 μm but can merge to form vacuoles as large as 200 μm in advanced cases.[126] Such extreme vacuolation becomes extracellular in the form of microcysts and has been referred to as *status spongiosis*. The spongiform degeneration can be found in both gray and white matter but is usually most pronounced in the gray matter neuropil. Areas of the brain often affected include the cerebral neocortex, subiculum of the hippocampus, caudate, putamen, thalamus, and the molecular layer of the cerebellar cortex.[126] Spongiform change occurs in the cerebral cortex in almost all cases of sCJD. Accompanying the spongiform change is a reactive astrocytic gliosis and varying degrees of neuronal loss. An inflammatory response is conspicuously absent. PrP amyloid plaques can be seen in a minority of patients and usually are associated with an M/V or V/V129 genotype.[127] Newer immunocytochemistry techniques that are specific for PrP^{Sc} have been developed to complement traditional histologic analysis of pathologic specimens. These techniques, when performed properly, can show the presence and distribution of PrP^{Sc} throughout the brain and can be very helpful in establishing a diagnosis of prion disease. PrP^{Sc} is detected easily by immunoblot of brain homogenate in all cases of sCJD. Transmission of disease through inoculation of infected brain homogenate into an experimental animal is considered the gold standard in prion disease diagnosis, and transgenic animals expressing human PrP show nearly 100 percent transmission efficiency.[22,63] Unfortunately, the long incubation time required before expression of disease—currently 150 to 200 days—limits the usefulness of this assay as a rapid diagnostic test.

Iatrogenic CJD (iCJD)

Infection via exposure to human biologicals contaminated with prions is classified as *iatrogenic CJD* (iCJD). To date, most such cases have resulted from exposure to contaminated cadaveric hGH. The first recognized hGH case was in a young boy with idiopathic hypopituitarism in 1985.[128] Since that time, at least three separate contaminated sources of hGH from France, the United Kingdom, and the United States have been linked to over 130 cases of CJD,[129–136] with the majority occurring in France. Direct evidence for this was provided by transmission of prion disease to squirrel monkeys following injection of hGH from the contaminated lots.[135] Among those who have received hGH, the risk of CJD is about 1 in 200 and correlates with the duration of therapy, with a mean incubation time of about 13 years.[134] With the advent of recombinant DNA technology, human pituitary extracts were replaced with recombinant hGH as a pure source of hGH in 1985. However, because of the prolonged incubation time of up to 30 years, CJD cases due to contaminated hGH are still being observed.

The second most common route of exposure has been through contaminated dura mater homografts, with the first case report in 1987.[137] At least 110 cases have now been reported worldwide, mostly from Japan.[138] These cases were attributed to a single manufacturer whose preparative procedures were inadequate to remove the infectious agent.[137,139–143] In this exposed population, the mean time to disease after implantation of the graft was 7.4 years, ranging from 1.3 to 16.1 years.[138] Many countries have withdrawn use of human dura mater grafts, but in those countries where dura mater grafts are still used, it is recommended that they be treated with at least 1 N NaOH for 1 hour to reduce possible infectivity.[144–147] Other preventive measures include stringent donor screening and individual processing to eliminate cross-contamination.

Other documented iatrogenic routes of exposure have been through contaminated gonadotropin hormone,[148–150] corneal transplants,[151] and contaminated depth electrodes used for seizure focus determination.[152] Transmission through neurosurgical procedures probably has occurred for some time. Attention was focused on this problem after the first study documenting this risk was published in 1977,[152] and no cases of iatrogenic exposure through neurosurgical instruments has been documented since 1980. In one of the contaminated depth electrode cases, the electrodes were sterilized with ethanol and formaldehyde vapor before being used subsequently for stereotactic EEG recordings,[152] and one was able to transmit spongiform encephalopathy to a chimpanzee 18 months after intradural implantation.[153] Given the difficulty of properly decontaminating tissue and surgical instruments,[154] many countries now require disposal of surgical instruments after use on CJD patients.

Iatrogenic exposure through blood transfusion is also of current concern. While a few animal model studies have suggested that transmission can occur via blood,[155–158] no convincing evidence has been presented that transmission through blood can occur in primates.[159,160] Case-control and epidemiologic studies have failed to show a risk of prion disease transmission through blood products, and no patients who require repeated blood transfusions, such as hemophiliacs, have developed CJD.[30,161,162] Presently, it appears that whole blood, plasma, and transplant organs do not present a significant risk of exposure to prions, presumably because titers in such tissue are very low or zero. Nevertheless, many countries now exclude individuals at high risk for CJD, such as those treated previously with hGH and those who have a family history of CJD, from blood donation.

Interestingly, the clinical picture of iCJD seems to depend on the route of inoculation. In cases of intracerebral inoculation, such as through contaminated depth electrodes and other surgical instruments, dura mater grafts, and corneal transplants, the clinical features are almost indistinguishable from sCJD, with rapidly progressive dementia an important early component of the disease. In a few dura mater cases where a posterior fossa graft was placed near the cerebellum after cerebellar tumor removal, the presentation was one of a cerebellar syndrome. Thus the site of intracerebral inoculation may influence the clinical presentation of the disease. In cases where the route of inoculation is peripheral, such as treatment with contaminated hGH, cerebellar ataxia is the predominant feature, with dementia presenting late in the course, if at all. This is similar to the presentation of kuru, a disease caused by peripheral exposure to prions through ingestion of infected human brain material (discussed below). The EEG, in cases of peripheral inoculation, shows a diffuse slow wave pattern rather than the periodic triphasic waves characteristic of sCJD.[153] The pathologic findings also depend on the route of inoculation. In cases of direct intracerebral inoculation, the neuropathology is nearly identical to sCJD, with spongiform change, astrocytosis, and neuronal loss the predominant findings. In hGH cases, the cerebellum is most affected, which shows gross atrophy, widespread neuronal loss, spongiform change, and the presence of PrP amyloid plaques.

The most important factor in diagnosing iCJD is the presence of a nongenetic risk factor for contracting CJD, such as cadaveric-derived hGH treatment, dura mater homograft, or another known risk, such as corneal transplant or application of depth electrodes. While questions have been raised regarding organ transplants, no causal relationship has been proven. Recently, however, a concern that certain general surgical procedures have been associated with iCJD has been raised.[161,163] A patient who presents with cerebellar ataxia and who received hGH treatment prior to 1985 should undergo a workup for CJD. Such patients can vary in age from adolescence to adulthood because the incubation period has now been documented to be up to 30 years. Most patients who are affected by iCJD are homozygous at the polymorphic codon 129.[50]

Variant CJD (vCJD)

The first vCJD cases were reported as an unusual form of sCJD that occurred in teenagers with clinical signs and neuropathology atypical of sCJD. Given the unusual clinical and pathologic features of this disease, it was classified as a new form of CJD, simply labeled *variant CJD* (vCJD).[20] The temporal association of the rise of vCJD with an epidemic of BSE in the United Kingdom originally gave rise to suspicion of a causal link between the two diseases. Epidemiologic and experimental evidence now supports the hypothesis that vCJD is caused by the consumption of beef products contaminated with bovine prions. It is widely believed that less stringent conditions in the rendering of cows for preparation of meat and bone meal that was fed to healthy cows enabled the survival of prions, which led to the BSE epidemic in the United Kingdom in the late 1980s and 1990s. At the peak of the BSE epidemic in 1989, more than 300 herds per month were becoming infected.[164] Initiation of the specified bovine offals (SBO) ban in late 1989 and the eventual slaughter of millions of cattle led to a sharp reduction of BSE in the United Kingdom.[165] To monitor the potential health consequences of the BSE epidemic to humans, a surveillance unit was instituted in 1990 to track changes in the incidence of CJD. The general expectation was that BSE in cattle would pose no greater threat to humans than scrapie, a known prion disease of sheep, which over the previous 40 years had not been identified as a risk factor for development of CJD.[24]

With over 150 cases now documented, a picture of vCJD has emerged that supports its distinction as a separate prion disease subtype. Unlike sCJD, which occurs most often in the sixth to seventh decades, vCJD occurs more often in younger individuals ranging in age from 18 to 74 years, with the average age at onset of 29 years. Why younger adults are more susceptible is not known, but it may reflect, in part, different dietary patterns in younger individuals. The disease course is also prolonged, averaging 16 months (range 9 to 38 months). Unique to vCJD are the initial symptoms of disease, consisting primarily of psychiatric disturbances (especially depression and paranoia), as well as sensory changes (e.g., dysesthesia) that are unrelated to anxiety levels. Such symptoms may persist for several months before overt signs of disease appear, consisting primarily of progressive gait and limb ataxia, followed much later by dementia. Myoclonus is observed in many cases. As with most other forms of prion disease, the patient progresses to a state of akinetic mutism before death. No risk factor for vCJD other than age has been identified, with the exception of living in a country with BSE. In contrast to sCJD, the EEG of vCJD does not show PSWCs,[20] and the CSF 14-3-3 protein is positive in less than 50 percent of cases. Putaminal hyperintensity in DWI, T_2-weighted, or proton-density-weighted MRIs can be seen in many cases. A definite diagnosis of vCJD cannot be made in the absence of the characteristic pathologic findings. These findings are surprisingly reproducible from patient to patient and are easily distinguished from sCJD.[20] The most remarkable finding is dense-core PrP plaques surrounded by a halo of spongiform change, termed *florid plaques,* most often present in the cerebral cortex. Similar plaques also are found in other parts of the cerebrum and cerebellum and are readily revealed by immunocytochemistry. Spongiform change is seen throughout the brain but especially intense in the basal ganglia and thalamus. Severe thalamic astrocytosis is also common. The PrP^{Sc} detected in the brain of a vCJD patient has a different electrophoretic mobility than PrP^{Sc} from a sCJD patient and is predominantly diglycosylated rather than monoglycosylated.[35] To date, all vCJD patients have been shown to be homozygous for methionine at codon 129, and therefore, genetic testing of *PRNP* may be informative for research purposes.

Kuru

Although largely of historical significance, the study of kuru has contributed enormously to our understanding of the infectious nature of prions, and its clinical course has been well described.[1,166,167] Kuru has been observed to occur in people aged 5 to over 60, with a mean duration of 1 year (range 3 months to 3 years). In stark contrast to sCJD, the clinical phenotype of kuru is of a cerebellar syndrome, with dementia occurring rarely. The prodromal stage of the disease lasts for several months and is characterized by headache, joint pain, and muscle aching of the limbs. Truncal ataxia predominates in the ambulatory stage, and the patient often develops a severe depression. As the ataxia progresses, the patient enters the sedentary stage of the disease, where he or she is unable to walk. Uncontrollable laughter also may develop at this point. Unlike sCJD, myoclonus is a rare feature of kuru, and the EEG is usually normal. In the tertiary and final stage of the disease the patient develops flaccid muscle weakness, and death eventually occurs from aspiration pneu-

monia or respiratory arrest. In concert with the clinical signs, the pathology is focused in the cerebellum, which shows macroscopic atrophy and microscopic amyloid plaques concentrated in the granule cell layer that stain positive for PrP.[2,168] These plaques are spherical in shape with radiating spicules extending from their peripheries. In a very small percentage of CJD and GSS, similar plaques, often described by neuropathologists as "kuru" or "kuru-like," may be evident.

Fatal Insomnia (FI)

FI, formerly known as *pure thalamic dementia,* was described originally in familial form in 1986 and identified as a prion disease by virtue of the presence of a dominant mutation of *PRNP* in 1992.[19,169–178] A sporadic form of this disease also has been described.[94,179–182] In the typical presentation, the patient develops untreatable insomnia, followed by dysautonomia, ataxia, and variable pyramidal and extrapyramidal signs and symptoms with relative sparing of cognitive function until late in the course. Age at disease onset averages 48 years (range 25 to 61 years), and the time to death averages 1 to 2 years (range 7 to 33 months).[176,177] Neuropathology shows neuronal loss and astrogliosis confined mainly to the thalamus and inferior olives, with little or no spongiform change and unusually small amounts of PrP^{Sc} present. The bizarre clinical and pathologic characteristics of FI, as well as the small amount of PrP^{Sc} present, obscured identification of this disease as a prion disease, and it is possible that other prion diseases exist that are yet unidentified. Familial fatal insomnia (FFI) occurs in the presence of an aspartate-to-asparagine substitution at codon 178 but only when methionine at codon 129 is allelic to this mutation.

Gerstmann-Sträussler-Scheinker Syndrome (GSS)

GSS is a strictly familial disease occurring only in the presence of particular mutations of the *PRNP* gene. The most common presentation consists of ataxia and dysarthria, followed by variable degrees of pyramidal and extrapyramidal symptoms, with dementia developing late in the disease.[183,184] Onset is usually before age 50, and the course is anywhere from 2 to 10 years. Because ataxia and discoordination of swallowing are early problems in GSS, aspiration pneumonia is a significant complication of death in these subjects. The defining pathologic feature of GSS is the numerous PrP-positive plaques deposited regionally or diffusely throughout the cortex. Vacuolation is not as conspicuous as in CJD, and neurofibrillary tangles are sometimes present. Given the preceding description, it is not surprising that some cases of GSS have been misdiagnosed as familial Alzheimer disease.[185]

▶ **TABLE 18-4.** MUTATIONS AND POLYMORPHISMS OF *PRNP*

Codon Affected	Amino Acid Change	Phenotype
Disease-Associated Point Mutations		
102	Pro (P) → Leu (L)	GSS
105	Pro (P) → Leu (L)	GSS
117	Ala (A) → Val (V)	GSS
131	Gly (G) → Val (V)	GSS
145	Tyr (Y) → Stop	GSS
160	Gln (Q) → Stop	GSS
178	Asp (D) → Asn (N)	CJD or FFI[†]
180	Val (V) → Ile (I)	CJD
183	Thr (T) → Ala (A)	CJD
187	His (H) → Arg (R)	CJD
198	Phe (F) → Ser (S)	GSS
200	Glu (E) → Lys (K)	CJD
208	Arg (R) → His (H)	CJD
210	Val (V) → Ile (I)	CJD
211	Glu (E) → Gln (Q)	CJD
217	Gln (Q) → Arg (R)	GSS
232	Met (M) → Arg (R)	CJD/GSS
Polymorphisms		
23	Pro (P) → Ser (S)	—
129	Met (M) → Val (V)	Modifier
171	Asn (N) → Ser (S)	Schizophrenia[‡]
188	Thr (T) → Arg (R)	—
219	Glu (E) → Lys (K)	Protective?
Insertional Mutations		
Octarepeat number*	−1	Normal
Octarepeat number*	+1	CJD
Octarepeat number*	+2	CJD
Octarepeat number*	+4	CJD
Octarepeat number*	+5	CJD
Octarepeat number*	+6	CJD
Octarepeat number*	+7	CJD
Octarepeat number*	+8	GSS/HD-like
Octarepeat number*	+9	GSS

*[Pro-(His/Gln)-Gly-Gly-Gly-(-/Gly)-Trp-Gly-Gln] × 5.
†FFI is seen when codon 129 is Met, and fCJD occurs when 129 is Val.
‡Polymorphism reported in normal controls and some patients with schizophrenia.

Familial CJD (fCJD)

Familial prion diseases, by definition, are due to a mutation in the *PRNP* gene. Because the mutations that lead to prion disease are autosomal dominant, identification of affected first-degree relatives is important in the diagnosis of familial prion disease, although reduced penetrance of certain mutations, misdiagnosis, or death due to other causes may complicate the pedigree. Mutations known to give rise to familial prion disease are shown in Table 18-4 and have been reviewed extensively elsewhere.[98] Many of these patients show a protracted course and have been misdiagnosed with Alzheimer disease or other form of dementia. Clinical and diagnostic features vary with mutation.

▶ DIFFERENTIAL DIAGNOSIS

From the preceding discussion one can appreciate the extremely variable clinical signs and symptoms associated with prion disease, and this results in considerable clinical overlap with other diseases. The potential for a movement disorder, psychiatric symptoms, and dementia (as well as other symptoms) to occur in prion disease, often contemporaneously, makes the list of potential diseases large and varied. Most prominent are other neurodegenerative diseases, in particular Alzheimer disease but also including the frontotemporal dementias, dementia with Lewy bodies, Huntington disease, Parkinson disease, amyotrophic lateral sclerosis, cortical basal degeneration, and the spinocerebellar ataxias. Typically, the rapid rate of progression of symptoms in nonfamilial prion disease argues against many of these neurodegenerative disorders. A PET scan may help to rule out some neurodegenerative disorders that show specific perfusion deficits, such as Alzheimer disease and the frontotemporal dementias, rather than the global hypoperfusion often seen in CJD. Metabolic disorders that can present with prion-like symptoms include ceroid lipufuscinosis (Kufs disease) and heavy metal toxicity. Ceroid lipufuscinosis can present with dementia and myoclonus and is usually easily diagnosed on brain biopsy. Heavy metal toxicity, especially lithium and bismuth toxicity, can show similar changes on EEG as prion disease. Cerebrovascular disease such as stroke and multiple-infarct dementia can mimic some of the symptoms of prion disease, but onset is usually much more rapid. The same is true for viral encephalitides and bacterial causes that, in addition to their very rapid onset, also elicit an easily identifiable immune response. CNS vasculitis also may present with rapid cognitive changes, but as with cerebrovascular disease, neuroimaging usually can identify this disease. Other autoimmune diseases that have overlapping symptoms with prion disease include immune thyroiditis, systemic vasculitides, limbic encephalitis, cerebellar degeneration, and other paraneoplastic syndromes. Immune thyroiditis often presents with periodic confusion and cerebellar ataxia, and elevated levels of antithyroglobulin and antithyroperoxidase antibodies, even in the presence of normal thyroid-stimulating hormone (TSH) levels, strongly suggest this disease. Testing for other autoantibodies, such as anti-Yo in cerebellar degeneration, can help to identify these syndromes. If the symptoms are due to an autoimmune reaction, they often will subside after corticosteroid treatment, unlike the symptoms of prion disease. Multiple sclerosis (MS) may present with an ataxia that is similar in some respects to that found in some cases of sCJD and GSS, but the presence of white matter lesions on MRI and periodic partial remission of symptoms will distinguish MS from prion disease. The dearth of specific markers for prion disease usually makes it a diagnosis of exclusion. Obtaining a *PRNP* genotype in suspected cases of familial prion disease may be helpful in the diagnosis, but a positive result should not preclude a careful and thorough workup to exclude other potentially treatable diseases.

▶ THERAPY FOR PRION DISEASE

In general, therapy for prion disease remains largely symptomatic and supportive. The myoclonus and seizures that may develop can be treated with clonazepam or other standard anticonvulsants. Unfortunately, there are no approved therapies that effectively treat prion disease. Several compounds have demonstrated promising results in a cell culture model of prion disease, most recently quinacrine and chlorpromazine,[186] but their utility has not been proven in animal models.[187] An open trial of quinacrine in the United Kingdom has begun. Other compounds that have been tried either in cell culture models, in vitro conversion models, or animals include pentosan polysulfate, Congo red, amphotericin B, acyclovir, suramin, dapsone, synthetic peptides that interact with PrP, and antibodies to PrP (see ref. 188 for review). In most cases these compounds appear much more promising in cell culture and in vitro than they do in animal studies. In those which appeared promising in ex vivo models, administration prior to or at the time of inoculation was necessary to delay the inevitable onset of disease in animals challenged with prions. When administered after inoculation or at the time symptoms were already present, they were ineffective. Currently in vogue as a research effort are antibodies that bind to and protect PrP^C from PrP^{Sc}.

REFERENCES

1. Gajdusek DC, Zigas V: Degenerative disease of the central nervous system in New Guinea: The endemic occurrence of "kuru" in the native population. *New Engl J Med* 257:974, 1957.
2. Gajdusek DC, Zigas V: Clinical, pathological and epidemiological study of an acute progressive degenerative disease of the central nervous system among natives of the eastern highlands of New Guinea. *Am J Med* 26:442, 1959.
3. Zigas V, Gajdusek DC: Kuru: Clinical study of a new syndrome resembling paralysis agitans in natives of the Eastern Highlands of Australian New Guinea. *Med J Aust* 2:745, 1957.
4. Gajdusek DC, Gibbs CJ Jr, Alpers M: Experimental transmission of a kuru-like syndrome to chimpanzees. *Nature* 209:794, 1966.
5. Gibbs CJ Jr, Gajdusek DC, Asher DM, et al: Creutzfeldt-Jakob disease (spongiform encephalopathy): Transmission to the chimpanzee. *Science* 161:388, 1968.
6. Sigurdsson B: Rida, a chronic encephalitis of sheep with general remarks on infections which develop slowly and some of their special characteristics. *Br Vet J* 110:341, 1954.
7. Chandler RL: Encephalopathy in mice produced by in-

oculation with scrapie brain material. *Lancet* 1:1378, 1961.

8. Gordon WS: Advances in veterinary research. *Vet Res* 58:516, 1946.

9. Zlotnik I: The pathology of scrapie: A comparative study of lesions in the brain of sheep and goats. *Acta Neuropathol (Berl) Suppl* 1:61, 1962.

10. Alper T, Haig DA, Clarke MC: The exceptionally small size of the scrapie agent. *Biochem Biophys Res Commun* 22:278, 1966.

11. Alper T, Cramp WA, Haig DA, et al: Does the agent of scrapie replicate without nucleic acid? *Nature* 214:764, 1967.

12. Prusiner SB: Novel proteinaceous infectious particles cause scrapie. *Science* 216:136, 1982.

13. McKinley MP, Bolton DC, Prusiner SB: A protease-resistant protein is a structural component of the scrapie prion. *Cell* 35:57, 1983.

14. Prusiner SB, McKinley MP, Groth DF, et al: Scrapie agent contains a hydrophobic protein. *Proc Natl Acad Sci USA* 78:6675, 1981.

15. Bolton DC, McKinley MP, Prusiner SB: Identification of a protein that purifies with the scrapie prion. *Science* 218:1309, 1982.

16. Oesch B, Westaway D, Walchli M, et al: A cellular gene encodes scrapie PrP 27-30 protein. *Cell* 40:735, 1985.

17. Hsiao K, Baker HF, Crow TJ, et al: Linkage of a prion protein missense variant to Gerstmann-Sträussler syndrome. *Nature* 338:342, 1989.

18. Goldfarb LG, Mitrova E, Brown P, et al: Mutation in codon 200 of scrapie amyloid protein gene in two clusters of Creutzfeldt-Jakob disease in Slovakia. *Lancet* 336:514, 1990.

19. Medori R, Tritschler HJ, LeBlanc A, et al: Fatal familial insomnia, a prion disease with a mutation at codon 178 of the prion protein gene. *New Engl J Med* 326:444, 1992.

20. Will RG, Ironside JW, Zeidler M, et al: A new variant of Creutzfeldt-Jakob disease in the UK. *Lancet* 347:921, 1996.

21. Scott M, Foster D, Mirenda C, et al: Transgenic mice expressing hamster prion protein produce species-specific scrapie infectivity and amyloid plaques. *Cell* 59:847, 1989.

22. Telling GC, Scott M, Hsiao KK, et al: Transmission of Creutzfeldt-Jakob disease from humans to transgenic mice expressing chimeric human-mouse prion protein. *Proc Natl Acad Sci USA* 91:9936, 1994.

23. Kretzschmar HA, Prusiner SB, Stowring LE, et al: Scrapie prion proteins are synthesized in neurons. *Am J Pathol* 122:1, 1986.

24. Brown P, Cathala F, Raubertas RF, et al: The epidemiology of Creutzfeldt-Jakob disease: Conclusion of a 15-year investigation in France and review of the world literature. *Neurology* 37:895, 1987.

25. Goldfarb LG, Korczyn AD, Brown P, et al: Mutation in codon 200 of scrapie amyloid precursor gene linked to Creutzfeldt-Jakob disease in Sephardic Jews of Libyan and non-Libyan origin. *Lancet* 336:637, 1990.

26. Brown P, Galvez S, Goldfarb LG, et al: Familial Creutzfeldt-Jakob disease in Chile is associated with the codon 200 mutation of the *PRNP* amyloid precursor gene on chromosome 20. *J Neurol Sci* 112:65, 1992.

27. Chatelain J, et al: Cluster of Creutzfeldt-Jakob disease in France associated with the codon 200 mutation (E200K) in the prion protein gene. *Eur J Neurol* 5:375, 1998.

28. Will RG, Alperovitch A, Poser S, et al: Descriptive epidemiology of Creutzfeldt-Jakob disease in six European countries, 1993–1995. *Ann Neurol* 43:763, 1998.

29. Will RG, Matthews WB, Smith PG, Hudson C: A retrospective study of Creutzfeldt-Jakob disease in England and Wales 1970–1979: II. Epidemiology. *J Neurol Neurosurg Psychiatry* 49(7):749, 1986.

30. Wientjens DP, Davanipour Z, Hofman A, et al: Risk factors for Creutzfeldt-Jakob disease: A reanalysis of case-control studies. *Neurology* 46:1287, 1996.

31. Kitamoto T, Iizuka R, Tateishi J: An amber mutation of prion protein in Gerstmann-Sträussler syndrome with mutant PrP plaques. *Biochem Biophys Res Commun* 192:525, 1993.

32. Bateman D, Hilton D, Love S, et al: Sporadic Creutzfeldt-Jakob disease in a 18-year-old in the UK (letter). *Lancet* 346:1155, 1995.

33. Britton TC, al-Sarraj S, Shaw C, et al: Sporadic Creutzfeldt-Jakob disease in a 16-year-old in the UK (letter). *Lancet* 346:1155, 1995.

34. Lasmezas CI, Deslys JP, Demaimay R, et al: BSE transmission to macaques. *Nature* 381(6585):743, 1996.

35. Collinge J, Sidle KC, Meads J, et al: Molecular analysis of prion strain variation and the aetiology of "new variant" CJD. *Nature* 383:685, 1996.

36. Bruce ME, Will RG, Ironside JW, et al: Transmissions to mice indicate that "new variant" CJD is caused by the BSE agent. *Nature* 389:498, 1997.

37. Hill AF, Desbruslais M, Joiner S, et al: The same prion strain causes vCJD and BSE. *Nature* 389:448, 1997.

38. Cousens SN, Vynnycky E, Zeidler M, et al: Predicting the CJD epidemic in humans. *Nature* 385:197, 1997.

39. Miller MW, Williams ES, McCarty CW, et al: Epizootiology of chronic wasting disease in free-ranging cervids in Colorado and Wyoming. *J Wildlife Dis* 36(4):676, 2000.

40. Gajdusek DC, Gibbs CJ Jr, Asher DM, et al: Precautions in medical care of, and in handling materials from, patients with transmissible virus dementia (Creutzfeldt-Jakob disease). *New Engl J Med* 297:1253, 1977.

41. Shaked GM, Shaked Y, Kariv-Inbal Z, et al: A protease-resistant prion protein isoform is present in urine of animals and humans affected with prion diseases. *J Biol Chem* 276(34):31479, 2001.

42. Owen F, Poulter M, Collinge J, Crow TJ: Codon 129 changes in the prion protein gene in Caucasians. *Am J Hum Genet* 46:1215, 1990.

43. Palmer MS, Dryden AJ, Hughes JT, Collinge J: Homozygous prion protein genotype predisposes to sporadic Creutzfeldt-Jakob disease. *Nature* 352:340, 1991.

44. Windl O, Dempster M, Estibeiro JP, et al: Genetic basis of Creutzfeldt-Jakob disease in the United King-

dom: A systematic analysis of predisposing mutations and allelic variation in the *PRNP* gene. *Hum Genet* 98:259, 1996.

45. Laplanche JL, Delasnerie-Laupretre N, Brandel JP, et al: Molecular genetics of prion diseases in France. *Neurology* 44:2347, 1994.

46. Salvatore M, Genuardi M, Petraroli R, et al: Polymorphisms of the prion protein gene in Italian patients with Creutzfeldt-Jakob disease. *Hum Genet* 94:375, 1994.

47. Collinge J, Beck J, Campbell T, Estibeiro K, Will RG: Prion protein gene analysis in new variant cases of Creutzfeldt-Jakob disease. *Lancet* 348:56, 1996.

48. Will R: New variant Creutzfeldt-Jakob disease. *Biomed Pharmacother* 53(1):9, 1999.

49. Doh-ura K, Kitamoto T, Sakaki Y, Tateishi J: CJD discrepancy. *Nature* 353:801, 1991.

50. Deslys JP, Marcé D, Dormont D: Similar genetic susceptibility in iatrogenic and sporadic Creutzfeldt-Jakob disease. *J Gen Virol* 75:23, 1994.

51. Parchi P, Castellani R, Capellari S, et al: Molecular basis of phenotypic variability in sporadic Creutzfeldt-Jakob disease. *Ann Neurol* 39:767, 1996.

52. Monari L, Chen SG, Brown P, et al: Fatal familial insomnia and familial Creutzfeldt-Jakob disease: Different prion proteins determined by a DNA polymorphism. *Proc Natl Acad Sci USA* 91:2839, 1994.

53. Dlouhy SR, Hsiao K, Farlow MR, et al: Linkage of the Indiana kindred of Gerstmann-Sträussler-Scheinker disease to the prion protein gene. *Nature Genet* 1:64, 1992.

54. Shibuya S, Higuchi J, Shin RW, et al: Codon 219 Lys allele of *PRNP* is not found in sporadic Creutzfeldt-Jakob disease. *Ann Neurol* 43:826, 1998.

55. Zulianello L, Kaneko K, Scott M, et al: Dominant-negative inhibition of prion formation diminished by deletion mutagenesis of the prion protein. *J Virol* 74(9):4351, 2000.

56. Perrier V, Kaneko K, Safar J, et al: Dominant-negative inhibition of prion replication in transgenic mice. *Proc Natl Acad Sci USA* 99(20):13079, 2002.

57. Knaus KJ, Morillas M, Swietnicki W, et al: Crystal structure of the human prion protein reveals a mechanism for oligomerization. *Nature Struct Biol* 8(9):770, 2001.

58. Donne DG, Viles JH, Groth D, et al: Structure of the recombinant full-length hamster prion protein PrP(29-231): The N terminus is highly flexible. *Proc Natl Acad Sci USA* 94:13452, 1997.

59. Safar J, Roller PP, Gajdusek DC, Gibbs CJ Jr: Conformational transitions, dissociation, and unfolding of scrapie amyloid (prion) protein. *J Biol Chem* 268:20276, 1993.

60. Büeler H, Fischer M, Lang Y, et al: Normal development and behaviour of mice lacking the neuronal cell-surface PrP protein. *Nature* 356:577, 1992.

61. Büeler H, Aguzzi A, Sailer A, et al: Mice devoid of PrP are resistant to scrapie. *Cell* 73:1339, 1993.

62. Sailer A, Bueler H, Fischer M, et al: No propagation of prions in mice devoid of PrP. *Cell* 77:967, 1994.

63. Telling GC, Scott M, Mastrianni J, et al: Prion propaga-

tion in mice expressing human and chimeric PrP transgenes implicates the interaction of cellular PrP with another protein. *Cell* 83:79, 1995.

64. James TL, Liu H, Ulyanov NB, et al: Solution structure of a 142-residue recombinant prion protein corresponding to the infectious fragment of the scrapie isoform. *Proc Natl Acad Sci USA*, 94:10086, 1997.

65. Kaneko K, Zulianello L, Scott M, et al: Evidence for protein X binding to a discontinuous epitope on the cellular prion protein during scrapie prion propagation. *Proc Natl Acad Sci USA* 94:10069, 1997.

66. Kretzschmar HA, Stowring LE, Westaway D, et al: Molecular cloning of a human prion protein cDNA. *DNA* 5:315, 1986.

67. Raeber AJ, Race RE, Brandner S, et al: Astrocyte-specific expression of hamster prion protein (PrP) renders PrP knockout mice susceptible to hamster scrapie. *EMBO J* 16:6057, 1997.

68. Kurschner C, Morgan JI: Analysis of interaction sites in homo- and heteromeric complexes containing Bcl-2 family members and the cellular prion protein. *Mol Brain Res* 37:249, 1996.

69. Brown DR, Schulz-Schaeffer WJ, Schmidt B, et al: Prion protein-deficient cells show altered response to oxidative stress due to decreased SOD-1 activity. *Exp Neurol* 146:104, 1997.

70. Liao YC, Lebo RV, Clawson GA, et al: Human prion protein cDNA: Molecular cloning, chromosomal mapping, and biological implication. *Science* 233:364, 1986.

71. Stahl N, Borchelt DR, Hsiao K, et al: Scrapie prion protein contains a phosphatidylinositol glycolipid. *Cell* 51:229, 1987.

72. Bendheim PE, Brown HR, Rudelli RD, et al: Nearly ubiquitous tissue distribution of the scrapie agent precursor protein. *Neurology* 42:149, 1992.

73. Perini F, Vidal R, Ghetti B, et al: PrP$_{27-30}$ is a normal soluble prion protein fragment released by human platelets. *Biochem Biophys Res Commun* 223:572, 1996.

74. Askanas V, Sarkozi E, Bilak M, et al: Human muscle macrophages express β-amyloid precursor and prion proteins and their mRNAs. *Neuroreport* 6:1045, 1995.

75. Westaway D, DeArmond SJ, Cayetano-Canlas J, et al: Degeneration of skeletal muscle, peripheral nerves, and the central nervous system in transgenic mice overexpressing wild-type prion proteins. *Cell* 76:117, 1994.

76. Jendroska K, Heinzel FP, Torchia M, et al: Proteinase-resistant prion protein accumulation in Syrian hamster brain correlates with regional pathology and scrapie infectivity. *Neurology* 41:1482, 1991.

77. Borchelt DR, Rogers M, Stahl N, et al: Rapid anterograde axonal transport of the cellular prion glycoprotein in the peripheral and central nervous systems. *J Biol Chem* 269:14711, 1994.

78. Collinge J, Whittington MA, Sidle KC, et al: Prion protein is necessary for normal synaptic function. *Nature* 370:295, 1994.

79. Whittington MA, Sidle KC, Gowland I, et al: Rescue of neurophysiological phenotype seen in PrP null mice by transgene encoding human prion protein. *Nature Genet* 9:197, 1995.

80. Manson JC, Hope J, Clarke AR, et al: PrP gene dosage and long term potentiation (letter). *Neurodegeneration* 4:113, 1995.

81. Brown DR, Qin K, Herms JW, et al: The cellular prion protein binds copper in vivo. *Nature* 390:684, 1997.

82. Stöckel J, Safar J, Wallace AC, et al: Prion protein selectively binds copper(II) ions. *Biochemistry* 37(20):7185, 1998.

83. Tobler I, Gaus SE, Deboer T, et al: Altered circadian activity rhythms and sleep in mice devoid of prion protein. *Nature* 380:639, 1996.

84. Sakaguchi S, Katamine S, Nishida N, et al: Loss of cerebellar Purkinje cells in aged mice homozygous for a disrupted PrP gene. *Nature* 380:528, 1996.

85. Moore RC, Lee IY, Silverman GL, et al: Ataxia in prion protein (PrP)–deficient mice is associated with upregulation of the novel PrP-like protein doppel. *J Mol Biol* 292(4):797, 1999.

86. Peoc'h K: Prion-like protein doppel expression is not modified in scrapie-infected cells and in the brains of patients with Creutzfeldt-Jakob disease. *FEBS Lett* 536(1–3):61, 2003.

87. Schroder B, Franz B, Hempfling P, et al: Polymorphisms within the prion-like protein gene (*PRND*) and their implications in human prion diseases, Alzheimer's disease and other neurological disorders. *Hum Genet* 109(3):319, 2001.

88. Bessen RA, Marsh RF: Distinct PrP properties suggest the molecular basis of strain variation in transmissible mink encephalopathy. *J Virol* 68:7859, 1994.

89. Bessen RA, Marsh, RF: Identification of two biologically distinct strains of transmissible mink encephalopathy in hamsters. *J Gen Virol* 73:329, 1992.

90. Collinge J: Biochemical typing of scrapie strains (reply). *Nature* 386:564, 1997.

91. Scott MR, Safar J, Telling G, et al: Identification of a prion protein epitope modulating transmission of bovine spongiform encephalopathy prions to transgenic mice. *Proc Natl Acad Sci USA* 94:14279, 1997.

92. Safar J, Wille H, Itri V, et al: Eight prion strains have PrP^Sc molecules with different conformations. *Nature Med* 4(10):1157, 1998.

93. Telling GC, Parchi P, DeArmond SJ, et al: Evidence for the conformation of the pathologic isoform of the prion protein enciphering and propagating prion diversity. *Science* 274:2079, 1996.

94. Mastrianni JA, Nixon R, Layzer R, et al: Prion protein conformation in a patient with sporadic fatal insomnia. *New Engl J Med* 340(21):1630, 1999.

95. Deleault NR, Lucassen, RW, Supattapone S: RNA molecules stimulate prion protein conversion. *Nature* 425(6959):717, 2003.

96. Weissmann C: A "unified theory" of prion propagation. *Nature* 352:679, 1991.

97. DeArmond SJ, Sanchez H, Yehiely F, et al: Selective neuronal targeting in prion disease. *Neuron* 19:1337, 1997.

98. Mastrianni JA: The prion diseases: Creutzfeldt-Jakob, Gerstmann-Straussler Scheinker, and related disorders. *J Geriatr Psychiatry Neurol* 11:78, 1998.

99. Gomori AJ, Partnow MJ, Horoupian DS, et al: The ataxic form of Creutzfeldt-Jakob disease. *Arch Neurol* 29:318, 1973.

100. Brown P, Cathala F, Castaigne P, et al: Creutzfeldt-Jakob disease: Clinical analysis of a consecutive series of 230 neuropathologically verified cases. *Ann Neurol* 20:597, 1986.

101. Sadeh M, Goldhammer Y, Chagnac Y: Creutzfeldt-Jakob disease associated with peripheral neuropathy. *Isr J Med Sci* 26:220, 1990.

102. MacGowan DJ, Delanty N, Petito F, et al: Isolated myoclonic alien hand as the sole presentation of pathologically established Creutzfeldt-Jakob disease: A report of two patients. *J Neurol Neurosurg Psychiatry* 63(3):404, 1997.

103. Heidenhain A: Klinische und anatomische utersuchungen uber eine eigenartige erkrankung des zentralnervensystems im praesenium. *Z Ges Neurol Psychiatry* 118:49, 1929.

104. Brownell B, Oppenheimer DR: An ataxic form of subacute presenile polioencephalopathy (Creutzfeldt-Jakob disease). *J Neurol Neurosurg Psychiatry* 28:350, 1965.

105. Salazar AM, Masters CL, Gajdusek DC, et al: Syndromes of amyotrophic lateral sclerosis and dementia: Relation to transmissible Creutzfeldt-Jakob disease. *Ann Neurol* 14:17, 1983.

106. Brown P, Gibbs CJ Jr, Rodgers-Johnson P, et al: Human spongiform encephalopathy: The National Institutes of Health series of 300 cases of experimentally transmitted disease. *Ann Neurol* 35:513, 1994.

107. Connolly JH, Allen IV, Dermott E: Transmissible agent in the amyotrophic form of Creutzfeldt-Jakob disease. *J Neurol Neurosurg Psychiatry* 51(11):1459, 1988.

108. Worrall BB, Rowland LP, Chin SS, et al: Amyotrophy in prion diseases. *Arch Neurol* 57:33, 2000.

109. Brandel JP, Delasnerie-Laupretre N, Laplanche JL, et al: Diagnosis of Creutzfeldt-Jakob disease: Effect of clinical criteria on incidence estimates. *Neurology* 54(5):1095, 2000.

110. Brown P, Gibbs CJ Jr, Rodgers-Johnson P, et al: Creutzfeldt-Jakob disease of long duration: Clinicopathological characteristics, transmissibility, and differential diagnosis. *Ann Neurol* 16:295, 1984.

111. Chiafalo N, Fuentes AN, Galvez S: Serial EEG findings in 27 cases of Creutzfeldt-Jakob disease. *Arch Neurol* 37:143, 1980.

112. Will RG, Matthews WB: A retrospective study of Creutzfeldt-Jakob disease in England and Wales 1970–1979: I. Clinical features. *J Neurol Neurosurg Psychiatry* 47:134, 1984.

113. Tateishi J, Kitamoto T, Hoque MZ: Experimental transmission of Creutzfeldt-Jakob disease and related diseases to rodents. *Neurology* 46:532, 1996.

114. Harrington MG, Merril CR, Asher DM, et al: Abnormal proteins in the cerebrospinal fluid of patients with Creutzfeldt-Jakob disease. *New Engl J Med* 1986 315:279, 1986.

115. Blisard KS, Davis LE, Harrington MG, et al: Premortem diagnosis of Creutzfeldt-Jakob disease by detection of abnormal cerebrospinal fluid proteins. *J Neurol Sci* 99(1):75, 1990.

116. Hsich G, Kenney K, Gibbs CJ, et al: The 14-3-3 brain

protein in cerebrospinal fluid as a marker for transmissible spongiform encephalopathies. *New Engl J Med* 335:924, 1996.

117. Rosenmann H, Meiner Z, Kahana E, et al: Detection of 14-3-3 protein in the CSF of genetic Creutzfeldt-Jakob disease. *Neurology* 49:593, 1997.

118. Zerr I, Bodemer M, Gefeller O, et al: Detection of 14-3-3 protein in the cerebrospinal fluid supports the diagnosis of Creutzfeldt-Jakob disease. *Ann Neurol* 43:32, 1998.

119. Zerr I, Bodemer M, Racker S, et al: Cerebrospinal fluid concentration of neuron-specific enolase in diagnosis of Creutzfeldt-Jakob disease. *Lancet* 345:1609, 1995.

120. Kropp S, Zerr I, Schulz-Schaeffer WJ, et al: Increase of neuron-specific enolase in patients with Creutzfeldt-Jakob disease. *Neurosci Lett* 261(1–2):124, 1999.

121. Aksamit AJ: Cerebrospinal fluid 14-3-3 protein: Variability of sporadic Creutzfeldt-Jakob disease, laboratory standards, and quantitation. *Arch Neurol* 60(6):803, 2003.

122. Geschwind MD, Martindale J, Miller D, et al: Challenging the clinical utility of the 14-3-3 protein for the diagnosis of sporadic Creutzfeldt-Jakob disease. *Arch Neurol* 60(6):813, 2003.

123. Beck E, Daniel PM, Davey AJ, et al: The pathogenesis of transmissible spongiform encephalopathy: An ultrastructural study. *Brain* 105:755, 1982.

124. Chou SM, Payne WN, Gibbs CJ Jr, et al: Transmission and scanning electron microscopy of spongiform change in Creutzfeldt-Jakob disease. *Brain* 103:885, 1980.

125. Lampert PW, Gajdusek DC, Gibbs CJ Jr: Subacute spongiform virus encephalopathies: Scrapie, kuru and Creutzfeldt-Jakob disease: a review. *Am J Pathol* 68:626, 1972.

126. DeArmond SJ, Prusiner SB: Prion diseases. In Lantos P, Graham D (eds): *Greenfield's Neuropathology,* 6th ed. London: Edward Arnold, 1997, pp 235–280.

127. Hauw JJ, Sazdovitch V, Laplanche JL, et al: Neuropathologic variants of sporadic Creutzfeldt-Jakob disease and codon 129 of PrP gene. *Neurology* 54(8):1641, 2000.

128. Koch TK, Berg BO, De Armond SJ, et al: Creutzfeldt-Jakob disease in a young adult with idiopathic hypopituitarism: Possible relation to the administration of cadaveric human growth hormone. *New Engl J Med* 313:731, 1985.

129. Anderson JR, Allen CMC, Weller RO: Creutzfeldt-Jakob disease following human pituitary-derived growth hormone administration (abstract). *Neuropathol Appl Neurobiol* 16:543, 1990.

130. Billette de Villemeur T, Beauvais P, et al: Creutzfeldt-Jakob disease in children treated with growth hormone. *Lancet* 337:864, 1991.

131. Billette de Villemeur T, Gelot A, et al: Iatrogenic Creutzfeldt-Jakob disease in three growth hormone recipients: A neuropathological study. *Neuropathol Appl Neurobiol* 20:111, 1994.

132. Billette de Villemeur T, Deslys JP, Pradel A, et al: Creutzfeldt-Jakob disease from contaminated growth hormone extracts in France. *Neurology* 47:690, 1996.

133. Brown P, Gajdusek DC, Gibbs CJ Jr, et al: Potential epidemic of Creutzfeldt-Jakob disease from human growth hormone therapy. *New Engl J Med* 313:728, 1985.

134. Fradkin JE, Schonberger LB, Mills JL, et al: Creutzfeldt-Jakob disease in pituitary growth hormone recipients in the United States. *JAMA* 265:880, 1991.

135. Gibbs CJ Jr, Asher DM, Brown PW, et al: Creutzfeldt-Jakob disease infectivity of growth hormone derived from human pituitary glands. *New Engl J Med* 328:358, 1993.

136. Croxson M, Brown P, Synek B, et al: A new case of Creutzfeldt-Jakob disease associated with human growth hormone therapy in New Zealand. *Neurology* 38:1128, 1988.

137. Thadani V, Penar PL, Partington J, et al: Creutzfeldt-Jakob disease probably acquired from a cadaveric dura mater graft: Case report. *J Neurosurg* 69:766, 1988.

138. Anonymous, from the Centers for Disease Control and Prevention: Creutzfeldt-Jakob disease associated with cadaveric dura mater grafts—Japan, January 1979–May 1996. *JAMA* 279(1):11, 1998.

139. Otto D: Jacob-Creutzfeldt disease associated with cadaveric dura. *J Neurosurg* 67:149, 1987.

140. Nisbet TJ, MacDonaldson I, Bishara SN: Creutzfeldt-Jakob disease in a second patient who received a cadaveric dura mater graft. *JAMA* 261:1118, 1989.

141. Masullo C, Pocchiari M, Macchi G, et al: Transmission of Creutzfeldt-Jakob disease by dural cadaveric graft. *J Neurosurg* 71:954, 1989.

142. Miyashita K, Inuzuka T, Kondo H, et al: Creutzfeldt-Jakob disease in a patient with a cadaveric dural graft. *Neurology* 41:940, 1991.

143. Willison HJ, Gale AN, McLaughlin JE: Creutzfeldt-Jakob disease following cadaveric dura mater graft. *J Neurol Neurosurg Psychiatry* 54:940, 1991.

144. Anonymous: Precautions in handling tissues, fluids, and other contaminated materials from patients with documented or suspected Creutzfeldt-Jakob disease. Committee on Health Care Issues, American Neurological Association. *Ann Neurol* 19(1):75, 1986.

145. Taguchi F, Tamai Y, Uchida K, et al: Proposal for a procedure for complete inactivation of the Creutzfeldt-Jakob disease agent [erratum appears in *Arch Virol* 122(3–4):411, 1992]. *Arch Virol* 119(3–4):297, 1991.

146. Taylor DM, Fraser H, McConnell I, et al: Decontamination studies with the agents of bovine spongiform encephalopathy and scrapie. *Arch Virol* 139:313, 1994.

147. Brown P, Rohwer RG, Gajdusek DC: Newer data on the inactivation of scrapie virus or Creutzfeldt-Jakob disease virus in brain tissue. *J Infect Dis* 153(6):1145, 1986.

148. Cochius JI, Burns RJ, Blumbergs PC, et al: Creutzfeldt-Jakob disease in a recipient of human pituitary-derived gonadotrophin. *Aust NZ J Med* 20:592, 1990.

149. Cochius JI, Hyman N, Esiri MM: Creutzfeldt-Jakob disease in a recipient of human pituitary-derived gonadotrophin: A second case. *J Neurol Neurosurg Psychiatry* 55:1094, 1992.

150. Healy DL, Evans J: Creutzfeldt-Jakob disease after pituitary gonadotrophins. *Br J Med* 307:517, 1993.

151. Duffy P, Wolf J, Collins G, et al: Possible person to person transmission of Creutzfeldt-Jakob disease. *New Engl J Med* 290:692, 1974.

152. Bernouilli C: Danger of accidental person to person transmission of Creutzfeldt-Jakob disease by surgery. *Lancet* 1:478, 1977.

153. Brown P, Preece MA, Will RG: "Friendly fire" in medicine: Hormones, homografts, and Creutzfeldt-Jakob disease. *Lancet* 340:24, 1992.

154. Brown P, Gibbs CJ Jr, Amyx HL, et al: Chemical disinfection of Creutzfeldt-Jakob disease virus. *New Engl J Med* 306:1279, 1982.

155. Kuroda Y, Gibbs CJ Jr, Amyx HL, et al: Creutzfeldt-Jakob disease in mice: Persistent viremia and preferential replication of virus in low-density lymphocytes. *Infect Immun* 41:154, 1983.

156. Casaccia P, Ladogana A, Xi YG, et al: Levels of infectivity in the blood throughout the incubation period of hamsters peripherally injected with scrapie. *Arch Virol* 108:145, 1989.

157. Brown P, Rohwer RG, Dunstan BC, et al: The distribution of infectivity in blood components and plasma derivatives in experimental models of transmissible spongiform encephalopathy. *Transfusion* 38:810, 1998.

158. Diringer H: Sustained viremia in experimental hamster scrapie: Brief report. *Arch Virol* 82:105, 1984.

159. Gajdusek DC: Subacute spongiform encephalopathies: Transmissible cerebral amyloidoses caused by unconventional viruses. In Fields BN, et al (eds): *Virology*, 2d ed. New York: Raven Press, 1990, pp 2289–2324.

160. Brown P: Can Creutzfeldt-Jakob disease be transmitted by transfusion? *Curr Opin Hematol* 2:472, 1995.

161. Collins S, Law MG, Fletcher A, et al: Surgical treatment and risk of sporadic Creutzfeldt-Jakob disease: A case-control study. *Lancet* 353(9154):693, 1999.

162. Esmonde TF, Will RG, Slattery JM, et al: Creutzfeldt-Jakob disease and blood transfusion. *Lancet* 341:205, 1993.

163. Ward HJ, Everington D, Croes EA, et al: Sporadic Creutzfeldt-Jakob disease and surgery: A case-control study using community controls (comment). *Neurology* 59(4):543, 2002.

164. Bradley R: Bovine spongiform encephalopathy (BSE): The current situation and research. *Eur J Epidemiol* 7:532, 1991.

165. Matthews D: BSE: A global update. *J Appl Microbiol* 94(suppl):120S, 2003.

166. Alpers M: Kuru: A clinical study. In mimeographed manuscript, reissued. Bethesda MD: U.S. Department of Health and Human Services, National Institutes of Health, 1964 pp 1–38.

167. Alpers M: Epidemiology and clinical aspects of kuru. In Prusiner SB, McKinley MP (eds): *Prions: Novel Infectious Pathogens Causing Scrapie and Creutzfeldt-Jakob Disease*. New York: Academic Press, 1987, pp 451–465.

168. Klatzo I, Gajdusek DC, Zigas V: Pathology of kuru. *Lab Invest* 8:799, 1959.

169. Gambetti P, Parchi P, Petersen RB, et al: Fatal familial insomnia and familial Creutzfeldt-Jakob disease: Clinical, pathological and molecular features. *Brain Pathol* 5:43, 1995.

170. Medori R, Montagna P, Tritschler HJ, et al: Fatal familial insomnia: A second kindred with mutation of prion protein gene at codon 178. *Neurology* 42:669, 1992.

171. Petersen RB, Tabaton M, Berg L, et al: Analysis of the prion protein gene in thalamic dementia. *Neurology* 42:1859, 1992.

172. Bosque PJ, Vnencak-Jones CL, Johnson MD, et al: A PrP gene codon 178 base substitution and a 24-bp interstitial deletion in familial Creutzfeldt-Jakob disease. *Neurology* 42:1864, 1992.

173. Reder AT, Mednick AS, Brown P, et al: Clinical and genetic studies of fatal familial insomnia. *Neurology* 45:1068, 1995.

174. Silburn P, Cervenakova L, Varghese P, et al: Fatal familial insomnia: A seventh family. *Neurology* 47:1326, 1996.

175. Nagayama M, Shinohara Y, Furukawa H, et al: Fatal familial insomnia with a mutation at codon 178 of the prion protein gene: First report from Japan. *Neurology* 47:1313, 1996.

176. Gambetti P: Fatal familial insomnia: A new human prion disease. In *Prion Diseases in Humans and Animals Symposium*. London: 1991.

177. Manetto V, Medori R, Cortelli P, et al: Fatal familial insomnia: Clinical and pathological study of five new cases. *Neurology* 42:312, 1992.

178. Lugaresi E, Medori R, Montagna P, et al: Fatal familial insomnia and dysautonomia with selective degeneration of thalamic nuclei. *New Engl J Med* 315:997, 1986.

179. Mastrianni J: Fatal sporadic insomnia: Fatal familial insomnia phenotype without a mutation of the prion protein gene. *Neurology* 48(suppl):A296, 1997.

180. Kawasaki K, Wakabayashi K, Kawakami A, et al: Thalamic form of Creutzfeldt-Jakob disease or fatal insomnia? Report of a sporadic case with normal prion protein genotype. *Acta Neuropathol* 93:317, 1997.

181. Parchi P, Capellari S, Chin S, et al: A subtype of sporadic prion disease mimicking fatal familial insomnia. *Neurology* 52(9):1757, 1999.

182. Gambetti P, Parchi P: Insomnia in prion diseases: Sporadic and familial. *New Engl J Med* 340:1675, 1999.

183. Gerstmann J: Über ein noch nicht beschriebenes reflex-phanomen bei einer Erkrankung des zerebellaren systems. *Wien Med Wochenschr* 78:906, 1928.

184. Gerstmann J, Sträussler E, Scheinker I: Über eine eigenartige hereditär-familiäre Erkrankung des Zentralnervensystems zugleich ein Beitrag zur frage des vorzeitigen lokalen Alterns. *Z Neurol* 154:736, 1936.

185. Heston LL, Lowther DLW, Leventhal CM: Alzheimer's disease: A family study. *Arch Neurol* 15:225, 1966.

186. Korth C, May BC, Cohen FE, et al: Acridine and phenothiazine derivatives as pharmacotherapeutics for prion disease. *Proc Natl Acad Sci USA* 98(17):9836, 2001.

187. Collins SJ, Lewis V, Brazier M, et al: Quinacrine does not prolong survival in a murine Creutzfeldt-Jakob disease model. *Ann Neurol* 52(4):503, 2002.

188. Brown P: Drug therapy in human and experimental transmissible spongiform encephalopathy. *Neurology* 58(12):1720, 2002.

CHAPTER 19

Rickettsial and Ehrlichial Infections

Daniel J. Sexton and Gregory A. Dasch

Although the term *rickettsia* has been applied loosely to a wide range of gram-negative bacteria that are, apparently, obligately intracellular and have associations with arthropods or other invertebrate hosts, this assemblage is highly polyphyletic, and the pathogenic potential of many of these agents is unknown. Here we will discuss only the neurologic symptoms occurring during classic and newly emerging rickettsioses and ehrlichioses that are caused by monophyletic closely related alphaproteobacterial species in the order Rickettsiales in the families Rickettsiaceae and Anaplasmataceae. The clinical features of many of the emerging diseases remain poorly defined.

Patients with severe neurologic symptoms with rickettsial and ehrlichial infections may die, recover completely, or rarely, develop long-term neurologic sequelae. This chapter will discuss the epidemiology, microbiology, pathology, diagnosis, treatment, prevention, and outcome of patients with rickettsial and ehrlichial infections. Discussions of the clinical features and se-

quelae will focus on the neurologic aspects of these arthropod-borne infections.

▶ EPIDEMIOLOGY AND MICROBIOLOGY

The genus *Rickettsia* includes 23 named species and at least 40 genotypes that are associated with hematophagous and phytophagous arthropods and leeches.[1] At least 15 of these species are pathogenic for humans (Table 19-1), and the potential for causing disease by others may be limited by a lack of a mechanism for human exposure, as well as microbial factors.[2,3] The rickettsial diseases are transmitted by ticks, fleas, lice, or mites, and the global distribution of these vectors accounts for the distribution of these diseases. With the exception of louse-borne epidemic typhus, in which humans are a primary reservoir for its etiologic agent, *Rickettsia prowazekii*, pathogenic rickettsioses generally are

▲ **TABLE 19-1.** FEATURES OF HUMAN DISEASES CAUSED BY RICKETTSIACEAE AND ANAPLASMATACEAE

Species	Human Disease Name or Effect	Principal Associated Vector	Geographic Distribution
Rickettsiaceae			
Typhus group			
R. prowazekii	Epidemic typhus	Pediculus human body louse	Worldwide
	Brill-Zinsser disease	None	Worldwide
	Sylvatic typhus	Neohaematopinus squirrel louse	East to Midwest (USA)
R. typhi	Endemic (murine typhus)	Xenopsylla and Ctenocephalides fleas	Worldwide
Spotted fever group			
R. rickettsii	Rocky Mountain spotted fever	Dermacentor and Amblyomma ticks	The Americas
R. amblyommii	Lone star tick spotted fever	Amblyomma ticks	East to Midwest (USA)
R. parkeri	Maculatum tick spotted fever	Amblyomma ticks	Southeast (USA)
R. akari	Rickettsialpox	Liponyssoides mouse mite	Worldwide
R. felis	Cat flea rickettsiosis	Ctenocephalides flea	Worldwide
R. africae	African tick typhus	Amblyomma ticks	Sub-Saharan Africa, Caribbean
R. conorii	Mediterranean spotted fever	Rhipicephalus and Haemaphysalis ticks	Africa, Southern Europe to Indian subcontinent
R. helvetica	Chronic perimyocarditis	Ixodes tick	Europe
R. slovaca	Tick-borne lymphadenopathy	Rhipicephalus ticks	Mediterranean
R. sharonii	Israeli tick typhus	Dermacentor ticks	Europe, Asia
R. caspiensis	Astrakhan spotted fever	Rhipicephalus ticks	Astrakhan (Russia)
R. mongolotimonae	Unnamed spotted fever	Hyalomma ticks	Mongolia, France
R. sibirica	North Asian tick typhus	Dermacentor ticks	Indian subcontinent to Russia
R. heilongjiangensis	Unnamed spotted fever	Dermacentor ticks	China
R. japonica	Oriental tick typhus	Hemaphysalis and Dermacentor ticks	Japan
R. honei	Flinders Island fever	Aponomma and Haemaphysalis ticks	Australia, Thailand
R. australis	Queensland tick typhus	Ixodes ticks	Australia
Orientia tsutsugamushi	Scrub typhus	Leptotrombidium mites	Australia, Asia-Pacific Region to Afghanistan
Anaplasmataceae			
Ehrlichia chaffeensis	Human monocytic ehrlichiosis	Amblyomma ticks	East (USA), worldwide?
Ehrlichia ewingii	Unnamed ehrlichiosis	Amblyomma ticks	East (USA)
Ehrlichia muris	Unnamed ehrlichiosis	Ixodes and Haemaphysalis ticks	Japan, Russia
Anaplasma phagocytophilum	Human granulocytic ehrlichiosis (anaplasmosis)	Ixodes ticks	USA, Europe
Neorickettsia sennetsu	Sennetsu ehrlichiosis	Unknown	Asia, Japan
Wolbachia sp.	Filariasis	Symbiont of species of filaria	Worldwide

zoonotic diseases. However, in most cases, the arthropod vectors are the primary reservoirs for maintenance of the respective agents because the agents are maintained by both transovarial and transtadial passages, and any stage of ectoparasite encountering humans can transmit the disease. Transmission does not occur solely by arthropod bite but can include self-inoculation into irritated bite sites or conjunctivae of infected crushed arthropods or arthropod feces or inhalation of aerosolized infected feces.

In the Americas, the most prevalent severe rickettsiosis, Rocky Mountain spotted fever caused by *Rickettsia rickettsii*, is transmitted by the dog tick, *Dermacentor variabilis,* in the central and eastern United States; by the wood tick, *D. andersoni,* in the western United States; and by *Amblyomma cajennense* in the rest of the Americas. Recently, *R. parkeri,* which is associated with the Gulf Coast tick, *Amblyomma maculatum,* was isolated from a patient with an eschar[4] that occurs only rarely in infections with *R. rickettsii. R. amblyommii* is widespread in the common human biting lone-star tick, *A. americanum*[5]; it has been implicated as a cause of mild spotted fever with flulike symptoms[6] similar to those described for African tick-bite fever infections with *R. africae.* This agent commonly causes illness in visitors to sub-Saharan Africa, where it is transmitted by *A. hebraeum* and *A. variegatum,* but this disease also can occur in the Caribbean in areas where *A. variegatum* has been introduced. Rickettsialpox, caused by *R. akari* and which is transmitted by mites from house mice, is largely an urban or suburban disease in the United States, although other hosts and vectors have been described; it often occurs after rodent control measures reduce host populations for the mite.[7] Recent concern about cases of suspected cutaneous anthrax or smallpox have increased identification of cases of this mild rickettsiosis. Murine typhus, caused by *R. typhi,* is associated worldwide with the Oriental rat flea, *Xenopsylla cheopis* and *Rattus,* in coastal and tropical areas.[8] However, endemic areas for murine typhus in the United States include California, Texas, and Hawaii, and this agent has been associated with other hosts, including the cat flea, *Ctenocephalides felis,* and opossums. *R. felis,* an atypical spotted fever group agent related to *R. akari,* is also found in cat fleas worldwide and has been shown to cause a murine typhus–like disease in a few cases.[9,10] Finally, although primary louseborne epidemic typhus is rare in the United States, it may occur as recrudescent typhus or Brill Zinsser disease in those experiencing typhus abroad many years earlier. A sylvatic cycle of *R. prowazekii* is also present in the eastern United States, where it is maintained in the southern flying squirrel, *Glaucomys volans,* and its lice. Humans may come in contact with infected louse feces through the squirrels inhabiting homes or by handling of these squirrels, which sometimes are maintained as pets or in wildlife conservation projects.[11]

Scrub typhus, caused by *Orientia tsutsugamushi,* is transmitted by infected larval mites (chiggers) of several genera of trombiculid mites, particularly *Leptotrombidium* spp.[12] *Orientia* originally was a species of *Rickettsia* but differs from it significantly in biologic, genetic, and antigenic properties. This monospecific genus exhibits a very wide range of biologic and genetic variation, and multiple types can be present in very local regions. Heterologous and homologous protective immunity does not persist very long, so secondary infections can occur. Human infections exhibit tremendous variations in severity and presentation, probably due to both host and microbial factors. The disease occurs in a large geographic region from Australia to Korea and from the Philippines to Afghanistan and in very diverse habitats from desert to tropical regions to semiurban environments and from coral atolls to rice paddies to arid riverine valleys in the mountains. Travelers to these regions often are exposed to the mites and may become infected.

Three human ehrlichioses are known to occur in the United States,[13] and these represent newly emergent zoonotic diseases, whereas some of the many chronic veterinary ehrlichioses, such as canine ehrlichiosis (*Ehrlichia canis*), heartwater (*E. ruminantium*) and ruminant ehrlichioses (*Anaplasma marginale* and *A. phagocytophilum*), and Potomac horse fever (*Neorickettsia risticii*), have been recognized for many years. The taxonomy of these ehrlichial agents in the family Anaplasmataceae was reorganized recently[14] to emphasize the common biologic and molecular traits of the four major clades, although additional groups may be necessary in the future. *A. phagocytophilum,* transmitted by the tick vector of Lyme disease, *Ixodes scapularis,* in the northern United States, by *I. pacificus* on the West Coast, and by other species of *Ixodes* ticks in Europe and Asia, was discovered to cause human granulocytic ehrlichiosis (anaplasmosis) in 1994.[15] *E. chaffeensis* (human monocytic ehrlichiosis) was discovered in 1986,[16] and *E. ewingii* was first recognized as a cause of human disease in 1999.[17] Both of the latter agents are transmitted by the tick *Amblyomma americanum* in the United States. DNA from agents similar to *E. chaffeensis* has been detected in other ticks in other regions of the world, but isolates have not been characterized to clarify their identity.[18] *E. muris* also may be an agent of human disease in Asia and possibly Europe. Like *N. risticii,* which involves a fluke–freshwater snail maintenance cycle, the human disease agent *N. sennetsu* appears to be maintained in a fish fluke in Asia and may infect humans who have eaten uncooked fish products. Unlike species of *Orientia* and *Rickettsia,* the tick-transmitted ehrlichial agents require persistent infection of one or more vertebrate reservoirs for maintenance because they cannot be maintained transovarially in ticks; they must be acquired from a host in the larval or nymph stage, persist transstadially, and then be transmitted to naive hosts in subsequent feedings.

Pathogenic *Rickettsia, Orientia,* and *Ehrlichia* cause transient or even chronic infections of humans in some cases, and prolonged survival in blood products has been demonstrated.[19,20] Consequently, blood transfusion– or organ transplantation–mediated transmission of these agents is not only possible theoretically but also has occurred in several cases, particularly during the eclipse phase following infection before onset of disease.[21–25] Screening donor individuals for these infections by polymerase chain reaction (PCR) when they are from endemic areas with high seasonal risk of exposure for these diseases may be prudent but is done rarely.[26] Because both rickettsial and ehrlichial agents may be present in animal tissues, exposure to infected animal tissues and blood also may pose a risk of infection, even when ectoparasites are not present.

▶ PATHOLOGY

In a classic paper[27] published over 50 years ago, Wolbach summarized the necropsy findings on patients dying of epidemic typhus, scrub typhus, and Rocky Mountain spotted fever, including his own seminal studies on typhus and Rocky Mountain spotted fever from 30 years earlier.[28,29] Pathologic abnormalities in the central nervous systems of patients with these three diseases were similar. All had varying degrees of diffuse cerebral edema, sharply circumscribed focal lesions consisting of clusters of microglial cells, and inflammatory infiltrates consisting of mononuclear cells in a perivascular pattern in the meninges. These clusters of microglial cells in the white and gray matter were termed *typhus nodules.* Wolbach noted that such nodules were more common and larger in patients with epidemic typhus and scrub typhus and less common and smaller in patients with Rocky Mountain spotted fever. Patients with Rocky Mountain spotted fever tended to have lesions involving larger blood vessels, which in some instances resulted in thrombosis and small infarctions. Moreover, Wolbach noted that microglial nodules were unlikely to be seen unless the patient had survived for at least 10 days after onset of symptoms. Military pathologists during World War II observed that patients with fatal scrub typhus typically have diffuse or focal mononuclear cell exudates in their leptomeninges, as well as clusters of microglial cells (known as *typhus nodules*) throughout their white and gray matter; occasionally, focal hemorrhages also are present.[30,31]

Experimental studies in guinea pigs confirmed that typhus nodules began as focal lesions around capillaries and then evolved into discrete focal lesions ranging in size from 60 to 180 mm. Such lesions were shown to enlarge and persist in guinea pigs even after fever had resolved and to persist for weeks after recovery. In human, such nodules were found up to 8 weeks after recovery from typhus.

Subsequent pathologic studies have largely confirmed Wolbach's descriptions of Rocky Mountain spotted fever. Modern pathologists have emphasized that focal brain lesions in patients with Rocky Mountain spotted fever are of three general types: perivascular inflammatory cells, glial nodules, and arteriolar thrombonecrosis with small infarcts. Microinfarcts are seen predominately in the white matter in patients surviving more than 10 days; such lesions tend to be more numerous in the brain stem.[32] The reason why some patients with RMSF develop severe encephalitis and others do not is unknown. Occasionally, patients dying of RMSF will have inflammatory changes largely confined to the central nervous system (CNS). For example, Katz and colleagues[33] described a 40-year old man who died of Rocky Mountain spotted fever after developing severe pulmonary edema. At autopsy, changes characteristic of Rocky Mountain spotted fever were found only in the CNS. This fact is important clinically and suggests that necropsy examination should include the CNS in fatal cases in which Rocky Mountain spotted fever is suspected. In fact, necropsy may be the only way to confirm the diagnosis of Rocky Mountain spotted fever in patients who die within the first 10 days of illness because serologic evidence of a rickettsial infection is unlikely to occur in such patients.[34] *Rickettsia* often are difficult to visualize and may be missed when tissues obtained at necropsy are examined using conventional histologic staining methods such Giemsa or Macchiavello's stains. However, immunologic staining techniques are highly sensitive for detecting rickettsiae in tissue samples. Although the sensitivity of such staining techniques decreases with increasing time following the institution of effective antirickettsial therapy, rickettsiae occasionally may be detected for up to 72 hours after doxycyline therapy has been initiated.[34]

Several pathologists have noted that patients dying of Rocky Mountain spotted fever often have prominent abnormalities in the brainstem.[35] Brainstems with microvascular lesions identical to those described originally by Wolbach also have been seen in patients who died of murine typhus and scrub typhus.[36] The mechanism by which *O. tsutsugamushi* produces CNS abnormalities is not well understood. CNS invasion by rickettsial organisms inside mononuclear cells and/or invasion of endothelial cells lining the meninges are both possible explanations for the finding of positive PCR amplification of rickettsial DNA in cerebrospinal fluid (CSF) samples from patients with clinical findings compatible with meningitis.[37]

Because Mediterranean spotted fever generally is a much milder disease than Rocky Mountain spotted fever, there have been only a few reports of postmortem examination of neural tissue in patients with this disease. However, when such examinations are done, findings similar to those seen in the CNS of patients with Rocky Mountain spotted fever have been reported.[38]

Autopsy studies of two patients dying of human monocytic ehrlichiosis failed to show significant pathologic abnormalities in the brain.[39] In another report, a patient dying of ehrlichiosis was found to have perivascular cuffing with plasma cells in the brain tissue.[40]

► CLINICAL FEATURES

Common Aspects of Neurologic Disease

Human infections by spotted fever group rickettsiae, typhus group rickettsiae, and *O. tsutsugamushi* (scrub typhus) almost invariably are associated with prominent and severe headaches. However, children, especially those younger than 5 years of age, may not complain of headache or be able to describe this symptom even if it is present. In addition to headache, an array of neurologic symptoms and complications may occur in all these rickettsial infections. Individual patients may have one or more of the following: delirium, confusion, seizures, coma, focal neurologic abnormalities, aseptic meningitis, and incontinence of bowel and bladder. Papilledema also may be present in patients with severe Rocky Mountain spotted fever.[41]

Patients with rickettsial or ehrlichial infections may develop neurologic symptoms on a continuum ranging from mild lethargy to coma. Neurologic signs in individual patients with Rocky Mountain spotted fever have included all the following as isolated findings or in various combinations: stupor, lethargy, delirium, coma, cranial nerve palsies, hearing loss, dysarthria, complete paralysis, hemiplegia, seizures, spasticity, athetosis, and neurogenic bladder.[36,42]

Severe CNS symptoms correlate with a poor outcome in patients with Rocky Mountain spotted fever.[41,43] Conlon and colleagues[44] retrospectively reviewed the records of 114 patients with Rocky Mountain spotted fever in order to determine predictors of prognosis. Neurologic involvement and an elevevated serum creatinine concentration at the time of hospitalization both were associated independently with an increased mortality using multivariate analysis.

Neurologic symptoms tend to be more severe in patients with Rocky Mountain spotted fever than in those with other spotted fever group rickettsial infections. However, occasionally, patients with Mediterranean spotted fever have a fulminant or malignant course. In such cases, the neurologic findings may be identical to those seen in patients with severe Rocky Mountain spotted fever.[45] Neurologic complications were reported in 6 of 227 patients with Mediterranean spotted fever reviewed by Font-Creus and colleagues.[46] Individual patients in this case series had seizures or decreased hearing, and 10 percent were described as having impaired consciousness at some point in their illness. Rosenthal and Michaeli[47] described a single patient who developed diplopia and ptosis as a complication of Mediterranean spotted fever.

Murine typhus is also generally a milder disease than Rocky Mountain spotted fever, but neurologic complications similar to those seen in Rocky Mountain spotted fever may occur rarely. In one case series involving 137 patients from Thailand with murine typhus, 3 of 137 patients had neurologic complications that included seizures, an intracerebral hemorrhage, and/or signs of meningoencephalitis.[48] Other authors have described individual cases of murine typhus with neurologic complications such as coma, hemiplegia, hallucinations, ataxia, aphasia and transient deafness, and facial paralysis[36,49,50]

Unlike murine typhus, epidemic typhus is accompanied commonly by neurologic complications that may include coma, stupor, delirium, focal cranial nerve abnormalities, spasticity, and incontinence.[51] Twenty-three percent of 60 patients with epidemic typhus admitted to a single hospital in Addis Ababa, Ethiopia, had tinnitus, 1 patient developed ptosis, and another patient developed transient hemiparesis.[52]

Similarly, neurologic complications are well known to occur in patients with scrub typhus. Complex or serious neurologic symptoms in individual patients with scrub typhus can result in clinical confusion with other infectious diseases that also cause cerebritis, meningoencephalitis, or meningitis.[36]

Infections with *R. rickettsii, R. conorii, R. prowazeki,* and *O. tsutsugamushi* all may produce signs, symptoms, and laboratory abnormalities typical of aseptic meningitis. In some cases, nuchal rigidity and stupor may be striking, and when polymorphonuclear cells are predominant in the CSF, all these findings may mimic bacterial meningitis. The range of abnormalities seen in the CSF of such patients is discussed later in this chapter.

The neurologic symptoms of patients with ehrlichial infections (including those infected with *A. phagocytophilum*) are similar in many ways to those with rickettsial infections, although the number of reports on neurologic manifestations and complications of ehrlichial infections is limited. As in rickettsial infections, headache is the most common neurologic symptom in patients with both human monocytic ehrlichiosis and *A. phagocytophilum* infection. Often the headache is intense. Confusion, lethargy, ataxia, and focal neurologic findings such as cranial nerve abnormalities, hyperreflexia, photophobia, and seizures also may occur in a small percentage of patients.[39,53] Brachial plexopathy was described in a single patient in a case series of 18 patients with *A. phagocytophilum* infection from New York.[54]

Unusual Neurologic Manifestations

Unusual CNS symptoms described in individual case reports of patients with rickettsial infections include tinnitus and hallucinations,[55] buccofacial dyskinesia,[56] and deafness.[57–59] Scott and colleagues[56] reported that a 63-year-old nurse developed transient tardive dyskinesia during the early convalescent phase of Rocky Mountain spotted fever. This patient developed purposeless lip smacking soon after becoming afebrile. Thereafter she developed oral facial dyskinetic movments characteristic of tardive dyskinesia and then transiently developed coma. Subsequently, she recovered fully and had no residual neurologic sequelae. Verbiest and colleagues[60] reported that a single patient with Mediterranean spotted fever developed subacute progressive sensory ataxic neuronopathy that began 1 week after apparent recovery from a mild case of *R. conorii* infection. This patient developed disabling progressive symptoms, and a biopsy of a peripheral nerve confirmed axonal degeneration. The authors speculated the pathogenesis of this unusual complication was immune mediated because a similar illness has been reported to occur rarely in patients with cancer, HIV infection, and as a residual disability in patients with Guillain-Barré syndrome. Guillain-Barré polyneuropathy also has been described in individual patients following infection with *R. conorii* and *R. rickettsii*.[61–63]

Short- and Long-Term Sequelae

A number of authors have described short-term neurologic sequelae in patients with Rocky Mountain spotted fever. Deafness is one of the most common of these sequelae. Deafness may be unilateral or bilateral. The mechanism of deafness is presumed to be vasculitis-induced cochlear damage.[64] Transient deafness also has been reported in patients with murine typhus.[36] Transient mononeuropathy or polyneuropathy producing symptoms such as foot drop has been reported in patients with Rocky Mountain spotted fever.[65]

Archibald and Sexton[66] reported that 9 of 20 patients with severe Rocky Mountain spotted fever (defined as having nonfatal illness requiring a hospital stay of 2 weeks of greater) had one or more long-term sequelae (defined as lasting more than a year). Six of these 9 patients had long-term neurologic complications, including spastic paraparasis, urinary incontinence, dysarthria, deafness, ataxia, hemiparesis, and persistent peripheral neuropathy. Other authors have

reported similar complications. Rosenblum and colleagues[67] reexamined 37 patients with Rocky Mountain spotted fever 1 to 7 years after their recovery from the disease. Six of these 37 patients had neurologic abnormalities such as intellectual impairment, ataxia, or signs of spasticity or muscle weakness. Other authors have described similar long-term neurologic complications, including spastic parasis of one arm,[55] seizures,[43] and persistent third nerve palsy.[68] Thomas and Berlin[69] described the autopsy findings in an adult who had severe Rocky Mountain spotted fever and then developed multiple neurologic complications including deafness, spastic paraplegia, a neurogenic bladder, and intellectual impairment. This patient died 18 months after his acute illness with Rocky Mountain spotted fever. Autopsy disclosed numerous old infarcts of the brain and spinal cord, widespread demyelination, gliosis of the white and gray matter, and thickened arterioles.

To our knowledge, long-term sequelae are uncommon in ehrlichial infections. Ratnasamy and colleagues[39] reported that 1 of 57 patients with human monocytic ehrlichiosis from their institution developed a facial nerve palsy that "resolved over 6 months after she recovered." However, since this patient also had a positive enzyme immunoassay (EIA) for *Borrelia burgdorferi* in serum and an equivocal serologic response to the same organism in her CSF, the possibility of coinfection with Lyme disease could not be ruled out. A case-control study of 85 patients with *A. phagocytophilum* infection and 102 age- and sex-matched controls found that patients with *A. phagocytophilum* infection were more likely to report recurrent fever, chills, and sweats up to 24 months after acute illness, but no patient had long-term neurologic sequelae, and there was no difference between general health functioning in cases and controls.[70]

▶ DIFFERENTIAL DIAGNOSIS

Rocky Mountain spotted fever, other spotted fever group rickettsial infections, murine and epidemic typhus, scrub typhus, human monocytic ehrlichiosis, and human granulocytic ehrlichiosis (anaplasmosis) all can be exceedingly difficult to diagnose. Indeed, even experienced physicians practicing in endemic regions may misdiagnose these potentially life-threatening diseases and confuse them with numerous infectious and noninfectious mimics.

The reasons for misdiagnosis are multiple.[71] First, all these diseases often begin with nonspecific symptoms that can be confused easily with benign viral or other self-limiting diseases. For example, Kirkland and colleagues[72] reported that over half of all patients with Rocky Mountain spotted fever were misdiagnosed during their first physician visit even though these physicians were practicing in North Carolina where the occurrence of Rocky Mountain spotted fever is well known to physicians and patients. Moreover, the earlier that patients sought medical care after the onset of symptoms, the more likely they were to be misdiagnosed.

Misdiagnosis is also common because the clinical features of rickettsial and ehrlichial diseases are often atypical and because the classic clinical features (such as skin rash and eschar, which are the hallmarks of some but not all of these diseases) may be absent or delayed in onset. For example, approximately 10 percent of patients with Rocky Mountain spotted fever do not develop a skin rash, and in an additional small percentage of patients skin rash may appear only hours before death or only at a focal location.[73] Misdiagnosis also may occur because of the absence of consistent and distinctive symptoms such as an eschar. Such eschars, which are important clues to the presence of scrub typhus, Mediterranean spotted fever, Queensland tick typhus, and Siberian tick typhus, may be absent in a substantial proportion of patients, leading to misdiagnosis. To make the diagnosis even more difficult, some patients with rickettsial and ehrlichial infections are given ineffective antibiotics early in the course of illness. Later, when a skin rash appears, such rashes are presumed incorrectly (and sometimes tragically) to represent drug allergies, further delaying recognition and treatment based on the correct diagnosis.

Finally, misdiagnosis may occur when patients acquire a rickettsial or ehrlichial infection and then travel to a nonendemic region in the same or a different country (or even continent). Hundreds of cases of "imported" rickettsial diseases have been described. In the last decade there have been numerous reports of imported cases of African tick bite fever, scrub typhus, and Mediterranean spotted fever into the United States, and cases of Rocky Mountain spotted fever, epidemic typhus, scrub typhus, and African tick bite fever have been imported into Europe.

The differential diagnosis of patients with rickettsial diseases depends on location and the prevalence of other diseases that can mimic their clinical features. For example, malaria and dengue are endemic in many of the regions where scrub typhus occurs. Thus misdiagnosis of scrub typhus as dengue and malaria is common, particularly when typical dermatologic manifestations of scrub typhus are absent or delayed in onset. Similarly, Rocky Mountain spotted fever has been confused with all the following diseases: measles, infectious mononucleosis, a host of nonspecific viral illnesses, drug reactions, staphylococcal bacteremia, herpes encephalitis, viral and bacterial meningitis, and streptococcal infections. Also, because some patients with Rocky Mountain spotted fever develop severe gastrointestinal symptoms in the first several days of illness, some patients with *R. rickettsii* have undergone

laparotomy and cholecystectomy on the mistaken impression that they had an acute abdomen.[74] The rickettsioses also frequently are mistaken for cases of typhoid fever in much of the world.

As mentioned previously, some patients with rickettsial and ehrlichial infections present with signs and symptoms suggestive of meningitis. Lumbar puncture in such cases often reveals a lymphocytic or neutrophilic pleocytosis that, in turn, can lead to erroneous assumptions that a viral or other bacterial infection is present.

Occasionally, other neurologic signs may dominate the clinical presentation and lead to misdiagnosis. For example, Horney and Walker[32] described a patient with Rocky Mountain spotted fever who became ill in October and lacked a skin rash. The patient underwent brain biopsy because the primary clinical symptoms suggested herpetic encephalitis. The biopsy actually revealed rickettsiae when special stains were used. Kirk and colleagues[55] described a patient with Rocky Mountain spotted fever who was admitted to a psychiatric hospital because her primary initial symptoms were hallucinations. The correct diagnosis was delayed until an infectious disease specialist evaluated her because of the unexplained fever and made the correct diagnosis.

► LABORATORY DIAGNOSIS

Isolation, Direct and Indirect Staining, and Immunohistochemistry

A number of methods for isolation of different species of rickettsiae and ehrlichiae from patients are available,[1,75] including shell vial culture, primary monocyte culture or inoculation of susceptible tissue culture cells, and inoculation into the yolk sacs of embryonated chicken eggs or animals. These procedures are restricted largely to specialized laboratories and are not suitably rapid to provide results that are useful for immediate patient care. Isolation of rickettsiae and ehrlichiae may not be possible in all cases of serologically proven infections. Several factors contribute to this failure. First, these agents have very slow generation times, typically 8 to 12 hours. Growth in culture does not occur initially at this rate because the agents first appear to go through an adaptation phase. The number of organisms in blood also can be rather low, so biopsy samples of the rash or eschar, when present, are preferred. However, while low concentrations of penicillin-steptomycin can be used to suppress the growth of contaminating skin flora with spotted fever rickettsiae and *Orientia*, antibiotic-free cell cultures generally are used for growth of rickettsiae and ehrlichiae. When rickettsial and ehrlichial infections are suspected, doxycycline treatment often is initiated before collection of whole blood or biopsies are considered. Although viable bacteria can persist in properly collected and stored samples, delays in shipment can reduce the probability that isolates are obtained. Consequently and unfortunately, many isolates are obtained primarily from autopsy specimens in which the number of organisms and/or amount of samples are much greater than are found in conventional specimens. Shell vial procedures, in which a concentrated sample (e.g., buffy coat) is inoculated by centrifugation onto a small cover-slip culture, can provide results in 48 to 72 hours in some cases,[76] but the number of organisms in primary cultures usually is sparse and requires confirmation of the identify of the agent involved by fluorescent microscopy with specific antisera or by PCR (see below). Nonetheless, efforts to make isolates are essential because only with such stocks can detailed biologic, physiologic, and immunologic investigations of both known and novel agents be done. Isolates also provide definitive information to the physician about the etiology of the clinical presentations that were observed and thus aid in defining criteria for differential diagnosis and for recognizing the occurrence of unusual clinical presentations.

A general stain used for *Rickettsia* is Gimenez. Giemsa stains, particularly rapid Diff-Quik versions, are suitable for detecting *Orientia* and the ehrlichiae. Acridine orange is a suitable stain when fluorescent microscopes are available. These stains permit convenient recognition of characteristic morphologies, size, and cell associations of the agent in well-established cell cultures but have relatively little value in primary patient samples because of the paucity of organisms present. However, in some cases it has been possible to detect *Orientia* in buffy coat cells and *R. conorii* in sloughed endothelial cells that had been concentrated by use of an endothelial cell–specific monoclonal antibody coated on magnetic beads.[77,78] Similarly, although ehrlichiae can be detected as rare characteristic morulae (mulberry-shaped microcolonies) in Giemsa-stained blood smears in 10 to 15 percent of patients with confirmed etiologies, care must be taken to distinguish these bodies from other structures with similar appearance.[15–18] Consequently, specific staining with labeled or unlabeled polyclonal or monoclonal antibodies specific for each agent is recommended. Directly labeled antibodies are usually fluorescein isothiocyanate (FITC)–labeled for fluorescent microscopy, whereas indirect conjugate detection of the primary antibody can employ FITC or light microscope stains for alkaline phosphatase– or horseradish peroxidase–labeled conjugates. The indirect light microscopy staining procedures have been employed widely in specific immunohistochemical (IHC) procedures for the detection of rickettsiae, ehrlichiae, and *Orientia* in histopathology slides.[4,7,79,80] When IHC results are positive in a tissue, there is a good likelihood that PCR and isolation from those tissues can be effected when a parallel unfixed sample has been processed properly. Unfortunately, not all IHC tests are positive, even in serologically confirmed cases. Such false-negative IHC tests may occur because bacterial burdens may be very low, inappropriate samples were collected, inadequate sample or sectioning was employed, or appropriate antibiotic therapy was initiated prior to specimen collection.

Serology and Molecular Microbiology

Most suspected cases of rickettsial or ehrlichial infections are confirmed by serologic procedures using indirect fluorescent antibody (IFA) procedures.[75] Not only have these procedures been available for the longest time, but they are also technically the least demanding for nonspecialty laboratories because they only require appropriate slide antigens that can be purchased from a number of commercial sources. The Centers for Disease Control and Prevention (CDC) also serves as a national diagnostic reference center for rickettsial and ehrlichial infections.[81] Nonetheless, because of the infrequency with which cases of these diseases are observed in regions that are not highly endemic, and because of the variation in morphology and antigen quality of different preparations, as well as the number of agents involved, operator training and assay validation and quality control are very important. Consequently, most samples are referred to specialty laboratories. Although a strong presumption of disease may be made when a significant IgG titer is obtained with a single serum sample obtained at presentation with clinical symptoms, it is strongly recommended that a second serum sample be obtained from all patients 10 to 20 days after initial presentation in order to detect a clear rise in antibodies or to confirm that high stationary titers are present.[82] In many cases patients will not yet have detectable antibodies in the acute sample, or borderline positive serologic tests will occur that do not offer confirmation of disease because of cross-reacting antibodies from genetically unrelated bacteria or previous rickettsial antigen exposure (even to nonpathogenic rickettsiae). Such false-positive serologic reactions are particularly likely to occur when low-level IgM antibodies against spotted fever and typhus group rickettsiae are detected in acute-phase serologic testing. In contrast, IgM tests are very specific for *Orientia*.[83]

Unfortunately, not all patients with rickettsial or ehrlichial infections exhibit clear seroconversions during their infections. This may be due to a number of factors. Some patients may be immunosuppressed or immunologically unresponsive to the major antigenic components of the specific etiologic agent. Some individuals mount very strong cell-mediated immune responses in the absence of significant antibody titers. Finally, specific antibody responses may be ablated by early antibiotic therapy, presumably because agent replication is suppressed before or during the development of humoral immunity.

In addition to IFA tests, dot and flow immunoassays and specific enzyme-linked immunosorbent assays (ELISAs) are now available to detect some rickettsial and ehrlichial agents. Dot and flow immunoassays are rapid and have a good shelf life but provide minimal information about the titers of positive reactions; thus presumptive positive reactions should be confirmed by more specific serology, and negative acute sample immunoassays need reconfirmation with later sera if rickettsial or ehrlichial etiologies are still suspected.[84–86]

A number of recombinant antigen–based ELISA antibody assays have been developed to detect infections by ehrlichiae and *Orientia*.[87–89] While the performance of these tests in comparison with IFA tests has been good, the significance of the signals obtained, particularly those close to cutoffs for positive reactions, is less well established. As for IFA tests, it is best for paired sera to be run at the same time. The general lack of availability of validated positive control sera continues to be a problem for standardization of serologic assays between laboratories. Because of the technical and biologic barriers to serologic detection of ehrlichial and rickettsial infections we have described, it is axiomatic that patient care and treatment should never be predicated only on serologic results.

It is important to understand that serologic reactions depend on the specific antigens and tests being employed.[90] Such limitations in the meaning of serologic test results are particularly relevant when an individual encounters a novel rickettsial or ehrlichial agent either in the United States or while traveling abroad and for which no tests are being conducted. While typhus and spotted fever group (SFG) rickettsial antigens generally react as group-specific tests based on two types of lipopolysaccharide (LPS) and the shared protein epitopes in rOmpB and/or rOmpA surface antigens, individuals vary greatly in their reactions to these two components, and the SFG LPS exhibits antigenic variations among species. Individual patients may vary relative to other individuals in the titers of their antibodies that are directed against the species-specific domains on the rOmpB/rOmpA proteins, and the quality of the sera from a single individual also may change over time. It is this group of antibodies that must be present for identification of the specific rickettsial etiologic agent (e.g., *R. prowazekii* versus *R. typhi*, *R. rickettsii* versus *R. amblyommii* or *R. akari*) eliciting the antibodies, presuming that appropriate absorption antigens are available. Consequently, while a positive group-reactive test may indicate that a rickettsial infection has occurred, higher titers may be detected when the correct specific antigen is employed.

The IFA test may provide clues that antibodies to another agent are being detected when specular rather than corpuscular staining is observed. About 20 percent of serum samples from patients with rickettsial infections show cross-reacting antibodies to both spotted fever group and typhus group antigens; thus both types of antigens should be tested routinely in order to ensure that the correct agent causing the infection is identified. Similarly, while *A. phagocytophilum* and *E. chaffeensis* antigens also are genus-reactive, they may share some cross-reactivity. These cross-reactions are examined more readily with higher-titered convalescent sera, although more specific reactions may be obtained in the acute serum. The identification of specific etiologies for rickettsial and ehrlichial infections may be important in characterizing the specific epidemiology of a case and in detecting clusters of cases so that public education efforts are appropriate. Finally, *Orientia* exhibits a wide range of antigenic types owing to the variability of its major 50- to 63-kDa antigen. Convalescent sera show greater cross-reactivities among different antigenic types and stronger reactions to conserved 47-, 60-, and 70-kD a group antigens.

Numerous PCR assays for genus- and species-specific genes have been developed for *Rickettsia, Anaplasma, Ehrlichia,* and *Orientia*.[1,18,37,91] Such assays are now used commonly to detect these agents in appropriate patient specimens and in their arthropod vectors. Increasingly, these assays are also being evaluated for suitability in testing fixed specimens submitted for histopathologic examination because they are very rapid tests and can provide specific and accurate identification of the etiologic agent when amplicons are obtained. Importantly, such amplification can occur even when no viable agent can be isolated from a specimen or when it is contaminated with other adventitious flora. Host-attached vector specimens often contain much higher concentrations of the etiologic agent than the patient specimens, and specific DNA often persists even in dead vectors. Similarly, DNA may persist in the absence of viable organisms in patients following initiation of antibiotic treatment. Specific agent identication can be made by amplification of specific gene regions or by using conserved primers to amplify variable regions that are analyzed with restriction enzymes or by DNA sequencing. Such testing can be done directly on the PCR products or on cloned amplicons. Because of the low numbers of organisms present in specimens from patients with rickettsial and ehrlichial infections, two sets of nested PCR reactions often are done.[91] Quantitative PCR assays are capable of detecting single copies of individual genes in a test aliquot; these assays are done in a single tube so that they are less subject to false-positive reactions than nested PCR reactions and provide a precise measure of the number of DNA copies in the sample. Quantative PCR are now available for all the major rickettsial and ehrlichial pathogens of humans.[92–95] The major sensitivity and technical limitation of these assays are the requirement to recover, purify, and concentrate small amounts of agent DNA from the patient materials into that small test volume that is assayed and to avoid copurification of PCR assay inhibitors. The presence of inhibitors can be evaluated by using a multiplexed assay that contains PCR controls to confirm that normal PCR amplification has occurred along with primers used in the specific-agent PCR assay. Similarly, DNA from a number of different agents can be detected simultaneously in multiplexed PCR assays that employ different fluorescent probes for each agent and the test control DNA.

Lumbar Puncture

Because nuchal rigidity was present in 13 to 33 percent of patients in several large case series, lumbar puncture is performed frequently as part of the initial diagnostic evaluation of patients with Rocky Mountain spotted fever.[96] A predominantly mononuclear CSF pleocytosis is present in approximately a third of patients with Rocky Mountain spotted fever who undergo lumbar puncture. Most patients with abnormal CSF have 10 to 100 cells/mm^3, but occasionally patients have more than 100 cells/mm^3. Rarely polymorphonuclear cells predominate when differential cell counts are performed.[42,97] In such cases, a misdiagnosis of bacterial meningitis can lead to erroneous therapy and delays in making the correct diagnosis.[32] The CSF glucose concentration usually remains normal even when patients have elevated CSF white blood cell counts and protein concentrations. Massey and colleagues[98] reported that CSF glucose concentrations were normal in 12 of 13 patients with severe Rocky Mountain spotted fever who underwent a total of 20 lumbar punctures; however, a single patient in this case series had a CSF glucose concentration of 17 mg/dl.

Crennan and colleagues[99] described a patient with Rocky Mountain spotted fever who underwent lumbar puncture and was found to have 112 white blood cells/mm^3 in the CSF. Sixty percent of these cells were eosinophils, 21 percent were lymphocytes, and 19 percent were monocytes. Recovery was uneventful, and when the lumbar puncture was repeated 5 days after commencement of therapy, the CSF white blood cell was 21 cells/mm^3, and no eosinophils were present.

CSF abnormalities in patients with scrub typhus are similar to those seen in patients with Rocky Mountain spotted fever; a mild CSF pleocytosis is common. Approximately a third of patients have elevated levels of protein in their CSF, but virtually all patients have normal CSF glucose concentrations. Pai and colleagues[37] studied 25 consecutive cases of serologically confirmed scrub typhus from a single hospital in Korea. A CSF pleocytosis typical of aseptic meningitis was found in 48 percent of patients. CSF white blood cell counts ranged from 0 to 110 cells/mm^3 (mean count 16.3). The mean lymphocyte proportion was 52 percent. CSF protein concentrations were elevated in 7 of 25 patients. As in other rickettsial infections, the CSF glucose concentration in patients with scrub typhus usually is normal even when a striking pleocytosis and/or an elevated CSF protein concentration is present. However, rarely, hypoglycorrhacia and a predominance of polymorphonuclear cells may be present simultaneously in the CSF.[100] Because some patients with scrub typhus lack a characteristic rash and/or eschar, such patients can be misdiagnosed easily as having viral or even bacterial meningitis when headache, stiff neck, and fever prompt a clinician to perform a lumbar puncture.[37]

Ratnasamy and colleagues[39] described the results of lumbar puncture in 15 of 57 patients with human monocytic ehrlichiosis from a single institution in Missouri. CSF was abnormal in 8 of these 15 patients. CSF abnormalities in these 8 patients and in 13 additional patients from the literature usually consisted of a lymphocytic pleocytosis, an elevated protein concentration, and a normal glucose concentration, although 23 percent of patients had greater than 50 percent segmented neutrophils in the CSF, and 5 patients had slightly decreased or borderline CSF glucose concentrations. In 2 of 8 patients, morulae were seen in white blood cells in the CSF. A mild CSF pleocytosis also has been reported to occur in patients with human granulocytic anaplasmosis.

Imaging

Computed tomographic (CT) scanning in patients with Rocky Mountain spotted fever may reveal normal findings, generalized cerebral edema, or cerebral infarction.[32,101] In one patient with severe Rocky Mountain spotted fever, magnetic resonance imaging (MRI) showed increased signal intensity in an apparent perivascular space distribution on T_2-weighted images. These punctate areas of increased signal to T_2-weighted images markedly improved when a second study was repeated on the eighteenth day of hospitalization, after clinical improvement had occurred.[102] Bonawitz and colleagues[103] compared the CT scan and MRI features with clinical outcomes in 34 patients with Rocky Mountain spotted fever. CT images were abnormal in only 4 of 44 CT scans, but abnormalities were seen in 4 of 6 MRI studies. Seventeen percent of patients had abnormal imaging features. Most abnormalities disappeared after clinical recovery in a small group of patients who had follow-up studies. Abnormalities that were noted in this study were similar to those reported by others. Imaging studies variably demonstrated changes suggestive of diffuse cerebral edema, diffuse meningeal enhancement, and/or focal cerebral infarctions. In one patient, MRI of the spine showed abnormal enhancement of surfaces of the distal spinal cord and cauda equina.

There is little information on imaging studies in patients infected with other spotted fever group rickettsiae. CT scanning in a patient with severe Mediterranean spotted fever disclosed ischemic changes in the internal capsule.[104] In one case series, CT scanning showed no abnormalities in the brains of 11 patients with human monocytic ehrlichiosis.[39] MRI with gadolinium enhancement showed nonspecific enhancement of the meninges in a single patient.

▶ TREATMENT

Doxycyline is remarkably effective in treating all the rickettsial and ehrlichial diseases. Antibiotic treatment in Rocky Mountain spotted fever and other spotted fever group rickettsial infections should be continued for at least 3 days after the patient has become afebrile. Most patients can be cured with 5 to 7 days of antibiotics. Most patients become afebrile within 48 hours of the institution of therapy, although patients with severe illness may take a longer time to improve clinically. The treatment of scrub typhus is slightly different. Courses of therapy with doxycycline as short as 1 day (400 mg given in two divided doses) have been advocated for the therapy of scrub typhus.[105] However, some experts have suggested that short courses of doxycycline or chloramphenicol are associated with an increased risk of relapse. For example, one study of the efficacy of 3-day therapy found that relapse occurred in 3 of 7 patients with scrub typhus treated with chloramphenicol and 3 of 6 treated with doxycycline; in comparison, no relapses were noted in 37 patients treated with either regimen for 5 days or longer.[106] A larger, more recent study found short-course therapy to be effective.[107] In this multicenter treatment trial, 116 patients with scrub typhus were randomized to receive 7 days of oral tetracycline (500 mg four times daily) or 3 days of doxycyline (100 mg twice daily). The patients were followed for 4 weeks after the completion of therapy. The cure rate was 100 percent in the tetracycline group and 94 percent in the doxycycline group. There were no relapses with either regimen.

Similar short courses of doxycycline have been effective in the treatment of epidemic typhus. In a small study from Rwanda, for example, a single 200-mg oral dose of doxycycline cured 35 of 37 patients; the 2 remaining patients had a relapse 6 and 7 days after initial response.[108] Despite these findings, most experts recommend that typhus be treated with a 5-day course of either doxycyline or chloramphenicol.

The same regimens used to treat rickettsial infections are thought to be effective for ehrlichial infections, although there have been no controlled trials examining the efficacy of different regimens of specific antimicrobial therapy in either human monocytic ehrlichiosis (HME). Both tetracycline and chloramphenicol appear to be effective clinically. In one study of 237 patients, 6 percent of 49 outpatients treated only with tetracycline were hospitalized compared with 92 percent of 38 patients treated only with antibiotics other than tetracycline or chloramphenicol.[109] Among hospitalized patients, recovery was faster for those treated initially with tetracycline or chloramphenicol than for those initially treated with other antibiotics; furthermore, severe illness or death was more probable in patients who did not receive tetracycline or chloramphenicol until 8 days or more after the onset of symptoms.

These clinical findings are different from those observed in vitro: *E. chaffeensis* is susceptible only to doxycline; chloramphenicol does not appear to be active.[110] In one study of hospitalized patients with HME, those who were treated with doxycycline defervesced 1 day sooner than those treated with chloramphenicol (2 versus 3 days).[111] Although these data are not conclusive, most experts believe that doxycyline is the drug of choice for treatment of adults and children because of its low risk of toxicity, low cost, and ready availability throughout the world.

Similar beneficial results of doxycycline therapy are seen in patients with *A. phagocytophilum* infection.[112] Rifampin also has been used to treat individual cases of *A. phagocytophilum* infection. For example, Krause and colleagues[113] reported the successful treatment of two children, ages 4 and 6, using a 5- to 7-day course of rifampin. These results are consistent with in vitro studies on the antimicrobial susceptibility of *A. phagocytophilum*. In one such study involving eight strains of *A. phagocytophilum* isolated from American patients, all strains were susceptible to doxycyline, rifampin, and levofloxacin.[114]

Doxycycline is currently the drug of choice for the treatment of all rickettsial and ehrlichial infections in both adults and children. However, there are a few exceptions to this general rule: Pregnant women and patients allergic to tetracyclines should be treated with chloramphenicol, the only other acceptable alternative to tetracycline-class drugs. In some areas of Southeast Asia, strains of *O. tsutsugamushi* cause disease that is resistant or unresponsive to therapy with doxycycline and other tetracyclines.[115] Azithromycin appears to have in vitro activity against such *O. tsutsugamushi* isolates, but only limited laboratory and clinical data are available to validate its efficacy. Despite this paucity of data, some authorities believe that azithromycin is an acceptable alternative treatment for scrub typhus in pregnant women and in patients with refractory disease from locations where doxycycline-resistant strains of *O. tsutsugamushi* have been found.[116] A randomized trial performed in an area of northern Thailand where strains of *O. tsutsugamushi* with reduced susceptibility to doxycyline are prevalent compared the efficacy of doxycycline alone with that of the combination of doxycycline and rifampin in 86 patients with mild scrub typhus infection.[117] The median duration of fever was significantly shorter in 24 patients treated with daily doses of 900 and 600 mg of rifampin (mean fever clearance times 22.5 and 27.5 hours, respectively) than in 52 patients treated with doxycycline therapy alone (mean fever clearance time 52 hours).

▶ PREVENTION

There is no effective commercially available vaccine to prevent Rocky Mountain spotted fever or any other rickettsial or ehrlichial disease. However, early detection and removal of attached ticks may prevent infection with spotted fever rickettsiae and ehrlichiae. Several hours of feeding is required for an infected tick to transmit these agents; thus disease will not occur if infected ticks are removed during this "activation" period.

Prophylactic therapy with doxycycline or another antibiotic is not recommended following tick exposure because only a small percentage of ticks (less than 1 percent) in endemic areas are infected with *R. rickettsii*,[42] and tick removal is an effective preventive measure. Patients who report attached engorged tick bites should be advised to inform their physicians if any systemic symptoms, especially fever and headache, occur in the following 14 days.

Eradication of human infestation with body lice will prevent transmission of epidemic typhus. Since people who live and work in close proximity to louse-infested individuals may acquire lice secondarily even if they wash their clothes regularly and have good hygiene, all louse-infested persons and workers in close contact with such persons should use long-acting insecticides. Human lice can be treated with agents such as DDT, malathion, and lindane; however, reports of resistance to one or more of these agents have appeared recently. Pyrethroid permethrin, when applied as a dust or spray to clothing or bedding, is highly effective against lice and is the delousing agent of choice. Fabric treated with permethrin retains toxicity to lice even after numerous washings, thereby offering significant long-term passive protection against epidemic typhus. The use of doxycyline as prophylaxis may be highly effective in interrupting typhus outbreaks. Since even a single dose of doxycycline offers protection against epidemic typhus, some experts recommend the use of one 200-mg dose of doxycycline once weekly by travelers or health care workers residing in areas in which epidemic typhus is present. Prophylaxis generally is continued for 1 week after leaving such areas. Protective clothing, masks, and gloves are recommended if direct handling of flying squirrels is necessary, but minimizing contact with these animals is desirable.

Studies also have demonstrated that chemoprophylaxis with doxycyline is effective when used by nonimmune individuals living or working in areas in which scrub typhus is endemic.[118] In a prospective, randomized, double-blind study involving 1125 military subjects in a hyperendemic focus in Taiwan, a single dose of doxycycline given once weekly reduced the incidence rate of scrub typhus compared with a control group treated with placebo. The incidence of scrub typhus was 2.5 times greater in the group receiving placebo ($p = 0.11$), and when subjects who failed to comply with scheduled administration of doxycycline were removed from the analysis, the incidence rate of scrub typhus in the control group was five times greater than that in the drug group ($p = 0.04$).

The use of repellants such as *N,N*-diethyl-3-methylbenzamide (DEET) and toxicants for mites is highly effective in preventing scrub typhus when applied to both clothing and skin.[119] Permethrin and benzyl benzoate are also useful agents when applied to clothing and bedding. Focal areas such as military camps or specialized work areas can be treated with chlorinated hydrocarbons such as lindane, dieldrin, or chlordane.

Control measures that are directed at peridomestic area reductions in infestation of deer with *Amblyomma americanum* and *Ixodes scapularis* by use of "four-poster" self-treatment devices are very promising. Acaricides that are applied to the deer while they are feeding on supplied whole kernel corn significantly reduce tick populations in the vicinity of the devices and coincidentally reduce the risk of tick transmission of *Borrelia* and ehrlichial infections.[120]

REFERENCES

1. Eremeeva ME, Dasch GA: *Rickettsia* and *Orientia*, in Sussman M (ed): *Molecular Medical Microbiology,* Vol 3. London: Academic Press, 2001, p 175.
2. Raoult D, Roux V: Rickettsioses as paradigms of new or emerging infectious diseases. *Clin Microbiol Rev* 10:694, 1997.
3. Parola P, Raoult D: Ticks and tickborne diseases in humans: An emerging infectious threat. *Clin Infect Dis* 32:897, 2001.
4. Paddock CD, Sumner JW, Comer JA, et al: *Rickettsia parkeri*: A newly recognized cause of spotted fever rickettsosis in the United States. *Clin Infect Dis* 38:805, 2004.
5. Childs JE, Paddock CD: The ascendancy of *Amblyomma americanum* as a vector of pathogens affecting humans in the United States. *Annu Rev Entomol* 48:307, 2003.
6. Dasch GA, Kelly DJ, Richards AL, et al: Western blotting analysis of sera from military personnel exhibiting

serological reactivity to spotted fever group rickettsiae. *Am J Trop Med Hyg* 49(suppl):220, 1993.

7. Paddock CD, Zaki SR, Koss T, et al: Rickettsialpox in New York City: A persistent urban zoonosis. *Ann NY Acad Sci* 990:36, 2003.

8. Azad AF: Epidemiology of murine typhus. *Annu Rev Entomol* 35:553, 1990.

9. Boostrom A, Beier MS, Macaluso JA, et al: Geographic association of *Rickettsia felis*–infected opossums with human murine typhus, Texas. *Emerg Infect Dis* 8:549, 2002.

10. Raoult D, La Scola B, Enea M, et al: A flea-associated rickettsia pathogenic for humans. *Emerg Infect Dis* 7:73, 2001.

11. Reynolds MG, Krebs JS, Comer JA, et al: Flying squirrel-associated typhus, United States. *Emerg Infect Dis* 9:1341, 2003.

12. Watt G, Parola P. 2003. Scrub typhus and tropical rickettsioses. *Curr Opin Infect Dis* 16:429, 2003.

13. Olano JP, Walker DH: Human ehrlichioses. *Med Clin North Am* 86:375, 2002.

14. Dumler JS, Barbet AF, Bekker CP, et al: Reorganization of genera in the families Rickettsiaceae and Anaplasmataceae in the order Rickettsiales: Unification of some species of *Ehrlichia* with *Anaplasma*, *Cowdria* with *Ehrlichia* and *Ehrlichia* with *Neorickettsia*, description of six new species combinations and designation of *Ehrlichia equi* and "HGE agent" as subjective synonyms of *Ehrlichia phagocyophila*. *Int J Syst Evol Microbiol* 51:2145, 2001.

15. Chen S, Dumler JS, Bakken JS, et al: Identification of a granulocytotrophic *Ehrlichia* species as the etiologic agent of human disease. *J Clin Microbiol* 32:589, 1994.

16. Maeda K, Markowitz N, Hawley C, et al: Human infection with *Ehrlichia canis*, a leukocytic rickettsia. *New Engl J Med* 316:853, 1987.

17. Buller RS, Arens M, Hmiel SP, et al: *Ehrlichia ewingii*, a newly recognized agent of human ehrlichiosis. *New Engl J Med* 341:148, 1999.

18. Paddock CD, Childs JE: *Ehrlichia chaffeensis*: A prototypical emerging pathogen. *Clin Microbiol Rev* 16:37, 2003.

19. McKechnie DB, Slater KS, Childs JE, et al: Survival of *Ehrlichia chaffeensis* in refrigerated, ADSOL-treated RBSs. *Transfusion* 40:1041, 2000.

20. Casleton BG, Salata K, Dasch GA, et al: Recovery and viability of *Orientia tsutsugamushi* from packed red blood cells and the danger of scrub typhus from blood transfusion. *Transfusion* 38:680, 1998.

21. Arguin PM, Singleton J, Rotz LD, et al: An investigation into the possibility of transmission of tick-borne pathogens via blood transfusion. Transfusion-Associated Tick-Borne Illness Task Force. *Transfusion* 39:828, 1999.

22. McQuiston JH, Childs JE, Chamberland ME, et al: Transmission of tick-borne agents of disease by blood transfusion: A review of known and potential risks in the United States. *Transfusion* 40:274, 2000.

23. Antony SJ, Dumler JS, Hunter E: Human ehrlichiosis in a liver transplant recipient. *Transplantation* 60:879, 1995.

24. Wells GM, Woodward TE, Fiset P, et al: Rocky Moun-

tain spotted fever caused by blood transfusion. *JAMA* 239:2763, 1978.

25. Eloubeidi MA, Burton CS, Sexton DJ: The great imitator: Rocky Mountain spotted fever occurring after hospitalization for unrelated illnesses. *South Med J* 90:943, 1997.

26. Leiby DA, Chung APS, Cable RG, et al: Relationship between tick bites and the seroprevalence of *Babesia microti* and *Anaplasma phagocytophila* (previously *Ehrlichia* sp.) in blood donors. *Transfusion* 42:1585, 2002.

27. Wolbach SB: The pathology of the rickettsial diseases of man, in Mouton FR (ed): *The Rickettsial Diseases of Man*. Washington: American Association of Advances in Science, 1948, p 118.

28. Wolbach SB: Studies on Rocky Mountain spotted fever. *J Med Res* 41:1, 1919.

29. Wolbach SB, Todd JL, Palfrey FW. *The Etiology and Pathology of Typhus*. Cambridge, MA: Harvard University Press, 1922.

30. Allen AC, Spitz S: A comparative study of the pathology of scrub typhus (tsutsugamushi disease) and other rickettsial diseases. *Am J Pathol* 21:603, 1945.

31. Settle EB, Pinkerton H, Corbett AJ: A pathologic study of tsutsugamushi disease (scrub typhus) with notes on clinicopathologic correlation. *J Lab Clin Med* 30:639, 1945.

32. Horney LF, Walker DH: Meningoencephalitis as a major manifestation of Rocky Mountain spotted fever. *South Med J* 81:915, 1988.

33. Katz DA, Dwarzack DL, Horowitz EA, et al: Encephalitis associated with Rocky Mountain spotted fever. *Arch Pathol Lab Med* 109:771, 1985.

34. Paddock CD, Greer PW, Ferebee TL, et al: Hidden mortality attributable to Rocky Mountain spotted fever: Immunohistochemical detection of fatal, serologically unconfirmed disease. *J Infect Dis* 179:1468, 1999.

35. Miller JQ, Price TR: The nervous system in Rocky Mountain spotted fever. *Neurology* 22:561, 1972.

36. Shaked Y: Rickettsial infection of the central nervous system: The role of prompt antimicrobial therapy *Q J Med* 79:301, 1991.

37. Pai H, Sohn S, Seong Y, et al Central nervous system involvement in patients with scrub typhus. *Clin Infect Dis* 24:436, 1997.

38. Walker DH, Herrero-Herrero JI, Ruiz-Bertan R, et al: The pathology of fatal Mediterranean spotted fever. *Am J Clin Pathol* 87:669, 1987.

39. Ratnasamy N, Everett ED, Roland WE, et al: Central nervous system manifestations of human ehrlichiosis. *Clin Infect Dis* 23:314, 1996.

40. Walker DH, Taylor JP, Buie JS, et al: Fatal human ehrlichiosis (abstract D76), in *Abstracts of the 89th Annual Meeting of the American Society for Microbiology*. Washington: American Society for Microbiology, 1989.

41. Kaplowitz LG, Fischer JJ, Sparling FP: Rocky Mountain spotted fever a clinical dilemma, in Remington JS Swartz MN (eds): *Current Clinical Topics in Infectious Diseases*, Vol 2. New York: McGraw-Hill, 1981, p 89.

42. Walker DH: Rocky Mountain spotted fever: A seasonal alert. *Clin Infect Dis* 20:1111, 1995.

43. Haynes RE, Sanders DY, Cramblett HG: Rocky Mountain spotted fever in children. *J Pediatr* 76:685, 1970.

44. Conlon PJ, Procop GW, Fowler V, et al: Predictors of prognosis and risk of acute renal failure in patients with Rocky Mountain spotted fever. *Am J Med* 101:621, 1996.

45. Devriendt J, Staroukine M, Amson R, et al: Malignant Mediterranean spotted fever. *Arch Intern Med* 145:1319, 1985.

46. Font-Creus B, Bella-Ceuto F, Espejo-Arenas E, et al: Mediterranean spotted fever. *J Infect Dis* 153:128, 1986.

47. Rosenthal T, Machaeli D: Murine typhus and spotted fever in Israel in the seventies. *Infection* 5:82, 1977.

48. Silapojakul K, Chayakul P, Krisanapan S, et al: Murine typhus in Thailand: Clinical features, diagnosis and treatment. *Q J Med* 86:43, 1993.

49. Dumler JS, Taylor JP, Walker DH: Clinical and laboratory features of murine typhus in south Texas, 1980–1987. *JAMA* 266:365, 1991.

50. Vander T, Medvodovsky M, Valdman S, et al: Facial paralysis and meningitis caused by *Rickettsia typhi* infection. *Scand J Infect Dis* 35:886, 2003

51. McDade JE, Sheppard CC, Redus M, et al: Evidence of *Rickettsia prowazekii* infection in the United States. *Am J Trop Med Hyg* 29:277, 1980.

52. Perine PL, Chandler BP, Krause DK, et al: A clinicoepidemiological study of epidemic typhus in Africa. *Clin Infect Dis* 14:49, 1992.

53. Bakken JS, Krueth J, Wilsn-Nordskog C, et al: Clinical and laboratory characteristics of human granulocytic ehrlichiosis. *JAMA* 275:199, 1996.

54. Aguero-Rosenfeld ME, Horowitz HW, Wormser GP, et al: Human granulocytic ehrlichiosis: A case series from a medical center in New York State. *Ann Intern Med* 125:904, 1996.

55. Kirk JL, Fine DP, Sexton DJ, et al: Rocky Mountain spotted fever: A clinical review based on 48 confirmed cases. *Medicine* 69:35, 1990.

56. Scott T, Haggerty PF, Green SL: Tardive dyskinesia due to Rocky Mountain spotted fever: Case report. *Virginia Med* 114:417, 1987.

57. Garg P, Blass DA: Rocky Mountain spotted fever manifested by cerebritis and pneumonitis *Maryland Med J* 36:343, 1987.

58. Steinfeld HJ, Silverstein J, Weisburger W, et al: Deafness associated with Rocky Mountain spotted fever. *Maryland Med J* 37:287, 1988.

59. Reimann HA, Ulrich HL, Fisher LC: Differential diagnosis between typhus and spotted fever. *JAMA* 98:1875, 1932.

60. Verbiest HBC, van Woerkom TCAM, Dumas AM, et al: Subacute progressive sensory ataxic neuronopathy after *Rickettsia conorii* infection. *Clin Neurol Neurosurg* 92:81, 1990.

61. Popivanova N, Hristova D, Hadjipetrova E: Guillain-Barré polyneuropathy associated with Mediterranean spotted fever: Case report. *Clin Infect Dis* 27:1549, 1998.

62. Bonduelle M, Giroud P, Lourmeau G, et al: Polyradiculoneuritis with hyperalbuminorachitis and pleocytosis after insect bites: Positive reacton for *Rickettsia conorii*. *Rev Neurol (Paris)* 119:244, 1968.

63. Toerner JD, Kumar PH, Garagusi VF: Guillain-Barré syndrome associated with Rocky Mountain spotted fever: Case report. *Clin Infect Dis* 22:1090, 1992.

64. Dolan S, Everett ED, Renner L: Hearing loss in Rocky Mountain spotted fever. *Ann Intern Med* 104:285, 1986.

65. Missirliu C, Missirliu MF, Etteldorf JN: Rocky Mountain spotted fever in children. *J Pediatr* 53:303, 1958.

66. Archibald LK, Sexton DJ: Long-term sequelae of Rocky Mountain spotted fever. *Clin Infect Dis* 20:1122, 1995.

67. Rosenblum MJ, Masland RL, Harrell GT: Residual effects of rickettsial disease on the central nervous system: Results of neurologic examination and electroencephalograms following Rocky Mountain spotted fever. *Arch Intern Med* 90:444, 1952.

68. Gorman RL, Saxon S, Snear OC III: Neurologic sequelae of Rocky Mountain spotted fever. *Pediatrics* 67:354, 1981.

69. Thomas MH, Berlin L: Neurologic sequelae of Rocky Mountain spotted fever. *Arch Neurol Psychiatr* 60:574, 1948.

70. Ramsey AH, Belongia EA, Gale CM, et al: Outcomes of treated human granulocytic ehrlichiosis. *Emerg Infect Dis* 8:398, 2002.

71. Masters EJ, Olson GS, Weiner SJ, et al: Rocky Mountain spotted fever: A clinician's dilemma. *Arch Intern Med* 163:769, 2003.

72. Kirkland K, Wilkerson W, Sexton DJ: Therapeutic delay in Rocky Mountain spotted fever. *Clin Infect Dis* 20:1118, 1995.

73. Sexton DJ, Corey GR: Rocky Mountain spotless and almost spotless fever: A wolf in sheep's clothing. *Clin Infect Dis* 15:439, 1992.

74. Walker DH, Lesesne HR, Varma VA, et al: Rocky Mountain spotted fever mimicking acute cholecystitis. *Arch Intern Med* 145:2194, 1985.

75. La Scola B, Raoult D: Laboratory diagnosis of rickettsioses: Current approaches to diagnosis of old and new rickettsial diseases. *J Clin Microbiol* 35:2715, 1997.

76. La Scola B, Raoult D: Diagnosis of Mediterranean spotted fever by cultivation of *Rickettsia conorii* from blood and skin samples using the centrifugation-shell vial technique and by detection of *R. conorii* in circulating endothelial cells: A 6-year follow-up. *J Clin Microbiol* 34:2722, 1996.

77. Walsh DS, Myint KS, Kantipong P, et al: *Orientia tsutsugamushi* in peripheral white blood cells of patients with acute scrub typhus. *Am J Trop Med Hyg* 65:899, 2001.

78. Drancourt M, Georges F, Brouqui P, et al: Diagnosis of Mediterranean spotted fever by indirect immunofluorescence of *Rickettsia conorii* in circulating endothelial cells isolated with monoclonal antibody-coated immunomagnetic beads. *J Inf Dis* 166:660, 1992.

79. Dawson JE, Paddock CD, Warner CK, et al: Tissue diagnosis of *Ehrlichia chaffeensis* in patients with fatal ehrlichiosis by use of immunohistochemistry, in situ hybridization, and polymerase chain reaction. *Am J Trop Med Hyg* 65:603, 2001.

80. Paddock CD, Greer PW, Ferebee TL, et al: Hidden mortality attributable to Rocky Mountain spotted fever: immunohistochemical detection of fatal, serologically unconfirmed disease. *J Infect Dis* 179:1469, 1999.

81. Comer JA, Nicholson WL, Olson JG, et al: Serologic testing for human granulocytic ehrlichiosis at a national referral center. *J Clin Microbiol* 37:558, 1999.

82. Fournier PE, Jensenius M, Laferl H, et al: Kinetics of antibody responses in *Rickettsia africae* and *Rickettsia conorii* infections. *Clin Diagn Lab Immunol* 9:324, 2002.

83. Jang WJ, Huh MS, Park KH, et al: Evaluation of an immunoglobulin M capture enzyme-linked immunosorbent assay for diagnosis of *Orientia tsutsugamushi* infection. *Clin Diagn Lab Immunol* 10:394, 2003.

84. Kelly DJ, Chan CT, Paxton, et al: Comparative evaluation of a commercial enzyme immunoassay for the detection of human antibody to *Rickettsia typhi*. *Clin Diagn Lab Immunol* 2:356, 1995.

85. Weddle JR, Chan TC, Thompson K, et al: Effectiveness of dot-blot immunoassay of anti-*Rickettsia tsutsugamushi* antibodies for serologic analysis of scrub typhus. *Am J Trop Med Hyg* 53:43, 1995.

86. Ching WM, Rowland D, Zhang Z, et al: Early diagnosis of scrub typhus with a rapid flow assay using recombinant major outer membrane protein antigen (r56) of *Orientia tsutsugamushi*. *Clin Diagn Lab Immunol* 8:409, 2001.

87. Land MV, Ching WM, Dasch GA, et al: Evaluation of a commercially available recombinant-protein enzyme-linked immunosorbent assay for detection of antibodies produced in scrub typhus rickettsial infections. *J Clin Microbiol* 38:2701, 2000.

88. Magnarelli L, Ijdo J, Wu C, et al: Recombinant protein-44-based class-specific enzyme-linked immunosorbent assays for serologic diagnosis of human granulocytic ehrlichiosis. *Eur J Clin Microbiol Infect Dis* 20:482, 2001.

89. Alleman AR, Barbet AF, Bowie MV, et al: Expression of a gene encoding the major antigenic protein 2 homolog of *Ehrlichia chaffeensis* and potential application for serodiagnosis. *J Clin Microbiol* 38:3705, 2000.

90. Pradutkanchana J, Silpapojakul K, Paxton H, et al: Comparative evaluation of four serodiagnostic tests for scrub typhus in Thailand. *Trans R Soc Trop Med Hyg* 91:425, 1997.

91. Massung RF, Slater KG: Comparison of PCR assays for detection of the agent of human granulocytic ehrlichiosis, *Anaplasma phagocytophilum*. *J Clin Microbiol.* 41:717, 2003.

92. Eremeeva ME, Dasch GA, Silverman DJ. Evaluation of a PCR assay for quantitation of *Rickettsia rickettsii* and closely related spotted fever group rickettsiae. *J Clin Microbiol* 41:5466, 2003.

93. Jiang J, Chan TC, Temenak JJ, et al: Development of a quantitative real-time polymerase chain reaction assay specific for *Orientia tsutsugamushi*. *Am J Trop Med Hyg* 70:351, 2004.

94. Loftis AD, Massung RF, Levin ML: Quantitative real-time PCR assay for detection of *Ehrlichia chaffeensis*. *J Clin Microbiol* 41:3870, 2003.

95. Hunfeld KP, Bittner T, Rodel R, et al: New real-time PCR-based method for in vitro susceptibility testing of *Anaplasma phagocytophilum* against antimicrobial agents. *Int J Antimicrob Agents* 23:563, 2004..

96. Sexton DJ. Burgdorfer W: Clinical and epidemiologic features of Rocky Mountain spotted fever in Mississippi 1933–1973. *South Med J* 68:1529, 1975.

97. Peterson JC, Overall JC, Shapiro JL: Rickettsial diseases of childhood: A clinical pathologic study of tick typhus, "Rocky Mountain spotted fever" and murine typhus "endemic typhus." *J Pediatr* 30:495, 1947.

98. Massey EW, Thames T, Coffey CE, et al: Neurologic complications of Rocky Mountain spotted fever. *South Med J* 78:1288, 1985.

99. Crennan JM, Van Scoy RE: Eosinophilic meningitis caused by Rocky Mountain spotted fever. *Am J Med* 80:288, 1986.

100. Fang CT, Fern WF, Hwang JJ, et al: Life-threatening scrub typhus with meningoencephalitis and acute respiratory distress syndrome. *J Formosa Med Assoc* 96:213, 1997.

101. Case Records of the Massachusetts General Hospital Case 32-1997. *New Engl J Med* 337:1149, 1997.

102. Baganz MD, Dross PE, Reinhardt JA: Rocky Mountain spotted fever encephalitis: MR findings. *AJNR* 333:420, 1995.

103. Bonawitz CB, Castillo M, Mukherji SK: Comparison of CT and MR features with clinical outcome in patients with Rocky Mountain spotted fever. *AJNR* 18:459, 1997.

104. Benhammou B, Balafrej A, Mikou N: Mediterranean boutonneuse fever disclosed by severe neurological involvement. *Arch Fr Pediatr* 48: 635, 1991.

105. Brown GW, Saunders JP, Singh S, et al: Single dose doxycycline therapy for scrub typhus. *Trans R Soc Trop Med Hyg* 72:412, 1978.

106. Sheehy TW, Hazlett D, Turk RE: Scrub typhus: A comparison of chloramphenicol and tetracycline in its treatment. *Arch Intern Med* 132:7, 1973.

107. Song JH, Lee C, Chang WH, et al: Short-course doxycycline treatment versus conventional tetracycline therapy for scrub typhus: A multicenter randomized trial. *Clin Infect Dis* 21:506, 1995.

108. Huys, J, Kayihigi J, Freyens, P, et al: Single-dose treatment of epidemic typhus with doxycycline. *Chemotherapy* 18:314, 1973.

109. Fishbein DB, Dawson JE, Robinson LE: Human ehrlichiosis in the United States 1985 to 1990. *Ann Intern Med* 120:736, 1994.

110. Brouqui P, Raoult D: In vitro antibiotic susceptibility of the newly recognized agent of ehrlichiosis in humans, *Ehrlichia chaffeensis. Antimicrob Agents Chemother* 36:2799, 1992.

111. Everett ED, Evans KA, Henry RB, et al: Human ehrlichiosis in adults after tick exposure. *Ann Intern Med* 120:730, 1994.

112. Bakken JS, Dumler JS, Chen,S-M, et al: Human granulocytic ehrlichiosis in the upper midwest United States: A new species emerging? *JAMA* 272:212, 1994.

113. Krause PJ, Corrow CL, Bakken JS: Successful treatment of human granulocytic ehrlichiosis in children using rifampin. *Pediatrics* 112:e252, 2003.

114. Maurin M, Bakken JS, Dumler JS: Antibiotic susceptibilities of *Anaplasma (Ehrlichia) phagocytophilum* strains from various geographic areas in the United States. *Antimicrob Agents Chemother* 47:413, 2003.

115. Watt G, Chouriyagune C, Ruangweerayud R, et al: Scrub typhus infections poorly responsive to antibiotics in northern Thailand. *Lancet* 348:86, 1996.

116. Strickman, D, Sheer, T, Salata, K, et al: In vitro effectiveness of azithromycin against doxycycline-resistant and -susceptible strains of *Rickettsia tsutsugamushi*, etiologic agent of scrub typhus. *Antimicrob Agents Chemother* 39:2406, 1995.

117. Watt, G, Kantipong P, Jongsakul, K, et al: Doxycycline and rifampicin for mild scrub-typhus infections in northern Thailand: A randomised trial. *Lancet* 356:1057, 2000.

118. Olsen JG, Bourgeois AL, Fang RC, et al: Prevention of scrub typhus: Prophylactic administration of doxycyline in a randomized, double blind trial. *Am J Trop Med Hyg* 29:989, 1980.

119. Frances SP, Khlaimanee N: Laboratory tests of arthropod repellents against *Leptotrombidium deliense*—noninfected and infected with *Rickettsia tsutsugamushi*—and noninfected with *L. fletcheri* (Acari: Trombiculidae). *J Med Entomol* 33:232, 1996.

120. Carroll JF, Allen PC, Hill DE, et al: Control of *Ixodes scapularis* and *Amblyomma americanum* through use of the "4-poster" treatment device on deer in Maryland. *Exp Appl Acarol* 28:289, 2002.

CHAPTER 20
Spinal Infectious Diseases

Karen L. Roos and Avanee Shah

► TRANSVERSE MYELITIS

Transverse myelitis is an acute focal inflammatory disorder of the spinal cord resulting in motor, sensory, and autonomic dysfunction. Transverse myelitis may be due to an infectious or parainfectious disease, a connective tissue disease (systemic lupus erythematosus, Sjögren's syndrome), spinal cord ischemia, a demyelinating disease related to multiple sclerosis, neurosarcoidosis, or an idiopathic myelopathy. There are a number of infectious etiologies of transverse myelitis, including herpesvirus infections (herpes simplex virus type 1, herpes simplex virus type 2, varicella-zoster virus, cytomegalovirus, Epstein-Barr virus), enteroviruses, human immunodeficiency virus (HIV), human T-cell lymphotropic virus type 1 (HTLV-1), Lyme disease, *Mycobacterium tuberculosis* infection, and syphilis.

The thoracic cord is affected most commonly in transverse myelitis. Varicella-zoster virus establishes latent infection in the dorsal root ganglion (Fig. 20-1). Reactivation of the virus in the form of shingles is most common in a thoracic dermatomal distribution. Reactivation of varicella-zoster virus also may cause a transverse myelitis in the thoracic cord.

Clinical Features

The initial presentation often consists of back pain followed by a subacute progression of lower extremity weakness. Bowel and bladder dysfunction develops. The symptoms either may evolve over a few hours or may progress over a number of days. When the maximal level of deficit is reached, 50 percent of patients are paraplegic, 100 percent have bladder dysfunction, and 80 to 94 percent have numbness, paresthesias, or bandlike dysesthesias.[1,2]

On neurologic examination there is bilateral lower extremity weakness, hypotonia, absent or decreased deep tendon reflexes, Babinski signs, and a well-defined sensory level, often in the midthoracic area. The lower extremity weakness typically is asymmetric and evolves into a symmetric spastic paraparesis with pathologically brisk reflexes.

Figure 20–1. Dorsal root ganglion. Reactivation of varicella-zoster virus in the dorsal root ganglion can cause transverse myelitis.

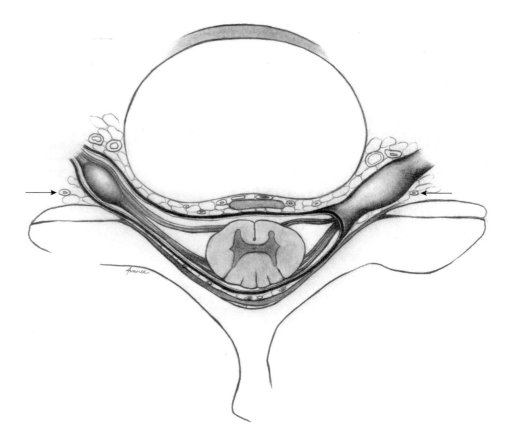

Diagnosis

An emergent neuroimaging procedure is performed to rule out a compressive extramedullary mass lesion. Gadolinium-enhanced magnetic resonance imaging (MRI) of the spinal cord is the neuroimaging modality of choice and should include images of the spinal cord several levels above and below the level of the lesion suggested by the finding of a sensory level on neurologic examination. Transverse myelitis causes swelling of the spinal cord that can be seen on MRI (Fig. 20-2).

If there is no evidence of an epidural abscess or a subdural empyema on MRI, examination of the cerebrospinal fluid (CSF) is indicated. The recommended CSF studies for transverse myelitis are listed in Table 20-1. Throat and stool cultures should be obtained for enteroviruses, as well as serology. Serum should be obtained for determination of cytomegalovirus (CMV) IgM and IgG, HIV, HTLV-1, angiotensin-converting enzyme, VDRL, FTA-ABS, Epstein-Barr virus (EBV) antiviral capsid antigen (VCA) IgG titers, EBV VCA IgM titers, and antibodies to EBV nuclear antigen (anti-EBNA IgG). In addition, diagnostic studies for connective tissue disease, including antinuclear antibodies (ANA), erythrocyte sedimentation rate (ESR), SS-A, and SS-B, should be performed.

Abnormal gadolinium enhancement of the spinal cord, CSF pleocytosis, or elevated CSF IgG index is required for a diagnosis of transverse myelitis. If these criteria are not met in the initial evaluation, repeat MRI and CSF analysis should be done 2 to 7 days after symptom onset.[3]

Differential Diagnosis

The primary disorder in the differential diagnosis is multiple sclerosis. Features suggestive of multiple sclerosis are predominantly sensory symptoms with relative sparing of motor symptoms, symmetric clinical findings, and an abnormal brain MRI. Occlusion of the anterior spinal artery also presents with the acute onset of paraplegia with loss of pain and temperature sensation below the level of the lesion. Posterior column function is spared. Since the CSF is noninflammatory, this disorder is more correctly classified as a myelopathy than as a myelitis. The Guillain-Barré syndrome presents with ascending weakness and areflexia, but a sensory level is not present, and examination of the CSF demonstrates an elevated protein concentration but no cells (an albuminocytologic dissociation). Meningovascular syphilis can present as a slowly evolving myelitis.

In HIV-infected individuals there are a number of spinal cord diseases, the most common of which is a slowly progressive myelopathy as a result of vacuolation of white matter of the spinal cord. This is discussed in detail in Chap. 8. Other viral etiologies of myeloradiculitis in HIV infection include herpes simplex virus type 2, CMV, and varicella-zoster virus. CMV radiculo-

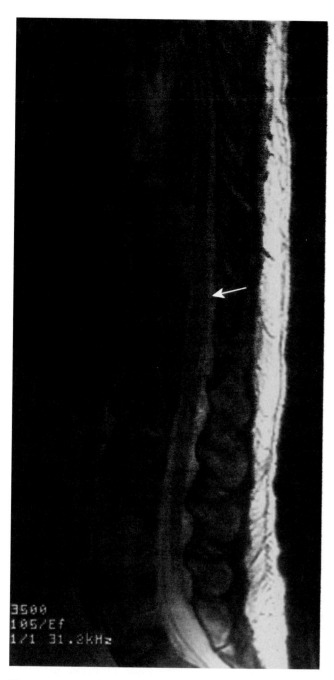

Figure 20–2. Sagittal MRI demonstrating swelling of the cord due to transverse myelitis in the midthoracic region.

▶ **TABLE 20-1.** CEREBROSPINAL FLUID STUDIES FOR TRANSVERSE MYELITIS

Cell count with differential
Protein and glucose concentration
PCR for herpes simplex virus 1 DNA
PCR for herpes simplex virus 2 DNA
Herpes simplex virus antibodies (with serum)
PCR for varicella-zoster virus DNA
Varicella-zoster virus antibodies (with serum)
Viral culture (for enteroviruses)
Reverse-transcriptase PCR for enteroviral RNA
PCR for HIV RNA
HTLV-1 antibodies (with serum)
PCR for cytomegalovirus DNA
PCR for Epstein-Barr virus DNA
VDRL, FTA-ABS
Borrelia burgdorferi antibodies
Oligoclonal bands (with serum)
IgG index (with serum)
Myelin basic protein
Angiotensin-converting enzyme

urinary urgency, incontinence, and impotence. Chapter 10 discusses HTLV-1-associated myelopathy/spastic paraparesis.

Treatment

Transverse myelitis of suspected infectious etiology is treated with intravenous acyclovir 10 mg/kg every 8 hours for 21 days and intravenous dexamethasone (10 mg every 6 hours) or methylprednisolone (1000 mg) for 3 to 5 days. Plasma exchange has been demonstrated to be efficacious in transverse myelitis of a noninfectious etiology.[5,6]

▶ SPINAL EPIDURAL ABSCESS

A spinal epidural abscess develops in the space outside the dura mater but within the spinal canal (Fig. 20-3). The clinical presentation is classic, beginning with back pain and followed by radicular pain and then signs of spinal cord compression. This infection is a neurosurgical emergency requiring surgical decompression of the epidural space combined with antimicrobial therapy.

Etiology

The most common causative organisms of spinal epidural abscess are *Staphylococcus aureus*, aerobic and facultative streptococci, and gram-negative bacilli (*Escherichia coli* and *Pseudomonas earuginosa*).[7,8] *S. epidermidis* is a causative organism of epidural abscess due to postoperative disk infection. In immunosuppressed patients, especially those with AIDS, and in intravenous drug abusers, *Mycobacterium tuberculosis* may be the etiologic organism.

myelitis is a distinct clinical entity that evolves over days to a few weeks and is characterized by leg weakness, hyporeflexia or areflexia, sacral dermatomal sensory loss, radicular pain, and bowel and bladder incontinence. CSF analysis reveals a polymorphonuclear pleocytosis, an elevated protein concentration, and CMV DNA by polymerase chain reaction (PCR). Other infectious causes of myelopathy in HIV-infected individuals include toxoplasmosis, tuberculosis, and cryptococcosis.[4]

Human T-cell lymphotropic virus type 1 (HTLV-1) causes a slowly progressive spastic paraparesis with

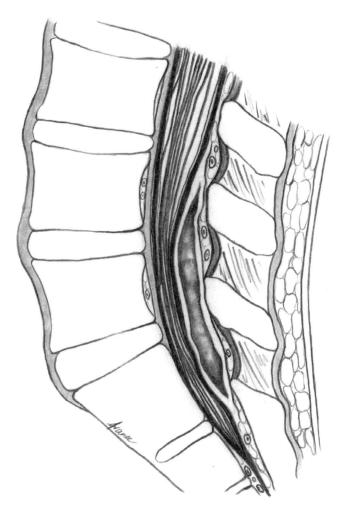

Figure 20-3. Sagittal view of spinal canal demonstrating the location of a spinal epidural abscess.

Pathophysiology and Pathogenesis

A spinal epidural abscess may develop as a result of the hematogenous spread of infection from a remote site of infection, including skin and soft tissue infections, urinary tract infections, pneumonia, endocarditis, and infected vascular lines. An epidural abscess also may develop by direct extension from a contiguous infection such as vertebral osteomyelitis. This is a particularly common etiology for spinal epidural abscess formation in intravenous drug abusers. Common predisposing factors for the formation of a spinal epidural abscess are diabetes mellitus, corticosteroid therapy, alcoholism, cancer, and chronic renal failure.[8] Infection of the epidural space also may occur from direct extension of infection from decubitus ulcers, infected abdominal wounds, or psoas abscesses. The formation of a small hematoma owing to mild blunt trauma also may provide a *locus minoris resistentiae* that allows for hematogenous seeding of infection, resulting in the formation of a spinal epidural abscess. Direct mechanical

compression of the spinal cord from the epidural abscess (Fig. 20-4) causes myelomalacia in the cord. The combination of myelomalacia and inflammatory thrombosis in the intraspinal vessels with subsequent ischemia and infarction is the cause of the neurologic deficits.

The spinal epidural space is only a true space posterior to the spinal cord and the spinal nerve roots. The anteroposterior width of the epidural space is greatest in the area where the spinal cord is smallest, i.e., from approximately T4 to T8 and from L3 to S2.[9,10] The anterior epidural space is only a potential space because the dura is virtually adherent to the posterior surface of the vertebral bodies along the ventral aspect of the spinal canal from the first cervical to the second sacral vertebrae. An epidural abscess may develop in the space anterior to or the space posterior to the cord.

Clinical Features

Heusner[11] described the classic presentation of a spinal epidural abscess in 1948. Back pain is the initial symptom, and fever is often present. Back pain is followed by radicular pain in the extremities or pain in an intercostal thoracic dermatomal distribution. As the disease progresses, signs of spinal cord compression de-

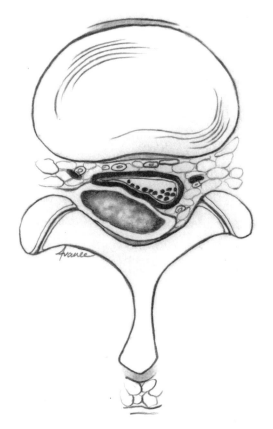

Figure 20-4. Axial view of spinal canal demonstrating a spinal epidural abscess compressing the spinal cord.

velop with paresis of appendicular musculature, loss of sensation below the level of the lesion, and loss of bowel and bladder control. Finally, there is complete paralysis of appendicular muscles and loss of all sensory modalities below the level of the lesion.

Diagnosis

MRI is the procedure of choice to demonstrate a spinal epidural abscess and the degree of spinal cord compression. An epidural abscess is isointense to CSF on MRI T_1-weighted images and enhances following the administration of gadolinium. Contiguous areas of infection also may be demonstrated by MRI and define the predisposing condition that led to formation of an epidural abscess (Fig. 20-5). Because spinal epidural abscess is usually the result of hematogenous seeding of the epidural space, there may be evidence of systemic illness with a peripheral leukocytosis.

Differential Diagnosis

Fever and back pain without associated signs of spinal cord compression may be due solely to pyogenic osteomyelitis and diskitis. Transverse myelitis has a similar clinical presentation to an epidural abscess. A subdural empyema is rare but is in the differential diagnosis. A subdural empyema forms in the space beneath the dura and can be distinguished from an epidural abscess by MRI. *Schistosoma mansoni* and *S. haematobium* can cause myelopathy due to a granulomatous intrathecal mass lesion and present with radicular pain, flaccid areflexic paraplegia, and bowel and bladder incontinence. Diagnosis is made by serum and CSF antibody tests, examination of stool, and rectal biopsy for ova. Pott's disease (tuberculous spondylitis) presents with fever and slowly progressive paraparesis. Non-Hodgkin's lymphoma and renal cell, lung, uterine, and thyroid carcinoma can metastasize to the epidural space. Lytic lesions typically are associated with epidural metastases.

Treatment

A spinal epidural abscess is a neurosurgical emergency requiring decompression of the spinal cord with the evacuation of pus and granulation tissue and antimicrobial therapy. Empirical therapy should include coverage for *S. aureus,* because this organism is the most common etiologic agent, gram-negative aerobic bacilli, and aerobic streptococci. A combination of vancomycin (pediatric dose: 60 mg/kg per day in a 6-hour dosing interval; adult dose: 500 mg every 6 hours) and a third-generation cephalosporin (ceftriaxone pediatric dose: 50 mg/kg every 12 hours; adult dose: 2 g every 12 hours) or fourth-generation cephalosporin (cefepime pediatric dose: 50 mg/kg every 8 hours; adult dose: 2 g every 8 hours) is recommended. Antimicrobial ther-

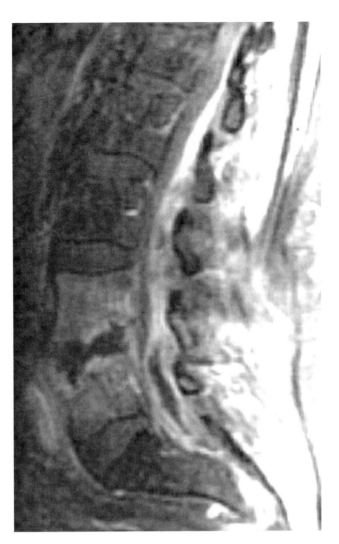

Figure 20–5. Sagittal T_1-weighted contrast-enhanced MRI demonstrates L4–L5 diskitis, osteomyelitis, epidural abscess, and inflammation.

apy can be modified when the infecting organism has been identified from abscess material and the results of antimicrobial sensitivity testing are known. Intravenous antibiotic therapy is continued for 4 to 6 weeks, followed by 2 to 3 months of oral antibiotic therapy. An epidural abscess due to *M. tuberculosis* is treated with a several-month course of isoniazid, rifampin, and pyrazinamide and intravenous and then oral corticosteroid therapy (see Chap. 13).

REFERENCES

1. Jeffery DR, MandlerRN, Davis LE: Transverse myelitis: Retrospective analysis of 33 cases, with differentiation of cases associated with multiple sclerosis and parainfectious events. *Arch Neurol* 50:532, 1993.
2. Lipton HL, Teasdall RD: Acute transverse myelopathy in adults: A follow-up study. *Arch Neurol* 28:252, 1973.

3. Transverse Myelitis Consortium Working Group: Proposed diagnostic criteria and nosology of acute transverse myelitis. *Neurology* 59:499, 2002.

4. Di Rocco A: Diseases of the spinal cord in human immunodeficiency virus infection. *Semin Neurol* 19:151, 1999.

5. Weinshenker BG, O'Brien PC, Petterson TM, et al: A randomized trial of plasma exchange in acute central nervous system inflammatory demyelinating disease. *Ann Neurol* 46:878, 1999.

6. Weinshenker BG: Plasma exchange for severe attacks of inflammatory demyelinating syndromes of the central nervous system. *J Clin Aphresis* 16:39, 2001.

7. Baker AS, Ojemann RG, Swartz MN, Richardson EP: Spinal epidural abscess. *New Engl J Med* 293(10):463, 1975.

8. Soehle M, Wallenfang T: Spinal epidural abscesses: Clinical manifestations, prognostic factors, and outcomes. *Neurosurgery* 51(1):79, 2002.

9. D'Angelo CM, Whisler WW: Bacterial infections of the spinal cord and its coverings, in Vinken PJ, Bruyn GW, Klawans HL (eds): *Handbook of Clinical Neurology*, Vol 33. Amsterdam: North-Holland, 1978, pp 187–194.

10. Dandy WE: Abscesses and inflammatory tumors in the spinal epidural space (so-called pachymeningitis externa). *Arch Surg* 13:477, 1926.

11. Heusner AP: Nontuberculous spinal epidural infections. *New Engl J Med* 239:845, 1948.

CHAPTER 21

Guillain-Barré Syndrome

Robert M. Pascuzzi

Guillain-Barré syndrome (GBS) is considered to be the prototypical "postinfectious" neurologic disorder. Most patients describe an antecedent febrile illness followed in days or weeks by the development of ascending paralysis that appears to be the basis of an acute inflammatory peripheral neuropathy. Although most skilled neurologists recognize GBS when they see it, the disorder is heterogeneous and diverse in its antecedent events, clinical presentations, and natural course. Even the name is diverse, with GBS, Landry-Guillain-Barré-Strohl syndrome, acute inflammatory demyelinating polyradiculoneuropathy (AIDP), and acute inflammatory neuropathy (AIN) all being synonymous.

▶ HISTORY

Octave Landry is credited with the earliest description of what has come to be recognized as Guillain-Barré syndrome.[1] In 1859, Landry reported a condition that he called "acute ascending paralysis," describing a patient who had a febrile illness in the springtime that was followed by the development of sensory symptoms within 2 months. One month later the patient developed subacute progressive inability to walk owing to leg weakness, followed by respiratory failure and then death. Landry pointed out that bowel and bladder function were spared, that sensory involvement was mild, and that muscles would respond to faradic electrical stimulation. The patient had an autopsy, but this apparently did not include the peripheral nerves. Landry reviewed four other cases from his own experience and five from the medical literature. He emphasized the absence of central nervous system (CNS) symptoms or signs, the occasional presence of muscle cramps, occasional relapsing course, and the tendency for a favorable outcome. He also noted that two of the cases occurred after an acute illness, two were associated with menstrual irregularities, one was postpartum, and one possibly was associated with syphilis. Westfall, in 1876, referred to this condition as "Landry's ascending paralysis."

Then, in 1916, Guillain, Barré, and Strohl reported two soldiers who developed an acute paralysis associated with loss of muscle stretch reflexes.[2] They emphasized the presence of elevated cerebrospinal fluid (CSF) protein concentration with a normal cell count (albuminocytologic dissociation). Their report did not recognize Landry's prior observations. Guillain, Barré, and Strohl state in their original paper that the illness

> . . . is characterized by motor difficulties, loss of the deep tendon reflexes with preservation of cutaneous reflexes, paresthesias with slight impairment of objective sensation, muscle tenderness, slight alteration in nerve conduction and electromyographic patterns, and a remarkable increase in cerebrospinal fluid albumin in the absence of a cellular reaction (albuminocytologic dissociation).

While the general clinical observations are attributed to Guillain and Barré, Andre Strohl probably was responsible for the electrophysiologic aspects. Guillain and Barré further developed their concept of the disease in subsequent publications, including the text *Travaux Neurologiques DeGuerre* in 1920.[3] Strohl's name largely was eliminated in the subsequent publications by Guillain and Barré. Death from respiratory failure remained a common outcome until the late 1940s, when the development of intensive care units and mechanical ventilation allowed for an overall reduction in mortality from GBS. Additional landmarks in clinical thinking on GBS include the observation by C. Miller Fisher of a variant associated with ophthalmoplegia, ataxia, and areflexia, published in 1956.[4]

► PATHOPHYSIOLOGY

In 1949, the classic clinical pathologic correlations were first reported by Hamaker and Kernohan.[5] In 50 cases of what was called "Landry-Guillain-Barré syndrome," they noted predominant inflammatory abnormalities in the anterior spinal roots. Since inflammatory cells were not present in more distal segments of peripheral nerves until late in the illness, they described the disorder as a "polyradiculoneuropathy." The subsequent seminal neuropathologic study by Asbury, Arnason, and Adams in 1969 described findings in 19 patients, noting abundant lymphocytic infiltration in spinal roots and nerves, leading them to conclude that "the pathologic hallmark of idiopathic polyneuritis is a perivascular mononuclear inflammatory infiltrate."[6]

Inflammatory Demyelinating Neuropathy

The pathology is classically that of a mononuclear inflammatory infiltrate in the endoneurium and myelin sheath. Patchy segmental multifocal demyelination is present along peripheral nerves, including nerve roots, whereas the axons themselves are relatively spared except in more severe cases.

Inflammatory infiltrates are comprised of lymphocytes, monocytes, and occasional plasma cells and tend to be perivascular. Less commonly, polymorphonuclear leukocytes are seen. The abnormalities are prominent around ventral roots and in the plexus and proximal nerve trunks but in some cases are present to an equal or greater extent distally along peripheral nerves. Similar inflammatory abnormalities also can be seen in dorsal roots and autonomic ganglia. In occasional patients there is axonal degeneration; in such cases, degeneration of anterior horn cells and dorsal root ganglia cells can be present, suggesting chromatolysis. While most of the pathology is found in the peripheral nervous system, there are occasional case reports of perivascular inflammation in the CNS. A few weeks after the onset of demyelination, Schwann cells are noted to proliferate. Several weeks later, as inflammation resolves, remyelination becomes evident.

Animal models resembling GBS were developed as early as 1955 by Waksman and Adams.[7] Experimental allergic neuritis (EAN) depends on the sensitivity of the P2 protein of peripheral nerve myelin and closely resembles human GBS in terms of clinical, electrophysiologic, and pathologic features. However, in humans, there is no clear evidence that the primary inflammatory attack is directed at the P2 protein.[8,9] A second animal model, galactocerebroside neuritis, involving antibodies against galactocerebroside, has been developed in rabbits. This animal model is not as similar pathologically as EAN because the cellular component of the nerve attack is not demonstrable. In addition, antigalactocerebroside antibodies are not present in human GBS.

Clearly, GBS is an inflammatory or immune-mediated condition. While most of the pathologic observations have emphasized lymphocyte-mediated delayed hypersensitivity as a possible mechanism, there is also evidence to suggest the role of circulating autoantibodies directed against the myelin sheath.[8–10] Perhaps GBS is a syndrome with a variety of immunologic mechanisms to account for an acute or subacute peripheral neuropathy.

Campylobacter jejuni Infection, GBS, and Axonal GBS

In 1984, Kaldor and Speed[11] reported serologic evidence for *Campylobacter jejuni* infection in 38 percent of a group of GBS patients from Australia. Subsequent reports supported this association, including that of Vriesendorp and colleagues,[12] in which 15 percent of 58 GBS patients had evidence for recent *C. jejuni* infection. Numerous additional studies confirm the association between *C. jejuni* infection and subsequent GBS.[13,14] Rees and Hughes[15] found *C. jejuni* in stool samples of 11 percent of GBS patients, along with serologic abnormalities in an additional 5 of 36 patients. Of the 25 percent of patients overall who had either stool culture or serologic evidence for *C. jejuni* infection, most had had an antecedent illness with diarrhea. In these series, there was a tendency for patients to have predominantly an axonal neuropathy as opposed to a demyelinating neuropathy, as well as the presence of IgG anti-GM$_1$ ganglioside antibodies.

While GBS is typically a demyelinating neuropathy, there is a subgroup of patients having clinical, electrophysiologic, and pathologic features indicating primarily an axonal injury, as opposed to loss of the myelin sheath. Feasby and colleagues[16,17] in 1986 noted a subgroup of GBS patients who had electrophysiologic findings of axonal degeneration, usually with severe paralysis and relatively slow recovery and pathologic changes in two cases indicating axonal degeneration without demyelination, and called this variant "axonal GBS." There has been disagreement about whether this represents an axonal variant of GBS or a truly distinct type of peripheral neuropathy.

Griffin and colleagues[18] reported four patients who died 7 to 60 days after the onset of clinically diagnosed GBS. Two of these patients had serologic evidence for recent *C. jejuni* infection. Autopsy findings in three patients studied 7 to 18 days after onset of symptoms showed ongoing wallerian degeneration of ventral and dorsal root fibers as well as peripheral nerves with relatively mild demyelination or lymphocytic infiltration. Macrophages were present in the periaxonal space of myelinated internodes, and occasional intraaxonal macrophages were present as well. The patients studied 60 days after the onset of symptoms showed extensive loss of large fibers in roots and peripheral nerves and only mild demyelination and remyelination. These carefully studied cases confirm that GBS, as defined clinically, can be associated with a severe sensorimotor neuropathy in which the predominant lesion involves axons of motor and sensory fibers and that an axonal form of GBS can follow *C. jejuni* infection.[18–20] A pure motor acute axonal neuropathy, a frequent cause of paralysis in China, also has been associated with antiganglioside antibodies.[21,22]

The prevailing theory for the association between *C. jejuni* infection and GBS is based on the bacterial lipopolysaccharide capsule that is rich in glycoconjugates. This lipopolysaccharide capsule has similarities to human glycoconjugates, and it may be that antibodies generated against the lipopolysaccharide capsule cross-react with glycoconjugates on peripheral nerves. Therefore, it may be that there is a shared epitope between the *C. jejuni* organism and human peripheral nerves[18] or so-called molecular mimicry.[22]

Illa and colleagues[23] reported axonal GBS in seven patients beginning 5 to 15 days after parenteral injection of gangliosides. These patients had high titers of IgG GM$_1$ antibodies with specificity for motor nerve terminals. Studies by Yuki and colleagues[24–27] indicate that the neuroepitope could be GM$_1$ ganglioside or GD$_{1a}$ ganglioside. The Fisher variant of GBS has been associated with antibodies against GQ$_{1b}$ gangliosides.[27–30] Therefore, it may be that glycolipids or glycoproteins having epitopes similar to GM$_1$ or GD$_{1a}$ are the immunologic attack site in the axonal forms of GBS.[18]

► CLINICAL FEATURES

Guillain-Barré Syndrome is the most common cause of acute nontraumatic generalized paralysis in young adults, with an annual incidence of 1.2 cases per 100,000 in developed countries. It can affect any age group from children to the elderly, although epidemiologic studies suggest that there is a peak in young adults and a second smaller peak in the fifth to seventh decades. It occurs in males slightly more often than in females.

Antecedent Events

A number of antecedent events have been reported to precede the development of acute ascending paralysis. Roper and colleagues[10,31] prospectively studied GBS patients at Massachusetts General Hospital, noting that 49 percent of patients had a prior upper respiratory tract infection, 10 percent had a diarrhea illness, and 3 percent had some form of pneumonia. In 3 percent of cases, Epstein-Barr virus infection was implicated, and cytomegalovirus infection occurred in 3 percent . Generalized malaise was noted in 3 percent , and another 3 percent had miscellaneous associated antecedent events, including Hodgkin's disease, surgery, systemic lupus erythematosus, or vaccination. In 27 percent of patients, there was no prior identifiable illness or antecedent event.[31] Other reported associations with GBS have included viral hepatitis, *Mycoplasma pneumoniae* infection, Lyme disease, and sarcoidosis. Reports of GBS in the setting of HIV infection suggest a stronger association than would be expected by chance occurrence.[32] *C. jejuni* infection as a cause of an acute diarrheal illness can be associated with subsequent GBS, as described earlier. Vaccinations have been implicated occasionally. Widespread public attention and notoriety occurred with the swine flu vaccination program in 1975 owing to the suggestion of an increased incidence of GBS associated with the vaccine.

Signs and Symptoms

Usually the patient experiences an acute respiratory or gastrointestinal illness that lasts for several days and then resolves. This is followed in 1 to 2 weeks by the development of "ascending paralysis." Typically, the legs are involved initially and, within a few days, the arms. Although described as an ascending paralysis, the weakness is usually about as marked in proximal limb muscles as in distal muscles. Patients often present with a complaint of difficulty walking; trouble arising from a chair or going up or down stairs; or simply instability of gait. Weakness tends to progress, usually over a course of 1 to 3 weeks. On occasion, patients have a fulminant rapidly progressive course in which paralysis becomes maximal within 1 or 2 days. Overall, about 50 percent of patients with GBS reach maximal weakness by 1 week, 70 percent by 2 weeks, and 80 percent by 3 weeks into the course of the illness. While symptoms are predominantly motor, patients commonly have mild paresthesias or mild objective sensory deficits on examination, particularly those involving position and vibration sense. Limb weakness is relatively symmetric, and there is symmetric loss of the muscle stretch reflexes. About one-third of patients develop respiratory involvement requiring mechanical ventilation, and 50 percent develop cranial nerve involvement that is expressed most often as facial weakness. One-half of patients develop oropharyngeal weakness, and 10 to 20 percent have some degree of ocular involvement. About 50 percent of patients develop autonomic dysfunction (including fluctuations of blood pressure, heart rate, ileus, and/or urinary retention). After progression of the weakness stops, patients tend to plateau for 2 to 4 weeks and then recover slowly. The recovery is such that by 6 months into the course of illness, 85 percent of patients are ambulatory. In 3 percent of patients there is recurrence of the paralytic illness, although some of these patients may have instead a chronic inflammatory neuropathy, as opposed to recurrent GBS.

Overall, the mortality from the acute illness is reported to be 2 to 5 percent. About 50 percent of patients have some degree of long-term residual symptomatic abnormality. Between 15 and 20 percent of patients have residual motor weakness at 1 year, and 5 percent remain severely disabled. This generally favorable natural history is the standard basis against which any therapeutic modality must be compared.

Laboratory Studies

Within the first few days most patients typically develop an abnormal cerebrospinal fluid (CSF) profile, with high CSF protein concentration in the absence of a pleocytosis (albuminocytologic dissociation). Glucose concentration is normal, as are cultures. The elevation of CSF protein concentration is presumed to result from an increased permeability of the blood-CSF barrier. In the first day or two, the CSF protein concentration commonly is normal. In Ropper's series, 34 percent of patients had normal CSF protein concentrations when measured in the first week, whereas in the second week only 18 percent were normal. Serial CSF studies may be necessary to demonstrate an abnormality. Up to 5 to 10 percent of GBS patients may have a lymphocytic pleocytosis with as many as 100 white blood cells (WBCs)/mm³. In patients with a CSF pleocytosis, the

possibility of GBS associated with HIV infection, Lyme disease, or sarcoidosis should be considered.

About 5 percent of GBS patients have abnormal liver function tests. Occasionally, patients have increased muscle enzymes, as is seen with many forms of acute denervation. In severe or sudden cases of paralysis, stool cultures for *C. jejuni* may be positive, and many of these patients have associated anti-GM₁ antibodies in serum.

Electromyography and nerve conduction studies (NCSs) can document the presence of a peripheral neuropathy that is of a demyelinating type.[33–37] A demyelinating neuropathy tends to produce very slow nerve conduction velocities, dispersed compound muscle action potentials (CMAPs), and multifocal conduction block. Early on, the abnormalities on nerve conduction studies may be limited to very prolonged F waves. Because the neuropathy is typically of a demyelinating type with sparing of the axons, there is usually relatively little fibrillation on electromyographic needle examination. In the first few days, the NCS may be normal or only mildly abnormal. The electrophysiologic abnormalities tend to lag behind the clinical examination. Severe reduction in the CMAP amplitude may predict the long-term outcome. Miller and colleagues[38] showed that CMAP amplitudes of less than 10 percent of normal were associated with a less favorable long-term prognosis.

Similarly, the North American Guillain-Barré Study Group noted a worse prognosis associated with CMAP amplitudes of less than 20 percent of normal. Such observations are not accepted universally because Triggs and colleagues[39] found that 50 percent of patients with severely reduced CMAP amplitudes were clinically normal at 1 year.

In patients with an "axonal form," the electrophysiologic picture is different in that the NCSs show low-amplitude responses, the conduction velocity is more mildly reduced, and the needle examination shows profuse fibrillation.

Fisher's Syndrome

In 1956, C. Miller Fisher reported "an easily recognizable syndrome . . . characterized among other features by total external ophthalmoplegia, severe ataxia and loss of the tendon reflexes."[4] This well-recognized variant of GBS has been given the eponym *Fisher's syndrome* and accounts for approximately 5 percent of the cases of acute GBS in most series. Patients typically present with diplopia followed within several days by ataxia or clumsiness of the limbs. Some patients describe dizziness. Over the first week of neurologic symptoms, hypoactive or absent muscle stretch reflexes develop. Fifty percent of patients describe paresthesias. Occasionally, other cranial nerves are involved, resulting in oropharyngeal or facial weakness. About one-third of patients develop associated severe limb weakness with respiratory failure. The ophthalmoplegia evolves over 1 to 3 days and is usually severe or complete and relatively symmetric.

Most patients have ptosis. Pupillary function tends to be normal. The presence of ataxia has raised the question of cerebellar involvement. There may be intention tremor, suggesting a cerebellar deficit. Some patients have unsteadiness, light-headedness, or dizziness. However, vertigo, nystagmus, cerebellar dysarthria, and scanning speech usually are absent. Patients with Fisher's syndrome most often have an elevated CSF protein concentration, but they are more likely than typical GBS to have normal CSF. A study comparing the increase in CSF protein concentration with anti-GQ_{1b} antibodies in 123 patients with Fisher's syndrome observed albuminocytologic dissociation (high CSF protein concentration) in 59 percent during the first 3 weeks of illness compared with serum anti-GQ_{1b} IgG antibody positivity in 85 percent.[30] The electrophysiologic studies show mild slowing of nerve conduction velocities compared with typical GBS and are more likely to be normal in the limbs than in GBS.

▶ DIFFERENTIAL DIAGNOSIS

The differential diagnosis includes the spectrum of illnesses causing acute or subacute paralysis. Spinal cord compression, transverse myelitis, and spinal cord infarction should be considered. Peripheral neuropathies from a variety of causes can mimic GBS, including critical-illness polyneuropathy; various toxins, including nitrofurantoin, chemotherapeutic drugs, and heavy metal poisoning, such as arsenic and thallium; autoimmune inflammatory diseases such as systemic lupus and polyarteritis nodosa; meningoradiculitis, as can be seen with Lyme disease, HIV infection, carcinomatous meningitis, and sarcoidosis; a paraneoplastic acute peripheral neuropathy; acute intermittent porphyria; and diphtheria. Hypokalemic periodic paralysis, myasthenia gravis, botulism, and poliomyelitis also should be considered. The presence of an acute or subacute flaccid paralysis in the setting of CNS signs and symptoms (such as encephalitis) should raise the question of West Nile virus infection.

▶ RECOMMENDED LABORATORY EVALUATION OF GBS

The following laboratory studies should be considered in a patient who presents with an acute or subacute paralytic syndrome resembling GBS:

1. If there is evidence of a focal spinal cord lesion, the patient should have emergent magnetic resonance imaging (MRI) of the involved level of the spine suggested by the history and examination findings. The presence of focal spinal pain, a discrete sensory level, prominent bladder and bowel dysfunction, paraparesis without arm involvement, or selective areflexia in the legs with normal reflexes in the arms mandates careful exclusion of a myelopathy by performing an emergency MRI.

2. CSF should be analyzed for evidence of a myelitis, as well as for the albuminocytologic dissociation typical for GBS. If the CSF is sampled within the first few days and is normal, a repeat study a week or two into the illness may be helpful if the diagnosis remains unclear.

3. Appropriate blood work includes a complete blood count (CBC), electrolyte determinations, and liver and renal function tests. With regard to underlying conditions that can mimic or be associated with GBS, serum tests for an autoimmune inflammatory disease such as systemic lupus and polyarteritis nodosa should be done. All patients should be screened for HIV infection, and selected patients should be screened for Lyme disease, sarcoidosis, and West Nile infection.

4. Urine collection for acute intermittent porphyria is indicated.

5. Tests for hypokalemic periodic paralysis, myasthenia gravis, botulism, poliomyelitis, and diphtheria depend on clinical evidence and suspicion and are not necessary in every patient.

6. Heavy metal poisoning can produce an acute or subacute peripheral neuropathy. In patients with a predominantly axonal form of GBS, heavy metal screens should be obtained, particularly for arsenic and thallium. Similarly, patients with pancytopenia, elevated liver function tests, and a history suggestive of a systemic illness also should be screened carefully for heavy metal poisoning. Patients with recurrent episodes of acute neuropathy also should be screened carefully for toxins.

7. When the antecedent illness is a gastrointestinal syndrome with diarrhea, stool cultures and serologic studies may reveal evidence of *C. jejuni* infection.

8. Screening for Epstein-Barr virus, cytomegalovirus, and hepatitis virus, as well as *Mycoplasma pneumoniae,* should be considered.

9. A careful review of the patient's prior medication list for any potentially neurotoxic drug, such as nitrofurantoin, may lead to a diagnosis of drug-induced toxic neuropathy, as might a history of recent cancer chemotherapy. Megadose vitamin exposure, particularly pyridoxine, also should be considered.

▶ MANAGEMENT

All patients with suspected GBS should be hospitalized for vigilant monitoring owing to the high risk of respiratory failure and the need for intubation and mechanical ventilation. Baseline spirometry, including forced vital capacity (FVC) and oximetry, should be obtained. Indications for intubation include an FVC dropping below 12 ml/kg or, in a normal-sized adult, FVC falling below 1 liter. Patients who are subjectively dyspneic or look to be struggling to breathe should be intubated, even if their FVC is above these levels. In general, one should err on the side of early intubation rather than late. A simple bedside estimate of FVC can be made by having the patient count out loud. If the patient can take a maximal inspiration and then can count up to 25, the FVC is probably about 2 liters. A patient who can count up to 10 probably has about a 1-liter FVC.

The cornerstone of treatment is that of meticulous general medical support.[40–42] There should be a low threshold for putting the patient in an intensive care unit. All patients who are having progression of their weakness should be in an intensive care unit. The common complications of GBS include respiratory failure, dysautonomia (especially cardiac arrhythmias, which may occur in 5 percent of patients), pneumonia, bladder dysfunction, pain, depression, phlebitis, pulmonary embolus, and the syndrome of inappropriate antidiuretic hormone (SIADH). Further complications from immobility and bed rest include decubiti, secondary compression neuropathy such as ulnar neuropathy and peroneal neuropathy, and the psychiatric sequelae associated with a prolonged immobilizing stay in the intensive care unit.[41] Intense back and limb pain improve with corticosteroids, as well as other drugs used for neuropathic pain.

Immunotherapy

Corticosteroids

To date, there have been no studies that demonstrate the effectiveness of corticosteroids in the treatment of GBS. There have been retrospective, nonrandomized studies, along with several small prospective, randomized studies, that have shown no clear benefit.[43] The use of high-dose intravenous methylprednisolone, as reported by Hughes and colleagues,[43] also has shown no benefit.[44] The Dutch GBS study group recently reported results of a prospective, randomized, controlled trial of intravenous methylprednisolone 500 mg/d for 5 days versus placebo.[45] All patients also received intravenous immunoglobulin (IVIG). In this large study of 225 patients, there was no significant difference between treatment with methylprednisolone and placebo.[45] In summary, to date there is no compelling evidence to support the use of corticosteroids in patients with GBS. The Quality Standards Subcommittee of the American Academy of Neurology published its "practice parameter" on immunotherapy for GBS syndrome, concluding that corticosteroid therapy is not beneficial.[46]

Plasma Exchange

In 1978, Brettle and colleagues[47] first reported the benefits of plasma exchange in the treatment of GBS. Several large randomized trials subsequently have demonstrated benefit of plasma exchange in treating GBS.[48–52] The North American GBS Study Group[49,50] and French[52] and Swedish[48] studies all have shown comparable benefit. In the North American GBS Study Group, the total volume of exchange was 200 ml/kg over 1 to 2 weeks, or about four to five exchanges of 3.5 to 4 liters on average.[49] There was no clear difference in the occurrence of complications in the plasma exchange versus the control group. The time to improve one clinical grade, which was defined as coming off the ventilator or being able to walk, decreased by 50 percent in the plasma exchange group (19 versus 40 days in the untreated group). The percentage of patients who were improved at 1 month, as well as the average clinical grade, was about 15 to 20 percent better in the plasma exchange group than in the control group. In addition, the time to regain independent walking was decreased by about 40 percent in the plasma exchange group (53 versus 85 days in the untreated patients). No benefit was shown in this study when plasma exchange was started later than 2 weeks from onset of symptoms, leading to the suggestion that it be used as early as possible after the diagnosis is made.[49] About 10 percent of patients are found to "rebound," and they often improve with repeat plasma exchange. The American Academy of Neurology "practice parameter" on immunotherapy for GBS is based on a meta-analysis of all six plasma exchange studies that revealed that the proportion of patients on the ventilator 4 weeks after randomization was reduced to 48 of 321 in the plasma exchange group compared with 106 of 325 in the control group (relative risk [RR], 0.56; 95 percent confidence interval [CI], 0.01–0.76; $p = 0.0003$). In a meta-analysis of four studies for which the outcome was available, 135 of 199 plasma exchange and 112 of 205 control patients had recovered full muscle strength after 1 year (RR, 1.24 in favor of plasma exchange; 95 percent CI, 1.07–1.45; $p = 0.005$). One class II trial demonstrated a convincing beneficial effect of plasma exchange (PE) in more mildly affected ambulatory patients. In the meta-analysis, the RR of serious adverse events was similar in the plasma exchange and control groups.[46] The "practice parameter" recommendation is as follows[46]:

> PE is recommended for nonambulant patients within 4 weeks of onset (level A, class II evidence) and for ambulant patients within 2 weeks of on-

set (level B, limited class II evidence). The effects of PE and IVIG are equivalent.[46]

Intravenous Immunoglobulin

High-dose IVIG was reported initially to be beneficial in GBS by Kleyweg and colleagues[53] in 1988. In 1992, the Dutch GBS Study Group reported a prospective, randomized trial comparing IVIG with plasma exchange.[54] In their study, IVIG was given at a dose of 0.4 g/kg per day for 5 days and was shown to be as beneficial as plasma exchange. The IVIG-treated patients showed a significantly shorter time to improve one disability grade, and somewhat fewer complications occurred in the IVIG group. Smaller series have suggested the greater possibility of clinical worsening during and following IVIG treatment,[57] along with an increase in the relapse rate of patients following treatment with IVIG.[57,58] Interestingly, the plasma exchange group in the Dutch study had outcome results similar to the control group (untreated group) of the North American Plasma Exchange Trial. Brill and colleagues[58] prospectively compared IVIG with plasma exchange in the treatment of 50 patients with GBS. Standard outcome measures did not differ between the two groups. Sixty-one percent of the plasma exchange–treated patients and 69 percent of the IVIG-treated patients improved by one disability grade at 1 month. The complication rate was found to be somewhat higher in the plasma exchange group. The authors concluded that the efficacy of IVIG in the treatment of GBS is similar to that of plasma exchange and that it can be used with safety. There was no difference in the relapse rate between the two therapies. This compares with the experience of the Dutch GBS Study Group, which reported 34 percent improvement of one disability grade within 1 month of receiving plasma exchange,[54] compared with 53 percent in those receiving IVIG and the reported 59 percent improvement rate of the plasma exchange–treated patients in the North American trial.[49] Brill and colleagues[58] also noted an increased frequency of complications in the plasma exchange group, including pneumonia, venous thrombosis, and line sepsis, compared with the IVIG group (19 versus 5). In the Dutch GBS Study Group, 68 complications were noted in the plasma exchange group compared with 39 in the IVIG group. A prospective multicenter trial revealed that plasma exchange followed by IVIG showed no significant benefit compared with plasma exchange alone in any measured outcome, indicating that combination therapy (plasma exchange followed by IVIG) is unlikely to be beneficial.[55] Studies of IVIG in children with GBS also indicate a beneficial effect.[56]

In general, IVIG is considered relatively safe. Mild side effects, including headache, nausea, myalgia, fever, and/or chills, are reported in 1 to 15 percent of patients.[57–62] However, there are sporadic anecdotal reports of more severe complications, including transmission of hepatitis C,[63] acute renal failure,[64] nephrotic syndrome,[65,66] stroke,[67,68] myocardial infarction,[69,70] aseptic meningitis,[71–73] and reversible encephalopathy with cerebral vasospasm.[74] Toxicity may be a result of sucrose toxicity, allergic phenomena, and effects of the high protein concentration on blood viscosity.

In the American Academy of Neurology "practice parameter" on immunotherapy for GBS, a meta-analysis of three trials comparing IVIG with plasma exchange revealed nonsignificant trends in favor of IVIG. There were no significant differences in the meta-analysis of time until discontinuation of mechanical ventilation and the proportions of patients dead or disabled after 1 year between the IVIG- and plasma excahnge–treated groups. In each trial, there were more adverse events in the plasma exchange group than in the IVIG group. The "practice parameter" recommendation is as follows[46]:

> IVIg is recommended for patients with GBS who require aid to walk within 2 (level A recommendation) or 4 weeks from the onset of neuropathic symptoms (level B recommendation derived from class II evidence concerning PE started within the first 4 weeks and class I evidence concerning the comparisons between PE and IVIg started within the first 2 weeks). The effects of IVIg and PE are equivalent.[46]

Presently, there is evidence to support the use of either plasma exchange or IVIG early in the course of GBS. Current data do not provide an indication of one therapy being clearly superior to the other.

▶ ACKNOWLEDGMENT

Mrs. Linda Hagan kindly helped prepare this manuscript.

REFERENCES

1. Landry O: Note sur la paralysie ascendante aigue. *Gaz Hebd* 6:472, 1859.
2. Guillain G, Barré JA, Strohl A: Sur un syndrome de radicu-lo-nevrite avec hyperalbuminose du liquide cephalo-rachidien sans reaction cellulaire. Remarques sur les caracteres clinques et graphiques des reflexes tendineux. *Bull Mem Soc Med Hop Paris* 40:1462, 1916.
3. Guillain G, Barré JA: *Travaux neurologiques de guerre.* Paris: Masson, 1920.
4. Fisher CM: An unusual variant of acute idiopathic polyneuritis (syndrome of ophthalmoplegia, ataxia and areflexia). *New Engl J Med* 255:57, 1956.
5. Haymaker W, Kernohan JW: The Landry-Guillain-Barré syndrome: A clinicopathologic report of fifty fatal cases and a critique of the literature. *Medicine* 28:59, 1949.

6. Asbury AK, Arnason BG, Adams RD: The inflammatory lesion in idiopathic polyneuritis. *Medicine* 48:173, 1969.

7. Waksman BH, Adams RD: Allergic neuritis: An experimental disease of rabbits induced by the injection of peripheral nervous tissue and adjuvants. *J Exp Med* 102:213, 1955.

8. Hartung HP, Pollard JD, Harvey GK, et al: Immunopathogenesis and treatment of the Guillain-Barré syndrome, part I. *Muscle Nerve* 18:137, 1995.

9. Hartung HP, Pollard JD, Harvey GK, et al: Immunopathogenesis and treatment of the Guillain-Barré syndrome, part II. *Muscle Nerve* 18:154, 1995.

10. Ropper AH: The Guillain-Barré syndrome. *New Engl J Med* 326:1130, 1992.

11. Kaldor J, Speed BR: Guillain-Barré syndrome and *Campylobacter jejuni*: A serological study. *Br Med J* 288:1867, 1984.

12. Vriesendorp FJ, Mishu B, Blaser M, et al: Serum antibodies to GM_1, peripheral nerve myelin, and *Campylobacter jejuni* in patients with Guillain-Barré syndrome and controls: Correlation and prognosis. *Ann Neurol* 34:130, 1993.

13. Enders U, Karch H, Toyka KV, et al: The spectrum of immune responses to *Campylobacter jejuni* and glycoconjugates in Guillain-Barré syndrome and in other neuroimmunological disorders. *Ann Neurol* 34:136, 1993.

14. Tam CC, Rodrigues LC, O'Brien SJ: Guillain-Barré syndrome associated with *Campylobacter jejuni* infection in England, 2000–2001. *Clin Infect Dis* 37:307, 2003.

15. Rees JH, Hughes RAC: *Campylobacter jejuni* and Guillain-Barré syndrome. *Ann Neurol* 35(2);248, 1994.

16. Feasby TE, Gilbert JJ, Brown WF, et al: An acute axonal form of Guillain-Barré polyneuropathy. *Brain* 109:1115, 1986.

17. Feasby TE, Hahn AF, Brown WF, et al: Severe axonal degeneration in acute Guillain-Barré syndrome: Evidence of two different mechanism? *J Neurol Sci* 116:185, 1993.

18. Griffin JW, Li CY, Ho TW, et al: Pathology of the motor-sensory axonal Guillain-Barré syndrome. *Ann Neurol* 39:17-28, 1996.

19. Griffin JW, Li CY, Ho TW, et al: Guillain-Barré syndrome in northern China: The spectrum of neuropathologic changes in clinically defined cases. *Brain* 118:577, 1995.

20. Ho TW, Mishu B, Li CY, et al: Guillain-Barré syndrome in northern China: Relationship to *Campylobacter jejuni* infection and anti-glycolipid antibodies. *Brain* 118:597, 1995.

21. McKhann GM, Cornblath DR, Griffin JW, et al: Acute motor axonal neuropathy: A frequent cause of acute flaccid paralysis in China. *Ann Neurol* 33:333, 1993.

22. Oomes PG, Jacobs BC, Hazenberg MPH, et al: Anti-GM_1 IgG antibodies and *Campylobacter* bacteria in Guillain-Barré syndrome: Evidence of molecular mimicry. *Ann Neurol* 38:170, 1995.

23. Illa I, Ortiz N, Gallard E, et al: Acute axonal Guillain-Barré syndrome with IgG antibodies against motor axons following parenteral gangliosides. *Ann Neurol* 38:218, 1995.

24. Yuki N, Taki T, Takahashi M, et al: Penner's serotype 4 of *Campylobacter jejuni* has a lipopolysaccharide that bears a GM_1 ganglioside epitope as well as one that bears a GD_{1a} epitope. *Infect Immun* 62:2101, 1994.

25. Yuki N, Yamada M, Sato S, et al: Association of IgG anti-GD_{1a} antibody with severe Guillain-Barré syndrome. *Muscle Nerve* 16:642, 1993.

26. Yuki N, Yoshino H, Sato S, et al: Acute axonal polyneuropathy associated with anti-GM_1 antibodies following *Campylobacter jejuni* enteritis. *Neurology* 40:1900, 1990.

27. Willison HJ, Veitch J, Patterson G, et al: Miller Fisher syndrome is associated with serum antibodies to GQ_{1b} ganglioside. *J Neurol Neurosurg Psychiatry* 56:204, 1993.

28. Yuki N, Sato S, Tsuji S, et al: Frequent presence of anti-GQ_{1b} antibody in Fisher's syndrome. *Neurology* 43:414, 1993.

29. Willison HJ, Veitch J: Immunoglobulin subclass distribution and binding characteristics of anti-GQ_{1b} antibodies in Miller Fisher syndrome. *J Neurochem* 50:159, 1994.

30. Nishimoto Y, Odaka M, Hirata K, et al: Usefulness of anti-GQ_{1b} IgG antibody testing in Fisher syndrome compared with cerebrospinal fluid examination. *J Neuroimmunol* 148:200, 2004.

31. Ropper AH, Wijdicks EFM, Truax BT: *Guillain-Barré Syndrome*. Philadelphia: Davis, 1991.

32. Cornblath DR, McArthur JC, Kennedy PGE, et al: Inflammatory demyelinating peripheral neuropathies associated with HTLV III infection. *Ann Neurol* 21:32, 1987.

33. Albers JW, Donofrio PD, McGonagle TK: Sequential electrodiagnostic abnormalities in acute inflammatory demyelinating polyradiculoneuropathy. *Muscle Nerve* 8:528, 1985.

34. Albers JW, Kelly JJ Jr: Acquired inflammatory demyelinating polyneuropathies: Clinical and electrodiagnostic features. *Muscle Nerve* 12:435, 1989.

35. Eisen A, Humphreys P: The Guillain-Barré syndrome: A clinical and electrodiagnostic study of 25 cases. *Arch Neurol* 30:438, 1974.

36. McLeod JG: Electrophysiological studies in the Guillain-Barré syndrome. *Ann Neurol* 9(suppl):20, 1981.

37. Olney RK, Aminoff MJ: Electrodiagnostic features of the Guillain-Barré syndrome: The relative sensitivity of different techniques. *Neurology* 40:471, 1990.

38. Miller RG, Peterson GW, Daube JR, et al: Prognostic value of electrodiagnosis in Guillain-Barré syndrome. *Muscle Nerve* 11:769, 1988.

39. Triggs WJ, Cros D, Gominak SC, et al: Motor nerve inexcitability in Guillain-Barré syndrome. *Brain* 115:1291, 1992.

40. Chalela JA: Pearls and pitfalls in the intensive care management of Guillain-Barré syndrome. *Semin Neurol* 21:399, 2001.

41. Henderson RD, Lawn ND, Fletcher DD, et al: The morbidity of Guillain-Barré syndrome admitted to the intensive care unit. *Neurology* 60:17, 2003.

42. Kieseier BC, Hartung HP: Therapeutic strategies in the Guillain-Barré syndrome. *Semin Neurol* 23:159, 2003.

43. Hughes RAC, Newsom-Davis JM, Perkin GD, et al: Controlled trial of prednisolone in acute polyneuropathy. *Lancet* October 7:750, 1978.

44. Guillain-Barré Syndrome Steroid Trial Group: Double-blind trial of intravenous methylprednisolone in Guillain-Barré syndrome. *Lancet* 341:586, 1993.

45. van Koningsveld R, Schmitz PI, Meche FG, et al: Dutch GBS Study Group. Effect of methylprednisolone when added to standard treatment with intravenous immunoglobulin for Guillain-Barré syndrome: Randomised trial. *Lancet* 363:192, 2004.

46. Hughes RA, Wijdicks EF, Barohn R, et al: Practice parameter: Immunotherapy for Guillain-Barré syndrome: Report of the Quality Standards Subcommittee of the American Academy of Neurology. *Neurology* 61:736, 2003.

47. Brettle RP, Gross M, Legg NJ, et al: Treatment of acute polyneuropathy by plasma exchange. *Lancet* 2(8099):1100, 1978.

48. Osterman PO, Lundemo G, Pirskanen R, et al: Beneficial effects of plasma exchange in acute inflammatory polyradiculoneuropathy. *Lancet* 2(8415):1296, 1984.

49. The Guillain-Barré Syndrome Study Group: Plasmapheresis and acute Guillain-Barré syndrome. *Neurology* 35:1096, 1985.

50. McKhann GM, Griffin JW, Cornblath DR, et al: Plasmapheresis and Guillain-Barré syndrome: Analysis of prognostic factors and the effect of plasmapheresis. *Ann Neurol* 23:347, 1988.

51. French Cooperative Group on Plasma Exchange in Guillain-Barré Syndrome: Efficiency of plasma exchange in Guillain-Barré syndrome: Role of replacement fluids. *Ann Neurol* 22:753, 1987.

52. French Cooperative Group on Plasma Exchange in Guillain-Barré syndrome. Plasma exchange in Guillain-Barré syndrome: One-year follow-up. *Ann Neurol* 32:94, 1992.

53. Kleyweg RP, van der Meche FGA, Meulstee J: Treatment of Guillain-Barré syndrome with high-dose gammaglobulin. *Neurology* 38:1639, 1988.

54. van der Meche FGA, Schmitz PIM, Dutch Guillain-Barré Study Group: A randomized trial comparing intravenous immune globulin and plasma exchange in Guillain-Barré syndrome. *New Engl J Med* 326:1123, 1992.

55. Plasma Exchange/Sandoglobulin Guillain-Barré Syndrome Trial Group: Randomised trial of plasma exchange, intravenous immunoglobulin, and combined treatments in Guillain-Barré syndrome. *Lancet* 349:225, 1997.

56. Koul R, Chacko A, Ahmed R, et al.: Ten-year prospective study (clinical spectrum) of childhood Guillain-Barré syndrome in the Arabian peninsula: Comparison of outcome in patients in the pre- and post-intravenous immunoglobulin eras. *J Child Neurol* 18:767, 2003.

57. Castro LHM, Ropper AH: Human immune globulin infusion in Guillain-Barré syndrome: Worsening during and after treatment. *Neurology* 43:1034, 1993.

58. Irani DN, Cornblath DR, Chaudry V, et al: Relapse in Guillain-Barré syndrome after treatment with human immune globulin. *Neurology* 43:872, 1993.

59. Bril V, Ilse WK, Pearce R, et al: Pilot trial of immunoglobulin versus plasma exchange in patients with Guillain-Barré syndrome. *Neurology* 46:100, 1996.

60. Mokrzycki MH, Kaplan AA: Therapeutic plasma exchange: Complications and management. *Am J Kidney Dis* 23:817, 1994.

61. Rodnitzky RL, Goeken JA: Complications of plasma exchange in neurologic patients. *Arch Neurol* 39:350, 1982.

62. Bouget J, Chevret S, Chastang C, et al: Plasma exchange morbidity in Guillain-Barré syndrome: Results from the French prospective, double-blind, randomized, multicenter study. *Crit Care Med* 21:651, 1993.

63. Thornton CA, Ballow M: Safety of intravenous immunoglobulin. *Arch Neurol* 50:135, 1993.

64. Duhem C, Dicato MA, Ries F: Side effects of intravenous immune globulins. *Clin Exp Immunol* 97(S1):79, 1994.

65. Bjoro K, Froland SS, Yun Z, et al: Hepatitis C infection in patients with primary hypogammaglobulinemia after treatment with contaminated immune globulin. *New Engl J Med* 331:1607, 1994.

66. Tan E, Hajinazarian M, Bay W, et al: Acute renal failure resulting from intravenous immunoglobulin therapy. *Arch Neurol* 50:137, 1993.

67. Silbert PL, Knezevic WV, Bridge DT: Cerebral infarction complicating intravenous immunoglobulin therapy for polyneuritis cranialis. *Neurology* 42:257, 1992.

68. Steg RE, Letkowitz DM: Cerebral infarction following intravenous immunoglobulin therapy for myasthenia gravis. *Neurology* 44:1180, 1994.

69. Woodruff RK, Grigg AP, Firkin FC, et al: Fatal thrombotic events during treatment of autoimmune thrombocytopenia with intravenous immunoglobulin in elderly patients. *Lancet* 328:217, 1986.

70. Dalakas MC: High-dose intravenous immunoglobulin and serum viscosity: Risk of precipitating thromboembolic events. *Neurology* 44:223, 1994.

71. Scribner CL, Kapit RM, Phillips ET, et al: Aseptic meningitis and intravenous immunoglobulin therapy. *Ann Intern Med* 121:305, 1994.

72. Sekul EA, Cupler EJ, Dalakas MC: Aseptic meningitis associated with high-dose intravenous immunoglobulin therapy: Frequency and risk factors. *Ann Intern Med* 121:259, 1994.

73. DeVlieghere FC, Peetermans WE, Vermylen J: Aseptic granulocytic meningitis following treatment with intravenous immunoglobulin. *Clin Infect Dis* 18:1008, 1994.

74. Voltz R, Rosen FV, Yousry T, et al: Reversible encephalopathy with vasospasm in a Guillain-Barré syndrome patient associated with intravenous immunoglobulin. *Neurology* 46:250, 1996.

CHAPTER 22

Polio and Postpolio Syndrome

Russell E. Bartt

▶ POLIO

History and Epidemiology

Humans are the only reservoir for poliovirus. From the mid-nineteenth and early twentieth centuries, epidemics of paralytic poliomyelitis (infantile paralysis, Heine-Medin disease) occurred in Europe and North America. In the centuries prior to that, accounts of paralytic disease caused occasional cases or clusters but not epidemics. It was realized that these epidemics were a modern phenomenon of improved hygiene and standards of living experienced in the Western world with a secondary drop in the level of "herd immunity."

Poliovirus and other enteroviruses often are referred to as "summer viruses," with 70 percent of the annual disease activity occurring from May through October.[1] Enteroviral disease does, however, occur throughout the year. During the summer peak of poliomyelitis, public beaches and parks would close. Family members often would be isolated from each other

(frequently children from their parents) to help contain poliomyelitis. In 1952, the U.S. epidemics peaked, with 57,879 cases reported that year.[2]

In 1954, an inactivated, injectable vaccine (IPV) developed by Dr. Jonas Salk was successful in field trials.[3] In April 1955, the vaccine was licensed to six companies that had produced vaccine for the trials in the preceding year. Inadequately killed virus was in two batches of vaccine at Cutter Laboratories, and cases of vaccine-induced paralytic disease followed, with 94 individuals and another 166 close contacts with infection eventually attributed to those vaccinations.[3] Vaccination was halted temporarily and then resumed later that year. The number of cases dropped and plateaued over the next 5 years. However, the "Cutter incident," coupled with a small upward trend in the number of cases in 1959–1960, compromised confidence in the safety and efficacy of IPV.[2] A live, attenuated monovalent oral vaccine (OPV) became available in 1961. A trivalent vaccine (for all three serotypes) followed in 1964. The ease of use, intestinal immunity, secondary immunity (shedding of attenuated virus to nonimmunized contacts), and long-lasting immunity all contributed to the widespread use of OPV.

Beginning in 1961, cases of paralytic disease that were temporally related to OPV recipients or their close contacts were reported to the Centers for Disease Control and Prevention (CDC). These cases of vaccine-associated paralytic poliomyelitis totaled 63 by 1965 and then decreased in number over subsequent years, probably as a result of a reduced number of susceptible contacts.[4] The rate of vaccine-associated paralytic poliomyelitis over three decades was 1 paralytic case per 2.4 to 3.2 million doses.[4–6] The risk is highest for the first dose (1 per 520,000 doses given) and lower for subsequent doses (1 per 12.3 million), the result of a protective effect of the first dose.[5] Overall, as many contacts as recipients of the vaccine developed vaccine-associated paralytic poliomyelitis despite the fact that many contacts had at least partial prior vaccination.[6,7] Annually, the number of vaccine-associated cases would average 8 per year in the United States.[6] Imported cases and the risk of reintroduction of wild-type virus to the United States justified the continued use of OPV.

The outbreaks in western Europe and the United States in the last 30 years have occurred mostly among "pockets" of unvaccinated individuals or members of religious groups objecting to vaccination. The last U.S. wild-type cases circulated among a religious group in the Midwestern states in 1979.[8] In 1992–1993, 68 cases of poliomyelitis in the Netherlands occurred, and members of an affiliated religious group in Alberta, Canada, had direct contact. Although no cases of paralytic disease occurred, 47 percent (21 of 45 persons) of the group in Alberta had the same poliovirus isolate as the Dutch cases.[8] These occurrences reinforce the need for maintaining awareness of possible polio importation.

With the last wild-type cases in the United States seen in 1979 and the last imported case seen in 1993, the risk of vaccine-associated paralytic poliomyelitis became less acceptable. Vaccine-associated paralytic poliomyelitis does not occur with IPV. To reduce the risk of vaccine-associated paralytic poliomyelitis, from 1996 to 1999, the Advisory Committee on Immunization Practices recommended a sequential IPV-OPV schedule with the first dose IPV followed by OPV.

As of January 1, 2000, the Advisory Committee on Immunization Practices officially recommended the exclusive use of IPV in routine childhood immunization in the United States.[9] The last vaccine-associated paralytic poliomyelitis case in the United States was in 1999.

Due to the vaccines and the focused efforts of governments and relief and health organizations, wild-type poliovirus now has been virtually eliminated from many areas of the world. The number of countries with endemic disease continues to drop. Currently, the Americas, Europe, and Australia have all been declared "polio-free nations."[10] In contrast, 15 years ago, endemic disease still occurred in most of the world.

At the end of 2003, endemic disease persisted in Nigeria, Niger, India, Pakistan, Afghanistan, and Egypt.[10] Cases reported in other countries have been imported from these few endemic countries. Occasional imported cases can lead to outbreaks due to a lack of consistent immunization campaigns to create a "barrier" to new cases. These importations from Nigeria and Niger to adjacent nations have occurred after 2 or more years of no paralytic disease.[11] Focused campaigns are ongoing in these "hotspots" to identify and overcome the obstacles that prevent satisfactory immunization coverage.[11]

The ratio of paralytic poliomyelitis to subclinical infection is in the range of 1:100 to 1:1000. Therefore, virus can circulate in a community for months before clinical disease occurs. Sewage studies have demonstrated that 0.27 to 0.4 percent of a community is excreting virus before paralytic disease occurs, and evidence of such may predict potential outbreaks.[12]

Pathophysiology and Pathogenesis

Poliovirus is one species of the genus *Enterovirus*, family Picornaviridae, a group that contains other significant human pathogens such as echovirus, the numbered enteroviruses, coxsackie A and B viruses, and hepatitis A.[13] These are all small, nonenveloped RNA viruses, and the family is named for these qualities (*pico* = "small," *virus* = "RNA").[1] The lack of a lipid membrane makes these viruses stable against detergents, ether, and ethanol; however, inactivation is achieved with ultraviolet light and chemical agents such as chlorine and formalin. These viruses can remain viable on surfaces if kept moist.[13] As the genus name suggests, all these agents are gastrointestinal pathogens with a fecal-oral route of transmission.

Poliovirus has three serotypes (serotypes 1, 2, and 3) based on its tendency to cause paralytic disease in primates and growth in cell culture.[13] Wild-type poliomyelitis is caused most frequently by all serotypes. Vaccine-associated disease is caused most often by serotype 3 virus, although immunosuppressed contacts of OPV vaccine recipients are more likely to have type 2.[5] In studies using OPV strains, serial passages of types 1 and 3 lead to a gradual loss of attenuation that is slower for type 1 than for type 3.[14] A point mutation of attenuated Sabin type 3 virus at codon 472 in the noncoding region of the genome, increases the neurovirulence and has a selective advantage in the gut, although not to the degree of the fully virulent type.[15]

Poliovirus and other enteroviruses replicate in the mucosa of the oropharynx and throughout most of the gastrointestinal tract.[1] The viral capsid is stable in acidic environments, ensuring its passage through the gas-

trum.[13] Replicated particles are in excreta within days, persist for weeks, and are infectious. Immunosuppressed hosts can secrete virus for many months or years.[16] Virus passes through intestinal lymphatics and then enters the bloodstream, resulting in a mild viremia (primary viremia). The initial viremia seeds other susceptible tissues such as the spleen and lymph nodes and may enter the central nervous system (CNS) at this stage, where a further cycle of replication can occur. This occurs in the first 5 days after initial exposure. A viremia of greater magnitude follows, and this viremia is more likely to result in neurologic disease.

The route of entry to the nervous system would appear to be hematogenous because viremia often precedes neurologic disease, although the precise mechanism has not been defined.[17,18] Direct entry to nerves of the intestinal plexus with retrograde transport to the nervous system is proposed, which would require transynaptic passage to enter motor neurons.[18] Invasion through the nerves of the oropharynx has been suggested and would be an explanation for cases with a primarily bulbar presentation. An increased incidence of vaccine-associated paralytic poliomyelitis has been observed in patients who have received intramuscular injections shortly after OPV exposure, a phenomenon known as *provocation paralysis*.[19] Of these mechanisms, viremic spread to the nervous system is the most generally accepted mechanism.[17,18]

The neurotropism of poliovirus, in particular for motor neurons of the anterior horn, Betz cells of the motor cortex (Brodman's area 4), and motor nuclei of the brain stem, has been recognized pathologically for some time.[20] An integral membrane protein present on motor cells acts as a cellular receptor for poliovirus, similar in structure to immunoglobulins.[21] The gene locus for this poliovirus receptor is located on chromosome 19q12-q13.2.[22] Transgenic mice can be rendered susceptible to paralytic disease, whereas only primates and humans are naturally susceptible to paralytic disease from poliovirus.[22]

Pathologic changes begin in the anterior horn cells a few days prior to paralysis with chromatolysis and intranuclear inclusions. This is followed by necrosis of the cell, and at this time, neutrophilic inflammatory cells are present coincident with clinical weakness.[20] The severity of the syndrome depends on the intensity of the lesions—cellular injury versus cell death.[17] Inflammation also involves the meninges. This may begin at the time of primary viremia and could represent initial CNS invasion because meningeal signs can be present clinically prior to paralysis.[23] Virus can be recovered from motor neurons only after the first several days of paralysis.[17] The presence of inflammatory cells in the spinal cord may persist for weeks and shift to a mononuclear predominance. Similar pathologic changes occur when lesions are in other infected motor nuclei of the medulla, motor cortex, and even cerebellar vermis and dentate nuclei.[18]

Clinical Features

Asymptomatic intestinal infection and replication without other clinically apparent disease occurs in more than 90 percent of those infected with poliovirus.[17,18,24] A "minor illness" is associated with the initial viremia, if it occurs, and systemic symptoms of fever, myalgias, and headache may be present. This syndrome typically lasts for 1 to 2 days and occurs in 4 to 8 percent of patients.[17] Gastrointestinal symptoms of nausea and diarrhea can occur. Most of the minor illness cases will resolve without further symptoms. In 1 to 2 percent of patients, 7 to 14 days after infection, a "major illness," occurs with abrupt onset of fever, headache, meningismus, or back pain. This major illness can merge with the minor illness, may be interrupted by a few afebrile days, or may occur without the minor illness as an antecedent.[17,18,23] A meningitis is associated with the major illness, and a nonparalytic poliomyelitis syndrome may be all that occurs.[17] The major illness lasts 5 to 10 days.

The onset of paralysis is with the major illness and occurs in fewer than 2 percent of patients.[24] Intense myalgias can occur in involved limbs. Generally, an ascending, asymmetric, and "patchy" distribution of weakness is seen. Legs are involved more often than the arms, although disease can range from unilateral leg weakness to tetraplegia. Muscle groups in an affected limb may be spared. The weakness generally is maximal within days as the fever resolves, and new weakness seen after day 5 is unlikely.[18,23]

Bulbar disease predominates in 10 to 15 percent of patients and is a more common syndrome in children than in adolescents or adults. Dysphagia, dysphonia, and facial weakness are described, with oculomotor or gaze dysfunction being rare.[18]

Respiratory failure is a significant cause of mortality, and about 10 percent of patients die during the acute phases of the disease. Dysautonomia may result in blood pressure abnormalities, dysrythmias, and urinary retention.[24]

Sensory symptoms are an uncommon but described phenomenon in poliomyelitis. Pain and cutaneous hyperalgesia can occur; however, sensory deficit is rare. Of the patients with a reported sensory deficit, a transverse myelitis is described.[25] Pathologically, the dorsal root ganglia do show destruction of varying numbers of sensory neurons.[20]

Recovery of motor function may begin at the end of the first week of weakness and generally improves over subsequent months.[23] Often there is acute dysfunction of muscle groups that does not persist. Atrophy in the more severely affected groups begins by the second week of paralysis.[24] Weakness of selected muscle groups may predispose to contractures and subluxation of joints. Asymmetric involvement of paraspinal muscles can result in scoliosis.[23]

Diagnosis

Etiologic diagnosis of flaccid paralysis relies on isolation of the pathogen and demonstration of a serologic response. Since asymptomatic carriers exist, with community OPV usage, stool isolates in cases of suspected polio are suspicious but not diagnostic. Viral particles often are present in the stool for several weeks, and collection of a few specimens should be performed because shedding of viral particles can be intermittent.[18] Oropharyngeal cultures are another source for culturable virus. A specific serologic response to one of the three serotypes, a fourfold (two-titer) rise, is considered diagnostic. Neutralization antibodies are the preferred method. The importance of serologic titers cannot be overemphasized in the diagnosis of polio, non-polio enteroviruses, and other viral infections. Even in the era of molecular diagnostic techniques such as polymerase chain reaction (PCR), the serologic response is considered diagnostic. It is important to collect and store acute sera in patients with potential neurologic infections and obtain convalescent sera in 4 weeks' time.

Lumbar puncture demonstrates a lymphocytic pleocytosis of typically a few hundred cells. Initially, the response may be neutrophilic, but after the first day or two, lymphocytes predominate. Protein concentration is elevated but usually not greater than 100 to 300 mg/dl.[18]

Glucose concentration is normal and with rare exception mildly decreased. All these findings are consistent with a viral meningitis that is typical for enteroviruses. The cerebrospinal fluid (CSF) pleocytosis drops rapidly after 2 weeks. It is difficult to demonstrate the virus in culture of the CSF. Enteroviruses all share a highly conserved region of the genome. This has been taken advantage of in the development of enteroviral PCR. Reported sensitivities have varied in the diagnosis of enteroviral meningitis but are much better than culture.[1,26]

Nerve conduction studies usually are normal.[27,28] Compound muscle action potentials may be of low amplitude in affected regions.[27] Electromyography demonstrates a reduced number of voluntary motor units initially, and denervation potentials emerge and are present for several weeks. In the convalescent phase, polyphasic motor units eventually organize to form very large motor unit potentials (giant MUPs) that are considered typical for polio.

The magnetic resonance imaging (MRI) characteristics of poliomyelitis have not been studied extensively because the last wild-type case in the United States pre-

ceded the widespread availability of MRI. The MRI appearance of a vaccine-associated case described a ventral spinal cord T_2-weighted intensity (nonenhancing) with expansion over several levels.[29,30] This appearance would not differ dramatically from that described in viral transverse myelitis. Figure 22-1 is an MRI of a woman who developed a febrile paralysis after her 3-month-old son was immunized with OPV. Stool isolate and serologic neutralization antibodies confirmed poliovirus type 2.

Treatment

The treatment of poliomyelitis is mainly supportive. Attention to respiratory function is essential, and monitoring of forced vital capacities is recommended to monitor and identify patients in need of ventilatory support. Intubation and mechanical ventilation may be necessary for airway protection. Pain and hyperalgesia can be treated with analgesics. Prophylaxis of deep venous thrombosis may be required if the patient is immobilized for any period of time. Passive range-of-motion

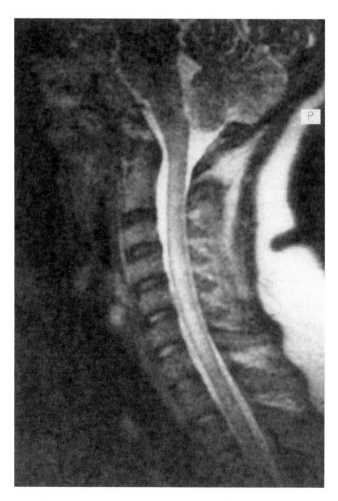

Figure 22–1. Sagittal T_2-weighted MRI of a case of vaccine-associated poliomyelitis.

exercises to prevent contractures can be started early in the care, with progression to the more demanding aspects of physical rehabilitation as tolerated as the condition improves.

Once a patient has recovered from the acute infectious stage, the convalescent titers and stool isolate should confirm the serotype responsible for the infection and the presence of antibodies to the other serotypes. Vaccination with IPV according to the Advisory Committee on Immunization Practices (ACIP) guidelines (in this chapter) may be indicated to ensure immunity against all three serotypes.

Complications

Acute complications of poliomyelitis are related to the weakness, possible respiratory failure, and complications of being bedridden. About half of all patients will suffer some residual weakness, with many recovering good function in partially weak muscles.[24] Ventilatory failure, usually with bulbar weakness, had a mortality that approached 50 percent in the polio epidemics of the 1950s, and modern mechanical ventilation would be expected to improve considerably on mortality. The overall mortality of poliomyelitis is less than 10 percent; however, 50 percent of all survivors have some chronic weakness.[17,24]

The outcome with regard to education, employment, and socioeconomic status has been evaluated in poliomyelitis survivors and compared with their siblings.[31] Education levels did not differ; however, fewer poliomyelitis survivors were employed full time, and they were more likely to live alone. The other late complication of poliomyelitis includes postpolio syndrome, which is discussed below.

Prevention

Vaccination programs have had a tremendous impact on the public health burden of poliovirus. The history and evolution of the recommended vaccination programs have been discussed. Current recommended vaccination practices in the United States are IPV alone for primary vaccination of children. The enhanced IPV vaccine used contains concentrated virus of all three serotypes in cell culture of monkey kidney cells (Vero cells), small amounts of phenoxyethanol and formaldehyde as preservative, and trace amounts of neomycin, streptomycin, and polymyxin B in the manufacturing process. Known sensitivity to any of these components is a contraindication to use. However, no serious adverse events have been reported. Four total doses are to be received beginning at 2 months, then 4 months, 6 to 18 months, and 4 to 6 years of age. The immunogenicity of the first dose is about 36 percent, it is 90 to 100 percent after two doses, and it is 99 to 100 percent after three doses.[32]

OPV should be used in children in the United States only if travel is to occur to an endemic area in less than 4 weeks (not enough time to receive two IPV vaccines). Parents who are unwilling to have their children receive the number of injections required for the full series can opt to receive OPV for the third and fourth doses if the risks of vaccine-associated paralytic poliomyelitis are understood and accepted.[32]

OPV remains the vaccine of choice for mass vaccinations in endemic areas. Control of outbreaks is superior because "intestinal immunity" is achieved, and the immunogenicity is high. During an outbreak in Albania in 1996, poliomyelitis cases decreased 90 percent within 2 weeks of a single-dose mass vaccination with OPV.[32]

Most adults in the United States are immune from childhood vaccination and are at minimal risk of exposure. However, travelers to endemic areas, laboratory and health care workers who might be in contact with polioviruses, and unvaccinated adults whose children are to receive OPV should be immunized. An uncertain or undocumented vaccination history should be considered as nonimmune. IPV is recommended, with the initial dose followed by a second dose at 4 to 8 weeks and another at 6 to 12 months, or if protection is needed sooner, then as many doses as can be given with a minimum 4-week interval between doses are recommended.[32]

In immunosuppressed patients, only IPV vaccination is recommended. Vaccination in pregnancy generally should be avoided, although if endemic area exposure is expected, OPV vaccination should be used.[32]

▶ POSTPOLIO SYNDROME

Postpolio syndrome (PPS) is defined as the development of new weakness, atrophy, and excessive fatigue that develops 15 years or more after a period of neurologic stability. It is important that another definable etiology cannot be detected after thoughtful evaluation. The term *postpolio syndrome* may be relatively recent; however, descriptions of slowly progressive weakness and atrophy as late complications of paralytic poliomyelitis date back to Charcot.[24]

Epidemiology

It is estimated that over 300,000 survivors of the polio epidemics are at risk for PPS according to the NIH/NINDS.[33] Most PPS patients were infected when endemic cases occurred, especially in the 1950s. Studies to estimate the frequency of PPS in poliomyelitis survivors have been performed. In one study, 64 percent of those who had poliomyelitis between 1935 and 1955 had symptoms of PPS, although in only 18 percent did it lead to a lifestyle change.[34] Another survey found the incidence of PPS to be 28.5 percent, peaking at 30 to 35 years after infection.[35] In that study, the level of prior weakness did not correlate with the likelihood of developing PPS. However, other series have reported that those with greater residual weakness were most at risk for the development of PPS.[36]

Pathogenesis

The current hypothesis is one of increased metabolic demands on surviving motor neurons that had increased their distal axonal sprouts to reinnervate muscle and maintain strength.[37] Evidence of motor unit instability, increased jitter, and reinnervation is present in patients previously affected by polio with or without current PPS.[38] This concept is also supported by muscle biopsy data.[38] Contrary or concurrent theories include persistent viral infection or autoimmune inflammation in the spinal cord. However, most of the evidence and expert opinions supports the concept of motor neuron dropout.[37,39]

Muscular and arthritic changes can result from altered biomechanical stresses over time. Scoliosis, asymmetric weight bearing in the lower extremities, and weight bearing upper extremity with canes, crutches, or wheelchair use can take their toll. Furthermore, PPS patients are subject to superimposed joint disease that occurs with increased incidence in the elderly.

Clinical Features and Diagnosis

New weakness and atrophy after years of neurologic stability has been termed *postpoliomyelitis progressive muscular atrophy* (PPMA).[40] Symptoms of cramps, fasiculations, and myalgias are common. Muscles with the greatest residual weakness are more likely to develop PPMA. Rarely, completely recovered muscles will develop atropy and weakness.[24]

PPS is relatively stable over substantial periods of time. In patients followed over a mean of 8.2 years, all developed new weakness, but at rate of decline that averaged about 1 percent per year using the MRC scale.[40]

Pain and fatigue in particular are subjective symptoms and raise the possibility of psychological symptoms, as opposed to organic dysfunction, although formal assessments have not supported this.[41] Nonetheless, identifying and treating a comorbid depression or mood disorder, if present, may improve somatic symptoms in selected patients.

Other investigations, including serologic studies and imaging, are recommended to look for other etiologies than PPS in these patients. Electromyography can be useful for finding other causes, such as carpal tunnel syndrome, radiculopathy, or myopathy that may be superimposed on the background of previous po-

liomyelitis.[39] In PPS specifically, electromyography has demonstrated increased jitter, a sign of inconsistent or unstable firing of motor unit fibers, which is present in all reinnervated postpolio muscles.[40] Patients with prior poliomyelitis and those with new weakness are not distinguished by electromyography or muscle biopsy evidence of reinnervation.[38]

Treatment

Treatment of PPS is managed with several approaches. Pharmacologic management of PPS itself has proved difficult. Pyridostigmine has been studied in a prospective, blinded, randomized trial and did not demonstrate any improvement despite improvement in jitter.[42] Prednisone has been evaluated to treat weakness and amantadine for fatigue, both in a controlled fashion, but without effect.[37] Management of musculoskeletal discomfort or neuropathic pain with conventional agents (e.g., nonsteroidal anti-inflammatory drugs, COX-2 inhibitors, and tricyclic antidepressants) is a reasonable approach in most patients.

Lifestyle changes and pacing of physical activities can help in the management of fatigue and diminished stamina. Weight loss is very important for some patients to help manage these symptoms. Assistive devices, bracing, and intermittent wheelchair use can help to conserve energy as well.

Exercise can improve function and is a prudent approach. Progressive resistance with isometric exercise has been shown to improve strength to a degree even greater than that of otherwise healthy elderly patients and without an adverse effect on motor unit survival.[43] Other studies have shown that nonfatiguing exercise programs, including dynamic water exercise, can improve conditioning and function.[44] Overall, short repetitions of maximal and submaximal effort but avoidance of exhaustion with appropriate rest in between are important. Dysphagia can be improved with speech therapy interventions.[44]

Respiratory sleep dysfunction should be evaluated and treated similarly to non-PPS patients, usually with positive-pressure ventilatory assistance.[44]

Reassurance of the relative stability over time is also important to alleviate substantially the concern these patients have of progressive weakness.

▶ CONCLUSION AND FUTURE OF POLIO

About 50 years ago, poliovirus infection and poliomyelitis were the dominant public health issue of the time. The success of the vaccines and the national and international public health efforts has reduced the incidence of disease dramatically. In 1988, there were over

350,000 cases in the world, and with a concerted effort, the number of cases in 2003 dropped to less than 800.[10] The number of cases of polio continues to decline, and those cases are restricted to a few geographic regions. As the world draws closer to potentially being free of poliomyelitis, new questions regarding polio may arise, such as the types of vaccination programs that need to be maintained, to whom; and if successful, when and how to withdraw the use of vaccines. Polio will be capable of reemergence for some time, and continued vigilance for case identification will be required. Six factors have been identified that shape the emergence (or reemergence) of a pathogen: human demographics and behavior, technology and industry, economic development and land use, international travel and commerce, microbial adaptation and change, and breakdown of public health measures.[45] Of these factors, the last has been a significant obstacle in the eradication of polio thus far in some parts of the world. This would be the most likely factor to contribute to a resurgence of paralytic disease. The continued awareness and identification of poliomyelitis therefore must remain in the consciousness of clinicians.

REFERENCES

1. Ropka SL, Jubelt B: Enteroviruses, in Nath A, Berger JR (eds): *Clinical Neurovirology.* New York: Marcel Dekker, 2003, pp 359–377.

2. Hinman AR, Koplan JP, Orenstein WA, et al: Live or inactivated poliomyelitis vaccine: An analysis of benefits and risks. *Am J Public Health* 78(3):291, 1988.

3. CBER, CfBEaR: *CBER Vision Newsletter,* commemorative issue (online); available at *www.fda.gov/cber/inside/centnews.htm;* accessed June 6, 2004.

4. Schohnberger L, McGowan JE, Gregg MB: Vaccine-associated poliomyelitis in the United States, 1961–1972. *Am J Epidemiol* 104(2):202, 1976.

5. Nkowane BM, Wassilak SGF, Orenstein WA, et al: Vaccine-associated paralytic poliomyelitis: United States, 1973–1984. *JAMA* 257(10):1335, 1987.

6. Strebel PM, Sutter RW, Cochi SL, et al: Epidemiology of poliomyelitis in the United States one decade after the last case of indigenous wild virus–associated disease. *Clin Infect Dis* 14:568, 1992.

7. Querfurth H, Swanson PD: Vaccine-associated paralytic poliomyelitis regional case series and review. *Arch Neurol* 47:541, 1990.

8. CDC: Isolation of wild poliovirus type 3 among members of a religious community objecting to vaccination—Alberta, Canada, 1993. *MMWR* 42(17):337, 1993.

9. Modlin J, Snider D, Clover R, et al: Poliomyelitis prevention in the United States: Updated recommendations of the Advisory Committee on Immunization Practices (ACIP). *MMWR* 49(RR05):1, 2000.

10. World Health Organization PEI: Polio eradication: Global progress (online); available at *www.polioeradication.org;* accessed June 3, 2004.

11. CDC: Wild poliovirus importations: West and Central Africa, January 2003–March 2004. *MMWR* 53(20):433, 2004.

12. Ramia S, Arif M: Paralytic poliomyelitis outbreak in Gizan, Saudi Arabia. *J Trop Pediatr* 37:202, 1991.

13. McKinney RE: The enteroviruses, in Joklik WK, Willett HP, Amos DB, Wilfert CM (eds): *Zinsser Microbiology,* 20th ed. Norwalk, CT: Appleton and Lange, 1992, pp 980–985.

14. Contreras G, Dimock K, Furesz J, et al: Genetic characterization of Sabin types 1 and 3 poliovaccine virus following serial passage in the human intestinal tract. *Biologicals* 20:15, 1992.

15. Evans DMA, Dunn G, Minor PD, et al: Increased neurovirulence associated with a single nucleotide change in a noncoding region of the Sabin type 3 poliovaccine genome. *Nature* 314:548, 1985.

16. MacLennan C, Dunn G, Huissoon AP, et al: Failure to clear persistent vaccine-derived neurovirulent poliovirus infection in an immunodeficient man. *Lancet* 363(9420):1509, 2004.

17. Modlin J, Coffey DJ: Poliomyelitis, polio vaccines and the post-poliomyelitis syndrome, in Scheld WM, Whitley RJ, Durack DT (eds): *Infections of the Central Nervous System,* 2d ed. Philadelphia: Lippincott-Raven, 1997, pp 57–72.

18. Lipton HL, Jubelt B: Enterovirus infections of the central nervous system, in Tyler KL, Martin JB (eds): *Infections of the Central Nervous System.* Philadelphia: Davis, 1993, pp 103–130.

19. Strebel PM, Ion-Nedelcu N, Baughman AL, et al: Intramuscular injections within 30 days of immunization with oral poliovirus vaccine: A risk factor for vaccine-associated paralytic poliomyelitis. *New Engl J Med* 332(8):500, 1995.

20. Sabin AB: Pathology and pathogenesis of human poliomyelitis. *JAMA* 120(7):506, 1942.

21. Mendelsohn CL, Wimmer E, Racaniello VR: Cellular receptor for poliovirus: Molecular cloning, nucleotide sequence, and expression of a new member of the immunoglobulin superfamily. *Cell* 56:855, 1989.

22. Online Mendelian Inheritance in Man (OMIM): MIM number (173850) (online); available at *http://www.ncbi.nlm.nih.gov/omim/.*

23. Brain WR: Poliomyelitis, in Brain WR (ed): *Diseases of the Nervous System,* 5th ed. London: Oxford University Press, 1955, pp 464–477.

24. Pascuzzi RM: Poliomyelitis and the postpolio syndrome, in Roos KL (ed): *Central Nervous System Infectious Diseases and Therapy.* New York: Marcel Dekker, 1997, pp 429–441.

25. Plum F: Sensory loss with poliomyelitis. *Neurology* 6(3):166, 1956.

26. Verstrepen WA, Bruynseels P, Mertens AH: Evaluation of a rapid real-time RT-PCR assay for detection of enterovirus RNA in cerebrospinal fluid specimens. *J Clin Virol* 25(suppl 1):S39, 2002.

27. So YT, Olney RK: AAEM case report no. 23: Acute paralytic poliomyelitis. *Muscle Nerve* 14(12):1159, 1991.

28. Agboatwalla M, Kirmani SR, Sonawalla A, et al: Nerve conduction studies and its importance in diagnosis of acute poliomyelitis. *Ind J Pediatr* 60(2):265, 1993.

29. Malzberg MS, Rogg JM, Tate CA, et al: Poliomyleitis: Hyperintensity of the anterior horn cells on MR images of the spinal cord. *AJR* 161:863, 1993.

30. Mermel L, Sanchez de Mora D, Sutter RW: Vaccine-associated paralytic poliomyelitis. *New Engl J Med* 329(11):810, 1993.

31. Farbu E, Gilhus NE: Education, occupation and perception of health amongst previous polio patients compared to their siblings. *Eur J Neurol* 9(3):233, 2002.

32. CDC: Poliomyelitis prevention in the United States: Updated recommendations of the Advisory Committee on Immunization Practices. *MMWR* 49(RR-5):1, 2000.

33. National Institutes of Health (NIH): Post-polio syndrome fact sheet (online); available at *http://www.ninds.nih.gov/health_and_medical/pubs/post-polio.htm;* accessed June 12, 2004.

34. Windebank A, Litchy W, Daube J, et al: Late effects of paralytic poliomyelitis in Olmsted County, Minnesota. *Neurology* 41(4):501, 1991.

35. Ramlow J, Alexander M, LaPorte R, et al: Epidemiology of the post-polio syndrome. *Am J Epidemiol* 136(7):769, 1992.

36. Trojan DA, Cashman N, Shapiro S, et al: Predictive factors for post-poliomyelitis syndrome. *Arch Phys Med Rehabil* 75:770, 1994.

37. Dalakas MC: Why drugs fail in postpolio syndrome. *Neurology* 53(6):1166, 1999.

38. Cashman N, Maselli R, Wollmann R, et al: Late denervation in patients with antecedent paralytic poliomyelitis. *New Engl J Med* 317(1):7, 1987.

39. Jubelt B, Agre JC: Characteristics and management of postpolio syndrome. *JAMA* 284(4):412, 2000.

40. Dalakas M, Elder G, Hallett M, et al: A long-term follow-up study of patients with post-poliomyelitis neuromuscular symptoms. *New Engl J Med* 314(15):959, 1986.

41. Clark K, Dinsmore S, Grafman J, Dalakas M: A personality profile of patients diagnosed with post-polio syndrome. *Neurology* 44(10):1809, 1994.

42. Trojan DA, Collet J-P, Shapiro S, et al: A multicenter, randomized, double-blinded trial of pyridostigmine in postpolio syndrome. *Neurology* 53(6):1225, 1999.

43. Ming Chan K, Amirjani N, Sumrain M, et al: Randomized controlled trial of strength training in post-polio patients. *Muscle Nerve* 27(3):332, 2003.

44. Jubelt B: Post-polio syndrome. *Curr Treat Opt Neurol* 6(2):87, 2004.

45. Johnson R: Emerging viral infections of the nervous system. *J Neurovirol* 9(2):140, 2003.

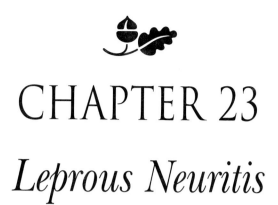

CHAPTER 23
Leprous Neuritis

Thomas D. Sabin and Thomas R. Swift

Leprosy (Hansen disease) is a chronic mycobacterial disease involving skin, mucous membranes, anterior portion of the eyes, testes, and most important, the peripheral nerves. It is in fact the only bacterial agent that regularly affects peripheral nerves, and it is nerve involvement that defines most of the clinical manifestations in all three major types of leprosy. *Mycobacterium leprae* has never been cultured satisfactorily but has been fully sequenced and found to have dropped out many metabolic functions in comparison with other mycobacteria.[1]

► EPIDEMIOLOGY

When the effectiveness of multidrug therapy (MDT) was established in the 1980s, international leprosy agencies set the goal of eliminating leprosy in the world by the year 2000. The number of registered cases was 5,069,232 in 1986 and dropped to 700,000 by 2001. This number is not as optimistic as it appears because change in case definitions account for most of the drop. Furthermore,

the number of new cases diagnosed each year in highly endemic countries is actually increasing. *Elimination* (not eradication) was defined as a reduction of prevalence to 1 case per 10,000 population, which experts believed would reduce the bacillary load below a critical level in a given population such that the disease eventually would disappear. The disease is now most common in the tropics, but historically and even at present the disease can occur in cold climates. While leprosy is not a major problem in the United States, immigration from Asia and South America requires that this diagnosis be kept in mind by American neurologists. The occurrence of new cases from the once-endemic areas around the Gulf Coast has been eliminated. Still, leprosy is not rare; there are at present 6000 cases in the United States.

The most likely portal of entry of the bacillus is the upper respiratory tract,[2] but other possibilities, such as inoculation via the skin, exist. Untreated patients with multibacillary disease daily produce nasal discharge containing millions of microorganisms that can remain viable outside the human host. Infected armadillos in the wild also have been proposed as an occasional source of cases in the United States.[3] Study of the problem is hampered by our inability to culture *M. leprae.* Over 95 percent of a given population probably are not susceptible to the disease after routine exposure, and although children appear more susceptible than adults, it may be more a matter of initial exposure usually occurring during childhood. Marital partners are at lower risk than household children,[4] and the disease is rare among visitors to endemic areas, including soldiers and missionaries.

The decline of leprosy that occurred in Europe and more recently in Hawaii correlates better with the changes generated by a rising standard of living than with any specific measures directed toward eradication of the disease. Where extreme public health measures such as enforced segregation were instituted in the past, a false decrease in incidence occurred because patients concealed the diagnosis out of fear of internment.

▶ CLINICAL MANIFESTATIONS

Leprosy occurs in three major forms and one minor form,[5] but the organism is the same for all: *M. leprae,* an acid-fast bacillus that is an obligate intracellular rod 1 to 8 μm long.[6] It is slow growing, having a division time of 12.5 days,[7] accounting for the often long incubation period and slow progression of the disease. A major problem has been the difficulty in culturing the organism. Infected armadillos and mouse foot pads are the most frequently used experimental hosts.[8,9] Which of the three forms of leprosy an individual will develop is related to the number of organisms present, which depends on the patient's ability to detect and destroy the bacilli. Where host immunity is highest, organisms are few and skin lesions sharply limited. This is referred to as *tuberculoid leprosy.* Where host immunity is lowest, bacilli are numerous and lesions widespread. This is referred to as *lepromatous leprosy. Immunity* as used here refers to host response specifically directed at *M. leprae* and may not relate to degrees of susceptibility to other infectious agents.[10,11] Between the extreme forms of tuberculoid and lepromatous leprosy is a middle ground where host response varies and may change over time. This form of leprosy is referred to as *intermediate, borderline,* or *dimorphous leprosy* and may be further subdivided.[5] Increasingly in leprosy research (e.g., as used in leprosy control programs) the terms *pauci-* and *multibacillary leprosy* are used because there is difficulty at times proving where intermediate leprosy ends and polar forms begin on either side of the spectrum. There is an early minor form of leprosy called *indeterminate* that may evolve into one of the three major forms or go on to self-healing.

Leprosy does not involve internal organs or the central nervous system because *M. leprae* reproduces poorly at core body temperature of 37°C, preferring instead a growth optimum of 32°C.[7,12,13] The temperature preference of *M. leprae* means that growth occurs in the cooler tissues of the body: skin on exterior surfaces of limbs and facial promontories, anterior portion of the eye,[14] mucous membranes in the upper airway, and testes. This was first suggested by Brand.[15] It is in the cool tissues that nerve damage first develops and develops most severely, producing a temperature-linked pattern of motor and sensory deficits that makes recognition possible.

Tuberculoid Leprosy

In tuberculoid leprosy, one or at most a few skin lesions are present, usually as sharply demarcated macules with raised red borders and central clearing. Nerve networks in the skin are destroyed by the granulomatous tissue reaction, and sweat glands and hair are lost. These skin lesions vary in size from 1 to 30 cm, vary in shape, and may occur anywhere on the body in cooler areas. There may be small satellite lesions nearby. Biopsy is best obtained from the active border and reveals epitheloid granuloma with foreign body and Langhans giant cells and may very rarely contain caseation. Bacilli are very few and may be fragmented. Underlying nerve trunks may be affected by direct continuity with the granuloma and may be grossly thickened. This form of leprosy usually goes on to self-healing, but antibiotic treatment is recommended.

Lepromatous Leprosy

In lepromatous leprosy there is unchecked bacterial multiplication and a constant bacteremia. Organisms are deposited throughout the body but multiply only in the cooler tissues. The disease rarely shows spontaneous arrest and after treatment may recur even where the bacterial index had fallen to zero.[16] Skin lesions are of variable appearance, including diffuse infiltrative, nodular, macular, and erythematous. Biopsy reveals a flattened rete separated by a clear space from foam-filled histiocytes laden with bacilli, particularly about skin appendages, blood vessels, and nerves. Patients may complain of rash, painless injury, nasal stuffiness, or if a leprosy reaction (see below) occurs, painful iritis,[17] neuritis, and orchitis.[18] Leprosy reaction may occur spontaneously but more often in association with antibacterial treatment in which large amounts of mycobacterial antigen become available from dead and decaying organisms. While most of the deformity in this type of leprosy is consequent to nerve damage, direct invasion by huge numbers of organisms may cause massive infiltration of the skin, destroy the nasal cartilage, deform the pinnae of the ears, and lead to upper airway obstruction. When this occurs, patients resort to mouth breathing with consequent cooling of the pharynx and larynx. Before the days of effective antibacterial treatment, patients with multibacillary disease eventually became blind, with facial diparesis, extremity ulceration, loss of digits, continued infiltration, scarring and discoloration of skin, multiple peripheral nerve palsies, airway obstruction, and secondary amyloidosis. Many patients also were deaf as a result of administration of streptomycin.

Intermediate (Borderline, Dimorphous) Leprosy

Intermediate leprosy is variable and constitutes a spectrum of disease from paucibacillary to multibacillary depending on the degree of host resistance to the bacilli. In the form on the tuberculoid end of the intermediate spectrum, organisms and skin lesions are few, although more numerous than in polar tuberculoid leprosy. In the form on the lepromatous end of the intermediate spectrum, organisms are numerous and skin lesions not as widespread or symmetric as in polar lepromatous leprosy. For purposes of classification and judging responses to drug therapy, there is increasing use of the terms *paucibacillary* (encompassing tuberculoid and high-resistance intermediate leprosy) and *multibacillary* (lepromatous and low-resistance intermediate leprosy). Clinically, intermediate leprosy is unstable, moving toward lepromatous leprosy without treatment (termed *downgrading*) or toward tuberculoid leprosy (termed *reversal reaction*) with treatment.

▶ DIAGNOSIS

The single most important factor in the diagnosis of leprosy, particularly in the United States and other countries where leprosy is rare, is for the physician to suspect the diagnosis. A high index of suspicion usually occurs as a result of a neurologic symptom or sign: skin lesions that are anesthetic, sensory loss that follows a temperature-linked pattern, the occurrence of painful neuritis, painless burns and wounds of other kinds, and ulceration on pressure areas of the hands and feet. However, nonneurologic symptoms also may be the presenting feature: nasal stuffiness, iritis, and orchitis. A tissue diagnosis depends on finding bacilli in skin smears or biopsies. The organisms are only weakly acid-fast, and skill is required in preparation of the tissue. Skin smears are obtained from affected areas (commonly the nasal mucosa or extensor surfaces of upper and lower extremities) by incising the skin and expressing tissue fluid onto slides that are stained. In patients with pau-

cibacillary leprosy, a biopsy and careful search for the often degenerating organisms must be done because bacilli are few. The percentage of intact bacilli to total bacilli is referred to as the *morphologic index* (MI) (varying from 1 to 10 percent prior to treatment), which indicates viability of bacilli.[19] Quantified counts of bacilli are also performed using light microscopy varying from 0 (no bacilli seen in 100 oil-immersion fields) to 6+ (over 1000 bacilli in each oil-immersion field). This is referred to as the *bacteriologic index* (BI). High values for both MI and BI are found in untreated lepromatous leprosy. Where skin scrapings are negative, the term *paucibacillary leprosy* is used to denote tuberculoid and high-resistance intermediate leprosy. Where skin scrapings are positive, the term *multibacillary* is used, referring to middle intermediate, borderline lepromatous, and lepromatous leprosy. Despite the relative ease of making a diagnosis of leprosy, failure to consider the diagnosis may lead to months and years of erroneous diagnoses and delay of treatment, during which further damage occurs.

▶ LEPROSY REACTIONS

Leprosy reactions occur in two types: those which occur in paucibacillary patients and are referred to as *type 1 reactions* and those which occur in multibacillary patients and are referred to as *type 2 reactions*. Type 1 reactions occur in tuberculoid and high-resistance intermediate leprosy. Existing skin lesions flare, become red and swollen, and occasionally ulcerate, and involved nerves may take part in the reaction. These events often follow the initiation of effective antibacterial therapy, with clearing of the organisms. Cell-mediated immunity appears to increase and the patient may progress to bacterial negativity, but permanent neurologic damage may occur unless the reaction is identified promptly and treated. At times, immune resistance to *M. leprae* appears to vary in intermediate leprosy, and bacilli and skin lesions become more numerous. These episodes have been referred to as *downgrading reactions*, but there is no erythema, edema, or fever. Downgrading reactions may be stimulated by concomitant medical conditions or occur spontaneously and indicate instability in the immune response of the patient on the intermediate spectrum.

Type 2 reactions occur in lepromatous leprosy and constitute a grave threat to the patient. Such reactions can result in blindness (from iritis), sterility and gynecomastia (from orchitis), painful arthritis, and paralysis (from neuritis). This form of reaction is referred to as *erythema nodosum leprosum* (ENL) and includes fever, prostration, and malaise, with the appearance of painful subcutaneous nodules (erythema nodosum).

This disorder affects about half of all patients with lepromatous leprosy and may occur spontaneously, in response to physical or psychological stress, but most often in association with effective antimycobacterial therapy. Lymph nodes and liver may become enlarged. Pathologically, this reaction is characterized by vasculitis involving medium-sized and small arteries and arterioles, with fibrinoid degeneration and cuffing with inflammatory cells. Antigens from *M. leprae* provoke an antibody response from the host, and antigen-antibody complexes appear to be involved in this complex process, with deposition of complement and cell lysis, provoking further polymorphonuclear infiltration, at times resulting in microabscess formation.[20,21] The reaction may be so severe in subcutaneous arteries that infarction of skin and underlying fat can occur with ulceration and eventual formation of thin "cigarette paper" scars.

▶ NEUROLOGIC MANIFESTATIONS

The neurologic features of leprosy are sufficiently characteristic that an accurate diagnosis of leprosy and of the type of leprosy present may be made confidently by neurologic examination alone. This is true even in patients in whom bacilli are no longer present because the nerve damage, once present, is permanent. The unique features of leprous neuritis are caused by two characteristics of leprosy bacilli: (1) the organisms have a predilection to invade and eventually destroy peripheral nerve, and (2) the organisms multiply in areas of cool temperature. How these two characteristics of the organism play out in individual patients depends on the immune response of the host. Nerve damage, however, is a constant feature of all forms of leprosy.

Tuberculoid Leprous Neuritis

In tuberculoid leprosy, the nerve involvement is sharply confined to a single or at most a few skin lesions. Within the skin lesion, cutaneous nerves are destroyed, and the skin is anesthetic (Fig. 23-1). Sympathetic nerves are also involved, and the lesions are anhydrotic and hairless. The circumscribed nature of the involvement dictates that nerve damage stops at the border of the skin lesion and sensation is normal beyond in unaffected skin. When a nerve trunk underlies a skin lesion, it too

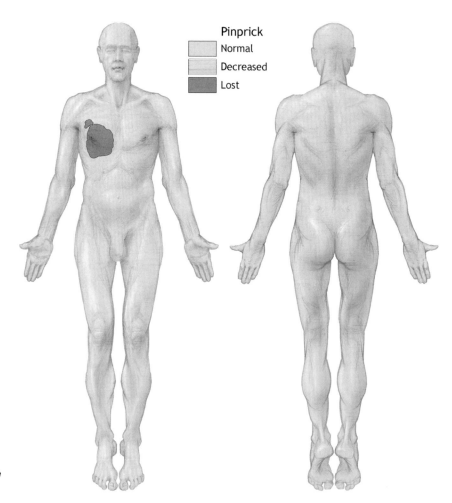

Pinprick
Normal
Decreased
Lost

Figure 23-1. Tuberculoid leprosy. The large skin lesion and a small satellite lesion are anesthetic. There are no other lesions.

may be involved and frequently is visibly and palpably thickened, and motor and sensory deficits from that nerve may be seen. "Cold" nerve abscesses may occur.[22] Calcification of nerves may be seen in long-standing cases of high-resistance leprosy and be visible on radiographs.[23,24] However, here too the process is limited. Such lesions may occur anywhere on the body but tend to spare the warm areas (under the scalp and in the axillae and groin). Simply mapping the area by checking sensation with a pin tells the physician that the area of anesthesia exactly conforms to the area of the skin lesion.

Lepromatous Leprous Neuritis

In lepromatous leprous neuritis, bacilli are deposited everywhere but multiply only in areas of cool temperature.[25,26] Where they grow, nerve involvement occurs; where they do not, neural involvement does not occur. Careful neuropathologic studies have been done on postmortem tissue of lepromatous leprosy patients. While a few organisms have been found in the brain and spinal cord, there appears to be no central nervous system (CNS) damage. Clinically, leprosy does not af-

fect the CNS; the neurologic manifestations are completely limited to peripheral nerves and possibly muscle.

In the early stages of the disease, the coolest areas of the body are symmetrically infiltrated by multiplying bacilli and are the first to manifest neurologic abnormalities: the extensor surfaces of the limbs, the pinnae of the ears, the skin overlying the zygoma, and the upper lip, nose, and chin (Fig. 23-2). This results in a purely sensory neuropathy. In these areas, pain and temperature sensations are lost. Deeper sensations such as deep pain, vibration, and joint position sense are preserved, reflecting the superficial nature of the neuropathy that affects nerve networks close to the skin surface. Motor nerve fibers tend to be in deep tissues throughout their course, and signs of muscle involvement do not occur early in the disease.

The superficial nature of the involvement of cutaneous nerves and nerve networks is manifest clinically by a temperature-linked sensory neuropathy,[25,26] easily distinguishable from the more common distal symmetric loss of most sensory polyneuropathies.[25]

As the disease progresses, the involved areas enlarge, now encroaching on slightly warmer areas of the

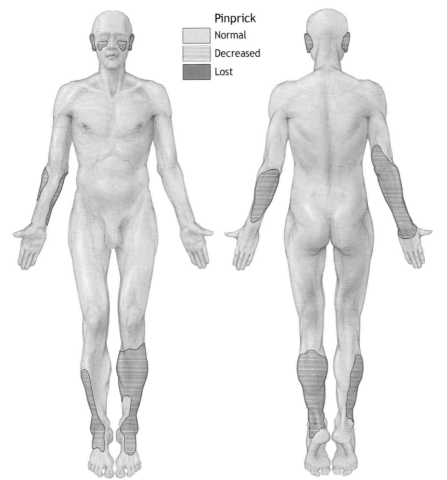

Figure 23-2. Early lepromatous leprosy. There is sensory loss symmetrically affecting extensor surfaces of the upper and lower extremities and the pinnae of the ears.

body, including breasts, central abdomen, and buttocks but sparing the warmest areas (under the scalp; in the axillae, antecubital fossae, and groins; and between the toes). Notably spared are preserved warm areas, including palms and soles, under frequently worn collars and watch bands, and in cutaneous vascular malformations. Certain peripheral nerve trunks are involved where they course close to the skin surface and are therefore cool: the ulnar nerve proximal to the elbow, the radial cutaneous nerve at the wrist, the great auricular nerve, facial nerve branches coursing over the face, the common peroneal nerve at the knee, and the superficial peroneal nerve at the ankle and dorsum of the foot (Figs. 23-3 through 23-5). Taken together, these nerve trunk lesions produce a pattern of temperature-linked involvement characterized at first by enlargement and hardening that may be palpated; the nerve trunks appear to be functioning normally.

Without treatment, the disease progresses inexorably. Large skin surfaces now are involved, with only the warmest spared. Nerve trunks may become grossly enlarged, and nerve trunk damage occurs with further sensory deficits that are now superimposed on the cutaneous nerve damage, producing complex sensory maps. In nerve trunks, the greatest bacillary density occurs in superficial portions.[27] Motor deficits now make their first appearance with facial muscle wasting and weakness, particularly affecting orbicularis oculi, corrugator, orbicularis oris, nasalis, depressor anguli oris, and platysma.[28] Interesting patterns of facial weakness are observed clinically. The lips and lids may become everted. The lateral portion of the frontalis may be spared because its nerve branch passes under the hairline, and when the patient attempts to wrinkle the brow, only the lateral portion of the frontalis contracts, raising the lateral portion of the eyebrows and resulting in a sinister, "devilish" appearance. The deep buccinator muscle is spared, resulting in "buccinator wrinkles" in an attempt to smile. In the extremities, a claw hand develops, as does a drop foot, and there are other signs of loss of intrinsic muscles, including cocked-up toes. New nerve trunk lesions appear: the radial nerve at the elbow, the median nerve proximal to the wrist,[29] and the tibial nerve in the popliteal fossa and at the ankle.

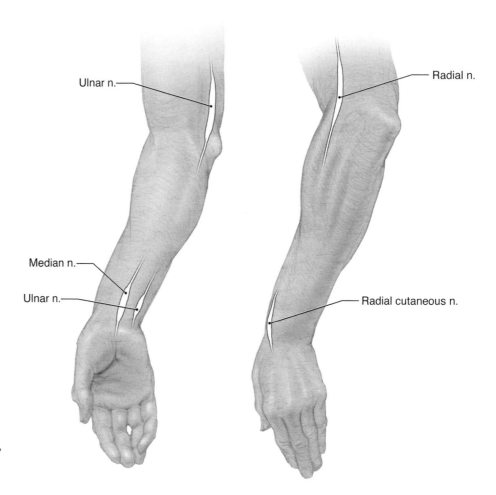

Figure 23-3. Lepromatous leprosy. Enlargement of ulnar, median, and radial nerves at cool locations.

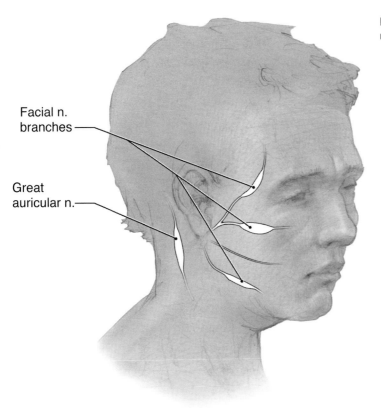

Figure 23-4. Lepromatous leprosy. Enlargement of facial nerve branches in the face.

Facial n.
branches

Great
auricular n.

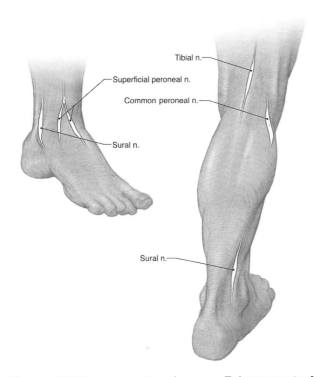

Tibial n.

Superficial peroneal n.

Common peroneal n.

Sural n.

Sural n.

Figure 23-5. Lepromatous leprosy. Enlargement of peroneal, tibial, and sural nerves at cool locations.

Deeper nerves such as circumflex, axillary, femoral, and sciatic are spared.

As a result of progressive intracutaneous and nerve trunk involvement, the patient eventually has sensory loss covering large portions of the skin surface and absolutely sparing only the scalp and deeper portions of the axilla, groin, and gluteal cleft, with relative sparing of a few areas on the extremities, including palms and soles, between toes, anticubital fossa, and midline of the back (Fig. 23-6). These areas also are spared the dermatologic lesions.[12] Searching for these areas of preserved sensation so close to anesthetic areas (e.g., the helices of the ears next to the scalp) allows one to make the diagnosis in long-standing cases of lepromatous leprosy. The temperature-linked pattern of motor deficits is likewise strongly suggestive of leprosy. Autonomic fibers are also damaged, and extremities become dusky, cool, and dry. Deep autonomic functions are not affected, and hypotension, diarrhea, impotence, and bladder problems do not occur. However, cardiac and genital systems reportedly may be affected.[30,31]

Intermediate Leprous Neuritis

Intermediate leprosy varies from pauci- to multibacillary disease and can be envisioned as a spectrum determined by the vigor of the host response. At either

Figure 23-6. Late lepromatous leprosy. Widespread cutaneous sensory loss sparing the warmest areas.

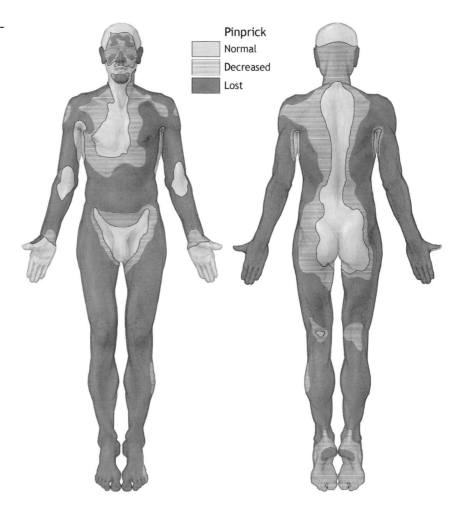

Pinprick
Normal
Decreased
Lost

extreme it may be difficult to differentiate from polar pauci- or multibacillary disease. However, the skin lesions and associated sensory loss vary from polar forms. Paucibacillary intermediate skin lesions are more numerous and widespread than in polar tuberculoid leprosy (Fig. 23-7). Multibacillary intermediate skin lesions are not as numerous, widespread, or symmetric as in polar lepromatous leprosy. All degrees of variability across the spectrum occur.

Whereas polar forms tend to be stable, intermediate leprosy is often unstable. In the older literature, worsening of intermediate leprosy was referred to as a *downgrading reaction,* where new skin lesions appeared and bacilli became more numerous. There also were *reversal reactions,* where lesions flared and bacilli were cleared, indicating an improvement in host immunity.

Reaction Neuritis

Reactive states play an important role in leprosy, superimposing new nerve lesions on established neuropathy due to the presence of bacilli. Reaction may occur at any time and in any form of leprosy. The most severe form occurs in patients with multibacillary dis-

ease either spontaneously or more often when treatment with antibiotics has resulted in death of the bacilli and liberation of large amounts of mycobacterial antigen. Since the heaviest bacillary loads are present in nerve trunks in areas of low temperature already dysfunctional, it is precisely in these areas that the reactive neuritis tends to be the most severe. A mild ulnar palsy suddenly may become severe, a foot drop may appear, and facial weakness worsens acutely. Associated with reactive neuritis, iritis, orchitis, and a severe form of erythema nodosum occurs, all of which are painful and associated with prostration and fever. At times, infarctions may occur in the skin. Recognition that reaction is occurring is important because reaction may be treated successfully, and nerve deficits may improve.[32] Reaction in multibacillary leprosy is believed to be an immunologically mediated process in which reactive T cells and immune complexes result in a complement-mediated vasculitis affecting skin, peripheral nerve, the anterior third of the eye, and the testes.[20,21] It is unfortunate that the circulating antibodies against *M. leprae* present in the blood, while not effective against the bacilli, are involved in a reaction that causes further damage to these tissues.

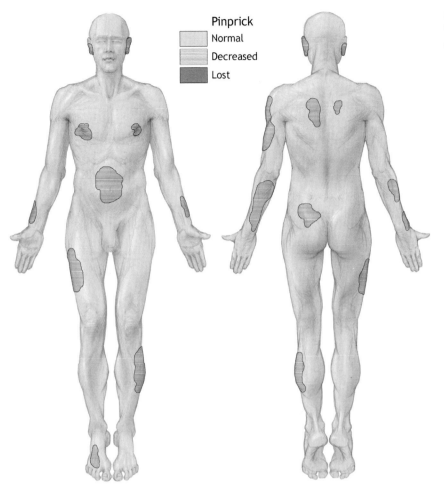

Pinprick
Normal
Decreased
Lost

Figure 23-7. Intermediate leprosy. Widespread discreet lesions with sensory loss.

▶ DEFORMITY

Deformity in leprosy is the defining feature of the disease in the public eye and to the patient the most distressing manifestation. Deformity occurs where bacilli are most numerous either by the destructive effects of proliferating bacilli themselves or, much more commonly, by the secondary effects of nerve damage. The picture of the advanced patient with leprosy, blind, with facial paralysis, everted lips and eyelids, infiltrated and scarred facial lesions, destroyed nasal cartilage, claw hands, foot drop, hand and foot wounds, shortened digits, and skin ulcers has been recognized since Biblical times and has resulted in ostracism from society and even family. Social isolation has made many patients, fearing that they have the disease, reluctant to come forward for treatment.

Bacillary proliferation accounts for facial infiltration (leonine facies), destruction of nasal and ear cartilage, and possibly invasion of articular cartilage, tendon, and bone in cool areas. Bacillary proliferation in the nasal cavity results at times in complete obstruction so that the patient resorts to mouth breathing and eventual infiltration of the oral cavity, pharynx, and hypopharynx.

Patients can become blind in several ways. Iritis may lead directly to blindness. Facial weakness may prevent eye closure with resulting corneal drying, secondary infection, and scarring. Corneal insensitivity may allow foreign bodies to cause extensive damage. Eyelashes may point directly at the cornea and produce mechanical trauma.

The pinnae of the ears become grossly deformed by the presence of large numbers of bacilli. When patients are treated successfully, the skin, previously distended, collapses and hangs in scarred folds.

The major deformity in leprosy occurs as a consequence of nerve injury. These deformities are not specific for leprosy and occur in other neurologic diseases where some degree of motor power remains in insensitive limbs. Leprosaria are a rich source of patients with hereditary sensory neuropathies, syringomyelia, a variety of diabetic neuropathy, insensitivity to pain, and so on. The major features that to the public constitute leprosy are produced by the peculiar nature of nerve lesions in these diseases: the ulcerated hands and feet, the short or lost digits, the amputations, and the many fresh lesions, particularly burns. It is not true that digits "drop off" in leprosy. It is now clear that repeated trauma with hematomas and secondary infection leads digits to shorten in little increments over many years. The bones and joints remain, but the phalanges become progressively shorter, and as the digit shortens, the nail rides down the shortening digit and may now appear at the metatarsal or metacarpal heads. Loss of protective pain and temperature senses allows these wounds to continue, the patient often using his or her hands as tools because he or she does not pay the price of pain. Involvement of autonomic fibers reduces sweating so that skin becomes hard and cracks in the flexion creases, becoming secondarily infected. Repeated pressure unfelt by the patient results in punched-out ulcers on weight-bearing portions of the soles and palms, so-called mal perforans common not just to leprosy but also to many of these diseases. Pressures on the hands and feet are made worse by the deformity attendant on the loss of intrinsic muscles, particularly the lumbricals, with cocked-up toes and clawed fingers.

▶ NEUROPATHOLOGY

In multibacillary leprosy, there is failure by the host to recognize *M. leprae* as foreign, and organisms proliferate to huge numbers.[33] It is still unclear why organisms show a predilection for Schwann cells that contain and may become distended by many bacilli.[27,34,35] Nerve damage is found in all cases of leprosy. The target of nerve invasion by *M. leprae* is the Schwann cell. Peripheral nerves are otherwise highly resistant to bacterial invasion so that recent contributions revealing how leprosy invades nerves are of special interest. A glycolipid designated as phenolic glycolipid 1 (PGL-1) is unique to *M. leprae* and binds to Schwann cell extracellular basal membrane protein laminin 2 and its associated α-dystroglycan membrane constituent.[36] The α-dystroglycan forms part of a transmembrane array that binds to intracellular actin and provides a potential route of entry for the bacilli. In cell culture systems, *M. leprae* does not invade Schwann cells that are actively forming myelin. PGL-1 attachment to Schwann cell basal membrane induces demyelination.[37,38] This in turn initiates dedifferentiation into a form of Schwann cell vulnerable to *M. leprae* invasion. The nonmyelinating Schwann cells associated with small autonomic and pain-temperature perception are readily invaded, and this correlates with the extensive pattern of intracutaneous nerve destruction that causes the loss of autonomic function and pain and temperature perception. These earliest stages of nerve damage occur in *M. leprae*–infected immunodeficient RAG-1 mice, indicating that early Schwann cell injury is not dependent on immune mechanisms that play an important role in nerve destruction later in the disease.[39]

An interesting association has been described between neurofibromatosis (in which Schwann cells proliferate) and leprosy.[40] Perineurial and endothelial cells also may contain bacilli,[41] but rarely have bacilli been seen intraaxonally.[42] Even while becoming enlarged due to the presence of large numbers of bacilli, edema, and the multiplication of Schwann cells, nerves may continue to function. When bacilli die and begin to disintegrate, releasing antigen, often reaction neuritis supervenes, and intraneural vasculitis and outpouring of periarterial inflammatory cells occurs, which may be the factor most important in causing dysfunction. Initially both axonal damage and segmental demyelination have been described.[43] In late stages of leprosy, there is loss of myelinated nerve fibers and intraneural fibrosis with huge amounts of collagen deposition. Schwann cell involvement leading to demyelination may be responsible for the slowing of nerve conduction velocity seen in involved segments.

In paucibacillary leprosy, the host is able to recognize the bacilli as foreign and to limit their proliferation so that few bacilli are found. The organisms are not as highly acid-fast as *M. tuberculosis*, and special techniques must be employed to prevent their decolorization. Immune techniques also have been used to identify bacilli in tissue sections. While organisms are fewer, the tissue response is more vigorous, and early and severe nerve damage occurs, albeit in an area limited to the skin lesion and possibly to underlying nerves. The tissue reaction consists of epithelioid granuloma with both foreign-body and Langhans giant cells. In the skin, intracutaneous nerve networks and adjacent subdermal nerves are destroyed by the granuloma. Both sensory and autonomic nerves are involved, and few intracutaneous nerves remain in biopsies stained for the presence of nerves. Sweat glands and hair follicles are lost permanently.

In intermediate leprosy, the damage to nerves varies depending on the degree of host resistance and contains features of pauci- and multibacillary disease. Some forms of leprosy reported as pure neural or polyneuritic are intermediate histologically. In this form, nerve trunk lesions are reported to occur in the absence of skin lesions.[44–46] Diagnosis in such cases requires the finding of *M. leprae* in nerve biopsy.

▶ ELECTROPHYSIOLOGIC STUDIES

There are no convincing abnormal electrophysiologic studies of brain or spinal cord in leprosy, reflecting the lack of involvement of these structures clinically; all abnormalities described involve the peripheral nervous system.[47,48] Motor and sensory nerve conduction studies have demonstrated slowing of velocity through clinically involved segments of nerve and improvement with treatment.[32,44,47] Brand operated on acutely swollen nerves in the course of reaction neuritis and found that when the epineurial sheath was incised and pressure released, segments previously unable to conduct an impulse now began to function, and muscle responses were observed. Several studies have shown reduction in conduction velocity during reactive episodes with neuritis that improved when treated with thalidomide.[48]

▶ DIFFERENTIAL DIAGNOSIS

Leprosy produces a temperature-linked neuropathy with intracutaneous sensory and autonomic loss, preserved reflexes, and enlarged nerves. Skin lesions are virtually always present. If the diagnosis is considered and the physician alerted by the proper epidemiologic setting, the diagnosis usually is obvious.

Nerve Enlargement

Diseases producing diffuse enlargement of nerve trunks include hereditary neuropathies, amyloidosis, neurofibromatosis, Refsum's syndrome, and certain dysimmune neuropathies. In leprosy, the nerve enlargements tend to be larger, firmer, more focal, and often are tender. With treatment, they may shrink but always remain hard. Chronically traumatized nerve segments may become enlarged but are more circumscribed than those in leprosy.

Polyneuropathy

Common causes of polyneuropathy include alcoholic-nutritional, diabetic, hereditary, and toxic. With few exceptions, polyneuropathies tend to involve first and most severely the longest nerves, and as the disease progresses, sequentially shorter nerves are affected.[26,49] Sensory loss occurs first in the toes and ascends gradually up the leg in a symmetric fashion. When the knee is reached, the fingertips begin to be affected because all nerves involved at a given stage of the disease are of the same length. Eventually, in severe cases, the longest nerves of the torso are affected, producing numbness on the anterior chest and abdomen that the unwary observer may mistake for a spinal cord sensory level. In rare cases, sensory loss occurs on the face and scalp. Motor polyneuropathies evolve similarly with a distal-to-proximal progression.

In contrast, sensory loss in low-resistance leprosy may involve proximal areas severely while sparing very distal parts, according to temperature. For example, the pinnae of the ears may be anesthetic, whereas sensation is spared between the toes. In contrast to stocking loss in polyneuropathies, in leprosy the sole may be spared, whereas the leg is anesthetic. Also in contrast to polyneuropathies, in low-resistance leprosy, vibration and position senses are maintained. In polyneuropathies muscle stretch reflexes are lost, whereas in leprosy they are preserved.

Weakness, when it occurs in low-resistance leprosy, is in the distribution of the named affected nerves. Ulnar nerve–innervated intrinsic hand muscles are affected before median, peroneal nerve–innervated muscles are affected before tibial, and so on.

Polyradiculopathies are easy to differentiate from low-resistance leprosy: Reflexes are lost early, both proximal and distal muscles are affected, and often little sensory loss occurs. When present, it tends to affect vibration and position senses, which are spared in leprosy.

Mononeuropathy and Mononeuropathy Multiplex

Leprosy does produce a mononeuropathy multiplex in a stereotyped fashion, which should be sought for.[50] In contrast to diseases such as diabetes, collagen diseases, and hereditary neuropathy with pressure palsies, in leprosy the nerves are large, hard, and usually accompanied by patches of anesthetic skin. Nerve involvement in leprosy occurs in predictable locations.

Chronic compression sites in the limbs are similar to areas of nerve involvement in leprosy, and traumatized nerves may become enlarged.[51] Again, a search for a patch of intracutaneous sensory loss is key.

Sensory perineuritis involves sensory nerves, producing pain, slight enlargement, and partial sensory loss.[52] However, there are no skin lesions. Sensory perineuritis may be migrant and recur in the same or other nerves. Biopsy reveals fascicle-specific inflammation.

A peculiar form of sensory loss occurs on the back of the torso in notalgia paresthetica. This occurs where the posterior primary sensory branch of spinal nerves, usually in the thorax, is entrapped by fascial layers. This results in pruritus and occasionally circumscribed sensory loss, usually partial. It may be mistaken for leprosy, but awareness of the condition combined with absence of a skin lesion makes the diagnosis.

▶ ANTIMYCOBACTERIAL TREATMENT

The aim of treatment is to stop the proliferation of bacilli and thus prevent or arrest nerve damage. While antibacterial treatment renders the patient noninfectious within days, clinical deficits, such as loss of sensation and motor power, and autonomic dysfunction are rarely restored unless they are due to reaction neuritis, when

▶ **TABLE 23-1.** LEPROSY TREATMENT

Drug	Side Effect	Frequency
Dapsone	Hemolysis	Common
	Agranulocytosis	Rare
	Rash	Rare
	Peripheral neuropathy[54,55]	Rare
Clofazimine	Skin pigmentation	Universal
	Gastrointestinal discomfort	Uncommon
Rifampin	Hepatotoxicity	Uncommon
	Accelerates metabolism of other drugs	Common

some improvement may occur with treatment. The many systems and body tissues affected by leprosy often require a team of internists, neurologists, orthopedic surgeons, ophthalmologists, rehabilitation specialists, public health officials, social workers, and vocational specialists. A problem in leprosy treatment is that in many parts of the world where leprosy is well known, patients often are afraid to accept treatment for fear of being identified and ostracized.

Before 1940, the treatment used was chaulmoogra oil, which has little antimycobacterial activity. Sulfones were introduced for treatment of leprosy at Carville, Louisiana, in 1940 and were the first treatment that could result in bacterial negativity.[53] However, both primary and secondary bacterial resistance emerged and required the use of new agents and combinations of drugs. Many drugs have been shown to have efficacy against *M. leprae* in the mouse foot pad and in the armadillo, the experimental animal most closely resembling human disease.

Drugs effective against *M. leprae* include dapsone, clofazimine (B663, Lamprene), rifampin, ethionamide, streptomycin, and ofloxacin (the last is used experimentally). The first three drugs are the most widely used, and side effects, with a few exceptions, are rare for these drugs (Table 23-1).

There is some controversy about optimal regimens for the treatment of leprosy in its various forms. For paucibacillary patients, suggested treatment in the United States is dapsone 100 mg daily with rifampin 600 mg daily for 6 months, followed by dapsone monotherapy for 3 to 5 years. For multibacillary patients, the combination is given for 3 years, followed by dapsone monotherapy for 10 years (for life in polar lepromatous leprosy). Where dapsone resistance is suspected or demonstrated in mouse foot pad tests, clofazimine 50 mg daily is substituted for dapsone in the multibacillary regimen.

Twenty years ago the World Health Organization suggested different protocols with shorter periods of treatment, and these approaches appear promising.[2] For paucibacillary patients, dapsone 100 mg daily and rifampin 600 mg monthly are continued for 6 months

and then discontinued. For multibacillary patients, dapsone 100 mg and clofazimine 300 mg once monthly (both supervised) are continued until bacteria have disappeared on skin scrapings but in any case for at least 2 years. Since patients rapidly become noninfectious, and since the great majority of people are not susceptible to leprosy, there is no need for isolation or hospitalization of patients undergoing treatment.

Experimental immunotherapy has reported some success using interferon[58] and transfer factor,[57] but results are not sufficiently studied to recommend widespread use. Vaccination with a mixture of heat-killed *M. leprae* and bacilli Calmette-Guérin (BCG) has been used and may be applicable to large populations to prevent multibacillary leprosy but is not a form of treatment.[58]

▶ TREATMENT OF REACTIONS

Reactions must be identified and treated promptly if damage to the patient's nerves, eyes, skin, joints, and testes is to be avoided. Type 1 reactions, which are severe or involve nerves or threaten skin ulceration, must be treated with corticosteroids in large doses. Typically this requires prednisone 60 to 80 mg/day, and even higher doses may be required depending on the severity of the reaction. Therapy at times may need to be prolonged, although in most patients symptoms clear rapidly, and corticosteroids may be tapered. For prolonged therapy, attempts to use alternate-day dosing and reductions in dose are necessary to manage side effects. Type 2 reactions are treated according to severity. Very mild reactions may be treated symptomatically, but for more severe reactions, the drug of choice is thalidomide, which may be obtained from the Gillis Long Hansen's Disease Center, Carville, Louisiana. Because of its teratogenicity, thalidomide is not approved for any condition except ENL, and even here stringent controls are necessary to prevent pregnancy during its administration. Thalidomide in a dose of 300 to 400 mg/day usually clears reaction within 36 to 48 hours, after which the dose is tapered to an average maintenance dose of 100 mg daily for several weeks. Thalidomide itself is reported to cause peripheral neuropathy, although in our experience this has not been a troubling side effect in leprosy patients. ENL often is recurrent, and thalidomide may need to be restarted.

Corticosteroids also rapidly control ENL and always should be used if neuritis or iritis occurs. Clofazimine, in addition to being antibacterial, also helps control ENL in a dose of 200 to 300 mg/day. Chloroquine and stibophen also have been used. Iritis is treated with corticosteroid eye drops in addition to the preceding measures. Mydriatics are required to prevent scarring with iris fixation and glaucoma.

Neuritis may occur as the sole manifestation of type 2 reactions and always should be treated with high-dose corticosteroids, as for type 1 reactions. Intraneural injections of corticosteroids have been advocated for acute neuritis,[59] but we have noted complete and permanent nerve palsies as a result and do not recommend its use.

Surgical Treatment

Nerve abscesses must be drained by carefully incising the epineurium and draining the abscess.[60,61] Fascicular dissection of nerve trunks has been advocated in patients with endoneurial edema, and ulnar nerve transposition has been performed, but the results of such surgeries are uncertain. Nerve grafting has been employed with limited improvement. Neurovascular island pedicle transfers have been reported to restore protective sensation to fingers. Plastic surgical procedures involve reconstruction of the nasal septum, removal of excess skin from the ears and eyelids, and implantation of scalp hair to replace lost eyebrows. Surgery on the hand includes tendon transfers to restore abduction-opponens action of the thumb and to correct the effects of loss of lumbrical muscle function. Lagophthalmos is corrected with a sling of temporalis muscle inserted through the lower lid to the inner canthus. Foot dorsiflexion can be corrected using the posterior tibial tendon inserted onto the dorsum of the foot.

► MINIMIZING THE COMPLICATIONS OF INSENSITIVITY

Here the physician may be of great help to the patient to correct existing problems, prevent future complications, and provide the patient with insight into the nature of the process that is destroying his or her hands, feet, and eyes. Not just in leprosy but also in other diseases where loss of protective pain sensation occurs in limbs capable of movement, there occur problems that may be eradicated completely through proper education and preventative measures. In leprosy, as in other conditions producing insensitivity, the skin heals normally. Wounds must be splinted. Inspection of the eyes, hands, and feet must be done daily to ensure that minor problems do not become major ones through recurrent trauma. Red areas on the hands and feet indicative of high pressure must be noted, and measures must be taken to reduce trauma or ulceration that may occur. Modifications of shoes and tools, and indeed even occupations, need to be made at times. Gloves should be worn. Goggles prevent eye drying and the introduction of foreign matter. Corrective tarsorrhaphy may be necessary. Sympathetic denervation with resulting drying and cracking of the skin on the hands and feet can lead to secondary infections. Soaking the hands and feet and then applying occlusive ointment help to conserve moisture.

Plantar ulcers (mal perforans) may be associated with purulent discharge, swollen lymph nodes, and fever. In such cases, the foot is soaked in warm water and elevated, and antibiotics are given. After this acute phase is over, the foot and ankle are placed in a total-contact plaster cast. Healing over several weeks to months is the rule, after which suitable footwear must be found that alleviates points of high pressure; otherwise, ulceration redevelops.

► SOCIAL REHABILITATION

Many leprosy patients come from the lower socioeconomic strata of society, and the presence of this stigmatizing disease may produce apparently insurmountable barriers to treatment, rehabilitation, and life adjustment. However, the disease is caused by a bacterium. It is treatable, and the patient poses no threat to others because most people are immune naturally. Patient education plays a big role in informing and counteracting prevalent misconceptions about the disease. Experts in vocational rehabilitation are needed where insensitivity or damage to eyes, hands, and feet are present. Social service helps to find health resources, financial support, and adequate housing.

► ACKNOWLEDGMENTS

We wish to thank Robert Jacobson, M.D., Ph.D., for his valuable insights into leprosy and its treatment and Victoria Morales and Teresa Chaney for typing the manuscript. The medical illustrations were provided by Andrew Swift.

REFERENCES

1. Vdand V, Brennan PJ: The genome of *Mycobacterium leprae:* A minimal mycobacterial gene set. *Genome Biol* 2(8):1023, 2001.

2. World Health Organization: *A Guide to Leprosy Control,* 2d ed. Geneva: World Health Organization, 1988.

3. Lumpkin LE III, Cox GF, Wolf JD Jr: Leprosy in five armadillo handlers. *J Am Acad Dermatol* 9:899, 1983.

4. Kluth FC: Leprosy in Texas: A study of occurrence. *Texas State J Med* 51:199, 1955.

5. Ridley DS, Jopling WH: A classification of leprosy for research purposes. *Lepr Rev* 39:19, 1962.

6. Carpenter CM, Miller JN: The bacteriology of leprosy. In Cochrane RG, Davey TF (eds): *Leprosy in Theory and Practice,* 2d ed. Baltimore: Williams & Wilkins, 1964, p 13.

7. Shepard CC: Experimental chemotherapy in leprosy, then and now. *Int J Lepr* 41:307, 1973.

8. Shepard CC: Multiplication of *Mycobacterium leprae* in the foot-pad of the mouse. *Int J Lepr* 30:291, 1962.

9. Kirchheimer WF, Storrs EE: Attempts to establish the armadillo *(Dasypus novemcinctus)* as a model for the study of leprosy: I. Report of lepromatoid leprosy in an experimentally infected armadillo. *Int J Lepr* 39:693, 1971.

10. Harboe M: The immunology of leprosy. In Hastings RC (ed): *Leprosy.* Edinburgh: Churchill Livingstone, 1987, pp 53–87.

11. Seghal VN: Immunology of leprosy: A comprehensive survey. *Int J Dermatol* 28:574, 1989.

12. Hastings RC, Brand PW, Mansfield RE, Ebner JD: Bacterial density in the skin in lepromatous leprosy as related to temperature. *Lepr Rev* 39:71, 1968.

13. Shepard CC: Temperature optimum of *Mycobacterium leprae* in mice. *J Bacteriol* 90:1271, 1965.

14. Pendergast JJ: Ocular leprosy in the United States. *Arch Ophthalmol* 23:112, 1940.

15. Brand PW: Temperature variation in leprosy deformity. *Int J Lepr* 27:1, 1959.

16. Jacobson RR, Trautman JR: Treatment of leprosy with the sulfones: I. Faget's original 22 patients: A thirty year follow-up on sulfone therapy for leprosy. *Int J Lepr* 39:726, 1971.

17. Harrell JD: Ocular leprosy in the Canal Zone. *Int J Lepr Rev* 39:197, 1968.

18. Job CK: Gynecomastia and leprous orchitis. *Int J Lepr* 29:423, 1961.

19. Ridley DS: Bacterial indices. In Cochrane RG, Davey TF (eds): *Leprosy in Theory and Practice.* Baltimore: Williams & Wilkins, 1965, p 620.

20. Cooper CL, Mueller C, Sinchaisri T, et al: Analysis of naturally occurring delayed-type hypersensitivity reactions in leprosy by in situ hybridization. *J Exp Med* 169:1565, 1989.

21. Wemambu SNC, Turk JL, Waters MFR, Rees RJW: Erythema nodosum leprosum: A clinical manifestation of the Arthus phenomenon. *Lancet* 2:933, 1969.

22. Seghal VN: Nerve abscesses in leprosy in northern India. *Lepr Rev* 37:109, 1966.

23. Lictman DM, Swafford AW, Kerr DM: Calcified abscess in the ulnar nerve in a patient with leprosy. *J Bone Joint Surg* 61A:620, 1979.

24. Selby RC: Neurosurgical aspects of leprosy. *Surg Neurol* 2:165, 1974.

25. Sabin TD, Ebner JD: Patterns of sensory loss in lepromatous leprosy. *Int J Lepr* 37:239, 1969.

26. Sabin TD: Neurologic features of lepromatous leprosy. *Am Fam Phys* 4:84, 1971.

27. Job CK, Desikan KV: Pathologic changes and their distribution in peripheral nerves in lepromatous leprosy. *Int J Lepr* 36:257, 1968.

28. Monrad-Krohn GH: *The Neurological Aspect of Leprosy.* Christiana, Norway, Jacob, Dybwad, 1923.

29. Sabin TD, Hackett R, Brand PW: Temperatures along the course of certain nerves affected in leprosy. *Int J Lepr* 42:33, 1974.

30. Kyriskidis MD, Noutsis CG, Robinson-Kyriakidid CA, et al: Autonomic neuropathy in leprosy. *Int J Lepr Other Mycobact Dis* 51:331, 1983.

31. Ramachandran A, Neelan PN: Autonomic neuropathy in leprosy. *Ind J Lepr* 49:277, 1987.

32. Naafs B, Pearso JMH, Baar AJM: A follow-up of nerve lesions in leprosy during and after reaction using motor nerve conduction velocity. *Int J Lepr* 44:188, 1976.

33. Powell CS, Swan LL: Leprosy: Pathologic changes in 50 consecutive necropsies. *Am J Pathol* 31:1131, 1955.

34. Hansen GA: Under sogeiser angaende spedalskhedens arasger tiedels ud forte sammem med forstander Hartwig. *Norske Mag Laegevidensk* 4(suppl):1, 1874.

35. Job CK: Pathology of peripheral nerve lesions in lepromatous leprosy: A light and electron microscopic study. *Int J Lepr* 39:251, 1973.

36. Rambukkana A, Yamada H, Zanazzi , et al: Role of α-dystroglycan as a Schwann cell receptor for *Mycobacterium leprae. Science* 282:2076, 1998.

37. Brophy PJ: Subversion of Schwann cells and the Leper's bell. *Science* 296:862, 1998.

38. Weinstein DE, Freedman VH, Kaplan G: Molecular mechanism of nerve infection in leprosy. *Trends Microbiol* 7(5):185, 1999.

39. Rambukkana A, Zanazzi G, Tapinos N, Salzer JL: Contact-dependent demyelination of *Mycobacterium leprae* in the absence of immune cells. *Science* 296:927, 2002; discussion 1475.

40. Swift T: Neurofibromatosis and leprosy. *J Neurol Neurosurg Psychiatry* 34:743, 1971.

41. Boddingius J: Unstractural and histophysiological studies on the blood-nerve barrier and perineurial barrier in leprosy neuropathy. *Acta Neuropathol (Berl)* 64:282, 1984.

42. Yoshizumi MO, Asbury AK: Intra-axonal bacilli in lepromatous leprosy. *Acta Neuropathol (Berl)* 27:1, 1974.

43. Gibbels E, Henke U, Klingmuller G, Haupt WF: Myelinated and unmyelinated fibers in sural nerve biopsy of a case lepromatous leprosy: A quantitative approach. *Int J Lepr* 55:333, 1987.

44. Jopling WH, Morgan-Hughes JA: Pure neural tuberculoid leprosy. *Br Med J* 2:788, 1965.

45. Jacob M, Mathai R: Diagnostic efficacy of cutaneous nerve biopsy in primary neuritic leprosy. *Int J Lepr Other Mycobact Dis* 56:56, 1988.

46. Uplekar MW, Anita NH: Clinical and histopathological observations on pure neuritic leprosy. *Ind J Lepr* 48:513, 1986.

47. Sheskin J, Magora A, Sagher F: Motor conduction velocity studies in patients with leprosy reaction treated with thalidomide and other drugs. *Int J Lepr* 37:359, 1969.

48. Sohi AS, Kandheri KC, Singh N: Motor nerve conduction studies in leprosy. *Int J Dermatol* 10:151, 1971.

49. Sabin TD: Peripheral neuropathy: The long and the short of it. *Muscle Nerve* 9:711, 1986.

50. Rosenberg RN, Lovelace RE: Mononeuritis multiplex in lepromatous leprosy. *Arch Neurol* 19:310, 1968.

51. Dawson DM, Hallett M, Millender LH: *Entrapment Neuropathies.* Boston: Little Brown, 1983.

52. Asbury AK, Picard EH, Baringer JR: Sensory perineuritis. *Arch Neurol* 26:302, 1972.

53. Faget GH, Pogge RC, Johansen FA, et al: The promin treatment of leprosy, a progress report. *Public Health Rep* 38:1729, 1943.

54. Saqueton AC, Lorinez AL, Vick NA, Homer RD: Dapsone and peripheral motor neuropathy. *Arch Dermatol* 100:214, 1969.

55. Sebille A, Cordoliani G, Raffalli MJ, et al Dapsone-induced neuropathy compounds in Hansen's disease nerve damage: An electrophysiological study in tuberculoid patients. *Int J Lepr Other Mycobact Dis* 55:16, 1987.

56. Nathan CF, Keplan G, Lewis WR, et al: Local and systemic effects of intradermal recombinant interferon in patients with lepromatous leprosy. *New Engl J Med* 315:6, 1986.

57. Hastings RC: Transfer factor as a probe of the immune defect in lepromatous leprosy. *Int J Lepr* 45:281, 1977.

58. Convit J, Aranzaau N, Ulrich M, et al: Immunotherapy with a mixture of *Mycobacterium leprae* and BCG in different forms of leprosy and in Mitsuda-negative contacts. *Int J Lepr* 50:415, 1985.

59. Tio TH: Neural involvement in leprosy: Treatment with intraneural injections of prednisolone. *Lepr Rev* 37:93, 1966.

60. Pandaya JJ, Anita NH: Elective surgical decompression of nerves in leprosy. *Lepr Rev* 49:53, 1978.

61. Enna CD, Brand PW: Peripheral nerve abscess in leprosy. *Lepr Rev* 41:175, 1970.

CHAPTER 24

Infectious Etiologies of Movement Disorders

Alberto J. Espay and Anthony E. Lang

A significant number of infectious etiologies are associated with movement disorders at their onset or some time during the course of the illness. Chorea in Sydenham disease is the classic abnormal involuntary movement associated with infection. At the hypokinetic end of the movement disorders spectrum, sporadic cases of parkinsonism can still complicate viral encephalitides even though the classic form, postencephalitic parkinsonism from Von Economo disease (encephalitis lethargica), is regarded as a nearly extinct disease. Other infectious diseases associated with movement disorders include Whipple's disease, Creutzfeldt-Jakob disease, subacute sclerosing panencephalitis, and acquired immunodeficiency syndrome (AIDS) [either from human immunodeficiency virus (HIV) toxicity or from opportunistic infections such as toxoplasmosis]. Whipple's disease and, to a lesser extent, AIDS are treatable conditions whose recognition is critical for favorable outcome or prolonged survival. Subacute sclerosing panencephalitis and Creutzfeldt-Jakob disease are ultimately fatal, but their identification is important for accurate prognosis and continued research efforts. Antimicrobial and antiemetic agents used to treat central nervous sys-

tem (CNS) infectious diseases and their complications also may cause involuntary movements. Table 24-1 is a comprehensive list of these drugs and the infectious etiologies associated with movement disorders.

▶ SYDENHAM DISEASE

History/Overview

Although it is Thomas Sydenham (1624–1689) on whom the eponymic honor is conferred, credit for recognition of "chorea minor" is given to the Dutch physician Steven Blankaart, who described *Chorea Sancti Viti* (St. Vitus' dance) as a separate nosologic entity in his *Lexicon Medicum* (1696).[1] The firm relationship between this disorder and streptococcal exposure would have to wait until the second part of the last century.[2] Since chorea is but one manifestation of a spectrum that includes tics, dysarthria, several behavioral abnormalities, and gait impairment, the term *Sydenham disease* (SD) has been proposed to replace the widely used *Sydenham's chorea*.

▶ **TABLE 24-1.** INFECTIOUS DISORDERS AND DRUGS ASSOCIATED WITH MOVEMENT DISORDERS

Disorder	Infection	Causative Drugs
Tremor (postural and/or kinetic)	HIV +/− *Toxoplasma gondii* Arboviruses Several infections may nonspecifically increase a physiologic tremor	*Antimicrobial drugs* Ciprofloxacin,[161] imipenem[162] gentamicin,[163] trimethoprim-sulfamethoxazole,[140,157] and pentavalent antimonials[164]*
Parkinsonism	HIV +/− *Toxoplasma gondii* Influenza virus Arboviruses Enteroviruses Measles virus Varicella-zoster virus Epstein-Barr virus *Mycoplasma pneumoniae* *Taenia solium* cysts Prions	*Antifungal drug* Amphotericin B[153]* *Antiemetics* *Phenothiazines:* Thiethylperazine,[165] prochlorperazine[166] *Substituted benzamides:* Metoclopramide,[154,167] sulpiride,[168] tiapride,[169] clebopride,[170] cisapride[171,172]
Chorea, athetosis, and/or hemiballism	Group A streptococcus (SD) HIV and *Toxoplasma gondii*, *Mycoplasma pneumoniae*, *Mycobacterium tuberculosis*, or *Treponema pallidum* *Treponema pallidum* (alone) CMV, VZV, HSV Epstein-Barr virus Influenza virus Measles and rubella viruses Enteroviruses Paramyxovirus (mumps) *Plasmodium falciparum* *Taenia solium* cysts *Mycoplasma pneumoniae* *Legionella* spp. Prions	*Antimicrobial drugs* Cyclizine[173] Pentamidine (causing hypoglycemia in AIDS patients)[174] Sulfasalazine[175] *Antiemetics* Metoclopramide[176] *Phenothiazines* are reported to cause choreoathetosis
Myoclonus	HIV +/− herpes zoster virus HIV + JC virus encephalitis Lyme disease Other encephalitides can result in multifocal myoclonus Measles virus (SSPE) *Schistosoma mansoni* Prions	*Antimicrobial drugs* Cefmetazole (cephalosporin),[177] pefloxacin (fluoroquinolone),[178] penicillin,[179] imipenem,[180] and isoniazid[181]
Tics	Herpes simplex virus Group A streptococcus	All *phenothiazines* can induce tardive tics
Dystonia	HIV +/− *Toxoplasma gondii* *Taenia solium* cysts *Mycoplasma pneumoniae*	All *phenothiazines* and *substituted benzamides* are capable of causing dystonia and/or akathisia
Akathisia	HIV and toxoplasmosis	

NOTE: CMV = cytomegalovirus; VZV = varicella-zoster virus; HSV = herpes simplex virus; SSPE = subacute sclerosis panencephalitis; SD = Sydenham disease.
*Pentavalent antimonials are first-line drugs in the treatment of leishmaniasis and are used often with amphotericin B, the second-line agent of choice for that condition.

Epidemiology

Chorea is a component of the spectrum of rheumatic fever (RF) that constitutes SD. The acute phase of RF, which develops soon after a streptococcal infection, is characterized by the common signs of arthritis and carditis, whereas chorea and neurobehavioral symptoms are a delayed and less common occurrence.[3,4] Chorea appears in one-fourth of affected children (usually younger than age 15) diagnosed with RF, on average 6 months after the infection, resulting in an estimated incidence of 0.2 to 0.8 cases of SD per 100,000 individuals. Males and females are equally affected, although after age 10, females predominate. RF is a significant public health problem in developing countries, where the prevalence may reach 20 per 1000 children 12 to 14 years of age (Soweto, South Africa).[5] In industrialized nations there has been a steady decline in the rate of RF over the second half of the twentieth century; more recently, it has been restricted to sporadic outbreaks that, interestingly, have occurred among children of high- to middle-income families.[6] Such decline, often attributed to the use of prophylactic penicillin therapy, has not resulted from a reduction in the incidence of streptococcal pharyngitis but rather from the disappearance of rheumatogenic strains in developed countries. The adult form of RF manifests primarily with arthritis instead of with chorea or other neurobehavioral symptoms. Worldwide, SD remains the most common cause of acute chorea among children.

Pathophysiology and Pathogenesis

SD may be a component or the sole manifestation of RF and most likely represents a self-limited autoimmune response to an infection with group A β-hemolytic streptococcus (GABHS) that typically causes pharyngitis. It is important to note that extrapharyngeal infections with group A streptococci, notably pyodermas, do not cause SD or other features of RF (i.e., they are nephritogenic strains associated with acute glomerulonephritis and not rheumatogenic ones).[3] It follows that SD-causing strains are primarily tropic for the throat rather than the skin. However, not all pharyngeal GABHS infections are capable of causing RF. In fact, most serotypes of group A streptococci are not associated with rheumatic fever. True rheumatogenic strains are limited to certain M serotypes, most commonly M5. The streptococcal M protein serves as an important antigen against which antistreptococcal antibodies are produced during GABHS infections. Because of the proposed shared homology between the M protein and the basal ganglia, these M type–specific antibodies are believed to cross-react with epitopes on neurons of the basal ganglia[7] in the process of molecular mimicry, causing the motor and behavioral deficits characteristic of SD. Presumably the same type of antibody cross-reaction with cardiac and synovial tissues results in rheumatic carditis and arthritis, respectively. Unfortunately, serologic evidence supporting a recent streptococcal infection may be absent in about a third of patients with SD because this is a relatively late manifestation of RF. On an experimental basis, the monoclonal antibody D8/17, which reacts with epitopes expressed on B-lymphocytes, has been consistently present in patients with acute RF and exhibits a transient increase above an already high baseline during rheumatic exacerbations.[8,9]

Interestingly, childhood-onset obsessive-compulsive disorder and Tourette's syndrome also have B cells expressing the D8/17 antigen, whereas these are absent in poststreptococcal glomerulonephritis and other autoimmune diseases.[10,11] It is unclear how the antigen D8/17 is related to the disease process, but its presence is now considered a marker for genetic susceptibility to RF and pediatric autoimmune neuropsychiatric disorders associated with streptococcal infection (PANDAS) (see later). The pathologic end result of the poststreptococcal process is diffuse small-vessel vasculitis and widespread cell loss in the basal ganglia and frontal and temporal cortices, according to the scant autopsy literature.[12,13]

Clinical Features

Chorea refers to random, erratic, purposeless movements that occur in any body part. The first suspicion of chorea arises when parents describe unprecedented "fidgetiness" and inattention in their affected child. Although the movements are often bilateral, chorea may be asymmetric, and up to 20 percent of patients have been described with pure unilateral involvement (hemichorea and, less commonly, hemiballism). The motor impersistence of chorea can be appreciated in the tongue during volitional protrusion (*chameleon* or *darting tongue*) and the hands in attempting to maintain a firm grip (*milkmaid grip*). The ability to draw and write is compromised as a result (Fig. 24-1). In addition to chorea, the neurologic examination may show nonspecific deficits such as dysarthria with reduction in verbal output, hypometric saccades, decreased muscle tone, and pendular muscle stretch reflexes (hung-up reflexes).[4] The increased emotional lability of these individuals is part of the neurobehavioral spectrum of the disorder, which includes obsessive-compulsive disorder, attention deficit, and anxiety. These symptoms develop within a few weeks of the onset of the abnormal movements and wax and wane in parallel with the motor manifestations. Obsessive-compulsive symptoms may be present in as many as 70 percent of patients with SD within the first 2 months of illness but are absent in acute RF without chorea.[14] The diverse array of neurologic and behavioral symptoms has supported the argument that SD should be considered a form of childhood autoimmune neuropsychiatric disorder, as discussed below (see "Differential Diagnosis"). Regardless of treatment, the course of the illness is classically restricted to 4 to 6 weeks, but "full" remission (which often implies resolution of the chorea and behavioral symptoms with mild residual tremor or clumsiness) may take up to 6 months. Approximately 20 percent of patients will have at least one recurrence.[15] Although the average time between symptomatic episodes has not been defined, recurrences may be seen at intervals as short as 4 months apart.[16] Multiple recurrences due to

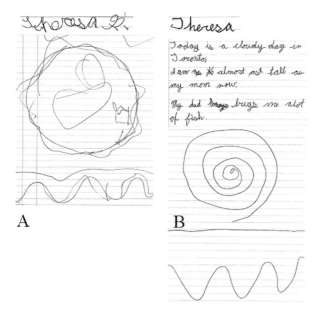

A   B

Figure 24-1. Writing in Sydenham disease. Handwriting and drawing examples from an 11-year-old girl who had gradual onset of right arm and leg chorea 8 months after a documented episode of GABHS pharyngitis. These samples were obtained 2 weeks (*A*) and 3 months (*B*) after onset of the movement disorder. The remarkably improved handwriting shown in *B,* regarded as normal by both the patient and her mother, took place while she was on concurrent treatment with valproic acid (for 10 weeks) and haloperidol (2 weeks, added given insufficient control with valproate). Both medications subsequently were tapered and withdrawn without recurrence.

the same presumed immunologic pathophysiology are extremely rare and need to be differentiated from the chorea complicating pregnancy and contraceptive use in adult women (see below).

Diagnosis

There are two major components of the diagnostic strategy for SD: ascertainment of a preceding infection with GABHS and the search for other associated disorder(s) supporting the diagnosis of RF (Table 24-2). Echocardiography is a high-yield procedure for the latter, given the frequency of concurrent silent carditis, which may be as common as overt carditis.[17] The most widely available test, although likely the least sensitive and specific, is a throat culture for group A streptococcus. Serology is more reliable because several antibodies can be detected and quantified in serum. Antistreptolysin-O (ASO) is measurable immediately following the onset of the infection, but titers decrease rapidly, often to a nondetectable range prior to the onset of chorea or other SD-related symptoms. In only 65 percent of cases of symptomatic SD are ASO titers elevated. Anti-DNase B antibodies are present for several weeks after the

GABHS infection and therefore often are elevated when the ASO titers have normalized, although these too may have declined by the time that symptoms of SD arise. The recent report that anti–basal ganglia antibodies (ABGAs) were detected by Western immunoblotting in all acute SD patients and nearly 70 percent of those with persistent disease has suggested that this test may be more sensitive than the ASO titer.[18] Given the high prevalence of otherwise uncomplicated GABHS infections in the pediatric population, the combined measurement of ASO, anti-DNase, and ABGA may increase the sensitivity and specificity of diagnosis. Obviously, when other manifestations of RF such as carditis and/or migratory polyarthritis are present in addition to positive serology, the diagnosis of SD can be established with confidence. The American Heart Association (AHA) in the updated 1992 version of the Jones criteria, however, accepts that "chorea may occur as the only manifestation of rheumatic fever."[19] Magnetic resonance imaging (MRI) of the brain may, in some cases, demonstrate transient hyperintensity in, and enlargement of, the basal ganglia during choreic bouts[20,21] (Fig. 24-2). Unfortunately, significant overlap in basal ganglia size between patients and controls exists.

Differential Diagnosis

Systemic lupus erythematosus (SLE) is the most common systemic cause of chorea that may be misinterpreted as SD. Since this presentation is often associated with a "secondary" antiphospholipid antibody syn-

▶ **TABLE 24-2.** REVISED JONES CRITERIA FOR RHEUMATIC FEVER[19] APPLIED TO THE DIAGNOSIS OF SYDENHAM DISEASE (BOTH A AND B ARE REQUIRED FOR DIAGNOSIS)

A. Chorea or other neurobehavioral deficits	*Or two of the following* ("minor" manifestations)
	Arthralgia
And one of the following:	Fever
Carditis*	Prolonged P/R interval
Polyarthritis	Acute phase reactants
Erythema marginatum	Increased ESR
Subcutaneous nodules	Increased CRP

B. Evidence of preceding streptococcal infection
Increased antistreptolysin (ASO) titers (>200 IU/ml)
Increased anti-DNase B titers (>300 IU/ml)
Increased antihyaluronidase and antistreptokinase titers
Positive throat culture for GABHS
M protein serotype determination (experimental)

*Echocardiography is recommended for all suspected SD cases because subclinical carditis, which would confirm the diagnosis of rheumatic fever, is often a coexisting condition. Anti-basal ganglia antibodies (ABGAs) by ELISA[182] have been found in acute and, to a lesser extent, persistent SD but are not included in the laboratory-based criteria because their role in SD pathology (autoimmune hypothesis) awaits confirmation (ESR = erythrocyte sedimentation rate; CRP = C-reactive protein).

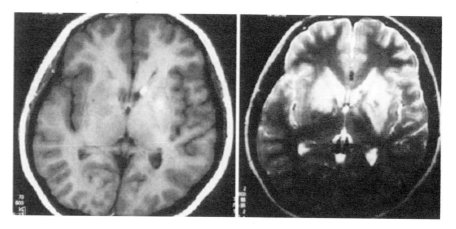

Figure 24-2. MRI in Sydenham disease. T_1-weighted MRI sequence (*left*) demonstrates swelling of the caudate nucleus and putamen, especially on the right. T_2-weighted sequence (*right*) shows increased signal intensity in the putamen, globus pallidus, and head of the caudate nucleus bilaterally. Three months later the T_1W study demonstrated resolution of the swelling but continued hyperintensity in the putamen, globus pallidus, and head of the caudate nuclei (not shown). *(Used with permission from Ikuta N et al: High-signal basal ganglia on T_1-weighted images in a patient with Sydenham's chorea. Neuroradiology 40:659, 1998.)*

drome, any atypical case of suspected SD should be screened for lupus anticoagulant (LA) and anticardiolipin (aCL) antibody, as well as anti-DNA antinuclear antibodies. The pathogenesis of these disorders is unknown, but hypercoagulability may play a role because another hypercoagulable disorder, polycythemia vera, also may cause chorea. Other factors such as hormonal status also play an important yet poorly understood role. Women of reproductive age may develop chorea during pregnancy (*chorea gravidarum*) and during the use of estrogen-containing oral contraceptives, interestingly in a higher proportion in those with either a past history of SD or SLE (sometimes previously undiagnosed) and aCL antibodies. The contraceptive-related chorea begins months after drug initiation and ends within weeks of its withdrawal, whereas chorea gravidarum tends to appear in the first trimester of pregnancy and ceases in 30 percent before delivery and within a few days thereafter in the remainder.[22] Other drugs with potential for causing choreiform movements include stimulants (such as amphetamines), antiepileptic agents (phenytoin and carbamazepine), tricyclic antidepressants, and neuroleptics. Two endocrinopathies cause choreiform movements: hyperthyroidism and hypoparathyroidism. Acute herpes simplex virus (HSV) encephalitis,[23] Lyme disease,[24] *Mycoplasma pneumoniae* infection,[25] and AIDS rarely cause chorea in the pediatric population. Although usually a more chronic condition, Wilson's disease should be considered in any child or young adult presenting with chorea given the therapeutic implications.

Treatment

Given the usual short-lived disease course and the relatively mild restriction in activities of daily living that the chorea and other manifestations tend to impose on the affected child, treatment of the chorea is often discouraged. When either severity or persistence of symptoms becomes disabling, therapy with haloperidol can be initiated.[26] Doses as low as 0.5 mg twice per day may decrease the chorea significantly without a substantial incidence of side effects. The usual regimen consists of 1.5 to 3 mg twice per day given over 4 to 6 weeks to limit the appearance of tardive side effects. The drug is only restarted if and when chorea returns. Valproic acid has been used successfully without significant side effects in doses of 15 to 25 mg/kg per day given in a twice-daily schedule. Valproic acid is considered by some as the current drug of choice given its comparatively favorable side-effect profile. The evidence for its efficacy in the literature is largely anecdotal.[27–30] Small observational studies have suggested that carbamazepine (15 to 20 mg/kg per day divided in two doses) can provide similar benefit to valproic acid.[31,32] Tetrabenazine can be considered in patients requiring longer-term treatment. Given the promising outcome of a small randomized, placebo-controlled trial of intravenous immunoglobulin (IVIg) and plasma exchange in children with another poststreptococcal, presumably autoimmune, disorder causing exacerbations of tics and obsessive-compulsive disorder (see PANDAS below),[33] IVIg and plasma exchange may become an option for severe refractory SD in the future. Thus far, however, the demonstration of a clear autoimmune etiology in SD, akin to that of myasthenia gravis, awaits further evidence. Finally, in adults in whom a recurrence of SD is considered in the differential diagnosis of later-onset chorea, discontinuation of oral contraceptives and other possible causative medications should be considered before initiating any of the preceding symptomatic treatments.

Complications

Residual mild tremor and impairment of fine motor control may persist beyond the usual 6-month resolution period. Persistent SD (defined as chorea lasting 2 or more years despite adequate treatment with neuroleptics and/or valproic acid) is associated with female gender and comorbid carditis.[34] Chorea may occur in as many as 50 percent of those who require cardiac surgery for management of rheumatic valvular disease. Neither the severity of chorea nor the presence of a hemichoreic distribution predicts persistence of symptoms. As emphasized earlier, recurrences of chorea are likely in patients with a history of SD during pregnancy, exposure to oral contraceptives, or GABHS reinfection.[35] Presumably the mechanism whereby hormonal triggers or drugs precipitate chorea in these patients differs from the autoimmune pathogenesis postulated for those whose recurrence is due to GABHS reinfection. The risk of chorea from oral contraceptives is an alarming 25 percent in women who have had SD.

Prevention

SD is the classic disorder in which primary prevention can be accomplished by antistreptococcal treatment as soon as a GABHS tonsillitis and/or pharyngitis has been confirmed. Oral penicillin V 2 g per day divided in two doses for 10 days is recommended. This regimen has proven efficacy, tolerability, cost-effectiveness, and absence of reported resistant organisms.[36] Children who have had an attack of rheumatic chorea or carditis are at very high risk of developing recurrences after subsequent pharyngitides and need a continuous antimicrobial drug regimen (secondary prevention) to prevent recurrences, particularly to prevent the complication of late carditis. For this group, penicillin G benzathine given intramuscularly at a dose of 1.2 million IU per month is preferred over 10-day oral penicillin largely because of compliance issues. The length of prophylaxis is subject to local conditions of endemicity, but a 5-year course has been suggested as adequate.[37] Cephalosporins, erythromycin, and amoxicillin-clavulanate are alternatives for prophylaxis in penicillin-allergic individuals.

Other Poststreptococcal Complications Possibly Related to SD

Pediatric autoimmune neuropsychiatric disorders associated with streptococcal infection (PANDAS) is a disorder proposed to be analogous in pathogenesis to SD (immunologic complication of streptococcal infection) in which the predominant symptoms are motor tics and obsessive-compulsive disorder, clinically indistinguishable from Tourette's syndrome.[38] A recent report demonstrating an association between Tourette's syndrome and GABHS infections (ABGA and increased ASO titers, as demonstrated in SD)[39] has increased support for the hypothesis that PANDAS and SD are ends of the same nosologic spectrum, as suspected clinically by the overlapping symptoms of tics and obsessive-compulsive disorder in the two disorders. The diagnosis of PANDAS has been applied to the occurrence of neurobehavioral symptoms in addition to, or instead of, chorea that appears or episodically exacerbates in close relationship to GABHS infections in prepubertal children. However, the status of PANDAS as a distinct nosological entity remains uncertain given the common occurrence of both GABHS infections and otherwise typical Tourette's syndrome in the general population. The tentative pathophysiology is centered on a similar cross-reactive antibody-mediated inflammation of the basal ganglia as in SD that occurs in genetically susceptible individuals. Application of morphometric imaging techniques has shown significantly greater average sizes of the caudate, putamen, and globus pallidus in children with SD[20] and poststreptococcal obsessive-compulsive disorder and tics.[40] With currently available evidence, however, SD and PANDAS still remain clinically separable conditions[41] (Table 24-3). It is unclear whether a given genetic predisposition is required for the development of a poststreptococcal neurobehavioral disorder and/or for its ultimate clinical presentation (i.e., SD versus PANDAS versus PSADEM; see below).

Poststreptococcal acute disseminated encephalomyelitis (PSADEM) is a recently described form of acute disseminated encephalomyelitis (ADEM) in children following an acute streptococcal pharyngitis (mean latency of 12 days) with prominent involvement of the basal ganglia manifesting with extrapyramidal and behavioral symptomatology and accompanied by the presence of anti–basal ganglia antibodies.[42] PSADEM is readily distinguished clinically from SD and PANDAS by its acute onset and the presence of dystonia or rigidity rather than chorea or tics. The disease may lead to somnolence, stupor, and coma but is considered to be largely monophasic, with recurrence triggered by a repeat GABHS pharyngitis reported in only 2 of 10 patients. Most children make a complete recovery, especially rapid, after a 3-day course of intravenous methylprednisolone. Hyperintensity of the caudate and putamen is observed on T_2-weighted brain MRI sequences (see Fig. 24-3).

▶ POSTENCEPHALITIC PARKINSONISM

History and Overview

Although it has been proposed that the pandemic of von Economo's disease ("sleeping sickness," 1917–1927)

▶ **TABLE 24-3.** SIMILARITIES AND DIFFERENCES BETWEEN SD AND PANDAS

Similarities	Differences
1. Symptom exacerbations are often (PANDAS) or always (SD) correlated with GABHS infections	1. Manifestations of rheumatic fever such as carditis or polyarthritis are exclusionary in PANDAS
2. Presence of anti-basal ganglia antibodies in SD and PANDAS (and Tourette syndrome)	2. Presentation is predominantly psychiatric in PANDAS (with tics) and motor in SD (chorea)
3. Presence of monoclonal antibody D8/17 in RF as well as PANDAS, childhood-onset obsessive-compulsive disorder, and Tourette syndrome	3. Antibiotic prophylaxis is effective in SD but unproven in PANDAS[183]
4. Common neurobehavioral symptoms (anxiety, obsessive-compulsive behavior, hyperactivity, emotional lability)	4. Course is often chronic ("sawtooth") in PANDAS but self-limited in SD (controversial)
5. Transient hyperintensity in, and enlargement of, the basal ganglia (inconsistent; other areas may be involved in SD)	

and its major sequela, postencephalitic parkinsonism, was caused by influenza, the viral etiology was never confirmed. Despite the fact that pandemic-related patients with parkinsonism are no longer seen, sporadic

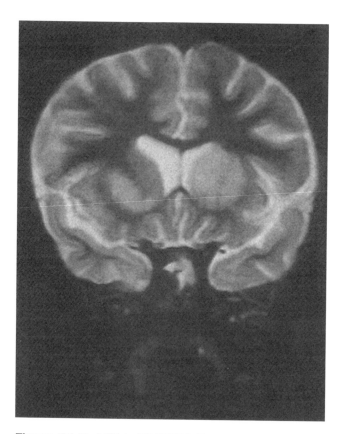

Figure 24-3. MRI in PSADEM. T_2-weighted coronal MRI sequence demonstrates lesions involving the left caudate and bilateral putamen nuclei. *(Used with permission from Dale RC, et al: Poststreptococcal acute disseminated encephalomyelitis with basal ganglia involvement and auto-reactive antibasal ganglia antibodies. Ann Neurol 50:588, 2001.)*

cases with the nosologic entity of encephalitis lethargica continue to be recognized. Several primary viral encephalitides have been associated with parkinsonism, including influenza, arboviruses, enteroviruses, varicella-zoster virus, and measles virus. Postencephalitic parkinsonism caused by neurotropic viruses and its clinical presentations will be compared with those seen during the pandemic of von Economo.[43]

Epidemiology

After becoming the most common form of parkinsonism in the 1920s and 1930s, postencephalitic parkinsonism has steadily declined in incidence. Currently, not only are the cases reported few in number, but the condition lacks the highly contagious nature attached to the original pandemic form. For instance, despite thousands of new cases of Japanese encephalitis annually (the most common arthropod-borne human encephalitis worldwide), postencephalitic parkinsonism following this infection remains a rare event. As with other neurotropic viruses, particularly the less common but greatly feared eastern equine encephalitis, postencephalitic parkinsonism is a potential but quite uncommon complication. St. Louis encephalitis virus, enteroviruses (especially coxsackie B2), measles, and varicella-zoster virus have been associated with clinical features compatible with the classic descriptions of encephalitis lethargica. For a list of postencephalitic and other infectious causes of parkinsonism, see Table 24-1.

Pathophysiology and Pathogenesis

The akinetic-rigid syndrome of postencephalitic parkinsonism results from preferential inflammatory involvement of the gray matter of the cerebral peduncles in the midbrain, which damages the substantia nigra and relatively spares other regions of the basal ganglia. Although Japanese encephalitis virus equally may involve the substantia nigra and the basal ganglia and thalamus, no full parkinsonian syndrome has been reported even with combined lesions of the substantia nigra and thalamus.[44] In postencephalitic parkinsonism, perivascular lymphocytic infiltration with diffuse neuronal loss and astrocytic reaction is observed in the brain stem and, to a lesser extent, in the spinal cord and cerebral cortex. Neurofibrillary tangles (NFTs) without Lewy bodies or senile plaques are widespread in the brain but predominate in the substantia nigra.[45] The presence of these tau-positive neural and glial fibrillary tangles is indistinguishable from that of those found in such tauopathies as progressive supranuclear palsy (PSP) and parkinsonism-dementia complex of Guam,[46] suggesting a possible common pathogenesis. The mechanism responsible for the prolonged latency between acute encephalitis and clinical parkinsonism that was characteristic of most patients with postencephalitic parkinsonism following encephalitis lethargica is not understood.

Clinical Features

Two distinct phases are recognized in the development of the classic form of postencephalitic parkinsonism: the acute encephalitic phase and the chronic parkinsonian phase. The acute phase classically was divided into three syndromes according to their main clinical features: *somnolent ophthalmoplegic*, *hyperkinetic* (acute catatonic schizophrenia with motor restlessness and visual hallucinations), and *amyostatic akinetic* [catalepsy ("waxy flexibility") and mutism]. The somnolent-ophthalmoplegic form is considered the most characteristic of encephalitis lethargica and consisted of alterations in the level of consciousness with excessive sleepiness and stupor (lethargica), as well as oculomotor deficits, including external ophthalmoplegia, nystagmus, oculogyric crises, and ptosis. Vertical supranuclear gaze palsy and eyelid-opening apraxia also were recognized.[47] The oculogyric crises were the hallmarks of von Economo postencephalitic parkinsonism. They were described as "tonic visual convulsions, occurring in fits and generally lasting only a few minutes, during which the patients as a rule look upwards and sideways."[43] The amyostatic-akinetic state was the acute equivalent of the later-appearing parkinsonism, which developed following a latency measured in months or even years after the acute encephalitic illness of von Economo. Other neurologic deficits observed in the classic and, to a lesser extent, recent forms of postencephalitic parkinsonism include dysarthria and palilalia, cervical and facial dystonia (particularly blepharospasm and jaw-opening dystonia), motor tics, and behavioral disorders (obsessive-compulsive disorder, disinhibition). Tachypnea and erratic breathing seem to be as common as excessive sleepiness or sleep-wake-cycle disruptions and

are the usual manifestations of brain stem and hypothalamic involvement, respectively.[48] The entire classic presentation can still be recognized today, albeit rarely. Once the deficits are established, the clinical course is considered to be largely nonprogressive, although late-stage deterioration is not uncommon. From the original cohort of von Economo's encephalitis, one-third died in the acute phase, another third survived with chronic disability, and the remainder apparently recovered, although many of these later developed postencephalitic parkinsonism with latencies as long as over 20 years. It also was not uncommon to see patients with classic features of postencephalitic parkinsonism (including oculogyric crises) who lacked a history of previous encephalitis.

The more recent cases of postencephalitic parkinsonism differ from those due to Von Economo's encephalitis mainly by the shorter latency of parkinsonian deficits, the less common occurrence of oculogyric crises, and the gradual improvement rather than continued deterioration after the initial viral encephalitis.[49] A summary of the published cases in which there has been clear documentation of encephalitis preceding parkinsonism and where there is predominant nigral involvement is presented in Table 24-4. Other rare encephalitides that preferentially affect the basal ganglia and/or thalami while sparing the substantia nigra are eastern equine encephalitis,[50] measles,[51] mumps,[52] and echovirus 25 infection (which has been associated with hemichorea instead of parkinsonism).[53]

Diagnosis

The diagnosis of encephalitis lethargica is predominantly clinical. Howard and Lees[48] proposed that seven clinical features associated with an acute or subacute encephalitic illness be used as major criteria: (1) signs of basal ganglia involvement, (2) oculogyric crisis, (3) ophthalmoplegia, (4) obsessive-compulsive behavior, (5) akinetic mutism, (6) central respiratory abnormalities, and (7) somnolence and/or sleep inversion. In the acute phase, cerebrospinal fluid (CSF) studies are crucial in supporting a viral etiology of the encephalitic process. For a detailed approach to diagnosing each specific viral agent, the reader is referred to Chapter 6 on viral encephalitis. Often a specific infectious etiology is not established, and only a mild lymphocytic pleocytosis or oligoclonal IgG banding will suggest the viral encephalitic process. Bilateral substantia nigra hyperintensities on T_2-weighted and fluid-attenuated inversion recovery (FLAIR) MRI sequences have been described in patients with parkinsonism occurring within days of the acute encephalitic illness[54,55] (Fig. 24-4). Lesions to the lentiform nuclei are documented occasionally (Fig. 24-5). In cases of postencephalitic parkin-

▶ **TABLE 24-4.** VIRAL ENCEPHALITIS WITH PREDOMINANT INVOLVEMENT OF SUBSTANTIA NIGRA (LATENCY OF PARKINSONISM RANGED BETWEEN 2 AND 20 DAYS)

Virus	Parkinsonian Features	Other Features	Outcome
Japanese B (5 patients, ages 7–16 years)[44]	Masklike face, bradykinesia, resting tremor, rigidity, sialorrhea, and postural instability	Restricted eye movements, opsoclonus, upbeating nystagmus	Complete recovery in 3/5 at 1-year follow-up, "substantial" recovery in 2/5 after 2 months from regaining consciousness
St. Louis (2 patients, ages 21 and 37 years)[184]	Postural tremor	Ataxia, absent gag, spasticity, bilateral Babinski	Complete recovery in 4 weeks
St. Louis (2 of 11 patients from epidemic in Dallas, Texas)[185]	Tremor in one patient	Ataxia of gait in one, confusion and paraparesis in the other	Complete recovery in one patient, residual paraparesis in the other (unclear follow-up)
Coxsackie B3 (21-year-old man)[55]	Cogwheel rigidity, catatonia, akinetic mutism, sialorrhea, hyperhidrosis	"Few" oculogyric crises, gait and limb ataxia, dysarthria	Continued but milder parkinsonism and less SN intensity on MRI after 50 days
Coxsackie B4 (33-year-old immunosuppressed woman)[186]	Cogwheel rigidity	Hypereflexia, ankle clonus, marked dysarthria, equivocal Babinski	Death from pneumonia, anasarca, deep venous thrombosis, and ventricular fibrillation
Post-measles vaccination (5-year-old boy)[187]	Bradykinesia, rigidity, inability to walk	Severe dysarthria, totally dependent on help for feeding and hygiene	Still moderate rigidity and mild bradykinesia with little dysarthria and hypomimia after 2 years
No virus identified (33-year-old woman)[54]	Bradykinesia and cogwheel rigidity, coarse tremor in the tongue, lips, and upper limbs	Dysarthria, ophthalmoplegia (no further details provided)	Almost full recovery by 3 months, "except facial bradykinesia"
No virus identified (21-year-old man)[188]	Bradykinesia, rigidity, resting and postural tremor, hypomimia	Dysarthria, dystonia in upper and lower limb, akathisia	Complete recovery in 3 weeks

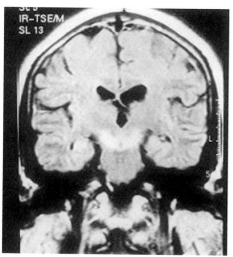 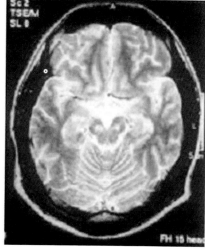

Figure 24-4. MRI in PEP. T_1-weighted coronal (*left*) and T_2-weighted axial (*right*) MRIs demonstrating hyperintensity within the substantia nigra. (*Used with permission from Savant CS, et al: Substantia nigra lesions in viral encephalitis. Mov Disord 18:213, 2003.*)

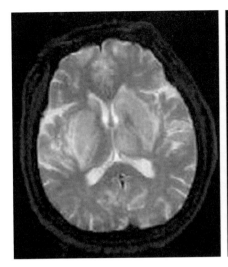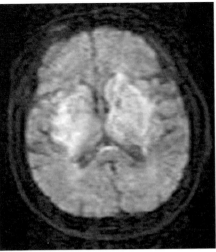

Figure 24-5. MRI in presumed viral encephalitis with parkinsonism as a major sequela. T_2-weighted (*left*) and FLAIR (*right*) axial MRI sequences obtained from a 72-year-old woman within 48 hours of rapid onset of ataxia, dysarthria, right facial paresis, and reduced level of consciousness. There is significant edema in the caudate nuclei and putamen bilaterally, as well as the left thalamus. Her initial CSF studies showed mild lymphocytic pleocytosis. She underwent a 2-week treatment with multiple antiviral and antibiotic agents. Her clinical condition improved within 1 month, but severe gait difficulties persisted, including gait ignition failure, short steps with hesitation and festination, freezing, and postural instability. A 3-month MRI follow-up study showed resolution of edema and mild to moderate third ventricular enlargement secondary to parenchymal atrophy.

sonism following presumed encephalitis lethargica, positron-emission tomography (PET) has demonstrated increased glucose metabolism in the putamen and lack of the typical anteroposterior putaminal gradient on [^{18}F]fluorodopa seen in idiopathic Parkinson's disease (IPD),[56] suggesting a more diffuse involvement of the substantia nigra pars compacta than that of IPD.

Differential Diagnosis

Oculogyric crises have been considered pathognomonic of the acute and chronic phases of encephalitis lethargica but in fact may occur as an idiosyncratic reaction to certain drugs, especially metoclopramide and phenothiazines. Moreover, the induction of acute dystonic reactions or neuroleptic malignant syndrome by these drugs may "superficially" mimic postencephalitic parkinsonism.[48] Herpes simplex virus encephalitis with behavioral disturbances and confusional states preceding coma may resemble encephalitis lethargica. However, the extrapyramidal features, oculogyric crises, and respiratory disturbances rarely are present during the course of herpes simplex virus encephalitis. The pathologic and clinical similarities (especially supranuclear gaze palsy and eyelid apraxia) between postencephalitic parkinsonism and progressive supranuclear palsy has led to the suggestion that progressive supranuclear palsy may have been missed among presumed cases of postencephalitic parkinsonism prior to its formal description in 1963.[57] In patients with supranuclear gaze palsy,

progressive supranuclear palsy is best distinguished from postencephalitic parkinsonism by the absence of a preceding encephalitic illness, the presence of early falls, and its inexorably progressive course.[47]

Treatment and Complications

Symptomatic benefit is often obtained from therapy with low-dose levodopa or a dopamine agonist given the relative preservation of the postsynaptic striatal neurons.[48,58] The main difficulty in managing postencephalitic parkinsonism is the very narrow therapeutic window with frequent development of drug-related motor and psychiatric complications such as dyskinesias and hallucinations. Methylprednisolone has been used successfully in the acute phase of presumed encephalitis lethargica.[59]

▶ WHIPPLE'S DISEASE

History/Overview

The pathologist George Hoyt Whipple in 1907 described a 36-year-old medical missionary with episodes of arthritis that were followed, during a 5-year course, by diarrhea, abdominal pain, increased skin pigmentation, fever, and weight loss and in whom prominent deposition of fat within the intestinal mucosa and mesenteric lymph nodes was observed on autopsy.[60] He therefore suggested the name "intestinal lipodystrophy" to indicate the possible derangement of fat metabolism believed to cause the disorder. The gastrointestinal symptoms were later found to occur primarily from malabsorption, and the causative agent was aptly named *Tropheryma* (from the Greek *trophi*, meaning "nourishment," and *eryma*, meaning "barriers").[61] It is now clear that any organ system can be affected, including the heart, lungs, skin, joints, and CNS. Despite its relative rarity in neurology, the importance of this disease resides in the challenges in establishing an accurate diagnosis, its potential treatability, and the fatal outcome that occurs without treatment.

Epidemiology

Whipple's disease occurs in about 1 in 100,000 people, of whom only 5 to 10 percent develop CNS involvement as the initial or predominant manifestation. Its rarity is the main reason that Whipple's disease is rarely considered in the absence of gastrointestinal symptoms. The clear male preponderance of 8:1 has not been explained but may be related to work or environmental exposures because many affected patients are farmers, construction workers, and machinists. Most reported patients are Caucasians, but the overall number of cases in the literature is too low to ascertain any racial susceptibility.

Pathophysiology and Pathogenesis

Tropheryma whippelii is an aerobic gram-positive, argyrophilic, rod-shaped actinomycete that may be either a commensal ubiquitous organism or an environmental pathogen present in sewage water.[62,63] In fact, it may be a rare member of the normal microbial flora, as judged by its presence in saliva in 35 percent of healthy subjects,[64] in 15 percent of biopsy specimens from elective gastrointestinal surgeries, and by the detection of bacillus-specific IgG antibodies in almost 75 percent of unaffected individuals.[65] The term *asymptomatic carrier state* is now used when referring to the relatively large group of normal individuals with positive *T. whippelii* polymerase chain reaction (PCR) in saliva or stools.[66] The pathogenicity is restricted to a small proportion of those presumably exposed to strains of different virulence or as yet unidentified genetic susceptibility factors. The tropism of *T. whippelii* for the gray matter, although with apparent little specificity, accounts for the varied neurologic presentations (discussed below). Besides the current certainty that humans are the only known host for the disease, little is known of its occurrence in nature, its mode of transmission to humans, the mechanism of disease production, or even whether the same actinomycete is responsible for the multisystemic manifestations of Whipple's disease.

Clinical Features

Extraintestinal Whipple's disease may present exclusively (5 percent) or at least concomitantly (up to 43 percent) with neurologic deficits.[67] The pathognomonic presentation is that of oculomasticatory myorhythmia,[68] which consists of rhythmic myoclonic movements of the tongue, mandible, and occasionally other skeletal muscles synchronized with convergent-divergent pendular nystagmus oscillating at about 1 Hz (oculofacial-*skeletal* myorhythmia[69]). These rhythmic movements may occur in one limb in isolation (limb myorhythmia or rhythmic myoclonus).[70] Because many patients do not develop these classic abnormalities, careful motor examination and evaluation of vertical saccades are the most important aspects of the neurologic examination. A common presentation is that of parkinsonism associated with abnormal vertical gaze, features that could be confused with progressive supranuclear palsy. Careful assessment of saccades may show mild restrictions in vertical gaze, correcting with oculocephalic maneuvers, or slow and hypometric ocular movements without restriction in their range.[71,72] Although supranuclear ophthalmoparesis may occur in the absence of oculomasticatory myorhythmia, when the latter is present, a supranuclear vertical gaze palsy is always obvious clinically.[69] In patients lacking the oculomasticatory myorhythmia, a diagnostic triad of skeletal rhythmic myoclonus, dementia, and ophthalmoplegia has been proposed. In a review of 84 confirmed cases, the diagnostic triad occurred in about 10 percent of neurologic Whipple disease, whereas isolated cognitive changes or supranuclear gaze palsy was present in 81 percent of the cohort, and 42 percent manifested both.[69] Among the less common manifestations of Whipple's disease are ocular features (uveitis, retinitis, and optic neuritis), hypothalamic involvement (insomnia, hyperphagia, and polydipsia), lymphadenopathy, and a sarcoidosis-like syndrome affecting the mediastinal nodes.[62] Obviously, when gastrointestinal (diarrhea, abdominal pain, weight loss), rheumatic (especially migratory polyarthralgias), or cardiovascular symptoms (murmurs from aortic or mitral valve insufficiency) antedate the neurologic presentation, the index of suspicion must increase exponentially. Although Whipple's disease usually has an insidious onset and slow progression, taking years to evolve fully, on occasion rapid deterioration occurs over weeks to months.

Diagnosis

A duodenal or, preferably, jejunal biopsy obtained through upper endoscopy is a high-yield diagnostic test that demonstrates periodic acid–Schiff (PAS)–positive, diastase-resistant foamy macrophages in the lamina propria on light microscopy and the characteristic intracellular rod-shaped bacilli on electron microscopy. PAS-

▶ **TABLE 24-5.** GUIDELINES FOR DIAGNOSIS OF WHIPPLE'S DISEASE

Definite CNS WD	Possible CNS WD
Must have any one of the following criteria: 1. Oculomasticatory or oculofacial-skeletal myorhythmia 2. Positive tissue biopsy 3. Positive PCR analysis If histologic or PCR analysis was not performed on CNS tissue, the patient must demonstrate neurologic signs	Must have any one of the following unexplained systemic symptoms: 1. Fever of unknown origin 2. Any gastrointestinal symptom(s) 3. Chronic migratory polyarthralgias 4. Lymphadenopathy, night sweats, or malaise Also must have any one of the following unexplained neurologic signs: 1. Supranuclear vertical gaze palsy 2. Rhythmic myoclonus 3. Dementia with psychiatric symptoms 4. Hypothalamic manifestations

SOURCE: *Adapted from Louis et al.[69]*

positive macrophages and characteristic bacilli also have been found in nonintestinal tissues, including liver, lung, heart, lymph nodes, synovium, and brain. Since the availability of PCR, the sensitivity of diagnosis has increased dramatically. *T. whippelii* DNA has a unique 1321-base sequence of a bacterial 16S ribosomal RNA that allows the unequivocal identification of this gram-positive actinomycete by PCR in most affected tissues (pleural, synovial, vitreous, neural), nondiagnostic intestinal tissue specimens,[72,73] CSF, and even peripheral blood.[74] Precisely because the PCR test may be more sensitive than tissue biopsy in some cases, the suggested guidelines for the diagnosis of *definite* CNS Whipple's disease "should be based on the presence of pathognomonic signs (oculomasticatory myorhythmia or oculofacial-skeletal myorhythmia) *or* positive biopsy *or*

polymerase chain reaction results"[69] (Table 24-5). One could argue, given the feasibility of PCR-based testing in most centers, that any unexplained neurologic dysfunction associated with ocular findings warrants 16S ribosomal RNA of *T. whippelii* PCR testing, particularly given the prospect for cure that treatment offers.

The few available imaging studies demonstrate hyperintensity on T_2-weighted (T_2W) and FLAIR MRI in the middle cerebellar peduncles either alone[72] (Fig. 24-6) or involving such diverse areas as the medial temporal lobe, anterior commissure, hypothalamus, mammillary bodies, optic chiasm, cerebral peduncles, and rarely, cervical spinal cord.[69,75–77] The scarcity of neuroradiologic descriptions is related to the high estimated frequency of normal brain imaging in confirmed CNS Whipple's disease patients (up to 50 percent).[69] The im-

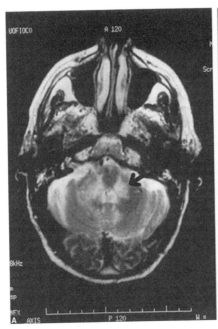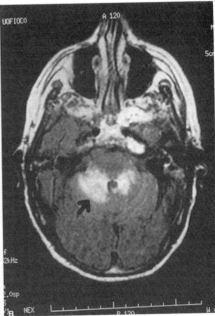

Figure 24-6. MRI in Whipple's disease. T_2-weighted (*left*) and FLAIR (*right*) axial MRI sequences of a patient with positive CSF *T. whippelii* PCR demonstrating hyperintense signal in the middle cerebellar peduncles bilaterally (*arrows*). *(Used with permission from Lee AG: Whipple disease with supranuclear ophthalmoplegia diagnosed by polymerase chain reaction of cerebrospinal fluid. J Neuroophthalmol 22:18, 2002.)*

ages published by Kremer and colleagues[76] also appear to show signal abnormalities within the periaqueductal gray area, which would strengthen the proposed anatomic substrate for the impairment of vertical saccades in the rostral interstitial nucleus of the medial longitudinal fasciculus.[71] Parkinsonism presumably arises largely from disease of the substantia nigra in the region of the cerebral peduncles and to a much lesser degree from lesions elsewhere in the basal ganglia.

Differential Diagnosis

Because of the varied brain and cerebellar gray matter involvement, a wide number of clinical presentations are possible. Whipple's disease may present with a clinical picture similar to that of a variety of encephalopathies, cerebral vasculitis, paraneoplastic syndromes, dementias, chronic meningitides, a range of focal lesions of the brain, and even a relapsing-remitting myelopathy suggestive of a demyelinating or neoplastic process.[77,78] Given such a wide differential, a high index of suspicion is critical. Individuals with parkinsonism and abnormal vertical gaze may be mistakenly thought to have progressive supranuclear palsy. In contrast to progressive supranuclear palsy, patients with Whipple's disease lack squarewave jerks and impairments in smooth pursuit and visual fixation.[71] In those with rhythmic myoclonus localized to muscles innervated by spinal nerves, the phenomenologic distinction with segmental spinal myoclonus may be difficult. Regarding the pathologic differential, it must be mentioned that PAS-positive macrophages and intracellular bacilli are also found in the intestinal lamina propria in patients with AIDS and *Mycobacterium avium* complex infection, although the bacilli of this infection are acid-fast.

Treatment

Treatment with trimethoprim-sulfamethoxazole is recommended both for initial therapy and for relapses of neurologic Whipple's disease. This antibiotic is given intravenously for 2 weeks and orally twice daily thereafter for 12 months. The treatment is long because of the high tendency for neurologic relapse and deterioration that occurs after antibiotics are withdrawn, sometimes months or years later.[79] A combination of parenteral penicillin and streptomycin, followed by 1 or 2 years of oral trimethoprim-sulfamethoxazole, also has been used successfully. Treatment with penicillin or tetracycline alone is associated with the highest rate of neurologic relapse.[79] In general, the use of single-drug therapy and antibiotics with poor blood-brain barrier penetration is discouraged. On occasion, the oculomasticatory myorhythmia may continue despite successful antibiotic therapy. The addition of oral valproate may effectively control this symptom.[80] Since PCR test

becomes negative within 4 to 6 months in patients treated for Whipple's disease, it may be a better tool than intestinal biopsy for monitoring response to treatment and detecting relapse.[81,82]

Complications

Death can occur due to CNS or cardiac complications and is a certain outcome when the disease goes undiagnosed or an untreated relapse occurs. Neurologic Whipple's disease is associated with a relatively high rate of relapse and is the most difficult form to eradicate. Relapses are more likely to occur with single-drug therapy and with antibiotics with poor or absent blood-brain barrier penetration. Despite treatment, some patients do not improve fully, and a small minority progress to death.[83,84] Given the scarcity of concentrated experience for this relatively rare infectious disease, adequate knowledge about its natural history, latency from infection to symptoms, and neurologic or systemic prognostic factors is lacking.

▶ PRION INFECTIONS

Chapter 18 provides an in-depth discussion of this topic. This section will concentrate almost exclusively on the movement disorders that are seen in the sporadic and new variant forms of Creutzfeldt-Jakob disease.

History/Overview

The discovery of prion diseases is one of the most fascinating stories of neurology. This was the ultimate result of both serendipity and a relatively intense interest in an obscure "degenerative disease" affecting the Fore people of the highlands of New Guinea. Anthropologic interest in the cannibalistic tribe and description of its unique illness (kuru)[85] were followed by an initially frustrating search for its genetic, infectious, and environmental etiologies.[86,87] Then a veterinarian neuropathologist, William Hadlow, while casually browsing a pictorial exhibit on kuru, observed the "uncanny resemblance" of brain preparations (vacuolated neurons) with those of scrapie, a progressive neurodegenerative disorder of sheep that could be induced experimentally by intracerebral or subcutaneous inoculation of affected brain tissue suspensions.[88] The similarity to scrapie opened the door to the possibility of a transmissible agent that was highly resistant to heat and formalin, had a long incubation period, and more important, replicated in the absence of nucleic acid.[89] This scrapie agent, a proteinaceous molecule, also was found to be responsible for kuru and a number of other disorders collectively known as *transmissible spongiform encephalopathies* (TSEs). The understanding that these disorders were caused by agents subsequently termed *prions* (*in*fectious nucleic acid-free *pro*teins) earned Stanley Prusiner the 1997 Nobel prize.[90]

Epidemiology

Prion infections include Creutzfeldt-Jakob disease [CJD, and new variant CJD related to bovine spongiform encephalopathy (BSE)], Gerstmann-Sträussler-Scheinker disease (GSS), fatal familial insomnia (FFI), and a number of animal diseases (scrapie, chronic wasting disease of elk, and BSE). Kuru has virtually disappeared after the practice of cannibalism stopped in New Guinea. Both GSS and FFI are familial disorders and will not be considered here. About 85 percent of CJD cases, the main focus of this subsection, and the bulk of all human prion diseases are largely sporadic (sCJD), with the familial form (fCJD) accounting for most of the remainder. Iatrogenic CJD has been described following treatment of growth hormone–deficient children with human growth hormone and surgical exposure to contaminated brain depth electrodes, corneal transplants, and dural cadaveric grafts. Iatrogenic CJD has become an extremely rare occurrence now that the risks and causes are known. The worldwide incidence of CJD is about 1 case per 1 million persons or 1/10,000 that of Alzheimer's disease.[91]

Although much alarm was raised in the late 1990s about the new variant Creutzfeldt-Jakob disease (vCJD), less than 150 cases have been reported, including two in North America. The number of new cases from the United Kingdom declined from a peak of 28 in 2000 to 17 in 2002,[92] suggesting that the "epidemic" may be disappearing, although it is also possible that this simply has represented the initial wave involving individuals with a much greater genetic predisposition (see below).

Pathophysiology and Pathogenesis

The main derangement in prion infections is in the metabolism of prion proteins. The normal isoform of these proteins (PrP^c, cellular) is expressed predominantly in the brain and is encoded by the prion gene (*PRNP*) on the short arm of chromosome 20. The disease-related isoform (PrP^{sc}, *scrapie*) is generated by a posttranslational change from the predominantly α-helical structure of PrP^c to a β-pleated sheet configuration.[93] This conformational change from PrP^c to PrP^{sc} is self-perpetuating and leads to the increasing neuronal deposition of β-pleated sheets, which are insoluble and resistant to proteases. This is the presumed mechanism that explains how prion diseases can be both inherited and infectious. All patients with familial CJD have mutations in the *PRNP* gene. Although the factors that determine the change from PrP^c to PrP^{sc} are not understood, genetics do play an important role. A polymorphism at codon 129 of the *PRNP* gene codes for either the presence of a methionine (met) or valine (val). The met/val combination clearly influences both clinical and pathologic manifestations of the disorder.[94] Bewteen 80 and 90 percent of patients with sCJD exhibit homozygosity for either methionine or valine (met/met or val/val) at codon 129, and this, combined with two different PrP^{sc} types, determines six major phenotypic variations.[94] On the other hand, all cases of vCJD described to date have been homozygous for methionine at codon 129 of the *PRNP* gene. Evidence supports consumption of bovine meat products contaminated with BSE as the mechanism of transmission, but this has not been firmly established. For further discussion on these and other related topics, including neuropathology, please consult Chapter 18 on prion infections.

Clinical Features

Movement disorders in prion diseases generally develop on a superimposed picture of rapidly progressive cognitive and behavioral impairment. Widespread neuronal degeneration in the cerebellum, pyramidal cortex and extrapyramidal tracts, and lower motor neurons creates a diverse and nonspecific array of signs and symptoms. What allows for heightened suspicion of a prion disease is the tempo of progression and the rapid succession of deficits from onset to death, often preceded by a late stage of akinetic rigid mutism. The mean age of patients with sCJD is 60 years. Only less than 10 percent of patients with pathologically confirmed CJD live more than 2 years after disease onset, and the mean interval between onset and death is 8 months. Myoclonus is the most common associated movement in typical cases, present eventually in nearly 90 percent of patients.[95] These movements are semiperiodic and cortical in origin, may affect any body area, and often are stimulus-sensitive (pathologic startle reflex). The most common presenting abnormal movement, however, is choreoathetosis (chorea and athetosis differ mainly in speed of movements and are largely considered part of the same hyperkinetic phenomenology). Choreoathetosis, dystonia, and even hemiballism may develop in approximately 25 percent of patients during the course of the disease.[96] Cerebellar dysfunction, as part of the Brownell-Oppenheimer variant, is perhaps the second most common presentation. Patients have prominent ataxia and limb dysmetria with a relatively longer course and less cognitive impairment. Ataxia is noted initially in approximately one-third of patients and develops ultimately in up to two-thirds. Patients with a prolonged course tend to have less myoclonus and more seizures and behavioral abnormalities. Visual abnormalities, especially cortical blindness, are particularly common in individuals with ataxia.[97] Parkinsonism is also a relatively common manifestation and, when parkinsonian features are combined with limb apraxia, alien limb phenomenon, and other symptoms may mimic corticobasal degeneration (CBD), albeit with a much more rapid course than is typical for idiopathic CBD.

The more recently described vCJD has a younger age at onset (mean age of 26 years), a slower clinical course, early psychiatric and sensory (paresthesia, pain) symptoms, absence of characteristic electroencephalographic abnormalities, and widespread kuru-type plaques (florid plaques) on neuropathology. Myoclonus and dystonia are conspicuously absent until the terminal stages. Chorea may occur as an early manifestation.

Diagnosis

Electroencephalography (EEG) is one of the most useful tests in supporting the presumptive diagnosis of CJD. When dementia and myoclonus are associated with the classic triphasic waves on EEG, the diagnosis is almost certain. Initially intermittent, these complexes become continuous with a periodicity of 1 Hz but eventually may disappear in patients with prolonged survival. Less specific EEG features observed at different stages include focal slowing, periodic lateralized epileptiform discharges, spike-and-wave complexes, and bisynchronous high-voltage periodic sharp-wave discharges. Both FLAIR and diffusion-weighted MRI often show increased signal in the basal ganglia and cortical ribbon, especially in the occipital lobe, in sCJD and the thalamic pulvinar region in vCJD patients.[98] Other noninvasive tests are less helpful. Elevation of 14-3-3 protein in CSF is a sensitive (95 percent) but nonspecific (~50 percent) marker of neuronal death and therefore cannot discriminate different forms of dementia or acute brain insults.[99] Single-photon-emission computed tomographic (SPECT) scans may show a nonspecific bifrontal decrease in blood flow that may be useful in identifying the best site for brain biopsy. In the proper clinical setting with the classic EEG and MRI abnormalities, it is generally unnecessary to consider a more invasive study such as brain biopsy. However, when diagnostic uncertainty remains, brain biopsy is a required step for definitive diagnosis. To establish the diagnosis, the biopsy must show spongiform degeneration, neuronal loss, astrogliosis, and confirmatory immunohistochemistry.[100] Indeed, biopsy material should demonstrate prion protein immunoreactivity with monoclonal antibodies that recognize PrP^{sc}-specific epitopes.[101] Circumventing the challenges of obtaining brain tissue has become possible recently by the identification of peripheral markers for both sCJD and vCJD. Immunoblot, another immunologic technique sensitive for the detection of PrP^{sc},[102] has been applied to olfactory biopsy specimens in sCJD [102,103] and tonsillar biopsy specimens (rich in lymphoreticular tissues) in vCJD,[104] correctly diagnosing CJD in all cases.

Differential Diagnosis

Rapidly progressive cognitive impairment and/or focal neurologic deficits with myoclonus and rigidity may be features of other dementing illnesses such as Alzheimer disease (AD), dementia with Lewy bodies (DLB), and frontotemporal dementia (FTD). In general, AD and FTD become a more likely consideration when the disease course is longer and DLB if parkinsonism or fluctuations in cognition are present, but significant clinical overlap can exist.[97,105] In both AD and certain forms of FTD, the microtubule-associated protein tau becomes hyperphosphorylated. Preliminary evidence has shown that discriminating the phosphorylated (P-tau) versus the nonphosphorylated forms of tau in CSF may be useful in distinguishing AD and FTD from CJD.[106] The P-tau/total tau ratio is lower in subjects with CJD compared with those with AD and FTD. CJD also can be confused with conditions capable of causing similar EEG abnormalities. Sharp-wave complexes can be seen in the dementias just described, whereas triphasic waves are also observed in drug toxicities (lithium, tricyclic antidepressants, barbiturates, phencyclidine, and bismuth intoxication), metabolic or anoxic encephalopathies, and other infections (subacute sclerosing panencephalitis and herpes simplex encephalitis).

Treatment

There is no effective treatment for CJD. A significant number of antiviral agents, interferon, anticonvulsants, antibiotics, and corticosteroids, among others, have not been efficacious in the treatment of CJD. Ongoing clinical studies are assessing the value of quinacrine and chlorpromazine and acridine and phenothiazine derivatives, respectively, as potential inhibitors of the PrP^c-to-PrP^{sc} conversion. Interference with this conversion is currently the target of active experimentation with transgenic mouse models. Active immunization with recombinant PrP and antiprion monoclonal antibodies can prolong the incubation period of scrapie in mice, suggesting that immune modulation may have a role in the treatment of CJD.[107,108]

► SUBACUTE SCLEROSING PANENCEPHALITIS (SSPE)

Overview/History

Subacute sclerosing panencephalitis (SSPE) is a late cerebral complication of a previous measles infection. Apart from acute encephalitis at the time of the initial infection, measles infection may result in two delayed cerebral syndromes: subacute measles encephalitis (SME) or subacute sclerosing panencephalitis (SSPE). The latency following the acute infection is the critical distinguishing element between these complications (months in SME and years in SSPE). Such a long interval between the initial infection and the development of these complications is intriguing and has never been well understood. The immune system likely has a role in at least modulating the clinical expression because

SME exhibits a similar though accelerated clinical picture when compared with SSPE, except that it occurs in immunosuppressed patients. The successful immunization strategies implemented in the last part of the twentieth century dramatically reduced the number of individuals with SSPE.

Epidemiology

Relatively rare in the western hemisphere, SSPE occurs with greater prevalence in adolescents and young adults of developing countries where measles is still endemic. SSPE is estimated to occur in 2 to 10 per 100,000 population in India and Pakistan, respectively, but less than 1 per million in the United States. In endemic areas, SSPE follows measles infection after an average latency of 8 years.[109] The incidence of SSPE among nonimmunized children is almost 200 times higher than the incidence among those who have been immunized effectively. Despite high rates of immunization, small measles epidemics can still develop from imported virus or waning immunity after insufficient immunization (e.g., measles vaccination before 12 months of age may result in primary vaccine failure because of maternal antibodies).[110] In contrast to children, older individuals with SSPE did not have measles at a later age but instead have had a longer interval before the onset of symptoms.[111] The main risk factor now as well as in the preimmunization era is acquiring the infection at or before the age of 2 years.[112]

Pathophysiology and Pathogenesis

The measles virus has six major structural proteins, of which the matrix (M) protein is critical. Defects in the M protein due to major mutations are associated with persistent measles infection in SSPE patients.[113] The M protein is attached to the membrane and interacts with the viral nucleocapsid, essential for controlling viral replication and transcription. Enhancement in viral replication results in the spread of a defective measles virus throughout the brain, possibly through axonal pathways.[114] Coexisting immunosuppression may result in a shorter disease latency and/or more aggressive disease course, as occurs in pregnant women,[115,116] but this remains speculative. The end result of the viral infection includes widespread demyelination and neuronal loss, perivascular inflammatory infiltration at cortical and subcortical levels, glial proliferation, and neuronal and glial intranuclear and intracytoplasmic inclusions. The occipital lobes, thalamus, and putamen are the structures with the greatest burden of pathology.[117]

Clinical Features

Behavioral and personality changes with cognitive regression nearly always precede the onset of visual and motor abnormalities. The ophthalmologic deficits include papilledema, chorioretinitis, homonymous visual field deficits, and cortical blindness. Monocular blindness is the most common visual abnormality, whereas myoclonus is the most prominent motor deficit. Limb and axial myoclonus usually is followed by a predominantly rigid phase and a final spastic phase prior to the end stage of akinetic mutism and death, all occurring in a "stuttering," or staged fashion. Initially paroxysmal and quasi-periodic in nature, myoclonus has been described as "slow" or "hung up."[117] The duration of these paroxysmal movements may be longer than the allowed myoclonus range of less than 0.5 s in duration, and the terms *paroxysmal dystonia*[118] and *periodic dystonic myoclonus*[119] have been suggested to describe this phenomena. When the myoclonic or dystonic movements appear, cerebellar and other extrapyramidal deficits such as choreoathetosis may become apparent to a greater degree in the most affected side. Frank dementia invariably is present at this stage, and its progression is accompanied by a comparable reduction in the myoclonic jerks.[117] A stage of autonomic instability, rigidity, and decreasing level of consciousness culminates in quadriparesis, akinetic mutism, neurovegetative state, and finally, death.

Diagnosis

When the clinical features are suggestive, EEG and CSF analysis are the critical tests for confirmation. The typical EEG shows periodic synchronous and symmetric high-amplitude delta waves every 5 to 10 seconds (often synchronous with the paroxysmal movements), suggesting a burst-suppression type of pattern (Fig. 24-7). In fact, periodic movements may be so subtle that they are missed until the patient is observed carefully at the time of EEG recording. The CSF examination is the current gold standard for diagnosis because it demonstrates the presence of antimeasles antibody titers and increased gammaglobulin (hyperglobulinorrachia greater than 20 percent of the total protein) in the setting of an otherwise noninflammatory fluid. CSF restricted oligoclonal IgG bands directed against measles nucleocapsid protein can also be detected. Brain MRI offers little help because prominent basal ganglia involvement is seen rarely and only tends to appear in advanced clinical stages, when the diagnosis should have been established by CSF measles antibody titers.[120] Brain MRI also may show periventricular and subcortical white matter hyperintense lesions in T_2 weighted sequences, but the extent and location of these lesions do not seem to correlate with clinical status.[121,122]

Differential Diagnosis

Other encephalitides due to herpes simplex virus, varicella-zoster virus, cytomegalovirus, Lyme disease, HIV infection (AIDS-dementia complex), and perhaps

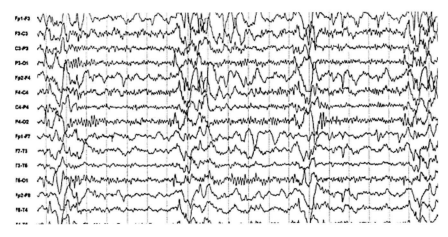

Figure 24-7. EEG in SSPE. Periodic synchronous and symmetric high-amplitude polyphasic discharges with disordered background activity, predominantly over the frontocentral region and associated with clinical myoclonus. These complex and relatively slow discharges occur every 7 seconds in this example (the intercomplex interval is usually reported to range between 4 to 15 seconds). *(Courtesy of Dr. Omkar Markand, Department of Neurology, Indiana University.)*

rubella (see below) may resemble SSPE. As mentioned earlier, SME may have a similar clinical presentation. When the MRI demonstrates hyperintense multifocal subcortical white matter lesions on T_2 weighted sequences, progressive multifocal leukoencephalopathy and ADEM must be considered. An extremely rare "slow virus" neurodegenerative disorder that reportedly mimics SSPE is progressive rubella panencephalitis (PRP). This has been reported in fewer than 20 persons between the ages of 8 and 21 years. Most have had signs of congenital rubella syndrome, antirubella antibody titer and IgG in CSF, and a more benign clinical course than SSPE. Finally, despite clinical and EEG similarities, CJD is rarely considered in the differential diagnosis of SSPE given the dissimilar ages at which these conditions occur, even though outliers in both have been reported.

Treatment

Treatment with IVIg, plasmapheresis, cytarabine, ribavirin, isoprinosine, amantadine, and beta and alpha interferon have not significantly altered the natural history of the disease. A treatment protocol consisting of oral isoprinosine (100 mg/kg per day), subcutaneous interferon-α2a (10 mU/m^2 three times per week), and oral lamivudine (10 mg/kg per day) resulted in higher remission rates and longer survival periods but without a decrease in the mortality rate.[123] The concurrent use of IVIg (bolus of 0.4 g/kg per day for 5 days, followed by 0.4 g/kg for 1 day each month) and isoprinosine was reported recently to produce significant motor and cognitive improvement in four patients followed for a period ranging from 6 to 60 months.[124] The authors propose that IVIg should be considered first-line treatment for SSPE. Long-term follow-up will be necessary

to determine whether IVIg alters the universally bad prognosis of SSPE to date (see below).

Complications

The prognosis for SSPE is very poor, and remissions are rare. Survival time varies from 4 weeks to 16 years and is shorter when measles occurred over the age of 2.5 years.[112] In about 10 percent of patients the disease lasts up to 10 years, and in another 10 percent death occurs within 3 months. Any observations of "spontaneous long-term improvement"[125,126] or remission need to take into account this pronounced variability in the natural history of the disorder. To date, virtually all patients have died within 10 years of the onset of symptoms.

Prevention

Early childhood immunization against rubeola remains the only known preventive measure.

▶ MOVEMENT DISORDERS IN AIDS PATIENTS

Overview

The specific involvement of the basal ganglia by opportunistic infections, direct neurotoxic effects of the HIV itself, and drug-induced side effects are all potential causes of movement disorders in patients with AIDS. These include choreoathetosis, hemiballism, dystonia, and less commonly, parkinsonism. Although any of these can occur during the course of established HIV infection, occasionally chorea and parkinsonism are the presenting symptoms of AIDS.

Epidemiology

Movement disorders are relatively rare in HIV infection or AIDS without concomitant opportunistic infections. Estimates of prevalence range from 2 to 8 percent of all HIV-infected individuals, mostly due to *Toxoplasma* infection. Population-based, controlled epidemiologic studies, however, are lacking. Methodologic shortcomings inherent to case reports and retrospective case series compromise accurate ascertainment of the entire spectrum of the nature and severity of movement abnormalities in HIV infection.[127] Prospective clinical examinations detect tremor and parkinsonian signs in nearly 50 percent of patients.[128,129] Most studies, however, suggest that hemichorea-hemiballism, one of the least common of all movement disorders, is the most common clinically symptomatic movement disorder associated with HIV infection, followed by an akinetic-rigid syndrome. Toxoplasmosis is both the most common opportunistic infection and the main cause of the hemichorea-hemiballism syndrome. With potent antiretroviral therapy there has been a decline in neurologic complications and related movement disorders in patients with AIDS.

Pathophysiology and Pathogenesis

Abnormal movements occurring in the context of HIV infection may result from the neurotoxicity of the virus itself, a regional encephalitic lesion, focal opportunistic infections (toxoplasmosis, cryptococcosis, cytomegalovirus, tuberculosis, and progressive multifocal leukoencephalopathy), or primary CNS lymphoma.[130–134] Hemichorea-hemiballism may occur as a consequence of focal involvement of the contralateral subthalamic nucleus, striatum, or less often, other sites. Parkinsonism due to focal lesions however, is relatively rare and often requires bilateral basal ganglia involvement.[135] HIV-related parkinsonism is more likely due to primary cerebral involvement by the HIV virus associated with ex vacuo hydrocephalus from generalized brain atrophy.[128] Hypermetabolism of the basal ganglia on positron-emission tomography (PET) as the earliest abnormality in asymptomatic HIV-positive patients (with hypometabolism developing when symptoms arise)[136,137] and an exquisite sensitivity to neuroleptic-induced parkinsonism suggest early involvement of the basal ganglia as a common feature of HIV encephalopathy.[138]

Drug-related complications are an important cause of abnormal movements in these patients. As mentioned earlier, HIV encephalopathic patients are highly susceptible to neuroleptics. These drugs may precipitate parkinsonism in up to three-fourths of patients treated with them, and this argues for the preferential use of atypical neuroleptics in patients requiring antipsychotic therapy.[131] The causal association between tremor and trimethoprim-sulfamethoxazole in patients with AIDS is well established.[139,140] It has been postulated that this is due to a disruption of dopamine production through glutathione or tetrahydrobiopterin depletion.

Clinical Features

While most of the abnormal movements develop as complications of established AIDS, hemichorea-hemiballism[35,134] or postural tremor[129,141] may be presenting symptoms of HIV infection and the AIDS-defining illness. The choreiform movements may begin in a restricted area (including the face) and progress to involve the entire contralateral hemibody, the amplitude reaching ballistic proportions.[142] Different types of tremor may occur due to HIV encephalopathy or strategically located focal opportunistic infections. These include a classic pill-rolling resting tremor, most often as a feature of drug-induced parkinsonism, postural and action tremor either in isolation or associated with other features including levodopa-resistant parkinsonism, and finally, a prominent kinetic tremor (Holmes tremor) that typically occurs in conjunction with other focal midbrain signs such as oculomotor paresis. In most patients the movements are either very asymmetric or strictly unilateral. Less common abnormal movements reported in association with HIV infection include focal dystonia (associated with *Toxoplasma* abscesses in the lenticular nucleus and thalamus),[143] segmental spinal myoclonus,[128] painful legs and moving toes syndrome (from painful peripheral neuropathy),[144] reversible myoclonic encephalopathy,[145] and focal, multifocal, or hemidystonic paroxysmal dyskinesias (from neuronal injury and loss in the subcortical gray matter).[146] Psychogenic movement disorders also occur, further confounding the clinical spectrum.

Diagnosis

The approach to diagnosis is to search for opportunistic infections or primary CNS lymphoma in the case of well-established HIV infection and to test for HIV itself when chorea, for instance, is suspected to be heralding AIDS. Since toxoplasmosis is the most common opportunistic infection, a CT scan or preferably MRI typically shows contrast-enhancing lesions with mass effect and surrounding edema in the basal ganglia contralateral to the symptomatic side (Fig. 24-8). If not contraindicated due to mass effect from structural lesions, a lumbar puncture is critical in further defining the etiology. The recommended CSF panel consists of PCR testing for Epstein-Barr virus (EBV) DNA, JC virus DNA, and *Toxoplasma gondii* DNA, assessing for primary CNS lymphoma (PCNSL), progressive multifocal leukoencephalopathy (PML), and toxoplasmic encephalitis (TE), respectively.[147] When toxoplasmosis serology is negative, a focal imaging abnormality with mass effect makes PCNSL highly likely (74 percent). When focal brain le-

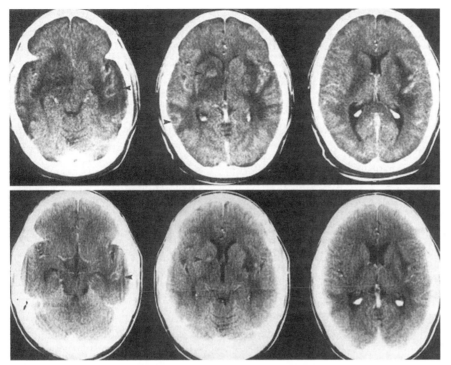

Figure 24-8. CT scan in cerebral toxoplasmosis. Contrast-enhanced head CT before (*upper row*) and 10 days after (*lower row*) antitoxoplasmosis therapy in a 32-year-old bisexual HIV-1-positive man with left facial and upper extremity chorea. Note the causative ring-enhancing lesion affecting the right globus pallidus (*center, upper row*), which improved following treatment with sulfadiazine and pyrimethamine. *(Used with permission from Nath A, et al: Movement disorders with cerebral toxoplasmosis and AIDS. Mov Disord 8:107, 1993.)*

sions do not exhibit mass effect, the probability of PML becomes more likely.[147] Interestingly, neither the absence of *T. gondii* serology nor the use of *Toxoplasma* prophylaxis excludes the possibility of TE. Seronegative patients with mass-occupying lesions receiving *Toxoplasma* prophylaxis have TE in nearly 60 percent of cases. Cerebral biopsy is restricted to selected EBV DNA–positive patients and seronegative individuals with focal brain lesions with mass effect when the risks are acceptable and empirical therapy has not resulted in clinical benefits.

Differential Diagnosis

Although much less common, the same HIV-related opportunistic infections can occur in immunocompetent individuals. Toxoplasmosis may result in neuroimaging abnormalities similar to those seen in primary CNS lymphoma and other opportunistic infections, although cryptococcosis usually presents with diffuse meningoencephalitis.[148]

Treatment

Managing movement disorders presenting in HIV-positive individuals requires the recognition and treatment of opportunistic infections, the use of potent antiretroviral therapy to address the primary infection, and symptomatic treatment of the particular movement abnormality if it interferes with function and is not improved by the preceding measures. The reader is referred to Chapter 7 for an in-depth discussion of the management of HIV and complicating opportunistic infections.

Disabling movement disorders complicating AIDS require symptomatic therapy. Hemichorea-hemiballism may respond to dopamine receptor–blocking agents (such as haloperidol) or dopamine-depleting agents (reserpine and tetrabenazine), as well as valproic acid. However, the neuroleptic sensitivity of these patients increases the likelihood of such medication-related complications as parkinsonism and tardive syndromes. Tremor is the least responsive of all HIV-related abnormal movements. The response to anticholinergics, clonazepam, propranolol, and primidone is often disappointing. Fortunately, tremor is rarely severe enough to require symptomatic treatment. In rare patients who remain disabled from a persistent movement disorder complicating a relatively static CNS process and whose underlying disease is stable, consideration might be given to a functional neurosurgical procedure (e.g., thalamotomy for unilateral Holmes tremor).

Complications

Rarely, HIV causes a rapidly progressive encephalopathy with generalized chorea that is fatal.[133] Besides the complications stemming from potent antiretroviral therapy, the only available study that correlates motor abnormalities and prognosis[149] indicated that HIV-infected patients with movement disorders, especially tremor-predominant symptoms, have a mortality rate of 76 percent within 2 years of the movement disorder presentation.

▶ ANTIEMETIC- AND ANTIMICROBIAL AGENT-INDUCED MOVEMENT DISORDERS

Overview

Prochlorperazine and metoclopramide are two commonly used antiemetics that are used often to treat vomiting in patients with CNS infections. These agents have dopamine receptor-blocking properties and are capable of inducing a variety of movement disorders, including acute dystonic reactions, akathisia, tardive dyskinesia, parkinsonism, and even neuroleptic malignant syndrome. For practical purposes, these detrimental effects are similar in appearance and severity to those occurring during treatment with typical antipsychotic agents such as haloperidol. Antimicrobial agents, on the other hand, generally are safer than antiemetics, and their association with the development of abnormal movements is largely anecdotal.

Epidemiology

Parkinsonism, tardive dyskinesia, and dystonia are the most frequent iatrogenic movement disorders found in clinical practice.[150] The prevalence of drug-induced parkinsonism, for instance, is approximately 33 per 100,000 individuals (about eight times less than that of idiopathic Parkinson's disease),[151] and between 20 and 40 percent of individuals exposed to chronic neuroleptic therapy develop tardive dyskinesia.[152] Most studies, however, do not distinguish antipsychotic- from antiemetic-induced parkinsonism. Most of the antiemetic- and antimicrobial-induced movement disorders associations are postmarketing case reports for which no careful analysis of the populations at risk are available (see Table 24-1). The epidemiologic factors associated with the likelihood of drug toxicity have not been elucidated.

Pathophysiology and Pathogenesis

Most antiemetics induce movement disorders through their ability to block dopamine D_2 receptors, for which they are termed *neuroleptics*. Drugs in this category include the phenothiazines, thiethylperazine and prochlorperazine, as well as the substituted benzamides, metoclopramide, sulpiride, tiapride, and clebopride. Blockade of D_2 receptors, largely in the striatum, is believed to account for acute dystonic reactions and especially drug-induced parkinsonism. Akathisia and neuroleptic malignant syndrome are likely due to more widespread dopamine antagonistic effects. The pathogenesis of tardive dyskinesia, which typically requires long-term drug use, is not well understood but probably involves factors distinct from pure D_2 receptor blockade.

Certain antibiotics have been reported to induce movement disorders. These are largely isolated cases, perhaps with the exception of the antifungal amphotericin B (particularly after intraventricular administration in the treatment of cryptococcal meningitis), which has been associated consistently with parkinsonism.[153] The pathogenesis of this uncommon side effect is poorly understood. Presumably, no preexisting nigral or basal ganglia dysfunction is required for the development of these disorders.

Clinical Features

The range of neuroleptic-induced movement disorders includes acute dystonic reactions, acute akathisia, parkinsonism, neuroleptic malignant syndrome, and tardive syndromes (including tardive dyskinesia, dystonia, tics, and akathisia) organized according to the order of appearance after drug initiation. It is also not uncommon for two or more of these drug-induced movement disorders (i.e., parkinsonism and tardive dystonia) to occur simultaneously in the same patient.[154] Acute dystonic reactions tend to occur shortly after introduction of a neuroleptic drug and include oculogyric crises and dystonia, especially of the craniocervical region. Subtle symptoms may be limited to dysarthria and dysphagia. Acute akathisia is an extremely common but underrecognized side effect of drugs with neuroleptic properties. Subjective restlessness and dysphoria are the principal complaints, often resulting in an inability to remain still and a need to move about and pace or perform a variety of stereotypic movements (e.g., hand rubbing, foot tapping) in order to relieve the restlessness. Drug-induced parkinsonism can be indistinguishable from idiopathic Parkinson's disease. A relatively prominent postural component of the tremor and the presence of low-frequency, high-amplitude facial tremor (rabbit syndrome) may raise suspicion as to the drug-related nature of the disorder. Neuroleptic malignant syndrome presents with marked rigidity, fever, autonomic instability, and alterations in the level of consciousness.[155] Finally, tardive dyskinesia usually develops only after chronic treatment with dopamine-blocking agents. It consists of stereotypic facial and oral dyskinesias producing most commonly lip smacking, intermittent brief tongue protrusion, or grimacing.[156] Other tardive disorders may be combined with these more common dyskinetic movements or occur in isolation, including tardive dystonia (e.g., retrocollis, internal rotation of the arms, and wrist flexion) and/or tardive akathisia (restlessness, pelvic rocking motions, moaning, rapid movements of the fingers). Occasionally, disabling persistent dystonia, comparable to tardive dystonia, occurs after only a very brief exposure to neuroleptic drugs, emphasizing the need to limit their use to well-established indications and to regularly reevaluate the need for ongoing therapy.

Among the antimicrobial agents, trimethoprim-sulfamethoxazole has been reported to cause postural tremor primarily, but not exclusively, in individuals with AIDS without known HIV-related CNS involvement (i.e., using the drug for *Pneumocystis carinii* pneumonia prophylaxis). The tremor is completely reversible after drug reduction or withdrawal.[140,157] For a full list of anti-microbial-related movement disorders, see Table 24-1.

Diagnosis and Differential Diagnosis

An accurate drug history is the best way to ascertain the possibility of an iatrogenic disorder. If the clinical picture is suggestive but the patient's medical history is unrevealing, direct contact with the pharmacy is critical in providing accurate documentation of the use of potentially causative agents. Always consider alternative diagnostic explanations, particularly the presence of additional underlying CNS disease that could serve as a predisposing factor for the development of a drug-induced movement disorder.

Treatment

Slow tapering instead of abrupt removal of the offending agent(s) is generally the best strategy in drug-induced movement disorders. However, in life-threatening drug-induced disorders, e.g., neuroleptic malignant syndrome, a more rapid or abrupt withdrawal is appropriate. The same applies to the acute side effects that begin shortly after drug initiation, such as acute dystonic reactions or akathisia. Abrupt withdrawal of chronically used neuroleptic-type antiemetics may be associated with the emergence of a tardive dyskinetic syndrome. If these symptoms are bothersome or disabling, then it may be necessary to reintroduce the causative drug followed by a more gradual dose tapering. Patients with disabling drug-induced parkinsonism may not improve sufficiently from withdrawal of the offending neuroleptic, and temporary symptomatic treatment with a dopamine agonist or levodopa may be necessary. More persistent symptoms suggest the possibility of an underlying primary parkinsonian disorder (possibly occult at the time of drug initiation) that could have predisposed the patient to this complication. The management of tardive dyskinesia is complex, and the reader is referred to more in-depth discussions of the topic.[158,159]

Prevention

Avoidance of potentially offending agents may not always be feasible but is the only way of preventing these iatrogenic disorders. For antiemetic control and motility disorders of the upper gastrointestinal tract, where available, domperidone, a peripheral dopamine antagonist, is the drug of choice. Ondansetron, a selective serotonin 5-HT3 receptor antagonist and a well tolerated treatment for patients with nausea and vomiting associated with cancer chemotherapy, radiotherapy, and

surgery, has proven safe when used in patients with Parkinson's disease and dystonic syndromes given the lack of dopamine receptor–blocking properties.[160]

REFERENCES

1. Rektor I: Chorea Sancti Viti in Lexicon medicum anno 1696. *J Neurol* 250:7, 2003.
2. Taranta A, Stollerman GH: The relationship of Sydenham's chorea to infection with group A streptococci. *Am J Med* 20:170, 1956.
3. Stollerman GH: Rheumatic fever. *Lancet* 349:935, 1997.
4. Cardoso F, Eduardo C, Silva AP, et al: Chorea in fifty consecutive patients with rheumatic fever. *Mov Disord* 12:701, 1997.
5. McLaren MJ, Markowitz M, Gerber MA: Rheumatic heart disease in developing countries: The consequence of inadequate prevention. *Ann Intern Med* 120:243, 1994.
6. Ayoub EM: Resurgence of rheumatic fever in the United States: The changing picture of a preventable illness. *Postgrad Med* 92:133, 1992.
7. Bronze MS, Dale JB: Epitopes of streptococcal M proteins that evoke antibodies that cross-react with human brain. *J Immunol* 151:2820, 1993.
8. Zabriskie JB, Lavenchy D, Williams RC Jr, et al: Rheumatic fever–associated B-cell alloantigens as identified by monoclonal antibodies. *Arthritis Rheum* 28:1047, 1985.
9. Feldman BM, Zabriskie JB, Wilverman ED, Laxer RM: Diagnostic use of B-cell alloantigen D8/17 in rheumatic chorea. *J Pediatr* 123:84, 1993.
10. Murphy TK, Goodman WK, Fudge MW, et al: B-lymphocyte antigen D8/17: A peripheral marker for childhood-onset obsessive-compulsive disorder and Tourette's syndrome? *Am J Psychiatry* 154:402, 1997.
11. Swedo SE, Leonard HL, Mittleman BB, et al: Identification of children with pediatric autoimmune neuropsychiatric disorders associated with streptococcal infections by a marker associated with rheumatic fever. *Am J Psychiatry* 154:110, 1997.
12. Greenfield JG, Wolfsohn JM: The pathology of Sydenham's chorea. *Lancet* 2:603, 1922.
13. Colony S, Malamud N: Sydenham's chorea, a clinicopathologic study. *Neurology* 6:672, 1956.
14. Asbahr FR, Negrao AB, Gentil V, et al: Obsessive-compulsive and related symptoms in children and adolescents with rheumatic fever with and without chorea: A prospective 6-month study. *Am J Psychiatry* 155:1122, 1998.
15. Marques-Dias MJ, Mercadante MT, Tucker D, Lombroso P: Sydenham's chorea. *Psychiatr Clin North Am* 20:809, 1997.
16. Terreri MT, Roja SC, Len CA, et al: Sydenham's chorea: Clinical and evolutive characteristics. *Sao Paulo Med J* 120:16, 2002.
17. Ozkutlu S, Ayabakan C, Saraclar M: Can subclinical valvitis detected by echocardiography be accepted as evidence of carditis in the diagnosis of acute rheumatic fever? *Cardiol Young* 11:255, 2001.

18. Church AJ, Cardoso F, Dale RC, et al: Anti-basal ganglia antibodies in acute and persistent Sydenham's chorea. *Neurology* 59:227, 2002.

19. Dajani AS, Ayoub E, Bierman FZ, et al: Guidelines for the diagnosis of rheumatic fever: Jones criteria, updated 1992. Special Writing Group of the Committee on Rheumatic Fever, Endocarditis, and Kawasaki Disease of the Council on Cardiovascular Disease in the Young, American Heart Association. *JAMA* 268:2069, 2003.

20. Giedd JN, Rapoport JL, Kruesi MJP, et al: Sydenham's chorea: Magnetic resonance imaging of the basal ganglia. *Neurology* 45:2199, 1995.

21. Ikuta N, Hirata M, Sasabe F, et al: High-signal basal ganglia on T_1-weighted images in a patient with Sydenham's chorea. *Neuroradiology* 40:659, 1998.

22. Golbe LI: Pregnancy and movement disorders. *Neurol Clin* 12:497, 1994.

23. Wang HS, Kuo MF, Huang SC, et al: Choreoathetosis as an initial sign of relapsing of herpes simplex encephalitis. *Pediatr Neurol* 11:341, 1994.

24. Piccolo I, Thiella G, Sterzi R, et al: Chorea as a symptom of neuroborreliosis: a case study. *Ital J Neurol Sci* 19:235, 1998.

25. Beskind DL, Keim SM: Choreoathetotic movement disorder in a boy with *Mycoplasma pneumoniae* encephalitis. *Ann Emerg Med* 23:1375, 1994.

26. Shenker DM, Grossman HJ, Klawans HL: Treatment of Sydenham's chorea with haloperidol. *Dev Med Child Neurol* 15:19, 1973.

27. Steinberg A, Reifen RM, Leifer M: Efficacy of valproic acid in the treatment of Sydenham's chorea. *J Child Neurol* 2:233, 1987.

28. McLachlan RS: Valproic acid in Sydenham's chorea. *Br Med J (Clin Res Ed)* 283:274, 1981.

29. Dhanaraj M, Radhakrishnan AR, Srinivas K, et al: Sodium valproate in Sydenham's chorea. *Neurology* 35:114, 1985.

30. Alvarez LA, Novak G: Valproic acid in the treatment of Sydenham chorea. *Pediatr Neurol* 1:317, 1985.

31. Genel F, Arslanoglu S, Uran N, et al: Sydenham's chorea: Clinical findings and comparison of the efficacies of sodium valproate and carbamazepine regimens. *Brain Dev* 24:73, 2002.

32. Pena J, Mora E, Cardozo J, et al: Comparison of the efficacy of carbamazepine, haloperidol and valproic acid in the treatment of children with Sydenham's chorea: Clinical follow-up of 18 patients. *Arq Neuropsiquiatr* 60:374, 2002.

33. Perlmutter SJ, Leitman SF, Garvey MA, et al: Therapeutic plasma exchange and intravenous immunoglobulin for obsessive-compulsive disorder and tic disorders in childhood. *Lancet* 354:1153, 1999.

34. Cardoso F, Vargas AP, Oliveira LD, et al: Persistent Sydenham's chorea. *Mov Disord* 14:805, 1999.

35. Cardoso F: Infectious and transmissible movement disorders. In Jankovic J, Tolosa E (eds): *Parkinson's Disease and Movement Disorders*. Baltimore: Williams & Wilkins, 1998, pp 945–966.

36. Dajani A, Taubert K, Ferrieri P, et al: Treatment of acute streptococcal pharyngitis and prevention of rheumatic fever: A statement for health professionals. Committee on Rheumatic Fever, Endocarditis, and Kawasaki Disease of the Council on Cardiovascular Disease in the Young, the American Heart Association. *Pediatrics* 96:758, 1995.

37. Berrios X, del Campo E, Guzman B, et al: Discontinuing rheumatic fever prophylaxis in selected adolescents and young adults; A prospective study. *Ann Intern Med* 118:401, 1993.

38. Swedo SE: Sydenham's chorea: A model for childhood autoimmune neuropsychiatric disorders. *JAMA* 272:1788, 1994.

39. Church AJ, Dale RC, Lees AJ, et al: Tourette's syndrome: A cross-sectional study to examine the PANDAS hypothesis. *J Neurol Neurosurg Psychiatry* 74:602, 2003.

40. Giedd JN, Rapoport JL, Garvey MA, et al: MRI assessment of children with obsessive-compulsive disorder or tics associated with streptococcal infection. *Am J Psychiatry* 157:281, 2000.

41. Murphy TK, Goodman WK, Ayoub EM, et al: On defining Sydenham's chorea: Where do we draw the line? *Biol Psychiat* 47:851, 2000.

42. Dale RC, Church AJ, Cardoso F, et al: Poststreptococcal acute disseminated encephalomyelitis with basal ganglia involvement and autoreactive antibasal ganglia antibodies. *Ann Neurol* 50:588, 2001.

43. von Economo C: *Encephalitis Lethargica: Its Sequelae and Treatment*. Oxford, England: Oxford University Press, 1931.

44. Pradhan S, Pandey N, Shashank S, et al: Parkinsonism due to predominant involvement of substantia nigra in Japanese encephalitis. *Neurology* 53:1781, 1999.

45. Miyasaki K, Takayoshi F: Parkinsonism following encephalitis of unknown etiology. *J Neuropathol Exp Neurol* 36:1, 1977.

46. Geddes JF, Hughes AJ, Lees AJ, et al: Pathological overlap in cases of parkinsonism associated with neurofibrillary tangles: A study of recent cases of postencephalitic parkinsonism and comparison with progressive supranuclear palsy and Guamanian parkinsonism-dementia complex. *Brain* 116:281, 1993.

47. Wenning GK, Jellinger K, Litvan I: Supranuclear gaze palsy and eyelid apraxia in postencephalitic parkinsonism. *J Neural Transm* 104:845, 1997.

48. Howard RS, Lees AJ: Encephalitis lethargica: A report of four recent cases. *Brain* 110(pt 1):19, 1987.

49. Casals J, Elizan TS, Yahr MD: Postencephalitic parkinsonism: A review. *J Neural Transm* 105:645, 1998.

50. Deresiewicz RL, Thaler SJ, Hsu L, et al: Clinical and neuroradiographic manifestations of eastern equine encephalitis. *New Engl J Med* 336:1867, 1997.

51. Ochi J, Okuno T, Uenoyama Y, et al: Symmetrical low density areas in bilateral thalami in an infant with measles encephalitis. *Comput Radiol* 10:137, 1986.

52. Tarr RW, Edwards KM, Kessler RM, et al: MRI of mumps encephalitis: Comparison with CT evaluation. *Pediatr Radiol* 17:59, 1987.

53. Peters AC, Vielvoye GJ, Versteeg J, et al: ECHO 25 focal encephalitis and subacute hemichorea. *Neurology* 29:676, 1979.

54. Kun LN, Yian SY, Haur LS, et al: Bilateral substantia nigra changes on MRI in a patient with encephalitis lethargica. *Neurology* 53:1860, 1999.

55. Verschueren H, Crols R: Bilateral substantia nigra lesions on magnetic resonance imaging in a patient with encephalitis lethargica. *J Neurol Neurosurg Psychiatry* 71:275, 2001.

56. Ghaemi M, Rudolf J, Schmülling S, et al: FDG- and Dopa-PET in postencephalitic parkinsonism. *J Neural Transm* 107:1289, 2000.

57. Litvan I, Agid Y, Jankovic J, et al: Accuracy of clinical criteria for the diagnosis of progressive supranuclear palsy (Steele-Richardson-Olszewski syndrome). *Neurology* 46:922, 1996.

58. Picard F, De Saint-Martin A, Salmon E, et al: Postencephalitic stereotyped involuntary movements responsive to L-dopa. *Mov Disord* 11:567, 1996.

59. Blunt SB, Lane RJM, Turjanski N, et al: Clinical features and management of two cases of encephalitis lethargica. *Mov Disord* 12:354, 1997.

60. Whipple GH: A hitherto undescribed disease characterized anatomically by deposits of fat and fatty acids in the intestinal and mesenteric lymphatic tissues. *Bull Johns Hopkins Hosp* 18:382, 1907.

61. Relman DA, Schmidt TM, MacDermott RP, et al: Identification of the uncultured bacillus of Whipple's disease. *New Engl J Med* 327:293, 1992.

62. Swartz MN: Whipple's disease: Past, present, and future. *New Engl J Med* 342:648, 2000.

63. Maiwald M, Schuhmacher F, Ditton HJ, et al: Environmental occurrence of the Whipple's disease bacterium (*Tropheryma whippelii*). *Appl Environ Microbiol* 64:760, 1998.

64. Street S, Donoghue HD, Neild GH: *Tropheryma whippelii* DNA in saliva of healthy people. *Lancet* 354:1178, 1999.

65. Raoult D, Birg ML, La Scola B, et al: Cultivation of the bacillus of Whipple's disease. *New Engl J Med* 342:620, 2000.

66. Amsler L, Bauernfeind P, Nigg C, et al: Prevalence of *Tropheryma whipplei* DNA in patients with various gastrointestinal diseases and in healthy controls. *Infection* 31:81, 2003.

67. Anderson M: Neurology of Whipple's disease. *J Neurol Neurosurg Psychiatry* 68:2, 2000.

68. Schwartz NA, Selhorst JB, Ochs AL, et al: Oculomasticatory myorhythymia: A unique movement disorder occurring in Whipple's disease. *Ann Neurol* 20:677, 1986.

69. Louis ED, Lynch T, Kaufmann P, et al: Diagnostic guidelines in central nervous system Whipple's disease. *Ann Neurol* 40:561, 1996.

70. Rajput AH, McHattie JD: Ophthalmoplegia and leg myorhythmia in Whipple's disease: Report of a case. *Mov Disord* 12:111, 1997.

71. Averbuch-Heller L, Paulson GW, Daroff RB, et al: Whipple's disease mimicking progressive supranuclear palsy: The diagnostic value of eye movement recording. *J Neurol Neurosurg Psychiatry* 66:532, 1999.

72. Lee AG: Whipple disease with supranuclear ophthalmoplegia diagnosed by polymerase chain reaction of cerebrospinal fluid. *J Neuroophthalmol* 22:18, 2002.

73. Dobbins WO III: The diagnosis of Whipple's disease. *New Engl J Med* 332:390, 1995.

74. Lowsky R, Archer GL, Fyles G, et al: Brief report: diagnosis of Whipple's disease by molecular analysis of peripheral blood. *New Engl J Med* 331:1343, 1994.

75. Schnider P, Trattnig S, Kollegger H, et al: MR of cerebral Whipple disease. *Am J Neuroradiol* 16:1328, 1995.

76. Kremer S, Besson G, Bonaz B, et al: Diffuse lesions in the CNS revealed by MR imaging in a case of Whipple disease. *Am J Neuroradiol* 22:493, 2001.

77. Messori A, Di Bella P, Polonara G, et al: An unusual spinal presentation of Whipple disease. *Am J Neuroradiol* 22:1004, 2001.

78. Clarke CE, Falope ZF, Abdelhadi HA, et al: Cervical myelopathy caused by Whipple's disease. *Neurology* 50:1505, 1998.

79. Keinath RD, Merrell DE, Vlietstra R, et al: Antibiotic treatment and relapse in Whipple's disease: Long-term follow-up of 88 patients. *Gastroenterology* 88:1867, 1985.

80. Simpson DA, Wishnow R, Gargulinski RB, et al: Oculofacial-skeletal myorhythmia in central nervous system Whipple's disease: Additional case and review of the literature. *Mov Disord* 10:195, 1995.

81. Ramzan NN, Loftus E Jr, Burgart LJ, et al: Diagnosis and monitoring of Whipple disease by polymerase chain reaction. *Ann Intern Med* 126:520, 1997.

82. Pron B, Poyart C, Abachin E, et al: Diagnosis and follow-up of Whipple's disease by amplification of the 16S rRNA gene of *Tropheryma whippelii*. *Eur J Clin Microbiol Infect Dis* 18:62, 1999.

83. Hausser-Hauw C, Roullet E, Robert R, et al: Oculofacioskeletal myorhythmia as a cerebral complication of systemic Whipple's disease. *Mov Disord* 3:179, 1988.

84. Schnider PJ, Reisinger EC, Gerschlager W, et al: Long-term follow-up in cerebral Whipple's disease. *Eur J Gastroenterol Hepatol* 8:899, 1996.

85. Berndt R: Reaction to contact in the eastern highlands of New Guinea. *Oceania* 24:190, 1954.

86. Gajdusek D, Zigas V: Degenerative disease of the central nervous system in New Guinea. *New Engl J Med* 257:974, 1957.

87. Klatzo I, Gajdusek D: Pathology of kuru. *Lab Invest* 8:799, 1959.

88. Hadlow W: Scrapie and kuru. *Lancet* 2:289, 1959.

89. Alper T, Haig DA, Clarke MC: The exceptionally small size of the scrapie agent. *Biochem Biophys Res Commun* 22:278, 1966.

90. Prusiner SB: Novel proteinaceous infectious particles cause scrapie. *Science* 216:136, 1982.

91. Tyler KL: Creutzfeldt-Jakob disease. *New Engl J Med* 348:681, 2003.

92. Andrews NJ, Farrington CP, Ward HJ, et al: Deaths from variant Creutzfeldt-Jakob disease in the UK. *Lancet* 361:751, 2003.

93. Prusiner SB: Prions. *Proc Natl Acad Sci USA* 95:13363, 1998.

94. Parchi P, Giese A, Capellari S, et al: Classification of sporadic Creutzfeldt-Jakob disease based on molecular and phenotypic analysis of 300 subjects. *Ann Neurol* 46:224, 1999.

95. Brown P, Cathala F, Castaigne P, et al: Creutzfeldt-Jakob disease: Clinical analysis of a consecutive series of 230 neuropathologically verified cases. *Ann Neurol* 20:597, 1986.

96. Hellmann MA, Melamed E: Focal dystonia as the presenting sign in Creutzfeldt-Jakob disease. *Mov Disord* 17:1097, 2002.

97. Tschampa HJ, Neumann M, Zerr I, et al: Patients with Alzheimer's disease and dementia with Lewy bodies mistaken for Creutzfeldt-Jakob disease. *J Neurol Neurosurg Psychiatry* 71:33, 2001.

98. Zeidler M, Sellar RJ, Collie DA, et al: The pulvinar sign on magnetic resonance imaging in variant Creutzfeldt-Jakob disease. *Lancet* 355:1412, 2000.

99. Burkhard PR, Sanchez JC, Landis T, et al: CSF detection of the 14-3-3 protein in unselected patients with dementia. *Neurology* 56:1528, 2001.

100. Budka H, Aguzzi A, Brown P, et al: Neuropathological diagnostic criteria for Creutzfeldt-Jakob disease (CJD) and other human spongiform encephalopathies (prion diseases). *Brain Pathol* 5:459, 1995.

101. Piccardo P, Langeveld JP, Hill AF, et al: An antibody raised against a conserved sequence of the prion protein recognizes pathological isoforms in human and animal prion diseases, including Creutzfeldt-Jakob disease and bovine spongiform encephalopathy. *Am J Pathol* 152:1415, 1998.

102. Wadsworth JD, Joiner S, Hill AF, et al: Tissue distribution of protease resistant prion protein in variant Creutzfeldt-Jakob disease using a highly sensitive immunoblotting assay. *Lancet* 358:171, 2001.

103. Hill AF, Zeidler M, Ironside J, et al: Diagnosis of new variant Creutzfeldt-Jakob disease by tonsil biopsy. *Lancet* 349:99, 1997.

104. Zanusso G, Ferrari S, Cardone F, et al: Detection of pathologic prion protein in the olfactory epithelium in sporadic Creutzfeldt-Jakob disease. *New Engl J Med* 348:711, 2003.

105. Haik S, Brandel JP, Sazdovitch V, et al: Dementia with Lewy bodies in a neuropathologic series of suspected Creutzfeldt-Jakob disease. *Neurology* 55:1401, 2000.

106. Riemenschneider M, Wagenpfeil S, Vanderstichele H, et al: Phospho-tau/total tau ratio in cerebrospinal fluid discriminates Creutzfeldt-Jakob disease from other dementias. *Mol Psychiatry* 8:343, 2003.

107. Sigurdsson EM, Brown DR, Daniels M, et al: Immunization delays the onset of prion disease in mice. *Am J Pathol* 161:13, 2002.

108. Sigurdsson EM, Sy MS, Li R, et al: Antiprion antibodies for prophylaxis following prion exposure in mice. *Neurosci Lett* 336:185, 2003.

109. Anlar B, Kose G, Gurer Y, et al: Changing epidemiological features of subacute sclerosing panencephalitis. *Infection* 29:192, 2001.

110. Wild TF: Measles vaccines, new developments and immunization strategies. *Vaccine* 17:1726, 1999.

111. Duclos P, Redd SC, Varughese P, et al:: Measles in adults in Canada and the United States: Implications for measles elimination and eradication. *Int J Epidemiol* 28:141, 1999.

112. Miller C, Farrington CP, Harbert K: The epidemiology of subacute sclerosing panencephalitis in England and Wales 1970–1989. *Int J Epidemiol* 21:998, 1992.

113. Cattaneo R, Schmid A, Spielhofer P, et al: Mutated and hypermutated genes of persistent measles viruses which caused lethal human brain diseases. *Virology* 173:415, 1989.

114. Sawaishi Y, Yano T, Watanabe Y, et al: Migratory basal ganglia lesions in subacute sclerosing panencephalitis (SSPE): Clinical implications of axonal spread. *J Neurol Sci* 168:137, 1999.

115. Wirguin I, Steiner I, Kidron D, et al: Fulminant subacute sclerosing panencephalitis in association with pregnancy. *Arch Neurol* 45:1324, 1988.

116. Joseph FG, Jacob J, Carrington D: SSPE: A forgotten disease? *Eur J Neurol* 9:542, 2002.

117. Singer C, Lang AE, Suchowersky O: Adult-onset subacute sclerosing panencephalitis: Case reports and review of the literature. *Mov Disord* 12: 342, 1997.

118. Ondo WG, Verma A: Physiological assessment of paroxysmal dystonia secondary to subacute sclerosing panencephalitis. *Mov Disord* 17:154, 2002.

119. Oga T, Ikeda A, Nagamine T, et al: Implication of sensorimotor integration in the generation of periodic dystonic myoclonus in subacute sclerosing panencephalitis (SSPE). *Mov Disord* 15:1173, 2000.

120. Akdal G, Baklan B, Cakmakci H, et al: MRI follow-up of basal ganglia involvement in subacute sclerosing panencephalitis. *Pediatr Neurol* 24:393, 2001.

121. Anlar B, Saatci I, Kose G, et al: MRI findings in subacute sclerosing panencephalitis. *Neurology* 47:1278, 1996.

122. Ozturk A, Gurses C, Baykan B, et al: Subacute sclerosing panencephalitis: Clinical and magnetic resonance imaging evaluation of 36 patients. *J Child Neurol* 17:25, 2002.

123. Aydin OF, Senbil N, Kuyucu N, et al: Combined treatment with subcutaneous interferon-alpha, oral isoprinosine, and lamivudine for subacute sclerosing panencephalitis. *J Child Neurol* 18:104, 2003.

124. Bejjani BP, Chemaly NR: Intravenous gammaglobulins in the treatment of subacute sclerosing panencephalitis. *Neurology* 60(suppl 1):A249, 2003.

125. Risk WS, Haddad FS, Chemali R: Substantial spontaneous long-term improvement in subacute sclerosing panencephalitis: Six cases from the Middle East and a review of the literature. *Arch Neurol* 35:494, 1978.

126. Solomon T, Hart CA, Vinjamuri S, et al: Treatment of subacute sclerosing panencephalitis with interferon-alpha, ribavirin, and inosiplex. *J Child Neurol* 17:703, 2002.

127. De Mattos JP, Rosso AL, Correa RB, et al: Involuntary movements and AIDS: Report of seven cases and review of the literature. *Arq Neuropsiquiatr* 51:491, 1993.

128. Mattos JP, Rosso AL, Correa RB, et al: Movement disorders in 28 HIV-infected patients. *Arq Neuropsiquiatr* 60:525, 2002.

129. Berger JR, Levy RM: The neurologic complications of human immunodeficiency virus infection. *Med Clin North Am* 77:1, 1993.

130. Maggi P, de Mari M, Moramarco A, et al: Parkinsonism

in a patient with AIDS and cerebral opportunistic granulomatous lesions. *Neurol Sci* 21:173, 2000.

131. Mirsattari SM, Power C, Nath A: Parkinsonism with HIV infection. *Mov Disord* 13:684, 1998.

132. Nath A, Jankovic J: Motor disorders in patients with human immunodeficiency virus infection. *Prog AIDS Pathol* 1:159, 1989.

133. Gallo BV, Shulman LM, Weiner WJ, et al: HIV encephalitis presenting with severe generalized chorea. *Neurology* 46:1163, 1996.

134. Pardo J, Marcos A, Bhathal H, et al: Chorea as a form of presentation of human immunodeficiency virus–associated dementia complex. *Neurology* 50:568, 1998.

135. Bhatia KP, Marsden CD: The behavioral and motor consequences of focal lesions of the basal ganglia in man. *Brain* 117:859, 1994.

136. Rottenberg DA, Moeller JR, Strother SC, et al: The metabolic pathology of the AIDS dementia complex. *Ann Neurol* 22:700, 1987.

137. von Giesen HJ, Antke C, Hefter H, et al: Potential time course of human immunodeficiency virus type 1–associated minor motor deficits: Electrophysiologic and positron emission tomography findings. *Arch Neurol* 57:1601, 2000.

138. Berger JR, Arendt G: HIV dementia: The role of the basal ganglia and dopaminergic systems. *J Psychopharmacol* 14:214, 2000.

139. Van Gerpen JA: Tremor caused by trimethoprim-sulfamethoxazole in a patient with AIDS. *Neurology* 48:537, 1997.

140. Slavik RS, Rybak MJ, Lerner SA: Trimethoprim/sulfamethoxazole–induced tremor in a patient with AIDS. *Ann Pharmacother* 32:1892, 1998.

141. Singer C, Weiner WJ: Tremor in the acquired immune deficiency syndrome. In Findley LJ, Koller WC (eds). *Handbook of Tremor Disorders*. New York: Marcel Dekker, 2003, pp 483–489.

142. Nath A, Hobson DE, Russell A: Movement disorders with cerebral toxoplasmosis and AIDS. *Mov Disord* 8:107, 1993.

143. Tolge CF, Factor SA: Focal dystonia secondary to cerebral toxoplasmosis in a patient with acquired immune deficiency syndrome. *Mov Disord* 6:69, 1991.

144. Pitagoras dM, Oliveira M, Andre C: Painful legs and moving toes associated with neuropathy in HIV-infected patients. *Mov Disord* 14:1053, 1999.

145. Thomas P, Borg M: Reversible myoclonic encephalopathy revealing the AIDS-dementia complex. *Electroencephalogr Clin Neurophysiol* 90:166, 1994.

146. Mirsattari SM, Berry ME, Holden JK, et al: Paroxysmal dyskinesias in patients with HIV infection. *Neurology* 52:109, 1999.

147. Antinori A, Ammassari A, De Luca A, et al: Diagnosis of AIDS-related focal brain lesions: A decision-making analysis based on clinical and neuroradiologic characteristics combined with polymerase chain reaction assays in CSF. *Neurology* 48:687, 1997.

148. Cardoso F: HIV-related movement disorders: Epidemiology, pathogenesis and management. *CNS Drugs* 16:663, 2002.

149. Arendt G, Hefter H, Hilperath F, et al: Motor analysis predicts progression in HIV-associated brain disease. *J Neurol Sci* 123:180, 1994.

150. Jimenez-Jimenez FJ, Garcia-Ruiz PJ, Molina JA: Drug-induced movement disorders. *Drug Saf* 16:180, 1997.

151. Morgante L, Rocca WA, Di Rosa AE, et al: Prevalence of Parkinson's disease and other types of parkinsonism: A door-to-door survey in three Sicilian municipalities. The Sicilian Neuro-Epidemiologic Study (SNES) Group. *Neurology* 42:1901, 1992.

152. Lang AE, Weiner WJ: *Drug-Induced Movement Disorders*. Mount Kisco, NY: Futura, 1992.

153. Fisher JF, Dewald J: Parkinsonism associated with intraventricular amphotericin B. *J Antimicrob Chemother* 12:97, 1983.

154. Grimes JD: Parkinsonism and tardive dyskinesia associated with long-term metoclopramide therapy. *New Engl J Med* 305:1417, 1981.

155. Samie MR: Neuroleptic malignant-like syndrome induced by metoclopramide. *Mov Disord* 2:57, 1987.

156. Goetz CG: Tardive dyskinesia. In Watts RL, Koller WC (eds): *Movement Disorders: Neurologic Principles and Practice*. New York: McGraw-Hill, 1997, pp 519–526.

157. Patterson RG, Couchenour RL: Trimethoprim-sulfamethoxazole–induced tremor in an immunocompetent patients. *Pharmacotherapy* 19:1456, 1999.

158. Casey DE: Tardive dyskinesia and atypical antipsychotic drugs. *Schizophr Res* 35:S61, 1999.

159. Shale H, Tanner C: Pharmacological options for the management of dyskinesias. *Drugs* 52:849, 1996.

160. Wilde MI, Markham A: Ondansetron: A review of its pharmacology and preliminary clinical findings in novel applications. *Drugs* 52:773, 1996.

161. Stahlmann R, Lode H: Fluoroquinolones in the elderly: Safety considerations. *Drugs Aging* 20:289, 2003.

162. Fujishita M, Kataoka R, Eguchi T, et al: [Seizure and tremor occurring in acute leukemia patients treated with imipenem/cilastatin.] *Rinsho Ketsueki* 30:392, 1989.

163. Lucas KH, Schliesser SH, O'Neil MG: Shaking, chills, and rigors with once-daily gentamicin. *Pharmacotherapy* 19:1102, 1999.

164. Laguna DE, Calabrese S, Zabala JA, et al: [Neurological toxicity from pentavalent antimonials during the treatment of visceral leishmaniasis.] *Med Clin (Barc)* 102:276, 1994.

165. Brennum J: [Extrapyramidal side effects after long-term treatment with thiethylperazine.] *Ugeskr Laeger* 150:2827, 1988.

166. Bateman DN, Darling WM, Boys R, et al: Extrapyramidal reactions to metoclopramide and prochlorperazine. *Q J Med* 71:307, 1989.

167. Bateman DN, Rawlins MD, Simpson JM: Extrapyramidal reactions with metoclopramide. *Br Med J* 291:930, 1985.

168. Mehta MA, Sahakian BJ, McKenna PJ, et al: Systemic sulpiride in young adult volunteers simulates the profile of cognitive deficits in Parkinson's disease. *Psychopharmacology (Berl)* 146:162, 1999.

169. Chouza C, Caamano JL, Romero S, et al: Extrapyramidal effects of benzamides. *Adv Biochem Psychopharmacol* 40:43, 1985.

170. Sempere AP, Duarte J, Palomares JM, et al: Parkinsonism and tardive dyskinesia after chronic use of clebopride. *Mov Disord* 9:114, 1994.

171. Sempere AP, Duarte J, Cabezas C, et al: Aggravation of parkinsonian tremor by cisapride. *Clin Neuropharmacol* 18:76, 1995.

172. Naito Y, Kuzuhara S: [Parkinsonism induced or worsened by cisapride.] *Nippon Ronen Igakkai Zasshi* 31:899, 1994.

173. Klawans HL, Moskovitz C: Cyclizine-induced chorea: Observations on the influence of cyclizine on dopamine-related movement disorders. *J Neurol Sci* 31:237, 1977.

174. Sweeney BJ, Edgecombe J, Churchill DR, et al: Choreoathetosis/ballismus associated with pentamidine-induced hypoglycemia in a patient with the acquired immunodeficiency syndrome. *Arch Neurol* 51:723, 1994.

175. Quinn AG, Ellis WR, Burn D, et al: Chorea precipitated by sulphasalazine. *Br Med J* 302:1025, 1991.

176. Patterson JF: Choreiform movement associated with metoclopramide. *South Med J* 79:1465, 1986.

177. Uchihara T, Tsukagoshi H: Myoclonic activity associated with cefmetazole, with a review of neurotoxicity of cephalosporins. *Clin Neurol Neurosurg* 90:369, 1988.

178. Durand JM, Telle H, Quiles N, et al: [Confusion syndrome, myoclonus and treatment with pefloxacin.] *Ann Med Interne (Paris)* 144:495, 1993.

179. Fossieck B Jr, Parker RH: Neurotoxicity during intravenous infusion of penicillin: A review. *J Clin Pharmacol* 14:504, 1974.

180. Frucht S, Eidelberg D: Imipenem-induced myoclonus. *Mov Disord* 12:621, 1997.

181. Destee A, Verrier A, Gelez P, et al: [Myoclonic encephalopathy caused by isoniazid-hydantoin combination.] *Lille Med* 24:41, 1979.

182. Church AJ, Dale RC, Cardoso F, et al: CSF and serum immune parameters in Sydenham's chorea: Evidence of an autoimmune syndrome? *J Neuroimmunol* 136:149, 2003.

183. Garvey MA, Perlmutter SJ, Allen AJ, et al: A pilot study of penicillin prophylaxis for neuropsychiatric exacerbations triggered by streptococcal infections. *Biol Psychiat* 45:1564, 1999.

184. Cerna F, Mehrad B, Luby JP, et al: St. Louis encephalitis and the substantia nigra: MR imaging evaluation. *AJNR* 20:1281, 1999.

185. Wasay M, Diaz-Arrastia R, Suss RA, et al: St Louis encephalitis: A review of 11 cases in a 1995 Dallas, Texas, epidemic. *Arch Neurol* 57:114, 2000.

186. Cree BC, Bernardini GL, Hays AP, et al: A fatal case of coxsackievirus B4 meningoencephalitis. *Arch Neurol* 60:107, 2003.

187. Alves RS, Barbosa ER, Scaff M: Postvaccinal parkinsonism. *Mov Disord* 7:178, 1992.

188. Savant CS, Singhal BS, Jankovic J, et al: Substantia nigra lesions in viral encephalitis. *Mov Disord* 18:213, 2003.

CHAPTER 25

Ophthalmic Disorders in Neurologic Infectious Diseases

Robert D. Yee

About 40 percent of the central nervous system (CNS) is involved with the visual system or the control of eye movements. About 50 percent of the afferent input to the CNS is related to vision. Therefore, it is understandable that ophthalmic signs and symptoms are encountered frequently in neurologic infections. Ophthalmic disorders are important in the diagnosis of neurologic infections and can become significant elements in the disability resulting from the infections. In addition, the eye, its adnexae, and the orbit can be the initial sites of infection that extend into the CNS. This chapter describes the disorders of the eye, its adnexae, and the orbit associated with CNS infections. The in-formation is organized into an initial section that describes the symptoms and signs of eye disorders at different anatomic locations and a second section that discusses the ophthalmic disorders according to the categories of infectious organisms. Chapters in textbooks of general ophthalmology[1,2] and neuroophthalmology[3,4] present similar information in more detail and use both an etiologic and an anatomic outline. Much of the information in this chapter relies on material written by authors of those chapters. The differential diagnosis and management of CNS infections and their ophthalmic disorders will not be discussed in detail in this chapter.

► SYMPTOMS AND SIGNS OF EYE DISORDERS

Eyelids

Infections of the eyelids can produce skin lesions and edema. Pain and hyperemia often accompany infectious blepharitis. Associated conjunctival and corneal inflammation causes conjunctivitis and keratitis. One of the functions of the eyelids is to spread the tears over the corneal surface and to protect the ocular surfaces from dryness and trauma. Therefore, blepharitis often causes irregularities of the corneal surface and blurring of vision. Cranial nerve palsies associated with CNS infections can impair eyelid motor functions. Impaired blinking can be caused by seventh nerve palsy from paresis of the orbicularis oculi muscles. The resulting exposure keratopathy also blurs vision and can lead to corneal ulceration. Paresis of the levator palpebrae superioris muscle from third nerve palsy produces ptosis of the upper eyelid.

Conjunctiva

Infections cause lesions in the conjunctiva. The accompanying inflammation produces dilation of the conjunctival vessels and a bright red appearance of the eye (Fig. 25-1). The type of infectious organism usually determines whether discharge from the eye is watery, mucoid, or purulent. Pain is variable, depending on the type of infectious organism. Conjunctival necrosis produces membranes that bleed when stripped from the surface of the eye. The accessory lacrimal glands open into the lower and upper conjunctival fornices and contribute to the aqueous layer of the tear film. Conjunctival goblet cells produce the mucus layer of the tear film. Therefore, scarring of the conjunctiva can cause abnormalities of the tear film, superficial ocular discomfort, dry eye, and blurred vision. Scarring of the opposed surfaces of the palpebral conjunctiva on the posterior eyelid surface and the bulbar conjunctiva on the surface of the globe causes adhesions called *symblepharon*. Clear edema fluid beneath the conjunctiva is called *conjunctival chemosis* and is produced by conjunctivitis or inflammation of the sclera, the intraocular tissues, or the orbit. Obstruction of venous blood flow from the orbit into the cavernous sinus produces chemosis and conjunctival injection.

Cornea

The cornea is the most important ocular tissue for refraction and image formation. Infectious keratitis can greatly impair image formation and blur vision in several ways. Roughening of the corneal surface from superficial keratitis, edema of the corneal epithelium, or ulceration causes irregular astigmatism. Light striking the corneal surface is scattered and refracted in various directions, which markedly degrades images on the retina. The cornea is normally transparent because of its relative dehydration and regular structure of its collagen lamellae. The cornea is avascular because limbal blood vessels normally end at the edges of the cornea. In keratitis, limbal vessels can extend into the cornea and leak plasma, causing opacification. Edema and scarring in the corneal stroma disrupt the regular pattern of the corneal lamellae causing loss of corneal transparency. The corneal endothelial cells at the posterior corneal surface pump water out of the cornea into the anterior chamber. Keratitis can damage the endothelial cells, leading to corneal edema and opacification (Fig. 25-2).

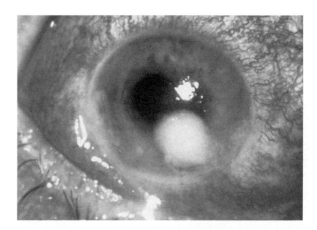

Figure 25-2. Bacterial corneal ulcer. Infection and inflammation produced white opacification of the ulcer. The surrounding cornea, especially the inferior one-half, is edematous and has lost some of its transparency. The irregular light reflex on the cornea above the ulcer shows that the corneal epithelium is also edematous and has lost its smooth surface. There is a small white hypopyon in the inferior anterior chamber.

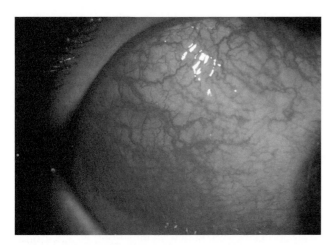

Figure 25-1. Viral conjunctivitis. The conjunctival blood vessels are dilated and tortuous.

Pain from keratitis is variable, depending on the infectious organism. Inflammation with hyperemia of the conjunctiva often accompanies keratitis.

Episclera and Sclera

The episclera is loose connective tissue between the sclera and conjunctiva that also contains blood vessels. Episcleritis produces focal or diffuse edema or opacification with dilatation of the episcleral vessels (Fig. 25-3). Accompanying pain is variable, depending on the severity of inflammation and the infectious organism. The hyperemia appears dark red rather than bright red as in conjunctivitis. Scleritis causes dilatation of scleral and episcleral blood vessels and produces a purple-red hyperemia (Fig. 25-4). Pain is often more intense than in episcleritis or conjunctivitis. Inflammation and thickening of the sclera can be localized or diffuse. Necrosis of scleral connective tissue causes a blue or brown discoloration of the sclera because the darkly pigmented ciliary body or choroid is seen beneath the thinned sclera (Fig. 25-5, Plate 1). Inflammation of adjacent cornea, iris, and ciliary body may cause keratitis and anterior uveitis.

Iris and Ciliary Body

The iris and ciliary body can be infected or inflamed when other ocular tissues are infected, such as in keratitis and scleritis. In anterior uveitis, veins that connect iris and ciliary vessels with vessels at the scleral surface become dilated, producing a deep red hyperemia at the edges of the cornea or limbus called *ciliary injection*. Pain is often deep in the eye and can be increased by exposure to light (photophobia and ciliary spasm). Iris and ciliary body veins dilate and leak plasma and white blood cells, producing flare and cells in the aqueous humor within the anterior chamber. Loss of trans-

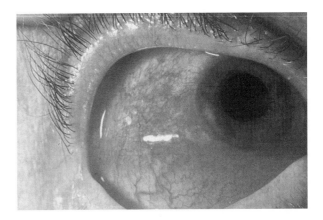

Figure 25-4. Scleritis. Diffuse inflammation of the sclera causes dilatation of blood vessels in the sclera, episclera, and conjunctiva and edema of those tissues.

parency of the aqueous humor and vitreous causes blurring. Accommodation is impaired because smooth muscles in the ciliary body are damaged. Anterior uveitis also can cause exudation of plasma from retinal blood vessels in the macula. Resulting macular edema also decreases visual acuity. The pupil can become small, and its light and near reactions are decreased. Adhesions between the iris and anterior lens surface (posterior synechiae) or between the iris and peripheral cornea (peripheral anterior synechiae and anterior synechiae) can develop. Necrosis of the iris causes iris atrophy with thinning and change in its color. Glaucoma can result from blockage of the trabecular meshwork by inflammatory cells that were suspended in the anterior chamber and move into the meshwork, inflammation of the trabecular meshwork itself, or peripheral and anterior synechiae mechanically blocking access of the aqueous humor to the meshwork.

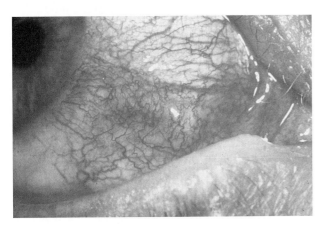

Figure 25-3. Nodular episcleritis. Focal inflammation of the episclera produces a nodular elevation. Both superficial conjunctival blood vessels and deeper episcleral vessels are dilated and tortuous.

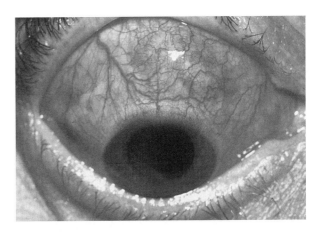

Figure 25-5. Scleritis and staphyloma. Scleritis produced necrosis of the sclera. The weakened sclera bulges outward (staphyloma), and the underlying bluish ciliary body and choroid are seen. See Plate 1.

Lens

The crystalline lens rarely becomes infected itself except after penetrating eye injuries. However, it can lose its transparency and become cataractous secondary to inflammation and infection elsewhere in the eye. Blurred vision and glare are the primary symptoms. Lens opacities can be seen easily with the direct ophthalmoscope as dark shadows in the bright red reflex from the fundus.

Vitreous

In vitritis, inflammatory cells, red blood cells, and plasma leak into the vitreous from blood vessels in the anterior uvea (iris and ciliary body), posterior uvea (choroids), retina, or optic disc. Loss of transparency causes blurred vision. Infectious organisms in the vitreous cavity can produce an abscess. Fibrous membranes and strands can develop between the vitreous cavity and the retina. If the retina is atrophic, weakened, and thin, traction between the vitreous and retina can cause retinal holes and tears, leading to a rhegmatogenous retina detachment. The traction also can detach the retina without a retinal break, producing tractional retinal detachment.

Retina and Choroid

The retina, which consists of the neurosensory retina and retinal pigment epithelium, and the choroid are closely approximated. Therefore, infection in either tissue often is accompanied by infection in the other. The type of visual loss produced by retinitis and choroiditis depends on the location of the lesion. Lesions affecting the macula or central retina cause blurring with loss of visual acuity, scotomas in the central parts of the visual field, and impairment of color vision. Lesions affecting the peripheral retina cause peripheral visual field loss. If the lesions damage the outer layers of the retina that contain the rod and cone photoreceptors, the visual field defects usually will be scotomas, with shape and size corresponding to the shape and size of the lesions themselves. If the lesions primarily damage the superficial layers of the retina that contain the ganglion cells and their axons, the visual field defects are often nerve fiber bundle defects, e.g., arcuate scotomas, or Bjerrum scotomas, and wedge-shaped sector visual field defects. Occlusions of the central retinal artery or its branches cause infarction of the inner half of the neurosensory retina that contains one-half of the bipolar cells, the ganglion cells, and ganglion cell axons. The infracted retina becomes opaque, blocking the red reflex from the retinal pigment epithelium and choroid. This produces the macular "cherry red spot" in central retinal artery occlusion. In branch retinal artery occlusions, visual field defects are altitudinal hemianopsias,

if superior or inferior branches are affected, or defects corresponding to the retinal areas supplied by nasal or temporal branches of the central retinal artery.

Lesions of the macula or optic nerve produce loss of visual acuity, impaired color vision, and central scotomas. However, macular lesions are not associated with a relative afferent pupillary defect found during the swinging-flashlight test unless the entire macula is affected. The macular photostress test will show delayed recovery of visual acuity after bright light has bleached the cone photoreceptors in the eye with the macular lesion. Macular lesions may cause distortion of images called *metamorphopsia*. The distortion can be demonstrated by asking the patient to look at an Amsler grid.

Optic Nerve and Visual Pathways

About 50 percent of axons in the human optic nerve come from ganglion cells in the macula. Therefore, damage to the optic nerve often produces loss of visual functions of the macula, including visual acuity, color vision, and central visual field. A number of visual field defects occur, including central scotomas, cecocentral scotomas, arcuate scotomas, altitudinal hemianopsias, quadrant defects, and peripheral rim defects. If the posterior portion of the intracranial optic nerve is damaged, a monocular temporal or nasal hemianopsia can occur. An afferent pupillary defect in the affected eye should be expected in the swinging-flashlight test unless both optic nerves are affected. If this occurs, decreased speed and amplitude of direct light reactions should be found in both eyes. Swelling of the optic disc with elevation of disc tissue and blurring of the disc margins can be caused by inflammation associated or not associated with direct infection (papillitis), infarction (anterior ischemic optic neuropathy), and increased intracranial pressure (papilledema). Papillitis (Fig. 25-6) and ischemic optic neuropathy usually impair the optic nerve's visual functions. Acute papilledema (Fig. 25-7) often only produces enlargement of the blind spot. Anterior uveitis and posterior uveitis often produce mild disc swelling. Optic atrophy is caused by any disorder that permanently damages optic nerve axons. Pallor of the optic disc is produced by loss of axons, reduction in small blood vessels, and decreased glial tissue. Damage to the retrobulbar, intracanalicular, and intracranial portions of the optic nerve produce delayed optic disc pallor days to weeks after the injury due to slow retrograde axonal degeneration and death of retinal ganglion cells.

The hallmark of damage to the optic chiasm is bitemporal hemianopsia with complete or partial loss of the temporal visual field in each eye. The border between the defective temporal field and the normal nasal field is along the vertical meridian. If the lesion damages the intracranial optic nerve and the junction of that

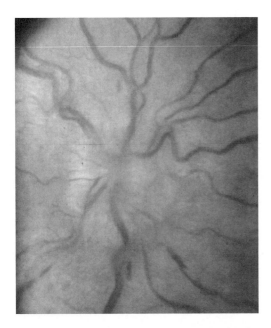

Figure 25-6. Papillitis. Swelling and opacification of optic nerve axons cause diffuse elevation of the optic disc and blurring of the disc margins. The optic cup is filled in. The retinal veins are tortuous and dilated, and several small splinter-shaped hemorrhages are in the peripapillary retina.

nerve and the chiasm, the affected eye has symptoms and signs of optic nerve damage, and the fellow eye has a partial superior temporal field defect (junctional scotoma). If damage to the optic chiasm includes the decussating retinal ganglion cell axons from the nasal halves of the retinas and the uncrossed axons from the temporal retinas, visual functions of both optic nerves are impaired.

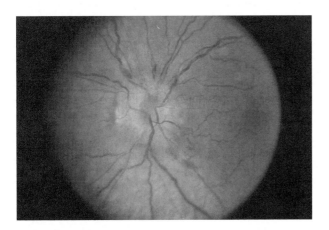

Figure 25-7. Papilledema. Optic disc swelling, dilatation of retinal veins, and splinter-shaped hemorrhages are similar to those seen in papillitis. However, typically both optic discs are swollen, and visual functions are normal, except for enlarged blind spots in papilledema.

Damage to the optic tracts, lateral geniculate bodies, visual radiations, and occipital lobes produce homonymous hemianopsias. The textbooks of ophthalmology and neuroophthalmology cited earlier present information about localization of lesions based on visual fields, pupil reactions in the swinging-flashlight test, and optic atrophy. Many of the CNS infections discussed below can cause blindness from bilateral lesions of the optic radiations or visual cortex in the occipital lobes (cortical blindness). Imaging of the visual pathways with magnetic resonance imaging (MRI) is often valuable. Thin slices of appropriate portions of the pathways with and without administration of gadolinium and with fat-suppression techniques (optic nerve and optic chiasm) are needed.

Orbit

Pain, periocular edema, and injection and proptosis usually accompany orbital cellulitis. Infectious organisms gain access to the orbit via the paranasal sinuses (Fig. 25-8), skin, vessels from the eyelids and face (Fig. 25-9),

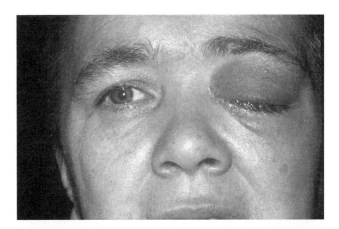

A

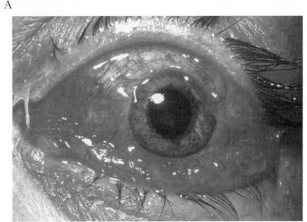

B

Figure 25-8. Orbital cellulitis and abscess. *A.* Bacterial ethmoiditis extended into the left orbit causing pain, periocular swelling, and proptosis. *B.* The conjunctiva is edematous and hyperemic.

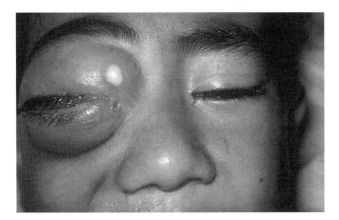

Figure 25-9. Orbital cellulitis. Bacterial cellulitis and abscess of the right upper eyelid caused orbital cellulitis with severe pain, proptosis, conjunctival edema and hyperemia, and periocular swelling.

the systemic circulation, and the eye (panophthalmitis). The direction of globe displacement can indicate the source of infection. For example, pyomucoceles of the frontal and ethmoid sinuses can displace the eye downward, temporally, and anteriorly (Figs. 25-10 and 25-11). Pyomucoceles of the maxillary sinus push the eye upward and anteriorly. An inflammatory mass in the muscle cone displaces the eye anteriorly (axial proptosis). Inflammation in the orbit can be diffuse or form abscesses and subperiosteal abscesses. Diplopia often is caused by ophthalmoplegia. Mechanical restriction from swelling of extraocular muscles and other orbital tis-

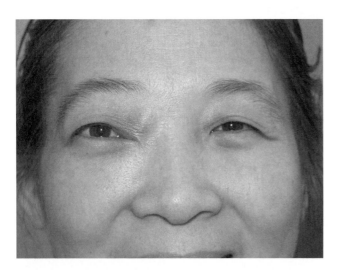

Figure 25-10. Pyomucocele of ethmoid, frontal, and maxillary sinuses. A large pyomucocele eroded through the medial orbital wall and caused slowly progressive displacement of the right eye laterally, downward, and anteriorly. The lesion can be palpated and seen beneath the skin at the medial canthus. Orbital cellulitis was not present.

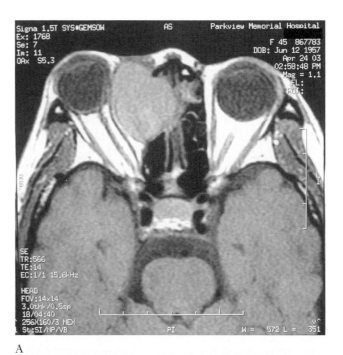

A

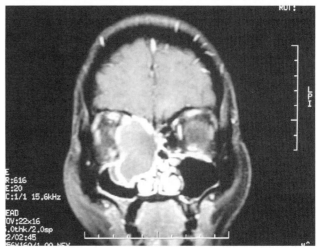

B

Figure 25-11. Pyomucocele of ethmoid, frontal, and maxillary sinuses. *A.* MRI coronal view through the anterior orbit shows the pyomucoceles eroding through the medial wall of the right orbit. The wall enhances with gadolinium. *B.* MRI axial view shows lateral displacement of the eye, extraocular muscles, and optic nerve.

sues, disruption of muscle fibers in the inflamed muscles themselves, and damage to the ocular motor cranial nerves in the orbit cause paresis of the extraocular muscles. Infection in the posterior orbit can produce the orbital apex syndrome. Multiple ocular motor nerve palsies cause ophthalmoplegia, and compression or inflammation of the optic nerve causes loss of vision. Computed tomographic (CT) scans and MRI are useful in imaging the orbit and its structures.

Cranial Nerves

The ocular motor cranial nerves (third, fourth, and sixth nerves), seventh nerve, and sensory divisions of the fifth nerve can be damaged at several locations, which include the peripheral, subarachnoid, and fascicular portions and their nuclei. Neuroophthalmic textbooks[3,4] describe the findings that help to localize the site of damage to these nerves. In many of the CNS infections discussed below, isolated or multiple cranial nerve palsies result from meningitis and inflammation of the nerves themselves. Increased intracranial pressure from meningitis and encephalitis often produces nonlateralizing and nonlocalizing sixth nerve palsies from damage to the subarachnoid portion of the nerve. Multiple palsies of ipsilateral third, fourth, and sixth nerves and loss of sensation in the first sensory division of the fifth nerve are indicative of cavernous sinus thrombosis or inflammation at the superior orbital fissure. Sparing or relative sparing of pupillary reactions in third nerve palsies also suggeset lesions at those locations. Ipsilateral Horner's syndrome and sixth nerve palsy are characteristic of cavernous sinus lesions. Cavernous sinus thrombosis often also produces signs of obstructed venous return from the orbits and bilateral cranial nerve palsies because of interconnections between the cavernous sinuses.

Other Ocular Motor Pathways and Higher Cortical Visual Functions

Pathways in the cerebral hemispheres, brain stem, and cerebellum are important in controlling eye movements. CNS infections that damage these pathways produce many ocular motor abnormalities. Textbooks describe these pathways and abnormalities in detail. Cerebral hemisphere lesions produce transient horizontal gaze palsy (volitional saccades), inability to suppress reflex saccades, impaired smooth pursuit, and decreased optokinetic nystagmus. Brain stem lesions cause supranuclear vertical and horizontal gaze palsies, internuclear ophthalmoplegia, skew deviation, and the ocular tilt reaction. They also produce various types of nystagmus, such as gaze-paretic nystagmus, upbeat nystagmus, pendular nystagmus, torsional nystagmus, and oculopalatal myoclonus. Cerebellar lesions cause impaired smooth pursuit, decreased optokinetic nystagmus, saccadic dysmetria, downbeat nystagmus, rebound nystagmus, periodic alternating nystagmus, and saccadic fixation instabilities (macro-square-wave jerks, ocular flutter, and opsoclonus).

The visual association areas in the occipital, parietal, and temporal lobes are important in interpretation of visual information for reading, identification of other symbols and objects, understanding of visuospatial relationships, reaching and grasping, perception of motion, and color vision. CNS infections that damage these areas produce several disorders, including the various elements of visual agnosia, optic ataxia, asimultanagnosia, akinetopsia, cerebral achromatopsia, and palinopsia.

▶ CATEGORIES OF INFECTIOUS ORGANISMS

Bacteria[5–7]

Gram-positive Cocci

STAPHYLOCOCCI

The staphylococci and other bacteria commonly cause blepharitis, conjunctivitis, and acute or chronic keratitis but rarely produce an endophthalmitis that extends into the CNS. Acute bacterial conjunctivitis caused by staphylococci and other bacteria usually produce lid edema, conjunctival injection, and a purulent discharge in one eye that involves the other eye in a few days. However, orbital cellulitis from these organisms can lead to CNS infection. They are the most common infectious causes of orbital cellulitis in adults. Sources of infection are paranasal sinusitis, eyelid or facial lesions, and septicemia. Pain, proptosis, diplopia with impaired range of eye movements, and visual loss from optic neuritis or compression can occur. Diffuse orbital infection or orbital abscesses can lead to cavernous sinus thrombosis, subdural empyema, and intracranial abscess by extension through the ophthalmic veins. When cavernous sinus thrombosis occurs, headache, nausea, vomiting, and decreased consciousness ensue.

Staphylococcus aureus, S. epidermidis, and other coagulase-negative staphylococci produce CNS infections in neonates, children, and adults associated with trauma, otitis media, paranasal sinus infection, septicemia, lumbar puncture, neurosurgical procedures including ventriculoperitoneal shunting, and osteomyelitis. They can cause meningitis, intracranial abscess, epidural and subdural empyema, and thrombosis of cerebral veins and dural venous sinuses. Staphylococcal infection is a rare cause of intracranial aneurysms. Meningitis, intracranial abscess, and cavernous sinus thrombosis can cause ocular motor cranial nerve palsies. Venous sinus thrombosis can cause papilledema from increased intracranial pressure.

STREPTOCOCCI

Streptococcal species, along with staphylococci and *Hemophilus influenzae,* can cause acute blepharitis and conjunctivitis with mucopurulent discharge and superficial keratitis (Fig. 25-12). These bacteria and others uncommonly cause anterior or posterior uveitis. When they do, the uveitis may be caused by endotoxins and exotoxins rather than by infection within the eye. Strep-

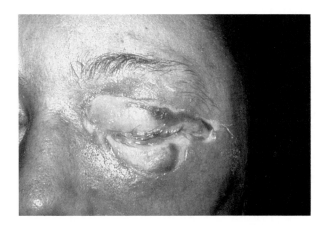

Figure 25-12. Streptococcal eyelid cellulitis. Necrosis of left upper and lower eyelids from beta-hemolytic streptococci.

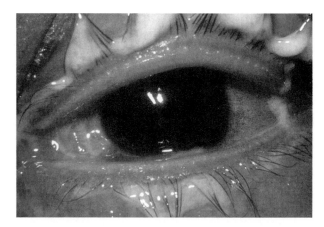

Figure 25-13. Gonococcal conjunctivitis. Hyperacute conjunctivitis with large amounts of white mucoid discharge. (*Courtesy of Fred M. Wilson II, M.D.*)

tococci, especially *Streptococcus pneumoniae,* can cause orbital cellulitis from paranasal sinus infection and meningitis. Pneumococcal meningitis produces ocular motor cranial nerve palsies, gaze palsies, and visual loss from vasculitis or infection of the optic nerves, optic chiasm, or posterior visual pathways. *S. viridans* and other streptococcal species also cause similar CNS infections. Iritis has been reported in rheumatic fever, in addition to the characteristic arthritis, carditis, rash, and neurologic manifestations. An immune reaction, rather than infection, probably produces the anterior uveitis.

ENTEROCOCCI

Enterococci normally are found in the gastrointestinal tract, oropharynx, and vagina. Bacteremia leads to infections of the eye and CNS. Keratitis with corneal ulceration, endophthalmitis, meningitis, brain abscess, empyema, septic aneurysm, and thrombosis of the cerebral and dural venous sinuses can occur.

Gram-Negative Cocci

NEISSERIA GONORRHOEAE

N. gonorrhoeae is of special importance to ophthalmologists because it causes a hyperacute conjunctivitis that can lead quickly to corneal ulceration and perforation of the globe. Newborns acquire the infection from passage through an infected mother's birth canal. Sexually active adults become infected by self-inoculation from their own infected urethra to the eye or from contact of their eye with secretions from their infected partners. The conjunctivitis is painful and produces copious purulent discharge, chemosis, and enlarged preauricular lymph node (Fig. 25-13). *N. gonorrhoeae,* along with *N. meningitides, Corynebacterium diphtheriae, H. aegyptium, Shigella* species, and *Listeria* species, can penetrate an intact corneal epithelium. That is, they can invade the cornea, causing keratitis and a

corneal ulcer, without a preexisting corneal abrasion. An ulcer in the peripheral cornea can perforate in days, leading to endophthalmitis (Fig. 25-14). In neonates, gonococcal conjunctivitis (ophthalmia neonatorum) must be differentiated from conjunctivitis caused by *Chlamydia trachomatis* and chemical conjunctivitis caused by topical silver nitrate, which previously was used commonly to prevent gonococcal conjunctivitis.

NEISSERIA MENINGITIDIS

N. meningitidis can cause conjunctivitis and keratitis, which are usually milder than those caused by *N. gonorrhoeae. N. meningitidis* is a leading causative organism of community-acquired acute bacterial meningitis. Basilar meningitis can cause cranial nerve palsies, including third, fourth, and sixth nerve palsies, optic neuritis, and optic chiasmitis. Optic neuritis is usually bilateral. Subarachnoid infection and inflammation over

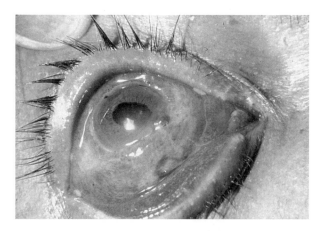

Figure 25-14. Gonococcal corneal ulcer. A corneal ulcer formed nasally at the edge of the right cornea. The ulcer perforated, causing prolapse of iris tissue into the ulcer and peaking of the pupil toward the perforation.

the brain convexities and in the basal cisterns produce communicating hydrocephalus, resulting in increased intracranial pressure and papilledema. Obstructive hydrocephalus also can occur. However, optic atrophy in most patients with this form of meningitis and others is often secondary to infection of the optic nerve rather than chronic papilledema. Optic disc swelling with normal optic nerve functions and normal opening pressure on lumbar puncture may be due to optic perineuritis. Nystagmus and other eye movement abnormalities from damage to the brain stem and cerebellum can develop. Cortical blindness that responds to antimicrobial therapy can occur.

Gram-Positive Bacilli

CLOSTRIDIUM BOTULINUM[8]

Spores of *C. botulinum* exist in soil and aquatic debris. Human diseases are produced when the spores germinate and the bacteria produce exotoxins, which are potent neurotoxins. Food botulism occurs after ingestion of contaminated food products that were not sterilized properly. Wound botulism results from neurotoxin released from bacteria growing in a wound that had been contaminated with spores. Bacteria colonizing the gastrointestinal tract cause infant botulism. In adults, botulism can come from colonization of diseased or surgically treated gastrointestinal tracts. In food botulism, blockage of peripheral cholinergic nerves can cause nausea; vomiting; extreme dryness of the mouth, pharynx, and eyes; urinary retention; constipation; and ileus within hours to a day after ingesting botulinum toxin. Diplopia from ophthalmoplegia and blurring from loss of accommodation develop. The lids are ptotic, and the pupils are dilated and poorly reactive. In wound botulism, spores are implanted in damaged tissues. Anaerobic conditions promote germination and production of neurotoxin. Within a few to several days, symptoms and signs similar to those in food botulism develop. In infant botulism, spores are ingested in contaminated food or soil and colonize the infant's gastrointestinal tract. A few to many weeks later, constipation, poor sucking, a weak cry, a poor gag reflex, and pooling of liquids and food in the mouth develop. Loss of head control, generalized weakness, hypotonia, and cranial nerve palsies, including ocular motor nerve palsies with poorly reactive pupils, develop. Crohn's disease and gastrointestinal bypass surgery for weight loss can be complicated by colonization of the gastrointestinal tract and botulism.

CLOSTRIDIUM TETANI

C. tetani also gains access to human hosts by contamination of wounds by its spores. Foreign bodies in the wounds contribute to the anaerobic environment required for germination of the spores. However, the spores can remain dormant for months or years. The incubation period is usually a few weeks. Tetanospasmin is released from lysis of bacteria, causing muscle spasms. Muscles near the wound develop weakness and stiffness; generalized symptoms ensue, often beginning with masticatory muscles, producing trismus. Reflex spasms in generalized tetanus produce opisthotonos and risus sardonicus. Wounds of the face, including the eyes, can cause early weakness and spasms of facial muscles and extraocular muscles. The most common ophthalmic sign of generalized tetanus is blepharospasm. Nuclear and infranuclear palsies of the ocular motor nerves can develop. Severe external ophthalmoplegia and internal ophthalmoplegia with dilated, poorly reactive pupils and loss of accommodation develop. Tonic divergence of the eyes and supranuclear vertical gaze palsy also can occur.

Other *Clostridium* species, e.g., *C. perfringens, C. septicum,* and *C. paraputrificum,* can cause brain abscesses and meningitis. They can cause ocular infections such as corneal ulcers and endophthalmitis (Fig. 25-15).

CORYNEBACTERIUM DIPTHERIAE

Infection with *C. diptheriae* is spread between humans by contact with respiratory secretions as inhaled droplets into the nasopharynx, by direct contact with the secretions, or by contact with infected skin lesions. Damage to surrounding tissues in the nose or pharynx is caused by exotoxins that inhibit protein synthesis and cause inflamed membranes. Systemic and neurologic symptoms are proportionate to the severity of the initial infection. Cough, hoarseness, stridor, and dyspnea are followed by prostration, respiratory failure, and myocarditis. Neurologic complications include polyneuritis that causes paralysis of the laryngeal and pharyngeal

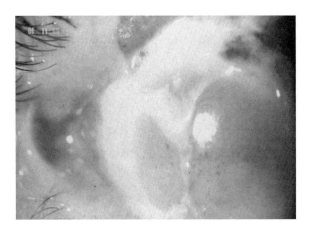

Figure 25-15. *Clostridia perfringens* endophthalmitis. Hematogenous spread of the bacteria caused an endophthalmitis. The cornea is opaque, and purulent discharge is seen on the corneal surface. (*Courtesy of John D. Sheppard, M.D.*)

muscles. Ophthalmic manifestations may be absent except for loss of accommodation. Pupillary light reactions can be intact, but near miosis may be decreased. Ocular motor cranial nerve palsies can occur. *C. diptheriae* can cause only localized ocular infection with conjunctivitis and keratitis.

LISTERIA MONOCYTOGENES

L. monocytogenes infections occur in individuals with impaired T-cell immunity, including neonates, elderly adults, pregnant women, patients treated with corticosteroids and other immunosuppressive drugs after organ transplantation, and patients with lymphoma, leukemia, and other neoplasms. *L. monocytogenes* can cause an acute meningitis, meningoencephalitis, or intracranial abscess. Brain stem encephalitis produces ocular motor cranial nerve palsies, internuclear ophthalmoplegia, skew deviation, gaze palsies, and nystagmus. *L. monocytogenes* also can cause keratitis.

PROPRIONIBACTERIUM ACNES

P. acnes is part of the normal flora of the skin and mucous membranes. Meningitis, encephalitis, and abscess due to *P. acnes* can complicate neurosurgical procedures, e.g., craniotomies and shunting procedures, or accompany trauma. An orbital cellulitis and frontal lobe abscess due to *P. acnes* can follow a penetrating orbital injury and fracture of the orbital roof. Interestingly, *P. acnes* can cause an indolent anterior uveitis after cataract surgery and intraocular lens implantation.

MYCOBACTERIUM TUBERCULOSIS

Mycobacteria, including *M. tuberculosis*, can cause a myriad of ocular and orbital infections, as well as CNS infections. The incidence of tuberculosis is increasing. Organisms disseminated from primary respiratory or gastrointestinal tract granulomas cause ocular manifestations. Conjunctivitis (phlyctenulosis), keratitis, and scleritis can occur. A phlyctenule is a raised, hyperemic lesion of the conjunctiva near the edge of the cornea (Fig. 25-16). Keratitis is sclerosing and interstitial. Granulomas of the conjunctiva, cornea, and sclera can lead to perforation of the eyes. Necrosis in the sclera leads to thinning and a blue color from the exposed underlying choroid. More often granulomatous or nongranulomatous anterior uveitis occurs (Fig. 25-17). Severe infection can spread to the ciliary body and sclera and cause endophthalmitis and panophthalmitis in which the infection and inflammation extend into the orbital tissues. Choroidal tuberculomas are single or multiple, elevated, white, yellow or gray lesions that may have an overlying exudative retinal detachment. Vasculitis of retinal vessels, Eales' disease, results from an immunologic response to the organism rather than to infection of the vessels. CNS infections include meningitis, intracranial tuberculoma, abscess, epidural tuberculomas,

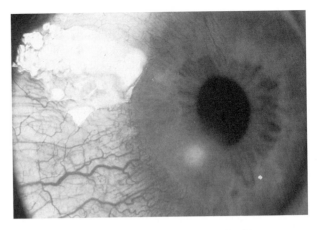

Figure 25-16. Tuberculous phlyctenule. The phlyctenule is a raised hyperemic lesion of the inferior conjunctiva. There is a round white corneal infiltrate in front of the phlyctenule.

and osteomyelitis of bones of the skull base. Tuberculous meningitis causes optic neuritis, optochiasmatic arachnoiditis, ocular motor nerve palsies, homonymous hemianopsia, and cortical blindness. Intracranial tuberculomas also can produce damage to the optic nerves, optic chiasm, and posterior visual pathways. Communicating and noncommunicating hydrocephalus results in papilledema and visual loss from chronic papilledema. Both isoniazid (INH) and ethambutol can cause a bilateral toxic optic neuropathy. The optic disc may be swollen or have a normal appearance. The visual loss is characterized by decreased visual acuity, impaired color vision, and visual field defects typical of optic nerve or optic chiasmal damage, e.g., central scotoma, cecocentral scotoma, constricted fields, and bitemporal hemianopsia. Pupillary light reactions are decreased, but there is usually no afferent papillary defect because both optic nerves are involved.

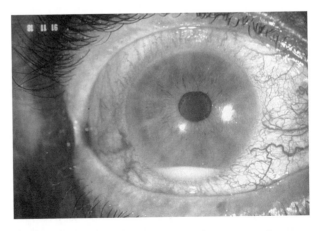

Figure 25-17. Tuberculous iritis. A nongranulomatous iritis produced a white hypopyon in the inferior anterior chamber. (*Courtesy of John D. Sheppard, M.D.*)

MYCOBACTERIUM LEPRAE

Infection by *M. leprae* involves the eyes and ocular adnexae in both the lepromatous and tuberculoid forms of the disease but much more frequently in the lepromatous form. In the lepromatous form, the distribution of the organism is widespread, and there is only a slight immune response. In the tuberculoid form, there is an intense immunologic response and only a few organisms. Many patients have intermediate forms. Involvement of the eyelids is common in lepromatous leprosy. Thickening of the eyelids causes ptosis, entropion (in-turning of the eyelid margin), and trichiasis (in-turning of the eyelashes), which abrades the cornea and causes scarring. Damage to the corneas also can result from exposure keratopathy secondary to seventh cranial nerve palsy. Corneal anesthesia caused by trigeminal nerve damage exacerbates keratopathy (neuroparalytic keratopathy). Lepromas consisting of macrophages, lymphocytes, and organisms can present as chalky white opacities under the corneal epithelium and in the anterior stroma. Lepromas also produce conjunctival nodules and episcleritis. A diffuse haziness of the corneal stroma and/or a vascularized pannus over the corneal surface can develop. Acute or chronic iridocyclitis, iris lepromas (creamy white iris pearls), and iris atrophy can occur. Patients with leprosy and erythema nodosum develop an acute bilateral iridocyclitis. Patients with lepromatous leprosy develop a chronic, more indolent anterior uveitis. Posterior uveitis in leprosy may be caused by infection by the organisms or immune reactions without organisms. Choroidal granulomas and retinal vaculitis occur rarely. Leprosy causes a peripheral neuropathy affecting sensory and motor nerves. Sensory loss from involvement of the trigeminal nerve is common. Facial nerve palsy frequently occurs, but ocular motor nerve palsies are rare.

ACTINOMYCES

Actinomyces most often affects the eyes as a cause of dacryocystitis with swelling of the lacrimal sac, obstruction of tear drainage into the nose, and conjunctivitis. Direct infection of the conjunctiva or eyelid is rare. Most instances of CNS infection are from hematogenous spread from infected dental, oral, gastrointestinal, or female genital tract sites. CNS infections produce meningitis and abscesses of the brain parenchyma, subdural space, and epidural space. Ocular motor nerve palsies and visual field defects from visual pathways lesions can occur.

NOCARDIA ASTEROIDES[10]

N. asteroides uncommonly causes infection of the eyelids, the lacrimal passages in the eyelids (canaliculitis), conjunctiva, cornea, and sclera. Most patients with CNS infections are debiliated or have immune deficiencies from other causes. The CNS infections originate from hematogenous spread from primary infected sites in the pulmonary tract. Orbital cellulitis can occur from hematogenous spread. The CNS lesions are brain abscesses and meningitis. Homonymous hemianopsias, ocular motor nerve palsies, and papilledema can develop.

TROPHERYMA WHIPPLEI[11]

T. whipplei causes Whipple disease. The organism has been found by light microscopy and electron microscopy in almost every tissue in the human body. However, isolated and cultured organisms have not yet caused a disease similar to the human disease in laboratory animals. The reticuloendothelial system cannot phagocytose the organisms sufficiently to eradicate them. The systemic manifestations include the insidious onset of migrating polyarticular arthralgias and nondeforming arthritis, pneumonitis, lymphadenopathy, and fever. Pericardial, pleural, or peritoneal effusions can occur, along with endocarditis and heart block. Gastrointestinal symptoms include indigestion, bloating, milk intolerance, abdominal pain, diarrhea, and bleeding. In later stages, malabsorption produces weight loss, hypotension, weakness, gray or brown skin pigmentation, and anemia. The multisystem symptoms and signs, especially arthritis, can persist for extended periods of time without gastrointestinal symptoms, or the latter may not occur. Ocular involvement occurs as keratitis, iritis, characteristic white, mulberry-like vitreous opacities, retinal opacities, and retinal vasculitis. Neurologic symptoms are variable and include drowsiness, confusion, memory loss, and disorientation. Pseudobulbar palsy, ataxia, trigeminal sensory loss, facial nerve palsy, and seizures can occur. Papilledema can occur in patients with encephalopathy. Whipple disease has characteristic neuroophthalmic manifestations. They include oculomasticatory myorhythmia consisting of low-frequency convergence oscillations of the eyes with simultaneous rhythmic movements of the eyelid, facial, mouth, and neck muscles and supranuclear palsy of vertical or horizontal gaze. The diagnosis is confirmed by a biopsy of the jejunum, which shows positive periodic acid–Schiff (PAS) intracellular staining of histiocytes or characteristic intracellular organisms on electron microscopy in biopsies of the jejunum or other tissues. A polymerase chain reaction (PCR)–based test for ribosomal RNA for cells in the jejunum, lymph nodes, pleural fluid, and blood can be diagnostic.

Gram-Negative Bacilli

Brucella species *B. abortus, B. melitensis,* and *B. suis* infect the genitourinary tract of cattle, goats, and swine, causing abortions, and are shed in milk. Humans become infected by direct contact with infected animals or contaminated tissues or dairy products. The acute human infection is characterized by fever that peaks in the afternoon, chills, sweating, arthralgias, generalized aching, anorexia, and weight loss. The systemic syndrome includes inflammation of the spleen, lymph nodes, lungs, liver, joints, endocardium, bone marrow, prostate, testicles, epididymis, meninges, and brain. The infection may become chronic and persist for years. All parts of the eye may be affected, but uveitis is the most common ocular manifestation. Iridocyclitis and choroiditis can be unilateral or bilateral. The anterior uveitis can produce a hypopyon, which is a white sediment of inflammatory cells in the inferior dependent part of the anterior chamber. The choroidal lesions are small and multifocal, confluent, or form a nodule. A vitritis or exudative retinal detachment can develop. Optic disc swelling can be produced by papilledema (increased intracranial pressure) or optic neuritis (papillitis) or can be secondary to the uveitis. Retrobulbar optic neuritis and arachnoiditis affecting the optic chiasm can occur. CNS infections include meningoencephalitis, meningitis, encephalitis, brain abscess, and subdural empyema. Sixth nerve palsy is usually the result of increased intracranial pressure.

BARTONELLA HENSELAE[12]

Bartonella species cause several human diseases, but *B. henselae* is of special interest because it produces cat-scratch disease with its neurologic and ocular manifestations. Kittens and adult cats are often asymptomatic reservoirs for *B. henselae* and transmit the disease to humans by scratches or bites. A papule or pustule develops at the site of contamination and is followed by regional lymphadenopathy, which can be chronic. Malaise, headache, fever, sore throat, and rashes also can develop. A few to several weeks after the injury and lymphadenopathy, CNS manifestations can develop, consisting of meningitis, encephalitis, myelitis, and radiculitis. Patients with encephalitis often have seizures. Ocular motor nerve palsies, homonymous visual field defects, and papilledema from increased intracranial pressure can occur. Other ocular manifestations include conjunctivitis associated with adenopathy of the preauricular lymph nodes, fever (Parinaud's oculoglandular syndrome), and retinitis. However, neuroretinitis is the most striking neuroophthalmologic manifestation of cat-scratch disease. A few weeks after the onset of systemic symptoms, painless visual loss occurs in one eye, and swelling of the optic disc and macular edema are found. The visual acuity loss can be mild to severe. Small hard yellow exudates form in the deep layers of the retina between the optic disc and the fovea (center of the macula), producing a partial macular star or part of a full macular star. The yellow dots form radii centered about the fovea (Fig. 25-18, Plate 2). Disc swelling resolves over several weeks, and the macular edema and macular exu-

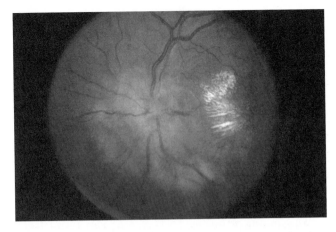

Figure 25-18. Neuroretinitis. *Bartonella henselae* (cat-scratch fever) produced swelling of the optic disc and peripapillary retina and a partial macular star in the left eye. Many small yellow-white dotlike exudates in the outer retinal layers form lines pointing toward the fovea. See Plate 2.

dates resolve over several months. Optic atrophy often results, but visual recovery is usually very good. The other eye can be affected later, and recurrences can occur. Other infections can cause neuroretinitis, including nondescript viral illnesses, syphilis (secondary and tertiary), toxoplasmosis, toxocariasis, Lyme disease, and disseminated histoplasmosis. The presence of the macular star with disc swelling is important in terms of neurologic prognosis. Whereas patients with acute idiopathic optic neuritis have a high likelihood of later developing definite multiple sclerosis, patients with neuroretinitis appear to have the same risk of developing multiple sclerosis as the general population.

BORDETELLA PERTUSSIS AND B. PARAPERTUSSIS

B. pertussis and *B. parapertussis* cause whooping cough or pertussis. Violent coughing during the paroxysmal phase of the disease can cause hemorrhages under the conjunctiva, in the vitreous and retina, and on the face due to elevation of intrathoracic and intraabdominal pressures. Ocular motor palsies and horizontal gaze palsy can develop. Papilledema, optic neuritis, retinal ischemia, and choroiditis can occur. Cerebral blindness is the most common cause of visual loss, although it is usually transient.

FRANCISELLA TULARENSIS

F. tularensis causes tularemia, which has several clinical forms. In the oculoglandular form, there is acute, painful conjunctivitis with purulent discharge. Conjunctival nodules and necrosis develop. The preauricular and cervical lymph nodes are swollen and painful. In all forms, meningitis and meningoencephalitis can develop.

FUSOBACTERIUM SPECIES

Fusobacterium species produce endotoxins and a co-agulase enzyme that causes thrombosis of arteries and veins. They can produce meningitis, brain abscess, subdural empyema, cavernous sinus thrombosis, and lateral sinus thrombosis. A brain abscess can cause a homonymous hemianopsia. Meningitis and cavernous sinus thrombosis can cause ocular motor nerve palsies.

HEMOPHILUS INFLUENZAE

H. influenzae can cause an acute unilateral conjunctivitis with mucopurulent discharge and eyelid edema that involves the other eye in a day or two. *H. influenzae* is the most common cause of orbital cellulitis in children.

PASTEURELLA MULTOCIDA

Animals, including domestic animals, have *P. multocida* in their respiratory and gastrointestinal tracts. Human infections arise from animal bites or inhalation of organisms. Conjunctivitis, endophthalmitis, and meningitis can occur.

PSEUDOMONAS AERUGINOSA

P. aeruginosa is a ubiquitous organism that is found in moist environments, including soil and water, moist parts of the human body, and moist locations in the hospital, such as respiratory equipment. Penetration of skin or mucous membranes and impaired immunity lead to infection. *P. aeruginosa* causes conjunctivitis, keratitis with corneal ulcers, scleritis, and endophthalmitis. It is a leading cause of gram-negative bacteremia, which can result in meningitis, brain abscess, and subdural empyema. Ocular motor cranial nerve palsies can result from meningitis and cavernous sinus thrombosis. Meningitis can cause optic neuritis and optic atrophy.

Viruses[13–15]

DNA Viruses

HERPES SIMPLEX VIRUS[16–18]

Almost all adults have positive serology for herpes simplex virus (HSV). The virus is transmitted by contact with skin or mucous membrane lesions that are shedding virus. The primary infection is usually asymptomatic. HSV type 1 and HSV type 2 can produce lesions in almost all ocular tissues and ocular adnexae. HSV type 2 causes ocular lesions in newborns, who are infected via the placenta (congenital herpes) or during passage through the birth canal (neonatal herpes), and in adults who have orogenital contact with an infected partner. Ocular involvement occurs in about 10 percent of newborns with disseminated infection. Primary HSV infection can produce skin lesions of the face and eyelids, follicular conjunctivitis, and epithelial keratitis (Fig.

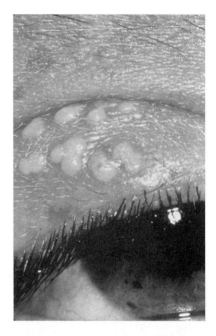

Figure 25-19. Herpes simplex blepharitis. Primary infection with herpes simplex virus produced white vesicles of the upper eye lid.

25-19). HSV conjunctivitis occurs primarily in children under the age of 5 years. It causes irritation, redness, watery discharge, and preauricular lymphadenopathy. Vesicular lesions of the eyelids and eyelid margins, coarse punctate epithelial keratitis, marginal corneal infiltrates, and dendritic corneal ulcers often are associated findings. Lesions from primary ocular infection usually heal without permanent damage. However, neonatal ocular HSV infection also can cause stromal keratitis, iris atrophy, cataract, chorioretinitis, and optic neuritis.

After the primary infection, HSV becomes latent in the trigeminal ganglion or autonomic ganglia. Many factors can trigger recurrent infection months to years later, including emotional stress, trauma, sun exposure, and menses. HSV is the leading cause of corneal blindness in developed countries. Corneal scarring and loss of visual acuity result from recurrent keratitis rather than from the primary infection. In reactivation, latent viruses in the neurons in the trigeminal, ciliary, or sympathetic ganglia or in the mesencephalic nucleus in the brain stem multiply, travel within the sensory axons to the cornea, and multiply further. Recurrent HSV keratitis characteristically produces thin branching ulcers in the epithelium (Fig. 25-20, Plate 3). Infected epithelial cells lyse, allowing virus to infect adjacent cells, producing the meandering dendritic corneal ulcer. The keratitis usually resolves spontaneously over 1 to 2 weeks. However, larger ulcers or additional recurrent ulcers can leave scarring of the underlying corneal stroma. Corneal

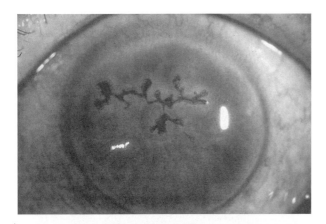

A

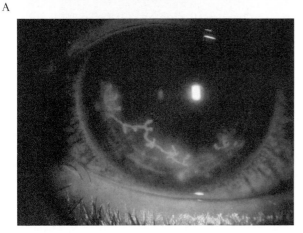

B

Figure 25-20. Dendritic herpes simplex virus keratitis. *A.* Superficial branching corneal ulcer has been stained with a red dye (rose bengal) and a green dye (fluorescein). (*Courtesy of Jerold S. Gordon, M.D.*) *B.* Another dendritic ulcer is stained with fluorescein and illuminated with cobalt blue light. See Plate 3. (*Courtesy of Herbert J. Ingraham, M.D.*)

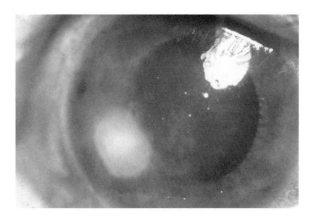

Figure 25-21. Herpes simplex virus disciform keratitis. Recurrent episodes of herpes simplex virus keratitis produced a dense white round opacity in the corneal stroma and a diffuse opacification of the stroma in the central cornea.

VARICELLA-ZOSTER VIRUS

Varicella-zoster virus (VZV) infection produces chicken pox as a primary infection (varicella) and shingles or zoster as a recurrent infection. The primary infection occurs in a congenital form in neonates or in a disseminated form in children. In the congenital form infection occurs in utero. Mothers have a history of chicken pox or zoster during pregnancy. The manifestations include dermatologically distributed cicatricial skin lesions, delayed development, cataract, chorioretinitis, and optic atrophy. About one-third of affected newborns have atrophic chorioretinal scars consistent with infection in utero. Microphthalmia, or congenitally small eyes, and optic nerve hypoplasia can occur.

In primary VZV infection in childhood there is a maculopapulovesicular rash that occurs in successive crops, fever, and malaise. Varicella is a relatively mild disease in normal children, lasting only several days. However, in immunocompromised children or adults, the manifestations are much more severe. In varicella, vesicular lesions can occur on the eyelids and conjunctiva. The cornea can have a superficial punctate keratitis or a dendritic keratitis. In contrast to the thin and delicate, arborizing, ulcerative dendrites in HSV keratitis, the dendrites in VSV keratitis are thicker and elevated. Anterior uveitis and cataract occur uncommonly. VZV can cause meningitis, myelitis (including Devic syndrome of transverse myelitis and bilateral optic neuritis), meningoencephalitis, acute cerebellar ataxia, and cerebral vasculitis with thrombosis. Ophthalmic manifestations of these CNS disorders include ocular motor nerve palsies, horizontal and vertical gaze palsies, bilateral and unilateral internuclear ophthalmoplegia, nystagmus, homonymous hemianopsia, optic neuritis, and papilledema.

sensation usually is depressed in the areas of the keratitis. Recurrent keratitis also can directly affect the corneal stroma, causing disciform edema, necrosis, and scarring (Fig. 25-21). Iridocyclitis can develop associated with recurrent keratitis or can occur in isolation. HSV also can cause posterior uveitis and retinitis. Along with varicella-zoster virus, HSV can produce acute retinal necrosis (ARN) and progressive outer retinal necrosis (PORN), often in immunocompromised adults. ARN and PORN will be described in a following section about varicella-zoster virus. HSV retinitis occurs rarely in congenital or neonatal HSV infections. When it occurs, it is usually bilateral and is associated with CNS infection. About 25 percent of neonates with HSV encephalitis have retinitis as well. Most adults with HSV retinitis also have bilateral ocular disease and encephalitis. Optic neuritis also occurs in patients with HSV encephalitis.

After the primary infection, VZV can remain dormant in sensory nerve ganglia for years. Although 90 percent of adults 60 years of age or older have serologic antibodies to VZV, only about 20 percent of them have had zoster. However, the incidence of zoster increases with age due to diminishing cellular immunity. Patients with impaired immune systems due to the acquired immune deficiency syndrome (AIDS), organ transplantation, and blood dyscrasias have a greater risk of developing zoster. The most frequent form of herpes zoster virus infection affects thoracic dermatomes. The second most common form is herpes zoster ophthalmicus, which affects the ophthalmic branch of the trigeminal nerve. All ocular tissues and adhexae can be affected. Headache, malaise, and fever are followed by pain, redness, and swelling of the periocular skin. Over the next few days, crops of vesicles occur in those areas, which form crusts. When the nasociliary branch of the ophthalmic nerve is affected and the vesicular rash involves the tip of the nose, Hutchinson's sign is produced (Fig. 25-22). A follicular conjunctivitis often develops. Rarely, necrotizing lesions of the conjunctiva, episclera, and sclera can lead to scleral thinning or perforation. Keratitis accompanies the skin lesions and conjunctivitis in about two-thirds of patients. As in chicken pox, a punctate superficial keratitis or dendritic keratitis can occur. The cornea can develop anterior stromal keratitis and disciform stromal keratitis. Damage to the corneal nerves can lead to neuroparalytic keratitis. Mild anterior uveitis often accompanies keratitis but can

occur separately. An acute or delayed scleritis can develop.

The pattern of affected tissues in zoster reflects recurrent infection from sensory nerves. However, tissues can be affected secondary to viremia. In immunocompromised patients, VSV can cause a fulminating retinitis and retinal vasculitis (Fig. 25-23). In AIDS patients, VSV and HSV cause acute retinal necrosis (ARN),[19]

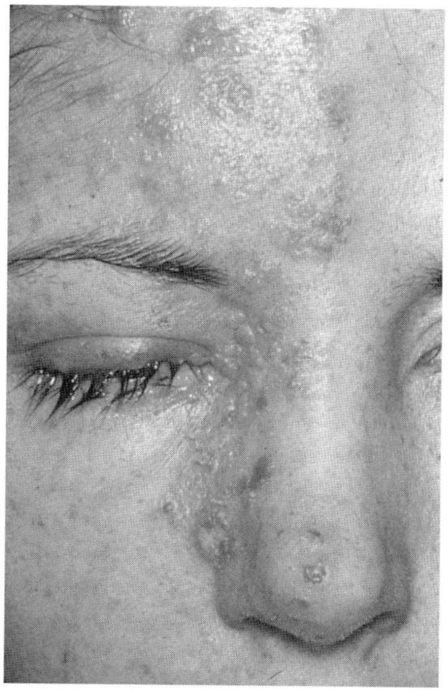

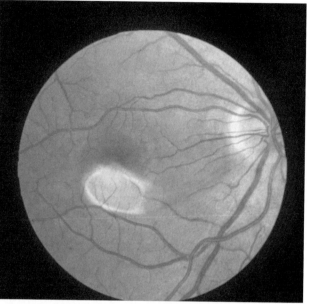

A

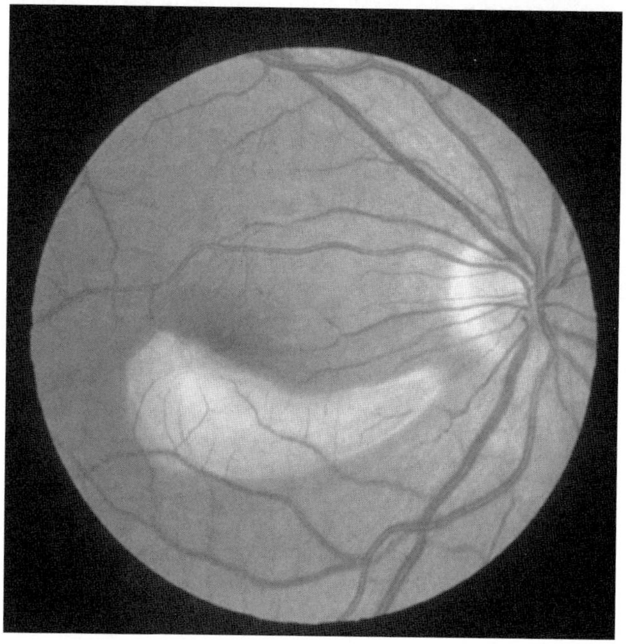

B

Figure 25-23. Varicella-zoster virus retinitis. *A.* VSV infection produced a white opacification of the retina below the fovea of the right eye. *B.* A few days later the infection spread along the tract of retinal ganglion cell axons toward the optic disc. Papillitis eventually developed.

Figure 25-22. Herpes zoster virus opthalmicus. Recurrent VSV infection caused a vesicular rash of the ophthalmic division of the right trigeminal nerve. The eyelids and tip of the nose are affected.

which is second only to cytomegalovirus (CMV) retinitis in incidence. Initially, patients who develop ARN have an anterior uveitis and vitritis. The retinitis begins in the peripheral retina as isolated, yellow-white, opaque areas of necrosis that involve the entire thickness of the neurosensory retina. They become confluent over a few days and spread toward the central retina over several days. ARN tends to spare the retina within the temporal vascular arcades. Retinal vasculitis and papillitis are often present. Four to eight weeks after the onset, scarring and thinning of the retina lead to retinal holes, retinal tears, and retinal detachment that often affects the central retina. Acute retinal necrosis may affect one eye initially but affects the other eye in 90 percent of patients unless it is treated successfully. Another form of fulminant retinitis occurs in immunocompromised patients. PORN occurs in more profoundly immunocompromised patients. It progresses more rapidly and has fewer signs of vitritis, retinitis, and papillitis than ARN. PORN begins in the peripheral retina or in the posterior retina as multifocal lesions of the outer retina that coalesce and spread rapidly. It initially spares retinal vessels. The whitish opacification from retinal necrosis affects the outer layers of the retina because the retinal blood vessels and retinal nerve fiber layer in the superficial retinal layers are not affected initially. The retina becomes thin and atrophic, which can lead to retinal detachment. There is probably a continuum between ARN and PORN reflecting gradations of impaired immunity. HSV infection also can cause PORN. Retinal vasculitis from zoster can cause occlusion of the central retinal artery and central retinal vein or their branches. Patients with zoster can develop optic neuritis, anterior ischemic optic neuropathy, and posterior ischemic optic neuropathy. Adie's tonic pupil and Horner syndrome can occur.

CNS disorders in zoster are more frequent and often more severe than in varicella. They include meningitis, encephalitis, encephalomyelitis, myelitis, cerebral vasculitis, multifocal leukoencephalitis, cranial neuropathies, herpes-zoster oticus (Ramsay Hunt syndrome), herpes-zoster ophthalmicus, postherpetic neuralgia, and segmental motor weakness. Zoster can cause ocular motor nerve palsies in association with the preceding CNS disorders or isolated ocular nerve palsies, in which case demyelination rather than infection or infarction may be the cause. Zoster also can produce an orbital apex syndrome, in which there are several ocular motor nerve palsies, optic nerve damage, and proptosis.

Epstein-Barr Virus

Epstein-Barr virus (EBV) infections in humans are ubiquitous. About 90 percent of adults have antibodies to EBV. EBV infection causes infectious mononucleosis. Epstein-Barr virus has been associated with nasopharyngeal carcinoma, Burkitt lymphoma, primary CNS lymphoma in AIDS patients, and chronic fatigue syndrome. The ocular manifestations of infectious mononucleosis are not common but can affect almost all ocular tissues. Blepharitis, dry eye syndrome, follicular conjunctivitis, episcleritis, and stromal keratitis can occur. In addition, anterior uveitis, macular edema, retinal hemorrhages, chorioretinitis, punctate outer retinitis, and panuveitis can develop. Subretinal hemorrhage from a choroidal neovascular net also can develop. These retinal and posterior uveal manifestations are usually mild, but permanent damage can occur with extensive chorioretinitis and panuveitis. Neuroophthalmic manifestations of CNS infection by EBV include ocular motor nerve palsies, opsoclonus-myoclonus syndrome in children, optic neuritis, and papilledema.

EBV also causes disorders not by direct infection but by its effect on the immune system. These include parainfectious optic neuritis and postinfectious demyelinating encephalomyelitis. *Parainfectious optic neuritis* occurs after systemic viral infection and after vaccinations (*postvaccination optic neuritis*). Optic neuritis has been reported in association with vaccination for influenza, measles, mumps, rubella, rabies, hepatitis B, tetanus, and diptheria. Characteristically, this disorder occurs in children 1 to 3 weeks after infection or vaccination. Inflammation and demyelination of the optic nerve produce unilateral or bilateral papillitis or retrobulbar optic neuritis. Parainfectious optic neuritis occurs with or without other CNS manifestations, such as meningitis and encephalitis. The prognosis for visual recovery is usually good, but visual recovery can be steroid-dependent for a period in some patients. EBV and many of the other viruses also can produce postinfectious encephalomyelitis or acute disseminated encephalomyelitis (ADEM). ADEM is a monophasic inflammatory demyelinating disease of the CNS. It occurs 1 to 3 weeks after nonspecific upper respiratory tract infections, a specific viral infection (most often measles), or vaccination. It also can occur after *M. pneumoniae* infection. ADEM usually causes drowsiness, seizures, coma, and multifocal deficits from lesions of the cerebral hemispheres, cerebellum, and spinal cord. It is also associated with demyelinative optic neuritis. The neuroophthalmic manifestations of ADEM are similar to those of multiple sclerosis, except that the manifestations are monophasic.

Cytomegalovirus

Cytomegalovirus (CMV) infection is commonly acquired in childhood and early adult life in developed countries. It can cause a congenital infection when mothers are infected in the first trimester and transfer the virus transplacentally and a disseminated perinatal infection acquired during passage through the infected genital tract. The most common ocular manifestations of congenital CMV infection are chorioretinitis and optic atrophy. The healed chorioretinal scars may resemble the scars of congenital toxoplasmosis. CMV is the most common ocular infection in AIDS patients. In adults, CMV ocular infection is usually a reactivation of a latent infection but can be a newly acquired infection, often through sexual contact. Conjunctivitis, an epithelial keratitis similar to that caused by VZV, and stromal keratitis can occur. However, the most serious vision-threatening infection is posterior uveitis. Before the advent of current highly effective antiretroviral treatment, systemic CMV infection occurred in about 45 percent of AIDS patients. The risk of CMV retinitis increases as the number of circulating CD4 lymphocytes decreases below 50 cells/mm³. Necrotizing retinitis begins as foci of white opacification in the retinal nerve fiber layer resembling cotton wool spots or white round granular lesions in the posterior or peripheral retina (Fig. 25-24, Plate 4). Lesions often occur along blood vessels. As full-thickness necrosis of the retina occurs, retinal hemorrhages may develop. The lesions enlarge as normal retina adjacent to them becomes infected (Fig. 25-25, Plate 5). Vitritis is usually mild but has become greater with the advent of immune reconstitution from potent antiretroviral therapy. As infection spreads and advances, white borders proceed from the edges of older lesions. There may be an angiitis that produces a frosted white appearance of retinal blood vessels. The necrotic retina is thin and develops holes and tears, which lead to retinal detachment in up to one-quarter to one-half of patients. Viro-static drugs given intravenously, orally,

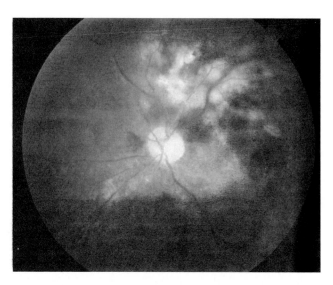

Figure 25-25. Cytomegalovirus retinitis. In the same patient, CMV retinitis has extended into the macula and peripapillary retina. The infection produced dense white infiltrates along the blood vessels and retinal hemorrhages. See Plate 5.

or intraocularly (ganciclovir implant) can ameliorate the retinitis. CMV can cause optic neuritis primarily by infecting the retrobulbar optic nerve or the optic disc or by spreading from adjacent infected peripapillary retina.

JC Virus

JC virus, a papillomavirus, causes progressive multifocal leukoencephalopathy (PML). A majority of adults have antibodies to the virus. The virus reactivates in individuals with impaired immunity from lymphoproliferative and myeloproliferative cancers, AIDS, chronic infections, and drugs. Infection of oligodendrocytes produces the CNS white matter lesions. Homonymous hemianopsia from unilateral lesions occur in about 45 percent of patients. Bilateral occipital lesions cause cortical blindness. Blindness may be the initial manifestation in some patients. PML also can produce visual agnosia and Balint syndrome (ocular apraxia, optic ataxia, and asimultanagnosia).

Variola and Vaccinia Viruses

One strain of variola virus causes smallpox. A maculopapular and vesicular rash often affects the eyelids and can involve the conjunctiva, resulting in scarring of both tissues. Keratitis, corneal ulcers, anterior uveitis, and panophthalmitis can occur. Ocular motor nerve palsies can occur. Vaccination with the vaccinia virus can cause a generalized vesicular rash. The eyelids can be affected. Conjunctivitis, keratitis, and anterior uveitis can develop. Vaccinia virus also can produce postvaccination encephalitis and encephalomyelitis. Optic neuritis and ocular motor cranial nerve palsies can occur.

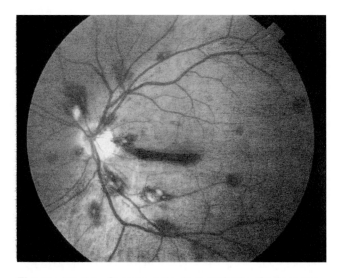

Figure 25-24. Cytomegalovirus retinitis. CMV retinitis developed in the peripheral retina in the left eye of a patient with AIDS. Areas of infection and retinal necrosis produce separate granular dense white infiltrates and confluent dense white infiltrates along blood vessels. There are small splinter-shaped hemorrhages in the superficial layers of the retina. See Plate 4.

RNA Viruses

INFLUENZA VIRUS

Influenza uncommonly is accompanied by encephalitis, meningoencephalitis, myelitis, Guillain-Barré syndrome, and isolated cranial nerve palsies. Influenza can produce keratitis involving the stroma with corneal ulcers at the edges of the cornea and anterior uveitis. Neuroretinitis with papillitis, macular edema, and perifoveal retinal exudates (macular star) can develop. Macular edema without optic disc swelling also can occur. Influenza vaccinations can cause postvaccination optic neuritis.

RUBEOLA VIRUS

Rubeola virus causes measles, whose frequency has decreased greatly due to vaccination. Conjunctivitis is part of its prodromal phase. Rubeola virus can cause papillitis or retrobulbar optic neuritis. The optic neuritis can be associated with severe macular edema. Visual function can recover with a normal-appearing optic disc or visual loss can persist with optic atrophy. As the macular edema decreases, a diffuse irregular pigmentation of the outer retina and choroid (salt-and-papper fundus) can develop. Eventually, a severe diffuse pigmentary retinopathy resembling retinitis pigmentosa can occur. Encephalitis, including involvement of the cerebellum, and encephalomyelitis can develop. Immunocompromised patients can develop acute or subacute measles inclusion-body encephalitis. Subacute sclerosing panencephalitis (SSPE) develops years after measles. Homonymous hemianopsia or cortical blindness can occur during the chronic progressive CNS disorder. Visual agnosia, visual illusions, papilledema, ocular motor nerve palsies, optic neuritis, retinal vasculitis, and retinitis also can occur. Single or multiple lesions in the macula can lead to visual loss before other symptoms and signs of SSPE. Infection by mutant measles virus and immune responses in the outer retina layers cause whitening of the macula and irregularity of pigmentation in the retinal pigment epithelium. Necrosis of the retina leads to a gliotic macular scar (Fig. 25-26).

MUMPS VIRUS

Follicular conjunctivitis and inflammation of the main lacrimal glands in the superotemporal orbits (dacryoadenitis) commonly accompany the other manifestations of mumps. Keratitis, anterior uveitis, retinal vasculitis, and central retinal vein occlusion occur less often. Rarely, cranial nerve palsies, myelitis, cerebellar ataxia, deafness, and vestibular neuronitis or labyrinthitis develop. Optic neuritis and papilledema also can occur.

COXSACKIEVIRUSES

A coxsackievirus can cause a highly infectious acute hemorrhagic conjunctivitis. Enterovirus 70 is more often the cause of this disorder. Painful swelling of the eye-

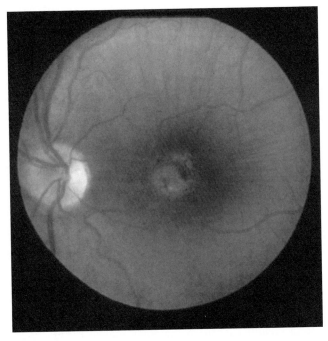

Figure 25-26. Macular scar in subacute sclerosing panencephalitis. Retinitis caused by rubeola virus produced a macular scar with loss of pigment in the retinal pigment epithelium and choroid and clumping of pigment.

lids and pinpoint or diffuse subconjunctival hemorrhages rapidly develop in both eyes and resolve without sequelae. A mild keratitis might occur. Chorioretinitis, panuveitis, optic neuritis, and neuroretinitis can develop. Aseptic meningitis, encephalitis, encephalomyelitis, and myelitis can occur. Coxsackieviruses can cause the opsoclonus-myoclonus syndrome in children and the Guillain-Barré syndrome.

POLIOVIRUS

Poliovirus produces a bulbar form of paralytic poliomyelitis in which cranial nerve palsies occur. About 10 percent of patients have paralysis of ocular motor nerves, and 50 percent have involvement of the facial nerve. Various types of nystagmus, saccadic oscillations, internuclear ophthalmoplegia, spasm of the near reflex, and Horner syndrome have been observed.

RABIES VIRUS

Human rabies is transmitted by bites of infected animals, but it also has been transmitted by corneal transplantation with donor tissue from persons with rabies encephalitis. The CNS is infected by centripetal spread from bites via peripheral nerves. Photophobia is one of the common initial symptoms of rabies. CNS manifestations include an acute hyperactive, furious, or encephalitic form or a progressive paralytic form. If the bite is on the face, ocular motor nerve paralysis can be part of the acute phase. Vaccination with phenol-inactivated adult animal nerve tissue vaccine has been followed by optic neuritis, neuromyelitis optica (Devic disease), neuroretinitis, and ocular motor nerve palsies.

RUBELLA VIRUS

The incidence of congenital rubella decreased dramatically due to widespread vaccination. The severity of effects of in utero infection depends on the fetus' stage of development at the time of maternal infection. Spontaneous abortion and multiple congenital defects occur more often with infection in the first 2 months of pregnancy. The ocular manifestations include microphthalmos (small eyes), strabismus, iris atrophy, cataract, glaucoma, and pigmentary retinopathy. CNS manifestations include meningoencephalitis and progressive panencephalitis in childhood. Children and adults with acquired rubella can have keratitis and dacryoadenitis. Rarely, they develop encephalitis. Ocular motor nerve palsies, supranuclear gaze palsies, optic disc swelling, and homonymous hemianopsia can occur.

Retroviruses

HUMAN IMMUNODEFICIENCY VIRUSES[20-22]

Ocular and neuroophthalmic manifestation of AIDS can be produced by human immunodeficiency virus (HIV) infection or opportunistic infection by other organisms. The most common ocular manifestation of AIDS is retinal microangiopathy (Fig. 25-27). Cotton wool spots in the retinal nerve fiber layer may be the initial sign of HIV infection. They represent microinfarctions in the nerve fiber layer caused by microvascular damage from HIV infection. They usually do not cause visual loss.

The retinal microangiopathy is associated with progression of HIV infection, decreasing CD4 lymphocyte numbers, and HIV-associated cognitive disorders. Unusually long eyelashes (trichomegaly) are associated with AIDS.

The impaired cellular immunity caused by AIDS produces many infections of the eye and the ocular adnexae, which are much less common in persons with normal immune systems. Some of these were discussed earlier, and some will be described below. Herpes simplex virus, varicella-zoster virus, and molluscum contagiosum (Fig. 25-28) can cause infection of the eyelids and conjunctiva. Keratitis caused by various viruses, bacteria, and fungi can occur. Certain neoplasms of the anterior segment also are associated with AIDS. Kaposi's sarcoma of the eyelid and conjunctiva are flat or raised bright red vascular lesions that are surrounded by dilated blood vessels. Conjunctival intraepithelial neoplasia (CIN) is a precursor of squamous cell carcinoma and appears as a flat, opaque lesion of the conjunctiva. Squamous cell carcinoma of the eyelid and conjunctiva usually occurs in older men but also occurs in younger patients with AIDS. It appears as a hyperemic nodular lesion with grayish overlying epithelium. The most severe ocular infections associated with AIDS cause retinitis and chorioretinitis. Herpes simplex virus and varicella-zoster virus can produce acute retinal necrosis and PORN. Retinitis and chorioretinitis from *Treponema pallidum* and *Toxoplasma gondii* also occur with increased frequency in AIDS. *M. tuberculosis, M. avium-intracellulare, Histoplasma capsulatum, Cryptococcus neoformans,* and *Acanthamoeba* can cause choroiditis.

Twenty percent of patients with AIDS and non-Hodgkin's lymphoma have extranodular lymphoma often affecting the CNS or eye. The incidence of ocular lymphoma is 100 times greater in immunocompromised patients than in nonimmunocompromised patients. Intraocular lymphoma produces anterior and/or posterior

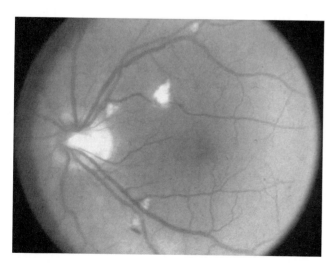

Figure 25-27. HIV retinopathy. The left eye of a patient with AIDS has several cotton wool spots, which are white lesions in the superficial retina with feathery edges. There is a small splinter-shaped retinal hemorrhage near the inferior temporal retinal vessels. (*Courtesy of Ronald Danis, M.D.*)

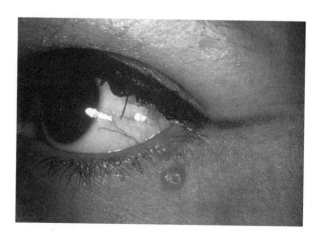

Figure 25-28. Molluscum contagiosum of eyelid. Two erythematous nodules in the left lower eyelid have umbilicated centers.

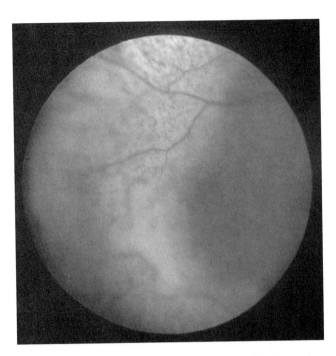

Figure 25-29. Intraocular lymphoma. Infiltration of the choroid produced an elevated white mass under the retina. See Plate 6.

uveitis. There may be peripapillary infiltrates with vitritis. Choroidal infiltrates may appear as yellow or white lesions below the retinal pigment epithelium (Fig. 25-29, Plate 6). Sheathing of retinal vessels and occlusion of central retinal arteries or veins can occur. Lymphoma also can present as an orbital infiltration. Orbital or cavernous sinus involvement may cause numbness of the face, proptosis, and diplopia. Ocular manifestations, such as ocular motor palsies and papilledema, may be the initial signs of primary CNS lymphoma in AIDS patients.

CNS disorders caused primarily by HIV infection include aseptic meningitis, meningoencephalitis, HIV-related headache, HIV-1-associated dementia complex, and HIV-1-associated minor cognitive/motor disorder. The latter two disorders can cause saccadic eye movement abnormalities such as ocular flutter, macro-square-wave jerks, and abnormal antisaccades. Impaired smooth pursuit eye movements also can be present. Neuroophthalmic manifestations in AIDS include a progressive retrobulbar optic neuropathy directly related to HIV infection and numerous other manifestations caused by secondary infections or neoplasms. The latter include papilledema, optic neuritis, neuroretinitis, optic perineuritis, infarction of the optic chiasm, homonymous hemianopsia, and cortical blindness. Many eye movement abnormalities can occur, such as ocular motor nerve palsies, internuclear ophthalmoplegia, dorsal midbrain syndrome, horizontal and vertical gaze palsies, various types of nystagmus, skew deviation, and ocu-

lar flutter. Pupillary abnormalities including Horner syndrome, tonic pupil, and light near dissociation of the pupil also can occur.

HUMAN T-CELL LYMPHOTROPIC VIRUS (HTLV) TYPES I AND II

HTLV-I infection is transmitted from mother to child through perinatal exposure or breast-feeding, by sexual contact, by contaminated needles, and by blood transfusion. It produces HTLV-I-associated myelopathy/tropical spastic paraparesis and adult T-cell leukemia. The former is rarely associated with uveitis, retinal vasculitis, papillitis, pigmentary retinopathy, optic atrophy, or nystagmus. The latter disorder can be associated with episcleritis, uveitis, and retinitis. Patients with HTLV-I infection without myelopathy can have uveitis, retinal vasculitis, and pigmentary retinopathy. HTLV-II transmission is similar to that of HTLV-I. HTLV-II infection can cause ataxia, spasticity, and peripheral neuropathy. Tonic pupil, retrobulbar optic neuritis, and abnormal saccadic eye movements have been described with this disorder.

Fungi[23-27]

CANDIDA ALBICANS

C. albicans is normally found in soil, food, and many locations in hospitals. It can be cultured in normal persons from skin, sputum, saliva, gastrointestinal tract, and female genitourinary tract. *Candida* infection is one of the most common nosocomial infections. In cold climates, *C. albicans* is a common cause of fungal keratitis, especially in patients with preexisting corneal disease, from use of topical corticosteroids and in immunocompromised patients from alcoholism, diabetes mellitus, and vitamin A deficiency. In warmer climates and in the tropics, *Fusarium* species and *Aspergillus* species are the most common causes of fungal keratitis. Corneal infiltrates are gray and elevated. They develop satellite lesions, ring-shaped infiltrates, and plaques on the corneal endothelium. *Candida* causes an endogenous endophthalmitis in patients with candidemia. Occasionally, *Candida* can enter the eye by direct inoculation. Patients often have chronic underlying systemic diseases and have been treated with broad-spectrum antibiotics and intravenous catheters. Immunosuppressed patients after organ transplantation, patients with AIDS, and intravenous drug abusers are at risk to develop candidemia.

Patients develop eye pain, visual loss, and floaters. The characteristic chorioretinal lesions are white and fluffy (Fig. 25-30). When the infection extends into the vitreous, snowball-like white opacities develop above the chorioretinal lesions (Fig. 25-31). The chorioretinal lesions enlarge and produce satellite lesions. Occasionally, scleritis, anterior uveitis with hypopyon, pa-

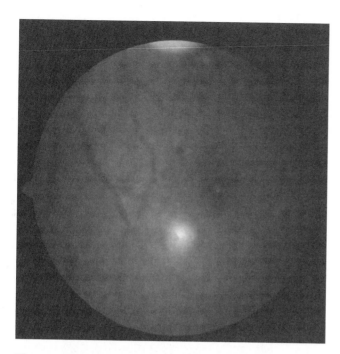

Figure 25-30. *Candida* chorioretinitis. A patient with candidemia developed a creamy white infiltrate in the macula. The infiltrate affects the choroid and overlying retina.

pillitis, or panophthalmitis occurs. The diagnosis of *Candida* chorioretinitis rests on the typical appearance of the lesions in addition to positive blood cultures and cultures of catheters, surgical wounds, or other lesions. Occasionally, vitreous biopsy and culture are needed.

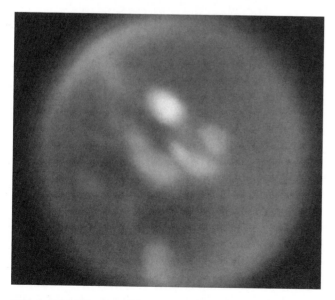

Figure 25-31. *Candida* endophthalmitis. In another patient with candidemia, infection extended from chorioretinal lesions into the overlying vitreous, producing white snowballs. (*Courtesy of Ronald Danis, M.D.*)

Other fungi can cause endogenous fungal uveitis. They include *Aspergillus flavus, A. fumigatus, C. neoformans, Sporothrix schenckii,* and *Blastomyces dermatitidis.* Amphotericin B, 5-fluorocytosine, and fluconazole have been used successfully to treat ocular and CNS *Candida* infections. The first two drugs also have been injected intraocularly.

ASPERGILLUS SPECIES

Aspergillus species are found commonly in the soil and decaying vegetation. *A. fumigatus* and *A. flavus* are the most common species causing human infections. Infections usually begin in the nose or paranasal sinuses after inhalation of spores, especially in debilitated or immunocompromised patients. *Aspergillus* infections cause allergic aspergillosis, aspergillomas, and invasive aspergillosis. In allergic aspergillosis, there is an immune reaction to carbohydrate and glycoprotein antigens of the organism. Rhinitis, asthma, and bronchopulmonary disorders develop. Paranasal sinusitis can develop and lead to orbital cellulitis. Aspergillomas are masses of lymphocytes, plasma cells, epithelioid cells, necrotic tissue, fibrous tissue, and fungal hyphae. Paranasal aspergillomas can extend into the orbit and brain, damaging the optic nerve, optic chiasm, and cavernous sinus. Aspergillomas at the skull base can cause sixth nerve palsy and other cranial nerve palsies. Immunosuppressed patients, e.g., AIDS patients, and debiliated patients may develop invasive aspergillosis. Fungal paranasal sinusitis can lead to invasion of the orbit or brain, and bronchopulmonary infection can spread hematogenously to the CNS. Endogenous posterior uveitis or endophthalmitis can occur (Fig. 25-32). Acute visual loss can be caused by direct infection or by thrombosis of blood vessels supplying the retrobulbar optic nerve. Orbital infection can produce an orbital apex syndrome, and cavernous sinus infection can cause multiple cranial nerve palsies. Invasive aspergillosis of the CNS presents as cerebral infarctions. Endogenous invasion of the internal carotid artery causes hemorrhagic infarctions. Septic infarctions with cerebritis, single or multiple abscesses, and brain swelling with transtentorial or tonsillar herniation can develop. Mycotic aneurysm, subarachnoid hemorrhage, subdural and epidural abscesses, and meningitis can occur. Treatment for allergic aspergillosis consists of antifungal drugs such as amphotericin B in standard or liposomal forms, itraconazole and flucytosine, and systemic corticosteroids. If there is no CNS involvement, antifungals may not be needed. Aspergillomas and invasive aspergillosis of the orbits and CNS require surgical debridement and antimicrobial therapy.

MUCORALES

Rhizopus species and *Rhizomucor* species cause human infections in the order Mucorales. Spores are spread

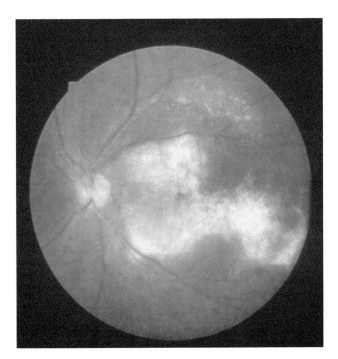

Figure 25-32. *Aspergillus* choroiditis. *Aspergillus* produced a large white subretinal mass in the macula of the left eye. (*Courtesy of Ronald Danis, M.D.*)

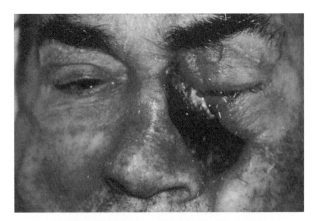

A

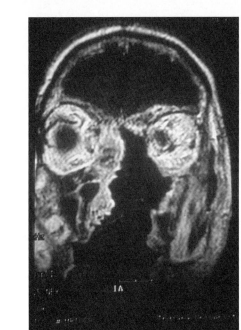

B

Figure 25-33. Mucormycosis. *A.* A patient with diabetic ketoacidosis developed mucormycosis of the nasal and maxillary sinus. The infection extended into the bones and skin, producing black necrotic ulcers, and into the left orbit. *B.* Coronal MRI shows necrosis of the nasal cavity and maxillary sinus and orbital cellulitis.

widely in decaying matter and are inhaled, residing in the nasal turbinates and lung aveoli. Spores can enter through breaks in the skin. However, germination of the spores in normal persons is prevented by humoral and cellular immune mechanisms, macrophages, and polymorphonuclear leukocytes. However, breakdown of these mechanisms in diabetic, immunocompromised, and debiliated patients permit germination. Hyphae invade tissues and grow along blood vessel walls. Thrombosis of the vessels leads to hemorrhagic necrosis. The most common forms of mucormycosis are cutaneous, gastrointestinal, pulmonary, rhinocerebral, and CNS. Rhinocerebral mucormycosis develops most often in patients with diabetes mellitus and ketoacidosis; infants with gastroenteritis, dehydration, and acidosis; intravenous drug abusers; patients treated with corticosteroids; organ transplant recipients; and patients with cancer. It occurs less often in AIDS patients because they are usually not neutropenic. The orbit and CNS are infected secondary to spread from lesions of the paranasal sinuses, nasal mucosa, skin of the face, and hard palate (Fig. 25-33). Thrombosis of arteries and veins in the eyes, orbits, neck, and brain causes hemorrhagic necrosis. Orbital cellulitis and the orbital apex syndrome cause pain, periorbital swelling, conjunctival injection and chemosis, proptosis, ophthalmoplegia, and visual loss. Visual loss can be due to thrombosis of choroidal and retinal arteries, endophthalmitis, infarction of the optic nerve and optic chiasm, and the ocular ischemic syndrome, in which occlusion of the

ophthalmic artery produces widespread ischemia of ocular tissues. Orbital cellulitis can lead to cavernous sinus thrombosis with thrombosis of the cavernous portion of the internal carotid artery. Isolated CNS mucormycosis is rare. Although the organism enters the CNS via the nose and paranasal sinuses, there are no signs or symptoms until neurologic manifestations develop. These include headache, seizures, decreased consciousness leading to coma, and multiple focal neurologic deficits. Ocular motor nerve palsies occur often. Patients often develop signs and symptoms of nasal, sinus, palate, and orbital lesions soon after their neurologic manifestations. Therapy of all forms of mucormycosis usually includes correction of the underlying metabolic and immune deficiencies, systemic and/or intralesional amphotericin B, and surgical debridement.

HISTOPLASMA CAPSULATUM

Humans become infected by *H. capsulatum* by inhaling spores in soil or particles of pigeon droppings. The spores germinate into yeast forms in the lungs. The yeasts are phagocytosed by macrophages, in which they grow. Eventually, foci of infection in the lungs, lymph nodes, liver, spleen, and other tissues become sites of inflammation with vasculitis, necrosis, calcification, and encapsulation. However, yeast can survive in the granulomas. The number of inhaled spores and the patient's immune status determine the severity and type of infection. Persons with intact immune systems are usually asymptomatic after their initial infection or when they become reinfected. Immunocompromised patients, such as AIDS patients, can develop disseminated histoplasmosis as a result of their initial infection or reinfection. With the development of immunodeficiency, dormant lesions can become reactivated. *H. capsulatum* produces three ocular syndromes: histoplasmic endophthalmitis, solitary chorioretinal histoplasmic granuloma, and the ocular histoplasmosis syndrome.

Histoplasmic endophthalmitis develops in immunocompromised patients. The initial symptoms include pain, floaters, and decreased vision. Conjunctival injection, anterior uveitis, yellow iris infiltrates, vitritis, and multiple creamy white chorioretinal lesions develop (Fig. 25-34). There is a diffuse granulomatous inflammation of the uveal tract and retinal infiltrates. Patients

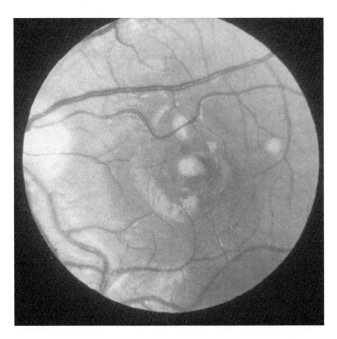

Figure 25-34. *Histoplasma* choroiditis. A patient with disseminated histoplasmosis has several creamy white subretinal lesions in the macula of the left eye.

are treated systemically with amphotericin B or itraconazole. Other fungi that cause endogenous endophthalmitis include *C. albicans* and *C. immitis*.

Solitary histoplasmic choroidal granuloma appears as a choroidal lesion with a variable amount of vitritis. Immunocompromised patients develop this form of histoplasmosis. The ocular histoplasmosis syndrome is the most common ocular form of histoplasmosis. Normal persons, who usually had initial infections in childhood, have small areas of chorioretinal atrophy around their optic discs and small, round, white, punched-out chorioretinal scars. These scars are often in the retinal periphery. When they are in the macula, they cause no visual loss. However, the macular scars can develop neovascularization spontaneously from the choroid decades after the initial infection. Leakage of plasma and bleeding under the retina from the small neovascular blood vessels cause painless loss of central vision (Fig. 25-35, Plate 7). Eventually, a much larger fibrotic subretinal scar develops with permanent damage to the overlying retina.

OTHER FUNGI

C. neoformans causes cryptococcosis. It is ubiquitous and causes opportunistic infections in immunocompromised patients. CNS infection produces meningitis and meningoencephalitis. The optic nerve is affected by infection from the adjacent meninges or by papilledema from increased intracranial pressure. The optic chiasm is damaged by infection or optochiasmatic arachnoiditis. Meningitis, increased intracranial pressure, and brain stem meningoencephalitis cause ocular motor cranial nerve palsies, internuclear ophthalmoplegia, skew deviation, nystagmus, supranuclear vertical gaze palsy, and Horner syndrome. The eyelids can have papules, nodules, plaques, and ulcers from localized or disseminated infection. Anterior uveitis with iris granulomas, spherical white superficial retinal lesions, multifocal choroiditis, and vitritis can develop. Ocular involvement usually occurs in patients with meningitis, but ocular trauma and corneal transplantation can cause intraocular infection. Orbital cellulitis occurs rarely.

C. immitis causes coccidioidomycosis with a mild pulmonary infection in normal persons and disseminated infection in patients with impaired T-cell immunity in endemic areas of the world, including the southwestern United States. CNS manifestations include meningitis, abscesses, granulomas, encephalitis, and vasculitis with multiple infarctions and aneurysms. The ocular manifestations include granulomas and abscesses of the eyelids, conjunctiva, cornea, and episclera and anterior uveitis, retinitis, multifocal choroiditis, and endophthalmitis (Fig. 25-36).

B. dermatitidis causes blastomycosis. It produces lung, skin, bone, and genitourinary infections. CNS infections cause meningitis, encephalitis, and myelitis. Oc-

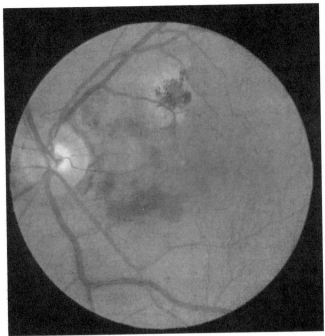
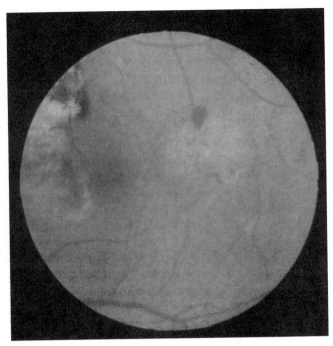

A   B

Figure 25-35. Ocular histoplasmosis syndrome. *A.* There is clumping of pigment of the retinal pigment epithelium and choroid around the edges of the left optic disc. Subretinal neovascularization from the choroid produces a whitish elevation of the retina temporal to the optic disc, which has subretinal hemorrhage at its edges. There is a chorioretinal scar above this lesion from laser treatment of a previous neovascular lesion. *B.* A few months later, the peripapillary lesion was photocoagulated producing a chorioretinal scar. There is a new lesion temporal to the fovea with a gray center and hemorrhages at its edges. See Plate 7.

ular infections occur in patients with normal immune systems. They include eyelid and conjunctival granulomas, keratitis, anterior uveitis, multifocal choroiditis, and endophthalmitis. Granulomas can form masses in the anterior chamber, iris, vitreous, and choroid.

Spirochetes[29]

TREPONEMA PALLIDUM[29–31]

The subspecies of *T. pallidum, T. pallidum pallidum,* causes syphilis. Other subspecies cause yaws and be-

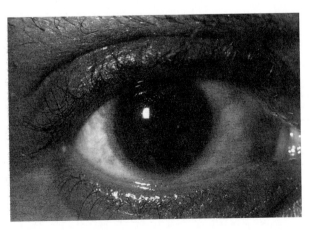

Figure 25-36. Coccidiodes uveitis. Iritis-produced posterior synechiae and an irregularly shaped pupil.

jel. The two major forms of syphilis are congenital and acquired. In congenital syphilis, infection of the fetus occurs in utero. However, infection of the newborn can occur during passage through the birth canal. Acquired syphilis is usually transmitted by sexual intercourse, but it also can be transmitted by contact with infected lesions outside the genital organs. Transmission by blood or blood products is rare. After gaining access through mucus membranes or abraded skin, the organisms spread to almost all tissues in the body via lymphatics and blood vessels. The stages of syphilis—incubation, primary, secondary, latent, and tertiary or late—are often overlapping. The number of organisms throughout the body and in the blood is greatest in the secondary stage. Organisms have been found in the aqueous humor in the secondary stage and in the cerebrospinal fluid (CSF) in the primary and secondary stages. Humoral antibodies and cellular immunity develop in the secondary stage but are only partially effective in controlling the infection. In the latent stage, patients have few, if any, manifestations of the infection, but relapses can occur. In the tertiary or late stage of syphilis, arteritis affects arteries in the CNS and vaso vasorum of the aorta, and gummas develop in various tissues and organs, including the CNS. Simultaneous infections with *T. pallidum pallidum* and HIV modify the manifestations of syphilis. Often the latent stage of syphilis is shortened, and the manifestations of neu-

THE COLOR PLATES

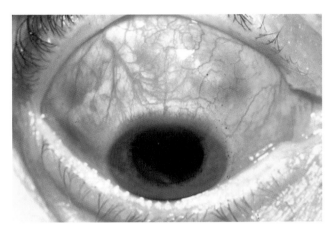

PLATE 1. Scleritis and staphyloma. Scleritis produced necrosis of the sclera. The weakened sclera bulges outward (staphyloma), and the underlying bluish ciliary body and choroid are seen.

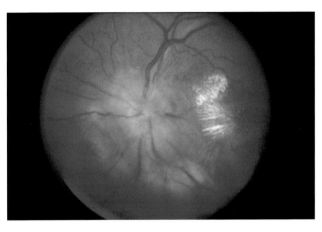

PLATE 2. Neuroretinitis. *Bartonella henselae* (cat-scratch fever) produced swelling of the optic disc and peripapillary retina and a partial macular star in the left eye. Many small yellow-white dotlike exudates in the outer retinal layers form lines pointing toward the fovea.

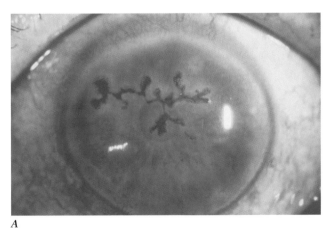

A

PLATE 3. Dendritic herpes simplex virus keratitis. (*A*) Superficial branching corneal ulcer has been stained with a red dye (rose bengal) and a green dye (fluorescein). (*Courtesy of Jerold S. Gordon, M.D.*)

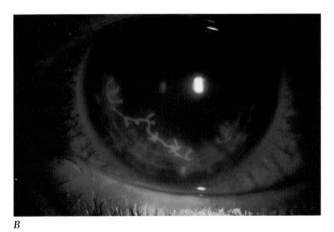

B

(*B*) Another dendritic ulcer is stained with fluorescein and illuminated with cobalt blue light. (*Courtesy of Herbert J. Ingraham, M.D.*)

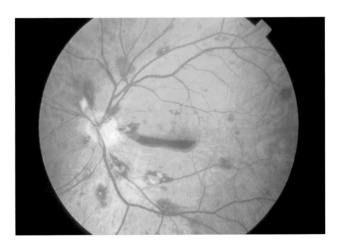

PLATE 4. Cytomegalovirus retinitis. CMV retinitis developed in the peripheral retina in the left eye of a patient with AIDS. Areas of infection and retinal necrosis produce separate granular dense white infiltrates and confluent dense white infiltrates along blood vessels. There are small splinter-shaped hemorrhages in the superficial layers of the retina.

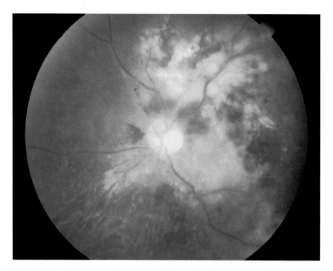

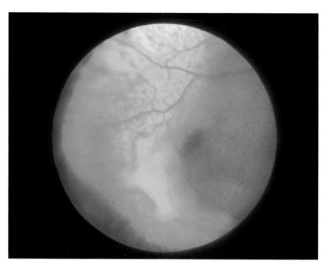

PLATE 5. Cytomegalovirus retinitis. In the same patient, CMV retinitis has extended into the macula and peripapillary retina. The infection produced dense white infiltrates along the blood vessels and retinal hemorrhages.

PLATE 6. Intraocular lymphoma. Infiltration of the choroid produced an elevated white mass under the retina.

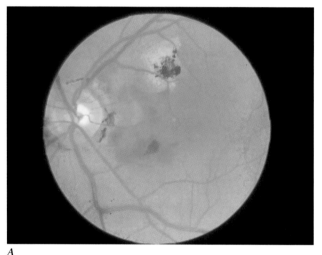

A

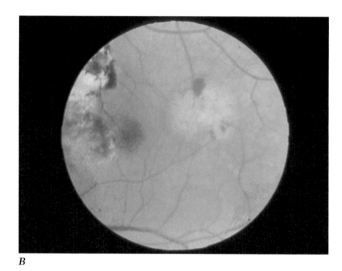

B

PLATE 7. Ocular histoplasmosis syndrome. (*A*) There is clumping of pigment of the retinal pigment epithelium and choroid around the edges of the left optic disc. Subretinal neovascularization from the choroid produces a whitish elevation of the retina temporal to the optic disc, which has subretinal hemorrhage at its edges. There is a

chorioretinal scar above this lesion from laser treatment of a previous neovascular lesion. (*B*) A few months later, the peripapillary lesion was photocoagulated producing a chorioretinal scar. There is a new lesion temporal to the fovea with a gray center and hemorrhages at its edges.

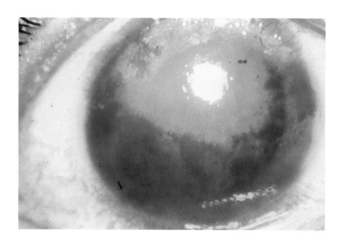

PLATE 8. Syphilitic interstitial keratitis. Large salmon patch inferiorly and small patch superiorly. Blood in blood vessels deep in the corneal stroma produce the red patches. There is diffuse edema of the corneal stroma centrally.

rosyphilis are more severe. Response to treatment often is reduced.

A chancre in the conjunctiva can result from direct contact with an infected lesion in primary syphilis. It is ulcerated and has rounded edges. Condylomata lata of the eyelids and alopecia of the eyebrow can occur in secondary syphilis. Conjunctivitis in this stage is usually nonspecific. The papillary conjunctivitis is usually mild but can lead to infection of the underlying sclera. Episcleritis and scleritis can occur in the secondary or tertiary stages. Conjunctival gummas can develop in tertiary syphilis. They are usually painful and are associated with necrotizing conjunctivitis. Gummas of the eyelid, sclera, cornea, iris, ciliary body, choroid, retina, orbit, optic nerve, and optic chiasm also can occur in tertiary syphilis. Gummas in the cerebral hemispheres, brain stem, and cerebellopontine angle produce a variety of neuroophthalmic findings including homonymous hemianopsia, papilledema, and ocular motor nerve palsies. Interstitial keratitis is often a delayed manifestation of congenital syphilis, but it can occur in acquired secondary syphilis. It might result from direct infection of the cornea and/or immune-complex reactions. In acquired syphilis, the keratitis is usually unilateral, whereas it is usually bilateral in congenital syphilis. Other forms of keratitis also occur in secondary syphilis. Interstitial keratitis begins as gray opacities in the deep stroma that begin in the periphery and then enlarge, coalesce, and spread (Fig. 25-37). There is usually pain, photophobia, tearing, and blurred vision. The cornea becomes edematous, and blood vessels from the limbus grow into the deep corneal stroma just anterior to Descemet's membrane as advancing reddish fronts called *salmon patches* (Fig. 25-38, Plate 8). As the corneal edema and stromal infiltrates decrease, corneal clarity improves, and the deep stromal blood vessels regress, becoming ghost vessels devoid of blood (Fig. 25-39).

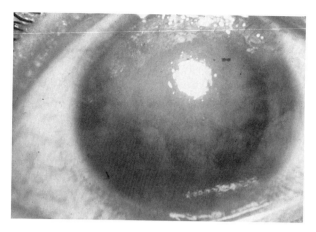

Figure 25-38. Syphilitic interstitial keratitis. Large salmon patch inferiorly and small patch superiorly. Blood in blood vessels deep in the corneal stroma produce the red patches. There is diffuse edema of the corneal stroma centrally. See Plate 8.

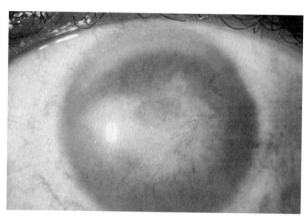

A

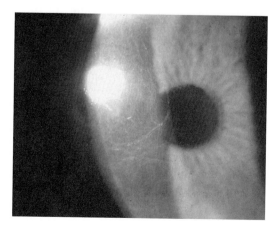

B

Figure 25-39. Syphilitic interstitial keratitis. *A.* Blood vessels in the deep corneal stroma are devoid of blood (ghost vessels). Scarring in the corneal stroma produces confluent white opacities. *B.* Ghost vessels are seen as white branching lines anterior to Descemet's membrane. (*Courtesy of James P. McCulley, M.D.*)

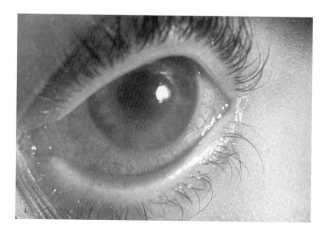

Figure 25-37. Syphilitic interstitial keratitis. Acute keratitis inferiorly in left eye. Edema of the corneal stroma clouds the cornea inferiorly. There is inferior ciliary injection.

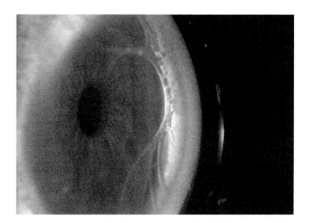

Figure 25-40. Syphilitic interstitial keratitis. Gonioscopic view of anterior chamber shows transparent tubelike scroll of Descemet's membrane in the anterior chamber behind the posterior surface of the cornea. (*Courtesy of James P. McCulley, M.D.*)

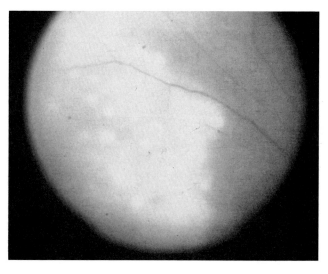

Figure 25-41. Syphilitic choroiditis. Confluent and round white infiltrates are in the choroid beneath retinal blood vessels. (*Courtesy of James Ganley, M.D.*)

Descemet's membrane often develops transparent ridges, tubes, scrolls, or webs extending into the anterior chamber (Fig. 25-40). Recurrent attacks of interstitial keratitis can occur.

Nonspecific iritis and iridocyclitis are the most common forms of syphilitic uveitis and usually occur in the secondary stage. The uveitis can be granulomatous or nongranulomatous. Dilatation of blood vessels in the iris stroma is characteristic. Cataracts develop but are not distinctive in appearance. Glaucoma can occur in congenital and acquired syphilis as a consequence of uveitis or maldevelopment of the tissues in the anterior chamber angle. Chorioretinitis occurs in both congenital and acquired syphilis. The periphery of the retina tends to be affected in the former, and the posterior pole tends to be involved in the latter. In secondary syphilis, the manifestations of syphilitic chorioretinitis are diverse. They include retinal vasculitis, macular edema with or without deep retinal exudates, diffuse chorioretinitis that produces a pigmentary retinopathy resembling retinitis pigmentosa, exudative retinal detachment, choroidal effusion, central retinal vein occlusion, retinal necrosis, and neuroretinitis (Figs. 25-41 and 25-42). In patients with HIV infection, acute syphilitic posterior placoid chorioretinitis appears as large yellow or grayish plaques in the retinal pigment epithelium next to the optic disc or in the macula. In secondary syphilis, unilateral and bilateral optic neuritis with papillitis can occur, often with a cellular reaction in the overlying vitreous. Syphilis also can cause a retrobulbar optic neuritis or perioptic neuritis. In the later disorder there is inflammation of the optic nerve sheath, often with sparing of the optic nerve itself. Visual acuity, color vision, and visual fields may be normal or mildly affected. Basilar meningitis in secondary syphilis can produce an opticochiasmatic arachnoiditis.

Homonymous hemianopsia results from meningitis affecting the optic tract and cerebral infarction from arteritis. Aseptic meningitis in secondary syphilis causes cranial nerve palsies, including ocular motor nerve palsies. Arteritis can cause cerebral infarctions.

In tertiary or late syphilis, CNS manifestations result from meningovascular neurosyphilis and paren-

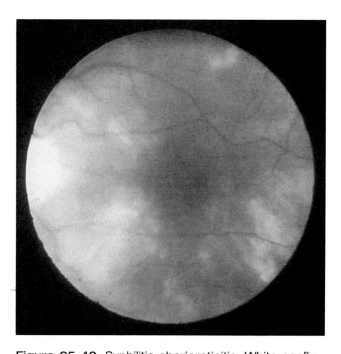

Figure 25-42. Syphilitic chorioretinitis. White confluent infiltrate temporal to the optic disc of the left eye obscures the retinal blood vessels (retinitis). White choroidal infiltrates are seen beneath the retinal blood vessels temporal to the fovea (choroiditis).

chymatous neurosyphilis. In contrast to meningitis in secondary syphilis, neurosyphilis develops months to years after the primary infection. Endarteritis of small blood vessels produces progressive ischemia. Papillitis, retrobulbar optic neuritis, and neuroretinitis can occur. Parenchymatous neurosyphilis is a degenerative process causing loss of neurons, which causes tabes dorsalis and general paresis. In tabes dorsalis there is damage to the spinal cord, especially the posterior columns, dorsal roots, and dorsal root ganglia. The Argyll Robertson pupil, optic atrophy, and ocular motor nerve palsies occur frequently with tabes dorsalis. The Argyll Robertson pupil is found commonly in the tertiary or late stage of syphilis but also can be an early sign of neurosyphilis. The pupils are characteristically small and irregular in shape. There is no constriction to light stimulation, but miosis during the near reflex is intact (light near dissociation). The syndrome results from interruption of afferent pupillomotor fibers in the dorsal mesencephalon. Other pupillary abnormalities are found in patients with tabes dorsalis. They include small, irregularly shaped pupils of unequal size that do not react normally to light or near and bilateral Adie's tonic pupil. Bilateral ptosis, optic atrophy, cranial nerve palsies, and various types of nystagmus can occur. Optic atrophy and similar pupillary abnormalities occur less often in patients with general paresis. Homonymous hemianopsia from cerebral infarction and visual hallucinations occur in general paresis.

BORRELIA BURGDORFERI

B. burgdorferi causes Lyme disease. The infection is transmitted to humans by bites of *Ixodes* ticks. In the early localized or primary stage, a rash (erythema chronicum migrans) develops at the site of the bite. The rash's erythematous annular margins expand gradually. Fever, arthralgias, myalgias, flulike symptoms, and adenopathy may develop. Conjunctivitis is the most common ocular manifestation. In the early disseminated or secondary stage there may be episcleritis, keratitis, vitritis, chorioretinitis, and endophthalmitis. Papillitis, retrobulbar optic neuritis, neuroretinitis, and anterior ischemic optic neuropathy can occur. In the chronic disseminated or tertiary stage, arthritis and a progressive encephalomyelitis can develop, which can produce ocular motor nerve palsies, homonymous hemianopsia, and cortical blindness. Stromal keratitis, vitritis, pigmentary retinopathy, and orbital myositis have been reported.

LEPTOSPIRA SPECIES

Leptospira species cause leptospirosis. Humans are infected from water or soil that is contaminated by urine of infected wild and domestic animals. Organisms penetrate the patient's mucous membranes or abraded skin, proliferate, and disseminate widely to all organs and tissues, including the eye and CSF. A less severe an-

icteric form and a more severe icteric form of the disease occur. In the former, conjunctivitis, conjunctival chemosis, interstitial keratitis, uveitis, vitritis, retinitis, and chorioretinitis develop. Aseptic meningitis, encephalitis, myelitis, peripheral neuritis, and the Guillain-Barré syndrome can occur. Severe kidney and liver damage develops in icteric leptospirosis. There is a widespread vasculitis that can produce subarachnoid, intracerebral, and gastrointestinal hemorrhages. Uveitis and retinitis with many cotton wool spots can be found.

Rickettsia[32]

Rickettsia are obligate intracellular, pleomorphic coccobacilli. Thirteen species cause various human infections, including several types of spotted fever, several types of typhus, erlichosis, Q fever, and acute febrile cerebrovasculitis. In each instance, organisms are injected into the host's blood by infected arthropods or by inoculation of infected feces of infected arthropods. Proliferating organisms in endothelial cells and vascular smooth muscle cells cause angiitis. Patients with Rocky Mountain spotted fever characteristically have fever and encephalitis with confusion, lethargy, insomnia, vertigo, stiff neck, and photophobia. They also can develop myelitis. Ocular manifestations include conjunctivitis, anterior uveitis, and diffuse and focal retinal vasculitis with retinal hemorrhages and cotton wool spots. Branch retinal artery occlusions can occur. Optic disc swelling is usually due to intraocular inflammation rather than increased intracranial pressure. CNS manifestations of Boutonneuse fever or Mediterranean spotted fever are less common and less severe than in Rocky Mountain spotted fever. Encephalitis, meningoencephalitis, polyradiculitis, and peripheral neuropathy can occur. Patients can have visual hallucinations, cerebral blindness, and ptosis. Ocular manifestations include conjunctivitis, uveitis, retinal vasculitis, branch retinal artery occlusion, and chorioretinopathy.

Protozoa[33,34]

Protozoa that cause CNS and ocular infections, especially uveitis and retinitis, include amebae, *T. gondii*, *Trypanosoma* species, *Plasmodium* species, *Babesia* species, and Microsporidia.

Amebae
ENTAMOEBA HISTOLYTICA

E. histolytica infects the human large intestine. Infections are transmitted between persons by ingestion of contaminated fecal material in water or vegetables or by direct fecal-oral contact. Therefore, there are high incidences of infection in developing countries and among homosexuals. Ingested cysts develop into trophozoites in the intestine and invade the intestinal mucosa. CNS infection usually results from hematogenous spread from the gastrointestinal tract, liver, or lungs. Encephalitis with intracranial abscesses causes focal neurologic manifestations. Horizontal gaze palsy from frontal lobe abscess, homonymous hemianopsia, nystagmus, and other eye movement abnormalities from cerebellar abscess and ocular motor nerve palsies can occur. *E. histolytica* also can cause meningoencephalitis. Ocular infections cause keratitis with corneal ulceration,[35,36] uveitis, retinal periphlebitis, and chorioretinitis.

NAEGLERIA FOWLERI, ACANTHAMOEBA SPECIES, AND BALAMUTHIA MANDRILLARIS

Three free-living amebae, *N. fowleri, Acanthamoeba* species and *B. mandrillaris,* cause CNS and/or ocular infections. *N. fowleri* causes primary amebic meningoencephalitis in persons swimming in warm freshwater lakes. Organisms in the trophozoite or flagellate form can invade the CNS through the nasal mucosa and cribiform plate and cause a fulminant, often fatal purulent meningoencephalitis with loss of taste and smell. In the late stages of disease, papilledema, ocular motor nerve palsies, and homonymous hemianopsia can occur. *Acanthamoeba* species cause chronic granulomatous amebic encephalitis in debilitated and immunocompromised persons. CNS infection results from hematogenous spread from skin or lung lesions. Patients develop slowly progressive focal neurologic deficits, seizures, and impairment of consciousness. Homonymous hemianopsia, papilledema, and ocular motor nerve palsies can occur. CNS infection also can produce intracranial abscess. *Acanthamoeba* species cause keratitis in contact lens wearers. Corneal trauma from contact lens wear and contaminated water or contact lens solutions can lead to an epithelial keratitis with pseudodendrites and elevated ridges. A stromal keratitis with ring infiltrate and anterior uveitis can develop (Fig. 25-43). Pain is often severe. Nodular or diffuse anterior or posterior scleritis with optic neuritis and chorioretinitis can occur. *B.*

mandrillaris also can cause granulomatous amebic encephalitis and intracranial abscess in debiliated or immunosuppressed individuals.

Toxoplasma gondii

T. gondii is an obligate intracellular parasite for which the cat is the most common definitive host. Humans and other animal species such as pigs, sheep, and cattle are intermediate hosts. Sexual reproduction occurs in the intestinal epithelium of the cat, and the asexual cycle occurs in the tissues of the intermediate hosts. Trophozoites, or tachyzoites, in the cat's intestine form oocysts, which are shed in the feces and ingested by intermediate hosts. Eating undercooked meat from other intermediate hosts that contains oocytes or tissue cysts also can infect humans. Trophozoites, which develop from the oocysts, are carried in macrophages to the thoracic duct and then into the general circulation and many organs of the intermediate host or can enter the blood directly from infected lesions and disseminate. The crescent-shaped trophozoites invade tissues and become intracellular parasites that cause inflammation and tissue necrosis. Because the trophozoites are intracellular, they are protected from the host's humoral immune system. The organisms form cysts that can remain dormant for years. Components of the cyst wall contain host antigens, making it difficult for the host's immune system to attack the cysts. When the cysts rupture, trophozoites are released, and recurrences are produced.

T. gondii is the most common protozoa to cause uveitis and retinitis in humans.[37,38] It is neurotrophic and commonly infects the CNS and retina. The vast majority of cases of uveitis in adults and children are recurrences of congenital infections. Maternal infections in the first trimester often leads to fetal death and spontaneous abortion. Most cases of congenital toxoplasmosis result from maternal infections in the second and third trimesters. If a mother acquires the infection prior to the pregnancy, the baby does not develop a congenital infection. A mother who has had one child with congenital toxoplasmosis usually does not have a second infected child. The retinal lesions are usually healed at birth. Although both eyes have atrophic chorioretinal scars, usually only one eye at a time has a recurrence. The chorioretinal scars are round or oval, have white centers from chorioretinal atrophy and baring of the sclera, and have pigmented edges. They cause localized scotomas. A central scotoma occurs if the scar is in the macula. Recurrences appear as fluffy elevated yellow-white retinal lesions adjacent to a scar (Fig. 25-44). Vitritis is often found over the active lesions and can be severe. The active retinal lesions are usually the size of the optic disc and lead to white-centered chorioretinal scars with pigmented edges when they heal. Ocular toxoplasmosis also can cause punctate inner reti-

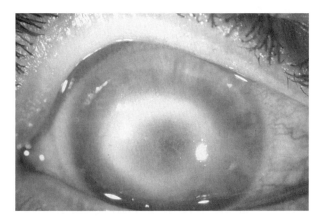

Figure 25-43. *Acanthamoeba* keratitis. Stromal keratitis with a ring-shaped infiltrate. (*Courtesy of Jerold S. Gordon, M.D.*)

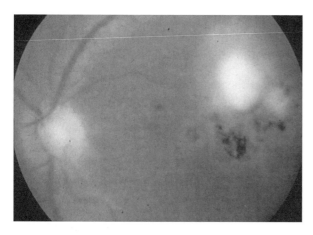

Figure 25-44. Recurrent toxoplasmic chorioretinitis. Two recurrent white round lesions arose near pigmented chorioretinal scars in the macula of the left eye.

nal lesions. These are small gray retinal lesions in the inner layers of the retina. Punctate outer retinal lesions are multiple gray lesions of the outer layers of the neurosensory retina and retinal pigment epithelium. There is usually mild or no vitritis over the latter two types of retinal lesions. Papillitis usually occurs as a result of reactivation of a juxtapapillary chorioretinal scar. However, papillitis and retrobulbar optic neuritis can develop without juxtapapillary scars (Fig. 25-45). Toxoplasmosis also can cause neuroretinitis.

Congenital toxoplasmosis may present as failure to thrive, seizures, mental retardation, microencephaly, microphthalmia, hydrocephalus, pneumonitis, fever, or rash. Acquired toxoplasmosis in immunocompetent per-

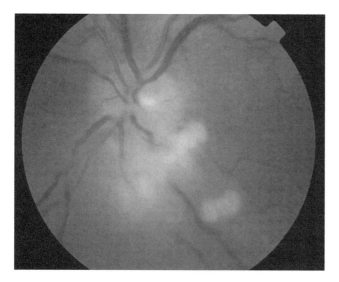

Figure 25-45. Toxoplasmic papillitis and retinitis. Confluent and round white retinal lesions are in the peripapillary retina and adjacent optic disc of the left eye. There is no antecedent chorioretinal scar.

sons causes flulike illness with fever, malaise, fatigue, and sore throat or mimics infectious mononucleosis. Pneumonitis, lymphadenopathy, splenomegaly, myocarditis, pericarditis, hepatitis, and encephalitis occur in severe primary infections. Ocular manifestations are rare. If chorioretinal lesions occur in acute acquired toxoplasmosis, they are usually unilateral, solitary, and nonpigmented. However, immunocompromised patients, including AIDS patients, have severe manifestations of acquired toxoplasmosis or reactivation of chronic or dormant infections.[39] Neuroophthalmic manifestations of CNS toxoplasmosis include ocular motor nerve palsies, vertical and horizontal gaze palsies, skew deviation, homonymous hemianopsia, and cortical blindness. Treatment of ocular toxoplasmosis may consist of antibiotics (sulfadiazine and/or clindamycin), systemic corticosteroids, and folic acid antagonists (pyrimethamine). Folinic acid is often given to prevent bone marrow suppression from pyrimethamine and sulfadiazine. In immunocompetent patients, treatment is used if the active lesion is in or near the macula or optic nerve. None of the antibiotics or pyrimethamine is completely safe to use during pregnancy. In neonates with systemic infection, treatment is continued until at least 1 year of age. In immunocompromised patients, treatment is given for any active lesion because of the threat of disseminated infection. These patients often need long-term suppressive treatment with antibiotics.

Trypanosoma
T. cruzi causes Chaga disease and *Trypanosoma* species cause African sleeping sickness. Feces from insects that have sucked blood from infected mammals transmit *T. cruzi* infections to humans through mucous membranes or skin abrasions. Transmission also can occur transplacentally and via transfusions. Trypomastigotes released from infected cells spread by the blood. In acute Chaga disease, an inflammatory lesion develops in the skin or conjunctiva. An acute meningoencephalitis can occur. In chronic Chaga disease, years after the initial infection, cardiac disease with arrhythmias and emboli can cause branch or central retinal artery occlusions, ischemic optic neuropathy, transient ischemic attacks, and strokes. Immunocompromised patients can develop meningoencephalitis in the chronic phase of the disease.

Plasmodium falciparum
Eyelid edema, conjunctival chemosis, subconjunctival hemorrhage, iritis, retinal hemorrhages, choroidal infarcts, and central retinal artery occlusion can occur in acute malaria.

Microsporidia
Infection from *Microsporidium* species occurs from ingestion of spores via the oral-fecal route and transpla-

centally. Most patients are immunocompromised, especially from HIV infection. Conjunctivitis, epithelial keratitis, and stromal keratitis can develop along with gastrointestinal, sinus, pulmonary, and renal manifestations. Myositis and encephalitis can occur.

Babesia

Babesia species cause human infection from bites of infected rodent ticks and by transfusion of contaminated blood. Sporozoites from infected saliva invade red blood cells, where they become trophozoites and merozoites. The latter disseminate in the blood when the red blood cells rupture. Babesiosis in European countries tends to occur in splenectomized patients and is severe. In the United States it occurs more often in previously healthy persons, is less severe, and is caused by different species. However, immunocompromised patients in the United States can have a more severe disease. Photophobia and conjunctival injection can occur. Hemolytic anemia is associated with retinal hemorrhages, cotton wool spots, ischemic optic neuropathy, homonymous hemianopsia, and stroke.

Helminths

TAENIA SOLIUM[41,42]

The parasite *T. solium* causes cysticercosis. When humans ingest food contaminated with *T. solium* eggs, larvae penetrate the intestinal mucosa and disseminate in blood to muscle, the CNS, and the eye. Years after cysticercosis begins, cysticerci can develop in the eyelids and eye, affecting the conjunctiva, anterior chamber, vitreous body, and subretinal space. Orbital cysticerci produce orbital inflammation with proptosis, eyelid edema, conjunctival hyperemia, and ophthalmoplegia. Cysticerci can develop in extraocular muscles and in the optic nerve. Neuroophthalmic manifestations of neurocysticercosis include homonymous hemianopsia; cortical blindness; ocular motor disorders from damage to cerebral, cerebellar, and brain stem pathways; various types of nystagmus; and ocular motor nerve palsies. Papilledema from increased intracranial pressure can occur due to the obstruction of the flow of CSF from subarachnoid and intraventricular cysts. A cysticercus in the suprasellar cistern can produce a chiasmal syndrome, and a cysticercus in the cavernous sinus can cause a cavernous sinus syndrome.

ECHINOCOCCUS SPECIES

Humans become infected by eating material contaminated with feces of dogs and foxes, which are the definitive hosts for *Echinococcus*. The ova hatch in the intestinal tract, and larvae penetrate the mucosa and spread by lymphatics and blood to the liver, lung, CNS, and eye. Oncospheres develop into hydatid cysts that are filled with other cysts and larvae. Symptoms usually develop years after the initial infection. Hydatid cysts can develop in the anterior chamber and vitreous cavity. They frequently occur in the orbit, causing proptosis, ophthalmoplegia, and visual loss from optic nerve compression or inflammation. Intracranial cysts form in the brain parenchyma, ventricles, brain stem, and cerebellum. Papilledema, homonymous hemianopsia, and ocular motor nerve palsies occur.

SCHISTOSOMA SPECIES

Humans are the definitive hosts for *Schistosoma* species. Adult worms in blood vessels produce fertilized eggs that are shed in feces and urine. Ciliated larvae infect freshwater snails, which in turn produce cercariae that penetrate human skin. The cercariae develop into schistosomula that infect the heart, lungs, and liver. In severe acute schistosomiasis, CNS manifestations can include papilledema, sixth nerve palsy from increased intracranial pressure, homonymous hemianopsia, cortical blindness, and optic neuritis. These result from inflammatory responses to the organisms. In chronic schistosomiasis, organisms can migrate to the lacrimal gland, eyelid, and eye, causing dacryoadenitis, lid nodules, conjunctivitis, subconjunctival hemorrhage, keratitis, iritis, choroiditis, and retinitis. CNS manifestations include encephalitis, meningitis, stroke, and intracranial masses. Neuroophthalmic manifestations include homonymous hemianopsia, cortical blindness, gaze palsies, ocular motor nerve palsies, papilledema, and optic neuritis. The ocular and CNS manifestations in chronic schistosomiasis result from inflammatory responses to the organisms and occlusion of blood vessels by adult worms and their eggs.

PARAGONIMUS SPECIES

Humans and other mammals are the definitive hosts for *Paragonimus* species. Mature worms reside in the lungs, and their eggs are released into the environment by their sputum and feces. Freshwater snails are intermediate hosts that become infected by larvae and release cercariae, which in turn infect crustacea. Humans eat infected crustacea. Metacercariae encyst in the intestine and penetrate the peritoneal cavity, pleural cavity, and lung. When organisms spread to the CNS hematogenously or directly along the jugular veins, they produce encephalitis and meningitis. Focal manifestations include seizures and strokelike disorders affecting the temporal and occipital lobes. Homonymous hemianopsia, papilledema, and sixth nerve palsy from increased intracranial pressure can occur.

ANGIOSTRONGYLUS CANTONENSIS

The definitive host for *A. cantonensis* is the rat. Adult roundworms in lungs produce larvae, which move from the trachea to the gastrointestinal tract, where they are excreted in feces. Humans are accidental hosts and become infected by eating raw snails or contaminated vegetables. *A. cantonensis* causes an eosinophilic meningitis or meningoencephalitis. Ocular motor palsies and optic neuritis can occur. Intraocular parasites can be found in the anterior chamber, vitreous cavity, and subretinal space.

GNATHOSTOMA SPINIGERUM

The definitive hosts for *G. spinigerum* are cats and dogs. Mature worms in the stomach shed eggs in their feces. The eggs develop into larvae and are eaten by freshwater crustacea. Fish, frogs, and snakes eat the crustacea and, in turn, are eaten by fowl. Humans, who are intermediate hosts, acquire infection by eating undercooked fowl containing cysts. The cysts develop into larvae and sexually immature worms, which form subcutaneous inflammatory lesions. Worms can migrate to the eye, appearing under the conjunctiva, in the anterior chamber, in the vitreous cavity, and in the retina (Figs. 25-46 and 25-47). CNS manifestations include meningitis, meningoencephalitis, intracerebral and sub-

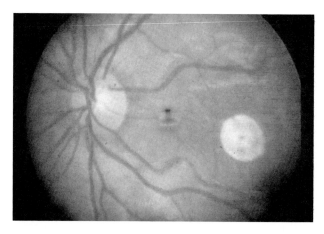

Figure 25-47. Subretinal nematode. White round nematode under the retina in macula of the left eye.

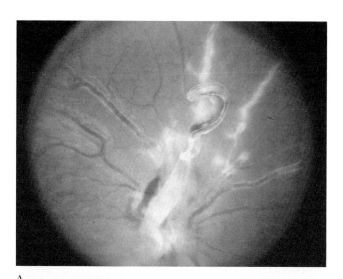

A

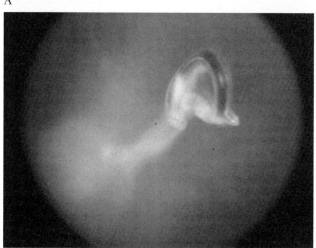

B

Figure 25-46. Nematode retinitis and vitritis. *A.* Retinitis appears as white inflammatory sheathing of retina vessels. *B.* Vitritis and nematode in vitreous above the optic disc. (*Courtesy of David W. Parke II, M.D.*)

arachnoid hemorrhage, and myelitis. Neuroophthalmic manifestations include homonymous hemianopsia, papilledema, ocular motor nerve palsies, and the dorsal midbrain syndrome.

LOA LOA

Adult *Loa loa* roundworms in vertebrate hosts produce circulating microfilaria. Deerflies become infected during a blood meal and develop larvae that migrate to the proboscis. The larvae infect human hosts during another blood meal. Local skin lesions, called *Calabar swellings,* and systemic infections occur. Such swellings can occur in the eyelids. Microfilaria can appear in the subconjunctival space and in retinal and choroidal blood vessels. In the retina and choroid, they produce hemorrhagic and inflammatory lesions that expand as the microfilaria migrate. CNS loiasis is caused by hematogenous spread of microfilaria into intracranial capillaries and severe inflammatory reactions when they die, producing symptoms of meningitis and encephalitis.

ONCHOCERCA VOLVULUS

Humans are the definitive hosts for *O. volvulus*. Adult worms produce microfilaria in the skin and subcutaneous tissues, which are ingested by *Simulium* flies during bites. Onchocerciasis occurs near fast-moving rivers in Africa because that is the habitat of the flies. Larvae migrate to the fly's proboscis and are deposited in the human's skin during a blood meal. Sexually mature adult worms and microfilaria develop and produce skin nodules and an itchy, erythematous dermatitis. Onchocerciasis causes river blindness from infiltration of microfilaria into ocular tissues. Tissue damage is caused by the inflammatory response to dying microfilaria and deposition of antigen-antibody complexes. Conjunctivitis, superficial keratitis with scarring, iridocyclitis, chorioretinitis, and optic neuritis can occur (Fig. 25-48). Although microfilaria are found in the CSF, there are no CNS manifestations of onchocerciasis.

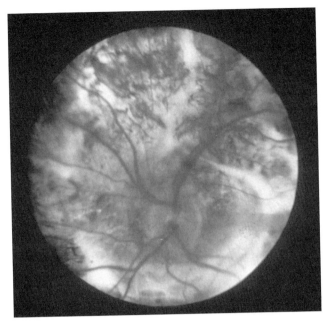

Figure 25-48. Onchocercal choroiditis. Chronic choroiditis produced diffuse, pigmented, and white fibrous scars under the retina of the left eye.

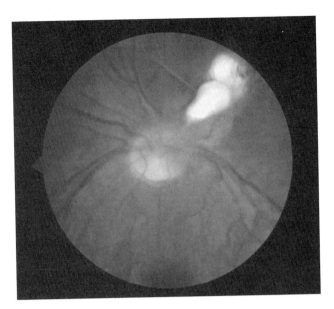

Figure 25-49. *Toxocara* vitreous abscess. White inflammatory mass in the posterior vitreous in front of the optic disc of the right eye.

TOXOCARA CANIS[43]

Adult *T. canis* roundworms in the intestinal tract of dogs deposit eggs in feces. Humans, especially children, ingest the eggs in contaminated soil. Larvae in the human intestinal tract migrate to the liver, lung, eye, and CNS (visceral larval migrans). Larvae that migrate to the eye produce white or yellow inflammatory masses or abscesses in the vitreous, retina, or choroid (Figs. 25-49 and 25-50). The retinal and subretinal lesions often affect the macula, causing loss of central vision. Because children are often affected, the visual loss can present as strabismus. Larvae may cause endophthalmitis with retinitis. Diffuse anterior and posterior uveitis, neuroretinitis, and retrobulbar optic neuritis can occur. CNS manifestations include encephalitis and myelitis. Larvae occlude small blood vessels causing hemorrhagic infarctions. Death of the larvae leads to granulomatous inflammation.

TRICHINELLA SPIRALIS

Humans become infected by *T. spiralis* by eating undercooked pork that contains encysted larvae. The larvae invade the intestinal mucosa and form adult male and female nematodes. The adult worms die after producing larvae, which penetrate the intestinal mucosa and spread to the thoracic duct and general circulation. The larvae migrate to skeletal muscles, including the extraocular muscles, where they encyst. The first phase of acute infection consists of gastrointestinal symptoms. The second phase includes fever, muscle pain, and muscle weakness. Edema of the face and eyelids can develop. When extraocular muscles are affected, ophthalmoplegia, proptosis, and pain with eye movements develop. Subconjunctival hemorrhage, conjunctival chemosis, retinal hemorrhages, chorioretinitis, and optic neuritis can occur (Fig. 25-51). The third stage of infection coincides with cyst formation. CNS trichinosis usually follows infection by large numbers of organisms and often accompanies myocarditis. CNS manifestations are caused by emboli from the heart, thrombosis of

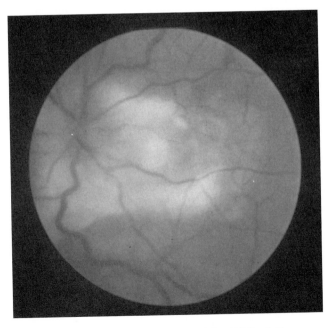

Figure 25-50. *Toxocara* choroiditis. White inflammatory mass beneath the retina and adjacent to the optic disc of the left eye.

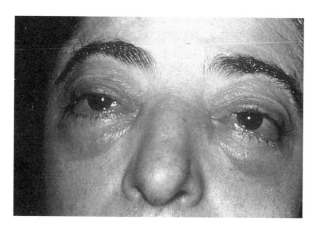

Figure 25-51. Orbital trichinosis. Proptosis, lid edema, conjunctival chemosis, and conjunctival injection from trichinosis of the extraocular muscles.

dural venous sinuses, and vasculitis with cerebral hemisphere and brain stem infarction. Ocular motor nerve palsies and cortical blindness can occur.

OTHER NEMATODES

Diffuse unilateral subacute neuroretinitis (DUSN) is caused by several nematodes, including *T. canis, Ancylostoma caninum,* and *Baylisascaris procyonis.* Multifocal gray-white lesions form in the outer retina that follow migration of worms in the subretinal space (Fig. 25-52). Depigmentation of the retinal pigment epithelium, retinal exudates, vitritis, and swelling of the optic disc occur. Visual loss can be severe. Photocoagulation of worms visible in the subretinal space can be performed. Meningitis and meningoencephalitis from *B. procyonis* infection can cause cortical blindness. *Dirofilaria immitis* has appeared in the vitreous cavity.

Mycoplasma[44]

Acute *M. pneumoniae* infections are caused by inhalation of infected respiratory secretions. *M. pneumoniae* usually produces a self-limited pneumonia in children and young adults. However, the pneumonia can be severe in immunocompromised patients, including those with AIDS. Papillitis, retrobulbar optic neuritis, and papilledema can develop. Other neuroophthalmic manifestations include ocular motor nerve palsies and various types of nystagmus. *M. hominis* infections are acquired in newborns by passage through an infected birth canal or in adults by sexual contact. Most often genitourinary disorders result, but disseminated infection can cause meningitis and orbital abscess.

Prions[45,46]

Prions are infectious protein particles that cause scrapie and bovine spongiform encephalopathy in animals and kuru, Creuzfeldt-Jakob disease, Gerstmann-Straussler-

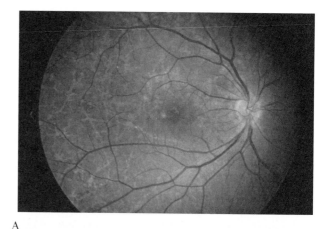

A

B

Figure 25-52. Binocular diffuse unilateral subretinal neuroretinitis. *A.* Migration of nematodes in the subretinal space caused multiple white tracks throughout the posterior pole of the right eye. *B.* Similar DUSN tracks in the left eye. (*Courtesy of Robert Kalina, M.D.*)

Scheinker disease, and fatal familial insomnia in humans. Kuru is transmitted by consumption of contaminated human tissues.[47] After many years it produces progressive cerebellar, brain stem, and cortical dysfunction with ataxia, tremor, dysphagia, dysarthria, choreoathetosis, and dementia. Patients usually die a few months to a few years after the onset of symptoms. Neuroophthalmic manifestations include various types of nystagmus, e.g., upbeat and downbeat nystagmus, skew deviation, internuclear ophthalmoplegia (INO), one-and-one-half syndrome (unilateral INO with ipsilateral horizontal gaze palsy), supranuclear vertical gaze palsy, and sixth nerve palsy.

Creutzfeldt-Jacob disease (CJD) occurs sporadically as an autosomal dominant inherited disease and a disease transmitted iatrogenically.[48,49] In the sporadic or nonfamilial form of CJD, symptoms of confusion are followed by ataxia and myoclonus with rapid progression (usually 4 to 5 months) to severe dementia. Iatrogenic transmission has occurred through injection of cadaveric pituitary gland extracts, tissue or organ grafts from cadavers (cornea, dura, pericardium and liver), improperly sterilized neurosurgical instruments, and contact with contaminated tissues by health care workers.[50,51] New-variant CJD manifests with changes in mood and behavior and impairment of memory that progress over several weeks to months.[52] In addition, patients develop myoclonus, aphasia, apraxia, pyramidal tract signs, and choreoathetosis. Patients are usually severely demented and bedridden several months after the onset of symptoms and die from respiratory or urinary tract infections within 1 year. In Heidenhain's variant of CJD, the initial manifestations are homonymous hemianopsia and cortical blindness. Dementia and myoclonus develop later. Cerebellar ataxia and diplopia are early signs in the Bronwell-Oppenheimer variant of CJD. Other neuroophthalmic manifestations include visual illusions, visual agnosia, eye movement disorders associated with cerebellar dysfunction, various types of nystagmus, ocular myoclonus, supranuclear vertical gaze palsy, and skew deviation.

Gerstmann-Straussler-Scheinker (GSS) disease is characterized by the gradual onset of cerebellar ataxia, dysarthria, dementia, and myoclonus in young adults and middle-aged adults. Several kindreds of GSS have been described. The neurologic deterioration progresses over a few to several years. Death is caused by urinary and respiratory infections in bedridden patients. Eye movement disorders include various types of nystagmus, abnormal smooth pursuit, saccadic and vestibular eye movements associated with cerebellar degeneration, and supranuclear vertical gaze palsy. Fatal familial insomnia (FFI) is a progressive autosomal dominantly inherited disorder with insomnia, dysautonomia, myoclonus, and ataxia. Dementia with delirium and hallucinations occurs. Two patients had unilateral sixth nerve palsies.

REFERENCES

1. Yanoff M, Duker JS: *Ophthalmology.* London: Mosby, 1999.

2. Albert DM, Jakobiec FA: *Principles and Practice of Ophthalmology,* 2d ed. Philadelphia: Saunders, 2000.

3. Miller NR, Newman NJ: *Walsh and Hoyt's Clinical Neuro-Ophthalmology,* 5th ed. Baltimore: Williams & Wilkins, 1998.

4. Tasman W, Jaeger EA: *Duane's Clinical Ophthalmology,* Vol. 2: *Neuro-Ophthalmology and Disease of the Orbit.* Philadelphia: Lippincott Williams & Wilkins, 2002.

5. Purvin VA: Bacteria and bacterial diseases. In Miller NR, Newman NJ (eds): *Walsh and Hoyt's Clinical Neuro-Ophthalmology.* Baltimore: Williams & Wilkins, 1998, pp 4065–4280.

6. McLeod SD: Bacterial keratitis. In Yanoff M, Duker JS (eds): *Ophthalmology.* London: Mosby, 1999.

7. Callegan MC, Engelbert M, Parke DW, et al.: Bacterial endophthalmitis: Epidemiology, therapeutics, and bacterium-host interactions. *Clin Microbiol Rev* 15:111, 2002.

8. Caya JG: *Clostridium botulinum* and the ophthalmologist: A review of botulism, including biological warfare ramifications of botulinum toxin. *Surv Ophthalmol* 46:25, 2001.

9. Rajeev B: Tuberculosis, leprosy and brucellosis. In Yanoff M, Duker JS (eds): *Ophthalmology.* London: Mosby, 1999.

10. Sridar MS, Gopinathan U, Garg P, et al.: Ocular *Nocardia* infections with special emphasis on the cornea. *Surv Ophthalmol* 45:361, 2001.

11. Knox DL: Bacterial posterior uveitis: Whipple's disease. In Yanoff M, Duker JS (eds): *Ophthalmology.* London: Mosby, 1999.

12. Cunningham ET Jr, Koehler JE: Ocular bartonellosis. *Am J Ophthalmol* 130:340, 2000.

13. Brazis PW, Miller NR: Virus (except retroviruses) and viral diseases. In Miller NR, Newman NJ (eds): *Walsh and Hoyt's Clinical Neuro-Ophthalmology,* 5th ed. Baltimore: Williams & Wilkins, 1998, pp 4945–5360.

14. McLeod SD: Viral keratitis. In Yanoff M, Duker JS (eds): *Ophthalmology.* London: Mosby, 1999.

15. Hudson HL, Boyer DS, Martin DF, et al: Viral posterior uveitis. In Yanoff M, Duker JS (eds): *Ophthalmology.* London: Mosby, 1999.

16. Chern KC Hwang DG: Herpetic uveitis. In Yanoff M, Duker JS (eds): *Ophthalmology.* London: Mosby, 1999.

17. Siverio Junior CD, Imai Y, Cunningham ET Jr: Diagnosis and management of herpetic anterior uveitis. *Int Ophthalmol Clin* 42:43, 2002.

18. Horton JC: Neurovisual manifestations of herpes viruses. *Int Ophthalmol Clin* 42:33, 2002.

19. Walters G, James TE: Viral causes of the acute retinal necrosis syndrome. *Curr Opin Ophthalmol* 12:191, 2001.

20. Currie J, Dwyer DD: Retroviruses and the acquired immune deficiency syndrome. In Miller NR, Newman NJ (eds): *Walsh and Hoyt's Clinical Neuro-Ophthalmology,* 5th ed. Baltimore: Williams & Wilkins, 1998, pp 5361–5464.

21. Dugel PU: Ocular infections related to human immunodeficiency virus. In Yanoff M, Duker JS (eds): *Ophthalmology.* London: Mosby, 1999.

22. Acharya NR, Cunningham ET Jr: Corneal, anterior segment, and adnexal manifestations of human immunodeficiency virus. *Int Ophthamol Clin* 38:161, 1998.

23. Arnold AC: Fungi and mycotic diseases. In Miller NR, Newman NJ (eds): *Walsh and Hoyt's Clinical Neuro-Ophthalmology,* 5th ed. Baltimore: Williams & Wilkins, 1998, pp 4281–4438.

24. Klotz SA, Penn CC, Negvesky GJ, Butrus SI: Fungal and parasitic infections of the eye. *Clin Microbiol Rev* 13:662, 2000.

25. McLeod SD: Fungal keratitis. In Yanoff M, Duker JS (eds): *Ophthalmology.* London: Mosby, 1999.

26. Moorthy RS, Fountain JA: Fungal uveitis. In Yanoff M, Duker JS (eds): *Ophthalmology.* London: Mosby, 1999.

27. Samiy N, D'Amico DJ: Endogeneous fungal endophthalmitis. *Int Ophthalmol Clin* 36:147, 1996.

28. Levin LA, Avery R, Shore JW: The spectrum of orbital aspergillosis: A clinicopathological review. *Surv Ophthalmol* 41:142, 1996.

29. Lesser RL: Spirochetes and the spirochetoses. In Miller

NR, Newman NJ (eds): *Walsh and Hoyt's Clinical Neuro-Ophthalmology,* 5th ed. Baltimore: Williams & Wilkins, 1998, pp 4779–4944.

30. Frohman L, Lama P: Annual update of systemic disease—1999: Emerging and re-emerging infections (part II). *J Neuro-Ophthalmol* 20:48, 2000.

31. Dugel PU: Syphilitic uveitis. In Yanoff M, Duker JS (eds): *Ophthalmology.* London: Mosby, 1999.

32. Miller NR: Rickettsiae and rickettsial diseases. In Miller NR, Newman NJ (eds): *Walsh and Hoyt's Clinical Neuro-Ophthalmology,* 5th ed. Baltimore: Williams & Wilkins, 1998, pp 4737–4778.

33. Cornblath WT: Protozoa and protozoal diseases. In Miller NR, Newman NJ (eds): *Walsh and Hoyt's Clinical Neuro-Ophthalmology,* 5th ed. Baltimore: Williams & Wilkins, 1998, pp 4613–4736.

34. Khanna A., Goldstein DA, Tessler HH: Protozoal posterior uveitis. In Yanoff M, Duker JS (eds): *Ophthalmology.* London: Mosby, 1999.

35. Illingworth CD, Cook SD: Acanthamoeba keratitis. *Surv Ophthalmol* 42:493, 1998.

36. Kumar R, Lloyd D: Recent advances in the treatment of *Acanthamoeba* keratitis. *Clin Infect Dis* 35:434, 2002.

37. Holland GN: Reconsidering the pathogenesis of ocular toxoplasmosis. *Am J Ophthalmol* 128:502, 1999.

38. Hovakimyan A, Cunningham ET Jr: Ocular toxoplasmosis. *Ophthalmol Clin North Am* 15:327, 2002.

39. Rodgers CA, Harris JR: Ocular toxoplasmosis in HIV infection. *Int J STD AIDS* 7:307, 1996.

40. Odel JG, Moazami G: Diseases caused by helminths. In Miller NR, Newman NJ (eds): *Walsh and Hoyt's Clinical Neuro-Ophthalmology,* 5th ed. Baltimore: Williams & Wilkins, 1998, pp 4439–4544.

41. Sabrosa NA, Zajdenweber M: Nematode infections of the eye: Toxocariasis, onchocerciasis, diffuse unilateral subacute neuroretinitis and cysticercosis. *Ophthalmol Clin North Am* 15:3515, 2002.

42. Pushker N, Bajaj MS, Betharia SM: Orbital and adnexal cysticercosis. *Clin Exp Ophthalmol* 30:322, 2002.

43. Sabrosa NA, de Souza EC: Nematode infections of the eye: Toxocariasis and diffuse unilateral subacute neuroretinitis. *Curr Opin Ophthalmol* 12:450, 2001.

44. Miller NR: Diseases caused by *Mycoplasma* (Mollicutes). In Miller NR, Newman NJ (eds): *Walsh and Hoyt's Clinical Neuro-Ophthalmology,* 5th ed. Baltimore: Williams & Wilkins, 1998, pp 4545–4560.

45. Eggenberger ER: Prions and prion diseases. In Miller NR, Newman NJ (eds): *Walsh and Hoyt's Clinical Neuro-Ophthalmology,* 5th ed. Baltimore: Williams & Wilkins, 1998, pp 4561–4612.

46. Collins S, McLean CA, Masters CL: Gerstmann-Straussler-Scheinker syndrome, fatal familial insomnia, and kuru: A review of these less common human transmissible spongiform encephalopathies. *J Clin Neurosci* 8:387, 2001.

47. Goldfarb LG: Kuru: The old epidemic in a new mirror. *Microbes Infect* 4:875, 2002.

48. Lueck CJ, McIlwaine GG, Zeidler M: Creutzfeldt-Jakob disease and the eye: I. Background and patient management. *Eye* 14:263, 2000.

49. Lueck CJ, McIlwaine GG, Zeidler M: Creutzfeldt-Jakob disease and the eye: II. Ophthalmic and neuro-ophthalmic features. *Eye* 14:291, 2000.

50. Lang CJ, Heckamann JG, Neundorfer B: Creutzfeldt-Jakob disease via dural and corneal transplants. *J Neurol Sci* 160:128, 1998.

51. Mehta JS, Franks WA: The sclera, the prion, and the ophthalmologist. *Br J Ophthalmol* 86:587, 2002.

52. Irani DN: The classic and variant forms of Creutzfeldt-Jakob disease. *Semin Clin Neuropsychiatr* 8:71, 2003.

CHAPTER 26

Neurologic Complications of Infective Endocarditis

Nina J. Solenski

► HISTORY

In 1885, Sir William Osler described to the Royal College of Physicians in London the classic triad of fever, heart murmur, and hemiplegia of "malignant endocarditis" in his now famous Gulstonian Lectures.[1] Since the nineteenth century, modern medical technological advancements and the formation of clinically operational criteria for defining infectious endocarditis have significantly advanced our study and treatment of this disease.[2,3] In particular, the emergence and use of the modified Duke criteria in 1994 have enhanced early detection and subsequent treatment of this sometimes occult disease.[4] Despite these advances, neurologic complications remain a major cause of morbidity and mortality during the course of infective endocarditis.

► INCIDENCE

Neurologic complications occur in 20 to 40 percent of patients with infective endocarditis, with stroke being the most common complication.[5–7] Meningitis, meningoencephalitis, intracranial mycotic aneurysm, seizures, encephalopathy, and psychiatric complications are also seen. Neurologic complications represent the heralding symptom in 12 to 23 percent of patients with infective endocarditis.[8,9] Usually, neurologic complications are diagnosed when the patient becomes symptomatic, e.g., with the development of hemiplegia from cerebral infarction or the onset of fever and confusion from meningoencephalitis. The true incidence of neurologic complications is likely higher if asymptomatic neuropathology is included.

The incidence of infective endocarditis has remained stable, but the clinical profile is changing, including peak mean age of incidence.[10,11] In some studies, more than 50 percent of cases of infective endocarditis are in the elderly (>60 years of age), especially in patients with severe comorbidities or heart disease.[7,12,13] The current peak incidence is between 70 and 74 years of age, an increase of a decade compared with the previous mean age of incidence of between 52 and 60 years of age. The increasing incidence of infective endocarditis, particularly in the elderly, may be due to the greater use of invasive techniques, to the naturally increasing size of the aging population (United States), or to advanced technology that has enhanced our diagnosis of infective endocarditis.[12,13] Certain procedures, especially intravascular monitoring, pacemaker insertion, chronic hemodialysis, gastrointestinal and oropharyngeal procedures, and genitourinary examination techniques, can increase the risk of infective endocarditis, particularly in the immunosuppressed or immunocompromised patient.

The overall incidence of neurologic complications in the setting of infective endocarditis reportedly has not changed over the last several decades;[5,7,14] however, no large patient series without intrinsic referral bias exists to determine this definitively. Patients with neurologic complications during infective endocarditis have a significant increase in mortality rate compared with those without neurologic complications. The overall reported fatality rate of infective endocarditis is approximately 20 percent. The overall percent mortality in patients with infective endocarditis and neurologic complications is greater than double this rate (approximately 50 percent), with the range from 16 to 87 percent.[15–18] Excluding fulminant *Staphylococcus aureus* infections, neurologic complications are responsible for up to 36 percent of the deaths in patients with native-valve infective endocarditis and for 10 to 45 percent in those with prosthetic-valve infective endocarditis.[2,16,18] Table 26-1 summarizes the potential neurologic complications associated with infective endocarditis, their relative incidence, pathophysiology, and other clinical features.

▶ PATHOPHYSIOLOGY

Pathogenesis of Infective Endocarditis

The actual mechanism of infection in humans is unknown; however, numerous animal models of infective endocarditis reveal that bacteria can adhere easily to and colonize damaged cardiac tissue even at low inocula. During infective endocarditis, the antithrombotic nature of the endothelial surface of the heart is lost, creating a prothrombotic surface.[20,21] Even minimal trauma (mechanical or inflammatory-mediated) leads to massive platelet-fibrin thrombus formation, which is susceptible to bacterial seeding. Repetitive bouts of bacteremia and thrombus formation lead to vegetations, which are an aggregate of fibrin, platelets, and white blood cells. As recently reviewed, in response to microbial invasion, endothelial cells produce tissue-factor activity and cytokines, triggering blood clotting and inflammation and promoting formation of the vegetation.[22,23] Traumatization of the endothelium can occur from cardiac conditions that favor a high-velocity jet stream, such as can occur across a narrow orifice or from a high- to low-pressure chamber.[24] Certain congenital or acquired cardiac lesions, such as a bicuspid aortic valve, patent ductus arteriosus, and ventricular septal defect, may produce a turbulent blood flow jet, damaging the endocardial lining. Infected valvular vegetations can result in serious local tissue damage with subsequent valvular regurgitation, paravalvular abscess, pericarditis, and fistula or aneurysm formation.[25] Streptococci are the most common causative organisms of infective endocarditis, followed by coagulase-positive and coagulase-negative staphylococci. In the past few decades, the number of cases of endocarditis due to *S. aureus*, especially hospital-acquired methicillin-resistant staphylococci, has increased significantly. During an acute infection with a virulent bacterial or fungal species, colonization of a preformed vegetation of platelet-fibrin and thrombin occurs quickly. The endocardial surface is damaged significantly, creating vegetations that tend to be soft, friable, and large, with a propensity for embolization. In subacute infections with "nonvirulent" organisms, the damaged endothelial surface may have adequate time to heal over, with reconstitution of the endothelial layer, fibrosis, and calcification over time.

The pathogenesis of infective endocarditis clearly involves perturbation of the cardiac tissue, with 70 percent of patients having a history of underlying cardiac valvular disease, congenital heart disease, or intravenous drug use.[26] Despite this propensity for cardiac disease in patients with infective endocarditis, there is no history of cardiac disease prior to presentation in 20 to 40 percent.[15,26] A decline in this number has been observed subsequently, which may be explained by better recognition of valvular heart disease and improved prophylactic and acute treatment of bacterial infections.[27]

Common Risk Factors for Neurologic Complications

S. aureus infection of either the mitral or aortic valve has been associated with a high incidence of neu-

▶ **TABLE 26-1.** NEUROLOGIC COMPLICATIONS OF INFECTIVE ENDOCARDITIS.

Neurologic Complication	Frequency	Pathophysiology	Clinical Comments
Central nervous system			
Cerebral ischemia/infarction	10–30%	• Cardioembolic source most common	• Can be initial sign of IE in up to 14% of patients
Ischemic		• Rarely global ischemia from cardiac failure	• Risk of recurrent stroke significantly decreases with antibiotic treatment, but strokes still can occur following initiation of treatment
Hemorrhagic		• TIA—can be embolic source from a mycotic aneurysm and harbinger of ICH	• Should prompt urgent examination for mycotic aneurysm formation
Intracranial or subarachnoid hemorrhage	3–8%	• Ruptured mycotic aneurysm	• Ipsilateral embolism precedes ICH in up to 30% of cases
		• Iatrogenic anticoagulation-related	• ICH in the setting of IE carries high mortality regardless of primary cause
Meningitis/meningoencephalitis	1–4%	• Multiple septic emboli to meningeal vessels	
Seizures	10–20%	• Cortical irritation from septic emboli, infarction, or hemorrhage	
Encephalopathy	25%	• Multiple microemboli	• Can be manifested by psychiatric symptoms, especially in the elderly
		• Metabolic disarray	
Macroabscess	<1%		
Movement disorders	Case reports	• Emboli to basal ganglia or connecting pathways	
Peripheral nervous system			
Peripheral neuropathy	25–43%	• Septic emboli to vasa vasorum	• Mononeuropathy (ulnar, median, peroneal, etc.), mononeuritis multiplex, and cranial neuropathy have all been reported
			• If occurs as the initial presentation of IE, suspect *Streptococcus viridans*
			• If critically ill and ventilatory weaning is difficult, suspect motor peripheral neuropathy
Ocular	Up to 25%	• Emboli to ophthalmic or central retinal artery results in sudden blindness (ophthalmologic emergency)	• Full fundal examination is mandatory in all IE patients

rologic complications.[28,29] The use of anticoagulant therapy has been found to have either no or a positive predictive value for the development of neurologic complications in infective endocarditis depending on the study. Similarly, there are conflicting data on the predictive value of echocardiographic evidence of vegetations and their association with a higher risk of neurologic complications in infective endocarditis patients.[28,30] Factors such as age, duration of prodrome, anticoagulation at the onset of symptoms, and the presence of atrial fibrillation were found to have no predictive value for the development of neurologic complications in one study of patients with infective endocarditis.[15] In another study, no correlation was demonstrated between the frequency of neurologic complication and gender, preexisting valvular disease, or cardiac dysrhythmias. The more common risk factors for the development of infective endocarditis and neurologic clinical implications are summarized in Table 26-2 and discussed in detail below.

Valvular Disease—Native

Neurologic complications are observed most frequently in left-sided infective endocarditis, most likely due to the direct access of the emboli through the aortic root into the internal carotid artery and more distal cerebral circulation. In right-sided endocarditis, vegetative emboli rarely gain access to the distal cerebral circulation, except in the setting of a patent foramen ovale (resulting in paradoxical emboli). It is unclear whether the aortic or mitral valves have different or similar rates of infection. Some studies report similar rates, whereas others demonstrate increased rates of either aortic or mitral valve disease.[28,31] There is a well-established association between rheumatic mitral valve disease and infective endocarditis. The overall incidence of rheumatic valve-related infective endocarditis is decreasing due to a decline in this disease in developed countries. As reviewed recently, degenerative valve lesions are a primary cause of senile aortic stenosis or mitral regurgitation and represent significant risk factors for infec-

▶ **TABLE 26-2.** RISK FACTORS FOR THE DEVELOPMENT OF INFECTIVE ENDOCARDITIS AND NEUROLOGIC COMPLICATIONS.

Valvular disease	Clinical comments
Native	• Left-sided infective endocarditis (mitral or aortic valve disease) most associated with neurologic embolic complication
Mitral and aortic valve	
Mitral valve prolapse	• Higher risk with valve redundancy or when associated with mitral regurgitation (murmur usually present)
Bicuspid or unicuspid aortic valve	
Prosthetic (mechanical and bioprosthetic)	• 25–40% of patients receiving prosthetic valve replacement experience a neurologic complication
Congenital heart disease	
Atrial septal defect	• Higher risk associated with conditions that create a high-velocity jet stream of blood or significant turbulence
Patent ductus arteriosis	
Ventricular septal defect	• Infective endocarditis with neurologic complications is rare in right-sided cardiac disease
Coarctation of the aorta	
Aortic stenosis	
Pulmonary stenosis/atresia	
Tetralogy of Fallot	
Marfan's syndrome	
Hypertrophic cardiomyopathy	
Idiopathic hypertrophic subaortic stenosis	
Iatrogenic	• Any process leading to systemic bacteremia
Invasive procedures	• See AHA and joint ACC-AHA recommendations (1997, 1998, respectively) for prophylaxis of invasive or high risk of inducing bacteremic states
Dental/orthodontic	
Chronic hemodialysis	
Indwelling catheters	
Surgical procedures	
Pulmonary/GU/GI instrumentation	
Personal habits	
Intravenous drug use	• IVDA is often associated with virulent *S. aureus* infections with increased risk of ICH
Poor dental hygiene	
Autoimmune disorders	
Inflammatory bowel syndrome	
Systemic lupus erythematosis	
Immunosuppression	
Chronic alcoholism	
Chronic steroid or immunosuppressant use	
HIV	

tive endocarditis, particularly in the elderly.[12,22] Degenerative valve lesions are present in up to 50 percent of patients with infective endocarditis who are older than age 60.[32]

Mitral valve prolapse has been implicated as a risk factor for infective endocarditis, particularly in mitral valve prolapse with redundant leaflets and significant mitral regurgitation. There is a five- to ninefold increased risk for infective endocarditis in patients with mitral valve prolapse.[33,34] Prolapsing valves are divided into *classic prolapse,* which is defined as prolapsing valves with leaflets greater than 5 mm thick, and *nonclassic prolapse,* in which the leaflets are less than 5 mm thick. Patients with classic prolapse have an incidence of 2.1 to 3.5 percent of developing infective endocarditis (4- or 5-year follow-up, respectively) or an absolute annual risk of 1:2000.[32,34–36] Despite the fact that the incidence of mitral valve prolapse in women is three times that of males, males with mitral valve prolapse may be at a higher risk for developing infective endocarditis than females.

Valvular Disease—Prosthetic-Valve Replacement

In prospective studies from 1980 to early 2000, the incidence of prosthetic valve infective endocarditis ranged from 10 to 16.5 percent,[7] with a high incidence of neurologic complications from both early and late (>60 days following surgery) infection. In other series it is estimated that 25 to 40 percent of patients with prosthetic valve–related infective endocarditis develop neurologic complications.[6,18,25,31] It is unclear if neurologic complications occur with the same frequency in native- and prosthetic-valve endocarditis because some series suggest similar and other series dissimilar rates of neurologic complications.[15,37–39] Patients with prosthetic valves requiring anticoagulation who are carefully anticoagulated may have a similar risk of neurologic complications as those with native-valve infective endocarditis. In a review by Jamieson of randomized clinical trials, the prevalence rates of thromboembolism, thrombosis, and prosthetic-valve endocarditis were the same for mechanical and biologic prostheses.[40] The overall mortality rate of prosthetic-valve endocarditis is high and estimated to be 25 to 73 percent.[40–43]

Congenital Cardiac Disease

The incidence of infective endocarditis in adults with congenital heart disease is greater than 10 times than that of the normal population.[44] Cardiac defects characterized by an abnormal pressure gradient of blood flow, from high to low, and those with a high-pressure jet stream are especially vulnerable for the development of infective endocarditis. This type of hemodynamic dysfunction occurs in a small interventricular septal defect, patent ductus arteriosus, and subaortic and valvular aortic stenosis.[23] As reviewed recently (2003), other forms of congenital cardiac disease associated with a higher risk of infective endocarditis include coarctation of the aorta, tetralogy of Fallot, transposition of the great vessels, Marfan disease, Eisenmenger syndrome, and idiopathic hypertrophic cardiomyopathy.[44] Since atrial septal defect of the secondum type involves no or minimal blood flow disruption, this cardiac defect does not carry a higher risk of infective endocarditis.

Iatrogenic

Recently, numerous invasive techniques have played a prominent role in promoting infective endocarditis and ultimately promoting neurologic complications. Dental procedures, including home oral irrigation devices and both major and minor invasive surgical procedures, including placement of intravascular lines and catheters, genitourinary instrumentation, and select gastrointestinal surgery or procedures, are capable of creating a transient bacteremia leading to infective endocarditis. Recognition of these sources of infection has led to the development of prophylactic antibiotic treatment guidelines for individual invasive procedures. The reader is referred to recent guidelines provided by the report of the Joint Task Force of the American College of Cardiology and the American Heart Association.[45–47]

Intravenous Drug Abuse (IVDA)

The subpopulation of patients using illicit intravenous (IV) drugs who subsequently contract infective endocarditis tends to be younger, with a mean age of 30 years, and are more likely to be chronic abusers and of male gender (3:1 male-to-female ratio).[48,49] In contrast to nonaddicts with infective endocarditis, patients with IVDA and infective endocarditis more commonly have right-sided cardiac disease, with overwhelming evidence that the tricuspid valve is the most frequently infected location, accounting for 40 to 60 percent of cases. Despite being the most common valve infected, tricuspid valve involvement in infective endocarditis may be underreported due to the frequent lack of a murmur and misdiagnosis with a pulmonary disease. Infective endocarditis with right-sided valvular involvement may present with fever, chest pain, cough, dyspnea, or even hemoptysis. Pulmonary symptoms predominate secondary to complications from septic emboli to the pulmonary vasculature. Since there is no direct arterial access to the brain or to the rest of the body, neurologic complications are rare in isolated right-sided infective endocarditis in IV drug abusers.[50,51] In patients with IVDA and left-sided infective endocarditis, there is a high frequency of neurologic complications ranging from 45 to 58 percent, which is higher than the nonaddict population with left-sided infective endocarditis.[9] Recent reports suggest that infective endocarditis involvement of left-sided valves is increasing.[51] This higher incidence of neurologic complications with left-sided infective endocarditis in the IVDA population may be due in part to a higher rate of failure to complete a course of antibiotics.[52] In addition, *S. aureus* is commonly the cause of infective endocarditis in IV drug abusers and is associated with a high incidence of neurologic complications.

Noncardiac Underlying Disease

Infective endocarditis can be associated with an immunosuppressed state, such as occurs with malignancy, diabetes, chronic alcoholism, and systemic infections, including human immunodeficiency virus (HIV). HIV infection associated with severe immunosuppression and left-side valvular infective endocarditis has a high risk for mortality.[53] Many of these same systemic illnesses are also associated with hypercoagulable states, further increasing the risk of thromboembolic complications, including brain embolic events. Poor dental hygiene, serious burns, and chronic hemodialysis are other important risk factors for infective endocarditis.[54,55] Patients on chronic immunosuppressive drugs for a variety of autoimmune diseases, such as systemic lupus erythematosus, rheumatoid arthritis, and myasthenia gravis, also may be at increased risk for developing infective endocarditis, particularly in the presence of a cardiac murmur or known cardiac defect.

Pathogenesis of Neurologic Complications

Overview

Neurologic complications of infective endocarditis most commonly involve the central nervous system (CNS), with the majority of pathology occurring from seeding of septic or nonseptic emboli within the cerebral vessels, the brain parenchyma, and/or within the meningeal lining (Fig. 26-1). For example, the acute onset of a focal neurologic deficit such as hemiplegia or aphasia may be due to embolic stroke, whereas global confusion with nuchal rigidity is typical of meningoencephalitis.

Cerebral emboli are by far the most frequent neurologic complication and are discussed in detail below. Some authors suggest that this complication is being identified more frequently than in previous years due to better diagnosis and increased survival. It is important to be aware that nearly half the patients with CNS emboli also may have peripheral emboli, thus requiring increased vigilance for renal dysfunction, limb ischemia, retinal ischemia, or other manifestations. Cerebral embolus is followed in decreasing frequency by meningitis, encephalopathy, headache, intracranial hemorrhage, seizure, abscess, and mycotic aneurysm. Rarely, neurologic complications can occur in the spinal cord and bony spinal canal in the form of spinal artery em-

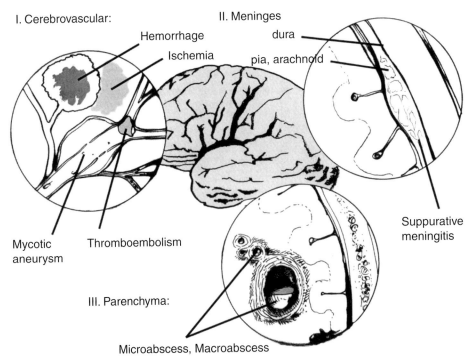

Figure 26–1. The pathogenesis of neurologic complications during infective endocarditis involves the cerebral blood vessels (mycotic aneurysm, arteritis, septic embolic occlusion), the meninges (meningitis), and the brain tissue (abscess, encephalitis). Thromboembolism and the formation of mycotic aneurysms can lead to ischemia or infarction and intracranial hemorrhage, respectively. Inflammation and infection of the meningitis and the brain tissue can lead to meningoencephalitis, microabscess, and rarely, macroabscess.

boli, space-occupying abscesses, or diskitis. In addition, there are case reports of various movement disorders, including dyskinesias, tremor, and myoclonus, implicating basal ganglia pathology. Psychiatric disorders, including psychosis, also have been reported infrequently.[56,57] Neurologic complications can occur in up to 30 percent of patients, usually within the first 2 weeks; therefore, monitoring for neurologic complications should be maximized during this time frame.

Role of Etiological Organism

Staphylococcal endocarditis is a more malignant disease than streptococcal endocarditis, with a case-fatality rate nearly seven times higher (40 verses 6 percent).[58] Over the last two decades, the incidence of antimicrobial-resistant staphylococcal endocarditis has been increasing. These staphylococci are virulent pathogens associated with significant morbidity and mortality, demanding rapid diagnosis and treatment. The clinical course tends to be acute, with rapid valvular damage and a frequently delayed antibiotic response. The risk of neurologic complications is increased significantly in endocarditis due to staphylococci.[28,29] For example, in one study limited to native-valve endocarditis, a neurologic presentation occurred in 54 percent of cases of *S. aureus* infective endocarditis compared with 19 percent of viridians streptococcal and enterococcal infective endocarditis.[59] In a larger retrospective review of patients with staphylococcal infective endocarditis, 35 percent of patients had neurologic complications. Patients with major neurologic manifestations had an extremely high mortality rate of 74 percent in comparison with a rate of 56 percent in patients without neurologic manifestations.[29] In this same series, most of the neurologic manifestations occurred on or shortly after presentation, with a low risk of recurrent embolism.[29] Other virulent organisms, including gram-negative bacilli, have been associated with cerebral emboli occurring within 2 weeks of the onset of the endocarditis.[15] It has been observed in autopsy cases that the more virulent organisms lead to extensive endocardial tissue damage without healing and thus form larger, friable, and potentially more mobile vegetations.

The group of fastidious gram-negative bacilli commonly referred to by the acronym HACEK is responsible for approximately 3 percent of all cases of infective endocarditis. Many of these organisms live in the oropharynx. In general, patients with a HACEK infection and infective endocarditis rarely have underlying heart disease.[60] This group of organisms includes *Hemophilus parainfluenzae, H. influenzae, H. aphrophilus, H. paraphrophilus, Actinobacillus actinomycetemcomitans, Cardiobacterium hominis, Eikenella corrodens,* and *Kingella* spp. HACEK group bacteria grow slowly and therefore should be considered in the differential diagnosis of culture-negative endocarditis. *Hemophilus*

spp. have been associated with larger vegetations and a high incidence of cerebral emboli.[61]

Enterobacteriaceae and anaerobic bacterial endocarditis has a high rate of neurologic complications.[62] The mortality rate for patients with anaerobic bacteria–related endocarditis is 21 to 43 percent and higher in untreated cases.[63] Most cases of anaerobic endocarditis are caused by anaerobic cocci, *Propionibacterium acnes,* and *B. fragilis.* A high incidence of embolic events is also seen in fungal endocarditis, especially endocarditis due to *Aspergillus* and *Candida* spp. Fungal emboli have a propensity to lodge in larger, more proximal arteries, such as the carotid or basilar artery. A fungal endocarditis should be considered in a patient taking steroids or with a known immunosuppressed state who develops fever and has negative cultures.

▶ CLINICAL PRESENTATION/COURSE

The more common "classic" symptoms or signs of infective endocarditis on presentation are, in decreasing frequency, fever, malaise, anorexia, weight loss, night sweats, and myalgia.[27] These classic symptoms are being replaced by more insidious and protean symptoms, many of which are neurologic in origin and lead to delay in diagnosis.[64] In a large patient series, the mean duration of prodrome, defined as the time interval between the first symptoms and confirmation of the diagnosis, was nearly 60 days.[15] In a large series (234 patients) of patients with bacterial endocarditis conducted in Finland from 1980 to 1996, 25 percent of patients presented with neurologic symptoms.[28] Of the patients with neurologic complications, in 76 percent a neurologic manifestation was present before antibiotic therapy and in 47 percent was the first sign of infective endocarditis.[28] In an earlier large series (218 patients) of patients with bacterial endocarditis at the Massachusetts General Hospital from 1964 to 1973, a total of 17 percent of patients had neurologic complaints as the first evidence of the underlying infective endocarditis[14] (Fig. 26-2). Figure 26-2 summarizes and compares the findings of these two studies conducted a decade apart. Morbidity is high in patients with infective endocarditis and neurologic complications; of patients surviving a neurologic complication, one-third will have permanent sequelae. The mortality rate is doubled for infective endocarditis patients with neurologic complications compared with those without neurologic complications (25 versus 12 percent, respectively).[28] Therefore, expedient evaluation of a neurologic sign or symptom in a patient suspected of having infective endocarditis can be lifesaving. A suggested patient management algorithm is illustrated in Fig. 26-3. A discussion of the clinical features of the most common neurologic complications associated with infective endocarditis follows.

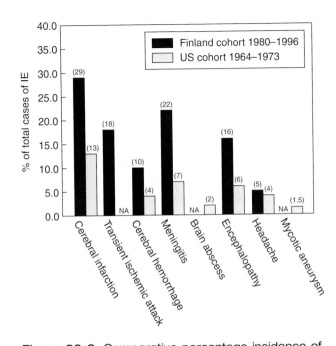

Figure 26–2. Comparative percentage incidence of the major neurologic complications in two studies conducted during different decades in patients with infective endocarditis (refs. 9 and 28).

Cerebral Embolism and Ischemic Stroke/Cerebral Infarction

Incidence/Risk Factors

Cerebral embolism is the most common neurologic complication of infective endocarditis, accounting for 30 to 50 percent of all neurologic complications of infective endocarditis. Frank cerebral infarction occurs in 10 to 42 percent of patients with infective endocarditis.[6,15,65] Ischemic strokes occur more frequently than hemorrhagic strokes; in one series, only 25 percent of the total strokes complicating infective endocarditis were hemorrhagic, which included intracranial hemorrhage, hemorrhagic infarctions, and subarachnoid hemorrhage.[65] More rarely, patients with infective endocarditis have strokes due to concurrent cardiac heart failure resulting in global cerebral ischemia. The presence of a prosthetic versus a native valve does not seem to influence the risk of stroke. For example, in one series, 5 percent of the infective endocarditis patient study population with cerebral embolism had a prosthetic valve in contrast to 10 percent who had a native valve.[65] The vast majority of embolic strokes occur in the territory supplied by the anterior cerebral circulation; multiple infarctions within a territory are common.[65] Table 26–3 reviews the common characteristics of infective endocarditis–related strokes. In a retrospective study conducted from 1978 to 1986, 62 percent of ischemic events involved the cortex or cerebellar hemisphere, whereas 16 percent were exclusively subcortical.[13] The remaining 22 percent of ischemic events involved the retina

or were of uncertain location. These same investigators noted that most infarcts were small (58 percent) or of moderate size (33 percent). Notably, however, current brain imaging techniques have higher sensitivity than those used in the 1970s and 1980s; thus the incidence of ischemic events may be underestimated. Although brain stem syndromes are considered rare, nearly 10 percent of major cerebral embolic infarctions in a small patient series were of this type.[13] In this same series, there were three cases of cerebral infarction due to hypotension (in the "watershed" areas).

Ischemic stroke can be an isolated presenting feature prior to the diagnosis of infective endocarditis in as many as 14 percent of cases of infective endocarditis. In one large prospective series of infective endocarditis, patients with CNS embolization tended to be older (>60 years), and the mitral valve was the most common suspected source of embolization.[7] During uncontrolled infection, there is a propensity for clustering of embolic phenomena at presentation, making immediate therapy imperative. The high initial rate of stroke can be reduced from 14 to 2 to 5 percent following 48 hours of appropriate antibiotic therapy.[13] The risk of recurrent stroke decreases significantly after starting antibiotics; however, neurologic complications can occur after initiation of antibiotic treatment, with a median onset of 4 days following antibiotic therapy.[15] It has been suggested that when embolic events occur or recur during later hospitalization, inadequate antibiotic therapy should be considered.[18]

As discussed previously, cerebral embolism occurring within 2 weeks of the onset of the endocarditis tends to be associated with the more virulent organisms, including *S. aureus* and gram-negative bacilli. In a retrospective review by Hart and colleagues,[13] moderate to large infarctions were five times more frequent with *S. aureus* endocarditis than with nonvirulent *Streptococcus* spp. endocarditis. Emboli in *S. aureus* endocarditis tended to occur early, to be multiple, and to carry a poorer prognosis.

Some studies suggest that aortic valve endocarditis is associated with a higher risk of stroke compared with mitral valve endocarditis,[28,31] wheeras other studies conclude the opposite.[65] One study comparing stroke incidence in mitral versus aortic valve endocarditis reported a higher association with mitral valve endocarditis, but there were no differences in stroke severity or subtype, vascular territory, length of hospitalization, or survival rate.[65] This higher association of stroke with mitral valve infective endocarditis may be due to larger vegetation formation (analyzed by either transthoracic or transesophageal echocardiography).[30] Recent data also suggest that up to 14 percent of patients with infective endocarditis have elevated antiphospholipid antibodies.[66,67] When antiphospholipid antibodies and soluble adhesion molecules are present

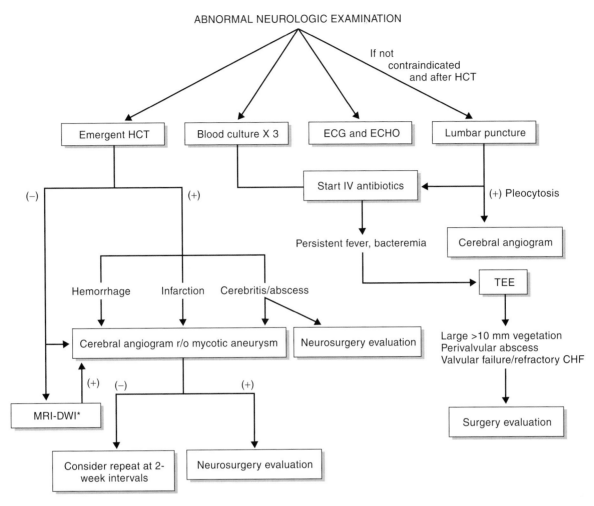

Figure 26–3. Suggested management for the treatment of patients with infective endocarditis and a neurologic symptom or deficit. HCT = head computed tomography; IV = intravenous, SAH = subarachnoid hemorrhage; TEE = transesophageal echocardiogram; r/o = rule out; MRI-DWI = magnetic resonance imaging with diffusion-weighted images. *If available. See text for details concerning TEE considerations and abnormal findings prompting further surgical evaluation.

in patients with infective endocarditis, they are 2.5 times more prone to embolization.[66]

Clinical Presentation

Most patients with non-IVDA infective endocarditis presenting with cerebral infarction have vegetative emboli originating from the left side of the heart. The majority of infarctions or transient ischemic attacks (TIAs) are in the middle cerebral artery (MCA) distribution and less often in the anterior cerebral artery (ACA) distribution. Rarely, posterior cerebral artery (PCA) occlusions occur. The typical dominant or nondominant hemispheric stroke syndrome from an MCA occlusion consists of contralateral hemiparesis or hemiplegia associated with hemisensory deficits and language dysfunction (dominant side). Occlusion of the ACA results in lower limb weakness and frontal lobe dysfunction. PCA occlusion results in occipital lobe dysfunction, including visual deficits such as, for example, homonymous hemianop-

sia. The more common anterior circulation cerebral infarction syndromes are summarized in Table 26-4. The onset of a TIA in a febrile patient with a murmur should alert the physician to neurologic complications of infective endocarditis. TIA, in addition to being the result of septic emboli with increased risk of infarction, can portend a fatal mycotic aneurysm rupture or intracranial hemorrhage.

Multiple cerebral microemboli can lead to significant neurologic sequelae as well. In one series of 45 patients with infective endocarditis undergoing postmortem examination, approximately 50 percent of patients had evidence of multiple microinfarctions (presumably from small-vessel emboli). Microscopic infarctions have been associated with neurologic complications, including encephalopathy (with a spectrum from confusion and decreased alertness to frank coma), focal or generalized seizures, personality changes, delirium, and psychosis. The elderly may be more prone to

▶ **TABLE 26-3.** COMMON STROKE CHARACTERISTICS IN INFECTIVE ENDOCARDITIS

Stroke Type	Description % of Total	Clinical Comments
Ischemic	74	More common in mitral versus aortic valve infective endocarditis
Hemorrhagic	26	More common in mitral versus aortic valve infective endocarditis
Intracranial	3	
Hemorrhagic infarction	15	
Subarachnoid	2	
Combination	6	
Perioperative	8	Stroke occurred on the day of or within 30 days of undergoing valve replacement for IC
Ischemic stroke by vascular territory		
Anterior	92	The majority of anterior ischemic strokes were partial territory (70%), while the remaining (30%) involved the entire anterior territory
Posterior	9	No lacunar-type infarctions were identified
Single	47	
Multiple	53	
Outcome (all strokes)	52	
Mortality		Mortality rate did not differ in patients with mitral valve IE compared to those with aortic valve IE
acutely	35	
by 12-month follow-up	17	

SOURCE: *Data based on ref. 65.*

▶ **TABLE 26-4.** ANTERIOR CIRCULATION CEREBRAL INFARCTION SYNDROMES.

Occluded Cerebral Artery	Neurologic Deficits	Clinical Comments
MCA Proximal	Contralateral: Weakness/sensory loss Visual field deficit Head/eye deviation Global aphasia (dominant side)	Observe closely for signs of increased cerebral edema with neurologic deterioration Risk of hemorrhagic conversion
Superior	Contralateral: Weakness > sensory loss Visual field deficit Motor language deficit*	Oral motor dysfunction leads to increase risk aspiration
Inferior	Contralateral: Sensory loss Visual field deficit Apraxia (neglect) Comprehension deficit*	If nondominant side, neglect can significantly impede rehabilitation
ACA	Contralateral: Leg weakness ± apraxia Mild leg sensory loss Apathy, abulia, incontinence	Behavioral changes can result in significant morbidity requiring education of the family of its organic nature

*Dominant-side lesion.

neuropsychiatric complications. These symptoms can occur in isolation of other more typical symptoms of infective endocarditis, making misdiagnosis common in the elderly population.

Diagnosis

At minimum, a computed tomographic (CT) scan of the brain (with and without contrast material) is required for the initial evaluation of any patient with fever and evidence of a fixed or transient focal or multifocal neurologic deficit. Life-threatening neurologic complications, including cerebral abscess and hemorrhage, need to be identified emergently and potentially treated. Cra-

nial CT scan remains the best choice as an initial imaging study because of its high sensitivity for detecting acute hemorrhagic pathology. In the setting of known infective endocarditis and cerebral infarction, the cranial CT scan may reveal signs of subacute cortical, subcortical, unifocal, or multifocal cerebral infarction (Fig. 26-4). Intracranial hemorrhage may be from hemorrhagic transformation of an ischemic infarction or from a primary parenchymal hemorrhage from a ruptured mycotic aneurysm (Fig. 26-5). Hemorrhagic conversion following cerebral infarction can be seen in 6.2 percent of patients from 1 to 4 days, 27.5 percent by 10 days, and 40.6 percent by 1 month.[68] Clinically, the occur-

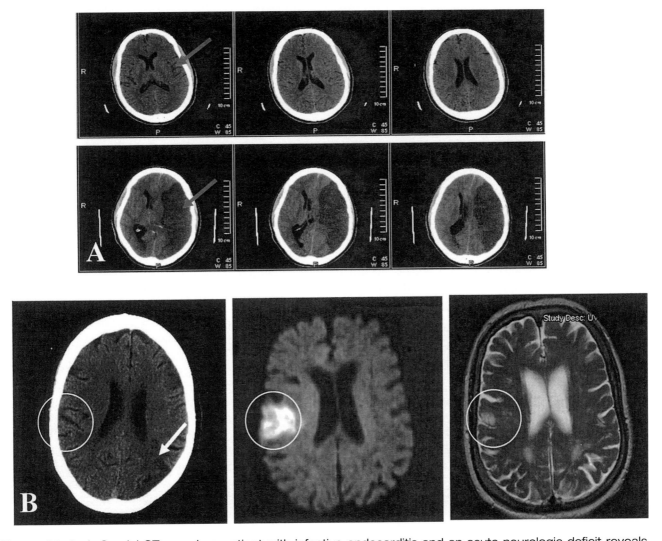

Figure 26–4. *A.* Cranial CT scan in a patient with infective endocarditis and an acute neurologic deficit reveals (less than approximately 6 hours) no lesions as seen in top panel in multiple cuts through the brain. However, over time a hypodensity is clearly demonstrated (*bottom panel*) in the same patient 48 hours later. There is a large hypodensity involving the left hemisphere of the brain consistent with infarction (*bottom panel*). *B.* An initial cranial CT scan in a patient with infective endocarditis and left-sided sensory complaints reveals a left-sided hypodensity (*arrow*) but no abnormality in the right hemisphere (*circled area*). A follow-up MRI with DWI sequences, however, reveals a high signal abnormality along the right temporopariental lobe consistent with an acute brain infarction (*circled area*).

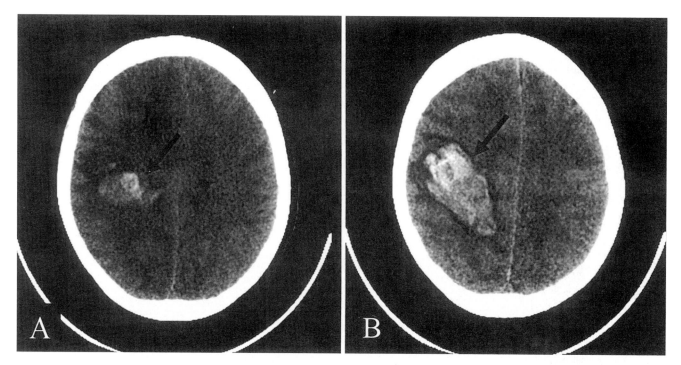

Figure 26–5. Cranial CT scan in a patient with known infective endocarditis who presented with acute left-sided hemisensory and motor signs reveals a large, homogeneous hyperintensity consistent with an intracranial hemorrhage or hematoma.

rence of a secondary hemorrhagic transformation may be suspected when the neurologic deficit is large or the patient has a sudden neurologic deterioration.

Many patients with infective endocarditis and a neurologic deficit require additional studies, including magnetic resonance imaging (MRI) with diffusion-weighted imaging (DWI), that allow for rapid determination of an acute stroke in the setting of infective endocarditis, which can prompt close neurologic monitoring and expeditious workup (Fig. 26-6). Cranial MRI has a higher sensitivity than a cranial CT scan for detecting small infarctions, especially in the posterior fossa (cerebellum and brain stem), making it a superior choice in patients with evidence of posterior circulation deficits (following an initial cranial CT scan to identify any potential hemorrhage). In addition, certain MRI sequences with contrast media may help to distinguish abscess from infarction. MRI therefore can be helpful in diagnosing the patient with infective endocarditis, especially when the initial cranial CT scan findings are "normal" and the patient has neurologic deterioration.

Therapy

Prompt organism-specific antimicrobial therapy remains the most important intervention for prevention of further embolic phenomena once cerebral infarction or ischemia has occurred during the course of infective endocarditis. In a 12-year retrospective follow-up study of neurologic complications following infective endo-

carditis, Salgado and colleagues[15] found that recurrent ischemic episodes were uncommon after initiation of antibiotic therapy (22 percent of all patients who developed neurologic complications). In this series of 175 patients, recurrent neurologic events occurred acutely in only 2 patients; both patients had mechanical valves and had their episode prior to antibiotic therapy.[15] The incidence of emboli is highest within the first 48 hours, especially during the acute, uncontrolled infectious state. Following this period, the risk of recurrent emboli falls significantly during adequate treatment.

In uncomplicated cases of infective endocarditis, valve replacement is rarely indicated, especially following a single initial cerebral embolic event. Exceptions are the presence of fungal endocarditis, cardiac hemodynamic failure due to valve incompetence, resistance to antibiotic therapy, and significant recurrent emboli. Under these life-threatening conditions, decisions surrounding surgical intervention and its timing in patients with infective endocarditis and stroke are complicated. The replacement of failing valves early in the course of complicated infective endocarditis is associated with improved survival, yet there is significant surgical risk associated with cardiopulmonary bypass. Despite the increased risk, some data suggest that surgical patients under these grave conditions can fare as well as medically treated patients with no significant differences in mortality between the groups.[69,70] A cranial CT scan prior to surgery should be obtained to en-

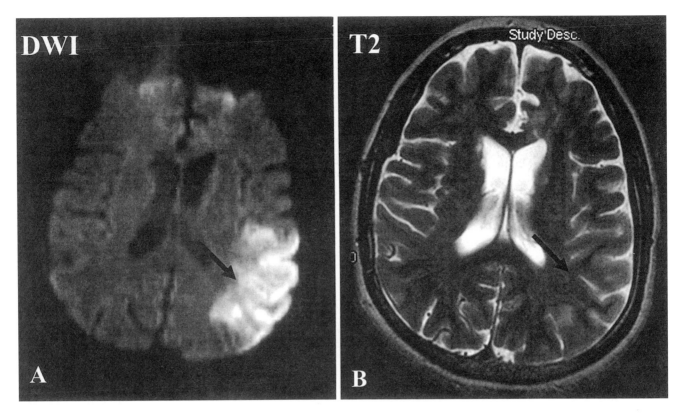

Figure 26–6. A cranial MRI of a young patient with a history of intravenous drug abuse who presented with fever, murmur, and acute difficulty with speech. The DWI sequence demonstrates a high signal abnormality in the territory of the left MCA (inferior division). The corresponding T_2 sequence demonstrates mild edematous changes in the same region.

sure that no poststroke hemorrhage is present, which would significantly increase the risk of a CNS bleed during surgery and would be a contraindication to surgery.[71]

ANTICOAGULATION IN NATIVE-VALVE ENDOCARDITIS

In the patient with native-valve endocarditis who survives the first episode of cerebral embolism, the recurrence rate is low following initiation of antibiotic therapy. The use of anticoagulation in this setting is difficult to justify. In general, it is felt that anticoagulation in native-valve endocarditis is hazardous, with the increased risk of intracerebral hemorrhage far outweighing any potential benefit.[72]

ANTICOAGULATION IN PROSTHETIC-VALVE ENDO-CARDITIS

The overall rate of cerebral infarction in prosthetic-valve endocarditis is approximately 25 percent. The use of anticoagulation in prosthetic-valve endocarditis is controversial, particularly once a stroke has occurred. The current trend is to anticoagulate the patient with a newly infected prosthetic valve mainly based on aggregate evidence suggesting that anticoagulation decreases the incidence of stroke in general. Some experts suggest the use of heparin sodium as soon as the diagnosis of prosthetic-valve endocarditis is sus-

pected and continuing during the course of antibiotic therapy.[73] In a recent study of 52 patients with stroke and infective endocarditis, the authors found that the use of anticoagulant drugs was not statistically significantly associated with an increase in mortality in the acute phase of infective endocarditis versus those taking aspirin.[65] If a large cerebral infarction is detected on cranial CT scan, it is recommended that heparin be discontinued and restarted at or later than 48 to 72 hours to decrease the risk of intracerebral hemorrhage formation.[73] In contrast, some investigators recommend discontinuing anticoagulation at the time of the embolic event, with reinstitution following resolution of the infection; one author reported that anticoagulation was an independent risk factor for mortality in patients with prosthetic-valve endocarditis caused by *S. aureus*.[40] The potential for serious complications, including cerebral hemorrhage and its associated mortality, has led other authors to question and/or disfavor the use of anticoagulation during prosthetic-valve endocarditis. Until data from adequate prospective, randomized clinical trials are reported, the true risk-benefit ratio of anticoagulation therapy both as a prophylaxis and as a therapy for recurrent cerebral ischemia is not known; therefore, a wide spectrum of use of anticoagulation in this patient subpopulation will be tolerated. Despite the controversial role of anticoagulation in the stroke patient with infective endocarditis, most physicians agree that anticoagulation should be discontinued in the event of known intracerebral hemorrhage or of a large stroke. There is also agreement that if anticoagulation is deemed beneficial, careful and frequent monitoring of the International Normalized Ratio (INR) is mandatory.

Aspirin and other antiplatelet drugs are being evaluated currently for prevention of embolic stroke during infective endocarditis. In a recent randomized, placebo-controlled study, the incidence of embolic events was compared in antibiotic-treated infective endocarditis patients randomized to either daily aspirin (325 mg) or no aspirin with a 4-year follow-up period.[74] Aspirin at this dosage did not appear to reduce the risk of embolic events and likely was associated with an increased risk of bleeding.[74]

Prognosis

A recent large study of patients with infective endocarditis and stroke determined a high overall 1-year case-fatality rate of 53 percent.[65] In patients surviving the acute cerebral event and in those with controlled infection, the risk of recurrent stroke is low.[14] Risk of embolization seems to increase with increasing vegetation size,[30] especially with mitral valve endocarditis and staphylococcal endocarditis. Therefore, patients with these conditions even during antimicrobial treatment should be monitored carefully for recurrent cerebral or systemic embolism.[71]

Encephalopathy

Incidence/Risk Factors

Encephalopathy is the second most frequent neurologic complication during infective endocarditis.[28] The term *encephalopathy* is nonspecific; therefore, a wide spectrum of CNS dysfunction is included within this diagnosis. Mild encephalopathy may be manifest by confusion and disorientation, whereas more severe encephalopathy may present as stupor or coma. Exacerbating factors for encephalopathy include advanced age, iatrogenic causes (mainly from drug therapy), hypoxia, and metabolic abnormalities such as metabolic acidosis, renal dysfunction, or electrolyte abnormalities, including hyponatremia. Hyponatremia, if present, can be a manifestation of the syndrome of inappropriate antidiuretic hormone secretion (SIADH), a condition seen commonly with serious CNS disorders. Acute renal dysfunction in the form of focal glomerular nephritis can occur from multiple septic renal infarctions.

Pathogenesis

The etiology of encephalopathy in most cases is multifactorial. Encephalopathy is attributed to microemboli, resulting in cerebral microinfarctions with petechial hemorrhage and microabscesses. These pathologic features are not seen typically on routine cranial CT scans but can be demonstrated by cranial MRI.[75,76] A total of 4 percent of the infective endocarditis patients in the Massachusetts General Hospital patient series had abscesses of less than 1 cm^3 (microscopic) in size in the absence of focal neurologic findings.[15] Patients with microabscesses frequently had a fulminant course of infective endocarditis and were infected with *S. aureus, Enterococcus,* or *Serratia marcescans.* In one series, in 40 percent of infective endocarditis patients presenting with "encephalopathy," MRI-DWI sequences demonstrated significant abnormalities.[75] DWI is useful for detecting the presence of cerebral infarctions in the patient with a nonfocal encephalopathic presentation. As discussed earlier, secondary exacerbating metabolic and drug-associated causes of encephalopathy also can occur, particularly in fulminant cases of infective endocarditis.

Diagnosis

Some series define a type of encephalopathy known as *acute* or *toxic encephalopathy* in which psychiatric manifestations predominate, including personality change, hallucinations, and paranoid ideations. Disorientation and confusion are prominent.[17,77] Similarly, cases of meningoencephalitis also have been described as "toxic encephalopathy" or as an "acute confusional syndrome." It is important to have an accurate diagnostic assessment of the extent of disease to better tailor treatment and define prognosis. Encephalopathy due to infective endocarditis occurs mainly in older adults and may be the predominant or presenting feature of endocarditis in 27 percent of elderly patients, often leading to misdiagnosis and delayed therapy.[77] In addition, the diagnosis of infective endocarditis can be difficult in elderly patients because many present with nonspecific complaints associated with confusion but in the absence of fever or leukocytosis. In addition, blood cultures may be negative.[28]

Therapy

Nearly any type of infectious encephalopathy will be improved with aggressive antibiotic treatment of the primary infection. Diligent correction of metabolic abnormalities and careful administration of sedating medications is recommended. In general, sedation should be minimized in order to assess changes in the neurologic examination adequately, which could signify worsening disease. Carefully monitoring for frequent metabolic complications of systemic infection, including changes in serum electrolytes and liver and renal function, can prevent the development of additional causes for encephalopathy.

Prognosis

Prognosis depends on early diagnosis and initiation of antimicrobial therapy. Treatment of reversible causes of encephalopathy such as hyponatremia, azotemia, and drug reactions can result in significant neurologic improvement. In one series, nearly 30 percent of patients with infective endocarditis presenting with encephalopathy died.[28] Elderly patients presenting with mental changes may have a poorer prognosis due to errors in diagnosis or to delay in initiating appropriate therapy, both contributing to morbidity and death. In one series of elderly patients with infective endocarditis, an initial error in diagnosis was made in 11 of 16 patients who ultimately died.[77]

Cerebral Hemorrhage

Incidence/Risk Factors

In this section, *cerebral hemorrhage* refers to intracerebral hematoma, subarachnoid hemorrhage, or hemorrhagic infarction. Evaluation of results from studies of cerebral hemorrhage in infective endocarditis is confounded by a lack of definition of the type of hemorrhage or the presence of more than one type of hemorrhage occurring simultaneously. In general, the incidence of intracranial hemorrhage (ICH) is in the range of 3 to 8 percent of patients with infective endocarditis.[8,78] There is increased risk of developing infective endocarditis–related ICH if the patient has a known cerebral infarction, a mycotic aneurysm, or a bleeding diathesis (such as secondary to chronic anticoagulation use). Although not always recognized clinically, antecedent embolism is most likely a prerequisite for ICH. Clinically recognized ipsilateral embolism precedes ICH in approximately 30 to 40 percent of patients.[78,79] Preceding severe headache also can occur and should prompt immediate evaluation of the cerebrovasculature. Hemorrhagic transformation of a cerebral infarction occurs in 6 to 24 percent of infarctions associated with native-valve endocarditis and in 8 to 36 percent of those with prosthetic-valve endocarditis.[80] Rarely, infective endocarditis presents with subarachnoid hemorrhage (1 percent or less), usually from rupture of a mycotic aneurysm. Identification of the aneurysm may be difficult even with routine cerebral arteriography, suggesting that the true incidence of ICH from this cause could be higher than reported.

The role of anticoagulation as a risk factor for ICH is well recognized and has presented a serious therapeutic dilemma in the patient with infective endocarditis and a prosthetic valve. In a large study of patients with infective endocarditis, it was noted that 23 percent of the hemorrhagic events occurred in the 3 percent of the patients who were on anticoagulation therapy.[15] In another series of patients who developed ICH in the setting of infective endocarditis, anticoagulation potentially contributed to intracranial hemorrhage in 24 percent of patients.[78]

Symptomatic ICH also can occur due to hemorrhagic conversion of an infarction associated with the use of anticoagulant or thrombolytic therapies. Rarely, the undiagnosed infective endocarditis patient presents to the emergency room with signs of acute myocardial infarction for which standard thrombolytic therapy can result in ICH.[79]

The abrupt onset of severe neurologic deficit and ICH is commonly associated with infective endocarditis due to *S. aureus*. These hemorrhages occur early in the clinical course (within 48 hours of admission) and during uncontrolled infection. There is evidence that patients on anticoagulant therapy, especially with prosthetic valve infective endocarditis due to *S. aureus*, have a significant risk of death from ICH within the first 72 hours of presentation.[40]

Potentially reversible medical conditions predisposing to a bleeding diathesis include disseminated intravascular coagulation, thrombocytopenia, and vitamin K deficiency states. These conditions need to be treated expeditiously.

Clinical Presentation

There is a wide spectrum of neurologic presentations with ICH in the setting of infective endocarditis. The patient may present with mild confusion or encephalopathy, coma, meningismus, headache, generalized seizure, or focal signs and symptoms such as hemiparesis or aphasia. Frequently, there is a combination of both focal and generalized neurologic deficits. As mentioned earlier, the occurrence of a TIA may precede intracerebral hemorrhage and can be a critical harbinger for worsening neurologic status. In one small patient series, 25 percent of infective endocarditis patients with TIA subsequently had a fatal intracerebral hemorrhage.[79] ICH in the setting of infective endocarditis can occur from a leaking or ruptured mycotic aneurysm. In one small series of patients with known intracranial mycotic aneurysms, there was an average of 10 days between the onset of warning signs or symptoms and subsequent hemorrhage.[80] If the signs and symptoms of impending ICH are not recognized early on, rapid neurologic deterioration, including death, can occur.

As with nonseptic emboli, hemorrhagic transformation of septic embolic infarction also can occur but tends to be asymptomatic and occurs more often with a large cerebral infarction.

Pathogenesis

Bleeding can occur in the subarachnoid space, in the brain parenchyma, or within the ventricular system. Two distinct mechanisms result in intracranial hemorrhage in the patient with infective endocarditis: (1) hemorrhagic transformation of a bland infarction and (2) primary intracerebral hematoma formation; importantly, the two forms of hemorrhage can coexist. The formation of an intracerebral hematoma during infective endocarditis can be the result of (1) acute cerebral vessel rupture,

(2) iatrogenic-related anticoagulation or thrombolytic administration, or (3) an acquired infection-related coagulation disorder, including disseminated intravascular coagulation (DIC) or thrombocytopenia.

In one small study analyzing ICH complications in patients with infective endocarditis, 24 percent were from hemorrhagic infarctions, 24 percent from necrotic arteritis, 12 percent from ruptured mycotic aneurysms, and the remaining 29 percent from unknown causes.[78] There is general agreement that most ICH is due to septic, necrotic arteritis (without aneurysm formation) from uncontrolled infection rather than from mycotic aneurysm rupture, which is a rare complication of infective endocarditis. In a recent histopathologic analysis of 16 patients with infective endocarditis and ICH, 15 examined at autopsy, 13 of 16 of the patients had evidence of either septic emboli and/or pyogenic arteritis.[83]

In the assessment of ICH, there is normally a distinction between intraparenchymal hematoma and hemorrhagic transformation of an infarction, which represent two different etiologies. In the infective endocarditis patient with intracranial bleeding, this distinction may be difficult, especially if anticoagulant therapy is in use, because one pathology can lead quickly to the other. The hemorrhage associated with infective endocarditis is usually lobar and either can remain confined within the parenchyma or can extend deeper into the subcortical tissue and even into the subarachnoid or intraventricular space. Devastatingly large CNS bleeds can result in cerebrospinal fluid flow obstruction with life-threatening acute hydrocephalus.

Diagnosis

Cranial CT scanning remains the initial neuroimaging test of choice to diagnose intracranial bleeding due to its high sensitivity for identifying hyperacute blood and extension of blood into the subarachnoid space. Most infective endocarditis–related cases of ICH are diagnosed by the finding of a noncalcific hyperdensity on a non-contrast-enhanced cranial CT scan. CT scanning of a parenchymatous hematoma reveals a homogeneous, hyperdense, usually well-demarcated lesion, sometimes with prominent mass effect (see Fig. 26-5). This radiologic finding is in contrast to a hemorrhagic infarction, which appears on CT scan as a more heterogeneous, patchy hyperdense signal usually following the anatomy of the gyri (Fig. 26-7). Regardless of the type of hemorrhage demonstrated on cranial CT scan, the finding of ICH should prompt a careful evaluation for a mycotic aneurysm. A small area of focal cortical enhancement adjacent to the hyperdense clot on a contrast-enhanced CT scan is suspicious for a mycotic aneurysm. If the neuroimaging studies are nondiagnostic for the cause of the ICH, early cerebral angiography is indicated to rule out a mycotic aneurysm.

Once ICH has been identified in the patient with infective endocarditis, the "gold standard" for the initial

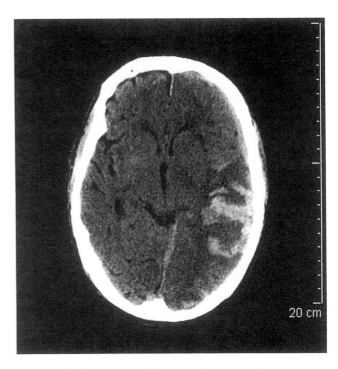

Figure 26–7. Cranial CT scan demonstrating a large left temporoparietal infarction with hemorrhagic conversion. Note the heterogeneity of the hyperintensity, which tends to follow the gyri formations of the brain (in contrast to a smooth, homogeneous hyperintenisty with mass effect as seen with an intracranial hematoma).

diagnostic workup is a four-vessel cerebral angiogram unless contraindicated (see "Cerebral Mycotic Aneurysm" below for details). For the patient who cannot tolerate conventional contrast cerebral angiography, MR-angiography (MRA) is an option. There is emerging experience using CT-angiography (CTA) imaging techniques for the assessment of aneurysm in general (Fig. 26-8). If available, it may be used as an alternative in the rare case of the patient who cannot tolerate a cerebral angiogram or an MRA. Notably, both MRA and CTA are significantly less sensitive than cerebral angiography for identifying mycotic aneurysms. If intracranial bleeding is suspected but neuroradiographic studies are negative, a lumbar puncture and cerebrospinal fluid analysis (if not contraindicated) may show evidence of subarachnoid hemorrhage, pleocytosis, or positive cultures.

Therapy

Patients with severe neurologic deficits or signs of impending neurologic deterioration should be transferred immediately to the intensive care setting, where constant hemodynamic and neurologic monitoring can be obtained. If infection is suspected, parental antibiotic therapy should be started immediately, particularly if the suspected organism is *S. aureus*. Any potential contributors to a bleeding diathesis such as antiplatelet ther-

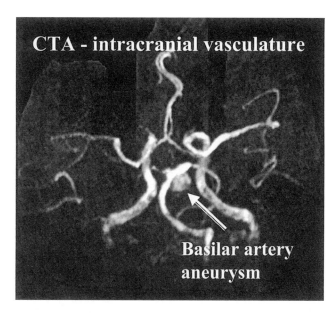

Figure 26–8. CT angiogram of a 74-year-old man with HIV infection presenting with encephalopathy, fever, dysarthria, and vertigo. A large basilar mycotic aneurysm was demonstrated. Blood cultures revealed a systemic fungal infection.

apy, vitamin deficiencies, thrombocytopenia, or DIC should be corrected or removed.

Craniotomy and evacuation of the hematoma in selected patients can be a lifesaving procedure, although no strict guidelines exist for the determination of when craniotomy is best performed for ICH. A few generally agreed on relative indications include (1) neurologic deterioration, in the case that there is potentially salvageable brain tissue if surgery is performed acutely, and (2) cerebellar hemorrhage, especially greater than 3 cm in size and if there is minimal deficit. Cerebellar hemorrhage in the setting of infective endocarditis is exceedingly rare, although there are case reports of mycotic aneurysms occurring in the vertebrobasilar system. Surgical treatment is advocated less frequently if there is a stable persistent neurologic deficit or initial coma.

Prognosis

Regardless of the mechanism of hemorrhage, the patient with symptomatic ICH in the setting of infective endocarditis has a high mortality in the range of 50 to 90 percent.[28,73,78] In patients surviving the initial hemorrhage, there is evidence that recurrent hemorrhage is infrequent both during and following antibiotic therapy.

Cerebral Mycotic Aneurysm

Incidence/Risk Factors

The reported incidence of mycotic aneurysm in infective endocarditis is 1 to 15 percent,[81–83] with approximately 20 percent being multiple. Mycotic aneurysm appears clinically in 2 percent of patients with diagnosed infective endocarditis and at autopsy in 5 to 10 percent.[5] The true incidence remains unknown due to obliteration on rupture and the fact that many patients remain asymptomatic (especially if treated with appropriate antibiotics) or die from rupture prior to hospital admission. With better treatment strategies, the overall incidence of mycotic aneurysm may be decreasing. In the early twentieth century, up to 30 percent of total intracranial aneurysms were infectious in origin compared with the current estimate of 2 to 6 percent.[82]

Clinical Presentation

The clinical presentation of mycotic aneurysm is protean. For example, an unruptured mycotic aneurysm can mimic an embolic stroke by presenting with a TIA or may be associated with a severe localized headache, suggesting subarachnoid hemorrhage (SAH). Unfortunately, the initial presentation may be the abrupt onset of a neurologic catastrophe (SAH or ICH) without a prior diagnosis of infective endocarditis.[84] In one large literature review of patients with infective endocarditis and the diagnosis of bacterial intracranial aneurysm, the clinical presentation included hemorrhage (52 percent), infarction (20 percent), unknown (20 percent), infarction with hemorrhage (6 percent), and headache only (2 percent).[85]

Pathogenesis

Cerebral mycotic aneurysms are formed when septic emboli migrate and lodge within the vasa vasorum or intraluminal space of the cerebral vasculature. Once stagnant, the septic emboli may produce an inflammatory destruction of the arterial wall, starting on the luminal side and working through the adventitial layer. An initial intraluminal septic clot may be the nidus for subsequent aneurysm formation, or alternatively, the embolus may become lodged within the vasa vasorum in the adventitial layer of the artery, leading to arterial dilatation. Mycotic aneurysms typically are located at bifurcation points within distal branches of the middle cerebral artery (MCA). This anatomic feature can help to distinguish mycotic aneurysms from congenital aneurysms because the latter occur commonly in the circle of Willis. Analysis of the location of the aneurysm in a total of 219 patients revealed involvement of the MCA in 39 percent, the ACA in 5 percent, the basilar artery in 5 percent, the intradural internal carotid artery (ICA) in 4 percent, and the PCA in 4 percent.[86] The most common pathogen is streptococci and less commonly staphylococci, enterococci, pneumococcus, and *Hemophilus* spp. Fungal aneurysms are rare but may be seen in immunocompromised patients and can occur in more proximal vessels.

Some investigators have suggested that IV drug abusers may be at increased risk for multiple mycotic aneurysm formation because of repeated episodes of bacteremia. Rarely, the mycotic aneurysm may be associated with an adjacent parenchymal abscess.

Diagnosis

There is general agreement that cerebral angiography is mandatory if new focal neurologic symptoms appear in the patient with infective endocarditis. Patients presenting with sterile meningitis and focal neurologic symptoms or with unilateral headache also should undergo cerebral angiography. Some authors suggest that cerebral angiography should be done expeditiously, with repeat angiography on completion of antibiotic therapy, because mycotic aneurysms can develop even during treatment and particularly if long-term anticoagulation is planned.[87] Cerebral angiographic findings in the patient with an unruptured aneurysm include irregularly shaped fusiform or saccular arterial wall dilatation or nonfilling or intraarterial filling defects with embolic clot (Fig. 26-9). Although MRA also can detect intracranial mycotic aneurysms, it is not the initial diagnostic test of choice because it is much less sensitive than cerebral angiography for detecting aneurysms, especially those less than 5 mm in size, and those located peripherally, as is often the case with mycotic aneurysms.

Therapy

The optimal therapeutic strategy for the unruptured aneurysm is uncertain. Bactericidal antibiotic therapy should be administered immediately on diagnosis for a standard 4- to 6-week course. In general, surgical intervention is favored when the aneurysm is symptomatic, resulting in bleeding, focal neurologic deficits, seizure, or severe headache. Chun and colleagues[88] presented a patient treatment algorithm based on review of 27 cases of mycotic aneurysms and suggested that endovascular therapy is the first option for patients in stable condition with ruptured aneurysms and that surgical therapy is the first option for patients in unstable condition with ruptured aneurysms. Surgery may not be an option if the aneurysm is not easily accessible. As an alternative to neurosurgery, investigative newer endovascular procedures have been reported for the treatment of mycotic aneurysm.[89-91] Endovascular interventions include either occlusion of the parent artery or preservation of the parent artery with more selective occlusion of the aneurysm with embolization materials, including coils or the inflation of balloons. More difficult management decisions arise in the patient with multiple lesions or with a lesion in a proximal eloquent location.

In the case of an unruptured mycotic aneurysm, many experts advocate initial antibiotic therapy for 4 to 6 weeks, with serial angiography as often as every 2 weeks, until the aneurysm disappears. If at any point the aneurysm appears to enlarge (which may occur despite initial shrinking in size) or fails to reduce after 4 to 6 weeks of antibiotic therapy, neurosurgical intervention may be needed. In a review of the literature of 81 patients with intracranial mycotic aneurysm treated medically, follow-up cerebral angiography revealed that the aneurysm disappeared in 30 percent, enlarged in 22 percent, decreased in 19 percent, remained unchanged in 15 percent, and increased in number in 15 percent.[85]

Prognosis

Rupture of a mycotic aneurysm is a catastrophic life-threatening event carrying a mortality rate of 30 to 90 percent depending on the organism. Fungal aneurysms carry the highest risk. One report suggests that the mortality rate of ruptured mycotic aneurysm can be lowered (25 percent) if surgery following angiography is performed early in the presence of deepening coma and an extensive lesion.[92] The risk of mortality in patients with unruptured mycotic aneurysm is less but still high at 30 percent.[93] Antibiotic therapy significantly lowers the risk of rupture; however, rupture has been reported as late as 6 months after a "cured" episode of infective endocarditis. Late rupture, as well as the potential for expansion, even during antimicrobial therapy, emphasizes the need for frequent follow-up cerebral angiography or MRA as indicated. In a small study of 14 patients with angiography-proven mycotic aneurysm, following 6 weeks of antibiotic treatment, 50 percent of patients had complete recovery, and the other half had permanent neurologic deficits.[94]

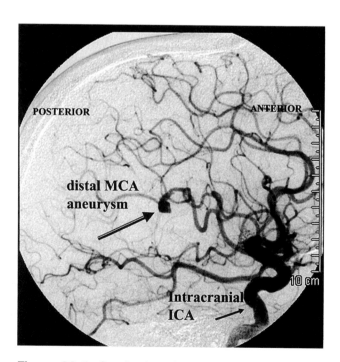

Figure 26–9. Cerebral angiogram (left sagittal view) of a 67-year-old woman with a diagnosis of infective endocarditis who presented with transient aphasia and right upper extremity weakness. The arterial angiographic films demonstrate a large mycotic aneurysm in the distal branch of the left middle cerebral artery (*arrow*).

Meningoencephalitis

Incidence/Risk Factors

The incidence of meningitis with infective endocarditis has been reported in large patient series as 1.4 to 3.5 percent,[1,59,83] with higher rates of 16 percent reported recently in a 17-year retrospective study in Finland.[28] The incidence may be higher in certain areas of the world where antibiotic use is not prevalent.[19] Virulent organisms such as *S. aureus*, enteric gram-negative bacilli, and *Streptococcus pneumoniae* are frequently associated with a purulent CSF, whereas viridans streptococci is associated with an aseptic or normal CSF.[14] In a large infective endocarditis patient series ($N = 218$), a total of 35 patients had a lumbar puncture (LP) on presentation of nuchal rigidity and/or disorientation; 46 percent had purulent CSF, 23 percent had aseptic CSF, and 6 percent had hemorrhagic CSF. Normal CSF was found in 26 percent of patients.[14] The clinical triad of *S. pneumoniae* pneumonia, meningitis, and endocarditis merits special attention. Also known as *Austrian's syndrome,* this is an especially serious disease associated with a high risk of morbidity and mortality.[95]

Pathogenesis

Multiple septic emboli can lodge in meningeal vessels, with direct vessel and CSF invasion creating significant inflammation of the meninges and brain tissue. This microbial seeding may lead to parameningeal lesions, including abscess. Infrequently, cerebral inflammation can be due to a secondary aseptic process, such as vasculitis or hemorrhage from a leaking mycotic aneurysm.

Diagnosis

The clinical presentation of meningoencephalitis can range from initial subtle confusion or personality changes to life-threatening coma. In the elderly population, milder symptoms of disorientation can be attributed inadvertently to fever alone, to an iatrogenic drug effect, or to a minor infection rather than to the initial stages of meningitis. Another confounding factor is that the elderly may develop meningitis without prominent meningeal signs.

A change in mental status and nuchal rigidity, fever, and headache are the more classic symptoms of meningoencephalitis. Headache, disorientation, and fever may progress slowly and insidiously or, in the case of virulent organisms, quickly to stupor, coma, and even death. Meningeal symptoms or signs have been noted in approximately 20 to 40 percent of patients with neurologic complications during infective endocarditis.[28] A heightened awareness of the possibility of meningoencephalitis and a low threshold for obtaining CSF analysis are mandatory. CSF should be examined for cell count, microscopic examination, culture and sensitivities, protein and glucose concentrations, antibodies, and polymerase chain reaction (PCR). A purulent profile consists of an increased number of white blood cells, predominantly polymorphonuclear leukocytes, low glucose concentration, and high protein concentration. Exceptions include partially treated meningitis, early *S. pneumoniae*, and if the patient is leukopenic or immunosuppressed. A cranial CT scan should be obtained prior to CSF examination in any patient with an altered level of consciousness or a focal deficit to rule out a space-occupying lesion, such as an associated abscess or hemorrhage. Blood cultures and chest x-ray also should be obtained.

Therapy

The mainstay of treatment is rapid administration of intravenous antibiotics that are specific for the suspected or isolated organism and can adequately cross the blood-brain barrier. Antibiotic choice and therapy are described in detail below. A cranial CT scan should be obtained urgently to rule out an associated abscess, hemorrhage, or embolic infarction. In the encephalopathic, stuporous, or comatose patient whose mental status does not improve with appropriate treatment, continuous subclinical seizures or nonconvulsive status epilepticus should be considered and diagnosed with an electroencephalogram. A potentially devastating complication of severe cases of meningoencephalitis is the development of cerebral edema, which can be treated temporarily with a hyperosmolar agent such as mannitol. Other serious complications include dural venous thrombosis, hydrocephalus with increased intracranial pressure, and CNS vasculitis with secondary cerebral ischemia or frank infarction. Cerebral vasculitis can be associated with infection with many pathogens, including unusual species, such as viridans streptococci or fungi. In severe cases of purulent meningoencephalitis, inflammatory cellular infiltrates lead to thickened arterial intima that can occlude or stenose meningeal or cerebral vessels, a condition known as *obliterative endarteritis*. Recently, it has been reported that in addition to antibiotics, corticosteroids (dexamethasone and low doses of hydrocortisone and fludrocortisone) have been a successful therapy for managing meningitis and septic shock.[95]

Prognosis

Acute purulent meningoencephalitis from a virulent organism such as *S. aureus, S. pneumoniae,* or gram-negative bacilli carries a poor prognosis; in some patient series, mortality in this setting is as high as 80 to 90 percent.

Headache

A diffuse, mild headache is a common complaint, occurring in 25 to 43 percent of patients with infective endocarditis. In contrast, an unrelenting, severe or localized headache may indicate the presence of mycotic aneurysm, SAH, or meningoencephalitis. This type of headache should prompt emergent cranial CT scanning and, if negative, a follow-up LP with CSF analysis to rule out an early-warning leak or infection in the subarachnoid space. Some experts suggest obtaining a cerebral angiogram to look for a mycotic aneurysm. In the elderly, the onset of a severe headache and elevated erythrocyte sedimentation rate may be confused with temporal arteritis, obscuring the diagnosis of infective endocarditis, especially if the patient is afebrile.[96] Headache is a common presentation of CNS vasculitis, which is a potential secondary complication of meningitis and can be responsible for transient focal neurologic deficits mimicking ischemic stroke.[97]

Seizure

During the course of infective endocarditis, 10 to 21 percent of patients experience a seizure, including a seizure as the initial symptom.[12,28] Focal seizures can occur following embolic cerebral infarction or from microemboli or acute ICH. Primary generalized seizures may occur as a result of metabolic abnormalities such as azotemia, hypoxia, and hyponatremia or as a result of medication reactions, including antibiotic therapy. High-dose penicillin, imipenem-cilastatin, haloperidol, wellbutrin, and meperidine may lower the seizure threshold. Careful attention should be paid to the patient with renal dysfunction in the administration of renally excreted drugs, such as penicillin, which should be dose-adjusted. As mentioned previously, subclinical seizure activity or "nonconvulsive status" should be suspected particularly in the elderly patient with a change in mental status and infective endocarditis who does not improve on appropriate antibiotic therapy. An electroencephalogram can be diagnostic.

Abscess

Brain microabscess (diameter < 1 cm) occurs in 0.9 to 3.8 percent of patients with infective endocarditis and presents clinically as encephalopathy. A higher incidence may be found at autopsy or if neuroimaging is performed. A macroabscess (diameter > 1 cm) develops rarely during infective endocarditis, accounting for less than 1 percent of all neurologic complications of infective endocarditis.[98] Presenting symptoms include meningismus, focal neurologic deficits, and seizures. Macroscopic abscesses have been documented 1 to 3 weeks following stroke; presumably the septic emboli provides the infectious nidus. Abscess also can form as an extension of purulent meningoencephalitis. The usual isolate from the abscess is *S. aureus* or streptococci. Recent data suggest a role for neurosurgical management of brain abscess, particularly in patients in whom the abscess is likely to rupture into the ventricular system, which is associated with an 80 percent mortality.[99,100]

Diagnosis is made most commonly by contrast-enhanced cranial CT scan or MRI (Fig. 26-10). If the CT scan is negative and MRI is not available, brain scan with technetium-99m is a very sensitive (but not specific) supplementary test for detecting brain abscess or cerebritis. LP can be hazardous and does not add important diagnostic information because the CSF cultures typically are negative.

Neuropathy

Mononeuropathy or multiple mononeuropathies (mononeuritis multiplex) occur in 1 to 2 percent of patients with infective endocarditis.[101] Specific reported peripheral neuropathies include ulnar, median, peroneal, and sciatic nerves. Rarely, there is involvement of cranial nerves IV, VI, VII, IX, X, and XII. Manifestations are specific to the cranial nerve involved and include paralysis of the face, and weakness of the palate, tongue, larynx, and ocular muscles. Rarely, neuropathy is the initial manifestation of infective endocarditis, with viridans streptococci the causative organism in nearly all cases. Both septic embolic occlusion of the vasa vasorum and immune-mediated vasculitis are suspected etiologies. The neurologic deficit usually resolves following antibiotic therapy.

Critically ill patients can develop a severe sensorimotor peripheral neuropathy also known as *critical-care polyneuropathy*. It has been reported during infective endocarditis with sepsis and may be associated with difficulty weaning from ventilatory support.[102] Clinical signs include weakness, especially in the lower limbs, and symmetrically decreased or absent deep tendon reflexes. Electromyography and nerve conduction studies usually demonstrate an axonal polyneuropathy with fibrillations, reduced motor compound action amplitudes, normal or near-normal motor nerve conductions, and normal distal latencies. Potential unproven etiologies include septic microemboli in the microvasculature, a bacterial toxin effect, and an immuno-mediated vasculitis. Also common in the intensive care setting are drug-induced neuropathies. A drug-induced myopathy also can occur in the critical care setting; high-dose steroids, both alone or with muscular relaxant drugs such as pancuronium bromide, are associated with a myopathy and may be responsible for difficulty to wean from ventilatory support.

Ocular

Visual system involvement during infective endocarditis has been reported in up to 25 percent of patients, with 35 percent of patients demonstrating fundal findings. Ophthalmic or central retinal artery occlusion due

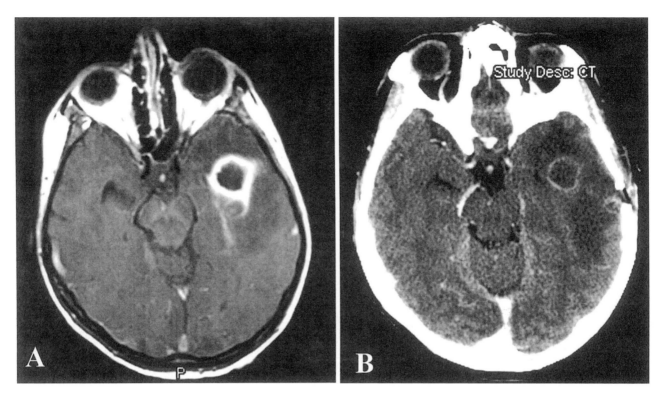

Figure 26–10. *A.* MRI with contrast administration demonstrating large ring-enhancing left temporal macroabscess. *B.* Corresponding sequence of a contrast-enhanced cranial CT scan. Note the mass effect with large surrounding hypodensity consistent with edema.

to emboli is a rare consequence of infective endocarditis but important to recognize. Symptoms of sudden monocular blindness in the infective endocarditis patient represent an ophthalmologic emergency.

Immediate funduscopic evaluation occasionally reveals the embolus in place, interruption, or box-carring of retinal arteriolar flow or venous dilatation. If recognized immediately, encouraging the embolus to break up and move distally may salvage residual vision. This usually consists of a retrobulbar injection of anesthesia and digital massage to intermittently raise and then lower the intraocular pressure. Anterior chamber paracentesis also may be effective. More distal vascular infarction can result in retinal hemorrhages or soft exudates (representing localized edema of the nerve fiber layer). As the blood in retinal hemorrhages separates, the elevated white blood cell count in patients with endocarditis may cause a central collection or whitening, resulting in so-called Roth spots. These are nonspecific and may be encountered in other causes of local retinal infarction. Vascular involvement along the afferent visual pathways, usually from mycotic aneurysms, can produce various forms of field defect. Septic emboli may cause an acute focal retinitis, followed by extension into the vitreous and endophthalmitis. Infective endocarditis represents one of the more common causes of the infrequently seen endogenous enophthalmitis. Extension of the infection to involve other orbital tissues can produce a panophthalmitis. Because of the frequency of ocular and visual involvement, a detailed ophthalmologic evaluation, including funduscopic examination, should be part of the evaluation of any patient with suspected infective endocarditis.

Other

Lumbar pain and diskitis occur in 3 to 10 percent of patients with infective endocarditis. An associated osteomyelitis and soft tissue abscess have been reported. Myalgia can occur either diffusely or limited to one muscle location such as to the thigh or calf. Musculoskeletal or vertebral complications typically resolve with appropriate antibiotic therapy. Rarely, neurologic manifestations develop due to spinal cord ischemia from emboli or parameningeal abscesses compromising the vascular supply to the spinal cord. Movement disorders such as chorea and dyskinesia also have been reported. The etiology may be due to embolic infarction of the basal ganglia.

▶ DIFFERENTIAL DIAGNOSIS

Noninfectious Etiology

In the febrile patient with neurologic complications and repeatedly negative blood cultures, other considerations include atrial myxoma, primary cholesterol emboli, vasculitis, and nonbacterial thrombotic endocarditis (NBTE).[18] NBTE is associated with overt and occult carcinoma, uremia, connective tissue disease, and surrounding vascular incision sites. Similar to endocarditis, the erythrocytic sedimentation rate and body temperature frequently are elevated in both carcinoma and connective tissue disease, complicating the diagnosis.

▶ DIAGNOSTIC CONSIDERATIONS

Echocardiography

Any patient suspected of having infective endocarditis should have an emergent echocardiographic study (ECHO). Two-dimensional echocardiography is a sensitive test for detecting cardiac vegetations. It is especially useful if vegetations are found when the diagnosis is in question prior to positive blood cultures; however, the lack of vegetation does not exclude the diagnosis of infective endocarditis. Echocardiographic evidence for infective endocarditis in order of specificity includes mobile mass on the endocardial surface, perivalvular abscess, mobile mass on a prosthetic valve, perforation or aneurysm of a valve leaflet, intracardiac or paravalvular fistula, nodular valve thickening, diffuse valve thickening, ruptured chordae, or unexplained valvular regurgitation.[103] Serial ECHO examinations during an uncomplicated course of infective endocarditis are not necessary unless the diagnosis is unconfirmed or in question. Vegetations can persist for months and are not necessarily an indicator of clinical course. In addition to imaging potential vegetations and the extent of infection, ECHO is crucial for quickly determining the hemodynamic state of the heart and for elucidating the cause of hemodynamic failure, if present. Congestive heart failure due to left ventricular dysfunction has grave prognostic implications and is the most common cause of death in patients with infective endocarditis. Acute mortality rates are as high as 85 percent for patients with refractory congestive heart failure. Rapidly progressive heart failure or the presence of valvular abscess (e.g., aortic root abscess) may mandate surgical intervention (see "Role of Cardiac Surgery" section).

Role of TTE versus TEE

Transthoracic echocardiography (TTE) detects vegetations in 40 to 80 percent of cases.[104–106] The transesophageal echocardiogram (TEE) has superior resolution, detecting vegetations in more than 90 percent of cases.[103] Frequently, TEE is performed following equivocal or poorly obtained TTE results or in patients with persistent fever despite antibiotic therapy in order to rule out possible perivalvular abscess. In general, TEE is superior to TTE for demonstrating prosthetic-valve infective endocarditis because detection of cardiac abnormalities is more difficult in patients with prosthetic valves. The AHA Science and Advisory Committee suggests that the decision of which type of ECHO to perform initially depends on the degree of clinical suspicion of infective endocarditis, with low suspicion favoring TTE and moderate to high suspicion favoring TEE.[72]

The role of ECHO in predicting risk of embolization in infective endocarditis remains controversial. There are increasing data suggesting that TEE is predictive of embolism and that certain morphologic characteristics of vegetations can predict risk of embolization.[107] The majority of data currently suggest that mitral or aortic vegetations larger than 10 mm and that are mobile on early initial ECHO predict embolic events.[103] In a large study of patients with definite *S. aureus* endocarditis (by the Duke criteria), Di Salvo and coleagues[107] found that right-sided valve endocarditis and vegetation length and mobility correlated to a higher risk of embolization. In this same study, infective endocarditis patients with large (>10 mm) and mobile vegetations were at particularly high risk for subsequent embolization. It is important to emphasize that the results represent both symptomatic and "silent" emboli that were identified with aggressive CT thoracoabdominal and cerebral scans. The main limitation of the study is that 61 percent of the patients underwent surgery, which can alter the natural history of embolization. Other earlier studies have failed to detect this relationship between vegetation size and mobility and the risk of embolization. For example, in one study involving 77 patients, small vegetations were as likely to embolize as larger vegetations.[108] Furthermore, there was no relationship between change in lesion size or morphology during antimicrobial therapy and the incidence of emboli. The disparities between studies may be due to different experimental paradigms (TTE versus TEE), patient populations (some studies include patients with previous evidence of embolization), different pathogens, timing of the study, size of the study, or definition of infective endocarditis.

Data to determine the prognostic value of ECHO specifically for cerebral embolism are similarly inconclusive. Available data from a few studies reveal no higher incidence of neurologic complications from emboli based on the presence or absence of vegetative lesions.[15,28] In a 12-year review of neurologic complications in 175 patients with infective endocarditis, vegetations were seen on echocardiography in approximately 37 percent of the patients with neurologic complications (of all types) and in 28 percent of patients without neurologic complications ($p = 0.26$, NS).[15]

Laboratory

A total of three separate sets of sterilely drawn venous blood cultures should be drawn over 24 hours for both aerobic and anaerobic culture. Blood cultures should be drawn prior to initiating antibiotic therapy. Antibiotic therapy should not be delayed and can be initiated immediately after obtaining the first set of venous blood cultures. Fungal cultures should be sent in patients who are known to be immunosuppressed. In patients with prior exposure to antibiotics, blood should be collected in β-lactamase-supplemented tubes. In the majority of patients with infective endocarditis, blood cultures are positive, a direct result of the constant low-grade bacteremia that occurs. However, there is a 19 to 27 percent incidence of culture-negative infectious endocarditis, with only 50 percent of these cases diagnosed having had antecedent antibiotic therapy as a potential etiology for the negative cultures.[109] Negative cultures can occur due to low blood sampling volume, prior empirical antibiotic therapy, or the presence of certain fastidious organisms, such as *Chlamydia, Mycoplasma, Brucella,* and certain fungal species. Some gram-negative organisms grow poorly and may require long incubation periods, including *Hemophilus, Actinobacillus, Cardiobacterium, Eikenella,* and *Kingella* spp. (also known as the HACEK group). If the pathogen is slow-growing or difficult to culture, PCR molecular methods can be the method of choice for diagnosis.[110] Baseline serum hematology and chemistries should be obtained, including total red and white cell counts (with indices and a differential, respectively), platelet count, renal and liver function, and prothrombin time. Leukocytosis occurs most often in acute infective endocarditis and is present in 20 to 30 percent of patients. Commonly, a normochromic, normocytic anemia is present. Erythrocyte sedimentation rate (ESR) and rheumatoid factor are elevated frequently, although this is a nonspecific finding and may depend on length of disease state and other unrelated factors, such as age. Immunologic abnormalities, including low circulating complement and/or elevated immune complexes such as anti-antiphospholipid antibodies, can occur.

Neuroimaging

As discussed previously in the section on ICH, a cranial CT scan is mandatory to distinguish hemorrhagic from nonhemorrhagic neurologic complications in any patient presenting with a transient or fixed neurologic deficit. A contrasted study can help to distinguish an abscess from meningoencephalitis in an encephalopathic patient with fever and meningitic signs. Infrequently, cranial CT scan also may suggest the presence of a mycotic aneurysm, prompting angiographic confirmation.

Particularly in the event that the cranial CT scan is unrevealing, brain MRI is very useful for the diagnosis of microemboli, microabscess, aseptic meningitis, and vasculitis associated with meningeal involvement in infective endocarditis. A more prominent role for MRI in infective endocarditis has been suggested, with MRI-angiography as a useful alternative to cerebral angiography for the serial follow-up of mycotic aneurysms in selected patients.

Cerebral Angiography

Four-vessel cerebral angiography is indicated in the patient with neurologic complications to rule out life-threatening mycotic aneurysm. Diagnostic sensitivity for the evaluation of mycotic aneurysm is approximately 90 percent. Cerebral angiography, if not otherwise contraindicated, is recommended in the following settings: (1) when the cranial CT scan demonstrates hemorrhage (regardless of cause), (2) when the cranial CT scan is normal but the history suggests an embolic phenomenon (e.g., TIA), and (3) when CSF examination reveals a pleocytosis and/or hemorrhage. The optimal timing of cerebral angiography is unknown. Some experts suggest that angiography should be performed without delay because in some patients mycotic aneurysm can rupture within 24 hours of the onset of neurologic symptoms. If cerebral angiography is contraindicated, MRA is a second choice to evaluate for mycotic aneurysm but has significantly less sensitivity.

Lumbar Puncture

A wide spectrum of CSF abnormalities can occur in the patient with infective endocarditis depending on the type of neurologic presentation. For example, in the patient with meningoencephalitis, the CSF most commonly reveals abnormalities. However, up to 60 percent of patients can have either a "normal" or an aseptic CSF with modest lymphocytic pleocytosis, moderately elevated protein concentration, normal glucose concentration, and a negative Gram's stain. Less commonly, the CSF is grossly purulent or hemorrhagic (>200 red blood cells/mm³). Purulent CSF occurs with more virulent organisms, including *S. aureus*, enteric gram-negative bacilli, and *S. pneumoniae*, whereas aseptic or normal CSF tends to occur with less virulent organisms such as viridans streptococci.

▶ TREATMENT CONSIDERATIONS

Antimicrobial Therapy

Effective antibiotic therapy requires timely administration, appropriate specificity of the drug to achieve maximal bactericidal effects with adequate penetration of the blood-brain barrier, and sufficient length of treatment. Initiating antibiotic therapy is associated with a sharp reduction in the number of embolic events, underscoring the need for prompt diagnosis and therapy. During therapy, the patient should be monitored vigilantly for improvement of neurologic signs and symptoms. Deterioration may warrant measurement of serum bactericidal titers and reevaluation of antibiotic choice.

The chosen antibiotic must be bactericidal and usually is administered parentally initially for 6 to 8 weeks (Table 26-5). Multiple antibiotics may be necessary for certain organisms, such as enterococci or gram-negative bacilli. Fungal infections may require both antifungal drugs and surgery. If cultures are negative, broad-spectrum antibiotic coverage is necessary. For a detailed description of antimicrobial therapy in the various forms of infective endocarditis, the reader is referred to excellent recent reviews.[25,111–114]

Anticoagulation

Based on evidence from both retrospective clinical studies and animal models of septic brain embolism, it is generally agreed that the routine use of anticoagulation is not recommended in patients with native-valve infective endocarditis due to the increased risk of CNS hemorrhagic transformation. Management of the patient with cerebral infarction and prosthetic-valve infective endocarditis can create a therapeutic dilemma. In patients with prosthetic-valve infective endocarditis, anti-coagulation is known to decrease the risk of stroke significantly.[38,115] The incidence of CNS thromboembolism in patients with prosthetic-valve infective endocarditis not receiving anticoagulation therapy is high, ranging from 46 to 71 percent.[115–117] This increased incidence of brain embolism must be weighed against the fact that the incidence of hemorrhage in the same patient population while on anticoagulation therapy is as high as 36 percent.[118] No large randomized trials exist to answer key questions concerning the risks and benefits of anticoagulation in this setting. Aggregate data represent a wide spectrum of therapeutic factors, including varying times of initiating antibiotic therapy, varying effectiveness of antibiotic therapy, type of anticoagulation chosen (warfarin versus heparin), and extent of anticoagulation (as assessed by INR and partial thromboplastin time). In a retrospective review of 61 patients with infective endocarditis and prosthetic valve replacement, no protective effect of anticoagulation therapy with warfarin was observed.[18] In certain clinical settings, anticoagulation can be detrimental; for example, in left-sided *S. aureus* endocarditis, anticoagulant therapy is closely associated with death due to neurologic complications.[40] The decision to use anticoagulants in the patient with prosthetic valve endocarditis is best made on a case-by-case basis because certain virulent organisms such as *S. aureus* carry a higher incidence of hemorrhage. Careful consideration of the use of anticoagulation therapy in the patient with a neurologic complication and prosthetic-valvular endocarditis

▶ **TABLE 26-5.** ANTIBIOTIC THERAPY FOR BACTERIAL ENDOCARDITIS

Pathogen	Antibiotic, Total Adult Daily Dose (Dosing Interval)
Streptococcus spp.	Penicillin G 20–24 million units/d (every 4–6 h) *or* Ceftriaxone 4 g/d (every 12 h) *or* Cefepime 4 g/d (every 12 h) *or* Cefotaxime 12 g/d (every 4 h)
Staphylococci Methicillin-susceptible	Nafcillin or oxacillin 12 g/d (every 4–6 h)
Methicillin-resistant	Vancomycin 2–3 g/d (every 6 h)
Gram-negative enterobacteriaceae (*Klebsiella* spp., *E. coli*, *Proteus* spp.)	Ceftriaxone or cefepime or cefotaxime
HACEK organisms*	Ceftriaxone

*Hemophilus spp., Actinobacillus actinomycetemcomitans, Cardiobacterium hominis, Eikenella corrodens, and Kingella spp.

is necessary in the presence of a large cerebral infarction, evidence of ICH, history of blood dyscrasia, mycotic aneurysm, and uncontrolled infection. When anticoagulation is indicated, intravenous heparin sodium rather than warfarin is the drug of choice due to its easy reversal. The extent of anticoagulation requires close monitoring because excessive anticoagulation can convert a bland infarction into a hemorrhagic one, with potential neurologic worsening. The reader is directed to recent (2001) American College of Cardiology guidelines for the appropriate use of anticoagulation in patients with prosthetic valve replacement.[116] Despite the potential benefit of anticoagulation in preventing thromboembolic events during infective endocarditis, the single most important measure is timely, effective antibiotic therapy.

Role of Cardiac Surgery

Traditional indications for cardiac surgery include refractory heart failure, suppurative intracardiac disease (such as myocardial or perivalvular abscess), ineffective antibiotic therapy with repeated relapses of infective endocarditis, the presence of an unstable prosthesis, and most cases of fungal endocarditis.[72] Multiple embolic episodes (excluding cutaneous) and the presence of virulent organisms such as staphylococci and gram-negative bacilli are considered a relative indication. More aggressive surgical intervention may be needed during the course of infective endocarditis when medical therapy is ineffective for infections by fungi, *Pseudomonas aeruginosa, Brucella* spp., or *Coxiella burnetti.* Cardiac valve replacement in patients who have had a single embolic event is controversial. The benefit of surgery is maximal during the initial acute phase when there exists a higher risk of embolic complications, but the decision to operate depends on patient circumstances. In the setting of medically refractive cardiac failure, some authors advocate surgery for all patients who do not respond promptly and completely to medical therapy within 24 hours.[112]

As recently reported by the American Heart Association statement guidelines on the diagnosis and management of infective endocarditis and its complications, echocardiographic features suggesting potential surgical intervention include certain characteristics of observed vegetations and/or evidence of valvular dysfunction or perivalvular extension. Table 26-6 reviews the clinical parameters of infective endocarditis patients in whom early surgery should be considered. The reader is also referred to a more comprehensive discussion on each of these findings and other pertinent clinical events.[72] In patients with preoperative cardioembolic cerebral infarction, the optimal timing of cardiac surgery is controversial. Since the first 3 to 5 days following cerebral infarction represent a vulnerable time for

▶ **TABLE 26-6.** INDICATIONS FOR SURGERY IN INFECTIVE ENDOCARDITIS

Clinical Feature	Echocardiographic Findings
Congestive heart failure (unresponsive to medical therapy)	Severe valvular dysfunction from: Valvular perforation Aortic or mitral valve regurgitation Ruptured chordae
Recurrent embolic events	Large vegetation (>10 mm) or a mobile or enlarging vegetation despite antimicrobial therapy
Perivalvular extension of infection	Annular abscess Valvular dehiscence, rupture or fistula (with heart failure)
Persistent bacteremia (refractory to treatment)	

SOURCE: *Data based on refs. 72 and 103.*

the development of cerebral edema, it has been recommended that surgery be delayed, especially in patients with a large stroke. In a retrospective study of patients with infective endocarditis and cerebral complications, it was found that delaying cardiac surgery decreased postoperative neurologic deterioration.[119] Other authors suggest that infective endocarditis patients with a nonhemorrhagic neurologic complication who undergo early cardiac surgery[69] do as well as or in some cases better than a similar medically treated group.[120]

▶ SUMMARY

A substantial number of patients will experience a neurologic complication during or following infective endocarditis. Despite recent innovations in antibiotic therapy, neurologic complications continue to contribute significantly to the overall morbidity and mortality of this disease. Mortality rates are higher in infective endocarditis patients with neurologic complications than in those without neurologic complications. Rupture of a mycotic aneurysm, intracerebral hemorrhage, and purulent meningoencephalitis are each associated with a mortality rate of 80 percent. This high mortality rate accentuates the need for early recognition of predisposing factors and institution of appropriate preventive measures, where possible. Equally important is early diagnosis. Cerebral embolic infarction remains the most common neurologic complication, followed by encephalopathy, intracranial hemorrhage, cerebral mycotic aneurysm, and meningoencephalitis. Other less common complications are headache, seizure, abscess, neuropathy, and ocular complications. Neurologic complications frequently can occur acutely but also can be delayed by months. Management of the patient with neurologic complications frequently involves a multidisciplinary team approach involving the cardiologist, neurologist, infectious disease specialist, ophthalmologist, and neurosurgeon. The optimal treatment strategy is determined with the results of echocardiograms, neuroimaging studies, laboratory tests, and occasionally, cerebral angiography, all costly interventions. While some therapies, including the use of anticoagulants, are controversial, the expeditious initiation of specific antimicrobial therapy remains the undisputed single most important treatment that can be administered.

REFERENCES

1. Osler W: Malignant endocarditis (Gulstonian Lecture). *Lancet* 1:1415, 1885.
2. Pelletier LL, Petersdorf RG: Infective endocarditis: A review of 125 cases from the University of Washington Hospitals, 1963–1972. *Medicine* 56:287, 1977.
3. Von Reyn CF, Levy BS, Arbeit RD, et al: Infective endocarditis: An analysis based on strict case definitions. *Ann Intern Med* 94:505, 1981.
4. Durack DT, Lukes AS, Bright DK: New criteria for diagnosis of infective endocarditis: Utilization of specific echocardiographic findings. Duke Endocarditis Service. *Am J Med* 96:200, 1994.
5. Lerner PI: Neurologic complications of infective endocarditis. *Med Clin North Am* 69:385, 1985.
6. Selky AK, Roos KL: Neurologic complications of infective endocarditis. *Semin Neurol* 12(3):225, 1992.
7. Bouza E, Menasalvas A, Munoz P, et al: Infective endocarditis: A prospective study at the end of the twentieth century. New predisposing conditions, new etiologic agents, and still a high mortality. *Medicine* 80:298, 2001.
8. Salgado AV: Central nervous system complications of infective endocarditis. *Stroke* 22:1461, 1991.
9. Tunkel AR, Kaye D: Neurologic complications of infective endocarditis. *Neurol Clin* 11:419, 1993.
10. Mylonakis E, Calderwood SB: Medical progress: Infective endocarditis in adults. *New Engl J Med* 345:1318, 2001.
11. Dhawan VK: Infective endocarditis in elderly patients. *Curr Infect Dis Rep* 5:285, 2003.
12. Gregoratos G: Infective endocarditis in the elderly: Diagnosis and management. *J Geriatr Cardiol* 12:183, 2003.
13. Hart RG, Foster JW, Luther MF, et al: Stroke in infective endocarditis. *Stroke* 21(5):695, 1990.
14. Pruitt AA, Rubin R, Karchmer A: Neurologic complications of bacterial endocarditis. *Medicine* 57:329, 1978.
15. Salgado AV, Fural AJ, Keys TF, et al: Neurologic complications of endocarditis: A 12-year experience. *Neurology* 39:173, 1989.
16. Steckelberg JM, Murphy JG, Ballard D, et al: Emboli in infective endocarditis: The prognostic value of echocardiography. *Ann Intern Med* 114:635, 1991.
17. Jones HR Jr, Siekert RG, Geraci JE: Neurologic manifestations of bacterial endocarditis. *Ann Intern Med* 71:21, 1969.
18. Davenport J, Hart RG: Prosthetic valve endocarditis, 1976–1987: Antibiotics, anticoagulation and stroke. *Stroke* 21:993, 1990.
19. Murenha E, Stein CM: Chemoprophylaxis of bacterial endocarditis: A survey of current practice in Zimbabwe. *J Antimicrob Chemother* 25(2):291, 1990.
20. Ferguson DJP, McColm AA, Savage TJ, et al: A morphological study of experimental rabbit staphylococcal endocarditis and aortitis: I. Formation and effect of infected and uninfected vegetations on the aorta. *Br J Exp Pathol* 67:667, 1986.
21. Weinstein L, Schlesinger JJ: Pathoanatomic, pathophysiologic and clinical correlations in endocarditis. *New Eng J Med* 291:832, 1974.
22. Moreillon P, Que YA: Infective endocarditis. *Lancet* 363:139, 2004.
23. Moreillon P, Que YA, Bayer AS: Pathogenesis of streptococcal and staphylococcal endocarditis. *Infect Dis Clin North Am* 16:297, 2002.
24. Rodbard S: Blood velocity and endocarditis. *Circulation* 27:18, 1963.
25. Murtagh B, Frazier OH, Letsou GV: Diagnosis and management of bacterial endocarditis in 2003. *Curr Opin Cardiol* 18(2):106, 2003.
26. Hoen B, Alla F, Selton-Suty C, et al: Changing profile of infective endocarditis: Results of a 1-year survey in France. *JAMA* 288(1):75, 2002.
27. Ako J, Ikari Y, Haori M, et al: Changing spectrum of infectious endocarditis: Review of 194 episodes over 20 years. *Circ J* 67:3, 2003.
28. Heiro M, Nikoskelainen J, Engblom E, et al: Neurologic manifestations of infective endocarditis: A 17-year experience in a teaching hospital in Finland. *Arch Intern Med* 160:2781, 2000.
29. Roder BL, Wandall DA, Espersen F, et al: Neurologic manifestations in *Staphylococcus aureus* endocarditis: A review of 260 bacteremic cases in nondrug addicts. *Am J Med* 102:379, 1997.
30. Cabell CH, Pond KK, Peterson GE, et al: The risk of stroke and death in patients with aortic and mitral valve endocarditis. *Am Heart J* 142(1):75, 2001.
31. Wallace SM, Walton BI, Kharbanda RK, et al: Mortality from infective endocarditis: Clinical predictors of outcome. *Heart* 88:53, 2002.
32. McKinsey DS, Ratts TE, Bisno AL: Underlying cardiac lesions in adults with infective endocarditis: The changing spectrum. *Am J Med* 82:681, 1987.
33. Clemens JD, Horwitz RI, Jaffe CC: A controlled evaluation of the risk of bacterial endocarditis in persons with mitral valve prolapse. *New Eng J Med* 307:776, 1982.
34. Freed LA, Levy D, Levine RA, et al: Prevalence and clinical outcome of mitral valve prolapse. *New Engl J Med* 341:1, 1999.
35. Marks AR, Choong CY, Sanfilippo AJ, et al: Identifica-

tion of high-risk and low-risk subgroups of patients with mitral valve prolapse. *New Engl J Med* 320:1031, 1989.

36. Playford D, Weyman AE: Mitral valve prolapse: Time for a fresh look. *Rev Cardiovasc Med* 2:73, 2001.

37. Keyser DL, Biller J, Coffman TT, et al: Neurologic complications of late prosthetic valve endocarditis. *Stroke* 21:472, 1990.

38. Leport C, Vilde JL, Bricaire F, et al: Fifty cases of late prosthetic valve endocarditis: Improvement in prognosis over a 15-year period. *Br Heart J* 58:66, 1987.

39. Madison J, Wang K, Gobel FL, et al: Prosthetic valve endocarditis. *Circulation* 51:940, 1975.

40. Jamieson WRE: Modern cardiac valve devices: Bioprostheses and prostheses; state of the art. *J Cardiac Surg* 8:89, 1993.

41. Tornos P, Almirante B, Mirabet S, et al: Infective endocarditis due to *Staphylococcus aureus:* Deleterious effect of anticoagulant therapy. *Arch Intern Med* 159:473, 1999.

42. Murphy JG, Foster-Smith K: Management of complications of infective endocarditis with emphasis on echocardiographic findings. *Infect Dis Clin North Am* 7(1):153, 1993.

43. Blackstone EH, Kirklin JW: Death and other time-related events after valve replacement. *Circulation* 72:753, 1985.

44. Thilen U: Infective endocarditis in adults with congenital heart disease. *Curr Infect Dis Rep* 5:300, 2003.

45. Seto TB, Kwiat D, Taira DA, et al: Physicians recommendations for use of antibiotic prophylaxis to prevent endocarditis. *JAMA* 284:68, 2000.

46. Bonow RO, Carabello B, de Leon AC, et al: ACC/AHA Guidelines for the Management of Patients with Valvular Heart Disease: Executive Summary. A report of the American College of Cardiology/American Heart Association Task Force on Practice Guidelines (Committee on Management of Patients with Valvular Heart Disease). *J Heart Valve Dis* 7(6):672, 1998.

47. Dajani AS, Taubert KA, Wilson W, et al: Prevention of bacterial endocarditis: Recommendations by the American Heart Association. *JAMA* 277:1794, 1997.

48. Levine DP, Crane LR, Zervos MJ: Bacteremia in narcotic addicts at the Detroit Medical Center: II. Infectious endocarditis: A prospective comparative study. *Rev Infect Dis* 8:374, 1986.

49. Chambers HF, Korzeniowski OM, Sande MA: Clinical manifestations in addicts and non-addicts. *Medicine* 62:170, 1983.

50. Ramsey RG, Gunnar RM, Tobin JR: Endocarditis in drug addicts. *Am J Cardiol* 25:608, 1970.

51. Brown PD, Levine DP: Infective endocarditis in the injection drug user. *Infect Dis Clin North Am* 16:645, 2002.

52. Openshaw H: Neurological complications of endocarditis in persons taking drugs intravenously. *West J Med* 124:276, 1976.

53. Cicalini S, Forcina G, De Rosa FG: Infective endocarditis in patients with human immunodeficiency virus infection. *J Infect* 42:267, 2001.

54. Strom BL, Abrutyn E, Berlin JA, et al: Risk factors for infective endocarditis: Oral hygiene and nondental exposures. *Circulation* 102:2842, 2000.

55. Cartotto RC, Macdonald DB, Wasan SM: Acute bacterial endocarditis following burns: Case report and review. *Burns* 24(4):369, 1998.

56. Antel JJ, Rome HP, Geraci JE, et al: Toxic organic psychosis as a presenting feature in bacterial endocarditis in the elderly. *Proc Mayo Clin* 30:45, 1955.

57. Traut EF, Carter JB, Gumbiner SH, et al: Bacterial endocarditis in the elderly. *Geriatrics* 4:205, 1949.

58. Sanabria TJ, Alpert JS, Goldberg R, et al: Increasing frequency of staphylococcal infective endocarditis. *Arch Intern Med* 150:1305, 1990.

59. Grandsden WR, Ekyn SJ, Leach RM: Neurological presentations of native valve endocarditis. *Q J Med* 73:1135, 1989.

60. Brouqui P, Raoult D: Endocarditis due to rare and fastidious bacteria. *Clin Microbiol Rev* 14:177, 2001.

61. Johnson RH, Kennedy RP, Marton KI, et al: *Hemophilus* endocarditis: New cases, literature review and recommendations for management. *South Med J* 70:1098, 1977.

62. Felner JM, Dowell VR Jr: Anaerobic bacterial endocarditis. *New Engl J Med* 283:1188, 1970.

63. Brook I: Endocarditis due to anaerobic bacteria. *Cardiology* 98(1–2):1, 2002.

64. Crawford MH, Durack DT: Clinical presentation of infective endocarditis. *Cardiol Clin* 21(2):159, 2003.

65. Anderson DJ, Goldstein LB, Wilkinson WE, et al: Stroke location, characterization, severity, and outcome in mitral vs aortic valve endocarditis. *Neurology* 61(10):1341, 2003.

66. Kupferwasser LI, Hafner G, Mohr-Kahaly S, et al: The presence of infection-related antiphospholipid antibodies in infective endocarditis determines a major risk factor for embolic events. *J Am Coll Cardiol* 33:1365, 1999.

67. Korkmaz S, Ileri M, Hisar I, et al: Increased levels of soluble adhesion molecules, E-selectin and P-selectin, in patients with infective endocarditis and embolic events. *Eur Heart J* 10:874, 2001.

68. Hornig CR, Dorndoff W, Agnoli AL: Hemorrhagic cerebral infarction: Prospective study. *Stroke* 17:179, 1986.

69. Parrino PE, Kron IL, Ross SD, et al: Does a focal neurologic deficit contraindicate operation in a patient with endocarditis? *Ann Thorac Surg* 67:59, 1999.

70. Piper C, Wiemer M, Schulte HD, et al: Stroke is not a contraindication for urgent valve replacement in acute infective endocarditis. *J Heart Valve Dis* 10:703, 2001.

71. Vilacosta I, Graupner C, San Roman JA, et al: Risk of embolization after institution of antibiotic therapy for infective endocarditis. *J Am Coll Cardiol* 39:1489, 2002.

72. Bayer AS, Bolger AF, Taubert KA, et al: Diagnosis and management of infective endocarditis and its complications. *Circulation* 98(25):2936, 1998.

73. Delahaye JP, Malquarti PV, Beaune J, et al: Cerebrovascular accidents in infective endocarditis: Role of anticoagulation. *Eur Heart J* 11:1074, 1990.

74. Chan KL, Dumesnil JG, Cujec B, et al: A randomized trial of aspirin on the risk of embolic events in pa-

tients with infective endocarditis. *J Am Coll Cardiol* 42:775, 2003.

75. Singhal AB, Topcuoglu MA, Buonanno FS: Acute ischemic stroke patterns in infective and nonbacterial thrombotic endocarditis. *Stroke* 33:1267, 2002.

76. Bakshi R, Wright PD, Kinkel PR, et al: Cranial magnetic resonance imaging findings in bacterial endocarditis: The neuroimaging spectrum of septic brain embolization demonstrated in twelve patients. *J Neuroimag* 9(2):78, 1999.

77. Terpenning MS, Buggy BP, Kauffman CA: Infective endocarditis: Clinical features in young and elderly patients. *Am J Med* 83:626, 1987.

78. Hart RG, Kagan-Hallet K, Joerns SE: Mechanisms of intracranial hemorrhage in infective endocarditis. *Stroke* 18:1048, 1987.

79. Siekert RG, Jones HR Jr: Transient cerebral ischemic attacks associated with subacute bacterial endocarditis. *Stroke* 1:178, 1970.

80. Frazee JG, Cahan LD, Winter J: Bacterial intracranial aneurysms. *J Neurosurg* 53:633, 1980.

81. Chukwedelunzu FE, Brown RD, Wijdicks EFM, et al: Subarachnoid haemorrhage associated with infectious endocarditis: Case report and literature review. *Eur J Neurol* 9:423, 2002.

82. Kumar M, Kitchen ND: Infective and traumatic aneurysms. *Neurosug Clin North Am* 9:577, 1998.

83. Ziment I: Nervous system complications in acute bacterial endocarditis. *Am J Med* 47:593, 1969.

84. Brust JCM, Taylor Dickinson PC, Hughes JEO, et al: The diagnosis and treatment of cerebral mycotic aneurysms. *Ann Neurol* 27:238, 1990.

85. Ojemann RG: Surgical management of bacterial intracranial aneurysms. In Schmideck HH, Sweet WH (eds): *Operative Neurosurgical Techniques, Indications, Methods, and Results.* New York: Grune & Stratton, 1982, p 933.

86. Weir B: Special aneurysms (nonsaccular and saccular). In Brown C, Eckhart C (eds): *Aneurysms Affecting the Nervous System.* Baltimore: Williams & Wilkins, 1987, p 134.

87. Salgado AV: Central nervous system complications of infective endocarditis. *Curr Concepts Cerebrovasc Dis Stroke* 26:19, 1991.

88. Chun JY, Smith W, Halbach VV, et al: Current multimodality management of infectious intracranial aneurysms. *Neurosurgery* 48:1203, 2001.

89. Watanabe A, Hirano K, Ishii R: Cerebral mycotic aneurysm treated with endovascular occlusion: Case report. *Neurol Med Chir (Tokyo)* 38(10):657, 1998.

90. Scotti G, Li MH, Righi C, et al: Endovascular treatment of bacterial intracranial aneurysms. *Neuroradiology* 38(2):186, 1996.

91. Chapot R, Houdart E, Saint-Maurice JP, et al: Endovascular treatment of cerebral mycotic aneurysms. *Radiology* 222(2):389, 2002.

92. Monsuez JJ, Vittecoq D, Rosenbaum A, et al: Prognosis of ruptured intracranial mycotic aneurysms: A review of 12 cases. *Eur Heart J* 10(9):821, 1989.

93. Bohmfalk GL, Bohmfalk GL, Story JL, et al: Bacterial intracranial aneurysm. *J Neurosurg* 48:369, 1978.

94. Corr P, Wright M, Handler LC: Endocarditis-related cerebral aneurysms: Radiologic changes with treatment. *AJNR* 16(4):745, 1995.

95. du Cheyron D, Lesage A, Le Page O, et al: Corticosteroids as adjunctive treatment in Austrian's syndrome (pneumococcal endocarditis, meningitis, and pneumonia): Report of two cases and review of the literature. *J Clin Pathol* 56(11):879, 2003.

96. Govindan S, Itani AL, Garcia JH: Inflammation of the temporal artery associated with subacute bacterial endocarditis and hepatitis B antigen. *Arch Neurol* 37:318, 1980.

97. Igarashi M, Gilmartin RC, Gerald B, et al: Cerebral arteritis and bacterial meningitis. *Arch Neurol* 41:531, 1984.

98. Kanter MC, Hart RG: Neurologic complications of infective endocarditis. *Neurology* 41:1015, 1991.

99. Turtz AR, Yocom SS: Contemporary approaches to the management of neurosurgical complication of infective endocarditis. *Curr Infect Dis Rep* 3:337, 2001.

100. Takeshita M, Kawamata T, Izawa M, et al: Prodromal signs and clinical factors influencing outcome in patients with intraventricular rupture of purulent brain abscess. *Neurosurgery* 48:310, 2001.

101. Jones HR Jr, Siekert RG: Embolic mononeuropathy and bacterial endocarditis. *Arch Neurol* 19:535, 1968.

102. Coronel B, Mercatello A, Couturier J, et al: Polyneuropathy: Potential cause of difficult weaning. *Crit Care Med* 18:486, 1990.

103. Lindner JR: Role of echocardiographic imaging in infective endocarditis. *ACC Curr J Rev* 2002.

104. Erbel R, Rohmann S, Dexler M: Improved diagnostic value of echocardiography in patients with infective endocarditis by transesophageal approach: A prospective study. *Eur Heart J* 1:43, 1988.

105. O'Brien JT, Geiser EA: Infective endocarditis and echocardiography. *Am Heart J* 108:386, 1984.

106. Buda AJ, Zotz RJ, LeMire MS, et al: Prognostic significance of vegetations detected by two-dimensional echocardiography in infective endocarditis. *Am Heart J* 112:1291, 1986.

107. Di Salvo G, Habib G, Pergola V, et al: Echocardiography predicts embolic events in infective endocarditis. *J Am Coll Cardiol* 37:1069, 2001.

108. Lutas EM, Roberts RB, Devereux RB, et al: Relation between the presence of echocardiographic vegetations and complication rate in infective endocarditis. *Am Heart J* 112:107, 1986.

109. Werner M, Andersson R, Olaison L, et al: A clinical study of culture-negative endocarditis. *Medicine* 82(4):263, 2003.

110. Lisby G, Gutschik E, Durack DT: Molecular methods for diagnosis of infective endocarditis. *Infect Dis Clin North Am* 16:393, 2002.

111. Le T, Bayer AS: Combination antibiotic therapy for infective endocarditis. *Clin Infect Dis* 36(5):615, 2003.

112. Sexton DJ, Spelman D: Current best practices and guidelines: Assessment and management of complications in infective endocarditis. *Cardiol Clin* 21(2):273, 2003.

113. Mylonakis E, Calderwood SB: Infective endocarditis in adults. *New Engl J Med* 345:1318, 2001.

114. Sanford JP: *Guide to Antimicrobial Therapy—2004.* West Bethesda, MD: Antimicrobial Therapy, Inc., 2004.

115. Wilson WR, Geraci JE, Danielson GK, et al: Anticoagulant treatment and central nervous system complications in patients with prosthetic valve endocarditis. *Circulation* 57:1004, 1978.

116. Stein PD, Alpert JS, Bussey HI, et al: Antithrombotic therapy in patients with mechanical and biological prosthetic heart valves. *Chest* 119(suppl 1):220S, 2001; erratum in *Chest* 120(3):1044, 2001.

117. Garvey CJ, Neu HC: Infectious endocarditis: An evolving disease. *Medicine* 57:105, 1978.

118. Carpenter JL, McAllister C: Anticoagulation in prosthetic valve endocarditis. *South Med J* 76:1372, 1983.

119. Gillinov AM, Shah RV, Curtis WE, et al: Valve replacement in patients with endocarditis and acute neurologic deficit. *Ann Thorac Surg* 61:1125, 1996.

120. Piper C, Wiemer M, Schulte HD, et al: Stroke is not a contraindication for urgent valve replacement in acute infective endocarditis. *J Heart Valve Dis* 10(6):703, 2001.

CHAPTER 27

Systemic and CNS Toxicities of Antimicrobial Agents

Sherry F. Queener

Antimicrobial agents are among the most widely used drugs in modern medicine, although many of the most useful drugs were developed over 40 years ago. For these older drugs, the purity of available preparations may have changed over time; thus some of the earliest reports of adverse reactions may not reflect the common experience for patients today who receive far purer preparations. In addition, some of the earlier drugs entered clinical use with less extensive clinical trials than what is required today; for these drugs, the most quantitative evidence for adverse reactions may come from later clinical trials where these older agents are used as comparators. For these reasons, the type of clinical evidence and the era in which it was collected are noted in the sections that follow for individual drugs. A thumbnail summary of systemic and CNS adverse effects of each drug class may be found in Table 27-1.

▶ ANTIBACTERIAL AGENTS

β-Lactam Antibiotics

β-Lactam antibiotics used in modern medicine include penicillins, cephalosporins, cephamycins, carbapenems,

carbacephems, and monobactams. The first β-lactams to be used clinically were penicillins. The penicillin preparations used in the earliest clinical trials in England in 1941 were primarily 2-pentenylpenicillin (also called *penicillin F*), but the penicillin produced in America by 1943 was primarily benzylpenicillin (*penicillin G*).[1] These early natural penicillins were mixtures of active compounds that also contained varying degrees of contaminants. The first preparations of penicillin V produced in 1948 also were prepared by direct fermentation, but 10 years later semisynthetic penicillins began to appear. By 1960 with the appearance of methicillin and subsequent semisynthetic penicillins, the purity of the compounds was greatly improved, and it was possible to assess the direct toxicity of the active compounds.

Systemic Adverse Effects

ALLERGIC REACTIONS AND RASHES
The most common adverse reaction to β-lactam antibiotics today is skin rash, with an incidence of up to 10 percent in various modern trials. In a 5-year study of 2488 courses of nafcillin or oxacillin therapy in 99 home care patients, the overall incidence of adverse drug re-

▲ **TABLE 24-1.** SUMMARY OF KEY SYSTEMIC AND CNS ADVERSE EFFECTS

Drug Class	Representatives	Systemic Adverse Effects	CNS Adverse Effects
Antibacterial drugs			
β-Lactams (penicillins and cephalosporins)	Amoxicillin, ampicillin, ceftriaxone, cephalexin, penicillin G, penicillin V	*Common:* Allergic reactions (fever, hives, itching, rash) biliary sludging (ceftriaxone), GI disturbances, superinfections *Infrequent:* Allergic reaction (anaphylaxis), antibiotic-associated colitis, blood dyscrasias, hepatotoxicity, nephritis, phlebitis (IV dosage)	Changes in mental status (procaine penicillin G), seizures
β-Lactams (carbapenems)	Ertapenem, imipenem, meropenem	*Common:* Allergic reactions (fever, hives, itching, rash), GI disturbances, phlebitis (IV dosage), superinfections *Infrequent:* Allergic reactions (anaphylaxis), antibiotic-associated colitis, blood dyscrasias	Agitation, anxiety, confusion, delirium, depression, dizziness, headache, insomnia, seizures, somnolence
Fluoroquinolones	Ciprofloxacin, levofloxacin, gatifloxacin, moxifloxacin, ofloxacin, trovafloxacin	*Common:* Cardiotoxicity, GI disturbances, phototoxicity *Infrequent:* Allergic reactions (anaphylaxis, rashes, Stevens-Johnson syndrome), antibiotic-associated colitis, hepatotoxicity, nephritis, phlebitis (IV dosage), tendonitis	CNS stimulation (agitation, confusion, hallucinations, insomnia, tremors), CNS depression (dizziness, drowsiness, headache, nervousness)
Macrolides	Azithromycin, clarithromycin, dirithromycin, erythromycin	*Common:* GI disturbances, cardiotoxicity, phlebitis (IV dosage), taste perversion *Infrequent:* Allergic reactions (anaphylaxis, rashes), blood dyscrasias, hearing loss, hepatotoxicity, nephritis, pancreatitis	Dizziness, headache (azithromycin) Confusion, hallucinations, psychosis (clarithromycin)
Tetracyclines	Demeclocycline, doxycycline, minocycline, tetracycline	*Common:* GI disturbances, phototoxicity, fungal superinfections (mouth, rectum, tongue, vagina), tooth discoloration (infants or children) *Infrequent:* Hepatotoxicity, nephrogenic diabetes insipidus (demeclocycline), pancreatitis, phlebitis (IV dosage)	Benign intracranial hypertension, bulging fontanel (infants), dizziness, unsteadiness, vestibular impairment (minocycline), visual changes
Glycopeptides	Vancomycin	*Common:* Nephrotoxicity, phlebitis (IV dosage) *Infrequent:* Allergic reactions (rash, "red man syndrome"), ototoxicity	Not reported
Aminoglycosides	Amikacin, gentamicin, kanamycin, streptomycin, tobramycin	*Common:* Hearing loss, nephrotoxicity, ototoxicity (hearing loss), peripheral neuropathy (streptomycin), vestibular disturbances (loss of balance) *Infrequent:* Allergic reactions (itching, rashes), neuromuscular blockade, optic neuritis (streptomycin)	Seizures (more common with concurrent IV and intrathecal dosing)

		Reactions	CNS effects
Acetamide	Chloramphenicol	*Common:* Bone marrow depression (reversible) *Infrequent:* Allergic reactions (fever, rash, shortness of breath), aplastic anemia (potentially fatal), cardiovascular collapse (Gray syndrome), GI disturbances, optic neuritis, peripheral neuropathy	Confusion, delirium, headache
Sulfonamides	Sulfamethoxazole, sulfisoxazole	*Common:* Allergic reactions (fever, itching, rash), GI disturbances, phototoxicity *Infrequent:* Blood dyscrasias, hepatotoxicity, nephrotoxicity (including crystal formation in urine), pancreatitis, thyroid dysfunction, serum sickness	Confusion, dizziness, euphoria, hallucinations, headache, lethargy
Antifolate	Trimethoprim	*Common:* Allergic reactions (anaphylaxis, itching, rash), GI disturbances *Infrequent:* Allergic reactions (erythema multiforme, exfoliative dermatitis, toxic epidermal necrolysis, Stevens–Johnson syndrome), blood dyscrasias, nephrotoxicity, phototoxicity	Aseptic meningitis, confusion, depression, dizziness, headache
Nitroimidazole	Metronidazole	*Common:* GI disturbances, peripheral neuropathy, superinfection (vaginal *Candida*), urinary discoloration *Infrequent:* Carcinogenicity, pancreatitis, taste perversion, thrombophlebitis	Aseptic meningitis, ataxia, dizziness, light-headedness, seizures, syncope
Lincosamine	Clindamycin	*Common:* Antibiotic-associated colitis, GI disturbances, superinfection (rectal, vaginal) *Infrequent:* Allergic reactions (rashes), blood dyscrasias, phlebitis (IV dosage)	Not reported
Streptogramins	Quinupristin/dalfopristin	*Common:* Arthralgia, cardiovascular, GI disturbances, infusion-site reactions, myalgia, thrombophlebitis *Infrequent:* Allergic reactions (itching, rashes)	Anxiety, confusion, dizziness, headache, insomnia
Oxazolidinone	Linezolid	*Common:* GI disturbances *Infrequent:* Allergic reactions (fever, itching, rash), blood dyscrasias, superinfection (oral or vaginal yeast infections)	Dizziness, headache, insomnia
Furantoin	Nitrofurantoin	*Common:* Allergic reactions (angioedema, arthralgia, chills, fever, rashes), GI disturbances, myalgia, pneumonitis *Infrequent:* Allergic reactions (anaphylaxis, erythema multiforme, exfoliative dermatitis, organ dysfunction, Stevens–Johnson syndrome), antibiotic-associated colitis, blood dyscrasias, hepatotoxicity, optic neuritis, pancreatitis, peripheral neuropathy, urinary discoloration	Confusion, dizziness, depression, drowsiness, headache, intracranial hypertension, psychotic reactions

(continued)

▶ **TABLE 24-1.** SUMMARY OF KEY SYSTEMIC AND CNS ADVERSE EFFECTS (*CONTINUED*)

Drug Class	Representatives	Systemic Adverse Effects	CNS Adverse Effects
Quinolones	Nalidixic acid	*Common:* Allergic reactions (rashes), GI disturbances, phototoxicity *Infrequent:* Allergic reactions (anaphylaxis, erythema multiforme, fever, hives, itching, Stevens-Johnson syndrome), antibiotic-associated colitis, blood dyscrasias, cholestatic jaundice, metabolic acidosis	Confusion, disorientation, dizziness, drowsiness, hallucinations, headache, intracranial hypertension, light-headedness, mental status change, restlessness, tremor, seizures, weakness
Antimycobacterial drugs			
Hydrazide	Isoniazid	*Common:* GI disturbances, peripheral neuropathy *Infrequent:* Allergic reactions (rash, lupus-like syndrome, organ dysfunction, vasculitis)	Seizures with high doses; therapy includes pyridoxal-5-phosphate
Rifamycins	Rifabutin, rifampin, rifapentine	*Common:* Allergic reactions (flulike syndrome, itching, rash, redness, organ dysfunction), blood dyscrasias, GI disturbances, nephrotoxicity *Infrequent:* Hepatotoxicity, uveitis	Confusion, dizziness, fatigue, headache, insomnia, mood change
Other first- and second-line TB drugs	Ethambutol, ethionamide, cycloserine, pyrazinamide	*Common:* GI disturbances, peripheral neuropathy, optic neuritis (ethambutol) *Infrequent:* Allergic reactions (fever, itching, rash), hepatotoxicity (pyrazinamide), hyperuricosemia (pyrazinamide and ethambutol)	Anxiety, aphasia, confusion, dizziness, drowsiness, depression, mood change, trembling, seizures, suicidal thoughts
First-line antileprotics	Clofazimine, dapsone, thalidomide	*Common:* Allergic reactions (rash), blood dyscrasias, GI disturbances, peripheral neuropathy, skin discoloration, tetratogenicity (thalidomide) *Infrequent:* Allergic reactions (erythema multiforme, sulfone syndrome), hepatotoxicity	Drowsiness, headache, insomnia, mood change
Antiviral drugs			
NRTI	Abacavir	*Common:* Allergic reactions (dyspnea, fever, rash, swelling), fatigue *Infrequent:* GI disturbances, hepatotoxicity (lactic acidosis), pancreatitis	Headache, insomnia
NRTI	Didanosine	*Common:* Blood dyscrasias, pancreatitis, peripheral neuropathy *Infrequent:* Allergic reactions (chills, fever, itching, rash), cardiomyopathy, GI disturbances, hepatitis, renal depigmentation	Anxiety, headache, insomnia, irritability, seizures
NRTI	Lamivudine	*Common:* Blood dyscrasias, cough, GI disturbances, pancreatitis, myalgia, peripheral neuropathy *Infrequent:* Allergic reaction (rash), alopecia	Dizziness, headache, insomnia
NRTI	Stavudine	*Common:* Blood dyscrasias, peripheral neuropathy	Headache, insomnia

Class	Drug	Systemic toxicity	CNS toxicity
		Infrequent: Allergic reactions (chills, fever, rash), arthralgia, asthenia, GI disturbances, myalgia, pancreatitis	
NRTI	Zalcitabine	*Common:* Peripheral neuropathy *Infrequent:* Allergic reactions (fever, rash), arthralgia, GI disturbances, hepatotoxicity (jaundice, lactic acidosis), myalgia, pancreatitis	Headache
NRTI	Zidovudine	*Common:* Blood dyscrasias (anemia, leukopenia, neutropenia), myalgia *Infrequent:* Bone marrow depression, GI disturbances, hepatotoxicity (lactic acidosis), myopathy, skin discoloration	Headache, confusion, insomnia, mental status change, seizures
NtRTI	Tenofovir	*Common:* GI disturbances *Infrequent:* Hepatotoxicity (lactic acidosis), nephrotoxicity	Not reported
NNRTI	Delavirdine, nevirapine	*Common:* Allergic reactions (fever, itching, rash), blood dyscrasias (nevirapine), GI disturbances *Infrequent:* Arthralgia (delavirdine), myalgia, ulcerative stomatitis	Headache
NNRTI	Efavirenz	*Common:* Allergic reactions (itching, rash), GI disturbances *Infrequent:* Allergic reactions (dyspnea, erythema multiforme, hives, Stevens-Johnson syndrome, ulceration), cardiac dysrhythmias, hematuria, hepatotoxicity, pancreatitis, peripheral neuropathy	Depression, dizziness, dream changes, headache, insomnia, mental function impaired (inability to concentrate), nervousness, psychosis, seizures, somnolence, suicidal thoughts, tremor, vertigo
HIV protease inhibitors	Amprenavir, atazanavir	*Common:* Allergic reactions (rash), GI disturbance, hepatotoxicity (atazanavir), hyperglycemia *Infrequent:* Allergic reactions (Stevens-Johnson syndrome), diabetes mellitus, fat redistribution, peripheral neuropathy, taste perversion (amprenavir)	Depression, mental status changes (amprenavir)
HIV protease inhibitor	Indinavir	*Common:* Asthenia, GI disturbances, nephrotoxicity (renal stones), taste perversion *Infrequent:* Fat redistribution, hyperglycemia, ketoacidosis	Dizziness, headache, insomnia, somnolence
HIV protease inhibitors	Lopinavir, nelfinavir, ritonavir	*Common:* GI disturbances, lipid metabolic changes (elevated cholesterol, triglycerides) *Infrequent:* Asthenia, diabetes mellitus, fat redistribution, hepatotoxicity (lactic acidosis), peripheral neuropathy	Anxiety, dream changes, confusion, mental status changes
HIV protease inhibitor	Saquinavir	*Common:* GI disturbances *Infrequent:* Allergic recations (rash), asthenia, diabetes mellitus (hyperglycemia, ketoacidosis), fat redistribution, peripheral neuropathy	Headache

(continued)

▲ **TABLE 24-1.** SUMMARY OF KEY SYSTEMIC AND CNS ADVERSE EFFECTS (*CONTINUED*)

Drug Class	Representatives	Systemic Adverse Effects	CNS Adverse Effects
Acyclic nucleosides	Acyclovir, adefocir, cidofovir, famiciclovir, ganciclovir, valacyclovir	*Common:* Allergic reactions (fever, itching, rash), blood dyscrasias (rare with acyclovir), GI disturbances, malaise, nephropathy including acute renal failure, thrombophlebitis (IV dosage) *Infrequent:* Allergic reactions (anaphylaxis, erythema multiforme, Stevens-Johnson syndrome, toxic epidermal necrolysis), GI disturbances, visual changes	Agitation, coma, delirium, dizziness, hallucinations, headache, light-headedness, mental status change, psychosis, somnolence, seizures, tremors
Neuraminidase inhibitors	Oseltamivir, zanamivir	*Common:* Allergic recations (facial edema, rash), GI disturbances, pulmonary dysfunction (zanamivir) *Infrequent:* Cardiac dysrhythmias, hepatotoxicity, hyperglycemia	Confusion, seizures
Amines	Amantadine, rimantadine	*Common:* Anticholinergic effects, GI disturbances, peripheral edema *Infrequent:* Cardiotoxicity, eye damage	Agitation, dizziness, headache, inability to concentrate, insomnia, nervousness, nightmares, psychiatric symptoms, seizures, suicide attempts; all more common with amantadine
IMP dehydrogenase inhibitor	Ribavirin	*Common:* Blood dyscrasias, GI disturbances, teratogenicity *Infrequent:* Allergic reactions (rash, redness)	Fatigue, headache, insomnia
Antifungal drugs Polyene	Amphotericin B	*Common:* Blood dyscrasias, fever and chills, GI disturbances, hypotension, nephrotoxicity, pulmonary dysfunction, thrombophlebitis *Infrequent:* Allergic reactions (rash), peripheral neuropathy, visual changes	Headache
Azoles	Fluconazole, itraconazole, ketoconazole, voriconazole	*Common:* GI disturbances, inhibition of steroidogenesis (ketoconazole) *Infrequent:* Allergic reactions, blood dyscrasias, hepatotoxicity, visual changes	Headache, dizziness
Cytosine analogue	Flucytosine	*Common:* Blood dyscrasias, GI disturbances, hepatotoxicity *Infrequent:* Allergic reactions	Not reported
Echinocandin	Caspofungin	*Common:* Allergic reactions (fever), liver enzyme elevation, phlebitis *Infrequent:* Allergic reactions (rash, redness), GI disturbances	Headache

Diamidine	Pentamidine	*Common:* Blood dyscrasias, GI disturbances, hepatotoxicity, hypoglycemia, hypotension, phlebitis, sterile abscesses *Infrequent:* Cardiac dysrhythmias, pulmonary dysfunction (inhalation route)	Anxiety, headache, nervousness, shakiness
Antiprotozoal drugs Aminoquinolones	Chloroquine, hydroxychloroquine, mefloquine, primaquine	*Common:* Eye damage, GI disturbances, skin discoloration *Infrequent:* Blood dyscrasias, hypotension (chloroquine overdose), ototoxicity	Depression, drowsiness, headache, irritability, mood change, seizures
Antimalarials	Atovaquone, proguanil, pyrimethamine	*Common:* Allergic reactions (atovaquone), cough (atovaquone), GI disturbances *Infrequent:* Blood dyscrasias, nephrotoxicity (proguanil)	Headache, insomnia; irritability, seizures (overdose of pyrimethamine)
Antihelminthic drugs First-line drugs	Ivermectin, mebendazole, oxamniquine, praziquantel, thiabendazole	*Common:* Allergies, GI disturbances, mutagenicity (oxamniquine) *Infrequent:* Cardiotoxicity, edema, hepatotoxicity, vision changes	Dizziness, headache, psychiatric symptoms, seizures (mostly with overdose)

actions in patients receiving nafcillin or oxacillin was 31.4 percent, but for those treated with penicillins other than nafcillin and oxacillin, the incidence was 4.1 percent, expressed as a percentage of the courses of therapy administered; for the group treated with nafcillin or oxacillin, rashes comprised about one-third of the total drug-related adverse reactions.[2] A retrospective study of 5923 pediatric patient records from a private-practice setting indicated that 7.4 percent of patients receiving penicillins developed rashes, but for all cephalosporins except cefaclor, the incidence of rashes was only 2.6 percent; in these pediatric patients, the incidence of rashes with cefaclor was 12.3 percent.[3] In an earlier study, the records of 15,438 consecutive medical inpatients were evaluated for evidence of cutaneous allergic reactions; in this study, the percentage of patients reacting to drugs was 2.1 percent for semisynthetic penicillins or cephalosporins, 1.8 percent for penicillin G, 3.3 percent for ampicillin, and 5.1 percent for amoxicillin.[4]

Interpretation of the studies reporting allergies to β-lactam antibiotics is clouded by the occurrence of rashes that may not be related to hypersensitivity reactions. The best documented cause of these apparently nonallergic rashes is exposure to the aminopenicillins ampicillin and amoxicillin. Ampicillin-induced rashes have been reported in 3 to 9.5 percent of treated patients in most studies,[5,6] but the incidence of these rashes may be dose-related. Studies in which patients received only 1 g daily of ampicillin showed a 4 percent incidence of rash, but doses of up to 3 g daily produced an incidence of 7 percent, and doses of 4 to 6 g daily produced a 22 percent incidence of rash.[6] Aminopenicillin-induced rashes often clear even while the drug therapy is continued, and the rash usually is not influenced by corticosteroid therapy, which differs from the course of a typical allergic rash. The aminopenicillin-specific rash also usually appears later in the course of therapy (around 5 days is the median time), and it is usually associated with less irritation or pruritus than typical allergic rashes. There is some evidence that rather than being mediated by IgE, reactions to aminopenicillins and rarely to other β-lactams such as ceftriaxone may involve T-cell mechanisms.[7,8] An additional complication with aminopenicillins is that the incidence of rash is very high when the drugs are used in patients with Epstein-Barr virus, cytomegalovirus, or lymphocytic leukemia.[5] The implication to be derived from these and many similar studies is that the appearance of an aminopenicillin-induced rash is not a good predictor of future IgE-mediated immediate allergic reactions to penicillins or other β-lactam antibiotics.

Early preparations of natural penicillins contained contaminants that caused a high incidence of fever, chills, and other allergic reactions.[1] Increasing purity of the clinical preparations reduced but did not eliminate all allergic reactions to this class of drugs because the mechanism producing many allergic reactions is directly related to the antibacterial mechanism; the same chemically labile β-lactam bond that is responsible for reacting with the bactericidal target transpeptidase is also involved with acylating other proteins that, in turn, act as haptens to generate an immunologic response to the drugs. With penicillins, this mechanism produces the so-called major antigens, the penicilloyl protein derivatives.

Less common determinants (also called *minor determinants*) of hypersensitivity to penicillins include a penicillanyl derivative that can be formed by amide bond formation between the free amino group of an amino acid within a protein and the carboxylic acid of the thiazolidine ring of the penicillin molecule.[9] A chemical rearrangement facilitated by the opening of both the β-lactam ring and the thiazolidine ring of the penicillin structure yields a penicillenate derivative linked through sulfhydryl bonds to a protein; this structure is also a minor determinant of hypersensitivity. Cephalosporins generate an even more diverse group of major and minor determinants because of the increased chemical complexity of the cephalosporin molecule.[9] Both the minor and major determinants are capable of producing serious or fatal reactions. Because these various reactions depend on the chemical nature of the individual β-lactam antibiotic administered, the purity of the preparation, and the variability of metabolism within each patient, it is difficult to assess population data to determine the mechanisms of allergic reactions with this class of drugs.

Skin testing with major and minor determinants has been reported to be of value in predicting who would be at risk for a fatal type I IgE-mediated allergic reaction to a β-lactam antibiotic when the tests are used with care.[5,10] Because patients tend to overreport penicillin allergy, a careful clinical history should be taken to help identify a true penicillin allergy.[5,11] Skin testing shows that up to 90 percent of persons who self-report a penicillin allergy do not have IgE antibodies for penicillin and may receive penicillins safely. Patients who have a positive skin test for penicillin allergy are likely to react to carbapenems as well as penicillins and should not receive either of these drugs. Cross-reactivity with other β-lactam antibiotics is less clear.

It has been suggested that patients with a history of penicillin allergy but a negative skin test for penicillins can receive cephalosporins safely,[10] provided they have not reacted previously to a cephalosporin. Patients who have a clinical history of a hypersensitivity reaction to a cephalosporin but a negative skin test to penicillin also have been treated successfully with penicillins. Generalizations about cross-reactivity between penicillins and cephalosporins cannot be made easily because the antibodies produced in patients may be generated to many different parts of these molecules. Antibodies generated to common portions of the ring systems will, of course, be cross-reactive, but antibodies generated to specific portions of the side chains will not react to β-lactams with other types of side chains. However, it must be remembered that some penicillins and cephalosporins share the same side chains. For example, ampicillin and cephalexin contain the same D-α-aminobenzyl side chain. Likewise, amoxicillin and cephadroxil contain the same *para*-hydroxy-D-α-aminobenzyl side chain. Thus antibodies generated to either of these side chains would react to both the related penicillins and the cephalosporins. These considerations point out the difficulties in predicting cross-reactivity in the clinical setting, where the specificity of the antibody generated in a patient is seldom known. A practical skin test to predict cephalosporin allergy has not been developed.

Serious allergic reactions, including anaphylaxis, occur much less often than rashes with β-lactam antibiotics. One study based on early clinical data suggested that the incidence of anaphylaxis was between 0.04 and 0.015 percent, with the greatest risk for adults aged 20 to 49 years.[12] The incidence of anaphylaxis is higher in patients who have positive skin tests for penicillin allergy when they are challenged with other penicillins[5] or with cephalosporins.[10] An international study with 1090 patients suggested that relatively well patients who were receiving monthly benzathine penicillin G injections to prevent rheumatic heart disease developed allergies at expected rates (3.2 percent), but the incidence of anaphylaxis was 0.2 percent[13]; one patient in this study died of anaphylaxis, generating a fatality rate of 0.05 percent. Penicillins have been reported to be the most common cause of drug-related fatal cases of anaphylaxis in the United States, with an estimated overall rate of 0.002 percent.[14] One study suggested that anaphylaxis was underreported for the period between 1992 and 1997 in the United Kingdom.[15] This report also included disturbing evidence that about half the previously unreported deaths occurred in patients who were known to be allergic to penicillin or amoxicillin and who died immediately on receiving a dose of cephalosporin intended as a substitute. These results reinforce the need for physicians to be highly cautious about cross-reactivity within the entire β-lactam family of drugs.

GASTROINTESTINAL (GI) DISTURBANCES AND SUPERINFECTIONS

Diarrhea, nausea, or vomiting may occur with any oral β-lactam antibiotic, as well as with some parenteral drugs. The mechanism often involves changes in the bacterial flora of the GI tract. Thus drugs with a broader spectrum, such as ampicillin or the cephalosporins, are more likely to produce these effects. The most serious form of GI disturbance is antibiotic-associated colitis, or

pseudomembranous colitis. This potentially fatal reaction occurs as a result of superinfection with *Clostridium difficile*, a β-lactam-resistant organism that produces a toxin that damages the intestinal epithelium. Although superinfection with *C. difficile* is relatively rare, up to 10 percent of patients receiving third-generation cephalosporins or imipenem may develop some form of secondary infection from resistant bacteria or yeast.

LOCAL INJECTION-SITE REACTIONS

Phlebitis or thrombophlebitis is a concentration-related adverse reaction with cephalosporins, nafcillin, or occasionally, other β-lactams administered intravenously. Symptoms include severe pain along the vein, redness, and swelling. Rarely, thrombi form along the inflamed vein. Strict adherence to the guidelines for diluting the drugs and for controlling rates of administration greatly lessen the incidence of this reaction.

NEPHROTOXICITY

Nephritis was an adverse reaction most closely linked with the now discontinued drug methicillin, but renal effects can be observed rarely with other β-lactam antibiotics. At high concentrations, some cephalosporins can damage renal tubular epithelium, but the effect is usually mild and reversible.

HEPATOTOXICITY

Jaundice and cholestasis linked to penicillin therapy is associated most often with the antistaphylococcal drugs. The incidences of hepatotoxicity with cloxacillin and dicloxacillin are reported in a modern Swedish study at 1.3 and 0.75 cases per million daily doses, respectively.[16] Flucloxacillin, another antistaphylococcal penicillin used in Australia and in Europe but not the United States, has a higher incidence of hepatotoxicity, which is reportedly greater in patients over 55 years of age.[17] Reports of hepatotoxicity with nafcillin are relatively rare.[18]

BILIARY DYSFUNCTION

Ceftriaxone therapy has been associated with biliary sludging in up to 43 percent of patients receiving the drug for long periods. The cause is thought to be a high concentration of relatively insoluble calcium-ceftriaxone complexes. In patients with sludging, about one-third will have biliary colic, but sludging typically resolves when the drug is discontinued.[19]

BLOOD DYSCRASIAS

Hypoprothrombinemia is linked most often to a subset of cephalosporins that contain the *N*-methyl-thiotetrazole side chain, i.e., cefamandole, cefmetazole, cefoperazone, and cefotetan. Other cephalosporins or broad-spectrum β-lactams such as carbenicillin, piperacillin, and ticarcillin also may prolong prothrombin time because they inhibit the intestinal bacteria that produce vitamin K. Eosinophilia also has been reported, especially with third-generation cephalosporins.

CNS Adverse Effects

INCIDENCE OF CNS EFFECTS

CNS effects of penicillins were reported in the early clinical trials of these drugs.[20] During this era, much of the therapy for bacterial meningitis involved intrathecal administration of the antibiotic because it was feared that the penicillins penetrated inadequately into the CNS when the drugs were administered intravenously. Occasional convulsions, irritability, meningeal irritation, and vomiting were observed with intrathecal administration of 3000 to 5000 units of penicillin in early trials for therapy of meningitis.[21] Increasing doses increased the likelihood and the severity of seizure activity with the intrathecal route. Muscular twitching and generalized seizure activity were reported with intrathecal doses of 200,000 to 500,000 units, as well as fatalities.[22,23] Penicillin itself was recognized as the convulsive agent in the antibiotic preparations being used in this way.[24]

Intravenously administered modern preparations of penicillins and cephalosporins are also associated with a significant risk of neurotoxicity. Symptoms range from agitation, confusion, dizziness, hallucinations, myoclonus, or nystagmus to seizures.[25] Although such symptoms have been associated with all β-lactam antibiotics, the highest incidence is with the carbapenems, including imipenem/cilastatin.[26] This outcome was noted in the summary of the phase I/III trials with imipenem/cilastatin, in which the frequency of seizures was 0.2 percent.[27] A more recent study that carefully controlled dosing and excluded patients with known risk factors for neurotoxicity still showed a relatively high incidence of seizures with either imipenem/cilastatin (0.38 percent) or with the newest carbapenem, meropenem (0.43 percent).[28]

MECHANISMS OF CNS EFFECTS

β-Lactam antibiotics cause excitability in the CNS by interfering with the function of γ-aminobutyric acid (GABA) A receptors, the most prevalent inhibitory regulator in the CNS. The result of inhibition of this system is that the natural inhibitory action of GABA is lost, and the tissue becomes more excitable and thus prone to seizure activity.[25,26,29,30] The level of inhibition produced by these antibiotics depends on the amount of drug that reaches the tissue.

Several studies have focused on identifying mechanisms of uptake and efflux of β-lactam antibiotics in the CNS. At least two processes are involved: direct movement of drug across the endothelial cells comprising the blood-brain barrier and active transport systems in the choroid plexus. As weak organic acids, most β-lactam antibiotics do not cross the blood-brain barrier very effectively. The more lipid-soluble members of the class, such as ceftriaxone or celsulodin, penetrate brain tissue more effectively than penicillin G, and a facilitated transport mechanism has been suggested.[31] A monocarboxylic acid transporter also has been offered as a possible mechanism.[32] Other studies using brain capillary endothelial cells in vitro failed to find evidence for carrier-mediated transport of penicillin G.[33] Likewise, there was no evidence that di- or tripeptide transporters for β-lactam antibiotics existed at the blood-brain barrier.[34] Whatever mechanisms turn out to be involved, it is clear that the efficiency of the uptake of β-lactam antibiotics across the blood-brain barrier in humans without infection is low.

The active transport systems in the choroid plexus are pumps that recognize weak organic acids and thus move β-lactam antibiotics from the cerebrospinal fluid (CSF) to the blood. This pump mechanism, unlike the putative transport mechanisms operating at the blood-brain barrier, has a high capacity and acts rapidly. Thus any β-lactam antibiotic that diffuses or is transported into the CNS ultimately is exposed to this robust export system and removed from the CSF, but not all β-lactam antibiotics have the same affinity for this export system. For example, ceftriaxone is a poor substrate for the organic acid pump in the choroid plexus and therefore achieves and maintains higher CNS tissue levels than penicillin G.[35]

RISK FACTORS FOR CNS ADVERSE REACTIONS

The most important risk factor for serious neurotoxicity with β-lactam antibiotics is a high concentration of drug in the brain.[25] As described earlier, these concentrations are low for most patients (usually 1 to 5 percent of serum levels) because of the relative impermeability of the blood-brain barrier to the drugs and the active transport of the drugs from CSF by the pumps in the choroid plexus. Despite these mechanisms, however, some patients develop very high levels of drug in the brain. In one study, three patients who developed seizures following intravenous doses of penicillin were evaluated for levels of drug at various sites.[36] The concentrations of penicillin in ventricular and cisternal fluids ranged from 74 to 221 mg/liter, which was well above both serum levels and the levels found in lumbar CSF. Thus the results of tests on fluid obtained by lumbar puncture may not necessarily reflect the exposure of brain tissue to the epileptogenic drug.

The mechanisms that may lead to high blood levels of these drugs have been explored in several studies. The most obvious is the dose of the drug. When high doses are given for prolonged periods, entry of the antibiotics into the CNS is promoted, and neurotoxicity may result. This effect has been well documented for imipenem/cilastatin in a study that was designed to intervene before physicians exceeded the recommended doses; under these conditions, the frequency of seizures was 0.2 percent. In contrast, in two studies in which dosages were not monitored, the frequency of seizures ranged from 3 to 6 percent, with an overall incidence of neurotoxicity of 11 percent.[37,38] Not only the total dose but also the dose relative to body weight is a factor determining the risk of neurotoxicity. For imipenem, doses above 4 g daily (or above 50 mg/kg) are not recommended. Meropenem is recommended at doses up to 6 g daily.

Another clear risk factor for neurotoxicity is impaired renal function.[25,29,30,39] Impaired renal function may contribute in several ways to altered pharmacokinetics of β-lactam antibiotics in the CNS. First, impaired renal function can elevate blood levels of the drug to higher than expected concentrations, driving drug into the brain. For this reason, dosages of most parenterally administered β-lactam antibiotics are adjusted based on creatinine clearance for individual patients; exceptions include nafcillin and ceftriaxone, drugs that are excreted primarily by biliary mechanisms. Uremia not only impairs the mechanisms for excreting drug from the body, but uremia also may lower protein binding of drugs, resulting in a higher proportion of unbound drug, which also facilitates entry into tissues. Second, uremia may increase the permeability of the blood-brain barrier itself, allowing a more extensive passage of drug from the blood into the brain tissue. Finally, the accumulation of organic acids in uremia may interfere with the pump mechanisms in the choroid plexus, with the result that export of the β-lactams may be impaired. Any or all of these factors may contribute to elevated concentrations of β-lactams in the brain and thus to neurotoxicity.

In addition, there are several other risk factors for neurotoxicity. For instance, increasing age has been suggested to increase the risk. It is not known to what degree decreasing renal function with age contributes to this correlation. Another factor identified in several studies is a history of previous CNS injury or disease.[25,39] Brain tumors, CNS radiation therapy, cerebral edema, and bacterial endotoxins or exotoxins are all known to increase permeability of the blood-brain barrier, which may increase entry of small molecules into the CNS. Hyperosmotic agents and organic acids used as contrast media also may affect the blood-brain barrier.

Fluoroquinolone Antibiotics

Fluoroquinolones began to appear in the 1980s but are related to older agents such as nalidixic acid. The key to the high antibacterial potency of the modern drugs is the fluorine substituent on the 6-position of the quinolone ring. The modern drugs generally are well tolerated, but some general and some serious drug-specific adverse reactions have been documented.

Systemic Adverse Effects

GI DISTURBANCES
GI disturbances are the most common adverse reaction reported for fluoroquinolones, with an incidence as high as 20 percent.[40] Anorexia, dyspepsia, and nausea are the most common symptoms, but abdominal discomfort, diarrhea, taste perversion, and vomiting also occur.

CARDIOTOXICITY
Prolongation of the corrected QT (QT_c) interval was noted in early clinical trials with both sparfloxacin and the now discontinued drug grepafloxacin. About 1.2 to 3 percent of patients who receive sparfloxacin have a prolongation of the QT_c interval that can be clinically significant, and the reaction may be dose-related.[40] Compromise of the cardiovascular system has been reported only rarely. The greatest significance of this potential adverse reaction is in creating the possibility for drug interactions; sparfloxacin should not be used with other drugs that cause bradycardia or additional prolongation of the QT_c interval. Levofloxacin rarely has been associated with adverse cardiac signs.

PHOTOTOXICITY
Fluoroquinolone antibiotics have the potential of generating free radicals when exposed to ultraviolet (UV) irradiation.[41] These reactive radicals may promote inflammation in skin exposed to sunlight or other sources of UV light. Phototoxic reactions are most likely with lomefloxacin and sparfloxacin, with incidence rates of around 2 percent.[40–42] Postmarketing surveillance suggests that phototoxic reactions are very rare with levofloxacin.[43]

ALLERGIC REACTIONS
Overall, allergic skin reactions occur with an incidence of less than 2 percent with the fluoroquinolones, although phototoxic reactions are relatively common (see preceding subsection); anaphylaxis has been observed in roughly 1 patient per 100,000.[40] Very rarely, a serious reaction, such as Stevens-Johnson syndrome or hypersensitivity vasculitis, has been reported. In an Italian study that evaluated 10,011 adverse drug reactions reported between January 1999 and December 2001, ciprofloxacin most often produced skin reactions (excluding phototoxicity); ciprofloxacin was also the only fluoroquinolone associated with Stevens-Johnson syndrome in this study.[42]

SUPERINFECTIONS

Antibiotic-associated colitis has been mentioned only rarely in clinical trials with fluoroquinolones. This class of antibiotics has less effect on anaerobic bacteria than do the β-lactams and therefore may cause less disruption of normal intestinal flora, decreasing the risk of overgrowth of *C. difficile*.

NEPHROTOXICITY

The risk for renal compromise is low with fluoroquinolones. A few serious reactions have been reported, but most were in older patients.[40] Crystallization in urine is possible for fluoroquinolones because the solubility of the drugs depends on pH. Under normal conditions, the fluoroquinolones remain soluble in the acidic pH of urine, but the fluoroquinolones are less soluble as the pH rises. Therefore, alkalinization of the urine should be avoided while patients are treated with these drugs, and water intake should be adequate to support an ample urine volume.

HEPATOTOXICITY

Hepatotoxicity evidenced by altered liver function tests is variable among the fluoroquinolones. Levofloxacin rarely causes increases in hepatic transaminase values, but sparfloxacin and ciprofloxacin may alter these values in 2 to 3 percent of patients. Trovafloxacin is the fluoroquinolone most likely to cause abnormalities in liver function. According to the manufacturer, the drug causes significant but asymptomatic increases in hepatic transaminase values in 9 percent of patients receiving the drug for 28 days or longer. Serious symptomatic liver toxicity, as well as acute pancreatitis, has been reported with trovafloxacin as more clinical experience has been gained with the drug. Patients receiving trovafloxacin should be monitored carefully for signs of liver dysfunction.

LOCAL INJECTION-SITE REACTIONS

Phlebitis and pain at the site of intravenous injections occurs with ciprofloxacin and ofloxacin.

CARTILAGE DAMAGE OR TENDON RUPTURE

In early evaluations of long-term toxicity of fluoroquinolones, young beagle dogs were noted to have altered gaits. Subsequent evaluation revealed that the drugs caused lesions within the cartilage in weight-bearing joints. Various studies report that about 1 percent of young adult humans receiving fluoroquinolones suffer arthopathy with pain, stiffness, or swelling of joints. Tendinitis or actual rupture of a tendon may occur. The incidence of this adverse reaction is difficult to assess fully but is thought to be about 1 in 100,000 patients. The risk is highest in those older than 50 years of age or in patients who are also receiving glucocorticoids. The fluoroquinolone that produced the highest incidence of musculoskeletal symptoms and serious tendon damage in a recent Italian study was levofloxacin.[42]

CNS Adverse Effects

INCIDENCE OF CNS EFFECTS

CNS effects are the second most common complaint of patients taking the fluoroquinolones; only GI disturbances are more common with these drugs.[40] Any of the fluoroquinolones may cause CNS effects, but the incidence seems lowest with levofloxacin (0.2 to 1.1 percent) or sparfloxacin (1.1 to 2.9 percent) and highest with trovafloxacin (3 to 11 percent).[44] The most common CNS adverse reaction with modern fluoroquinolones is headache, which usually appears on the first day of therapy. In addition, agitation, confusion, delirium, dizziness, drowsiness, insomnia, and psychosis have been noted. Seizures occur rarely but can occur with any member of the fluoroquinolone group.[40,45]

MECHANISMS OF CNS EFFECTS

Like the β-lactams, fluoroquinolones appear to block binding of GABA to the GABA-A receptors in the CNS.[46,47] Without the inhibitory action of GABA acting through the GABA-A receptors, the CNS is rendered more excitable and prone to seizure activity. Some studies also have suggested direct action of certain fluoroquinolones at receptors for excitatory amino acids (e.g., N-methyl-D-aspartate receptors) in the CNS.[48,49]

RISK FACTORS FOR CNS ADVERSE REACTIONS

In early clinical trials with ciprofloxacin, the concurrent use of the antibiotic with theophylline was associated with an increased risk of CNS adverse reactions. More recent studies suggest that simultaneous use of nonsteroidal anti-inflammatory drugs (NSAIDs) with fluoroquinolones increases the risk of CNS effects.[43,48]

As with other classes of antibiotics, the concentration of fluoroquinolone in the brain is related to toxicity. The concentration of drug in the brain depends on the dose administered and the lipophilicity of the drug, but the most important determinants of brain tissue concentration may be various efflux pumps active at the blood-brain barrier.[50] Well-known systems such as P-glycoprotein and multidrug-resistance-associated protein 1 recognize fluoroquinolones, such as sparfloxacin, and move this relatively lipid-soluble compound from brain back to blood. Levofloxacin is more water soluble and diffuses less readily into the brain, which may explain the relatively low incidence of CNS reactions with levofloxacin.

Macrolide Antibiotics

Macrolides were introduced into clinical medicine in the 1950s with the discovery of erythromycin and related agents that contain a complex 14-member substituted heterocyclic ring. The newer drugs of this class (azithromycin, clarithromycin, dirithromycin) have a broader clinical use and a different pattern of adverse reactions.

Systemic Adverse Effects

GI DISTURBANCES

Abdominal cramps, diarrhea, nausea, and vomiting are the most common adverse reactions to erythromycin, occurring in 15 to 20 percent of patients.[51] The adverse reactions are dose-related. Stomach acid causes erythromycin, but not clarithromycin or azithromycin, to form a hemiketal that is highly irritating to the GI tract. In addition, erythromycin is an agonist at motilin receptors. Both these actions stimulate intestinal motility. The new macrolides cause some of the same symptoms, but the incidence seems to be lower with these drugs. For example, in phase II and III trials with clarithromycin, the incidence of nausea, diarrhea, and abdominal pain was 3.8, 3.0, and 1.9 percent, respectively.[52] Clarithromycin also causes taste perversion in about 3 percent of patients.

CARDIOTOXICITY

Erythromycin administered intravenously prolongs the QT and QT_c intervals.[53] Reports based on the Food and Drug Administration (FDA) MEDWATCH database show that women are twice as likely as men to suffer a life-threatening ventricular arrhythmia following intravenous infusion of erythromycin lactobionate.[54,55] Prolongation of the QT interval, ventricular tachycardia, and torsades de pointes also occur with other macrolides.[56]

Macrolide effects on cardiac physiology have been well studied in attempts to explain the proarrythmogenic effects of the drug class. In particular, erythromycin blocks cardiac potassium channels, including the rapidly activating delayed rectifier current. This action prolongs the transmembrane action potential, which, in turn, is reflected in the prolonged QT interval. The gender difference in susceptibility to this adverse reaction may be related to a gender difference in expression of affected potassium channels.[54]

HEPATOTOXICITY

Erythromycin in various formulations has been linked to hepatotoxicity, although this is uncommon. The reactions have been described as cholestasis but also may resemble viral hepatitis or acute pancreatitis. Hepatox-icity with clarithromycin or azithromycin is less common than with erythromycin. Among the erythromycins, the lauryl salt of erythromycin propionate (erythromycin estolate) is the most common cause of hepatotoxicity. Erythromycin propionate is directly toxic to liver cells, but hepatotoxic reactions to this drug are now thought to have an allergic component as well.[57]

ALLERGIC REACTIONS

Allergic reactions to macrolides develop in less than 3 percent of patients.[58] Rash and eosinophilia are the expected reactions with erythromycin therapy, but anaphylaxis is also possible.[59] Immediate allergic reactions also have been reported with clarithromycin.[60] Skin testing is not helpful in predicting or explaining allergic reactions in most patients.

Hypersensitivity reactions with the macrolides may produce symptoms of organ toxicity, such as interstitial nephritis or hepatitis.[61,62] The allergic component of these reactions has not been well characterized but is suggested by the immediate return of symptoms on rechallenge with the macrolide that caused the original reaction.

LOCAL INJECTION-SITE REACTIONS

Erythromycin and other macrolides cause local tissue irritation. Thus intravenous administration of macrolides may lead to thrombophlebitis starting at the injection site. The drugs should be diluted carefully and administered by slow infusion according to the manufacturers' instructions because tissue irritation is concentration-dependent. The drugs should never be given by intramuscular injection.

OTOTOXICITY

Erythromycin has been associated with transient deafness in rare patients. This reaction is correlated with a high plasma concentration, usually exceeding 12 μg/ml. These levels are unlikely to be achieved except when daily doses of over 4 g are used in patients with renal or hepatic function impaired by age or disease. The reaction is usually reversible when the drug is discontinued.

PANCREATITIS

Pancreatitis is an uncommon adverse reaction to erythromycin.

CNS Adverse Effects

INCIDENCE OF CNS EFFECTS

CNS effects are rare with macrolides. Dizziness and headache have been reported with azithromycin; headache was reported in 1.7 percent of patients receiving clarithromycin.[52] More serious CNS reactions such as confusion, hallucinations, and psychosis were reported with clarithromycin use in the United Kingdom.[63] Clarithromycin also was identified as the antimicrobial agent most commonly associated with drug-induced mania.[64]

MECHANISMS OF CNS EFFECTS

At high concentrations, macrolide antibiotics may inhibit glutamate neurotransmission in the CNS. It has been hypothesized that this action may contribute to psychotic reactions.

RISK FACTORS FOR CNS ADVERSE REACTIONS

The primary risk factor for CNS effects with macrolides is concomitant administration of other drugs that interact with the CYP3A drug metabolism system in the liver. In one report, a neuropsychiatric reaction was tentatively linked to the accumulation of high levels of an active metabolite of clarithromycin; the accumulation may have been caused by nevirapine, a well-known inducer of CYP3A.[63]

Tetracycline Antibiotics

Tetracyclines were important broad-spectrum drugs when they were introduced in the late 1940s, but by the 1970s, overuse of the class had led to the development of widespread resistance. Other broad-spectrum drugs such as cephalosporins and extended-spectrum penicillins largely replaced tetracyclines for bacterial infections. The introduction of doxycycline and minocycline rejuvenated interest in the class because these newer, more lipophilic drugs had very different pharmacokinetics and resistance patterns than the older agents.

Systemic Adverse Effects

GI DISTURBANCES

As a class, the tetracyclines are irritative to the GI tract, commonly producing symptoms of cramping, diarrhea, heartburn, nausea, or vomiting. Dosage instructions for demeclocycline, oxytetracycline, and tetracycline advise taking these drugs with a full glass of water to avoid the risk of esophageal ulceration. Taking the drugs with food reduces GI symptoms but also reduces absorption, especially of the older drugs; doxycycline and minocycline may be taken with food with less effect on absorption.

SUPERINFECTIONS

As classic broad-spectrum antibiotics, the tetracyclines eliminate many components of the normal bacterial flora of the human body, increasing the risk of superinfections. Yeast infections of the oropharynx, vagina, and bowel are relatively common. Changes in intestinal flora contribute to diarrhea caused by these drugs.

Staphylococcal enterocolitis and pseudomembranous colitis caused by toxins from *C. difficile* are life-threatening conditions occasionally caused by tetracyclines.

PHOTOTOXICITY

Demeclocycline and doxycycline commonly cause phototoxic reactions resembling an exaggerated sunburn, as well as tingling sensations in skin exposed to sunlight. Other tetracyclines also may cause this effect, but the incidence is lower. Hyperpigmentation of the skin or mucous membranes is relatively common with minocycline when this drug is used at high doses for a year or longer. The mechanism of this reaction is unrelated to sensitivity to sunlight.

BONES AND TEETH

Tetracyclines strongly chelate calcium and thus bind avidly to the matrix of bones and teeth. When the drug is incorporated into teeth, it produces a permanent yellow discoloration that over time with exposure to sunlight may darken. Enamel formation also may be impaired in some children. This property has led to the precaution of limiting the ordinary use of tetracyclines to children older than 8 years and avoiding use in women who are breast-feeding because the drugs distribute into milk.

Tetracyclines also bind to bone and remain after therapy. The deposited bands of fluorescent drug in the bone have been used to assess bone growth in both fetuses and adults.[65,66] Some older reports suggest that long-bone growth may be depressed in premature infants exposed to tetracyclines, at least partially caused by the antianabolic effects of the drugs.[67]

NEPHROTOXICITY

Tetracyclines inhibit protein synthesis in some mammalian tissues and thus have an antianabolic effect that may create a negative nitrogen balance. As protein synthesis declines, the production of urea increases as amino acids are degraded. In patients with compromised renal function, tetracycline, oxytetracycline, or demeclocycline may accumulate to toxic levels, further damaging the kidneys.

Demeclocycline is associated with nephrogenic diabetes insipidus, with increased urine output. This reaction depends on the dose of drug and usually is reversible. Fanconi syndrome, associated with amino aciduria, glycosuria, hypocalcemia, and proteinuria, was reported in the earlier literature but is uncommon with modern preparations of tetracyclines.[68]

HEPATOTOXICITY

Jaundice or liver failure is rare in most patient populations treated with tetracyclines, but the risk increases in pregnant women or postpartum women with renal impairment. The drug-induced fatty liver degeneration can be rapidly fatal. For this reason, as well as to prevent changes in bones and teeth of the fetus, tetracyclines usually are avoided in the last half of pregnancy.

LOCAL INJECTION-SITE REACTIONS

Tetracyclines must be diluted properly and administered at rates recommended by the manufacturer in order to avoid phlebitis. Doxycycline and minocycline are administered by slow intravenous infusion and are not injected intramuscularly. A preparation of oxytetracycline for intramuscular injection includes 2% lidocaine to offset the intense pain and burning of tissues exposed to high concentrations of the drug.

PANCREATITIS

Pancreatitis is an uncommon adverse reaction to tetracyclines.

CNS Adverse Effects

INCIDENCE OF CNS EFFECTS

Diplopia, headache, nausea, or vomiting caused by increased intracranial pressure may occur rarely with tetracyclines. The syndrome has been called *benign intracranial hypertension* or *pseudotumor cerebri*. In infants, the only sign is usually a bulging fontanelle. Intracranial pressure returns to normal when the drug is discontinued, but permanent visual damage may occur if the syndrome is not recognized and the intracranial pressure reduced promptly.

Minocycline has been associated with vestibular impairment, producing symptoms of ataxia, dizziness, and vertigo. Minocycline is the only tetracycline that causes this adverse reaction.

MECHANISM OF CNS EFFECTS

The mechanism by which tetracyclines may elevate intracranial pressure is unknown.[69]

RISK FACTORS FOR CNS ADVERSE REACTIONS

Intracranial hypertension produced by tetracyclines is now known to be possible in any age group and in both sexes, although the syndrome was first recognized in infants.[69–71]

Vancomycin

Vancomycin is a glycopeptide antibiotic that was discovered nearly 50 years ago but recently has become an important tool to treat infections caused by resistant enterococci. Vancomycin is an example of a drug where formulations have changed over the long course of its clinical use, and modern preparations cause fewer adverse reactions than reported in the early literature. The first preparations used in the 1950s actually were dark brown and cloudy, earning the drug the nickname "Mississippi mud."[72]

Systemic Adverse Effects

NEPHROTOXICITY

Nephrotoxicity remains one of the most commonly reported reactions to vancomycin, with incidence rates from 8 to 11 percent.[72,73] The nephrotoxicity is generally asymptomatic and self-limiting. The appearance or degree of nephrotoxicity has not correlated well with peak serum concentrations of the drug, but trough levels above 10 μg/ml were associated with a greater risk.[72,74] Patients who were more seriously ill (i.e., had a higher APACHE score) also had a greater risk of nephrotoxicity with vancomycin.[72]

The risk of nephrotoxicity with vancomycin is greatly increased by coadministration of other nephrotoxic drugs. For example, 36 percent of cancer patients who received vancomycin with amphotericin B, aminoglycosides, cyclosporine, or cisplatin developed nephrotoxicity compared with 8 percent of patients who received no other nephrotoxic drugs combined with vancomycin.[72] Specific examples of synergistic toxicity also may include β-lactam antibiotics. An outbreak of acute renal failure among heart surgery patients was linked to an antibiotic regimen of vancomycin plus cefodizime.[75] Nephrotoxicity was detected in 50 percent of patients receiving vancomycin-cefodizime, but in that same facility the combination of vancomycin and ceftriaxone had a lower rate of nephrotoxicity, similar to the 8 percent expected. The cause of this synergistic toxicity was attributed to the potential of both cefodizime and vancomycin to induce acute tubular necrosis by effects on the tubular epithelium. Cefodizime is a third-generation cephalosporin not currently available in the United States, but other renally excreted cephalosporins have the same potential for renal tubular damage at high concentrations; ceftriaxone is excreted primarily by nonrenal mechanisms.

LOCAL INJECTION-SITE REACTIONS

Phlebitis remains a risk for patients receiving vancomycin but is highly dependent on how the drug is administered. Overall, 3 percent of cancer patients receiving vancomycin along with chemotherapy developed phlebitis, but the highest incidence was in patients who received vancomycin for longer than 1 week and who received the drug through a peripheral long line as opposed to a subclavian, jugular, or femoral line.[72]

ALLERGIC REACTIONS

Modern preparations of vancomycin cause fewer allergic reactions than reported in the earlier literature. For example, in a study of 742 cancer patients, rashes developed in 18 percent of patients who received vancomycin with a β-lactam antibiotic but appeared in only 1 percent of patients who received vancomycin with aminoglycosides, a class of agents with a much lower allergic potential than the β-lactam class.[72]

Rapid intravenous infusion of vancomycin produces intense flushing of the face, neck, or trunk. This reaction has been called "red neck" or "red man." Its development may be related in part to general histamine release induced by the drug. However, the reaction is prevented by slowing the rate of infusion. Only 1 percent of cancer patients receiving vancomycin developed this reaction; patients who developed this reaction were retreated without incident by increasing the infusion time from 1 hour to 2 to 3 hours.[72]

OTOTOXICITY

In modern trials, about 3 percent of patients receiving vancomycin develop signs of ototoxicity, including tinnitus or frank hearing loss, but the effects are reversible with discontinuation of the drug. This reaction is not well correlated with peak serum levels of vancomycin.[72]

CNS Adverse Effects

INCIDENCE OF CNS EFFECTS

Vancomycin does not penetrate into the CSF or the brain in appreciable amounts. There are no clinical reports of CNS toxicity.

Aminoglycoside Antibiotics: Amikacin, Gentamicin, Kanamycin, Streptomycin, Tobramycin

Aminoglycosides were among the most effective drugs for infections caused by gram-negative bacteria when they were first introduced, but the inconvenient pharmacokinetics of the drugs, coupled with their high potential for toxicity, has resulted in their being replaced by broad-spectrum β-lactam antibiotics for most applications. Despite some calls for their abandonment, the aminoglycosides remain important for specific infections in seriously ill patients.[76]

Systemic Adverse Effects

NEPHROTOXICITY

Nephrotoxicity is the dose-limiting toxicity for most patients receiving an aminoglycoside. Although cells of the renal tubular epithelium may be destroyed, the kidneys are capable of replacing at least part of the damaged cells so that over time many patients regain lost renal function. Reports of the incidence of nephrotoxicity vary widely in the literature. In carefully selected patients whose dose of aminoglycoside is based on individual patient monitoring, the incidence is generally low, but under less controlled conditions, incidence rates of 25 percent or higher are not uncommon.[77] The best predictor of aminoglycoside nephrotoxicity in most studies is the trough level of the drug; trough levels above 2.5 μg/ml have been associated with greater nephrotoxicity.[78] Dosing information supplied with the drugs suggests 2 μg/ml as the maximum tolerated trough level for aminoglycosides other than kanamycin or amikacin, for which trough levels are listed as 5 μg/ml. The risk of nephrotoxicity is greatly increased when other nephrotoxic drugs are also used with the aminoglycoside.[76,79] Older age and a longer duration of therapy also increase the risk of nephrotoxicity in most studies.[80]

Many hospitals have adopted once-daily dosing in an attempt to control aminoglycoside nephrotoxicity without resorting to individual patient monitoring. A meta-analysis of several studies comparing once-daily dosing with standard multiple dosing showed that nephrotoxicity still occurred with once-daily dosing, although the incidence was lower for gentamicin.[77] A more recent study in the elderly showed an incidence of nephrotoxicity of 9.3 percent and revealed no advantage with once-daily dosing.[81] A study that evaluated once-daily dosing in critically ill patients concluded that individual patient monitoring was still required because of the high interpatient variability in pharmacokinetics with these drugs.[82] A retrospective study involving records of 2405 patients at two teaching hospitals also supported the efficacy of individual patient monitoring in lowering the incidence of nephrotoxicity and in reducing total care costs by avoiding this adverse reaction.[80]

OTOTOXICITY

Hearing loss and vestibular dysfunction are associated with aminoglycoside antibiotics, with a reported incidence of 1 to 15 percent.[76,77] Unlike nephrotoxicity, which is usually reversible, ototoxicity induced by aminoglycosides is irreversible because hair cells in the inner ear are destroyed and not replaced.[77] Most patients receiving aminoglycosides are not evaluated rigorously for ototoxicity, and the actual incidence of damage may be much higher than the literature suggests.[39] The earliest signs of hearing loss are in the high-frequency range; these signs will not be noticed conversationally and should be evaluated by audiometry. Vestibular damage may be marked by awkwardness or loss of balance (especially with the eyes closed), as well as dizziness, nausea, and vomiting. As with nephrotoxicity, ototoxicity increases with longer duration of therapy; thus patients receiving an aminoglycoside as part of a therapeutic regimen for tuberculosis have an incidence of ototoxicity of 18 percent or higher.[83] High trough levels and the use of other ototoxic drugs also increase the risk of ototoxicity.

NEUROMUSCULAR BLOCKADE

Aminoglycoside antibiotics reduce acetylcholine release from motor nerve terminals and in addition also lower the response to acetylcholine on the postjunctional side of the synapse. These actions produce a nondepolarizing type of blockade that is reversed as the aminoglycoside is eliminated from the body. Historically, this effect was important for explaining respiratory arrest following intraperitoneal dosing or lavage with an aminoglycoside because the muscles used for breathing were paralyzed. In modern clinical practice, this potential for interfering with muscle function is of most concern in patients with predisposing conditions, such as myasthenia gravis, or in surgery patients receiving a neuromuscular blocker during anesthesia. Calcium reverses aminoglycoside neuromuscular blockade.

ALLERGIC REACTIONS

Allergic reactions are uncommon with this class of drugs, but itching, rash, redness, and swelling occur in some patients.

PERIPHERAL NEURITIS

Streptomycin has been associated with peripheral neuritis, producing a burning sensation on the face, numbness, or tingling. Streptomycin also has been associated with a risk of optic neuritis, with loss of vision.

CNS Adverse Effects

INCIDENCE OF CNS EFFECTS

Occasional reports in the early literature suggested that aminoglycosides could cause significant toxicity to the CNS.[22] The clearest example was a study in which gentamicin was administered intraventricularly to infants to treat meningitis. Those infants developed levels as high as 130 μg/ml in the intraventricular fluid; 42.9 percent of the infants died, compared with 12.5 percent in the control group that received parenteral antibiotics.[84] The mechanism for CNS toxicity of the aminoglycosides is unclear, but the risk factors most likely include elevated levels of drug. Seizures have been induced by concomitant intraventricular and intravenous dosing of the drugs.

Chloramphenicol

Chloramphenicol is an older drug that fell into relative disuse because the drug was associated with a rare but fatal adverse reaction in adults and a syndrome that was fatal for a number of infants who were treated with doses of drug too large for their immature livers and kidneys to eliminate. In recent years, chloramphenicol has taken on a limited but important role for specific infections in which its antimicrobial spectrum and unusual pharmacokinetics give a therapeutic advantage. In particular, this generally bacteriostatic drug penetrates well into the CNS and is bactericidal against important CNS pathogens.[85]

Systemic Adverse Effects

BLOOD DYSCRASIAS

The most important adverse reactions to chloramphenicol are blood dyscrasias, which are of two general types. The first is bone marrow suppression, a dose-related reaction usually seen in patients whose serum levels exceed 25 μg/ml. The symptoms include anemia, leukopenia, and thrombocytopenia.[86] With patient monitoring, this relatively common reaction can be detected early and usually is reversed when the drug is discontinued. The mechanism producing this reaction is thought to involve chloramphenicol inhibition of mitochondrial protein synthesis in human marrow cells.[87]

The second type of blood dyscrasia is aplastic anemia, which is an idiosyncratic reaction that is not related to dose or duration of therapy. Aplastic anemia usually appears weeks or months after therapy has ended and often is fatal. The incidence of aplastic anemia following chloramphenicol therapy has been variously reported in the older literature as 1 in 15,000 to 1 in 40,000 cases per course of therapy.[86] Most of the first cases reported involved the use of oral chloramphenicol, and involvement of a metabolite of the drug was hypothesized to cause aplastic anemia.[88] Modern studies have attempted to quantify the risk of aplastic anemia more precisely. The Thai Aplastic Anemia Study Group reported a 10-year population-based case-control study of aplastic anemia that determined an overall incidence rate of 3 to 5 cases of aplastic anemia per 1 million persons per year. Although this study showed a correlation of aplastic anemia with occupational exposure to solvents and agricultural pesticides, there was no association with chloramphenicol, a drug used more commonly in Thailand than in the United States.[89] Likewise, a recent Brazilian study of aplastic anemia showed an incidence of 2.4 cases per 1 million persons per year and a positive correlation of aplastic anemia with the use of acetone-containing solvents or of organophosphate pesticides; there was no positive association with chloramphenicol use.[90] A study designed to evaluate the risk of aplastic anemia from ocular administration of chloramphenicol concluded that it was less than 1 per 1 million treatment courses by ocular administration.[91] These studies taken together have confirmed the rarity of aplastic anemia associated with chloramphenicol administration; due to the rarity of this adverse effect, the incidence with modern usage patterns of the drug has not been determined.

PERIPHERAL NEUROPATHY

Peripheral neuropathy with burning, pain, tingling, or weakness in the extremities has been reported. Optic neuritis with eye pain, blurred vision, or visual loss is a rare and usually reversible complication of short-term chloramphenicol therapy.[39] The complication was seen in up to 13 percent of cystic fibrosis patients when the drug was used for months to years.[86]

GI DISTURBANCES

Diarrhea, nausea, and vomiting have been reported with oral use of chloramphenicol.

ALLERGIC REACTIONS

Allergic reactions are rare but do occur. Skin rash, fever, and difficulty breathing are the most likely allergic reactions, but contact dermatitis and even anaphylaxis are possible.[92,93]

CARDIOVASCULAR REACTIONS

Overdose with chloramphenicol is associated with uneven breathing, unresponsiveness, cardiovascular collapse, and death. This reaction originally was called the *gray-baby syndrome,* the name coming from the blue-gray color of the skin of these patients and the fact that it was first noted in neonates. Neonates are particularly sensitive to overdose because the livers of newborns do not readily form the glucuronide derivative of chloramphenicol, which is the first step to eliminating the drug. The kidneys of neonates are also less able to excrete unconjugated drug. The result is an accumulation of chloramphenicol to toxic levels. Modern drug monitoring can prevent this outcome by allowing doses to be adjusted to the excretory capacity of the infant.

CNS Adverse Effects

INCIDENCE OF CNS EFFECTS

Confusion, delirium, and headache have been reported rarely with chloramphenicol. Psychiatric symptoms also have been noted but are rare even during prolonged therapy with the drug.[22] The mechanism and risk factors are unknown. It is known that chloramphenicol penetrates readily into the CNS and for this reason is useful in treating various brain infections, including abscesses.[94,95]

Sulfonamide Antibiotics

Sulfonamides entered clinical use shortly before the advent of the first β-lactam antibiotics in the 1940s. The sulfonamide class has changed over the years with the introduction of more water-soluble drugs (e.g., sulfisoxizole) and the abandonment of relatively insoluble and more toxic agents (e.g., sulfanilamide).

Systemic Adverse Effects

ALLERGIC REACTIONS

Allergic reactions to sulfonamides are common, appearing in 2 to 4 percent of adults or children but in up to 60 percent of patients with acquired immune deficiency syndrome (AIDS).[3,9,96] Skin rashes include hives, itching, and redness. More serious cutaneous reactions such as Stevens-Johnson syndrome and toxic epidermal necrolysis are rare. Anaphylaxis is also rare unless the patient has a history of allergic reactions to this class of drugs. Drug-induced fever occurs in 1 to 2 percent of patients, usually appearing a few days after the start of therapy and often accompanied by headache, itching, and rash. A syndrome resembling serum sickness is also a delayed reaction to these drugs. Other delayed reactions may include effects on a variety of organ systems. These drugs have been associated with vasculitis, lupus-like syndrome, nephritis, and hepatitis, which all may have an allergic component.

The immunogenicity of sulfonamides is related to properties of the specific drugs and to the metabolic capacity of the patient. Acetylation is the primary route of metabolism of sulfonamides, but many individuals are slow acetylators, which exposes the drug to oxidative metabolic pathways that produce toxic nitroso compounds and hydroxylamine. If these toxic metabolites are not complexed with glutathione, they are free to interact with proteins and form haptens that are strongly immunogenic.[9] Slow acetylators thus are more likely to suffer hypersensitivity reactions.[96] The high incidence of hypersensitivity reactions in AIDS patients may be caused by the lower levels of glutathione found in these patients. Currently, there is no skin test or other diagnostic test that is useful in predicting allergic reactions to sulfonamides.

PHOTOTOXICITY

Patients receiving sulfonamides often show sensitivity to sunlight, with excessive reddening or blistering of the skin.

GI DISTURBANCES

GI disturbances are relatively common with these orally administered drugs. Symptoms include anorexia, diarrhea, nausea, and vomiting.

HEPATOTOXICITY

An acute fulminating hepatic necrosis has been reported with sulfonamides. This rare reaction may have an allergic basis.

NEPHROTOXICITY

Lack of solubility in the acidic pH of normal urine was a common property of the first sulfonamides used clinically, but modern drugs are much more soluble, and the formation of crystals in urine is relatively rare today. Sulfamethoxazole is one of the less soluble drugs of this class currently being used. Adult patients receiving sulfamethoxazole should receive sufficient fluids to produce about 1200 ml of urine a day. This strategy is adequate to prevent crystalluria in nearly all patients. Interstitial nephritis and tubular necrosis also have been reported with sulfonamides. Allergic mechanisms may be involved.

BLOOD DYSCRASIAS

Sulfonamides cause hemolytic anemia in patients lacking adequate glucose-6-phosphate dehydrogenase in red blood cells. This genetically determined trait is more common in western Asian, eastern Mediterranean, and certain African populations but also occurs in the United States among persons from these populations. Males are more likely to show the trait than females because the trait is carried on the X chromosome. Agranulocytosis and thrombocytopenia may occur with sulfonamides, but both appear reversible when the drug is discontinued. Sulfonamides are a rare cause of aplastic anemia.

ENDOCRINE EFFECTS

Sulfonamides are chemically related to antithyroid drugs and on occasion may themselves cause dysfunction of the thyroid gland. Goiter can occur.

PANCREATITIS

Pancreatitis is an uncommon adverse reaction to sulfonamides.

CNS Adverse Effects

INCIDENCE OF CNS EFFECTS

CNS effects such as dizziness, headache, and lethargy are relatively common with sulfonamides. CNS toxicity with symptoms of confusion, delirium, depression, disorientation, euphoria, hallucinations, or seizures are more rare.

MECHANISMS OF CNS EFFECTS

A syndrome of aseptic meningitis has been described with sulfonamides alone or with sulfamethoxazole with trimethoprim and is thought at least in part to have an allergic basis.[97] The mechanism for other forms of CNS adverse reactions is unclear.

RISK FACTORS FOR CNS ADVERSE REACTIONS

One report suggests that drug-induced encephalitis is more common in patients with connective tissue disorders, but other risk factors have yet to be identified.[97]

Trimethoprim and Cotrimoxazole

Trimethoprim is used in the United States primarily with sulfamethoxazole; this fixed combination is called *cotrimoxazole*. Trimethoprim is used alone occasionally, especially for urinary tract infections.

Systemic Adverse Effects

ALLERGIC REACTIONS

Cotrimoxazole commonly causes adverse skin reactions, including maculopapular exanthema, urticaria, and vasculitis. A study that monitored drug-induced skin reactions in 48,005 hospitalized patients over a 19-year period concluded that cotrimoxazole and sulfonamides alone were second only to β-lactams as a cause of skin reactions.[98] Most of the reactions appeared within the first day of therapy. Just as with sulfonamides alone, the incidence of skin reactions with cotrimoxazole is much higher in AIDS patients than in other groups of patients. In many studies, over half of AIDS patients treated with cotrimoxazole develop a drug-induced skin reaction.[3,9,96] Cotrimoxazole or trimethoprim has been associated with serious allergic reactions, including erythema multiforme, exfoliative dermatitis, Stevens-Johnson syndrome, and toxic epidermal necrolysis, but the incidence is low. Discontinuing the drug when a rash occurs may lessen the progression to these serious reactions.[98]

Allergic reactions to cotrimoxazole in the past often were attributed solely to the sulfonamide component in cotrimoxazole, but recent studies show that trimethoprim also contributes significantly to allergic reactions. In one patient who originally developed anaphylaxis to cotrimoxazole, IgE antibodies to trimethoprim were detected, and the patient did not react to challenge with sulfamethoxazole.[99,100] Fixed drug reactions consisting primarily of pigmented skin lesions also have been associated with cotrimoxazole. There is some evidence that the risk for fixed drug reactions with cotrimoxazole is increased for patients with certain HLA class I antigens, including A30 B13 Cw6.[101]

GI DISTURBANCES

Cotrimoxazole is used orally most often and has been associated with anorexia, cramping, diarrhea, nausea, and vomiting. These reactions are not uncommon and usually do not require cessation of therapy unless the symptoms are prolonged and intense.

BLOOD DYSCRASIAS

Trimethoprim, as a folic acid antagonist, can cause a variety of blood disorders, including megaloblastic anemia. Leukopenia, neutropenia, thrombocytopenia, and methemoglobinemia also have been observed. Except in cases of overdose, these are rare. A long-term study of drug-induced thrombocytopenia in Denmark showed that over the 24-year reporting period, cotrimoxazole was the single most common cause of drug-induced thrombocytopenia, although overall thrombocytopenia remained a rare drug reaction.[102]

PHOTOTOXICITY

Cotrimoxazole is associated with reddening or blistering of any skin exposed to sunlight, a reaction probably related to sulfamethoxazole.

NEPHROTOXICITY

Trimethoprim affects potassium balance. Like the potassium-sparing diuretic amiloride, trimethoprim competitively inhibits epithelial sodium channels in the distal nephron, which blocks potassium excretion. Trimethoprim acting in this way can cause potentially lethal hyperkalemia.[103] Because blockade of the sodium channels by trimethoprim is competitive, discontinuing the drug reverses the effect.

HEPATOTOXICITY

Hepatitis has occurred with sulfonamides; it also occurs rarely with cotrimoxazole, and in at least one patient hepatitis was accompanied by pancreatitis, both in the original episode and on rechallenge.[104]

CNS Adverse Effects

INCIDENCE OF CNS EFFECTS

CNS effects other than headache are relatively rare with trimethoprim. Cotrimoxazole can produce any of the CNS effects associated with sulfonamides (confusion, delirium, depression, disorientation, dizziness, euphoria, hallucinations, or seizures). Aseptic meningitis is a rare but increasingly recognized adverse reaction with either trimethoprim alone or cotrimoxazole. In a recent review of the literature of antibiotic-induced aseptic meningitis, trimethoprim was reported as the cause of 10 cases, cotrimoxazole was the cause of 20 cases, 2 cases were associated with other sulfonamides, and the remaining 7 cases were attributed to six different drugs.[105]

MECHANISMS OF CNS EFFECTS

The most commonly held view is that aseptic meningitis has an allergic basis. Immune complexes have been detected in sera from patients with cotrimoxazole-induced aseptic meningitis.[105] The proinflammatory cytokine interleukin 6 (IL-6) was elevated in patients with trimethoprim-induced aseptic meningitis; in one of these patients, IL-6 was elevated not only in serum but also in CSF.[106]

RISK FACTORS FOR CNS ADVERSE REACTIONS

Connective tissues disorders have been suggested as a risk factor for encephalitis with sulfonamides.[97] Suggestions of altered immune system function or undetected meningeal defects as risk factors for drug-induced aseptic meningitis have yet to be proven.[105] Slow acetylators of sulfonamides may be at higher risk of allergic reactions because they produce more oxidative metabolites of the drugs.[107]

Metronidazole

Metronidazole was used originally primarily as an antiprotozoal agent but is now used commonly to treat infections caused by anaerobic bacteria.

Systemic Adverse Effects

GI DISTURBANCES

GI symptoms are common with metronidazole, occurring in about 6 percent of treated patients. Nausea with or without vomiting is most common, but abdominal pain and diarrhea also occur frequently. Some patients report a taste perversion described as a bad metallic taste.

PERIPHERAL NEUROPATHY

Numbness, pain, tingling, or weakness in the hands occurs in about 2 percent of patients receiving metronidazole. Peripheral neuropathy is usually slowly reversible if the drug is discontinued promptly. This reaction is most common at high doses.

LOCAL INJECTION-SITE REACTIONS

Phlebitis and painful injection sites were common complaints in early trials with metronidazole. The drug is now supplied already diluted as an isotonic solution to help minimize these effects.

SUPERINFECTIONS

Because metronidazole destroys many anaerobic bacteria normally found in the bowel and elsewhere in the body, overgrowth with other resistant organisms is common. Yeast infections of the mouth or vagina occur most often. Diarrhea is a common adverse reaction with metronidazole that is most likely also related to changes in intestinal flora. Antibiotic-associated colitis caused by *C. difficile* is possible, although the drug has been used to treat this condition when it is caused by other antibiotics.

HEPATOTOXICITY

Metronidazole produces a disulfiram-like effect when taken with ethanol. The mechanism for this effect is unknown.

PANCREATITIS

Metronidazole occasionally has been associated with pancreatitis.[108]

NEPHROTOXICITY

Metronidazole may darken the urine, but this action is not associated with renal damage.

CARCINOGENICITY

One of the most troubling potential adverse effects of metronidazole is carcinogenicity or teratogenicity. The compound is mutagenic in the Ames test in bacteria, and either metronidazole or its metabolites have caused tumors in laboratory rodents given high doses for prolonged periods. Potentially carcinogenic metabolites have been detected in human urine after therapeutic doses of metronidazole.[109] The hydroxy metabolite of metronidazole is also carcinogenic in vitro.[110] Nevertheless, epidemiologic studies in humans failed to show a correlation between short-term metronidazole use and the incidence of any human cancer.[111,112] The caveat to these human studies is that the time for follow-up seldom exceeded 10 years, whereas the time to develop cancer can be decades, depending on the type of cancer. These studies also did not select out patients who may have received the drug for longer periods, which might be an increased risk for cancer. Thus the question of carcinogenicity for the drug as used in humans remains open. The drug is usually avoided in the first trimester of pregnancy, although a study of prenatal exposure to metronidazole at any stage of pregnancy failed to show a correlation with tumor development in children under 5 years of age.[112]

CNS Adverse Effects

INCIDENCE OF CNS EFFECTS

CNS effects are relatively uncommon with metronidazole. Dizziness or headache occurs in about 2 percent of patients; ataxia, light-headedness, seizures, or syncope also may occur. Metronidazole is a rare cause of aseptic meningitis and encephalopathy.[105] Seizures have been associated with high doses of metronidazole.[22]

MECHANISMS OF CNS EFFECTS

The exact mechanism by which metronidazole produces CNS effects is unknown, but the drug does penetrate the CNS readily, unlike many other agents. Very high doses of the drug in rats produced histologic changes similar to those associated with Wernicke's encephalopathy in humans,[113] as well as impaired balance and lesions in the cerebellum and brain stem.[22] Magnetic resonance imaging (MRI) studies of a single patient with metronidazole-induced encephalopathy showed lesions affecting both gray and white matter, which were at-tributed to axonal swelling secondary to acute toxic insult; the cerebral lesions in this patient were essentially reversed in 6 weeks, but the damage to peripheral nerves persisted for months.[114] This clinical course was similar to an earlier patient for whom MRI was not available.[22]

RISK FACTORS FOR CNS ADVERSE REACTIONS

Risk factors are not clearly documented, but many patients who develop encephalopathy with metronidazole also have preexisting organ impairment.[115–117] Common associated conditions include frank renal failure or serious liver disease, but altered renal or liver function tests are not associated with induction of seizures.[22] These conditions may alter the pharmacokinetics of the drug, but seizures or other CNS effects are not correlated with high levels of metronidazole.[22,114] Preexisting organ failure may contribute to CNS irritability by causing accumulation of ammonia or organic acids. Metronidazole usually is contraindicated in patients with existing CNS diseases, including epilepsy, to avoid additive effects of the drug.

Clindamycin

Clindamycin is an older antibacterial agent that has continued to find new uses through the years as its antibacterial use has waned. It is currently indicated primarily for anaerobic bacterial infections, for certain protozoal diseases, and for *Pneumocystis carinii* pneumonia (with primaquine).

Systemic Adverse Effects

GI DISTURBANCES

Clindamycin commonly causes GI symptoms, including abdominal pain, diarrhea, nausea, and vomiting. Diarrhea is the most common of these; the incidence has been up to 30 percent in some studies, but incidences of around 10 percent are more common.

SUPERINFECTIONS

Most cases of diarrhea produced by clindamycin are likely to arise from the profound effect the drug has on anaerobic microbial flora of the intestinal tract. As the normal anaerobic flora die off, other resistant organisms overgrow, producing mild to severe symptoms. At one time clindamycin was the leading cause of antibiotic-associated colitis, although more cases are currently produced by aminopenicillins because those drugs are used more widely than clindamycin. Oral doses of clindamycin are more likely to lead to colitis than are parenteral doses because the drug is relatively slowly absorbed from the intestine and undergoes enterohepatic circulation.

ALLERGIC REACTIONS

Allergic reactions are relatively uncommon with clindamycin, but itching, rashes, and redness have occurred. Just as with the sulfonamides, skin reactions to clindamycin may be more common in human immunodeficiency virus (HIV)–positive patients than in other patient groups. Very rarely, Stevens-Johnson syndrome, anaphylaxis, and erythema multiforme have occurred.

LOCAL INJECTION-SITE REACTIONS

Clindamycin can cause tissue irritation or thrombophlebitis at local injection sites, especially at high concentrations.

BLOOD DYSCRASIAS

Clindamycin occasionally causes neutropenia or thrombocytopenia.

CARDIOVASCULAR EFFECTS

Care must be taken to avoid giving clindamycin as an undiluted bolus injection because hypotension and cardiovascular collapse can occur when the drug is administered in this way.

CNS Adverse Effects

INCIDENCE OF CNS EFFECTS

CNS effects have not been reported with clindamycin.

Quinupristin/Dalfopristin

This new antibiotic combination comes from an old family of antimicrobials, the streptogramins. This new preparation represents an attempt to deal with nosocomial infections caused by organisms resistant to standard antibiotics by developing drugs from unusual classes of compounds. As a new clinical entity, the spectrum of adverse effects is likely to change as more patients are treated with these antibiotics.

Systemic Adverse Effects

LOCAL INJECTION-SITE REACTIONS

Quinupristin/dalfopristin is highly irritating to veins and surrounding tissues, making local reactions the most common adverse reaction. In the clinical trials reported by the manufacturer, up to 42 percent of patients had swelling, pain, or inflammation at the infusion site. The incidence was even higher if the infusion was at a peripheral site. Thrombophlebitis was reported in 2.4 percent of patients. Local reactions to quinupristin/dalfopristin may be minimized by diluting the drug to 500 or 750 ml rather than the standard 250 ml. Reactions are also reduced when the drug is administered via a peripherally inserted central catheter (PICC).

ARTHRALGIA/MYALGIA

Arthralgias and/or myalgias have been a common reaction, occurring in up to 7.8 percent of patients. The reaction can be severe and has led to discontinuation of therapy in 2 percent of patients.

GI DISTURBANCES

Nausea has been reported in up to 4.6 percent of patients. Diarrhea and vomiting also occur in 2.7 to 3.7 percent of patients.

ALLERGIC REACTIONS

Rash and itching have been reported in up to 3.1 percent of patients. There are also rare reports of angioedema and anaphylaxis.

HEPATOTOXICITY

Increased bilirubin levels are seen commonly in patients treated with quinupristin/dalfopristin. Jaundice or hepatitis was seen rarely in clinical trials.

CNS Adverse Effects

INCIDENCE OF CNS EFFECTS

Headache was reported in 1.6 percent of patients receiving quinupristin/dalfopristin. Anxiety, confusion, dizziness, insomnia, and paresthesias were seen in less than 1 percent of patients. Serious CNS reactions such as convulsions or encephalopathy were seen in less than 0.1 percent of patients.

Linezolid

Linezolid is the first member of the new antibiotic class the oxazolidinones. This drug, like quinupristin/dalfopristin, was developed primarily to deal with nosocomial infections caused by organisms resistant to conventional antibiotics.

Systemic Adverse Effects

GI DISTURBANCES

GI effects are among the most common reactions in patients receiving linezolid in clinical trials of the drug.[118] Symptoms included constipation (2.2 percent), diarrhea (8.3 percent), nausea (6.2 percent), and vomiting (3.7 percent). Localized abdominal pain also was reported by a few patients. In addition, 1.8 percent of patients reported an alteration in taste.

SUPERINFECTIONS

Candida infections have been reported in a few patients receiving linezolid, usually localized to the mouth or vagina.

ALLERGIC REACTIONS

Allergic reactions are relatively uncommon with linezolid, with rash, fever, or itching occurring in 2 percent or less of patients receiving the drug.

BLOOD DYSCRASIAS

Anemia is a rare adverse reaction with linezolid and is most likely produced by suppression of erythropoiesis. Thrombocytopenia may be an immune-mediated event.[119]

CNS Adverse Effects

INCIDENCE OF CNS EFFECTS

Headache was reported in 6.5 percent of patients in clinical trials, but the mechanism is unknown. More serious CNS adverse reactions have not been reported to date.

Nitrofurantoin

Nitrofurantoin is the only nitrofuran used systemically in the United States. The pharmacokinetics of the drug make it most useful for urinary tract infections.

Systemic Adverse Effects

GI DISTURBANCES

Nausea and vomiting are common with nitrofurantoin use. Although the drug can cause local GI irritation, nausea and vomiting may arise at least in part from effects in the CNS because intravenous doses of the drug also can cause nausea and vomiting.

ALLERGIC REACTIONS

Allergic reactions occur in about 4 percent of patients, with symptoms of angioedema, fever, itching, rash, and urticaria. Anaphylaxis is a rare event. Systemic allergic reactions occasionally may produce lupus-like symptoms, vasculitis, or other signs of organ inflammation, as noted in the sections that follow.

PULMONARY INJURY

Nitrofurantoin causes both acute and chronic lung injury. The risk for lung injury increases with age and is more common in women than in men.[120] Acute pneumonitis usually appears during the first week of therapy, with symptoms including chest pains, chills, cough, dyspnea, eosinophilia, and fever. These symptoms are thought to have an allergic basis related to deposition of immune complexes or to T-cell cytotoxicity. Radiographs of the lungs show pleural effusion or pulmonary infiltrates. These acute reactions often resolve when the drug is discontinued.

Patients who receive nitrofurantoin for prolonged periods are at risk of diffuse interstitial pneumonitis and fibrosis. The onset is gradual and characterized by cough and progressive exertional dyspnea. The reaction is thought to be due to the formation of free radicals (active oxygen species) in the lungs through metabolism of the drug and the high oxygen tension. The reversibility of these symptoms is less likely than for the acute reaction; up to 10 percent of patients with pulmonary fibrosis may die of this complication.[120]

CARDIOTOXICITY

Direct cardiotoxicity has not been noted, but occasionally in association with pulmonary complications from nitrofurantoin, bundle-branch block is seen on the electrocardiogram (ECG).

PERIPHERAL NEUROPATHY

Nitrofurantoin produces an ascending sensorimotor neuropathy. It is imperative that the drug be stopped when this complication appears because it can be progressive and is not fully reversible. Symptoms include burning, numbness, pain, or tingling in the extremities. This reaction is more common in the elderly and in those with impaired renal function.

ARTHRALGIA/MYALGIA

Joint and muscle pain are common reactions to nitrofurantoin and are thought to have an allergic basis.

HEPATOTOXICITY

Hepatotoxicity due to nitrofurantoin includes both acute and chronic conditions resembling hepatitis; both are thought to have an allergic basis. Antinuclear antibodies to smooth muscle may be present.[121] Hepatotoxicity usually resolves when the drug is discontinued. A high percentage of patients with pulmonary complications from nitrofurantoin also have elevated transaminases suggestive of liver damage.

PANCREATITIS

Pancreatitis is an uncommon adverse reaction to nitrofurantoin.

SUPERINFECTIONS

Candida or *Pseudomonas* superinfections have developed in the genitourinary tract of treated patients. Antibiotic-associated colitis has been reported rarely. Superinfections at other sites are unlikely because of low distribution of the drug outside the urinary tract or the bile.

BLOOD DYSCRASIAS

Granulocytopenia, leukopenia, megaloblastic anemia, or thrombocytopenia may occur with nitrofurantoin use. Aplastic anemia is rare. For patients with glucose-6-phosphate dehydrogenase deficiency, nitrofurantoin increases the risk of hemolysis by increasing active oxygen species and depleting glutathione from red blood cells.

NEPHROTOXICITY
Nitrofurantoin imparts a rusty or brown discoloration to urine, but this effect is harmless.

CNS Adverse Effects

INCIDENCE OF CNS EFFECTS
CNS symptoms such as dizziness, drowsiness, and headache are relatively common with nitrofurantoin. Less often patients have confusion, depression, intracranial hypertension, mood changes, or psychotic reactions. Blurred vision may be a sign of optic neuritis, which is a rare adverse reaction to nitrofurantoin.

MECHANISMS OF CNS EFFECTS
The mechanism of CNS toxicity has not been confirmed but may have an allergic basis, as seen for other drugs such as sulfonamides, trimethoprim, and metronidazole.

RISK FACTORS FOR CNS ADVERSE REACTIONS
Risk factors have not been clearly identified.

Nalidixic Acid

Nalidixic acid is related to the fluoroquinolones but has a low potency and is useful only for urinary tract infections.

Systemic Adverse Effects

GI DISTURBANCES
The most common adverse reaction to nalidixic acid is nausea, which may be accompanied by abdominal pain, diarrhea, or vomiting.

ALLERGIC REACTIONS
Common reactions to nalidixic acid include a variety of skin rashes. Severe allergic reactions, such as anaphylaxis, erythema multiforme, and Stevens-Johnson syndrome, occur more rarely. At least one case of hypersensitivity pneumonitis has been linked to nalidixic acid.[122]

PHOTOTOXICITY
Nalidixic acid is a relatively common cause of sunburn-like reactions in skin exposed for short periods to sunlight. Most reactions are quickly reversible, but some persist or recur after the drug is discontinued.

METABOLIC EFFECTS
Nalidixic acid can cause metabolic acidosis, marked by rapid breathing, nausea, vomiting, or weakness.

CNS Adverse Effects

INCIDENCE OF CNS EFFECTS
CNS effects are among the most common adverse effects of nalidixic acid. Dizziness, drowsiness, headache, vertigo, and weakness are common complaints. Signs of CNS stimulation are seen less often; symptoms include confusion, light-headedness, restlessness, and tremor. Rarely, intracranial hypertension occurs. Most CNS symptoms resolve when the drug is discontinued. Blurred vision, double vision, photophobia, and changes in color perception also may occur with nalidixic acid. These reactions disappear when the drug is discontinued.

MECHANISMS OF CNS EFFECTS
No mechanism has been proven for the CNS or visual changes caused by this drug.

RISK FACTORS FOR CNS ADVERSE REACTIONS
Patients with a history of seizure disorders or with cerebral arteriosclerosis are considered to be at higher risk for CNS symptoms caused by nalidixic acid.

▶ ANTIMYCOBACTERIAL AGENTS

Isoniazid

Isoniazid, one of the most important antimycobacterial drugs, is an older agent with a well-defined profile of adverse reactions. Because of its importance as a single agent, isoniazid is discussed separately, but it is in fact used most often in combination with one of the drugs in the following sections.

Systemic Adverse Effects

PERIPHERAL NEUROPATHY
Numbness and tingling of the legs caused by peripheral neuropathy is a common dose-related adverse reaction to isoniazid. At doses of 3 to 5 mg/kg per day, only about 1 percent of patients develop this reaction, but at higher doses it is much more common. Peripheral neuropathy can be prevented with pyridoxine supplementation, usually 10 to 25 mg/day. Peripheral neuropathy is more common in persons who receive inadequate pyridoxine in their diet (i.e., malnourished or alcoholic patients) or in slow acetylators of the drug, who tend to accumulate toxic metabolites of the parent drug.

HEPATOTOXICITY
Isoniazid commonly causes liver damage that may progress to chronic liver disease. Hepatotoxicity may begin with vague symptoms such as anorexia, nausea, vomiting, or weakness and progress to more obvious

signs such as darkened urine or jaundice. The incidence of this adverse reaction in persons under 20 years of age is about 0.3 percent, but the incidence increases about tenfold with age, with preexisting liver disease, and in persons who take ethanol daily.[123] Women are more likely than men to develop fatal hepatitis.[124] Patients receiving both rifampin and isoniazid are also at greater risk of liver damage.

Histology of the liver during overt hepatitis shows hepatocellular damage and necrosis. Two mechanisms may contribute to this liver damage. The first involves metabolism of isoniazid to monoacetylhydrazine, a compound known to cause liver cell necrosis in animal studies.[125] A second mechanism invokes an allergic process.

GI DISTURBANCES
Isoniazid commonly causes diarrhea, nausea, stomach pain, or vomiting. These symptoms are usually self-limiting.

ALLERGIC REACTIONS
Skin rashes are a rare reaction to isoniazid. The drug more commonly causes symptoms and signs similar to lupus erythematosus, with an increase in antinuclear antibodies.[126] Vasculitis, arthralgia, or organ involvement may occur.

CNS Adverse Effects

INCIDENCE OF CNS EFFECTS
Neurotoxicity is uncommon to rare with standard doses of isoniazid, although depression, mental status changes, seizures, and even aseptic meningitis have been noted.[105] Mania and psychotic symptoms also have been reported.[64] Poisoning with isoniazid is one of the most common causes of drug-induced seizures.[127] Overdose with isoniazid rapidly produces nausea and vomiting, usually followed within 1 to 2 hours by coma, disorientation, dizziness, hyperreflexia, lethargy, or slurred speech. Seizures usually occur within 3 hours of the overdose. Doses as low as 40 mg/kg may produce seizures, and serum levels above 10 μg/ml are considered toxic. Death from seizures or related metabolic acidosis is not uncommon with doses above 100 mg/kg.[128] Seizures may be refractory to treatment with standard anticonvulsants.

MECHANISMS OF CNS EFFECTS
Isoniazid interferes with the function of pyridoxal-5-phosphate, a critical cofactor for several important enzymes, including glutamic acid decarboxylase, an enzyme needed for the production of the inhibitory neurotransmitter GABA. Isoniazid depletes the body of pyridoxal-5-phosphate, thus inhibiting glutamic acid decarboxylase and lowering GABA production.[22,128] Without adequate levels of GABA, the CNS becomes ex-

citable, and seizures occur. Seizure control is greatly improved if intravenous pyridoxine is given to allow resynthesis of adequate pyridoxal-5-phosphate. A single dose of 5 g pyridoxine may be given, or the dose of pyridoxine may be adjusted to match gram for gram the dose of isoniazid taken. Acute massive doses of pyridoxine should be avoided because of the potential neurotoxicity of the vitamin in large doses.

RISK FACTORS FOR CNS ADVERSE REACTIONS
Risk factors have not been completely identified, but isoniazid is usually avoided, if possible, in patients who have a history of prior seizures.

Rifamycins: Rifampin, Rifabutin, Rifapentine

Rifampin is used in combination with other antimicrobial agents for treating tuberculosis and leprosy. Rifapentine is used in combination with other antimicrobial agents for tuberculosis. The related drug rifabutin may be used to treat tuberculosis in HIV-infected patients or for infections caused by *Mycobacterium avium*.

Systemic Adverse Effects

GI DISTURBANCES
Anorexia, cramping, diarrhea, dyspepsia, nausea, and vomiting are common reactions with rifamycins. Rifabutin also rarely has caused a perversion of taste.

ALLERGIC REACTIONS
Symptoms of itching, rash, or skin redness have occurred with rifamycins. They are most common with rifabutin and least common with rifapentine. Rashes caused by rifampin may be associated with developing anaphylaxis, which is thought to relate to the presence of IgE antibodies, but these are not always detected.[129] A flulike syndrome has been reported for rifampin, with fever, chills, and body aches. The condition is more likely to occur when the drug is used intermittently but is also more likely at higher doses.[129] For example, at doses of 1200 mg twice weekly, the incidence of flulike syndrome was 16 percent; at 900 mg twice weekly it dropped to 2.5 percent, and with 450 to 600 mg daily the incidence was 0 to 0.3 percent. This tendency to develop flulike symptoms on intermittent dosing schedules has been used to advantage by clinicians who switch patients who develop the flulike syndrome from intermittent dosage to daily doses, a strategy that allows the drug to be continued in most cases.

Allergic reactions such as the flulike syndrome, rashes, and acute renal failure are much more likely to occur in patients who have received rifampin previously. Patients with HIV infection are more likely to develop allergic reactions than HIV-seronegative patients.

BLOOD DYSCRASIAS

Neutropenia is a common reaction seen with rifabutin. Anemia, leukopenia, neutropenia, and thrombocytopenia are seen occasionally with the other rifamycins. Studies with rifampin indicate that the formation of IgM or IgG antibodies in response to the drug are likely to be responsible for thrombocytopenia and occasional hemolysis that is seen.[129]

NEPHROTOXICITY

Hematuria and proteinuria are reported commonly with rifapentine use. Rifampin occasionally causes interstitial nephritis, which is related to the formation of IgM or IgG antibodies to the drug, with subsequent binding of immune complexes to renal tubular epithelial cells. This reaction is most common with intermittent dosing regimens and usually reverses on discontinuation of the drug.[129] All the rifamycins are highly colored compounds that impart a red color to body fluids, including urine. This discoloration is harmless and does not signify toxicity.

HEPATOTOXICITY

Hepatitis occurs occasionally with rifampin or rifapentine.

OPTIC DAMAGE

Rifabutin has been associated rarely with uveitis. This reaction is dose-related, occurring most commonly when daily doses exceed 1050 mg. All the rifamycins are highly colored compounds that impart a red color to sweat and tears. This harmless discoloration may stain clothing or soft contact lens.

CNS Adverse Effects

INCIDENCE OF CNS EFFECTS

CNS effects are seen only occasionally with rifamycins. Reported symptoms include confusion, dizziness, fatigue, headache, insomnia, and mood changes. No mechanism has been proven for these reactions.

Antituberculosis Drugs Used in Multidrug Combinations: Ethambutol, Streptomycin, Pyrazinamide, Cycloserine, Ethionamide

These drugs are discussed together because they are often used together. When used in combination with isoniazid or with a rifamycin, the additional adverse reactions of those drugs have to be considered.

Systemic Adverse Effects

GI DISTURBANCES

Anorexia, cramping, diarrhea, dyspepsia, nausea, and vomiting are common adverse reactions to oral antituberculosis therapy. The drugs most likely to cause these effects are ethionamide and ethambutol.

PERIPHERAL NEUROPATHY

Peripheral neuropathy, with tingling or numbness in the extremities, is common with antituberculosis therapy. Ethambutol, streptomycin, and cycloserine are all associated with this complication.

OPTIC NEURITIS

Optic neuritis is a dose-related adverse effect of ethambutol. Optic neuritis is seen most commonly in patients taking daily doses above 25 mg/kg for periods longer than 2 months. Optic neuritis may be seen in only one or in both eyes and is usually reversible, but full recovery, if it occurs, may take months.

ALLERGIC REACTIONS

Fever, itching, and rash are uncommon reactions to these agents.

NEPHROTOXICITY/OTOTOXICITY

Streptomycin has the highest nephrotoxic and ototoxic potential of the aminoglycoside family.

HEPATOTOXICITY

Pyrizinamide causes dose-related hepatotoxicity. The risk is increased with doses of 40 to 50 mg/kg, with longer periods of therapy, and with age greater than 60 years.[130]

METABOLIC EFFECTS

Both pyrazinamide and ethambutol may produce hyperuricosemia. Symptoms may be mild or severe, with acute pain in the joints (gouty arthritis).

CNS Adverse Effects

INCIDENCE OF CNS EFFECTS

Anxiety, aphasia, confusion, dizziness, drowsiness, headache, irritability, depression, mood changes, muscle twitching, nightmares, trembling, and suicidal thoughts all have been reported with the use of these drugs. These effects are caused most often by cycloserine (up to 30 percent of patients receiving 500 mg bid), ethambutol, and ethionamide. Seizures are associated most commonly with cycloserine (8 percent of patients receiving 500 mg bid), but streptomycin also can contribute to their development.

MECHANISMS OF CNS EFFECTS

The high risk of CNS toxicity with cycloserine is related to the ability of cycloserine to antagonize the action of pyridoxal-5-phosphate in the brain, leading to reduced GABA production. Just as with isoniazid, pyridoxine supplementation can help reverse or prevent CNS toxicity due to cycloserine.

RISK FACTORS FOR CNS ADVERSE REACTIONS

Other factors that may increase the risk of seizures with cycloserine include the use of ethanol and a history of preexisting convulsive disorders. Other CNS effects of cycloserine may be dose-related and are more likely at daily doses above 500 mg or serum concentrations in excess of 30 μg/ml.

Drugs Used for Leprosy: Dapsone, Clofazimine, Thalidomide

These drugs have limited applications and are used most often for leprosy.

Systemic Adverse Effects

GI DISTURBANCES

Abdominal pain, anorexia, constipation, nausea, and diarrhea are most likely with thalidomide (11 to 59 percent) and least likely with dapsone. GI disturbances occur most likely with daily doses of clofazimine above 200 mg, affecting up to 60 percent of patients at higher doses. Thalidomide occasionally increases appetite or causes dry mouth.

PERIPHERAL NEUROPATHY

Thalidomide causes sensory fibers in the limbs to degenerate, leading to progressive and irreversible symptoms unless the drug is discontinued at the first signs of peripheral neuropathy. Initial signs include paresthesias of the feet or hands and burning or muscle cramps in the extremities. Peripheral neuropathy appears gradually over weeks or months. The incidence reported in the literature is variable in part because patients with drug-related neuropathy may show few clinical symptoms and only show signs of neuropathy if tested by electrophysiologic methods. In HIV-infected patients, the incidence of peripheral neuropathy due to thalidomide approaches 50 percent. Dapsone is a less common cause of peripheral neuropathy.

ALLERGIC REACTIONS

Dapsone commonly causes simple skin rashes but is also capable of causing much more serious allergic reactions such as erythema multiforme, exfoliative dermatitis, and toxic epidermal necrolysis. Delayed hypersensitivity reactions sometimes referred to as the *sulfone syndrome* include anemia, exfoliative dermatitis, fever, jaundice, lymphadenopathy, malaise, and methemoglobinemia. Skin rash has been seen with thalidomide and is most common in AIDS patients.

BLOOD DYSCRASIAS

Dapsone commonly causes hemolytic anemia or methemoglobinemia. The risk of hemolytic anemia is increased in patients with glucose-6-phosphate deficiency. Fatal aplastic anemia or agranulocytosis also has occurred. Neutropenia has been noted rarely with thalidomide.

CARDIOTOXICITY

Thalidomide rarely causes an irregular heartbeat or hypotension.

NEPHROTOXICITY

Thalidomide rarely causes signs of renal failure, with reduced urine output.

HEPATOTOXICITY

Jaundice has been seen with dapsone use.

SKIN EFFECTS

Both thalidomide and clofazimine can dry the skin. In addition, clofazimine is a highly colored compound that deposits in skin and other tissues, especially at high doses. The skin discoloration is distressing to many patients. The red color of urine, feces, sputum, sweat, and tears is an expected and harmless side effect of the drug. Up to 57 percent of patients also experience discoloration of the conjunctiva. Because clofazimine is highly tissue bound and excreted slowly, the discoloration of tissues and fluids may take weeks to months to clear after the drug is discontinued.

TERATOGENICITY

Thalidomide is a known teratogen in humans and must be avoided in any woman who is pregnant or able to become pregnant.

CNS Adverse Effects

INCIDENCE OF CNS EFFECTS

Thalidomide was introduced as a sedative, so drowsiness is a common and expected adverse reaction. Less commonly the drug may cause headache, dizziness, or mood alterations. Headache, insomnia, and nervousness are relatively common adverse reactions to dapsone and are considered dose-related.

MECHANISMS OF CNS EFFECTS

Thalidomide may activate the sleep centers in the thalamus or hypothalamus, leading to sedation.

RISK FACTORS FOR CNS ADVERSE REACTIONS

The risk of CNS side effects with thalidomide increases with the dose.

▶ ANTIVIRAL AGENTS

Nucleoside/Nucleotide HIV Reverse-Transcriptase Inhibitors (NRTIs): Abacavir, Didanosine, Lamivudine, Stavudine, Tenofovir, Zalcitabine, Zidovudine

Drugs used to treat HIV infection are commonly used in combinations, making assignment of adverse reactions to specific drugs a challenging task; most of the data for these drugs comes from complicated studies comparing two or more drug combinations with each other. Many of the adverse reactions noted below are more common in HIV-positive patients with more advanced disease.

Systemic Adverse Effects

BLOOD DYSCRASIAS
Zidovudine affects bone marrow function, thus making anemia or neutropenia a dose-limiting toxicity with this agent. Lamivudine combined with lower doses of zidovudine still cause neutropenia in about 8 percent of patients and anemia in about 3 percent. Stavudine also affects cells in the bone marrow, leading to loss of cells in the erythroid and granulocyte-macrophage lineages. Didanosine causes thrombocytopenia, anemia, or other blood dyscrasias in about 5 percent of patients, but the risk increases up to tenfold if patients have abnormal baseline levels when didanosine therapy is begun.

ALLERGIC REACTIONS
Abacavir causes a multiorgan hypersensitivity reaction in approximately 5 percent of patients. Symptoms include abdominal pain, diarrhea, dyspnea, fever, mouth ulcers, muscle pain or general malaise, numbness of face or extremities, rash, and swelling of feet and legs. If the drug is not withdrawn, anaphylaxis or multiorgan failure may be fatal. Didanosine, lamivudine, stavudine, and zalcitabine uncommonly cause chills, fever, itching, or rashes. Lamivudine with zidovudine rarely has been associated with erythema multiforme, Stevens-Johnson syndrome, and generalized vasculitis.

LIPODYSTROPHY
Patients on long-term therapy for HIV infection often show a redistribution of fat around the body, usually with a gain between the shoulders and around the waist but a loss in the face, legs, and arms. This syndrome has not been completely explained, but some studies show that these drugs damage mitochondria in fatty tissue, which can lead to fat loss.[131]

GI DISTURBANCES
Didanosine causes abdominal pain, nausea, and vomiting, but the most common GI effect is diarrhea, which

may be caused by the buffering agent in preparations of didanosine. Lamivudine given in combination with zidovudine also commonly causes GI distress, including nausea in about one-third of patients and diarrhea in nearly 20 percent. GI disturbances are less common with other NRTIs.

PERIPHERAL NEUROPATHY
Didanosine, stavudine, and zalcitabine cause neuropathy that can progress to axonal degeneration; this reaction is dose-limiting in up to 20 percent of patients. This reaction may be partly related to mitochondrial damage produced by these drugs, but other mechanisms are possible.[132] Early symptoms are tingling or burning in the hands and feet, but these sensations are replaced by pain as the condition progresses. Lamivudine with zidovudine has been associated with peripheral neuropathy in about 12 percent of treated patients.

MYOPATHY
Zidovudine causes muscle inflammation. Symptoms may be slow in developing and include weakness or tenderness of the muscles. This adverse reaction may be due to zidovudine effects on mitochondria. When zidovudine is given with lamivudine, about 12 percent of patients report muscle pain. Muscle or joint pain also is reported occasionally by patients receiving other NRTIs.

PANCREATITIS
Didanosine causes some degree of pancreatitis in about 25 percent of patients who receive the drug, and about 5 percent show serious signs of damage; the effect is dose-related, and fatalities have occurred. The clinical symptoms of abdominal pain, nausea, and vomiting are accompanied by elevated serum amylase and lipase levels. Didanosine must be withdrawn permanently if pancreatitis occurs, and the drug should be avoided in patients with known risk factors for pancreatitis (e.g., previous history of pancreas disease or record of diagnostic procedures on the pancreas, active alcohol abuse, gall stones, morbid obesity, or hypertriglyceridemia). Stavudine is also associated with pancreatitis, but the risk is less than with didanosine. Other NRTIs also may cause pancreatitis rarely.

RESPIRATORY TOXICITY
Lamivudine with zidovudine causes cough or nasal stuffiness in up to 20 percent of patients.

CARDIOTOXICITY
Cardiomyopathy is a rare adverse reaction to didanosine.

EYE DAMAGE
Didanosine rarely causes retinal damage, which has been reported in children receiving the drug.

HYPERGLYCEMIA

Lamivudine with zidovudine rarely causes hyperglycemia.

NEPHROTOXICITY

Tenofovir, a new nucleotide inhibitor of reverse transcriptase, is related to the nephrotoxic drugs cidofovir and adefovir. Little data exist to document nephrotoxicity with tenofovir, but a single case report describes a patient with stable chronic renal insufficiency who was receiving didanosine successfully but died of lactic acidosis when tenofovir was added to the regimen.[133] Two other patients showed typical signs of renal tubular necrosis associated with tenofovir, suggesting that this toxicity may be rare but is a possible complication with this relatively new agent.[134]

HEPATOTOXICITY

Enlargement of the liver, hepatitis, and fatty liver degeneration have occurred with zidovudine, abacavir, stavudine, and didanosine but are rare with other NRTIs. Metabolic acidosis or lactic acidosis also occurs and may be related to mitochondrial damage caused by these drugs. These adverse reactions have caused rare fatalities.

CNS Adverse Effects

INCIDENCE OF CNS EFFECTS

Anxiety, headache, irritability, insomnia, and restlessness are relatively common reactions to didanosine and resolve when the drug is discontinued. Seizures also have been reported but are rare. Zidovudine commonly causes severe headache and insomnia. Zidovudine with lamivudine causes headache in about 35 percent of patients. Insomnia, dizziness, and depression are reported in about 10 percent of patients receiving the combination. Seizures have been noted with the use of zidovudine either alone or in combination.

MECHANISMS OF CNS EFFECTS

Drugs of this class diffuse into the CNS and produce drug concentrations in the CSF that are 10 to 100 percent of serum concentrations. The exact mechanism producing CNS toxicity is unclear.

RISK FACTORS FOR CNS ADVERSE REACTIONS

HIV infection itself is a risk factor for CNS reactions because advanced cases of AIDS may show many neurologic complications even if anti-HIV drugs have not been used.[135]

Nonnucleoside HIV Reverse-Transcriptase Inhibitors (NNRTIs): Efavirenz, Delavirdine, Nevirapine

These drugs, acting by different mechanisms than the nucleoside or nucleotide inhibitors of reverse transcriptase, are valuable in combination therapy of HIV infection. Their use in combinations complicates assessment of adverse reactions.

Systemic Adverse Effects

ALLERGIC REACTIONS

Efavirenz has caused rashes in up to 40 percent of treated children and 27 percent of adults. The rashes range from simple erythema or pruritus to erythema multiforme or Stevens-Johnson syndrome. Delavirdine and nevirapine cause similar reactions. Skin rashes are one of the limiting toxicities with this class of drugs.

GI DISTURBANCES

Diarrhea, nausea, and vomiting are common adverse reactions to delavirdine and nevirapine. Sores in the mouth also have been reported.

MYALGIA

Muscle aches have been reported with delavirdine.

BLOOD DYSCRASIAS

Granulocytopenia is a common adverse reaction to nevirapine, especially in children. Symptoms include chills, fever, and sore throat.

CNS Adverse Effects

INCIDENCE OF CNS EFFECTS

Adverse CNS reactions are among the most common adverse events reported for efavirenz. In early trials, up to 52 percent of patients reported some CNS symptoms, which ranged from dizziness or headache to more serious psychiatric symptoms such as abnormal dreaming, confusion, depression, insomnia, loss of concentration, nervousness, and somnolence. Nevirapine and delavirdine cause fewer CNS effects, with headache being the most common symptom.

MECHANISMS OF CNS EFFECTS

Efavirenz is a highly lipophilic drug that readily penetrates into the CSF, producing therapeutically effective drug concentrations. The drug has not been shown to bind to known neuroreceptors or to interfere with known neurotransmitters; therefore, the mechanism for the CNS adverse reactions is unclear.

RISK FACTORS FOR CNS ADVERSE REACTIONS

HIV infection itself is a risk factor for CNS complications.[135]

HIV Protease Inhibitors: Amprenavir, Atazanavir, Indinavir, Lopinavir, Nelfinavir, Ritonavir, Saquinavir

These drugs are used only in combination with other anti-HIV drugs. Lopinavir is available only in fixed combination with ritonavir. Most of the data for these drugs come from studies comparing two or more drug combinations with each other, complicating the assignment of specific adverse reactions.

Systemic Adverse Effects

GI Disturbances
GI effects including abdominal pain, diarrhea, nausea, and vomiting are characteristic adverse reactions to this class of drugs. Diarrhea is reported by 20 percent of patients receiving nelfinavir. Atazanavir causes less diarrhea but still is associated with nausea and vomiting. Indinavir commonly causes taste perversion.

Metabolic Effects
Amprenavir commonly has been associated with development of hyperglycemia, which rarely progresses to diabetes mellitus. Atazanavir occasionally has been linked to diabetes mellitus, dyslipidemia, gout, and lactic acidosis. Other protease inhibitors also occasionally may cause hyperglycemia, diabetes mellitus, or ketosis. Indinavir and ritonavir cause generalized weakness or fatigue.

Allergic Reactions
Amprenavir commonly causes skin rashes. Rashes are also seen with atazanavir and occasionally with other protease inhibitors. Rash is a common adverse reaction to nelfinavir, and desensitization has been used on occasion.[136]

Peripheral Neuropathy
Amprenavir and ritonavir cause paresthesias, with tingling or prickling sensations in the arms and legs, as well as around the mouth. Early trials suggest that this reaction may be less common with atazanavir, but definitive conclusions await the long-term use of this drug in significant numbers of patients.

Cardiotoxicity
The combination of lopinavir with ritonavir has been associated occasionally with cardiac arrhythmias.

Lipodystrophy
Protease inhibitors contribute to fat redistribution in patients who receive the drugs for prolonged periods. This syndrome, in which fat increases between the shoulders (buffalo hump) and around the trunk while diminishing in the face, arms, and legs, may have several causes, including other drugs (e.g., NRTIs). However, the syndrome was first noted when indinavir was introduced; an early slang term for the syndrome was "crix belly," which is based on the trade name Crixivan for indinavir.

Nephrotoxicity
Indinavir causes kidney stones in about 4 percent of treated patients. This adverse reaction is dose-related and can be ameliorated with adequate hydration. Indinavir may also crystallize in renal tubules, leading to blockage and renal damage; this effect is worsened as urinary pH approaches neutrality.[134]

Hepatotoxicity
Atazanavir increases total bilirubin levels in about 35 percent of patients, and 7 to 8 percent may have jaundice or scleral icterus. Indinavir and saquinavir also increase bilirubin levels, usually without causing symptoms.

CNS Adverse Effects

Incidence of CNS Effects
Amprenavir causes depression and other mood changes in significant numbers of patients. Depression also has been noted with other protease inhibitors, as well as insomnia and dizziness.

Mechanisms of CNS Effects
HIV protease inhibitors as a group do not penetrate the CNS very well, the exception being indinavir.[137] The mechanism for CNS effects of protease inhibitors is unclear, but one case report suggests an unusual possibility. The oral formulation of amprenavir contains 55 percent polypropylene glycol; at high doses with this formulation, polypropylene glycol may cause CNS depression and seizures.[138]

Risk Factors for CNS Adverse Reactions
As noted for NRTIs, HIV infection itself is a risk factor for CNS complications.[135]

Acyclic Nucleoside Antivirals: Acyclovir, Adefovir, Cidofovir, Famciclovir, Ganciclovir, Valacyclovir

These drugs are all antimetabolites capable of inhibiting many viral as well as mammalian enzymes, but they differ in their clinical indications. Acyclovir, famciclovir, penciclovir, and valacyclovir are used against herpes simplex virus or varicella-zoster virus; cidofovir and ganciclovir, for cytomegalovirus; and adefovir, for hepatitis B.

Systemic Adverse Effects

Blood Dyscrasias
Cidofovir caused neutropenia in 20 percent of patients who received doses of 5 mg/kg in early clinical trials. Ganciclovir causes a reversible granulocytopenia in about 40 percent of patients; this adverse reaction is

dose-limiting in about 50 percent of patients with this complication. Ganciclovir also causes reversible thrombocytopenia in 20 percent of treated patients. Anemia is less common. Acyclovir rarely causes anemia or other blood dyscrasias such as neutropenia or thrombocytopenia. Hemolysis has occurred with acyclovir.

GI Disturbances

Parenterally administered acyclovir commonly causes anorexia, nausea, or vomiting; lower oral doses are less likely to cause these symptoms. Valacyclovir causes similar reactions to orally administered acyclovir. Adefovir and ganciclovir may cause abdominal pain, diarrhea, flatulence, nausea, and vomiting. Cidofovir commonly causes anorexia, diarrhea, nausea, and vomiting. Famicyclovir is well tolerated and only occasionally causes diarrhea or nausea.

Eye Damage

Visual changes have occurred with acyclovir. Adefovir has been associated with ocular hypotony, especially in patients with preexisting diabetes mellitus. Intravitreal injection of ganciclovir may cause conjunctival scarring, retinal detachment, scleral induration, or subconjunctival hemorrhage.

Allergic Reactions

Acyclovir causes a variety of allergic reactions, including anaphylaxis, hives, and rashes, that may include serious reactions such as erythema multiforme, toxic epidermal necrolysis, or Stevens-Johnson syndrome. Adefovir and ganciclovir have been associated with fever, itching, and rash.

Nephrotoxicity

Rapid infusion of high doses of acyclovir causes the drug to crystallize in renal tubules, leading to renal damage or acute renal failure.[134] Renal toxicity is treatment-limiting for cidofovir and adefovir. These drugs directly damage renal proximal tubular epithelial cells because they are concentrated in the cells, entering via an active transport system on the basolateral membrane. Although the drugs may exit via apical carriers or channels, they are present at high enough concentrations to impede cellular metabolism, which can directly kill the cells. Probenecid blocks uptake of these organic anions into the proximal tubular cells and reduces nephrotoxicity.[134] Adefovir has been approved for use in hepatitis B rather than in HIV because the lower doses required for hepatitis B are also associated with a lower incidence of renal toxicity.

Hepatotoxicity

Adefovir has a low potential for direct hepatotoxicity, but on discontinuation of hepatitis B therapy, about 25 percent of patients experience a rebound of hepatitis

symptoms accompanied by viral replication. Fatalities have occurred. Adefovir also has the potential to cause lactic acidosis.

Local Injection-Site Reactions

Acyclovir may cause severe inflammation at the injection site. With intravenous use, the drug has caused disseminated intravascular coagulation, which leads to oozing of blood at injections sites or elsewhere. Ganciclovir may cause phlebitis when used intravenously, unless the infusion is administered over at least 1 hour.

Whole-Body Reactions

Acyclovir may cause swelling of the lymph glands and edema throughout the body. Acyclovir also causes a general feeling of malaise in 11 percent of treated patients. Asthenia also has been noted with adefovir, cidofovir, and valaciclovir. Adefovir may cause excessive coughing, pharyngitis, or sinusitis.

CNS Adverse Effects

Incidence of CNS Effects

Acyclovir may cause coma, confusion, hallucinations, tremor, or seizures, as well as mood changes or psychosis. Cidofovir and valaciclovir commonly cause headache, but other CNS symptoms are rare. Famciclovir also causes headache and dizziness but few other symptoms. Ganciclovir may cause mood changes, nervousness, or tremor.

Mechanisms of CNS Effects

Acyclovir penetrates the CNS adequately to achieve antiviral concentrations. The exact mechanism by which acyclovir produces neurotoxic symptoms is unclear, and for most patients the results of CNS imaging were inconclusive.[139] CNS effects for other drugs in this group are mild and nonspecific.

Risk Factors for CNS Adverse Reactions

Acyclovir is more likely to cause adverse CNS effects when the drug is used at high concentrations or when it accumulates in patients with renal impairment; plasma levels above 25 μg/ml are commonly associated with toxicity. CNS effects are also more common in immunocompromised patients and the elderly.

Antiviral Phosphonate: Foscarnet

An analogue of pyrophosphate, foscarnet is used for cytomegalovirus and herpes simplex infections.

Systemic Adverse Effects

Nephrotoxicity

Nephrotoxicity is dose-limiting with this drug. Acute tubular necrosis, nephrogenic diabetes insipidus, and crystal formation in glomeruli have been reported.

GI DISTURBANCES

Abdominal pain, anorexia, nausea, and vomiting are common with foscarnet. The drug also occasionally causes stomatitis or sores on mucous membranes at various body sites.

BLOOD DYSCRASIAS

Anemia was seen in about 33 percent of patients in early clinical trials with foscarnet, and granulocytopenia or leukopenia was reported in nearly 20 percent; these reactions were rare reasons to discontinue therapy.

PERIPHERAL NEUROPATHY

Muscle twitching and tingling of the mouth and extremities have been noted. Muscle twitching may be caused by changes in calcium distribution.

CNS Adverse Effects

INCIDENCE OF CNS EFFECTS

Anxiety, confusion, dizziness, fatigue, and headache are common adverse reactions to foscarnet. Tremors and seizures also may occur. It is not known if these reactions are caused solely by changes in calcium distribution in the body.

Neuraminidase Inhibitors: Oseltamivir, Zanamivir

Both drugs are used to shorten the duration and severity of influenza. Oseltamivir is given orally, but zanamivir is inhaled. Because of this route of administration, systemic adverse reactions to zanamivir are uncommon.

Systemic Adverse Effects

GI DISTURBANCES

Oseltamivir caused an increase over placebo in nausea and vomiting in early clinical trials with adult patients who had naturally acquired influenza. Diarrhea was reduced by oseltamivir. These results were supported by phase III trials in children.

PULMONARY TOXICITY

Zanamivir may cause bronchospasm and may decrease pulmonary function, especially in patients with preexisting asthma or chronic obstructive pulmonary disease.

CARDIOTOXICITY

Arrhythmias have been reported in postmarketing monitoring with both oseltamivir and zanamivir.

ALLERGIC REACTIONS

Oseltamivir may cause rash, swelling of the face, or toxic epidermal necrolysis. Inhaled zanamivir also can cause oropharyngeal edema and skin rashes that may progress to serious reactions.

HEPATOTOXICITY

Oseltamivir has been associated with hepatitis and abnormal liver function tests.

METABOLIC REACTIONS

Oseltamivir may worsen diabetes mellitus.

CNS Adverse Effects

INCIDENCE OF CNS EFFECTS

Confusion and seizures have been noted for both oseltamivir and zanamivir in postmarketing surveillance. The mechanism and risk factors are unknown.

Antiviral Amines: Amantadine, Rimantadine

These drugs are used as antivirals, but amantadine is also used at higher doses to treat parkinsonism.

Systemic Adverse Effects

GI DISTURBANCES

Anorexia and nausea are relatively common with amantadine. Amantadine also has anticholinergic actions that lead to constipation and drying of mucous membranes. Rimantadine occasionally causes anorexia, dry mouth, nausea, stomach pain, or vomiting.

WHOLE-BODY REACTIONS

Amantadine causes peripheral edema and with chronic therapy can cause livedo reticularis, particularly on the legs of female patients.

NEPHROTOXICITY

The anticholinergic effects of amantadine may cause difficulty in urination.

CARDIOTOXICITY

Amantadine may cause hypertension and rarely is associated with congestive heart failure.

EYE DAMAGE

Amantadine rarely causes corneal depostis or otherwise affects vision.

CNS Adverse Effects

INCIDENCE OF CNS EFFECTS

CNS effects are the most common adverse reactions to amantadine. Doses of 200 mg daily cause symptoms such as agitation, dizziness, headache, inability to concentrate, insomnia, nervousness, nightmares, and somnolence. Confusion and seizures are less common. Psychiatric symptoms and suicide attempts have been reported. CNS effects are less common with rimantadine, although this difference may be due more to differences in pharmacokinetics than to the intrinsic CNS toxicity of the drugs.[140]

MECHANISMS OF CNS EFFECTS

The anticholinergic actions of amantadine may cause blurred vision, confusion, and hallucinations. In addition to these anticholinergic actions, amantadine has been recognized recently to act as an uncompetitive antagonist of the *N*-methyl-D-aspartate (NMDA) receptor in the CNS.[141] This highly lipophilic drug penetrates the brain readily and accumulates in tissues, probably associated with lysosomes.

RISK FACTORS FOR CNS ADVERSE REACTIONS

Serious adverse reactions to amantadine are more likely in elderly patients or those with preexisting psychiatric conditions.

Ribavirin

Ribavirin is used in the United States to treat respiratory syncytial virus, but the drug has activity against a number of other viruses.

Systemic Adverse Effects

BLOOD DYSCRASIAS

Ribavirin is associated with anemia, related to hemolysis and bone marrow suppression. These effects are dose-related and usually reversible.

GI DISTURBANCES

Anorexia and nausea may be caused by ribavirin.

TERATOGENICITY

Ribavirin is embryocidal in several animal species; the drug must be avoided in pregnant women.

ALLERGIC REACTIONS

Rashes or contact dermatitis may occur with prolonged contact with ribavirin. Redness of the eyes also may appear.

CNS Adverse Effects

INCIDENCE OF CNS EFFECTS

Ribavirin is associated with fatigue, headache, and insomnia. The drug has been used by intraventricular injection for control of viral encephalitis and has caused somnolence in 40 percent of treated patients and headache in 30 percent.[142] The lack of serious CNS effects by this route suggests that the drug is not significantly neurotoxic.

▶ ANTIFUNGAL AGENTS

Antifungal Polyenes: Amphotericin B (Fungizone), Amphotericin Lipid Complex (Abelcet), Amphotericin Liposomal (Ambisome)

Amphotericin B is the most powerful antifungal for systemic infections, but toxicity limits the total dose that may be used. Newer formulations in which amphotericin is complexed with various lipids alter tissue distribution and lower serum concentrations. At the same time, a significant reduction in toxicity is achieved. Therefore, doses of the lipid-containing formulations are higher than those possible with amphotericin alone. Amphotericin B is an older drug, and the data that follow for incidence of adverse reactions come from newer studies where it was used as the comparator.

Systemic Adverse Effects

NEPHROTOXICITY

Renal toxicity is dose-limiting with amphotericin B, and nearly all patients receiving the drug show signs of renal impairment. With total doses below 4 g, renal impairment may be slowly reversible, but above that dose permanent damage occurs. Good hydration helps to control azotemia but does not altogether prevent it. Amphotericin impairs renal function in several ways. The drug acutely lowers renal blood flow, impeding glomerular filtration. It is also directly toxic to renal tubular cells, changing membrane function and causing electrolyte disturbances. The most common of these is hypokalemia; intravenous potassium is required by many patients.

Lipid-containing formulations of amphotericin B are much less nephrotoxic than the parent drug. One explanation put forth for this reduced nephrotoxicity relates to the distribution of amphotericin B to lipoproteins in human serum. Uncomplexed amphotericin administered intravenously initially binds to high-density lipoproteins (HDL) but moves to low-density lipoproteins (LDL) in a process mediated by lipid-transfer protein. When amphotericin B is complexed with lipids or is in liposomes, this transfer to LDL is impeded. Amphotericin B bound to LDL is more nephrotoxic than when it is bound to HDL. Thus the lipid-containing formulations may lower the concentration of the nephrotoxic agent while still allowing distribution of the drug to the tissues.

BLOOD DYSCRASIAS

Hypochromic, normocytic anemia is an expected reaction to amphotericin B therapy because the drug lowers production of erythropoietin. Anemia occurs in only about 4 percent of patients receiving amphotericin lipid complex. Other blood dyscrasias such as thrombocytopenia or leukopenia are less common.

GI DISTURBANCES
Intravenous amphotericin B commonly causes anorexia (3.4 percent), diarrhea (11.2 percent), nausea (21.3 percent), or vomiting (13.5 percent). These reactions are less common with amphotericin lipid complex but still occur in up to 10 percent of patients.

WHOLE-BODY REACTIONS
Fever and chills are expected reactions to intravenous amphotericin B, occurring in up to 75 percent of patients; these reactions also occur in about 15 percent of patients who receive amphotericin B in lipid complex. The reaction occurs soon after the infusion is started and is usually over within 30 to 45 minutes. Meperidine, acetaminophen, and intravenous corticosteroids have been used to lessen this acute reaction. Patients also report generalized pain during infusion of amphotericin B.

CARDIOTOXICITY
Hypotension is a relatively common acute reaction to infusion of amphotericin B. If the drug is infused too rapidly, cardiac arrhythmias or shock may occur. Hypotension also was observed in 7 percent of patients receiving amphotericin B lipid complex; 5 percent developed cardiac arrest.

ALLERGIC REACTIONS
Although rashes may occur in small numbers of patients, dangerous allergic reactions are rare.

PULMONARY TOXICITY
Dyspnea or rapid respiration occurs commonly with amphotericin B infusion. Wheezing or tightness in the chest may signal a hypersensitivity reaction. Up to 10 percent of patients receiving amphotericin B lipid complex may develop respiratory failure.

EYE DAMAGE
Blurred or double vision is possible with either intravenous infusion or intrathecal injection of amphotericin B.

PERIPHERAL NEUROPATHY
Numbness, tingling, or weakness in the hands and feet may occur with amphotericin B infusion but is more likely with intrathecal injection.

LOCAL INJECTION-SITE REACTIONS
Thrombophlebitis is a common complication of amphotericin B therapy, occurring in about 22 percent of patients.

CNS Adverse Effects

INCIDENCE OF CNS EFFECTS
Headache is a common reaction (19 percent) to amphotericin B infusion, but seizures are rare. Headache was seen in 4 percent of patients receiving amphotericin B lipid complex in early clinical trials. The mechanism and risk factors for CNS reactions are not fully understood.

Antifungal Azoles: Fluconazole, Itraconazole, Ketoconazole, Voriconazole

Unlike the antifungal polyenes, the azoles are generally well-tolerated drugs.

Systemic Adverse Effects

GI DISTURBANCES
Nausea and other GI complaints are most common with fluconazole and itraconazole (about 8 percent of patients).

ALLERGIC REACTIONS
Allergic reactions are uncommon with this class of drugs, but serious reactions such as Stevens-Johnson syndrome have been reported with fluconazole.

HEPATOTOXICITY
Liver enzyme abnormalities may occur with these drugs, and rarely they may induce hepatitis. To avoid the risk of potentially fatal hepatic necrosis, these drugs must be discontinued if signs of hepatotoxicity develop; this reaction is best documented for ketoconazole.

METABOLIC TOXICITY
Ketoconazole inhibits steroidogenesis. As a result, the drug lowers testosterone levels. The most common symptom is gynecomastia in males. Testosterone levels are unaffected by other azoles.

BLOOD DYSCRASIAS
Fluconazole rarely causes agranulocytosis or thrombocytopenia.

EYE DAMAGE
Ketoconazole may rarely cause photophobia. The newest azole, voriconazole, has been linked to a dose-related transient visual disturbance that arises because the drug seems to slow deactivation of visual receptors.[143]

CNS Adverse Effects

INCIDENCE OF CNS EFFECTS
Headache and dizziness are reported occasionally by patients receiving an azole antifungal drug, but the class generally has little CNS activity.

Antifungal Antimetabolite: Flucytosine

Flucytosine conversion to fluorouracil within fungal cells is required for antifungal activity of this antimetabolite. Low levels of fluorouracil are also found in the sera of patients receiving flucytosine; this cytotoxic compound may account for some of the adverse reactions seen with flucytosine.

Systemic Adverse Effects

GI DISTURBANCES
About 5 percent of patients have nausea or diarrhea.

BLOOD DYSCRASIAS
Bone marrow depression is a dose-related toxicity with flucytosine. Neutropenia, which is usually reversible, may develop when serum levels of flucytosine exceed 100 μg/ml. Thrombocytopenia is less common; fatal bone marrow aplasia is rare.

ALLERGIC REACTIONS
Skin rashes occur occasionally.

HEPATOTOXICITY
Liver enzyme abnormalities occur in about 5 percent of patients.

CNS Adverse Effects

INCIDENCE OF CNS EFFECTS
CNS adverse reactions have not been reported.

Antifungal Echinocandin: Caspofungin

Caspofungin is the only member of its class currently available in the United States.

Systemic Adverse Effects

HEPATOTOXICITY
Liver enzymes are elevated in about 12 percent of patients receiving caspofungin.

LOCAL INJECTION-SITE REACTIONS
About 14 percent of patients develop signs of phlebitis or thrombophlebitis with infusion of caspofungin.

GI DISTURBANCES
Diarrhea, nausea, or vomiting occurs in about 3 percent of patients receiving 70-mg doses but is less with doses of 50 mg.

ALLERGIC REACTIONS
Erythema and rashes are possible during infusion with caspofungin; fever is relatively common. Anaphylaxis has not been observed

CNS Adverse Effects

INCIDENCE OF CNS EFFECTS
Headache is reported by about 8 percent of patients, but little is known about mechanisms behind this symptom.

Antifungal Diamidine: Pentamidine

Pentamidine is an old antiprotozoal drug that has become a mainstay in the treatment of *P. carinii* infections. Since *P. carinii* now has been recognized as an unusual fungus, the drug is considered among the antifungals. Toxicities become treatment-limiting for many patients receiving this drug.

Systemic Adverse Effects

METABOLIC TOXICITY
Hypoglycemia is a common reaction to pentamidine. The drug is directly toxic to beta cells of the pancreas, causing the cells to release insulin. This reaction usually appears late in the first week of therapy and may last days to weeks. The reaction is worsened by high drug doses, prolonged drug use, or possibly intermittent therapy. Weeks to months after therapy is completed, hyperglycemia and diabetes mellitus may occur.

WHOLE-BODY REACTIONS
Rapid infusion of pentamidine causes profound hypotension. The drug should be given by slow intravenous infusion over 1 to 2 hours.

BLOOD DYSCRASIAS
Leukopenia, neutropenia, and thrombocytopenia are common reactions to parenterally administered pentamidine. Anemia also may occur.

GI DISTURBANCES
Anorexia, diarrhea, nausea, and vomiting are common reactions. Taste perversions often described as a metallic taste also occur.

NEPHROTOXICITY
Pentamidine commonly causes nephrotoxicity manifested by decreased urinary output.

HEPATOTOXICITY
Liver enzymes are commonly elevated. Pancreatitis may occur with parenterally administered pentamidine.

CARDIOTOXICITY
Pentamidine has been associated with cardiac arrhythmias, especially ventricular and other tachyarrhythmias.

ALLERGIC REACTIONS
Pentamidine can cause itching, rashes, or redness of the skin.

LOCAL INJECTION-SITE REACTIONS

Pentamidine infusions can cause pain along the vein. The drug is highly irritating and causes sterile abscesses if released into tissues.

PULMONARY TOXICITY

When pentamidine is given by inhalation the drug may cause chest pain, coughing, difficulty breathing, pharyngitis, or wheezing. When administered by this route the drug does not distribute outside the lung, and extrapulmonary growth of *P. carinii* has developed in many patients.

CNS Adverse Effects

INCIDENCE OF CNS EFFECTS

Anxiety, headache, nervousness, and shakiness are common with pentamidine, but these symptoms arise from hypoglycemia and not from direct CNS toxicity.

▶ ANTIPROTOZOAL AGENTS

Antimalarial Aminoquinolones: Chloroquine, Hydroxychloroquine, Mefloquine, Primaquine

These antimalarial drugs have been used occasionally for other purposes. Chloroquine and hydroxychloroquine sometimes are used for rheumatoid disease, but doses are higher than antimalarial doses, and more toxicity results. Primaquine has been used with clindamycin as therapy for *P. carinii* infections.

Systemic Adverse Effects

EYE DAMAGE

Chloroquine commonly affects the function of ciliary muscles of the eye, making reading difficult. At doses exceeding 2.4 mg (base) per kilogram or with prolonged therapy, chloroquine may damage the retina. The changes are irreversible. For long-term use at higher doses, hydroxychloroquine may be preferred because this drug seems to cause fewer visual abnormalities.[144] Nevertheless, at doses exceeding 5 mg/kg, hydroxychloroquine also causes corneal opacities, keratopathy, and retinopathy.

GI DISTURBANCES

Anorexia, cramping, diarrhea, nausea, and vomiting are caused commonly by chloroquine, especially at higher doses. These reactions occur with similar incidence with other members of the class.

BLOOD DYSCRASIAS

Agranulocytosis, aplastic anemia, neutropenia, and thrombocytopenia are rare reactions to chloroquine, hydroxychloroquine, and mefloquine. Primaquine is more likely to cause hemolytic anemia, especially in patients deficient in glucose-6-phosphate dehydrogenase. Primaquine also is associated with methemoglobinemia, which may cause cyanosis in patients receiving high doses.

CARDIOTOXICITY

At normal antimalarial doses, chloroquine causes few cardiovascular abnormalities, but hypotension is possible, as well as prolongation of the QRS interval. With acute overdoses, cardiac complications become life-threatening. Hypotension may be profound, and conduction disturbances in the heart impair normal function; cardiac arrest, respiratory collapse, and death occur. These cardiovascular symptoms are related to the quinidine-like membrane-stabilizing effects of chloroquine. Similar cardiac symptoms have been noted with mefloquine or hydroxychloroquine.

WHOLE-BODY REACTIONS

With prolonged use, chloroquine or hydroxychloroquine may deposit in various tissues and cause discoloration, especially of the skin, fingernails, and inside the mouth. Hair may take on a bleached appearance, or hair loss may occur.

OTOTOXICITY

Hearing loss or ringing in the ears is a rare reaction to chloroquine or hydroxychloroquine.

ALLERGIC REACTIONS

Mefloquine rarely causes Stevens-Johnson syndrome.

CNS Adverse Effects

INCIDENCE OF CNS EFFECTS

At normal antimalarial doses, chloroquine only rarely causes headache, mood changes, or seizures. With acute overdose or with prolonged high doses, the risk of coma, drowsiness, headache, irritability, and seizures is greatly increased. At normal doses used for prophylaxis, mefloquine may cause more depression or altered thinking patterns than chloroquine.[145] CNS effects are among the most common adverse reactions reported for mefloquine.[146]

MECHANISMS OF CNS EFFECTS

The mechanism producing serious CNS effects with quinolone antimalarials is unknown.[147]

RISK FACTORS FOR CNS ADVERSE REACTIONS

Risk factors for CNS effects include preexisting seizure disorders.[148]

Antimalarials: Atovaquone, Proguanil, Pyrimethamine

Atovaquone and proguanil are currently available in the United States as a fixed combination for use in malaria. Atovaquone alone also has been used to treat *P. carinii* and *T. gondii* infections in immunocompromised patients. Pyrimethamine is combined most often with sulfadoxine for treating chloroquine-resistant malaria.

Systemic Adverse Effects

GI DISTURBANCES
Diarrhea, nausea, and vomiting occurred in more than 10 percent of patients receiving atovaquone, but many of the early studies with the drug were in AIDS patients, who may be more susceptible to adverse reactions. Proguanil or pyrimethamine at normal doses causes anorexia and generally mild gastrointestinal distress. Acute overdose of proguanil or pyrimethamine causes epigastric distress and vomiting.

ALLERGIC REACTIONS
Atovaquone commonly causes allergic skin rashes or fever. There is a single report of Stevens-Johnson syndrome associated with the combination of atovaquone and proguanil.[149] Allergic reactions are rare with pyrimethamine.

PULMONARY TOXICITY
Cough is a common adverse reaction to atovaquone.

NEPHROTOXICITY
Acute overdoses of proguanil may cause renal irritation or hematuria.

BLOOD DYSCRASIAS
As an antifolate, pyrimethamine is capable of causing agranulocytosis, leukopenia, and thrombocytopenia.

CNS Adverse Effects

INCIDENCE OF CNS EFFECTS
Headache and insomnia have been reported with atovaquone, but the mechanisms and risk factors have not been explored. Overdose with pyrimethamine causes hyperexcitability of the nervous system, which may lead to seizures, respiratory depression, and cardiovascular collapse.

Antihelminthic Agents: Ivermectin, Mebendazole, Oxamniquine, Praziquantel, Thiabendazole

These drugs are the preferred drugs in the United States for flukes, tapeworms, and roundworms. Adverse reactions may be difficult to assess because many reactions are caused by the dissolution of worms destroyed by therapy. Thus, for some of these drugs, the degree of side effects relates to the initial body burden of parasites.

Systemic Adverse Effects

ALLERGIC REACTIONS
Skin reactions such as itching or rash may occur with ivermectin and are related to reactions to components of dying worms. Similar reactions are noted with praziquantel. Thiabendazole is a rare cause of Stevens-Johnson syndrome but is associated more commonly with itching or rash.

GI DISTURBANCES
Mebendazole is poorly absorbed orally and may cause abdominal pain, diarrhea, nausea, or vomiting; other reactions are rare. Although well absorbed orally, oxamniquine and praziquantel also cause abdominal pain, diarrhea, nausea, and vomiting. Thiabendazole causes nausea in about 67 percent of patients receiving 25 mg/kg twice daily for 3 days.[150]

WHOLE-BODY REACTIONS
Edema is associated with ivermectin. Praziquantel often causes fever or sweating.

CARDIOTOXICITY
Ivermectin may cause tachycardia or postural hypotension.

EYE DAMAGE
Thiabendazole may cause vision changes, as well as drying of the eyes and other mucous membranes.

HEPATOTOXICITY
Thiabendazole has caused serious liver dysfunction, including intrahepatic cholestasis.

NEPHROTOXICITY
Oxamniquine creates an orange discoloration to the urine. This reaction is harmless and is not a sign of nephrotoxicity. Thiabendazole rarely causes crystalluria. Metabolites of thiabendazole impart an unpleasant odor to urine, but this reaction is harmless.

MUTAGENICITY
Oxamniquine is mutagenic and at high doses is embryocidal in animal studies. Other drugs in this class have low potential for mutagenicity.

CNS Adverse Effects

INCIDENCE OF CNS EFFECTS

These drugs are capable of causing a variety of dose-related CNS symptoms. Ivermectin does not cross the blood-brain barrier well and thus does not cause CNS effects at normal doses; however, acute overdose has been associated with dizziness, headache, and seizures. Mebendazole causes few symptoms other than GI disturbances, but high doses have been reported to cause dizziness or headache. Oxamniquine causes changes in the electroencephalogram, with spike and wave activity usually correlating with peak drug concentrations in serum.[151,152] About 33 percent of patients experience dizziness, drowsiness, or headache with oxamniquine. Rarely, oxamniquine induces seizures or psychiatric disorders. Praziquantel causes transient dizziness, drowsiness, or headache in up to 15 percent of patients receiving a single 20 mg/kg dose; up to 50 percent of patients are affected if that dose is repeated three times. Thiabendazole very commonly causes dizziness, drowsiness, or headache; less commonly the drug is associated with delirium, feelings of disorientation, or other psychiatric symptoms.

MECHANISMS OF CNS EFFECTS

The mechanisms behind the CNS effects of these drugs remain unclear.

RISK FACTORS FOR CNS ADVERSE REACTIONS

Patients with preexisting seizure disorders or neuropsychiatric disease are at increased risk for recurrence with oxamniquine therapy. Risk factors for reactions to the other drugs have not been thoroughly evaluated.

REFERENCES

1. Queener SF: History and origins of beta-lactam antibiotics. In: Queener SF, Webber JA, Queener SW (eds): *Beta-Lactam Antibiotics for Clinical Use.* New York: Marcel Dekker, 1986, pp 3–15.

2. Dahlgren AF: Adverse drug reactions in home care patients receiving nafcillin or oxacillin. *Am J Health Sys Pharm* 54:1176, 1997.

3. Ibia EO, Schwartz RH, Wiedermann BL: Antibiotic rashes in children: a survey in a private practice setting. *Arch Dermatol* 136:849, 2000.

4. Bigby M, Jick S, Jick H, Arndt K: Drug-induced cutaneous reactions: a report from the Boston Collaborative Drug Surveillance Program on 15,238 consecutive inpatients, 1975 to 1982. *JAMA* 256:3358, 1986.

5. Salkind RR, Cuddy PG, Foxworth JW: Is this patient allergic to penicillin? An evidence-based analysis of the likelihood of penicillin allergy. *JAMA* 285:2498, 2001.

6. Adcock BB, Rodman DP: Ampicillin-specific rashes. *Arch Fam Med* 5:301, 1996.

7. Renn CN, Straff W, Dorfmuller A, et al: Amoxicillin-induced exanthema in young adults with infectious mononucleosis: Demonstration of drug-specific lymphocyte reactivity. *Br J Dermatol* 147:1166, 2002.

8. Sicherer SH: Advances in anaphylaxis and hypersensitivity reactions to foods, drugs, and insect venom. *J Allergy Clin Immunol* 111:829S, 2003.

9. Gruchalla RS: Drug allergy. *J Allergy Clin Immunol* 111:548S, 2003.

10. Kelkar PS, Li JTC: Current concepts: Cephalosporin allergy. *New Engl J Med* 345:804, 2001.

11. Macy E, Mangat R, Burchette RJ: Penicillin skin testing in advance of need: Multiyear follow-up in 568 test-result-negative subjects exposed to oral penicillins. *J Allergy Clin Immunol* 111:1111, 2003.

12. Idsoe O, Guthe T, Willcox RR, de Weck AL: Nature and extent of penicillin side-reactions, with particular reference to fatalities from anaphylactic shock. *Bull WHO* 38:159, 1968.

13. Markowitz M, Kaplan E, Cuttica R, et al: Allergic reactions to long-term benzathine penicillin prophylaxis for rheumatic fever. *Lancet* 337:1308, 1991.

14. Neugut AI, Ghatak AT, Miller RL: Anaphylaxis in the United States: An investigation into its epidemiology. *Arch Intern Med* 161:15, 2001.

15. Pumphrey RSH, Davis S: Underreporting of antibiotic anaphylaxis may put patients at risk. *Lancet* 353:1157, 1999.

16. Olsson R, Wiholm BE, Sand C, et al: Liver damage from flucloxacillin, cloxacillin, and dicloxacillin. *J Hepatol* 15:154, 1992.

17. Fairley CK, McNeil JJ, Desmond P, et al: Risk factors for development of flucloxacillin associated jaundice. *Br Med J* 306:233, 1993.

18. Presti ME, Janney CG, Neuschwander-Tetri BA: Nafcillin-associated hepatotoxicity: Report of a case and review of the literature. *Dig Dis Sci* 41:180, 1996.

19. Ko CW, Sekijima JH, Lee SP: Biliary sludge. *Ann Inter Med* 130:301, 1999.

20. Rammelkamp CH, Keefer CS: The absorption, excretion and toxicity of penicillin administered by intrathecal injection. *Am J Med Sci* 205:342, 1943.

21. Edwards WM, Kellsey DC: Toxicity of intrathecal penicillin. *US Armed Forces Med J* 1:806, 1950.

22. Snavely SR, Hodges GR: The neurotoxicity of antibacterial agents. *Ann Intern Med* 101:92, 1984.

23. Cohen MM: Fatality following the use of intrathecal penicillin: Case report. *J Neuropathol Exp Neurol* 11:335, 1952.

24. Walker AE, Johnson HC: Convulsive factor in commercial penicillin. *Arch Surg* 50:69, 1945.

25. Schliamser SE, Cars O, Norrby SR: Neurotoxicity of beta-lactam antibiotics: Predisposing factors and pathogenesis. *J Antimicrob Chemother* 27:405, 1991.

26. Norrby SR: Neurotoxicity of carbapenem antibacterials. *Drug Saf* 15:87, 1996.

27. Calandra GB, Wang C, Aziz M, et al: The safety profile of imipenem/cilastatin: Worldwide clinical experience based on 3470 patients. *J Antimicrob Chemother* 18:193, 1986.

28. Norrby SR, Newell PA, Faulkner KL, et al: Safety pro-

file of meropenem: International clinical experience based on the first 3125 patients treated with meropenem. *J Antimicrob Chemother* 36:207, 1995.

29. Martinez-Rodriguez JE, Barriga FJ, Santamaria J, et al: Nonconvulsive status epilepticus associated with cephalosporins in patients with renal failure. *Am J Med* 111:115, 2001.

30. Barbey F, Bugnon D, Wauters J-P: Severe neurotoxicity of cefepime in uremic patients. *Ann Intern Med* 135:1011, 2001.

31. Spector R: Ceftriaxone transport through the blood-brain barrier. *J Infect Dis* 156:209, 1987.

32. Kang YS, Terasaki T, Tsuji A: Acidic drug transport in vivo through the blood-brain barrier: A role of the transport carrier for monocarboxylic acids. *J Pharmacobiodyn* 13:158, 1990.

33. Torok M, Huwyler J, Drewe J, et al: Transport of the beta-lactam antibiotic benzylpenicillin and the dipeptide glycylsarcosine by brain capillary endothelial cells in vitro. *Drug Metab Dispos* 26:1144, 1998.

34. Toyobuku H, Sai Y, Kagami T, et al: Delivery of peptide drugs to the brain by adenovirus-mediated heterologous expression of human oligopeptide transporter at the blood-brain barrier. *J Pharmaocl Exp Ther* 305:40, 2003.

35. Spector R: Ceftriaxone pharmacokinetics in the central nervous system. *J Pharmacol Exp Ther* 236:380, 1986.

36. Smith H, Lerner PI, Weinstein L: Neurotoxicity and "massive" intravenous therapy with penicillin: A study of possible predisposing factors. *Arch Intern Med* 120:47, 1967.

37. Donovan C, White ML, Cheung A, et al: Seizure incidence with imipenem use at a VA hospital. *Hosp Form* 30:172, 1995.

38. Townsend KA, Alaniz C, Stumpf JL, et al: Imipenem-cilastatin use: Evaluation of dosing and survey of adverse effects. *Hosp Pharm* 27:298, 1992.

39. Thomas RJ: Neurotoxicity of antibacterial therapy. *South Med J* 87:869, 1994.

40. Lipsky BA, Baker CA: Fluoroquinolone toxicity profiles: A review focusing on newer agents. *Clin Infect Dis* 28:352, 1999.

41. Ball P, Tillotson G: Tolerability of fluoroquinolone antibiotics: Past, present, and future. *Drug Saf* 13:343, 1995.

42. Leone R, Venegoni M, Motola D, et al: Adverse drug reactions related to the use of fluoroquinolone antimicrobials: An analysis of spontaneous reports and fluoroquinolone consumption data from three Italian regions. *Drug Saf* 26:109, 2003.

43. Yagawa K: Latest industry information on the safety profile of levofloxacin in Japan. *Chemotherapy* 47:38, 2001.

44. Stahlmann R, Lode H: Fluoroquinolones in the elderly: Safety considerations. *Drugs Aging* 20:289, 2003.

45. Melvani S, Speed BR: Alatrofloxacin-induced seizures during slow intravenous infusion. *Ann Pharmacother* 34:1017, 2000.

46. Takayama S, Hirohashi M, Kato M, Shimada. H: Toxicity of quinolone antimicrobial agents. *J Toxicol Environ Health* 45:1, 1995.

47. Tsuji A, Sato H, Kume Y, et al: Inhibitory effects of quinolone antibacterial agents on gamma-aminobutyric acid binding to receptor sites in rat brain membranes. *Antimicrob Agents Chemother* 32:190, 1988.

48. DeSarro A, DeSarro G: Adverse reactions to fluoroquinolones: An overview on mechanistic aspects. *Curr Med Chem* 8:371, 2001.

49. Lode H: Potential interactions of the extended-spectrum fluoroquinolones with the CNS. *Drug Saf* 21:123, 1999.

50. Tamai I, Yamashita J, Kido Y, et al: Limited distribution of new quinolone antibacterial agents into brain caused by multiple efflux transporters at the blood-brain barrier. *J Pharmacol Exp Ther* 295:146, 2000.

51. Periti P, Mazzei R, Mini E, Novelli A: Adverse effects of macrolide antibacterials. *Drug Saf* 9:346, 1993.

52. Guay DR, Patterson DR, Seipman N, Craft JC: Overview of the tolerability profile of clarithromycin in preclinical and clinical trials. *Drug Saf* 8:350, 1993.

53. Mishra A, Friedman HS, Sinha AK: The effects of erythromycin on the electrocardiogram. *Chest* 115:983, 1999.

54. Ebert SN, Liu XK, Woosley RL: Female gender as a risk factor for drug-induced cardiac arrhythmias: Evaluation of clinical and experimental evidence. *J Womens Health* 7:547, 1998.

55. Drici MD, Knollmann BC, Wang WX, Woosley RL: Cardiac actions of erythromycin: influence of female sex. *JAMA* 280:1774, 1998.

56. Kundu S, Williams SR, Nordt SP, Clark RF: Clarithromycin-induced ventricular tachycardia. *Ann Emerg Med* 30:542, 1997.

57. Dujovne CA, Showman D, Biachine J, Lasagna L: Experimental bases for the different hepatotoxicity of erythromycin preparations in man. *J Lab Clin Med* 79:832, 1972.

58. Demoly P, Benahmed S, Valembois M, et al: Allergy to macrolide antibiotics: Review of the literature. *Presse Med* 29:321, 2000.

59. Jorro G, Morales C, Braso JV, Pelaez A: Anaphylaxis to erythromycin. *Ann Allergy Asthma Immunol* 77:456, 1996.

60. Gangemi S, Ricciardi L, Fedele R, et al: Immediate reaction to clarithromycin. *Allerg Immunopathol* 29:31, 2001.

61. Cascaval RI, Lancaster DJ: Hypersensitivity syndrome associated with azithromycin. *Am J Med* 110:330, 2001.

62. Alvarez-Elcoro S, Ezler MJ: The macrolides: Erythromycin, clarithromycin, and azithromycin. *Mayo Clin Proc* 74:613, 1999.

63. Prime K, French P: Neuropsychiatric reaction induced by clarithromycin in a patient on highly active antiretroviral therapy (HAART). *Sex Transm Dis* 77:297, 2001.

64. Abouesh A, Stone C, Hobbs WR: Antimicrobial-induced mania (antibiomania): A review of spontaneous reports. *J Clin Psychopharmacol* 22:71, 2002.

65. Ott SM: Bone formation periods studied with triple tetracycline labels in women with postmenopausal osteoporosis. *J Bone Miner Res* 8:443, 1993.

66. Glorieux FH, Salle BL, Travers R, Audra PH: Dynamic

histomorphometric evaluation of human fetal bone formation. *Bone* 12:377, 1991.

67. Cohlan SQ, Bevlander G, Tiamsic T: Growth inhibition of prematures receiving tetracycline: Clinical and laboratory investigation. *Am J Dis Child* 105:453, 1963.

68. Appel GB, Heu HC: The nephrotoxicity of antimicrobial agents (second of three parts). *New Engl J Med* 296:722, 1977.

69. Digre KB: Not so benign intracranial hypertension: Condition needs to be diagnosed before patients develop visual symptoms. *Br Med J* 326:613, 2003.

70. Quinn AG, Singer SB, Buncic JR: Pediatric tetracycline-induced pseudotumor cerebri. *J Am Assoc Pediatr Ophthalmol Strabismus* 3:53, 1999.

71. Lochhead J, Elston JS: Doxycycline-induced intracranial hypertension. *Br Med J* 326:641, 2003.

72. Elting LS, Rubenstein EB, Kurtin D, et al: Mississippi mud in the 1990s: Risks and outcomes of vancomycin-associated toxicity in general oncology practice. *Cancer* 83:2597, 1998.

73. Wood MM: Comparative safety of teicoplanin and vancomycin. *J Chemother* 12:21, 2000.

74. Bhatt-Mehta V, Schumacher RE, Faix RG, et al: Lack of vancomycin-associated nephrotoxicity in newborn infants: A case-control study. *Pediatrics* 103:808, 1999.

75. Fiaccadori E, Maggiore U, Arisi A, et al: Outbreak of acute renal failure due to cefodizime-vancomycin association in a heart surgery unit. *Intensive Care Med* 27:1819, 2001.

76. English WP, Williams MD: Should aminoglycoside antibiotics be abandoned? *Am J Surg* 180:512, 2000.

77. Ferriols-Lisart R, Alos-Alminana M: Effectiveness and safety of once-daily aminoglycosides: A meta-analysis. *Am J Health Syst Pharm* 53:1141, 1996.

78. Susser Z, Raveh D, Yinnon AM: Safety of once-daily aminoglycosides in the elderly. *J Am Geriatr Soc* 48:857, 2000.

79. LeMoyec L, Racine S, LeToumelin P, et al: Aminoglycoside and glycopeptide renal toxicity in intensive care patients studied by proton magnetic resonance spectroscopy of urine. *Crit Care Med* 30:1242, 2002.

80. Streetman DS, Nafziger AN, Destache CJ, Bertino AS Jr: Individualized pharmacokinetic monitoring results in less aminoglycoside-associated nephrotoxicity and fewer associated costs. *Pharmacotherapy* 21:443, 2001.

81. Baciewicz AM, Sokos DR, Cowan RI: Aminoglycoside-associated nephrotoxicity in the elderly. *Ann Pharmacother* 37:182, 2003.

82. Buijk SE, Mouton JW, Gyssens IC, et al: Experience with a once-daily dosing program of aminoglycosides in critically ill patients. *Intensive Care Med* 28:936, 2002.

83. de Jager P, van Altena R: Hearing loss and nephrotoxicity in long-term aminoglycoside treatment in patients with tuberculosis. *Int J Tuberc Lung Dis* 6:622, 2002.

84. McCracken GH Jr, Mize SG, Threlkeld N: Intraventricular gentamicin therapy in gram-negative bacillary meningitis of infancy: Report of the Second Neonatal Meningitis Cooperative Study Group. *Lancet* 1:787, 1980.

85. Rahal JJ Jr, Simberkoff MS: Bactericidal and bacteriostatic action of chloramphenicol against meningeal pathogens. *Antimicrob Agents Chemother* 16:13, 1979.

86. Bartlett JG: Chloramphenicol. *Med Clin North Am* 66:91, 1982.

87. Alcindor T, Bridges KR: Sideroblastic anaemias. *Br J Haematol* 116:733, 2002.

88. Holt R: The bacterial degradation of chloramphenicol. *Lancet* 1:1259, 1967.

89. Issaragrisil S: Epidemiology of aplastic anemia in Thailand. Thai Aplastic Anemia Study Group. *Int J Hematol* 70:137, 1999.

90. Maluf EM, Pasquini R, Eluf JN, et al: Aplastic anemia in Brazil: Incidence and risk factors. *Am J Hematol* 71:268, 2002.

91. Laporte J-R, Vidal XBE, Ibanez L: Possible association between ocular chloramphenicol and aplastic anaemia: The absolute risk is very low. *Br J Clin Pharmacol* 46:181, 1998.

92. Sachs B, Erdmann S, al Masaoudi T, Merk HF: Molecular features determining lymphocyte reactivity in allergic contact dermatitis to chloramphenicol and azidamphenicol. *Allergy* 56:69, 2001.

93. Palchick BA, Funk EA, McEntire JE, Hamory BH: Anaphylaxis due to chloramphenicol. *Am J Med Sci* 288:43, 1984.

94. Thea D, Barza M: Use of antibacterial agents in infections of the central nervous system. *Infect Dis Clin North Am* 3:553, 1989.

95. Boom WH, Tuazon CU: Successful treatment of multiple brain abscesses with antibiotics alone. *Rev Infect Dis* 7:189, 1985.

96. Choquet-Kastylevsky G, Vial T, Descotes J: Allergic adverse reactions to sulfonamides. *Curr Allergy Asthma Rep* 2:16, 2002.

97. Blumenfeld H, Cha JH, Cudkowicz ME: Trimethoprim and sulfonamide-associated meningoencephalitis with MRI correlates. *Neurology* 46:556, 1996.

98. Hunziker T, Kunzi UP, Braunschweig S, et al: Comprehensive hospital drug monitoring (CHDM): Adverse skin reactions, a 20-year survey. *Allergy* 52:388, 1997.

99. Cabanas R, Caballero MT, Vega A, et al: Anaphylaxis to trimethoprim. *J Allergy Clin Immunol* 97:137, 1996.

100. Bijl AM, Van der Klauw MM, Van Vliet AC, Stricker BH: Anaphylactic reactions associated with trimethoprim. *Clin Exp Allergy* 28:510, 1998.

101. Ozkaya-Bayazit E, Akar U: Fixed drug eruption induced by trimethoprim-sulfamethoxazole: Evidence for a link to HLA-A30 B13 Cw6 haplotype. *J Am Acad Dermatol* 45:712, 2001.

102. Pedersen-Bjergaard U, Andersen M, Hansen PB: Thrombocytopenia induced by noncytotoxic drugs in Denmark 1968–1991. *J Int Med* 239:509, 1996.

103. Perazella MA: Trimethoprim-induced hyperkalaemia: Clinical data, mechanism, prevention, and management. *Drug Saf* 22:227, 2000.

104. Brett AS, Shaw SV: Simultaneous pancreatitis and hepatitis associated with trimethoprim-sulfamethoxazole. *Am J Gastroenterol* 94:267, 1999.

105. Moris G, Barcia-Monco JC: The challenge of drug-in-

duced aseptic meningitis. *Arch Intern Med* 159:1185, 1999.

106. Antonen J, Hulkkonen J, Pasternack A, Hurme M: Interleukin 6 may be an important mediator of trimethoprim-induced systemic adverse reaction resembling aseptic meningitis. *Arch Intern Med* 160:2066, 2000.

107. Theodorou AA, Barton LL, Rice SA, Rieder MJ: Trimethoprim-sulfamethoxazole-associated central nervous system disease. *Pediatr Infect Dis J* 14:76, 1995.

108. Kasten MJ: Clindamycin, metronidazole, and chloramphenicol. *Mayo Clin Proc* 74:825, 1999.

109. Koch RL, Beaulieu BB, Chrystal EJT, Goldman P: A metronidazole metabolite in human urine and its risk. *Science* 211:398, 1981.

110. Menendez D, Bendesky A, Rojas E, et al: Role of P53 functionality in the genotoxicity of metronidazole and its hydroxy metabolite. *Mutat Res* 501:57, 2002.

111. Falagas ME, Walker AM, Jick H, et al: Late incidence of cancer after metronidazole use: A matched metronidazole user/nonuser study. *Clin Infect Dis* 26:384, 1998.

112. Thapa PB, Whitlock JA, Worrell KGB, et al: Prenatal exposure to metronidazole and risk of childhood cancer: A retrospective cohort study of children younger than 5 years. *Cancer* 83:1461, 1998.

113. von Rogulja P, Kovac W, Schmid H: Metronidazole encephalopathy in rats. *Acta Neuropathol (Berl)* 25:36, 1973.

114. Ahmed A, Loes DJ, Bressler EL: Reversible magnetic resonance imaging findings in metronidazole-induced encephalopathy. *Neurology* 45:588, 1995.

115. Uhl MD, Riely CA: Metronidazole in treating portosystemic encephalopathy. *Ann Intern Med* 124:455, 1996.

116. Omotoso AB, Opadijo OG: Acute encephalopathy associated with metronidazole therapy. *Afr J Med Med Sci* 26:97, 1997.

117. Arik N, Cengiz N, Bilge A: Metronidazole-induced encephalopathy in a uremic patient: A case report. *Nephron* 89:108, 2001.

118. Paladino JA: Linezolid: An oxazolidinone antimicrobial agent. *Am J Health Syst Pharm* 59:2413, 2002.

119. Bernstein WB, Trotta RF, Rector JT, et al: Mechanisms for linezolid-induced anemia and thrombocytopenia. *Ann Pharmacother* 37:517, 2003.

120. Boggess KA, Benedetti TJ, Raghu G: Nitrofurantoin-induced pulmonary toxicity during pregnancy: Report of a case and review of the literature. *Obstet Gynecol Surv* 51:367, 1996.

121. Reinhart HH, Reinhart E, Korlipara P, Peleman R: Combined nitrofurantoin toxicity to liver and lung. *Gastroenterology* 102:1396, 1992.

122. Dan M, Aderka D, Topilsky M, et al: Hypersensitivity pneumonitis induced by nalidixic acid. *Arch Intern Med* 146:1423, 1986.

123. Garcia Rodriguez LA, Ruigomez A, Jick H: A review of epidemiologic research on drug-induced acute liver injury using the general practice research database in the United Kingdom. *Pharmacotherapy* 17:721, 1997.

124. Snider D, Caras G: Isoniazid-associated hepatitis

deaths: A review of available information. *Am Rev Respir Dis* 145:494, 1992.

125. Mitchell JR, Zimmerman HJ, Ishak KG, et al: Isoniazid liver injury: Clinical spectrum, pathology, and probably pathogenesis. *Ann Intern Med* 84:181, 1976.

126. Rothfield NF, Bierer WF, Garfield JW: Isoniazid induction of antinuclear antibodies. *Ann Intern Med.* 88:650, 1978.

127. Steinmann RA, Rickel MK: A 23-year-old with refractory seizures following an isoniazid overdose. *J Emerg Nurs* 28:7, 2002.

128. Shah BR, Santucci K, Sinert R, Steiner P: Acute isoniazid neurotoxicity in an urban hospital. *Pediatrics* 95:700, 1995.

129. Martinez E, Collazos J, Mayo J: Hypersensitivity reactions to rifampin: Pathogenetic mechanisms, clinical manifestations, management strategies, and review of the anaphylactic-like reactions. *Medicine* 78:361, 1999.

130. Yee D, Valiquette C, Pelletier M, et al: Incidence of serious side effects from first-line antituberculosis drugs among patients treated for active tuberculosis. *Am J Respir Crit Care Med* 167:1472, 2003.

131. Shikuma CM, Hu N, Milne C, et al: Mitochondrial DNA decrease in subcutaneous adipose tissue of HIV-infected individuals with peripheral lipoatrophy *AIDS* 15:1801, 2001.

132. Moyle G: Toxicity of antiretroviral nucleoside and nucleotide analogues: Is mitochondrial toxicity the only mechanism? *Drug Saf* 23:467, 2000.

133. Murphy MD, O'Hearn M, Chou S: Fatal adverse drug reactions after addition of Viread (tenofovir) to Videx (didanosine)–containing HIV treatment regimen. *Clin Infect Dis* 36:1082, 2003.

134. Perazella MA: Drug-induced renal failure: Update on new medications and unique mechanisms of nephrotoxicity. *Am J Med Sci* 325:349, 2003.

135. Goodkin K, Wilkie FL, Concha M, et al: Subtle neuropsychological impairment and minor cognitive-motor disorder in HIV-1 infection: Neuroradiological, neurophysiological, neuroimmunological, and virological correlates. *Neuroimag Clin North Am* 7:561, 1997.

136. Demoly P, Messaad D, Trylesinski A, et al: Nelfinavir-induced urticaria and successful desensitization. *J Allergy Clin Immunol* 102:875, 1998.

137. Haas DW, Johnson B, Nicotera J, et al: Effects of ritonavir on indinavir pharmacokinetics in cerebrospinal fluid and plasma. *Antimicrob Agents Chemother* 47:2131, 2003.

138. James CW, McNelis KC, Matalia MD, et al: Central nervous system toxicity and amprenavir oral solution. *Ann Pharmacother* 36:171, 2002.

139. Blohm ME, Nurnberger W, Aulich A, et al: Reversible brain MRI changes in acyclovir neurotoxicity. *Bone Marrow Transplant* 19:1049, 1997.

140. Hayden FG, Hoffman HE, Spyker DA: Differences in side effects of amantadine hydrochloride and rimantadine hydrochloride relate to differences in pharmacokinetics. *Antimicrob Agents Chemother* 23:458, 1983.

141. Kornhuber J, Quack G, Danysz W, et al: Therapeutic

brain concentration of the NMDA receptor antagonist amantadine. *Neuropharmacology* 34:713, 1995.

142. Tomoda A, Nomura K, Shiraishi S, et al: Trial of intraventricular ribavirin and interferon-alpha combination therapy for subacute sclerosing panencephalitis (SSPE) in Japan. *No to Hattatsu* 35:321, 2003.

143. Sheehan DJ, Hitchcock CA, Sibley CM: Current and emerging azole antifungal agents. *Clin Microbiol Rev* 12:40, 1999.

144. Easterbrook M: Detection and prevention of maculopathy associated with antimalarial agents. *Int Ophthalmol Clin* 39:49, 1999.

145. Petersen E, Ronne T, Ronn A, et al: Reported side effects to chloroquine, chloroquine plus proguanil, and mefloquine as chemoprophylaxis against malaria in Danish travelers. *J Travel Med* 7:79, 2000.

146. Schwartz E, Potasman I, Rotenberg M, et al: Serious adverse events of mefloquine in relation to blood level and gender. *Am J Trop Med Hyg* 65:189, 2001.

147. Vuurman EFPM, Muntjewerff ND, Uiterwijk MMC, et al: Effects of mefloquine alone and with alcohol on psychomotor and driving performance. *Eur J Clin Pharmacol* 50:475, 1996.

148. Bem JL, Kerr L, Stuerchler D: Mefloquine prophylaxis: An overview of spontaneous reports of severe psychiatric reactions and convulsions. *J Trop Med Hyg* 95:167, 1992.

149. Emberger M, Lechner AM, Zelger B: Stevens-Johnson syndrome associated with Malarone antimalarial prophylaxis. *Clin Infect Dis* 37:5e, 2003.

150. Grove DE: Treatment of strongyloidiasis with thiabendazole: An analysis of toxicity and effectiveness. *Trans R Soc Trop Med Hyg* 76:114, 1982.

151. Foster R: A review of clinical experience with oxamniquine. *Trans R Soc Trop Med Hyg* 81:55, 1987.

152. Krajden S, Keystone JS, Glenn C: Safety and toxicity of oxamniquine in the treatment of *Schistosoma mansoni* infections, with particular reference to electroencephalographic abnormalities. *Am J Trop Med Hyg* 32:1344, 1983.

CHAPTER 28

Rasmussen's Encephalitis

Riley Snook

Rasmussen's encephalitis is a rare progressive unilateral encephalopathy encountered almost exclusively in childhood. In 1958, Rasmussen described a new syndrome in children of 18 months to 5 years of age with focal seizures, progressive hemiparesis, and contralateral hemispheric brain atrophy.[1] While many cases of this syndrome have been reported since its description in 1958, the etiology and pathogenesis remain poorly understood. The typical clinical manifestations of the syndrome are a sudden onset of focal seizures in a young child that progresses over months to years into a refractory seizure disorder with hemiparesis, intellectual deterioration, and occasionally death. On histopathologic examination of brain tissue, there is perivascular inflammation, microglial nodules, gliosis, and astrocytosis, suggesting a focal viral encephalitis.[2] Aguilar and Rasmussen[2] hypothesized that the etiology of this syndrome was a viral infection. Brain involvement usually begins in a focal cortical region and progresses to involve the remainder of the cortex of the hemisphere. As a rule, the process does not involve the contralateral hemisphere and spares the thalamus, basal ganglia, and brain stem. The etiology of the syndrome remains a mystery. Various diagnostic techniques have found evidence of a variety of viral agents in brain material of affected patients, including enteroviruses, cytomegalovirus (CMV), Epstein-Barr virus (EBV), and herpes simplex virus (HSV). Thus far no consistent infectious agent has been identified. An autoantibody to the inotropic glutamate receptor subunit protein GluR3 has been identified in brain tissue and sera of many affected patients, suggesting an autoimmune mechanism. However, inconsistencies in the identification of this antibody and its absence in the cerebrospinal fluid (CSF) of affected patients continue to hinder a definitive description of an etiologic process. Recently, a derangement in cellular immunity has been proposed as the pathogenic process. A description of this disorder is included in this textbook because it was thought originally to be a viral encephalitis, and another etiology has not yet been determined.

▶ EPIDEMIOLOGY

The occurrence of Rasmussen's encephalitis is sporadic, with onset typically in childhood (mean 6.8 ± 5.1 years).[3] The estimated incidence in children is 1 per million.[4] Approximately 50 percent of patients will have had an infectious or inflammatory illness before the onset of epilepsy.[4] In approximately 40 percent, the illness occurs within a month of the first seizure, and in the remainder, within 6 months.[4] Over the past few years, cases of Rasmussen's encephalitis have been described in the literature in young adults as well as children, making it likely that Rasmussen's encephalitis is more prevalent than once thought.

▶ PATHOPHYSIOLOGY

The original description of the pathology by Rasmussen has remained the definitive pathologic criteria for diagnosing the syndrome and includes perivascular round cell infiltration, microglial nodules, astrocytosis, and spongy degeneration. While these findings generally are nonspecific, when placed in the clinical setting of intractable focal seizures, progressive hemiparesis, and isolated hemispheric atrophy, the features are virtually pathognomonic. The pathophysiology of the syndrome remains unknown, but technical advances have allowed the development of a few plausible hypotheses. In 1994, a link between antibodies against the inotropic glutamate receptor consisting of or containing GluR3, a glutamine subunit protein, and Rasmussen's encephalitis was observed. Some rabbits immunized with GluR3 subunits developed intractable focal epilepsy and had progressive decline in function leading to death, as has been described in Rasmussen's encephalitis.[5] After this discovery, GluR3 antibodies were found in human sera of several patients with classic Rasmussen's encephalitis. The role of the GluR3 antibody in the pathogenesis of Rasmussen's encephalitis remains unknown, however. A hypothesis has been proposed that anti-GluR3 antibodies gain entry to the brain via a compromised blood-brain barrier.[6] The anti-GluR3 antibodies then target antigens, causing neuronal injury. A vicious cycle is set in motion where neuronal injury leads to focal seizures that may produce focal permeability of the blood-brain barrier, and the cycle repeats itself.[6] The mechanism of how the anti-GluR3 antibody produces injury is debated. A direct role has been suggested for the GluR3 antibody binding to the glutamate receptor, causing overexcitement of the glutamate channel, and resulting in a massive cytotoxic response and subsequent neuronal and glial death. Another hypothesis is that the GluR3 antibody activates the complement cascade and indirectly causes a similar effect of glutamate channel overexcitement and cytotoxic neuronal death. However, a recent report implicates a direct effect of cytotoxic T cells as the mediator for the pathogenesis of Rasmussen's encephalitis.[7] In pathologic specimens of tissue of patients with Rasmussen's encephalitis, T-cell infiltration has been evident consistently. Early theories suggested that T-cell migration seen in pathologic specimens was induced by release of cytokines after GluR3-mediated cell damage had begun. The most recent reports, however, suggest that the cytotoxic T cells

may be the primary immunologic insult, possibly reacting to neuronal antigens presented secondary to a chronic viral infection.[7] The presence of the GluR3 antibodies may be a result of release of GluR antigens in the serum after cell death via an impaired blood-brain barrier. GluR3 autoantibodies have been identified in only approximately 50 percent of patients.[7] In an animal model of Rasmussen's encephalitis, approximately 50 percent of the rabbits immunized with anti-GluR3 developed symptoms.[5] It was proposed that a genetic susceptibility was required to develop symptoms. Anti-GluR3 antibodies have been identified in patients' sera only and not in the cerebrospinal fluid (CSF) or brain tissue. Therefore, GluR3 antibodies may be present as a secondary phenomenon in the sera of susceptible patients but not necessarily contribute to the pathogenesis of Rasmussen's encephalitis. The unihemispheric pathology in Rasmussen's encephalitis remains puzzling, but the recent cellular immune response hypothesis may provide an explanation. A single event, perhaps a viral infection, may cause a breach of the blood-brain barrier, and infection of a localized region of cortical tissue may occur. The antigens expressed in that region may, in turn, activate a specific class of T cells and cause the immune response in that region. The cellular immune response tends to be slower and localized and involves dysregulation of cellular metabolism leading to apoptosis. The course of initial inflammation leading to atrophy could be correlated with a decreasing number of T cells and reactive astrocytes, as assessed by quantitative histopathology.[8] These features of early active inflammation that "burns out" later on would fit with the clinical course and pathologic findings in Rasmussen's encephalitis.

Over the years, much work has gone into the search for an infectious agent responsible for Rasmussen's encephalitis. Efforts have been focused primarily on isolating viral particles in the cortex of affected individuals. Using brain tissue of affected patients and techniques such as in situ hybridization and polymerase chain reaction (PCR), investigators have identified viral DNA from multiple viruses, including: HSV-1, CMV, EBV, and human herpesvirus type 6 (HHV-6). However, viral particles have been identified in only a minority of patients with Rasmussen's encephalitis. Not only has no consistent viral etiology been found, but the majority of patients also have no virus detected by current techniques in their affected cortex. Furthermore, viral DNA has been isolated in patients with other epileptic syndromes and from normal individuals, the so-called normal brain flora.

It also has been proposed that a bacterial illness may be the inciting event in Rasmussen's encephalitis. The ligand-binding domains of glutamate receptors (GluRs) and bacterial periplasmic amino-acid-binding proteins have been shown to be structurally similar.[9]

The hypothesis proposed, then, is that a bacterial infection in a genetically susceptible individual induces the development of serum anti-GluR antibodies. A later focal disruption to the blood-brain barrier (i.e., trauma, surgery, or viral infection) allows the entrance of the anti-GluR antibodies and the subsequent syndrome of Rasmussen's encephalitis.[6]

▶ DIAGNOSIS

The diagnosis of Rasmussen's encephalitis typically is clinical, with support from neuroimaging, electroencephalography, and pathology when available. Most patients with Rasmussen's encephalitis will be previously healthy children younger than 6 years of age. The typical first signs are a focal seizure disorder that appears suddenly. Secondary generalization of seizures is not uncommon. In 20 percent of patients, generalized or focal status epilepticus will be the initial manifestation of disease.[4] The localization of attacks suggests a central cortical involvement, with temporal involvement less common and occipital involvement rare.[4] Motor involvement usually is evident by a loss of fine finger movements initially progressing to involve the arm and face. Leg involvement is less common initially.[4] Examination of the CSF shows abnormalities in approximately 50 percent of patients, with lymphocyte counts in the range of 6 to 70 cells/mm[3] and protein concentration between 50 and 98 mg/dl.[4] Children with Rasmussen's encephalitis often will be refractory to treatment and will develop gradual hemiparesis of one side. Intellectual decline is very common, and patients may begin to lose milestones as the syndrome progresses. Despite multidrug therapy, the patient will have more frequent and longer seizures, and up to 50 percent will develop epilepsia partialis continua, a continuous focal epilepsy.[4] Over several months to a few years, most children will be severely disabled and will lose much of their motor skills and cognitive ability. The prognosis is very poor, with most children dying from medical complications despite aggressive supportive care.

▶ NEUROIMAGING

Neuroimaging has been an important tool for diagnosing Rasmussen's encephalitis. A classic finding of Rasmussen's encephalitis is unihemispheric atrophy (Fig. 28-1) that progresses over time. In many cases the atrophy is initially focal and over time progressively involves a hemisphere. Serial magnetic resonance imaging (MRI) shows the spread of inflammation as an early increase in volume with hyperintense T_2/FLAIR signal to a final stage of atrophy without signal abnormality. However, the atrophy does not cross the midline, an

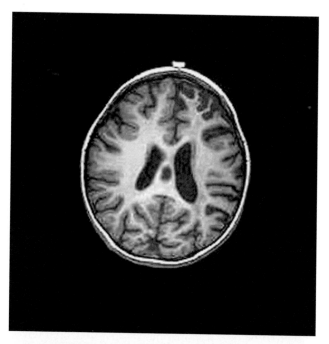

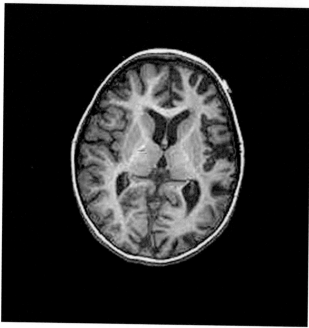

Figure 28–1. Cranial MRI demonstrating left focal atrophy in child with Rasmussen's encephalitis.

important point when making the diagnosis. MRI has been very useful in showing focal hemispheric atrophy, following progress, and planning for surgery.

More recently, single-photon-emission tomographic (SPECT) scanning has been used to show changes in regional cerebral blood flow (rCBF) in an affected hemisphere. Studies have shown that in patients with Rasmussen's encephalitis the affected brain regions are hyperperfused ictally and hypoperfused interictally.[10] Simultaneous electroencephalogram (EEG) and SPECT scanning are often performed to improve localization of the inflammatory focus. SPECT can be a useful adjunct to MRI when planning epilepsy surgery. SPECT has been useful as well in making early diagnosis of the syndrome. Before MRI changes are seen, SPECT scanning can show a change in rCBF in a hemisphere and can allow clinicians to begin treatment before significant atrophy or disability is evident. Positron-emission tomography (PET) has been used in an analogous fashion to SPECT in evaluating patients with Rasmussen's encephalitis. The major difference with PET scanning is that the parameter evaluated is the difference in glucose metabolism in affected brain regions instead of differences in regional blood flow as in SPECT. Both techniques are gaining popularity as adjunctive imaging modalities in diagnosing and managing Rasmussen's encephalitis.

Magnetoencephalography (MEG) has been used as an adjunct to imaging methods in localizing the focus of epileptiform activity in preoperative testing and was shown to be useful in mapping somatosensory evoked fields of eloquent regions of brain both pre- and postoperatively.[11]

▶ ELECTROENCEPHALOGRAPHY

EEG, although nonspecific, has been useful for many years in supporting a diagnosis of Rasmussen's encephalitis. A slowing of background activity may be bilateral but usually is asymmetric. When clinical seizures develop, EEG will show unilateral multiple active foci of epileptogenic activity in at least one-third of patients and bilateral synchronous epileptiform discharges in one-half.[4] In the early stages, interictal activity is localized to the affected hemisphere. As the disease progresses, increasingly frequent bilaterally synchronous and contralateral epileptiform activity may develop.[12] EEG is limited, therefore, because some patients will have secondary generalization of their seizures, and electrographic and clinical manifestations are poorly correlated (Fig. 28-2).

▶ DIFFERENTIAL DIAGNOSIS

Rasmussen's encephalitis is a diagnosis of exclusion; therefore, encephalitis and meningitis need to be ruled out first. Analysis of the CSF should be performed routinely in all patients who were previously healthy with new-onset focal seizures.

▶ TREATMENT

Treatment of Rasmussen's encephalitis has been difficult, with no current consensus on modalities or timing of treatment. Many different approaches have been attempted with varying success. McLachlan and colleagues[13] reported partial to complete responses in four patients with intravenous ganciclovir. Two of the patients had CMV identified in the CSF.[13] Zidovudine re-

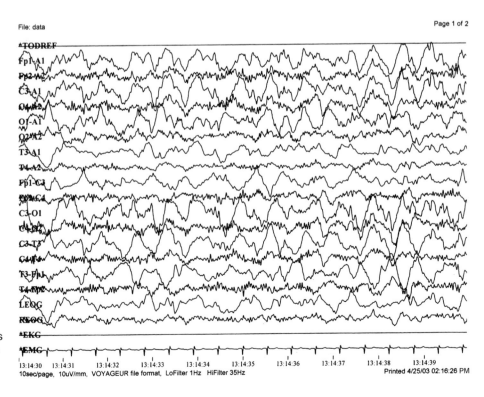

Figure 28-2. EEG of a child with Rasmussen's encephalitis demonstrating high-amplitude delta range activity in the left hemisphere.

portedly was effective in achieving complete seizure control in a patient with Rasmussen's encephalitis.[14] The trial was discontinued after 21 months, however, due to granulocytopenia. A single case report described success treating a 3-year-old girl with Rasmussen's encephalitis with intraventricular interferon-α (INF-α) via an Ommaya reservoir using a protocol for subacute sclerosing panencephalitis (SSPE).[15] The authors showed that after induction and maintenance therapy with INF-α over 6 months, the child was seizure-free. However, the child remained hemiparetic and functionally impaired after treatment. Also, the long-term outcome of the patient was not described. Conventional and newer antiepileptic medications, although used widely, are usually of little benefit. The use of corticosteroids has shown some temporary improvement in a few patients.[16]

Functional hemispherectomy remains the treatment of choice.[17] Recently, immunomodulatory methods such as immunoadsorption, plasmapheresis, and intravenous immunoglobulin have been used with encouraging success in Rasmussen's encephalitis. Selective immunoadsorption of IgGs was used in a 14-year-old girl with Rasmussen's encephalitis who was seropositive for anti-GluR3 IgG antibodies.[18] Immunoadsorption markedly reduced serum levels of anti-GluR3A and anti-GluR3B IgGs, and the child had a marked clinical response with a large reduction of seizures, intellectual stabilization, and improvement in verbal abilities. The clinical improvement was maintained over 2 years with monthly or bimonthly immunoadsorption treatments. The use of plasmapheresis techniques also has shown promise in the treatment of Rasmussen's encephalitis. In a series of four patients (three with documented anti-GluR3 antibody titers and one of unknown antibody status) who underwent treatment with multiple plasma exchange treatments for Rasmussen's encephalitis, marked improvement of clinical symptoms after initiation of plasma exchange was seen in three of the four patients. The patients began to show improvement as early as 5 days into treatment, and improvement persisted for 4 to 9 weeks. Immunomodulatory therapy is now used widely in an effort to prolong functional status in patients who are not disabled enough to warrant hemispherectomy.

Epilepsy surgery, including cerebral hemispherectomy, is the treatment most likely to produce a sustained remission in Rasmussen's encephalitis. Multiple surgical approaches have been undertaken, including partial cortectomy and multiple subpial transactions. These approaches may provide a temporary control of seizures, but the seizures typically relapse as the inflammatory process spreads to other brain regions.[19–21] Cerebral hemispherectomy can produce a sustained remission from seizures in a majority of patients. Early surgical intervention also can decrease the degree of

intellectual decline and other neurologic impairments.[22–24] A modification of the complete (anatomic) hemispherectomy procedure, the functional hemispherectomy, was developed to treat the widespread cerebral involvement in Rasmussen's encephalitis while minimizing the neurologic deficits caused by complete hemispherectomy. At present, functional hemispherectomy is the recommended treatment for young patients with intractable epilepsy and a rapidly disabling course.[23,24]

▶ CONCLUSION

Rasmussen's encephalitis remains a devastating syndrome of children and young adults of mysterious origin. While the etiology of the syndrome remains unknown, understanding of the immunologic abnormalities responsible for the pathologic changes seen in Rasmussen's encephalitis is increasing. Advances in neuroimaging techniques have allowed for earlier diagnosis and have improved the clinician's ability to make timely and accurate treatment decisions. Immunomodulatory treatment methods have shown some promise in palliating the effects of the syndrome and prolonging functional ability. Surgical hemispherectomy, however, remains the definitive treatment for halting the progression of seizures and disability.

REFERENCES

1. Rassmussen TB, Olsweski J, Lloyd-Smith DL: Focal seizures die to chronic localized encephalitis. *Neurology* 8:435, 1958.
2. Aguilar MJ, Rasmussen T: Role of encephalitis in pathogenesis of epilepsy. *Arch Neurol* 2:663, 1960.
3. Oguni H, Andermann F, Rasmussen TB: The natural history of the syndrome of chronic encephalitis and epilepsy: A study of the MNI series of 48 cases, in Andermann F (ed): *Chronic Encephalitis and Epilepsy: Rasmussen's Syndrome*. Stoneham, MA: Butterworth-Heinemann, 1991, pp 7–35.
4. Andermann F, Rasmussen T: Chronic encephalitis and epilepsy: an overview, in Andermann F (ed): *Chronic Encephalitis and Epilepsy: Rasmussen's Syndrome*. Stoneham, MA: Butterworth-Heinemann, 1991, pp 282–288.
5. Rogers SW, Andrews PI, Gahring LC, et al: Autoantibodies to glutamate receptor GluR3 in Rasmussen's encephalitis. *Science* 265:648, 1994.
6. Andrews PI, Dichter MA, Berkovic SF, et al: Plasmapheresis in Rasmussen's encephalitis. *Neurology* 46:242, 1996.
7. Bien CG, Bauer J, Deckwerth TL, et al: Destruction of neurons by cytotoxic T cells: A new pathogenic mechanism in Rasmussen's encephalitis. *Ann Neurol* 51:311, 2002.

8. Bien CG, Urbach H, Deckert M, et al: Diagnosis and staging of Rasmussen's encephalitis by serial MRI and histopathology. *Neurology* 58:250, 2002.

9. O'Hara PJ, Sheppard PO, Thogersen H, et al: The ligand-binding domain in metabotropic glutamate receptors is related to bacterial periplasmic binding proteins. *Neuron* 11:41, 1993.

10. Hartley LM, Gordon I, Harkness W: Correlation of SPECT with pathology and seizure outcome in children undergoing epilepsy surgery. *Dev Med Child Neurol* 44:676, 2002.

11. Hideaki I, Simos PG, Wheless JW, et al: Multimodality functional imaging evaluation in a patient with Rasmussen's encephalitis. *Brain Dev* 24:239, 2002.

12. Andrews PI, McNamara JO, Lewis DV: Clinical and electroencephalographic correlates in Rasmussen's encephalitis. *Epilepsia* 38:189, 1997.

13. McLachlan RS, Levin S, Blume WT: Treatment of Rasmussen syndrome with ganciclovir. *Neurology* 47:925, 1996.

14. DeToledo JC, Smith DB: Partially successful treatment of Rasmussen's encephalitis with zidovudine: Symptomatic improvement followed by involvement of contralateral hemisphere. *Epilepsia* 35(2):352, 1994.

15. Dabbagh O, Gascon G, Crowell J, et al: Intraventricular interferon-α stops seizures in Rasmussen's encephalitis: A case report. *Epilepsia* 39(9):1045, 1997.

16. Hart YM, Cortez M, Andermann F, et al: Medical treatment of Rasmussen's syndrome (chronic encephalitis and epilepsy): Effects of high-dose steroids or immunoglobulins in 19 patients. *Neurology* 44:1030, 1994.

17. Antel JP, Rasmussen T: Rasmussen's encephalitis and the new hat. *Neurology* 46:9, 1996.

18. Antozzi C, Granata T, Aurisano N, et al: Long-term selective IgG immunoadsorption improves Rasmussen's encephalitis. *Neurology* 51:302, 1998.

19. Andermann F, Freeman JM, Vigemano F, et al: Surgically remediable diffuse hemispheric syndrome, in Engle J Jr (ed): *Surgical Treatment of the Epilepsies*. New York: Raven Press, 1993, pp 87–101.

20. Gupta PC, Roy S, Tandon PN: Progressive epilepsy due to chronic persistent encephalitis: Report of four cases. *J Neurol Sci* 22:105, 1974.

21. Hufnagel A, Zentner J, Fernandez G, et al: Multiple subpial transaction for control of epileptic seizures: Effectiveness and safety. *Epilepsia* 38:678, 1997.

22. Honavar M, Janota I, Polkey CE: Rasmussen's encephalitis in surgery for epilepsy. *Dev Med Child Neurol* 34:3, 1992.

23. Vining EP, Freeman JM, Pillas DJ, et al: Why would you remove half a brain? The outcome of 58 children after hemispherectomy—the Johns Hopkins' experience: 1968 to 1996. *Pediatrics* 100:163, 1997.

24. Villemure JG, Andermann F, Rasmussen TB: Hemispherectomy for the treatment of epilepsy due to chronic encephalitis, in Andermann F (ed): *Chronic Encephalitis and Epilepsy: Rasmussen's Syndrome*. Stoneham, MA: Butterworth-Heinemann, 1991, pp 235–244.

CHAPTER 29

Neurologic Complications of Immunization

Hema Patel and Bhuwan P. Garg

MEASLES VACCINE

MUMPS VACCINE

RUBELLA (GERMAN MEASLES) VACCINE

POLIOMYELITIS VACCINE

DIPHTHERIA AND TETANUS VACCINES

PERTUSSIS VACCINE

HEMOPHILUS INFLUENZAE TYPE B VACCINE

HEPATITIS B VACCINE

INFLUENZA VACCINE

VARICELLA VACCINE

PNEUMOCOCCAL VACCINE

SMALLPOX VACCINE

Widespread vaccination practices have markedly reduced the incidence, morbidity, and mortality of many infectious diseases. A very effective immunization program resulted in the global eradication of smallpox in 1980. In the United States, major reductions in the incidence of other vaccine-preventable diseases such as diphtheria, measles, mumps, pertussis, poliomyelitis, congenital and acquired rubella, tetanus, and *Hemophilus influenzae* type b disease have occurred. The current schedule for childhood immunizations recommended by the Advisory Committee on Immunization Practices (ACIP), the American Academy of Pediatrics (AAP), and the American Academy of Family Physicians is outlined in Table 29-1.[1] Although immunization has successfully reduced the incidence of vaccine-preventable diseases, vaccinations can cause adverse effects. These are usually minor, rarely serious, and often neurologic in nature.[2] The frequency and severity of immunization-related complications are difficult to judge because most reports are anecdotal. The Moni-

toring System for Adverse Events Following Immunization (MSAEFI) of the Centers for Disease Control and Prevention (CDC) and the more recent Vaccine Adverse Event Reporting System (VAERS), an epidemiologic database maintained jointly by the CDC and the Food and Drug administration (FDA) in Atlanta, Georgia, since 1990, are passive surveillance systems for collecting data on illnesses temporally associated with immunization. However, because of the method of data collection, these systems are not very accurate in ascertaining the frequency of these complications.

Safer vaccines have been developed, and postmarketing surveillance of vaccine-related adverse events has been increased. As more vaccines are added to the recommended immunization schedule, it is very important to have an understanding of the risks and benefits and to be able to explain them to parents. Despite concerns about vaccine safety, vaccination is safer than the risks associated with the diseases these vaccines prevent.

▶ **TABLE 29-1.** CHILDHOOD IMMUNIZATION
SCHEDULE

Recommended Age	Immunization(s)*
Birth	Hepatitis-B
2 months	DTaP, IPV, Hib, hepatitis B, PCV
4 months	DTaP, IPV, Hib PCV
6 months	DTaP, Hib, hepatitis B, PCV
6–18 months	IPV
12–18 months	Varicella
15–18 months	DTaP
12–15 months	MMR, Hib, PCV
4–6 years	DTaP, IPV
11–12 years	MMR (may also be given at 4–6 years), Td
2–18 years	Hepatitis B and varicella (if not administered during infancy)

*DTaP = diphtheria, tetanus, acellular pertussis; Hib = *Hemophilus
influenzae* type b; DTP = diphtheria, tetanus, whole-cell pertussis;
MMR = measles, mumps, rubella; OPV = trivalent oral polio vaccine; Td = tetanus and diphtheria toxoid; PCV = pneumococcal
conjugate vaccine.
SOURCE: *Adapted from recommendations of the Advisory Committee on Immunization Practice (ACIP), the American Academy of Pediatrics (AAP), the American Academy of Family Physicians (AAFP),
and the American Medical Association.*[1]

▶ MEASLES, MUMPS, AND RUBELLA VACCINES

Immunization against measles, mumps, and rubella
(MMR) has been administered in a combined vaccine
in the United States since 1971.[3]

▶ MEASLES VACCINE

Measles is a viral infection caused by a member of
the paramyxovirus group. A live, highly attenuated
measles virus (Edmonston-Enders strain, formerly called
Moraten) vaccine, licensed in 1968, is the only measles
vaccine now available for general use. It is available as
a single-antigen preparation, combined with rubella vaccine, or combined with mumps and rubella vaccines
(MMR vaccine).[3] The ACIP recommends that MMR vaccine be used when any of the individual components
is indicated.[4] Approximately 2 to 5 percent of children
who receive only one dose of the MMR vaccine fail to
develop immunity (i.e., primary vaccine failure). Ninety-
nine percent of patients who receive two doses (with
the first dose received no earlier than the first birth-
day) develop serologic evidence of immunity.[5] This
vaccine-induced immunity appears to be lifelong in
most individuals.[6]

Before measles vaccine was licensed in 1963, an
average of 400,000 measles cases were reported each
year in the United States. In the late 1960s and early
1970s, the reported cases decreased to approximately
22,000 to 75,000 cases per year. With the initiation of
the Measles Elimination Program in 1978, the incidence
decreased further.[4] By 1982, 97 percent of all children
entering school in the United States had been vaccinated against measles. The incidence of measles had
fallen from almost 500 per 100,000 population in 1950
to 0.5 per 100,000 population in 1982. During that period, the reported annual deaths from measles declined
from 700 to 2, and reports of measles encephalitis declined from 300 to 1. It is estimated that during the first
20 years of the measles vaccine program, the vaccine
resulted in 52 million fewer cases of measles and prevented 5200 deaths and 17,400 cases of mental retardation.[7] However, there was a resurgence of measles
from 1989 to 1991, with more than 55,000 cases and
150 deaths.[8,9] With mobilization of efforts to increase
vaccination coverage, the incidence has now been reduced to less than 1000 cases each year since 1993,
with demonstration of "foreign origin" of all the strains
submitted for analysis to the CDC and absence of any
"United States strain" of measles virus.[10] The most common causes of death are pneumonia in children and
acute encephalitis in adults.

Complications

Local and Systemic Reactions

Mild measles-like symptoms such as fever, rash, conjunctivitis, cough, and rhinorrhea may occur 1 to 2
weeks following immunization in approximately 2 to
15 percent of patients.[11] Measles-containing vaccines
can cause thrombocytopenia within 2 months of vaccination. It is usually benign, resolving within 1 month
in most children,[12] although hemorrhagic complications
have been reported.[13,14] Thrombocytopenia occurs at a
rate of approximately 1 in 30,000.[13,15] The risk is higher
for persons who previously have had immune thrombocytopenic purpura, particularly those who had
thrombocytopenic purpura within 6 weeks after an earlier dose of the vaccine.[14]

Allergic Reactions

Allergic reactions after administration of MMR vaccine
are rare, consisting of wheal and flare or urticaria at the
injection site. Immediate anaphylactic reactions are extremely rare and are thought to be related to the gelatin
component and not associated with hypersensitivity to
egg antigens, as was suggested previously.[16,17] MMR
vaccine may be administered with relative safety to
children with egg allergy, and the value of prior skin

testing or use of special protocols is in question.[18,19] However, a previous anaphylactic reaction to a measles-containing vaccine remains a contraindication.[19]

Neurologic Complications

ENCEPHALOPATHY AND ENCEPHALITIS

The terms *encephalopathy* and *encephalitis* have been used interchangeably in the literature. Encephalitis develops in 1 per 1000 persons infected with measles virus. Many uncontrolled observational studies describe encephalitis/encephalopathy after the administration of measles vaccine.[20,21] In the period 1963–1971, 51 million doses of measles vaccine were distributed, and 84 patients with new-onset neurologic disease following vaccination without evidence of other causes were reported to the CDC. The onset of symptoms was clustered around 6 to 15 days after immunization. Diagnoses included encephalopathy (60 percent), encephalomyelitis, aseptic meningitis, and transverse myelitis. Although there was no way to prove that these complications were vaccine-related, the clustering of cases 6 to 15 days after immunization is significant. The incidence of encephalitis/encephalopathy was 1.16 cases per 1 million distributed doses, compared with a background incidence of encephalitis of 2 to 3 cases per 1 million children of similar age.[20] The incidence of postinfectious encephalomyelitis following natural measles infection is 1 per 1000 cases.[22]

Therefore, while a cause-and-effect relationship between measles immunization and encephalopathy has not been established conclusively,[23] the clustering of cases in the second week after immunization is worrisome. Two large studies since 1994 have continued to support the Institute of Medicine's conclusion that there is no evidence for an increased risk for either encephalopathy or sequelae after measles vaccination.[24,25] In contrast, a third study recently reported a positive association between measles vaccination and encephalopathy. On reviewing claims submitted to the U.S. National Vaccine Injury Compensation Program between 1970 and 1993, 48 children developed encephalopathy without determined cause within 15 days of receiving the first dose of measles vaccine, suggesting a causal relationship.[3] However, even if all these cases were caused by measles vaccination, the incidence still remains much lower than that following natural infection and comparable with that in healthy controls. Evidence is inadequate to establish a causal relationship between measles vaccine and Guillain-Barré syndrome, as well as transverse myelitis.

SUBACUTE SCLEROSING PANENCEPHALITIS (SSPE)

SSPE is a devastating form of measles panencephalitis that follows natural measles infection in 5 to 10 of every 1 million cases of measles.[26] SSPE has been extremely rare since the early 1980s. Development of SSPE following administration of the live, attenuated vaccine and a negative history of natural measles was first reported in 1968.[27] Thereafter, several additional reports of SSPE in individuals vaccinated against measles appeared,[20,26,28] with latency ranging from 3 weeks[20] to 5 years[28] between vaccination and the onset of SSPE. The National Registry for SSPE, founded in 1969, reported a decline in SSPE from 41.33 new cases per year between 1967 and 1975 to 4.2 new cases per year from 1982 to 1986.[29] Although there was a decline in the absolute number of cases of SSPE, there was an increase in the proportion of cases that occurred following measles vaccination from 13 percent of all reported cases of SSPE prior to 1976 to 24.75 percent after 1975.[29] It is thought that the live, attenuated measles virus vaccine may be capable of contributing to the pathogenesis of SSPE, with a shorter incubation period for SSPE following vaccination than after natural (wild) measles infection.[29] The risk of SSPE following vaccination is lower than following natural measles; the incidence of SSPE with natural measles infection was 8.5 per 1 million compared with 0.7 per 1 million vaccine recipients who had not had measles.[30] Therefore, the risk of SSPE is not a contraindication to routine immunization against measles.[23]

IMMUNOSUPPRESSIVE ENCEPHALOPATHY

Immunosuppressive encephalopathy is distinct from acute measles encephalitis and SSPE. It has been documented in two immunocompromised children postvaccination.[31,32] Measles virus of the vaccine strain was isolated from the cerebrospinal fluid (CSF) of a 7-year-old girl with acute lymphoblastic leukemia 10 weeks after she had received MMR vacccine.[31] Another case occurred in a child with leukemia who had been vaccinated with the Schwarz strain of measles vaccine.[32] Therefore, measles immunization should be administered with caution in immunosuppressed individuals.[4]

SEIZURES

Febrile and afebrile seizures may occur 7 to 14 days following measles or MMR vaccination.[33,34] The risk is approximately 1 case per 3000 doses of MMR vaccine administered.[15] Normal children who experience febrile or afebrile seizures following measles vaccination usually recover completely without sequelae. Children with a personal history or first-degree family history of seizures are at an increased risk, and their parents should be informed of this.[4,33] Prophylaxis with antipyretics initiated before the onset of fever and continued for 5 to 7 days has been suggested. Children with seizure disorders on anticonvulsants should continue these medications after measles vaccination.[4,19] There is no association between MMR vaccination and residual seizure disorder.[4,23,33]

AUTISM

Concern has been raised regarding a possible relationship between MMR vaccine and autism[35] and inflammatory bowel disease.[36,37] It was hypothesized that MMR vaccination leads to a nonspecific gut injury permitting the absorption of nonpermeable peptides, which in turn cause severe developmental disorders. However, these reports have many limitations and are noncomparitive and anecdotal. Symptoms of autism that are commonly first noted by parents in the second year of life may follow administration of the vaccine by weeks or months, and a close temporal association is expected by chance. In the United Kingdom, where these research findings were first published, MMR vaccine use declined.[38] Several studies thereafter have failed to show a relationship between the rate of autism and the administration of the MMR vaccine.[39,40] The AAP[41] concluded that the currently available evidence does not support such an association.

Ophthalmologic Complications

Two children have been reported with transitory oculomotor palsy associated with systemic symptoms of measles infection following immunization. One patient had ptosis, whereas the other had a complete third nerve palsy.[42,43] Isolated case reports of optic neuritis complicating MMR immunization also have been reported.[44,45] Bilateral measles retinitis associated with symptoms of systemic measles infection was reported in a 16-month-old girl following immunization. She presented with total blindness and had incomplete recovery of vision.[46]

▶ MUMPS VACCINE

Mumps is an acute viral illness with characteristic symptoms of parotitis and aseptic meningitis and caused by a paramyxovirus. Mumps vaccine is a live, attenuated virus vaccine introduced in 1967.[47] The Jeryl Lynn strain is used in the United States, and the Urabe strain is used in Japan. Clinical efficacy has been estimated to be approximately 95 percent. Neutralizing antibody response is usually detected within 2 weeks of the vaccination, although this may be delayed for up to 6 weeks in some recipients.[48] Immunity is assumed to last for greater than 25 years and is probably lifelong.[4] Since mumps vaccine is administered with measles and rubella in a combined vaccine as MMR vaccine, it is difficult to distinguish the adverse effects of the individual antigens.

Complications

Mumps is a very safe vaccine, with most adverse reactions following MMR vaccine being attributable either to the measles or the rubella component.

Local and Systemic Reactions

Fever, parotitis, and orchitis have been reported rarely. Allergic reactions, including rash, pruritus, and purpura, are uncommon and mild.[4] There is no evidence to establish a link between mumps and diabetes mellitus.[23]

Neurologic Complications

Fifteen percent of patients with mumps have an aseptic meningitis. Encephalitis is rare, occurring in less than 260 per 100,000 cases. Mumps virus (both wild type and vaccine strain) has been isolated from the CSF of patients with aseptic meningitis. This complication is firmly established for the Urabe strain, with an incidence of 1.1 cases per 1000 vaccine recipients. Aseptic meningitis occurs within 2 months of vaccination. There have been no reports of severe illness or long-term sequelae.[49] Data concerning aseptic meningitis in association with the Jeryl Lynn strain are scarce. Between 1988 and 1992, 13 cases of aseptic meningitis following MMR vaccination were reported in the United Kingdom that had occurred within 15 to 35 days of vaccination with the Urabe strain.[50] Eleven cases of meningitis occurring after MMR vaccination were reported in the United States to the VAERS from 1990 to 1992. In none of these was the strain identified or the virus isolated. Since 1992, only the Jeryl Lynn strain has been used, and no further cases of aseptic meningitis have been reported.[15,50] The incidence of encephalitis within 30 days of receipt of mumps-containing vaccine is approximately 0.4 per 1 million doses of the Jeryl Lynn vaccine, which is lower than the observed background rate of encephalitis of 2 to 6 cases per 10,000 persons in the normal population.[19] Ataxia has been reported infrequently following administration of MMR vaccine and has been thought to be related to the mumps component of the vaccine, but a causal relationship has not been established.[51]

Otologic Complications

Sensorineural deafness has been reported to occur in 4 percent of patients following natural mumps infection[52,53] and also has been reported following MMR vaccination.[52–55] A 7-year-old girl developed total deafness in the left ear 11 days after an injection of MMR vaccine without subsequent recovery,[52] and a 3-year-old girl who had received MMR vaccination at 15 months of age developed moderate to severe bilateral unremitting sensorineural deafness.[53] However, a causal relationship between MMR vaccination and sensorineural deafness has not been established.[23]

▶ RUBELLA (GERMAN MEASLES) VACCINE

Rubella is caused by a virus of the togavirus group. It is characterized by transient skin rash, postauricular or suboccipital lymphadenopathy, and fever. Transient polyarthralgia or polyarthritis occur frequently, more commonly among women.[56] Central nervous system (CNS) complications (i.e., encephalitis) occur at a rate of 1 per 6000 cases, usually in adults.[4] The most important consequence of rubella virus infection is congenital rubella syndrome. The original rubella vaccines containing live, attenuated virus were licensed for use in the United States in 1969 and were produced using three different cell cultures, namely, duck embryo (HPV-77:DK-12), dog kidney (HPV-77:DE-5), and rabbit kidney cells (Cendehill strain). In January 1979, all these vaccines were replaced by the current strain, which is Wistar RA 27/3 prepared in human diploid cell culture. Wistar RA 27/3 is associated with an increased and more persistent antibody response and fewer adverse effects. This new vaccine produces an immune response that closely parallels the natural infection and provides long-term, probably lifelong immunity in more than 95 percent of susceptible persons 1 year of age or older who receive a single dose of the vaccine.[57] Following introduction of the vaccine, the number of cases of rubella decreased from 57,600 cases (58 cases per 100,000 population) in 1969 to an annual average of fewer than 200 cases since 1992.[4]

Complications

Arthralgia and Arthritis

Up to 40 percent of people (adults more often than children, especially females), vaccinated with the current rubella vaccine develop arthralgias, and 10 percent develop transient arthritis beginning 1 to 3 weeks after immunization and lasting 1 to 3 weeks.[56,58,59] The joints most frequently affected include proximal interphalangeal and metacarpophalangeal joints, knees, ankles, and toes. Symptoms are mild following vaccination with RA 27/3 and rarely disrupt work.[58] The Institute of Medicine in 1991 reported that there is evidence to suggest a causal relationship between RA 27/3 rubella vaccine and acute and chronic arthritis.[60] However, other studies suggest that there is no evidence of an increased risk for chronic arthropathies due to the rubella vaccine.[61]

Neurologic Complications

PERIPHERAL NEUROPATHY

During the mass immunization program of children that began in 1969 and continued for several years thereafter, two fairly well-defined syndromes of peripheral neuropathy were recognized following immunization with all three of the original rubella vaccines: brachial radiculoneuritis (arm syndrome) and lumbosacral radiculoneuritis (leg syndrome).[62–65] The arm syndrome occurred 10 to 62 days after immunization and was characterized by nocturnal episodes of pain involving the wrists and hands associated with paresthesias and lasting up to 5 weeks. The leg syndrome occurred 29 to 70 days following immunization and was characterized by asymmetric popliteal pain and inability to straighten the legs or bear weight with worsening of the symptoms at night. The leg pain lasted for 2 to 14 days with periodic recurrences during two and a half years of follow-up.[62] These complications have not been described following vaccination with the current (RA 27/3) vaccine.[65]

DEMYELINATING DISEASES

There are isolated case reports of young women who developed transverse myelitis, sometimes associated with optic neuritis, following rubella immunization.[66,67] This complication is not seen in children and may represent the first manifestation of multiple sclerosis. The relationship between immunization and these symptoms may be coincidental, or the immunization may have triggered the first attack of multiple sclerosis.[67] Guillain-Barré syndrome and carpal tunnel syndrome also have been reported infrequently.[60]

Congenital Rubella Syndrome

Congenital rubella syndrome is caused by infection of the fetus via the maternal bloodstream. Six- to eight-year follow-up of infants born to mothers who were infected during the first 12 weeks of gestation revealed that 85 percent had the congenital rubella syndrome.[68] One of the most important reasons for rubella immunization is to protect the unborn child from acquiring congenital rubella syndrome.[4] The older vaccines (not the currently used RA 27/3) may cross the placenta and infect the fetus.[69,70]

Data collected by the CDC in the Vaccine in Pregnancy (VIP) Registry from 1971 through 1989 revealed no cases of congenital rubella syndrome in the 324 offspring of 321 women who had received rubella vaccine within 3 months before to 3 months after conception and continued pregnancy to term. Ninety-four of these women had received the older HPV-77 (Cendehill) vaccine, and 226 received the RA 27/3 vaccine. The estimated risk of RA 27/3 vaccine–induced malformation is 0 to 2 percent (1.6 percent for all types of rubella vaccines), significantly less than the more than 20 percent risk for congenital rubella syndrome associated with maternal infection in the first trimester.[71] While no cases of congenital rubella syndrome were noted in the CDC study, others have reported isolation of rubella virus in the products of conception from abortions following inadvertent immunization.[69,70] Approximately 1 to 2 percent of infants born to vaccinated mothers had serologic evidence of subclinical infection, with the rate of rubella virus isolation being much higher with the older vaccines. Data indicate that the risk of placental or fetal infection from the RA 27/3 vaccine is small.[72,73] Even though the risk of congenital rubella syndrome after vaccination appears to be minimal, this small risk should be avoided by vaccinating women only when not pregnant and advising them not to become pregnant for at least 3 months following vaccination.[73] Physicians should determine the immune status of all women of childbearing age in their care and vaccinate those who are inadequately immunized.

▶ POLIOMYELITIS VACCINE

Poliomyelitis is caused by an enterovirus. There are three types of polioviruses (types 1, 2, and 3) with no cross-immunity. Poliomyelitis reached a peak in the United States in 1952 with over 20,000 paralytic cases.[74] The Salk vaccine, an inactivated poliovirus vaccine (IPV) administered by the parenteral route, was developed in 1953 by Jonas Salk and licensed for use in 1955. This was replaced by the oral polio vaccine (OPV), a live, attenuated vaccine developed by Albert Sabin and licensed for use in 1963. Both IPV and OPV are trivalent and effective. OPV produces secretory mucosal immunity within the gastrointestinal tract, as well as serum humoral immunity. The live, attenuated virus is shed from the gastrointestinal tract and spreads to unvaccinated persons, leading to herd immunity. Also, as an oral preparation, it is better tolerated than the injectable form.[75] The oral polio vaccine was recommended for general use by the AAP in 1964, with the exception of adults and individuals who are immunocompromised or have immunocompromised contacts because of the risk of developing vaccine-associated paralytic poliomyelitis (VAPP). With the onset of widespread polio vaccination, the incidence of poliomyelitis declined dramatically. The last reported case of paralytic poliomyelitis caused by endemic transmission of wild virus in the United States was in 1979.[74] The elimination of wild-virus-associated poliomyelitis in the western hemisphere in 1991 and the rapid progress in global polio eradication efforts changed the risk-benefit ratio associated with the exclusive use of OPV for routine immunization. Following the development of an enhanced-potency IPV (which poses no risk of VAPP) in 1987, the CDC in September 1996 accepted the ACIP recommendation for a sequential IPV/OPV schedule to reduce the risk of VAPP.[76] On June 17, 1999, to eliminate the risk of VAPP, the ACIP recommended an ad-

ditional change to an all-IPV schedule for routine childhood polio vaccination in the United States.[77]

Complications

The inactivated poliovirus vaccine has an excellent safety record, producing only low-grade fever for the first 2 days in 14 percent of recipients and restlessness in 15 percent.[78] While the inactivated poliovirus vaccine is not known to cause VAPP, it is not as effective as the oral polio vaccine in preventing the spread of wild-type poliovirus among susceptible persons.[79]

Neurologic Complications of OPV

ACUTE PARALYTIC POLIOMYELITIS
There are two types of vaccine-related poliomyelitis: that occurring in vaccine recipients and that in the contacts of vaccinated persons, especially those with impaired immunity.[74] Acute paralytic poliomyelitis is a major complication seen only following OPV. The inactivated poliovirus vaccine does not contain live virus and cannot cause VAPP. VAPP is more likely to occur in persons 18 years of age or older and in immunosuppressed individuals, particularly those with B-lymphocyte disorders (e.g., agammaglobulinemia). VAPP has a low incidence, occurring approximately once in every 3.22 million doses of OPV.[80] The most recent cases of paralytic poliomyelitis in the United States have been vaccine-related. Between 1980 and 1996, a total of 142 confirmed cases of paralytic poliomyelitis were reported; 134 (94 percent) were attributable to the administration of OPV.[76] The risk of VAPP was estimated to be approximately 1 case per 2.4 million doses, with the majority of VAPP cases occurring after administration of the first dose (1 case per 750,000 first doses).[76,81] Ongoing surveillance is documenting a decrease in VAPP, with the last case of VAPP reported in 1999. These findings provide useful information to support the ACIP recommendation made in 1999 to shift to an all-IPV schedule.[81]

GUILLAIN-BARRÉ SYNDROME (GBS)
Following a nationwide immunization campaign with OPV for children and adults in Finland during a 5-week period between February 10 and March 15, 1985, there were 10 patients who developed the GBS. Six patients became symptomatic within the first 6 weeks of vaccination, and all the cases of GBS occurred within 10 weeks of vaccination. The crude annual incidence rate of GBS was estimated at 1 case per 100,000 population.[82] This evidence favors a causal relationship between OPV and GBS. If GBS occurs within 5 days to 6 weeks of a vaccination, subsequent vaccinations with

OPV may be associated with an increased risk of recurrent GBS.[83]

▶ DIPHTHERIA, TETANUS, AND PERTUSSIS VACCINES

Routine immunization against diphtheria, tetanus, and pertussis in infancy and early childhood since the 1940s has played a major role in reducing the incidence of cases and deaths from each of these diseases.

▶ DIPHTHERIA AND TETANUS VACCINES

Diphtheria is an acute toxin-mediated disease caused by *Corynebacterium diphtheriae* and most commonly involving the pharynx and the tonsils. In the United States, the incidence of diphtheria has decreased because of immunization from over 200,000 cases in 1921 to only 15 cases reported from 1990 to 1994.[84] No cases were reported in 1993 and 1995. Only one case was reported each year in 1998, 1999, and 2000. Most of these cases (55 percent) were in persons 40 years of age and older who were not immunized or inadequately immunized, corroborating the finding of inadequate levels of circulating antitoxin in many adults (up to 60 percent with less than protective levels).[85] Diphtheria continues to occur in other parts of the world. In 1990, a major epidemic of diphtheria occurred in countries of the former Soviet Union. By 1994, the epidemic had affected all the 15 newly independent states with more than 140,000 cases and more than 4000 reported deaths, comprising over 90 percent of all diphtheria cases reported to the World Health Organization from the entire world.[86]

Tetanus is an acute, often fatal disease caused by an exotoxin produced by the gram-positive spore-forming anaerobic bacillus *Clostridium tetani*. In the United States, tetanus has decreased dramatically from 560 reported cases in 1947 to an average of 57 cases reported annually from 1985 to 1994.[84] A provisional all-time low of 27 cases (0.02 cases per 100,000) was reported in 2001.[87] The increase in cases among younger persons in the last half of the 1990s is related in part to the increased number of cases among young drug users in California in the late 1990s. Although rare in the United States, tetanus occurs exclusively among unvaccinated or inadequately vaccinated persons. Neonatal tetanus is rare in the United states, with only 2 cases reported since 1989.[88,89] Neither of the infants' mothers had ever received tetanus toxoid.

Diphtheria and tetanus toxoid generally are administered together as Td in adults and DT or DTaP (a combination that includes acellular pertussis vaccine) in children. Diphtheria and tetanus toxoid (DT) should be used in children younger than age 7 years in whom pertussis vaccine is contraindicated. Tetanus and diphtheria toxoid (Td) should be used in individuals older than 7 years. Td has a lower concentration of diphtheria toxoid than DT. Monovalent tetanus toxoids are also available. After a primary series of three properly spaced doses in persons 7 years of age and older and four doses in children younger than 7 years of age, essentially all vaccinees achieve antitoxin levels considerably greater than the minimal protective level of 0.01 IU/ml.[90] Because of waning antitoxin titers, most individuals have antitoxin levels below optimal levels 10 years after the last dose. To maintain protective levels of antitoxin antibody, immunization with tetanus toxoid given with diphtheria toxoid as Td is suggested at 10-year intervals. Because of a possibility of developing serious neuropathy due to overimmunization with tetanus toxoid, a careful history of prior immunization should be taken before administrating routine booster injections.[91] Clean minor wounds require no booster in a fully immunized person (last booster within 10 years). Persons with contaminated wounds should receive a booster if more than 5 years have elapsed since the last dose. The only contraindication to the use of the toxoids is history of a neurologic or severe hypersensitivity reaction following a previous dose.[92]

Complications

Diphtheria and tetanus toxoids are administered together so frequently that it is difficult to analyze the adverse reactions of each separately. There are no known serious adverse reactions to diphtheria toxoid, although data are limited.

Local and Systemic Reactions

Erythema and induration with or without local tenderness are seen commonly after the administration of vaccines containing diphtheria antigen, are usually self-limited, and do not require therapy. Minor reactions, including local pain, erythema, and swelling, may occur within 48 hours of immunization with tetanus toxoid.[93] Severe local reactions characterized by extensive painful swelling, often from shoulder to elbow associated with systemic manifestations such as fever and malaise, are infrequent. This is an Arthus reaction in which immune complexes form locally in the walls of small arteries, and usually it is seen in persons who have received frequent doses of tetanus toxoid. These patients often have very high serum antitoxin levels.[94] They should not be given further routine or emergency doses of Td more frequently than every 10 years, even if they have a wound that is neither clean nor minor.[19]

Anaphylaxis

Rarely, anaphylactoid reactions can occur within 2 hours of immunization with tetanus toxoid. Symptoms include urticaria, angioedema, shortness of breath, pruritus, and hypotension.[93] However, no deaths caused by anaphylaxis following DTP vaccination have been reported to the CDC since the inception of vaccine adverse events reporting in 1978, a period during which more than 80 million doses of DTP vaccine were administered. No cases of anaphylaxis associated with the administration of diphtheria toxoid alone have been reported.

Neurologic Complications

DEMYELINATING DISEASES

Several case reports of acute disseminated encephalomyelitis (ADEM) have been described in association with tetanus toxoid administration.[95,96] Transverse myelitis[97,98] and optic neuritis also have been reported.[99] However, the evidence to date is inadequate to establish a causal relationship between tetanus toxoid, DT, or Td and demyelinating diseases of the CNS.

GUILLAIN-BARRÉ SYNDROME (GBS)

The risk of GBS after tetanus toxoid is extremely low. Most reported cases have occurred in adults who received either tetanus toxoid alone or a combination of tetanus toxoid and anti-tetanus toxin serum.[100–102] These case reports do not demonstrate a definite cause-and-effect relationship between tetanus toxoid and GBS. The most convincing exception is the case of a patient who received tetanus toxoid on three separate occasions over a period of 13 years and developed a well-documented polyneuropathy of the GBS type following each administration with latencies of 21, 14, and 10 days. He had minimal residual neurologic signs following the second episode and made a full functional recovery following the third.[103] A few cases of GBS following DT also have been reported. The MSAEFI lists four cases between 1979 and 1990 in relation to DT. The VAERS lists two cases of GBS between 1990 and 1992 with Td, both of whom received MMR vaccine simultaneously as well. The Institute of Medicine concluded that tetanus toxoid–containing vaccines can trigger the onset of GBS.[104] No increased risk of GBS has been observed with the use of DTP in children. In a study of 0.7 million children of preschool ages who were vaccinated with DTP during a 7-year period, only two cases of GBS were reported, whereas three cases of GBS were expected by chance alone.[105] If GBS occurs 5 days to 6 weeks after vaccination, subsequent vaccinations could be associated with a greater risk of GBS. A previous history of GBS unrelated to vaccination should be of concern but has not been established as a risk factor.

OTHER NEUROPATHIES

Administration of tetanus and diphtheria toxoids alone or in combination also has been linked to the occurrence of mononeuropathy due to nerve damage from injection of the vaccine directly into the nerve rather than due to the vaccine itself.[106] Cranial mononeuropathies and brachial neuritis also have been reported.[107–109] The latter is thought to be a result of an allergic or hypersensitivity reaction[107] and has a 1-month attributable incidence of approximately 0.5 to 1 case per 100,000 recipients of tetanus toxoid.[104]

ENCEPHALOPATHY

Tetanus and diphtheria toxoids have not been associated with an increased risk of encephalopathy or seizures.

▶ PERTUSSIS VACCINE

Pertussis is caused by a gram-negative coccobacillus, *Bordetella pertussis*. Pertussis, first described in 1579, became a nationally reportable disease in 1922. Reports of pertussis reached a peak of 265,269 cases and 7518 deaths in 1934. Following widespread immunization against pertussis, beginning in 1947 in the United States, the number of reported cases and associated mortality have declined.[110] However, since the 1980s, the incidence of pertussis has been increasing gradually. This may be due to increased awareness, improved diagnostic testing, or better reporting of cases to health departments.[111] A total of 27,826 cases of pertussis were reported to the CDC during 1980–1989, for an average annual incidence of 1.2 cases per 100,000 population, with the increase being disproportionately large among adolescents and adults. Infants younger than 2 months of age were at greatest risk for acquiring pertussis and for pertussis-related complications (average annual incidence 62.8 per 100,000). Infants younger than 2 months of age had the highest rates of hospitalizations (82 percent), seizures (4 percent), encephalopathy (1 percent), and death (1 percent). This may reflect poor rates of immunization because 64 percent of children 3 months to 4 years of age who were reported to have pertussis had not been immunized appropriately.[112] In 1997–2000, the highest annual pertussis incidence was among infants younger than 6 month old. Seizures and encephalopathy were reported among 0.8 and 0.1 percent, respectively, of all cases and among 1.4 and 0.2 percent, respectively, of infants younger than 6 months old. Whooping cough can occur in vaccinated persons but is less severe.[113] Also, immunization prevents the disease but not the infection, so immunized children may carry the organism and infect other children or adults.[114]

Whole-cell pertussis vaccine is composed of a suspension of formalin-inactivated B pertussis cells. It was used widely in clinical practice by the mid-1940s. Its efficacy varies from 65 to 95 percent, with the protection decreasing after 5 to 10 years.[115] It is being replaced increasingly by acellular pertussis vaccine (discussed below). However, since whole-cell pertussis vaccine is still being used worldwide, adverse events associated with its use are discussed.

Complications

Local and Systemic Reactions

Local reactions are seen more frequently following the use of combined DTP vaccine than with DT alone, occurring with almost 50 percent of the doses of whole-cell pertussis vaccine. These include local erythema, swelling, and pain. Systemic reactions such as fever, drowsiness, anorexia, vomiting, and persistent crying may also be seen.[116]

Hypotonic-Hyporesponsive Episodes

A hypotonic-hyporesponsive episode can occur within 4 hours of immunization and is characterized by the sudden onset of pallor or cyanosis, hypotonia, and unresponsiveness for a period usually ranging from 10 to 30 minutes, but full recovery may take up to 10 days.[117] The pathogenesis of hypotonic-hyporesponsive episodes is poorly understood.[118] The reported rate of hypotonic-hyporesponsive episodes following whole-cell pertussis vaccine varies from 57 to 250 episodes per 100,000 doses, being higher than the reported rates of 4 to 140 episodes per 100,000 doses of acellular pertussis vaccine.[118,119] Hypotonic-hyporesponsive episodes occur more commonly after the first dose.[116,117] They are not associated with permanent sequelae.[117] In 1991, the Institute of Medicine concluded that there was sufficient evidence to establish a causal relationship between whole-cell pertussis and hypotonic-hyporesponsive episodes.[120]

Although a hypotonic-hyporesponsive episode has been regarded as a contraindication to pertussis revaccination by many physicians, preliminary results from studies on a very small number of children who have been revaccinated suggest that the rate of recurrence is not high.[121] Also, no child who has had a hypotonic-hyporesponsive episode following whole-cell vaccine and who then received acellular pertussis vaccine has had a recurrence. Therefore, many health authorities now advocate revaccination in children with acellular pertussis vaccine who have experienced a hypotonic-hyporesponsive episode after pertussis vaccination.[121,122]

Neurologic Complications

SEIZURES

The incidence of seizures after pertussis vaccination has been estimated at 1 in every 1750 to 10,000 injections.[116,123] Febrile convulsions are the most common adverse neurologic reaction to pertussis vaccination and are not associated with permanent neurologic sequelae.[116] They usually occur within 48 hours of the third immunization, which is usually given at 6 months of age, an age when simple febrile convulsions are common.[124,125] More than half the children with postimmunization febrile convulsions have a personal or family history of febrile convulsions. Postimmunization nonfebrile convulsions occur less frequently, and these children may have a personal but not a family history of convulsions.[126] Since it is extremely difficult to differentiate a simple febrile seizure from one that is due to a reaction to pertussis vaccine, any seizure closely following pertussis vaccination should be considered a contraindication to further pertussis immunization.

INFANTILE SPASMS

Since the age at which DTP is administered is also the peak age of onset of infantile spasms, a cause-and-effect association had been suspected. Independent surveys from Denmark, Japan, and the United Kingdom have examined this association. The studies in Denmark and Japan did not support a causal relationship between pertussis immunization and infantile spasms.[127,128] The United Kingdom National Childhood Encephalopathy Study (NCES) received reports on 269 patients with infantile spasms. An excess risk of infantile spasms in the 28 days following immunization could not be demonstrated. However, there was an excess risk in the first 7 days following either DTP or DT immunization that was later offset by a decreased risk in the 21 days that followed. This suggests that vaccination may trigger the onset of infantile spasms and bring them to attention more quickly. Subsequent neurologic outcome is no different in children whose spasms are immunization-triggered from that in those in whom they began spontaneously.[129] The Institute of Medicine found no evidence to indicate a causal relationship between DTP vaccine and infantile spasms.[120]

ENCEPHALOPATHY

Postpertussis vaccination encephalopathy is characterized by seizures, altered mental status, and other signs of cerebral involvement beginning hours to days after immunization.[130] The absolute risk of an event is extremely small. Data from the CDC for the years 1978 through 1981 suggest a rate for severe reaction of 1 per 230,000 doses of vaccine but provide no information on long-term sequelae.[131] By comparison, 5 of 1277 children with natural pertussis infection between 1979 and 1981 had acute encephalopathy as a result of pertussis infection.[132] This suggests a much higher risk of encephalopathy due to natural infection than following pertussis vaccine. The diagnosis is based primarily on the temporal relationship between immunization and the onset of symptoms.

In 1974 in the United Kingdom, 50 children were evaluated for neurologic illness that may have been related to DPT immunization. Thirty-two suffered convulsions, and 22 were subsequently mentally retarded. The conclusion was made that "the clustering of cases in the first 24 hours after inoculation suggested a causal rather than a coincidental relation," and a prospective study was recommended.[133] Unfortunately, due to media sensationalization of this report, the vaccination rate in the United Kingdom fell to 31 percent, leading to the pertussis epidemic of 1977–1979.[134]

In 1976, the NCES assessed the risk of neurologic complications of immunization. The study identified all children aged 2 months to 3 years admitted during a 3 year period with encephalitis or encephalopathy, unexplained coma, convulsions lasting more than 30 minutes or followed by persistent neurologic complications, infantile spasms, or Reye's syndrome. A total of 1182 children were registered. Two controls matched for sex, age, and area of residence were selected for each child with encephalopathy. It was found that 3.5 percent of encephalopathies were temporally related to pertussis immunization. The attributable risk (difference between the incidence of encephalopathy in immunized versus nonimmunized children) was approximately 1 case per 110,000 injections. The difference between the encephalopathic and control groups was greatest during the first 72 hours following immunization. The NCES also estimated the risk of permanent brain damage in previously normal children to be 1 case per 310,000 injections. Of 11 children with permanent sequelae, possible alternative explanations were present in 6. Two patients had encephalitis, one due to coxsackievirus B5 and the other due to rhinovirus; three had infantile spasms; and one had Reye's syndrome.[134] Since no attempt has been made to provide a precise definition of the clinical syndrome or to exclude other causes of encephalopathy, predicted incidences just listed may be overestimates. A 10-year follow-up study showed that children who had a serious acute neurologic illness after DTP administration were more likely to have chronic nervous system dysfunction 10 years later than children in the control group. These children with chronic nervous system dysfunction were more likely to have received DTP within 7 days of the original acute neurologic illness than children in the control group (3.3 percent of 367 children versus 0.8 percent of 723 children).[135,136] The AAP's committee on infectious diseases concluded that there is an association between DTP vaccination and chronic nervous system dysfunction in children who earlier had severe acute illness after DTP vaccine.[19] There was no evidence to suggest that vaccines, in

particular DTP, are a cause of sudden infant death syndrome (SIDS).[137]

Acellular Pertussis Vaccine

Acellular pertussis (DTaP) vaccines were developed with the aim of achieving adequate protection against pertussis with fewer side effects. Acellular vaccines contain purified, inactivated *B. pertussis* antigens, including pertussis toxoid (PT), filamentous hemagglutinin (FHA), 69-kDa outer membrane proteins (pertactin), and agglutinogens (fimbriae). Acellular pertussis vaccines contain two or more of these denatured elements of *B. pertussis* required for immunity. The first DTaP vaccine was licensed in 1991 in the United States for use in children older than 15 months of age.[138] In 1996, DTaP was licensed for use in all age groups, including completion of the series in children who received one or more doses of the whole-cell DTP, and whole-cell pertussis vaccines are no longer manufactured.[139,140]

Approximately 15 percent of pertussis cases in the United States occur in adolescents and adults. Use of pertussis-containing vaccines in persons 7 years of age or older currently is not recommended because vaccine reactions are thought to be more frequent in older age groups, and pertussis-associated morbidity and mortality decrease with age.[139] Older children and adults with pertussis are often a source of infection for unimmunized children. It is not clear if administration of acellular vaccines to this age group will reduce the risk of their being infected with *B. pertussis* or reduce the risk of transmission to young children. However, the administration of acellular vaccines to older children and adults should be considered in order to reduce the reservoir and circulation of *B. pertussis*, thereby reducing the incidence of pertussis in infants too young to benefit from immunization.[140]

Acellular pertussis vaccines are more effective than the whole-cell vaccines, with an efficacy of 84 to 85 percent. The major advantage of the acellular or component vaccines is that they contain little or no endotoxin. Therefore, there is a reduction in the incidence of high fever, persistent crying, hypotonic-hyporesponsive episodes, and seizures in comparison with the whole-cell vaccine,[141] with a decline of nearly 45 percent in reports of these serious adverse events to the VAERS since 1996.[117] However, there is an increase in local reactions (pain, redness, swelling at injection site) and mild systemic reactions (fever) with the fourth and fifth doses of DTaP. Swelling at the injection site increased from 2 percent following the first dose to 20 to 30 percent after the fourth dose. Fever was seen in 5 to 25 percent. Approximately 2 percent experienced swelling of the entire extremity after receipt of the fourth dose without long-term sequelae.[142] Despite this increase in reactogenicity experienced with the fourth and fifth doses, DTaP is still the preferred vaccine. The ACIP and AAP contraindications for whole-cell pertussis vaccine also should be considered as contraindications for the use of acellular vaccine.

Contraindications

Guidelines for absolute contraindications and precautions to pertussis vaccination are given in Table 29-2.[143] Pertussis vaccination also should be deferred in children with progressive disorders (e.g., uncontrolled epilepsy, infantile spasms, progressive encephalopathy), a personal history of convulsions, and suspected neurologic conditions that predispose to seizures. The ACIP has concluded that a family history of convulsions in parents and siblings is not a contraindication to pertussis vaccination and that children with such family histories should receive pertussis vaccination according to the recommended schedule.[19,143] Stable or resolved neurologic conditions (e.g., cerebral palsy, controlled idiopathic epilepsy) are not contraindications as well. DTP vaccination may be postponed in the presence of ongoing febrile illness that is moderate or severe. Minor illness such as a mild upper respiratory infection with or without low-grade fever is not a contraindication.[19]

The Child Neurology Society issued the following conclusions in a consensus statement[144]:

1. Administration of pertussis vaccine is associated with a short-term increased risk of seizures, mostly febrile seizures, and complete recovery is expected.

2. The association between pertussis vaccine and progressive or chronic neurologic disorder raised by case reports has not been conclusively proven by controlled studies.

3. At present there is no means by which the diagnosis of pertussis vaccine encephalopathy can be established in an individual case.

In addition, there is a causal relationship between pertussis vaccine and an unusual shocklike state referred to as a *hypotonic-hyporesponsive episode*, as well as inconsolable crying, probably caused by pain at the injection site.

► HEMOPHILUS INFLUENZAE TYPE B VACCINE

Prior to introduction of *H. influenzae* type b (Hib) vaccines, an estimated 12,000 persons developed *H. influenzae* type b disease annually in the United States.[145] Nearly 75 percent of the cases occurred in children younger than 2 years of age. This susceptibility correlates with their lack of antibody to the type b capsular polysaccharide polyribosylribitol phosphate (PRP). Meningitis occurred in 50 to 65 percent of cases of invasive Hib disease, with a mortality rate of 2 to 5 percent. Permanent sequelae, including hearing loss, mental retardation, and seizures, occurred in 19 to 45 percent of survivors.[145] The incidence of Hib disease decreased dramatically in the late 1980s following routine immunization of infants, with only 341 confirmed cases reported during 1996–2000 (average of 68 cases per year).[146] In the 1970s, a plain polysaccharide vaccine composed of purified PRP was prepared. However, it had an age-related response and was not effective in children younger than 18 months of age. No boost in antibody titer was observed with repeated doses. In addition, a possible increased incidence of disease in the postimmunization period (7 days) had been noted.[147] Therefore, in the late 1980s, a series of vaccines using PRP conjugated with other compounds to increase vaccine efficacy was developed. These vaccines differ in the molecular size of the Hib polysaccharide, the protein used as the carrier, and the methods used to link the polysaccharide to the protein. Variations in the type or frequency of adverse effects may occur because of differences in the polysaccharide or protein content of these vaccines. Conjugated preparations include PRP-D (diphtheria toxoid), HbOC (*Corynebacterium diphtheriae* protein), PRP-OMP (*Neisseria meningitidis* outer membrane protein complex), and PRP-T (tetanus toxoid). The first Hib conjugate vaccine (PRP-D) was licensed in1987.

The plain PRP vaccines do not provide protective amounts of antibody until after age 2 years, whereas

---

► **TABLE 29-2.** CONTRAINDICATIONS AND PRECAUTIONS TO PERTUSSIS VACCINES[143]

Contraindications
1. Allergic hypersensitivity to the vaccine components
2. Encephalopathy within 7 days of vaccination not due to another identifiable cause

Precautions
These events were considered contraindications in previous ACIP recommendations. Pertussis vaccination may be considered only in circumstances (high incidence of pertussis) in which benefit of vaccination outweighs the risk.
1. Development of fever of 40.5°C (105°F) or higher not due to another identifiable cause within 48 hours after vaccination
2. Collapse or shocklike state (hypotensive-hyporesponsive episode) within 48 hours after vaccination
3. Persistent, inconsolable crying lasting 3 hours or longer within 48 hours after vaccination
4. Convulsions with or without fever occurring within 3 days of vaccination

the conjugate vaccines stimulate anti-PRP antibody responses in young infants and also produce larger amounts of these antibodies. Repeat doses elicit a booster response. In addition, they induce an anti–PRP antibody response in many individuals who do not respond well to natural infection with Hib or to the plain PRP vaccine, including patients with Hib disease before the age of 2 years and those with splenectomy, sickle cell disease, and malignancy.[148,149] Protective levels of antibody to Hib vaccine are seen within 1 month of immunization with the conjugate vaccines in more than 95 percent of patients.[150] The AAP and the ACIP recommend routine immunization of infants 2 months of age and older with a Hib conjugate vaccine, and this practice has resulted in a marked decrease in the incidence of Hib disease in the United States.[151] Two combination vaccines that contain Hib conjugate vaccine are also available: a DTaP-Hib (TriHIBit) and a hepatitis B–Hib combination (COMVAX).

Complications

Local and Systemic Reactions

Local reactions, including pain, tenderness, swelling, and erythema at the injection site, and systemic reactions, including low-grade fever and irritability, may occur within 24 to 72 hours of vaccination with Hib conjugate vaccine or PRP vaccine. These reactions are mild and transient. They are seen in approximately 2 to 25 percent of vaccine recipients, with overall reaction rates being lower following plain PRP vaccine than following conjugate vaccines.[152]

Neurologic Complications

GUILLAIN-BARRÉ SYNDROME (GBS)

Seven cases of GBS were reported following immunization with three different Hib conjugate vaccines during a period when several million doses of the vaccines were distributed (VAERS, November 1990 to July 1992).[153,154] Five of these fit the criteria for vaccine-related GBS. Hib conjugate vaccine was the only potential predisposing factor in three.[153,154] These data, with only 5 cases per several million doses, are insufficient to support a definite causal link between GBS and Hib vaccine.[155]

TRANSVERSE MYELITIS

There is inadequate evidence to support an association between Hib vaccines and transverse myelitis.

Early Susceptibility to H. influenzae Type B

Early-onset Hib disease following immunization is defined as a case of serious systemic infection caused by Hib that occurs within the 7-day interval following immunization for Hib. Anecdotal reports suggest that immunization of children over 18 months of age with unconjugated PRP vaccine is associated with an increased risk of disease for 7 days thereafter.[156] Since PRP vaccine contains purified capsular polysaccharide only, the early-onset cases of Hib infection could not have been caused by infectious material in the vaccine itself. This increased susceptibility might be related to a transient decrease in preexisting antibody level caused by the formation of antigen-antibody complexes; other mechanisms also have been postulated.[157] Cellulitis and epiglottitis, rather than meningitis, are more likely in early-onset Hib disease, developing within 72 hours of immunization. There is no evidence to suggest a causal relation between immunization with conjugate Hib vaccines and an increased risk of disease in the early post-vaccination interval.[158]

▶ HEPATITIS B VACCINE

Acute massive hepatic necrosis or chronic active hepatitis and cirrhosis of the liver may occur following hepatitis B virus infection. More than 170 million people in the world today are infected with hepatitis B virus, with an estimated 200 to 300 million chronic carriers worldwide. In the United States, an estimated 1 to 1.25 million persons are chronically infected, and an additional 5000 to 8000 persons become chronically infected each year.[159] The risk of becoming a carrier decreases with age. A plasma-derived hepatitis B vaccine was licensed for use in the United States in 1981. It was not well accepted because of unbased fears of transmission of live hepatitis B virus and other blood-borne pathogens (e.g., human immunodeficiency virus) and was removed from the U.S. market in 1992. Recombinant hepatitis B vaccine, the first vaccine using recombinant DNA technology, was licensed in the United States in 1986. It is produced by two manufacturers in the United States— Merck and Company Vaccine Division (Recombivax HB) and Glaxo Smith Kline Pharmaceuticals (Engerix-B). Both vaccines are available in pediatric and adult formulations. Both the pediatric and adult formulations of Recombivax can be used in any age group. Hepatitis B vaccine is indicated in persons of all ages, especially those who are at increased risk for exposure to hepatitis B virus infection. These include health care personnel, patients on hemodialysis or requiring frequent transfusions of blood or blood products, institutionalized patients and their close contacts, household members and sexual partners of hepatitis B virus carriers, intravenous drug abusers, homosexuals, heterosexuals with multiple partners, and adolescents, as well as infants born to mothers who are positive for hepatitis B surface antigen.[160]

Hepatitis B recombinant vaccines are given in a three-dose series. The sequence consists of two priming doses given 1 month apart, followed by a third dose given 6 months after the first dose. Those who have not been vaccinated against hepatitis B during infancy should complete the series during any childhood visit. However, there is an age-specific decline in immunogenicity. The maximal immune response is in children 2 to 19 years of age; by 60 years of age, only 75 percent of vaccinees develop protective antibody titers.[159] A diminished response is also seen in persons with immunosuppressive illnesses.[160] The vaccine is 80 to 100 percent effective in preventing infection or clinical hepatitis in those who complete the vaccination course.

Complications

Local and Systemic Reactions

Local reactions, including soreness, erythema, and local induration, are seen in approximately one-third of recipients of both the plasma-derived and recombinant vaccines; 10 to 15 percent may experience systemic reactions such as fatigue, headache, and fever.[161]

Anaphylaxis

Hepatitis B vaccines rarely may cause anaphylaxis (VAERS, November 1990 to July 1992). Subsequent vaccination with hepatitis B vaccine is contraindicated for persons who previously have had an anaphylactic response to a dose of this vaccine.

Neurologic Complications

DEMYELINATING DISEASES

Although there have been some reports of GBS following hepatitis B vaccination, the evidence is insufficient to support an association.[162] There are also reports of transverse myelitis and optic neuritis.[162] Hepatitis B vaccine has been alleged to cause or exacerbate multiple sclerosis.[163] However, large population-based studies have shown no association between hepatitis B vaccination and either the development or increased risk of exacerbation of multiple sclerosis.[164,165]

▶ INFLUENZA VACCINE

Influenza is characterized by an abrupt onset of fever, myalgia, sore throat, cough, malaise, and in severe cases, pneumonia. It is estimated that more than 10,000 influenza-associated deaths occurred during each of the 19 different U.S. epidemics from 1972 to 1995.[166] Currently licensed influenza vaccines available in the United States consist of inactivated split-virus preparations. The efficacy of influenza vaccine depends on the age and immunocompetence of the recipient, as well as on the degree of similarity between the vaccine virus strains and those which circulate during the influenza season.

Vaccines are effective in protecting up to 90 percent of healthy young adults and only 30 to 70 percent of the elderly. Among elderly nursing home residents, the vaccine can be 50 to 60 percent effective in preventing complications such as pneumonia and 80 percent effective in preventing death.[166] Immunity rarely exceeds a year.[166]

The vaccine is recommended for persons 50 years of age or older, residents of chronic care facilities with chronic medical conditions, and patients with cardiopulmonary disorders, diabetes, renal dysfunction, or immunosuppression, including HIV infection. Health care workers and close contacts of persons in chronic care facilities also should be vaccinated. In addition, influenza vaccine may be administered to any person who wishes to reduce the chance of becoming infected with influenza.[166] Each year the influenza vaccine contains strains representing the viruses that are likely to circulate in the United States during the influenza season (late December to early March). Currently, the most effective method of reducing the impact of influenza is by performing yearly vaccination of persons at high risk by vaccinating them no more than 2 to 4 months before the influenza season.

Complications

Local and Systemic Reactions

The most frequent side effect, reported by fewer than one-third of patients, is pain at the vaccination site lasting up to 2 days. Systemic reactions, including fever, malaise, and myalgias, are infrequent, occurring in less than 1 percent of vaccine recipients, and may last for 1 or 2 days.[166]

Allergic Reactions

Immediate allergic reactions, including hives, angioedema, and anaphylaxis, may result from hypersensitivity to a vaccine component, most commonly residual egg protein. Although persons with known immunoglobulin E–mediated hypersensitivity to eggs may be at increased risk for allergic reactions, some studies have indicated that these individuals can receive influenza vaccines safely without significant allergic reactions.[167] Protocols have been established for patients who have medical conditions that place them at increased risk for influenza infection or its complications. Persons with egg allergy should consult a physician for appropriate evaluation to determine if they can be vaccinated.[166]

Neurologic Complications

Neurologic complications of influenza immunization were rarely reported before 1976. In that year, a national immunization program was established against the "swine flu" (A/New Jersey) strain of influenza virus.

Over the next 2 months, an increase in cases of GBS was documented. The risk of GBS attributable to influenza immunization was estimated at 1 per 100,000 immunizations, with onset usually occurring 5 to 10 weeks following the immunization.[168] In 1992–1993 and 1993–1994 the CDC reported an increased incidence of this complication. However, further investigation of these claims found no such increased risk. The adjusted relative risk of 1.7 (95 percent confidence interval 1.0–2.8; $p = 0.04$) in the 6 weeks after vaccination suggested slightly more than 1 additional case of GBS per 1 million persons vaccinated against influenza as compared with a background incidence of 0.87 cases per 1 million persons per 6-week period. Subsequent vaccines prepared from other virus strains have not clearly been associated with GBS.[169] Regardless, vaccination should be avoided in any individual who developed GBS within 6 weeks of a previous influenza vaccination.

Neurologic disorders temporally associated with influenza vaccination, such as encephalopathy,[170–172] brachial plexus neuropathy or neuralgic amyotrophy,[173] acute transverse myelitis,[174] anterior ischemic optic neuropathy,[175] isolated cranial neuropathies,[176] vasculitis,[177] and giant cell arteritis,[178,179] have been reported. However, these complications are too infrequent to establish a causal relationship.

▶ VARICELLA VACCINE

Varicella is a highly communicable disease caused by the varicella-zoster virus. Herpes zoster (shingles) occurs when latent varicella-zoster virus reactivates, causing recurrent infection. In the United States, approximately 3.5 million cases of varicella occur annually, most frequently during winter and early spring, with a peak incidence in children between 5 and 9 years of age.[180] Natural varicella is more severe and complications more frequent in older individuals and infants younger than 1 year of age.[180] The fatality rate of varicella among children 1 to 14 years of age is approximately 1 per 100,000 cases compared with 25.2 per 100,000 cases in adults 30 to 49 years of age. Approximately 100 previously healthy individuals die of complications of varicella each year in the United States.[181] The incidence of varicella, as well as varicella-related hospitalizations, has fallen significantly since the licensure of a live, attenuated varicella virus (OKA strain) vaccine in the United States in March 1995.[182]

Vaccination is indicated in individuals 12 months of age and older who have not had varicella. Children between 12 months and 12 years of age should receive a single dose. When vaccination is given after 13 years of age, a second dose administered 4 to 8 weeks later is recommended. Severity of varicella after infection is much milder in vaccinated as compared with unvaccinated children.[183,184] Vaccine efficacy is estimated at 80 to 90 percent against infection and 95 percent against severe disease.[183] Immunity appears to be long lasting and probably permanent in the majority of vaccinees. Efficacy of the varicella vaccine may be reduced if a live viral vaccine was given immediately before the vaccination. Risk of breakthrough infection is 2.5 times higher if varicella vaccine is administered less than 30 days after MMR vaccination compared with administration of varicella vaccine before, simultaneously, or more than 30 days after MMR vaccination. Inactivated vaccines (DTaP, Hib, IPV, and hepatitis B) and OPV did not increase the risk of breakthrough varicella if administered less than 30 days prior to the varicella vaccine.[185] The ACIP strongly recommends that varicella vaccine be administered at 12 to 18 months of age.

Complications

Varicella vaccine is generally well tolerated. A mild maculopapular or varicelliform rash at the injection site or elsewhere may occur in approximately 4 percent of individuals, fever in approximately 14 percent, and local pain and redness in 15 to 20 percent. The risk of herpes zoster is four to five times higher from wild virus infection than following immunization; most of these cases have occurred in children, with the illness being mild and without complications.[183] Other reported adverse reactions include headache, irritability, fatigue, cough, diarrhea, anorexia, lymphadenopathy, myalgia, arthralgia, pneumonitis, and febrile seizures, but a causal link has not been established. Anaphylaxis, encephalitis, ataxia, and erythema multiforme also have been reported.[183,184]

Contraindications and Precautions

Varicella vaccine is contraindicated in patients with a history of hypersensitivity to any component of the vaccine or anaphylactoid reaction to neomycin. Other contraindications include immunodeficiency, family history of congenital or hereditary immunodeficiency, tuberculosis, active febrile illness, and pregnancy. Vaccination should be deferred for at least 5 months following blood or plasma transfusions or administration of immune globulin including varicella-zoster immune globulin. Immune globulin should not be administered for 2 months after immunization. Salicylates should be avoided for 6 weeks after vaccination because Reye's syndrome following the use of salicylates during natural varicella infection has been reported. Vaccine recipients should avoid close contact with susceptible high-risk individuals for up to 6 weeks, e.g., newborns, pregnant women, and immunocompromised individuals. Pregnancy should be avoided for 1 month following vaccination.[183,184]

► PNEUMOCOCCAL VACCINE

Streptococcus pneumoniae is a gram-positive diplococcus that can cause pneumonia, bacteremia, and meningitis. Encapsulated organisms are pathogenic, whereas organisms without capsular polysaccharides are not. The encapsulated pneumococcal strains have been subclassified into serotypes according to the chemical composition of the antigenic determinant sites (epitomes) they display within their capsular polysaccharide matrices. Of the 90 serotypes identified, 23 specific serotypes represent 85 to 90 percent of invasive pneumococcal disease in the United States. Pneumococcal infection is estimated to kill more than 1 million children younger than 5 years of age annually throughout the world, with the majority of the deaths occurring in developing countries.[186] The highest rates of invasive pneumococcal disease occur in young children, especially those younger than 2 years of age. In 1998, the estimated incidence rates were 165 and 203 cases per 100,000 population per year among children aged less than 12 months and 12 to 13 months, respectively.[187] The risk is increased in children of certain racial groups, particularly Native Americans or African-Americans, and in children attending day-care centers. Children with functional or anatomic asplenia, such as sickle-cell disease, and with immunosuppression (including HIV infection) are at a higher risk (>150 cases per 100,000 population per year). In the United States each year 5000 cases of meningitis, 500,000 cases of pneumonia, and 7 million cases of acute otitis media due to the pneumococcus occur in children younger than 5 years of age.[187]

Pneumococcal polysaccharide vaccine is composed of purified preparations of pneumococcal capsular polysaccharide. In 1983, a 23-valent capsular polysaccharide vaccine (PPV23) was licensed for use. It contains polysaccharide antigens from 23 types of pneumococcal bacteria that are epidemiologically the most important serotypes, accounting for 85 to 90 percent of invasive pneumococcal infection. Although the 23-valent vaccine provided adequate immunity in healthy persons older than 5 years of age, many of the pneumococcal serotypes are poorly immunogenic in younger children,[188,189] which is the age group with the highest incidence of infection.[186] Its immunogenicity is also suboptimal in some high-risk groups, including the geriatric population and the immunocompromised.

The first pneumococcal conjugate vaccine (PCV7) was licensed in the United States in 2000. It contains purified capsular polysaccharide of 7 serotypes of *S. pneumoniae* conjugated to an inert immunogenic variant of diphtheria toxoid known as CRM197 that is also used as the carrier in one *H. influenzae* type b vaccine conjugate. The serotypes included in PCV7 account for 85 to 90 percent and 68 to 81 percent of invasive pneumococcal disease in children younger than 6 years of age in North America and western Europe, respectively.[190] PPV23 is 60 to 70 percent effective in preventing invasive disease. However, it is not effective in children younger than 2 years of age. Children younger than 2 years of age (and immunocompromised individuals) are incapable of mounting a T-cell-dependent immune response to the polysaccharide macromolecules in the 23-valent vaccine formulation. However, the PCV7 vaccine, by coupling a polysaccharide antigen to an immunogenic carrier protein, is converted from a T-cell-independent antigen to a T-cell-dependent antigen with the induction of an amnestic response. It stimulates a T-cell-dependent immune response in children older than 6 weeks, whereas unconjugated vaccine formulations consisting of only the polysaccharide antigens stimulate T cell-independent immune responses in children younger than 5 years of age.[188,189] PCV7 is immunogenic in infants and children, including those with sickle-cell disease and HIV infection. In a large clinical trial it was shown to be more than 90 percent effective against invasive disease.[191] The duration of protection following PCV7 is currently unknown.

Pneumococcal polysaccharide vaccine PPV23 should be administered routinely to all adults 65 years of age or older. It is also indicated in persons aged 2 years and older with anatomic or functional asplenia (e.g., sickle-cell disease, Hodgkin's disease, lymphoma), immunocompromised individuals (e.g., chemotherapy, HIV infection), and those living in special environments or social settings (e.g., Native American populations). Pneumococcal conjugate vaccine PCV7 is used for the routine immunization of all children younger than 24 months of age and 25 to 59 months with high-risk medical conditions. It is not routinely recommended for persons older than 59 months of age.

Complications

Local Reactions

The most common adverse reactions following PPV7 and PPV23 are local reactions. For PPV23, 30 to 50 percent of vaccinees report pain, swelling, or erythema at the injection site persisting for 48 hours. Adverse reactions are less common following PCV7, occurring in 10 to 20 percent.[191]

Systemic Reactions

Systemic reactions such as fever and myalgias are uncommon (<1 percent of vaccinees) following PPV23 as compared with 15 to 24 percent following PCV7.[191] Serious adverse reactions are rare.

► SMALLPOX VACCINE

Smallpox is an acute infectious disease caused by the variola virus. No infectious disease in history has been more lethal. In the twentieth century, smallpox killed 300 million people worldwide. The last case of smallpox in the United States was reported in Texas in 1949. The last indigenous case of smallpox on earth occurred in Somalia in October 1977.[192] The World Health Assembly officially certified the global eradication of smallpox in May 1980. To facilitate the possible development of a less reactogenic smallpox vaccine, as well as an antiviral drug that could be used in the treatment of patients with smallpox, the Fifty-Second World Health Assembly authorized temporary retention of remaining stocks of variola virus in two designated laboratories: the CDC and Prevention in Atlanta and the Institute of Virus Protection in Moscow.[193] There has been a renewed interest in vaccinating populations against smallpox because it could be used for bioterrorism.

The smallpox vaccine currently licensed for use in the United States is Dryvax, a live-virus preparation of the infectious vaccinia virus prepared in the 1980s from calf lymph with a seed virus derived from the New York City Board of Health (NYCBOH) strain of vaccinia virus.[192] It does not contain smallpox (variola) virus. The U.S. military has a program to develop a new smallpox vaccine, but its testing and development are not expected to be completed before 2005 at the earliest.

Preliminary epidemiologic studies have demonstrated that a high level of protection (nearly 100 percent) against smallpox persists for up to 5 years after primary vaccination and substantial but waning immunity for 10 years or more.[192] The fatality rate among people vaccinated less than 10 years prior was 1.3 percent, 7 percent among those vaccinated 11 to 20 years prior, and 11 percent among those vaccinated 20 or more years prior to infection. In contrast, 52 percent of unvaccinated people died during a smallpox epidemic.[194] In the event of an intentional release of smallpox virus, the ACIP recommends vaccination of all persons who are exposed to the initial release of the virus, contacts of people who develop smallpox, and others at risk of exposure, including medical personnel involved in the care and transportation of smallpox patients, laboratory personnel involved in processing of clinical specimens, and persons likely to come into contact with infectious material from smallpox patients.[192]

Complications

Adverse Reactions Specific to the Vaccine

Inadvertent inoculation (transfer of vaccinia from the vaccination site to another part of the body) is the most frequent complication of smallpox vaccination, accounting for approximately half of all complications of primary vaccination and revaccination. Most common sites involved are face, eyelids, nose, mouth, genitalia, and rectum. More severe complications include eczema vaccinatum (EV), generalized vaccinia, progressive vaccinia, fetal vaccinia, and postvaccinal encephalitis (PVE).

EV is a generalized superinfection of the skin with vaccinia virus among vaccinees or in contacts with eczema or past history of eczema. It is usually mild and self-limited, but it can be fatal, especially in children younger than 2 years of age.[195] It is estimated to occur at a rate of 10.4 per 1 million primary vaccination doses.[196]

Generalized vaccinia results from vaccinia viremia, with vesicles or pustules appearing on normal skin distant from vaccination site in persons without preexisting skin disease. It is self-limited and occurs at a rate of 23.4 per 1 million primary vaccinations.[196]

Progressive vaccinia (vaccinia necrose) is a severe illness that is seen exclusively in persons with cellular immunodeficiency and is characterized by necrosis at the vaccination site often with metastatic lesions, sepsis, and death.[195,196] It occurs at a rate of 0.9 per 1 million primary vaccinations and requires treatment with vaccinia immune globulin and antiviral agents.[196]

Fetal vaccinia is a rare complication and follows primary vaccination of the pregnant mother in the first trimester. It usually results in stillbirth or death of the infant soon after delivery. Fewer than 50 cases have been reported.[196]

Neurologic Complications

POSTVACCINAL ENCEPHALITIS (PVE)

PVE was first recognized as a complication of the Jennerian cowpox inoculation in 1905 in France, and a second case was observed in London Hospital in 1912.[197] The incidence of postvaccinal encephalitis in the United States was 1.0 per 100,000 primary vaccinations in 1968.[198] In the majority of cases, PVE affects primary vaccinees younger than 12 months of age or adolescents and adults receiving primary vaccination. Most cases are believed to result from autoimmune or allergic reactions rather than from direct viral invasion of the nervous system. An incubation period of 6 to 12 days is followed by an abrupt onset of fever, headache, meningeal signs, ataxia, vomiting, and confusion. The illness could progress to seizures, stupor, and coma. CSF analysis revealed pleocytosis, increased protein, and normal glucose concentration.[199] In the United States, the case-fatality rate of PVE between 1959 and 1966 was approximately 25 percent.[195] Microscopic examination of brain specimens at autopsy showed mononuclear or lymphocytic perivascular infiltration involving white matter more than gray matter, focal areas of demyelination, and diffuse cortical petechial hemorrhages.[197,198] Antivaccinia gamma globulin (AGG) is not effective in treating PVE.

Antivaccinia gamma globulin is the only product currently available for the treatment of complications of smallpox vaccination. It is effective for the treatment of eczema vaccinatum and certain cases of progressive vaccinia but provides no benefit in the treatment of post-vaccinial encephalitis[200] and has no role in the treatment of smallpox. Certain antiviral compounds, such as cidofovir, have been reported to be active against vaccinia virus in vitro and in animal studies. Their safety and efficacy in humans are unknown, and they are not approved by the FDA.

OTHER NEUROLOGIC SYNDROMES

Other neurologic syndromes associated with smallpox vaccine include headache, fever, photophobia, and nuchal rigidity developing 5 to 7 days after vaccination and febrile convulsions associated with the febrile response to the vaccine.[201]

Other Complications

Certain smallpox vaccine reactions are similar to those caused by other vaccines and include fever, anaphylaxis, nonspecific erythematous or urticarial rashes which resolve spontaneously, and rarely, erythema multiforme and Stevens Johnson syndrome.[196]

Contraindications and Precautions

Smallpox vaccination generally is contraindicated for persons who have the following conditions or have a close contact with the following conditions: (1) a history of atopic dermatitis (commonly referred to as *eczema*) irrespective of disease severity or activity, (2) active acute, chronic, or exfoliative skin conditions that disrupt the epidermis, (3) pregnant women or women who desire to become pregnant within 28 days after vaccination, and (4) persons who are immunocompromised as a result of HIV infection or acquired immunodeficiency syndrome (AIDS), autoimmune conditions, cancer, radiation treatment, immunosuppressive medications, or other immunodeficiencies. It is also contraindicated for persons who have experienced a serious allergic reaction to a prior dose of vaccine or to a vaccine component, women who are breast-feeding, those taking topical ocular steroid medications, those with moderate to severe intercurrent illnesses, and persons younger than 18 years of age.[196]

REFERENCES

1. American Academy of Pediatrics: Active immunization. In Pickering LK (ed): *Red Book: 2003 Report of the Committee on Infectious Diseases,* 26th ed. Elk Grove Village, IL: American Academy of Pediatrics, 2003.
2. Patel H, Garg BP: Complications of immunization. In Biller J (ed): *Iatrogenic Neurology.* Boston: Butterworth-Heinemann, 1998, p 485.
3. Weibel RE, Caserta V, Benor DE, et al: Acute encephalopathy followed by permanent brain injury or death associated with further attenuated measles vaccines: A review of claims submitted to the National Vaccine Injury Compensation Program. *Pediatrics* 101(3):383, 1998.
4. Centers for Disease Control and Prevention. Measles, mumps and rubella–vaccine use and strategies for elimination of measles, rubella and congenital rubella syndrome and control of mumps: Recommendations of the Advisory Committee on Immunization Practices (ACIP). *MMWR* 47(RR8):1, 1998.
5. Watson JC, Pearson JA, Markowitz LE, et al: An evaluation of measles revaccination among school-entry-aged children. *Pediatrics* 97(5):613, 996.
6. Markowitz LE, Preblud SR, Fine PE, et al: Duration of live measles vaccine-induced immunity. *Pediatr Infect Dis J* 9:101, 1990.
7. Bloch AB, Orenstein WA, Stetler HC, et al: Health impact of measles vaccination in the United States. *Pediatrics* 76:524, 1985.
8. The National Vaccine Advisory Committee. The measles epidemic: The problems, barriers, and recommendations. *JAMA* 266:1547, 1991.
9. Atkinson WL: Epidemiology and prevention of measles. *Dermatol Clin* 3:553, 1995.
10. de Quadros CA, Olive JM, Hersh BS, et al: Measles elimination in the Americas: Evolving strategies. *JAMA* 275(3):224, 1996.
11. Peltola H, Heinonen OP: Frequency of true adverse reactions to measles-mumps-rubella vaccine. *Lancet* 1:939, 1986.
12. Jadavji T, Scheifele D, Halperin S, et al: Thrombocytopenia after immunization of Canadian children, 1992–2001. *Pediatr Infect Dis J* 22:119, 2003.
13. Neiminen U, Peltola H, Syrjälä MT, et al: Acute thrombocytopenic purpura following measles, mumps and rubella vaccination: A report on 23 patients. *Acta Pediatr* 82:267, 1993.
14. Beeler J, Varricchio F, Wise R: Thrombocytopenia after immunization with measles vaccines: Review of the vaccine adverse events reporting system (1990–1994). *Pediatr Infect Dis J* 15:88, 1996.
15. Farrington P, Pugh S, Colville A, et al: A new method for active surveillance of adverse events from diphtheria/tetanus/pertussis and measles/mumps/rubella vaccines. *Lancet* 345(8949):567, 1995.
16. Sakaguchi M, Nakayama T, Inouye S : Food allergy to gelatin in children with systemic immediate-type reactions, including anaphylaxis, to vaccines. *J Allergy Clin Immunol* 98:1058, 1996.
17. Annamari P, Mäkinen-Kiljunen S, Davidkin I, et al: Allergic reactions to measles-mumps-rubella vaccination. *Pediatrics* 107(2):27, 2001.
18. James JM, Burks AW, Roberson PK, et al: Safe administration of the measles vaccine to children allergic to eggs. *New Engl J Med* 332(19):1262, 1995.
19. Update: Vaccine side effects, adverse reactions, contraindications and precautions: Recommendations of the Advisory Committee on Immunization Practices (ACIP). *MMWR* 45(RR12):1, 1996.

20. Landrigan PJ, Witte JJ: Neurological disorders following live measles-virus vaccination. *JAMA* 223:1459, 1973.

21. Alderslade R, Bellman MH, Ross EM, et al: The National Childhood Encephalopathy Study: A report on 1000 cases of serious disorders in infants and young children from the NCES research team. In *Whooping Cough: Reports from the Committee on the Safety of Medicines and the Joint Committee on the Vaccination and Immunization*. London: Her Majesty's Stationary Office, 1981.

22. Miller DL: Frequency of complications of measles, 1963: Report on a national inquiry by the Public Health Laboratory Service in collaboration with the Society of Medical Officers of Health. *Br Med J* 2:75, 1964.

23. Measles and mumps vaccines. In Stratton KR, Howe CJ, Johnston RB (eds): *Adverse Events Associated with Childhood Vaccines: Evidence Bearing Causality*. Institute of Medicine. Washington: National Academy Press, 1994, p 118.

24. Miller D, Wadsworth J, Diamond J, et al: Measles vaccination and events. *Lancet* 349(9053):730, 1997.

25. Black S, Shinefield H, Ray P, et al: Risk of hospitalization because of aseptic meningitis after measles-mumps-rubella vaccination in one to two-year-old children: An analysis of the Vaccine Safety Datalink (VSD) Project. *Pediatr Infect Dis J* 16:500, 1997.

26. Modlin JF, Jabbour JT, Witte JJ, et al: Epidemiologic studies of measles, measles vaccine and subacute sclerosing panencephalitis. *Pediatrics* 59(4):505, 1977.

27. Schneck SA: Vaccination with measles and central nervous system disease. *Neurology* 18(part II):79, 1968.

28. Cho CT, Lansky LJ, D'Souza BJ: Panencephalitis following measles vaccination (letter). *JAMA* 224:1299, 1973.

29. Dyken PR, Cunningham SC, Ward LC: Changing character of subacute sclerosing panencephalitis in the United States. *Pediatr Neurol* 5:339, 1989.

30. Subacute sclerosing panencephalitis surveillance: United States. *MMWR* 31:585, 1982.

31. Valmari P, Lanning M, Tuokko H, et al: Measles virus in the cerebrospinal fluid in postvaccination immunosuppressive measles encephalopathy. *Pediatr Infect Dis J* 6:59, 1987.

32. Mitus A, Holloway A, Evans AE, et al: Attenuated measles vaccine in children with acute leukemia. *Am J Dis Child* 103:243, 1962.

33. Hirtz DG, Nelson KB, Ellenberg JH: Seizures following childhood immunizations. *J Pediatr* 102:14, 1983.

34. Griffin MR, Ray WA, Mortimer EA, et al: Risk of seizures after measles-mumps-rubella immunization. *Pediatrics* 88:881, 1991.

35. Wakefield AJ, Murch SH, Anthony A, et al: Ileal-lymphoid-nodular hyperplasia, nonspecific colitis and pervasive developmental disorder in children. *Lancet* 351(9103):637, 1998.

36. Thompson NP, Montgomery SM, Pounder RW, et al: Is measles vaccination a risk factor for inflammatory bowel disease? *Lancet* 345(8957):1071, 1995.

37. Wakefield AJ, Pittilo RM, Sim R, et al: Evidence of persistent measles virus infection in Crohn's disease. *J Med Virol* 39:345, 1993.

38. Begg N, Ramsay M, White J, et al: Media dents confidence in MMR vaccine. *Br Med J* 316:561, 1998.

39. Payne C, Mason B: Autism, inflammatory bowel disease and MMR vaccine (letter). *Lancet* 351(9106):907, 1998.

40. Taylor B, Miller E, Farrington CP, et al: Autism and measles, mumps and rubella vaccine: No epidemiological evidence for a causal association. *Lancet* 353(9169):2026, 1999.

41. Halsey NA, Hyman SL, and the Conference Writing Panel: Measles-mumps-rubella vaccine and the autistic spectrum disorder: Report from the New Challenge in Childhood Immunizations Conference, convened in Oakbrook, IL, June 12–13, 2000. *Pediatrics* 107(5):84, 2001.

42. Pampiglione G, Griffith AH, Bramwell EC: Transient cerebral changes after vaccination against measles. *Lancet* 2:5, 1971.

43. Chan CC, Sogg RL, Steinman L: Isolated oculomotor palsy after measles immunization. *Am J Ophthalmol* 89:446, 1980.

44. Kazarian EL, Gager WE: Optic neuritis complicating measles, mumps and rubella vaccination. *Am J Ophthalmol* 86:544, 1978.

45. Stevenson VL, Acheson JF, Ball J, et al: Optic neuritis following measles/rubella vaccination in two 13-year-old children. *Br J Ophthalmol* 80:1110, 1996.

46. Marshall GS, Wright PF, Fenichel GM, et al: Diffuse retinopathy following measles, mumps and rubella vaccination. *Pediatrics* 76(6):989, 1985.

47. Buynak ZB, Hilleman MR: Live attenuated mumps virus vaccine: I. Vaccine development. *Proc Soc Exp Biol Med* 123:768, 1966.

48. Hilleman MR, Buynak EB, Weibel RE, et al: Live attenuated mumps-virus vaccine. *New Engl J Med* 278(5):227, 1968.

49. Fujinaga T, Motegi Y, Tamura H, et al: A prefecture-wide survey of mumps meningitis associated with measles, mumps and rubella vaccine. *Pediatr Infect Dis J* 10:204, 1991.

50. Miller E, Goldacre M, Pugh S, et al: Risk of aseptic meningitis after measles, mumps and rubella vaccine in UK children. *Lancet* 341(8851):979, 1993.

51. Plesner A-M, Hansen FJ, Taudorf K, et al: Gait disturbance interpreted as cerebellar ataxia after MMR vaccination at 15 months of age: A follow-up study. *Acta Pëdiatr* 89:58, 2000.

52. Nabe-Nielsen J, Walter B: Unilateral deafness as a complication of the mumps, measles and rubella vaccination. *Br Med J* 297:489, 1988.

53. Brodsky L, Stanievich J: Sensorineural hearing loss following live measles virus vaccination. *Int J Pediatr Otorhinolaryngol* 10:159, 1985.

54. Healy CE. Mumps vaccine and nerve deafness (letter). *Am J Dis Child* 123:612, 1972.

55. Kaga K, Chimera K, Motoko I: Unilateral total loss of auditory and vestibular function as a complication of mumps vaccination. *Int J Pediatr Otorhinolaryngol* 43:73, 1998.

56. Geier DA, Geier MR: Rubella vaccine and arthritic adverse reactions: An analysis of the Vaccine Adverse Events Reporting System (VAERS) database from 1991 through 1998. *Clin Exp Rheumatol* 19(6):724, 2001.

57. Balfour HH, Groth KE, Edelman CK: RA27/3 rubella vaccine: A four-year follow-up. *Am J Dis Child* 134:350, 1980.

58. Polk BF, Modlin JF, White JA, et al: A controlled comparison of joint reactions among women receiving one of two rubella vaccines. *Am J Epidemiol* 115:19, 1982.

59. Tingle AJ, Mitchell LA, Grace M, et al: Randomized double-blind placebo controlled study on adverse effects of rubella immunization in seronegative women. *Lancet* 349(9061):1277, 1997.

60. Evidence concerning rubella vaccines and arthritis, radiculoneuritis, and thrombocytopenic purpura. In Howson CP, Howe CJ, Fineberg HV (eds): *Adverse Effects of Pertussis and Rubella Vaccines: A Report of the Committee to Review the Adverse Consequences of Pertussis and Rubella Vaccines.* Division of Health Promotion and Disease Prevention, Institute of Medicine. Washington: National Academy Press, 1991, p 187.

61. Ray P, Black S, Shinefield H, et al: Risk of chronic arthropathy among women after rubella vaccination. *JAMA* 278:551, 1997.

62. Kilroy AW, Schaffner W, Fleet WF, et al: Two syndromes following rubella immunizations: Clinical observations and epidemiological studies. *JAMA* 214(13):2287, 1970.

63. Gilmartin RC, Jabbour JT, Duenas DA: Rubella vaccine myeloradiculoneuritis. *J Pediatr* 80(3):406, 1972.

64. Speier JE: Complications of rubella vaccination (letter). *JAMA* 213:2272, 1970.

65. Schaffner W, Fleet WF, Kilroy AW, et al: Polyneuropathy following rubella immunization: A follow-up study and review of the problem. *Am J Dis Child* 127:684, 1974.

66. Holt S, Hudgins D, Krishnan KR, et al: Diffuse myelitis associated with rubella vaccination. *Br Med J* 2:1037, 1976.

67. Kline LB, Margulies SL, Oh SJ: Optic neuritis and myelitis following rubella vaccination. *Arch Neurol* 39:443, 1982.

68. Peckham CS: Clinical and laboratory study of children exposed in utero to maternal rubella. *Arch Dis Child* 47:571, 1972.

69. Wyll SA, Herrmann KL: Inadvertent rubella vaccination of pregnant women: Fetal risk in 215 cases. *JAMA* 225:1472, 1973.

70. Vaheri A, Vesikari T, Oker-Blom N, et al: Isolation of attenuated rubella-vaccine virus from human products of conception and uterine cervix. *New Engl J Med* 286:1071, 1972.

71. Preblud SR: Some current issues relating to rubella vaccine. *JAMA* 254:253, 1985.

72. Rubella vaccination during pregnancy: United States 1971–1983. *MMWR* 33(26):365, 1984.

73. Preblud SR, Stetler HC, Frank JA Jr, et al: Fetal risk associated with rubella vaccine. *JAMA* 246:1413, 1981.

74. Strebel PM, Sutter RW, Cochi SL, et al: Epidemiology of poliomyelitis in the United States one decade after the last reported case of indigenous wild virus-associated disease. *Clin Infect Dis* 14:568, 1992.

75. Nightingale EO: Recommendations for a national policy on poliomyelitis vaccination. *New Engl J Med* 297:249, 1977.

76. Centers for Disease Control and Prevention: Poliomyelitis prevention in the United States: Introduction of a sequential vaccination schedule of inactivated poliovirus vaccine (IPV) followed by oral poliovirus vaccine. *MMWR* 46(RR-3):1, 1997.

77. Centers for Disease Control and Prevention: Notice to readers: Recommendations of the Advisory Committee on Immunization Practices: Revised recommendations for routine poliomyelitis vaccination. *MMWR* 48:590, 1999.

78. Ruuskanen O, Salmi TT, Stenvik M, et al: Inactivated polio vaccine: Adverse reactions and antibody responses. *Acta Paediatr Scand* 69:397, 1980.

79. Willis E, Sherrod JL: Childhood immunizations: Position on the enhanced inactivated poliovirus vaccine and live attenuated oral poliovirus vaccine dilemma. *J Natl Med Assoc* 89:785, 1997.

80. Centers for Disease Control and Prevention: Poliomyelitis—United States, 1975–1984. *MMWR* 35(11):180, 1986.

81. American Academy of Pediatrics Committee on Infectious Disease: Poliomyelitis prevention: Recommendations for use of inactivated poliovirus vaccine and live oral poliovirus vaccine. *Pediatrics* 99(2):300, 1997.

82. Kinnunen E, Färkkilä M, Hovi T, et al: Incidence of Guillain-Barré syndrome during a nationwide oral polio virus vaccine campaign. *Neurology* 39:1034, 1989.

83. Polio vaccines, in Stratton KR, Howe CJ, Johnston RB (eds): *Adverse Events Associated with Childhood Vaccines: Evidence Bearing on Causality.* Institute of Medicine. Washington: National Academy Press, 1994, p 187.

84. Centers for Disease Control and Prevention: Summary of notifiable diseases—United States, 1994. *MMWR* 43(53):70, 1995.

85. Diphtheria. In Atkinson W, Wolfe C (eds): *Epidemiology and Prevention of Vaccine-Preventable Diseases,* 7th ed. Washington: Public Health Foundation, 2002, p 39.

86. Vitek CR, Wharton M: Diphtheria in the former Soviet Union: Reemergence of a pandemic disease. *Emerg Infect Dis* 4(4):539, 1998.

87. Wasilak SGF, Orenstein WA, Sutter RW: Tetanus toxoid. In Plotkin SA, Orenstein WA (eds): *Vaccines,* 3d ed. Philadelphia: Saunders, 1999, p 441.

88. Kumar S, Malecki JM: A case of neonatal tetanus. *South Med J* 84(3):396, 1991.

89. Craig AS, Reed GW, Mohon RT, et al: Neonatal tetanus in the United States: A sentinel event in the foreignborn. *Pediatr Infect Dis J* 16:955, 1997.

90. Peebles TC, Levine L, Eldred MC, et al: Tetanus toxic emergency boosters: A reappraisal. *New Engl J Med* 280(11):575, 1969.

91. Collier LH, Polakoff S, Mortimer J: Reactions and antibody responses to reinforcing doses of adsorbed and plain tetanus vaccines. *Lancet* 1:1364, 1979.

92. Acel-Imune package insert, Lederle laboratories, Division American Cyanamid Company, Pearl River, NY, issued January 3, 1997.

93. Jacobs RL, Lowe RS, Lanier BQ: Adverse reactions to tetanus toxoid. *JAMA* 247:40, 1982.

94. Facktor MA, Bernstein RA, Fireman P: Hypersensitivity to tetanus toxoid. *J Allergy Clin Immunol* 52:1, 1973.

95. Schlenska GK: Unusual complications following tetanus toxoid administration. *J Neurol* 215:299, 1977.

96. Schwarz G, Lanzer G, List WF: Acute midbrain syndrome as an adverse reaction to tetanus immunization. *Intensive Care Med* 15:53, 1988.

97. Whittle E, Roberton NRC: Transverse myelitis after diphtheria, tetanus and polio immunization. *Br Med J* 1:1450, 1977.

98. Read SJ, Schapel GJ, Pender MP: Acute transverse myelitis after tetanus toxoid vaccination (letter). *Lancet* 339:1111, 1992.

99. Topaloglu H, Berker M, Kansu T, et al: Optic neuritis and myelitis after booster tetanus toxoid vaccination (letter). *Lancet* 339:178, 1992.

100. Quast U, Hennessen W, Widmark RM: Mono- and polyneuritis after tetanus vaccination (1970–1977). *Dev Biol Stand* 43:25, 1979.

101. Reinstein L, Pargament JM, Goodman JS: Peripheral neuropathy after multiple tetanus toxoid injections. *Arch Phys Med Rehabil* 63:332, 1982.

102. Holliday PL, Bauer RB: Polyradiculoneuritis secondary to immunization with tetanus and diphtheria toxoids. *Arch Neurol* 40:56, 1983.

103. Pollard JD, Selby G. Relapsing neuropathy due to tetanus toxoid: Report of a case. *J Neurol Sci* 37:113, 1978.

104. Diphtheria and tetanus toxoids. In Stratton KR, Howe CJ, Johnston RB (eds): *Adverse Events Associated with Childhood Vaccines: Evidence Bearing Causality*. Institute of Medicine. Washington: National Academy Press, 1994, p 67

105. Rantala J, Cherry JD, Shields WD, et al: Epidemiology of Guillain-Barré syndrome in children: Relationship of oral polio vaccine administration to occurrence. *J Pediatr* 124:220, 1994.

106. Blumstein GI, Kreithin H: Peripheral neuropathy following tetanus toxoid administration. *JAMA* 198(9):1030, 1966.

107. Tsairis P, Dyck PH, Mulder DW: Natural history of brachial plexus neuropathy: Report on 99 patients. *Arch Neurol* 27:109, 1972.

108. Baust W, Meyer D, Wachsmuth W: Peripheral neuropathy after administration of tetanus toxoid. *J Neurol* 222:131, 1979.

109. Kiwit JC: Neurological amyotrophy after administration of tetanus toxoid (letter). *J Neurol Neurosurg Psychiatry* 47:320, 1984.

110. Immunization Practices Advisory Committee (ACIP): Diphtheria, tetanus and pertussis: Recommendations for vaccine use and other preventive measures. *MMWR* 40(RR-10.):1, 1991.

111. Summary of notifiable diseases—United States, 1998. *MMWR* 47(53):v, 1999.

112. Farizo KM, Cochi SL, Zell ER, et al: Epidemiological features of pertussis in the United States, 1980–1989. *Clin Infect Dis* 14:708, 1992.

113. Miller CL, Fletcher WB: Severity of notified whooping cough. *Br Med J* 1:117, 1976.

114. Cherry JD, Brunell PA, Golden GS, et al: Report of the Task Force on Pertussis and Pertussis Immunization—1988. *Pediatrics* 81:939, 1988.

115. Onorato IM, Wasilak SG, Meade B: Efficacy of whole-cell pertussis vaccine in preschool children in the United States. *JAMA* 267:2745, 1992.

116. Cody CL, Baraff LJ, Cherry JD, et al: Nature and rates of adverse reactions associated with DTP and DT immunizations in infants and children. *Pediatrics* 68:650, 1981.

117. DuVernoy TS, Braun MM: Hypotensive-hyporesponsive episodes reported to the Vaccine Adverse Events Reporting System (VAERS), 1996–1998. *Pediatrics* 106(4):52, 2000.

118. Gold MS: Hypotonic-hyporesponsive episodes following pertussis vaccination: A cause for concern? *Drug Saf* 25(2):85, 2002.

119. Rosenthal S, Chen RT, Hadler S: The safety of acellular pertussis vaccine vs whole-cell vaccine. *Arch Pediatr Adolesc Med* 150:457, 1996.

120. Evidence concerning pertussis vaccines and central nervous system disorders including infantile spasms, hypsarrhythmia, aseptic meningitis and encephalopathy. In Howson CP, Howe CJ, Fineberg HV (eds): *Adverse Effects of Pertussis and Rubella Vaccines. A Report of the Committee to Review the Adverse Consequences of Pertussis and Rubella Vaccines*. Institute of Medicine. Washington: National Academy Press, 1991, p 65

121. Vermeer-de Bondt PE, Labadie J, Rümpke HC: Rate of recurrent collapse after vaccination with whole cell pertussis vaccine: Follow-up study. *Br Med J* 316:902, 1998.

122. Australian College of Pediatrics Policy Statement: Contraindications to immunization against pertussis. *J Pediatr Child Health* 30:310, 1994.

123. Ouvrier RA: Whooping cough immunizations: A neurologist's viewpoint. *Med J Aust* 2:300, 1978.

124. Pollock TM, Morris J: A 7-year survey of disorders attributed to vaccination in northwest Thames region. *Lancet* 1:753, 1983.

125. Harker P: Primary immunization in febrile convulsions in Oxford in 1972–1975. *Br Med J* 2:490, 1977.

126. Stetler HC, Orenstein WA, Bart KJ, et al: History of convulsions and use of pertussis vaccine. *J Pediatr* 107:175, 1985.

127. Melchior JC: Infantile spasms and early immunization against whooping cough: Danish survey from 1970–1975. *Arch Dis Child* 52:134, 1977.

128. Matsumoto A, Watanabe K, Negoro T, et al: Infantile spasms: Etiological factors, clinical aspects and long term prognosis in 200 cases. *Eur J Pediatr* 135:239, 1981.

129. Bellman MH, Ross EM, Miller DL: Infantile spasms and pertussis immunization. *Lancet* 1:1031, 1983.

130. Berg JM: Complications of pertussis immunization. *Br Med J* 2:24, 1958.

131. Cherry JD: The epidemiology of pertussis and pertussis immunization in the United Kingdom and the United States: A comparative study. *Curr Probl Pediatr* 14:53, 1984.

132. Pertussis surveillance 1979–1981. *MMWR* 31(25):333, 1982.

133. Kulenkampff M, Schwartzman JS, Wilson J: Complications of pertussis inoculation. *Arch Dis Child* 49:46, 1974.

134. Miller DL, Ross EM, Alderslade R, et al: Pertussis immunization and serious acute illness in children. *Br Med J* 282:1595, 1981.

135. Madge N, Diamond J, Miller D, et al: The National Childhood Encephalopathy Study: A 10-year follow-up. A report on the medical, social, behavioral and educational outcomes after serious, acute illness in early childhood. *Dev Med Child Neurol Suppl* 68:1, 1993.

136. Miller DL, Madge N, Diamond J, et al: Pertussis immunization and serious acute illness in children. *Br Med J* 307:1171, 1993.

137. Evidence concerning pertussis vaccines and deaths classified as sudden infant death syndrome. In Howson CP, Howe CJ, Fineberg HV (eds): *Adverse Effects of Pertussis and Rubella Vaccines. A Report of the Committee to Review the Adverse Consequences of Pertussis and Rubella Vaccines.* Institute of Medicine. Washington: National Academy Press, 1991, p 125.

138. Centers for Disease Control and Prevention. Pertussis vaccination: Acellular pertussis vaccine for reinforcing and booster use. Supplementary ACIP statement: Recommendations of the Immunizations Practice Advisory Committee (ACIP). *MMWR* 41(RR-1):1, 1992.

139. Centers for Disease Control and Prevention. Pertussis vaccination: Use of acellular pertussis vaccines among infants and children. Recommendations of the Advisory Committee on Immunization Practices (ACIP). *MMWR* 46(RR-7):1, 1997.

140. Guris D, Strebel PM, Bardenheir B, et al: The changing epidemiology of pertussis in the United States: Increasing reported incidence in adolescents and adults, 1990–1996. *Clin Infect Dis* 28:1230, 1999.

141. Geier DA, Geier MR: Serious conditions following pertussis immunization: An analysis of endotoxin levels, the Vaccine Adverse Events Reporting System (VAERS) database and literature review. *Pediatr Rehabil* 5(3):177, 2002.

142. Use of diphtheria toxoid–tetanus toxoid–acellular pertussis vaccine as a five-dose series: Supplemental recommendation of the Advisory Committee on Immunization Practices (ACIP). *MMWR* 49(RR-13):1, 2000.

143. American Academy of Pediatrics: Pertussis. In Pickering LK (ed): *Red Book: 2003 Report of the Committee on Infectious Diseases,* 26th ed. Elk Grove Village, IL: American Academy of Pediatrics; 2003, p 472

144. Child Neurology Society Consensus Statement: Pertussis immunization and the central nervous system. *Ann Neurol* 29:458, 1991.

145. Cochi SL, Broome CV, Hightower AW: Immunization of US children with *Hemophilus influenzae* type b polysaccharide vaccine: A cost-effectiveness model of strategy assessment. *JAMA* 253(4):521, 1985.

146. Progress towards elimination of *Hemophilus influenzae* type B disease among infants and children—United states, 1998–2000. *MMWR* 51:234, 2002.

147. Shapiro ED, Murphy TV, Wald ER, et al: The protective efficacy of *Hemophilus* b polysaccharide vaccine. *JAMA* 260:1419, 1988.

148. Frank AL, Labotka RJ, Rao S, et al: *Hemophilus influenzae* type b immunization of children with sickle cell diseases. *Pediatrics* 82:571, 1988.

149. Feldman S, Gigliotti F, Shenep JL, et al: Risk of *Hemophilus influenzae* type b disease in children with cancer and response of immunocompromised leukemic children to a conjugate vaccine. *J Infect Dis* 161:926, 1990.

150. Kayhty H, Peltola H, Eskola J, et al: Immunogenicity of *Hemophilus influenzae* oligosaccharide-protein and polysaccharide-protein conjugate vaccination of children at 4, 6, and 14 months of age. *Pediatrics* 84:995, 1989.

151. Adams WG, Deaver KA, Cochi SL, et al: Decline of childhood *Hemophilus influenzae* type b (Hib) disease in the Hib vaccine era. *JAMA* 269:221, 1993.

152. Ahonkhai VI, Lukacs LJ, Jonas LC, et al: *Hemophilus influenzae* type b conjugate vaccine (meningococcal protein conjugate) (PedvaxHIB): Clinical evaluation. *Pediatrics* 85(4 pt 2):676, 1990.

153. D'Cruz OF, Shapiro ED, Spiegelman KN, et al: Acute inflammatory demyelinating polyradiculoneuropathy (Guillain-Barré syndrome) after immunization with *Hemophilus influenzae* type b conjugate vaccine. *J Pediatr* 115:743, 1989.

154. Gervaix A, Caflisch M, Suter S, et al: Guillain-Barré syndrome following immunization with *Hemophilus influenzae* type b conjugate vaccine. *Eur J Pediatr* 152:613, 1993.

155. Gross TP, Hayes SW: *Hemophilus* conjugate vaccine and Guillain-Barré syndrome (letter). *J Pediatr* 118:161, 1991.

156. Black SB, Shinefield HR, Hiatt RA, et al: Kaiser Permanente Pediatric Vaccine Study Group: Efficacy of *Hemophilus influenzae* type b capsular polysaccharide vaccine. *Pediatr Infect Dis J* 7:149, 1988.

157. Marchant CD, Band E, Froeschle JE, et al: Depression of anticapsular antibody after immunization with *Hemophilus influenzae* type b polysaccharide-diptheria conjugate vaccine. *Pediatr Infect Dis J* 8:508, 1989.

158. Santosham M, Wolff M, Reid R, et al: The efficacy in Navajo infants of a conjugate vaccine consisting of *Hemophilus influenzae* type b polysaccharide and *Neisseria meningitidis* outer-membrane protein complex. *New Engl J Med* 324:1767, 1991.

159. Hepatitis. In Atkinson W, Wolfe C (eds): *Epidemiology and Prevention of Vaccine-Preventable Diseases,* 7th ed. Washington: Public Health Foundation, 2002. p 169.

160. Centers for Disease Control and Prevention: Protection against viral hepatitis: Recommendations of the Immunization Practices Advisory Committee (ACIP). *MMWR* 39(S-2):1, 1990.

161. Andre FE: Summary of safety and efficacy data on a yeast-derived hepatitis B vaccine. *Am J Med* 87(3A):14S, 1989.

162. Shaw FE, Graham DJ, Guess HA, et al: Postmarketing surveillance for neurological adverse events reported after hepatitis B vaccination: Experience of the first three years. *Am J Epidemiol* 127(2):337, 1988.

163. Herroelen L, De Keyser J, Ebinger G: Central nervous system demyelination after immunization with recombinant hepatitis B vaccine. *Lancet* 338:1174, 1991.

164. Ascherio A, Zhang SM, Herman MA, et al: Hepatitis B vaccination and the risk of multiple sclerosis. *New Engl J Med* 344(5):327, 2001.

165. Confavreux C, Suissa S, Sadddier P, et al: Vaccinations and the risk of relapse in multiple sclerosis. *New Engl J Med* 344(5):319, 2001.

166. Prevention and control of influenza: Recommendations of the Advisory Committee on Immunization Practices (ACIP). *MMWR* 45(No RR-5):1, 1996.

167. James JM, Zeiger RS, Lester MR, et al: Safe administration of influenza vaccine to patients with egg allergy. *J Pediatr* 133(5):624, 1998.

168. Schonberger LB, Bregman DJ, Sullivan-Bolyal JZ, et al: Guillain-Barré syndrome following vaccination in the national influenza immunization program—United States, 1976–1977. *Am J Epidemiol* 110(2):105, 1979.

169. Lasky T, Terracciano GJ, Magder L, et al: The Guillain-Barré syndrome and the 1992–1993 and 1993–1994 influenza vaccines. *New Engl J Med* 339(35):1797, 1998.

170. Cherington M: Locked-in syndrome after "swine-flu" inoculation (letter). *Arch Neurol* 34:258, 1977.

171. Gens RD, Beecham HJ: Meningoencephalitis after influenza inoculation (letter). *New Engl J Med* 299:721, 1978.

172. Yahr MD, Lobo-Antunes J: Relapsing encephalomyelitis following the use of influenza vaccine. *Arch Neurol* 27:182, 1972.

173. Weintraub MI, Chia DTS: Paralytic brachial neuritis after swine flu vaccination (letter). *Arch Neurol* 34:518, 1977.

174. Wells CEC: A note on vaccination against influenza. *Br Med J* 3:755, 1971.

175. Kawasaki A, Purvin VA, Tang R: Bilateral anterior ischemic optic neuropathy following influenza vaccination. *J Neuro-Ophthalmol* 18(1):56, 1998.

176. Felix JK, Schwartz RH, Myers GJ: Isolated hypoglossal nerve paralysis following influenza vaccination. *Am J Dis Child* 130:82, 1976.

177. Kelsall JT, Chalmers A, Sherlock CH, et al: Microscopic polyangiitis after influenza vaccination. *J Rheumatol* 24:1198, 1997.

178. Perez C, Loza E, Tinture T: Giant cell arteritis after influenza vaccination. *Arch Intern Med* 160(17):2677, 2000.

179. Finsterer J, Artner C, Kladosek A, et al: Cavernous sinus syndrome due to vaccination-induced giant cell arteritis. *Arch Intern Med* 161(7):1008, 2001.

180. Preblud SR: Varicella: Complications and costs. *Pediatrics* 78(suppl):728, 1986.

181. Varicella. In Atkinson W, Wolfe C (eds): *Epidemiology and Prevention of Vaccine-Preventable Diseases,* 7th ed. Washington: Public Health Foundation, 2002, p 139.

182. Seward JF, Watson BM, Peterson CL, et al: Varicella disease after introduction of varicella vaccine in the United States, 1995–2000. *JAMA* 287(5):606, 2002.

183. American Academy of Pediatrics, Committee on Infectious Diseases: Recommendations for the use of live attenuated varicella vaccine. *Pediatrics* 95(5):791, 1995.

184. Varivax package insert, Merck and Company, West Point, PA, issued May 1996.

185. Centers for Disease Control and Prevention:. Simultaneous administration of varicella vaccine and other recommended childhood vaccines—United States, 1995–1999. *MMWR* 50(47):1058, 2001.

186. Shields B: Prevnar (heptavalent pneumococcal conjugate vaccine): Disease prevention in infants and children. *J Pediatr Health Care* 15(4):203, 2001.

187. Centers for Disease Control and Prevention, Advisory Committee on Immunization Practices: Preventing pneumococcal disease among infants and young children: Recommendations of the Advisory Committee on Immunization Practices (ACIP). *MMWR* 49(RR-9):1, 2000.

188. Douglas RM, Paton JC, Duncan SJ, et al: Antibody response to pneumococcal vaccination in children younger than 5 years of age. *J Infect Dis* 148(1):131, 1983.

189. Koskela M, Leinonen M, Häivä V-M, et al: First and second dose antibody response to pneumococcal polysaccharide vaccine in infants. *Pediatr Infect Dis* 5(1):45, 1986.

190. Hausdorff WP, Bryant J, Parasdiso PR, et al: Which pneumococcal serogroups cause the most invasive disease: Implications for conjugate vaccine formulation and use, part 1. *Clin Infect Dis* 30:100, 2000.

191. Black S, Shinefield H, Fireman B, et al: Efficacy, safety, and immunogenicity of heptavalent pneumococcal conjugate vaccine in children. *Pediatr Infect Dis J* 19(3):187, 2000.

192. Recommendations of the Advisory Committee on Immunization Practices (ACIP): Vaccinia (smallpox) vaccine. *MMWR* 50(RR10):1, 2001.

193. Henderson DA, Inglesby TV, Bartlett JG, et al: Smallpox as a biological weapon: Medical and public health management. *JAMA* 281(22):2127, 1999.

194. Mack TM: Smallpox in Europe, 1950–1971. *J Infect Dis* 122:303, 1970.

195. Lane JM, Ruben FL, Abrutyn E, et al: Deaths attributable to smallpox vaccination, 1959 to 1966, and 1968. *JAMA* 212(3):441, 1970.

196. Smallpox vaccination and adverse reactions: Guidance for clinicians. *MMWR* 52(RR-4):1, 2003.

197. Rivers TM: Viruses. *JAMA* 92:1147, 1929.

198. Lane JM, Ruben FL, Neff JM, et al: Complications of smallpox vaccination, 1968: National surveillance in the United States. *New Engl J Med* 281(22):1201, 1969.

199. Neff JM, Lane JM, Pert JH, et al: Complications of smallpox vaccination: I National Survey in the United States, 1963. *New Engl J Med* 276:125, 1967.

200. Johnson E: Studies on smallpox and complications of smallpox vaccine. *Pediatrics* 26:176, 1960.

201. Miravalle A, Roos KL: Encephalitis complicating smallpox vaccination. *Arch Neurol* 60:925, 2003.

INDEX

Page numbers followed by *t* or *f* refer to tables or figures, respectively.

Penicillium marneffei, 188
prevention of, 179
Sporothrix schenckii, 188
treatment of, 177–179
amphotericin B in, 177–178
caspofungin in, 179
fluconazole in, 178
flucytosine in, 178
itraconazole in, 178
ketoconazole in, 179
miconazole in, 179
neurosurgery in, 179
voriconazole in, 178–179
zygomycetes, 188–189
ophthalmic, 428–432. *See also*
Ophthalmic disorders, in
neurologic infections
Fusarium CNS infections, 176, 188. *See also* Fungal infections, CNS
Fusobacterium ophthalmic infections, 421

G

Gabapentin, for HIV-associated distal sensory polyneuropathy, 108, 108t
gag region, HIV, 117
Gammaglobulin, IV, for HTLV-1-associated myelopathy/tropical spastic paraparesis, 146
Ganciclovir
for cytomegalovirus infections
encephalitis, 72, 72t
with HIV, 95–96, 96t
neonatal, 38, 48, 50t
for HSV-1 encephalitis, 72
for human herpes virus-6 encephalitis, 72, 72t
for Rasmussen's encephalitis, 520
systemic and CNS toxicities of, 480t, 504–505
for varicella-zoster virus encephalitis with HIV, 72, 72t
for viral encephalitis, acute, 72, 72t
Gatifloxacin, systemic and CNS toxicities of, 476t, 485–486
General paralysis of the insane, 223
Gentamicin
for bacterial meningitis, 20–22, 21t, 22t
movement disorders from, 384t
systemic and CNS toxicities of, 476t, 490–491
German measles. *See* Rubella virus infections
Gerstmann-Sträussler-Scheinker (GSS) disease, 312t, 314t, 318, 396
differential diagnosis of, 319–320
ophthalmic disorders from, 441–442
treatment of, 320
Glasgow Coma Scale, 269t

Glaucoma, 411
from rubella virus, 427
syphilitic, 434
Glucose, in CSF, 4–5
Glycopeptide agents. *See* Vancomycin
Gnathostoma spinigerum infections (gnathostomiasis)
CNS, 242t, 250
ophthalmic, 439, 439f
Gonococcal infections
conjunctivitis, 416, 416f
corneal ulcer, 416, 416f
Granulomatous amebic encephalitis, 278–280
Grip, milkmaid, 385
Group A β-hemolytic streptococcus (GABHS) infection
chorea from, 385. *See also* Sydenham disease
Tourette's syndrome and, 388
GSK3β, for HIV dementia, 129–130
Guillain-Barré syndrome, 349–355
Campylobacter jejuni vs. axonal, 350–351
clinical features of, 351–353
differential diagnosis of, 353
from diphtheria and tetanus vaccines, 530
from *Hemophilus influenzae* type B vaccine, 534
history of, 349–350
laboratory evaluation of, 353
management of, 354–355
pathophysiology of, 350–351
Gummatous neurosyphilis, 225

H

H₂ receptor antagonist, with dexamethasone, 24
HAART (highly active antiretroviral therapy)
on HIV-associated distal sensory polyneuropathy, 107
for HIV dementia, 128–129, 128f
on progressive multifocal leukoencephalopathy with HIV, 85
HACEK (*Haemophilus, Actinobacillus, Cardiobacterium, Eikenella, Kingella*) bacilli, infective endocarditis from, 451
Haemophilus aphrophilus endocarditis, 451
Haemophilus brain abscess, 30. *See also* Brain abscess, bacterial
antimicrobials for, 32, 33t
Haemophilus influenzae infections
endocarditis, 451
ophthalmic, 415, 421
Haemophilus influenzae type b
conjugate vaccine, 14, 26

Haemophilus influenzae type b
meningitis, 14. *See also* Meningitis, bacterial
antibiotics for, 20, 21t
incidence of, 14
Haemophilus influenzae type b vaccine (Hib), 533–534
complications of, 534
Haemophilus parainfluenzae endocarditis, 451
Haemophilus paraphrophilus endocarditis, 451
Haloflantrin
adverse effects of, 273t
for cerebral malaria, 267
Haloperidol
for movement disorders in HIV, 401
for seizures with infective endocarditis, 464
for Sydenham disease, 387
Hansen disease. *See* Leprous neuritis
Headache
CSF diagnostic studies for, 8t
with infective endocarditis, 463–464
Helicephalobus deletrix CNS infection (micronemiasis), 242t, 253
Helminthic infections, 241–255
ascarioid, 253
cestode, 241–249. *See also* Cestode infections
dracontiasis, 253
loiasis, 253
micronemiasis, 253
nematode, 249–252. *See also* Nematode infections
ophthalmic, 438–441
trematode, 253–255
Hemianopsias
altitudinal, 412
bilateral, 412–413
homonymous, 413
from *Acanthamoeba* spp., 436
in AIDS, 428
from *Babesia,* 438
from Creutzfeldt-Jakob disease, 442
from *Echinococcus* spp., 438
from *Entamoeba histolytica,* 436
from *Gnathostoma spinigerum,* 439
from JC virus, 425
from Lyme disease, 435
from *Naegleria fowleri,* 436
from *Paragonimus* spp., 438
from rubella virus, 427
from *Schistosoma* spp., 438
from subacute sclerosing panencephalitis, 426
syphilitic, 434, 435
from *Taenia solium,* 438
from *Toxoplasma gondii,* 437
from varicella-zoster virus, 422
Hemiballism, infectious etiologies of, 384t